Foundations of Theory and Practice for the Occupational Therapy Assistant

Foundations of Theory and Practice for the Occupational Therapy Assistant

Amy Wagenfeld, PhD, OTR/L, SCEM, CAPS

Assistant Professor
Department of Occupational Therapy
Western Michigan University

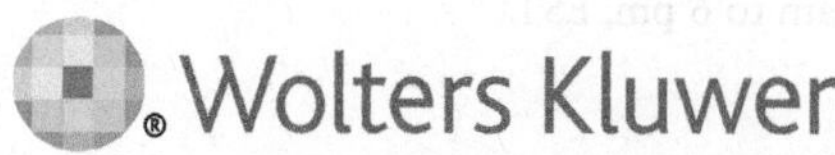

Philadelphia • Baltimore • New York • London
Buenos Aires • Hong Kong • Sydney • Tokyo

Acquisitions Editor: Michael Nobel
Product Development Editor: Linda G. Francis
Production Product Manager: Priscilla Crater
Senior Manufacturing Manager: Margie Orzech
Editorial Assistant: Tish Rogers
Marketing Manager: Shauna Kelley
Design Coordinator: Stephen Druding
Production Service: SPi Global

Two Commerce Square
2001 Market Street
Philadelphia, PA 19103 USA
LWW.com

Printed in the United States of America

Library of Congress Cataloging-in-Publication Data
Wagenfeld, Amy, author.
Foundations of theory and practice for the occupational therapy assistant / Amy Wagenfeld.
p. ; cm.
Foundations of theory & practice for the occupational therapy assistant
Includes bibliographical references and index.
ISBN 978-1-4963-1425-3 (alk. paper)
I. Title. II. Title: Foundations of theory & practice for the occupational therapy assistant.
[DNLM: 1. Occupational Therapy—ethics. 2. Occupational Therapy—methods. 3. Allied Health Personnel. WB 555]
RM735
615.8'515—dc23

2015018484

Care has been taken to confirm the accuracy of the information presented and to describe generally accepted practices. However, the authors, editors, and publisher are not responsible for errors or omissions or for any consequences from application of the information in this book and make no warranty, expressed or implied, with respect to the currency, completeness, or accuracy of the contents of the publication. Application of the information in a particular situation remains the professional responsibility of the practitioner.

The authors, editors, and publisher have exerted every effort to ensure that drug selection and dosage set forth in this text are in accordance with current recommendations and practice at the time of publication. However, in view of ongoing research, changes in government regulations, and the constant flow of information relating to drug therapy and drug reactions, the reader is urged to check the package insert for each drug for any change in indications and dosage and for added warnings and precautions. This is particularly important when the recommended agent is a new or infrequently employed drug.
Some drugs and medical devices presented in the publication have Food and Drug Administration (FDA) clearance for limited use in restricted research settings. It is the responsibility of the health care provider to ascertain the FDA status of each drug or device planned for use in their clinical practice.

To purchase additional copies of this book, call our customer service department at (800) 638-3030 or fax orders to (301) 223-2320. International customers should call (301) 223-2300.

Visit Lippincott Williams & Wilkins on the Internet: at LWW.com. Lippincott Williams & Wilkins customer service representatives are available from 8:30 am to 6 pm, EST.

10 9 8

Our role consists in giving opportunities rather than prescriptions.

—Adolf Meyer, 1921

To all occupational therapy assistants, past, present, and future.

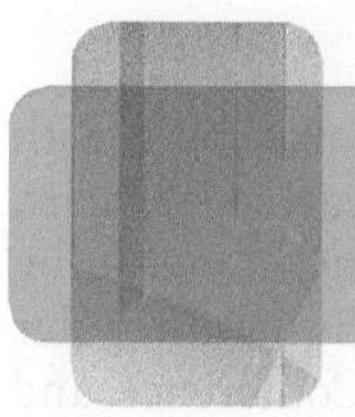

Contributor Biographies

Naomi Abrams, OTD, OTR/L, CEAS, is currently playing the roles of an occupational therapist, business owner, injury prevention consultant, lecturer, writer, and caretaker of one very cute dog, Charlie. Her company, Worksite Health & Safety Consultants, LLC, provides injury prevention services around the country. Her recent book, *Why is My Office a Pain in My…?*, has been well received as a therapy aid, client resource, and text book on office ergonomics. Contact: info@workinjuryfree.com.

Sue Berger, PhD, OTR/L, BCG, FAOTA, is a clinical associate professor at Boston University in the Department of Occupational Therapy. Her clinical practice has spanned the health care continuum, with experience working with adults in environments of acute care, rehabilitation, long-term care, hospice, and home care. She completed her doctoral work in gerontology focusing her research on understanding the challenges and barriers of engaging in occupations for older adults living with vision loss. Despite many years of schooling, she has learned the most from listening to stories and experiences from the older adults she has had the privilege to meet.

Karie Carbone is an occupational therapy student at Rush University in Chicago, Illinois, where she has completed practicum experiences in acute care, inpatient rehabilitation, and inpatient psychiatry settings. She received her Bachelor of Arts degree in Special Education from Seattle Pacific University in 2012. Karie worked in a community-based program for children and adults with developmental disabilities in Seattle. In Chicago, Karie was a one-on-one aide for a student with a behavior disability at a low-income elementary school. Karie finds meaning and purpose through serving at-risk populations including individuals who are refugees, homeless, and live in poverty. Karie is passionate about occupational therapy because it opens up an unlimited number of ways in which she can make an impact in the lives of others.

Vicki Case, OTR/L, has been an assistant professor for the Occupational Therapy Assistant Program at Adventist University of Health Sciences, in Orlando, Florida, since 1999. She has 24 years of experience as an occupational therapist and was a rehabilitation director for a large rehab company for 8 years. She has experience training therapists in the area of documentation and currently enjoys teaching students the value of excellence in documentation.

Ann Chapleau, DHS, OTR/L, is associate professor of occupational therapy at Western Michigan University. She has worked in the mental health and addictions field for over 25 years as a clinician, manager, and academician. Her research interests include interventions to prevent homelessness and reduce health disparities among people with severe mental illness. She is currently studying the use of *Goal Attainment Scaling* for interprofessional program evaluation. She serves on the editorial board of the *Open Journal of Occupational Therapy* (OJOT) and was the recipient of the 2012 Michigan Occupational Therapy Association's Award of Excellence.

Carla A. Chase, EdD, OTR/L, has been a practicing occupational therapist for 20 years and an educator for 15 years, first teaching occupational therapy assistants at a local community college and currently teaching occupational therapists at Western Michigan University. Her work in home care focuses on serving the needs of older adults in order to support continued participation in meaningful occupations and to create a safe and comfortable place for them in their home and community. Her health and wellness program includes relaxing to the sound of her alpaca chewing hay and exercising with a pitchfork and shovel while cleaning up after them.

Margaret Christenson, MPH, OTR/L, FAOTA, is founder of Lifease, a software company that linked product and idea solutions to potential problems in the homes of older people or those with disabilities. The company was sold in 2013, and the software will be developed in a different format. Margaret also developed a visual library that includes illustrations of environmental problems and solutions for aging changes with a focus on incorporation of universal design. Many of these images are available on the CD of AOTA's publication: *Occupational Therapy and Home Modifications: Promoting Safety and Supporting Participation.* Margaret was chair of AOTA's Gerontology Special Interest Section, its representative to the White House Council on Aging, and chair of the committee on Specialty Certification in Environmental Modifications. When she lived in Minnesota, she was the 1989 Minnesota Occupational Therapist of the Year.

Alice Gandell, MSMSP, OTR/L, graduated from the University of Illinois and has been a practicing occupational therapist for 45 years. She is a clinical instructor in the Nova Southeastern University Medical Professions Clinic and adjunct professor in the occupational therapy program. A Master's degree in marriage and family therapy has complemented her interactions with clients and their families facilitating positive therapeutic change. Alice has presented at local and regional workshops for parents, teachers, and other professionals. With Sheri Feldman, EdD, CCC-SLP, she authored a helpful book for parents and caregivers of special needs children entitled *PLAY, Partnership Learning Activities for the Young Child*. Alice remains involved with her family and her many art and craft projects using them to make things for her four grandchildren and others.

Debbie Grimes, COTA, has over 13 years of experience as an occupational therapy assistant. She received her associate degree in occupational therapy in 1999 from Amarillo College. Debbie's interest in occupational therapy began when she was working in the public school systems as a teaching assistant. She worked with special needs children for approximately 4 years in that position. Witnessing the OT practitioners' creativity and dedication to serving the children inspired Debbie to become an OTA. She began her career as an OTA working with the geriatric population. Her desire to work with children eventually led her to a career with pediatrics. She has been a foster parent to special needs children as well. Currently, she resides with her husband and dog with special needs in the Texas panhandle.

Lieutenant Colonel (RET) Sandra Harrison-Weaver, MHE, OTR/L, CHT, served 28 years in the U.S. Army before retiring in 2014. LTC(RET) Harrison-Weaver previously served as the Program Director for the Army Occupational Therapy Assistant Program and as Chief of the Occupational Therapy Department at Walter Reed National Military Medical Center in Bethesda, Maryland. She has presented nationally at the American Occupational Therapy Association and American Society of Hand Therapists annual meetings. She has been an item writer for the national OT exam and currently serves on the AOTA Roster of Accreditation Evaluators. Her passions are teaching and upper extremity rehabilitation.

Scott L. Homer, MS, OTR/L, is an assistant professor and program director of the Occupational Therapy Assistant Program at Maria College in Albany, New York. As a graduate of the program who returned to serve as a tutor and adjunct instructor, Scott has been involved with all aspects of the OTA curriculum. Scott's clinical experiences as a COTA include long-term care, inpatient brain injury rehabilitation, and school-based pediatric practice. Upon completing an MS degree in OT at Utica College, he practiced in the outpatient arena, both with hand therapy and pediatric clients. A teacher at heart, Scott finds the most purpose and meaning in educating current and future OT practitioners. He is a regular presenter at the New York State OT Conference and teaches workshops on neurology, anatomy, and kinesiology throughout the state. Scott remains dedicated to the Maria College OTA program where he was nurtured by the supportive and caring faculty whom he is now honored to call colleagues.

DeLana Honaker, PhD, OTR, FAOTA, has over 20 years of experience in early intervention, school-based, and pediatric practice. She received her BS, MA, and PhD degrees in occupational therapy from Texas Woman's University. Her specialty is in working with children with autism spectrum disorders, sensory processing disorders, feeding difficulties, and learning differences. DeLana worked as Lead Therapist for the Lubbock Independent School District from 1994 to 2004 and continues to work in Early Childhood Intervention, pediatric home health, and pediatric outpatient services. She is also an app developer and is currently developing a new multiprofessional pediatric assessment app for smart devices. DeLana is also a research scientist and professor with 14 years of experience in academia as an associate professor at Elizabethtown College and as an adjunct professor for Texas Woman's University and Texas Tech University Health Sciences Center. In 2010, she was appointed to the Texas Board of Occupational Therapy Examiners; she has also served as a Commissioner on Practice for the American Occupational Therapy Association from 2005 to 2008. She was named a Fellow of the American Occupational Therapy Association in 2014 in recognition of exceptional service, scholarship, teaching, and leadership for the profession in technology and pediatrics.

Tia Hughes, DrOT, MBA, OTR/L, is program director of the occupational therapy and occupational therapy assistant program at Adventist University in Orlando, Florida. She has been an occupational therapist since 1991 and worked primarily in physical dysfunction settings. She has been a manager of occupational therapists and occupational therapy assistants and is responsible for program development, employee supervision, and professional marketing. Her experience in education has allowed her to empower students to develop professional career goals that expand over time to meet the needs of the individual and the community of those whom we serve.

Tamera Keiter Humbert, DEd, OTR/L, is an associate professor at Elizabethtown College where she teaches both undergraduate and graduate courses. She started her career as an occupational therapy assistant and then transitioned into various roles as an occupational therapist. Her current areas of occupational practice include mental health and wellness, international practice, and spirituality. She conducts research related to women overcoming violence and international cross-cultural practice. Her work and research has taken her to Haiti, Rwanda, Kenya, Cuba, Costa Rica, and throughout the United States.

Jennifer Kaldenberg, MSA, OTR/L, SCLV, FAOTA, is a clinical assistant professor and academic fieldwork coordinator at Boston University in the Department of Occupational Therapy and an adjunct assistant professor of vision rehabilitation at the New England College of Optometry. She has clinical experience in rehabilitation, home care, and outpatient, primarily with adults. For the past 12 years, her practice and research has focused on older adults with visual impairment and the functional implications of vision loss. She has published and presented extensively on a variety of topics related to vision loss both nationally and internationally. Jennifer was involved in the development of a specialty certification in low vision through AOTA and in writing the *Occupational Therapy Practice Guidelines for Older Adults with Low Vision.*

Kevin Kunkel, PhD, MSPT, MLD-CDT, completed a BS at Stanford University. After graduating, he became a professional baseball player with the Oakland Athletics. Following his baseball career, Kevin attended The University of Miami and received an MS in physical therapy. Kevin's professional clinical career in physical therapy has covered various setting including acute inpatient rehabilitation, acute medical, orthopedics and neurologic inpatient, intensive care, home health, wound care, and outpatient rehabilitation. He developed and is the owner of a comprehensive outpatient rehabilitation facility in West Palm Beach called The Flagler Institute for Rehabilitation. Kevin completed a PhD program at the Miller School of Medicine at The University of Miami in 2010. In 2011, Kevin joined the faculty at Nova Southeastern University as an assistant professor in the department of physical therapy.

Helene Lieberman, MA, OTR/L, has been practicing occupational therapy for 24 years. After graduating Boston University's Sargent College of Allied Health Professions with a BS in occupational therapy, she worked in New York with a variety of pediatric diagnoses. After moving to Florida, Helene provided inpatient and outpatient pediatric rehabilitation occupational therapy services. Realizing the integral part of the family in pediatric therapy, Helene returned for a master's degree in family support services. She worked at the Baudhuin Preschool for children with autism for 12 years. While there, she supervised and lectured to the occupational therapy students at Nova Southeastern University. After venturing out on her own as well as providing occupational therapy services for a local home therapy company, Helene was an adjunct professor in the occupational therapy department at Nova Southeastern University. Helene is the proud mom to three very inquisitive boys and wife of a patient man.

Wanda J. Mahoney, PhD, OTR/L, is an assistant professor at Midwestern University in Illinois and has worked as an occupational therapist with children and adults with developmental disabilities for over 10 years. She provided early intervention services in children's homes and day care centers in urban New Orleans, worked at a special education school and residential program on the Navajo reservation in Arizona, practiced at specialized schools for children with autism in the Chicago area, and consulted with several programs for adults with developmental disabilities. She completed her doctorate in occupational therapy and has concentrated on obtaining the perspectives of people with significant disabilities in several research projects.

Diane L. Maxson, MHA, MS, OTR/L, is a graduate of the occupational therapy programs at Virginia Commonwealth University and Boston University with a specialty in Clinical Pediatrics. She has practiced in a wide variety of medical, educational, and community settings during her 30-year career. Following the completion of an LEND Fellowship and Master's degree in Healthcare Administration Diane founded the Therapeutic Learning Center in Canton, Massachusetts. Located in the Boston suburbs TLC provides a variety of therapy services and programs within one inclusive, supportive setting. She has presented nationally and internationally on a variety of topics and serves on the Executive Board of the Massachusetts Association of Occupational Therapists.

Kevin Piendak, EMBA, OTR/L, graduated from the occupational therapy program at Quinnipiac College in 1996. Since then, he has been employed at New England Rehabilitation Hospital in Woburn, Massachusetts, and has developed a large repertoire of clinical skills with multiple diagnostic populations. In 2002, Kevin earned his Executive Masters in Business Administration degree from Troy University's Sorrell College of Business. He has held several leadership and supervisory positions, mentored a large number of occupational therapy staff, advocated for program development, participated in research activities, and is a devoted coordinator of his facility's student program providing clinical education to the next generation of occupational therapy professionals. Recently, Kevin has served as a member of the Executive Board of the Massachusetts Association of Occupational Therapists and has focused his efforts on incorporating new treatment technologies into his facility to provide improved care for a variety of patient populations.

Sheri Purdy, OTR/L, CLT, graduated from Quinnipiac College in 1988 and became a certified lymphedema therapist in 2010. As the occupational therapy manager at New England Rehabilitation Hospital, she oversees more than 50 occupational therapy practitioners. She has spent her career working with the elderly in subacute nursing facilities and acute rehabilitation hospitals. Sheri thrives on helping clients gain independence and in promoting quality of life. Sheri has served as a board member of the Massachusetts Association for Occupational Therapy for the past 8 years. She is serving a 3-year term on the AOTA Roster for Accreditation Evaluators, assisting with credentialing processes for occupational therapy programs throughout the United States. Sheri published *Return to Work Information Sheet for People that have Cognitive Impairments* for AOTA and is involved with research looking at how Kinesio taping decreases pain in people who have had strokes and its correlation with subluxed shoulders.

Dawndra Meers Sechrist, OTR, PhD, is the program director for the Master of Occupational Therapy program at Texas Tech University Health Sciences Center. She has worked over 20 years in a wide variety of adult and older adult settings including acute care, skilled nursing, inpatient rehabilitation, and home health. She has been an assistant professor at Texas Tech University Health Sciences Center for over 13 years and continues to work PRN in an acute care county hospital setting. She received her Neuro-Developmental Treatment certification in 1997. Dawndra received her PhD from Texas Tech University with an emphasis on adult learning. Dawndra is currently an item writer for the National Board for Certification in Occupational Therapy, Inc. (NBCOT).

Sarah G. Sieradzki, OTR/L, HTR, CDP, is a native Hoosier, having attended Depauw University and graduated from Indiana University in 1976 with a BS in Occupational Therapy. She is a Clinical Specialist in mental health occupational therapy at University Hospitals, Case Medical Center in Cleveland, Ohio. She has over 35 years of experience in occupational therapy, mostly in mental health, and has mentored students from nine universities as a clinical supervisor. She became a Certified Dementia Practitioner in 2010. Sarah is the author of the chapter *Documentation: The Professional Process of Recording Outcomes* in *Horticultural Therapy Methods: Making Connections in Health Care, Human Service, and Community Programs*. Sarah is also an adjunct faculty member at Cuyahoga Community College and a part-time instructor/lecturer in the occupational therapy program at Cleveland State University.

Stacy Smallfield, DrOT, MSOT, OTR/L, FAOTA is a professor at the University of South Dakota in the Department of Occupational Therapy. She has taught graduate-level occupational therapy coursework related to adult physical rehabilitation, therapeutic adaptations, the environment, and evidence-based practice for over 10 years. In her clinical practice, she has worked with adults and older adults in subacute rehabilitation, long-term care, inpatient rehabilitation, long-term acute care, and ergonomic settings. She has also worked in a nontraditional occupational therapy position as an innovation designer developing new products and services that enhance the well-being of older adults and their families.

Lieutenant Colonel Matthew St. Laurent, MS, OTR/L, CHT, has served over 20 years in the U.S. Army to include one tour in Mosul, Iraq, and over 9 years of service at Walter Reed as an occupational therapist. He is currently the Chief of the Occupational Therapy Department at the Walter Reed National Military Center in Bethesda, Maryland. Walter Reed has the largest occupational therapy service of all military treatment facilities and recently integrated into a joint Army, Navy, and Air Force facility. Walter Reed serves all of our nations heroes returning from military conflicts around the world. LTC St. Laurent's specialty is upper extremity clinical rehabilitation.

Scott A. Trudeau, PhD, OTR/L, works as a research health scientist at the Geriatric Research Education and Clinical Center (GRECC) at the Edith Nourse Rogers Memorial VA Medical Center in Bedford, Massachusetts. He is also a senior lecturer at Tufts University. Scott's research explores topics of home safety, personal care, the dynamics of caregiving, factors contributing to successful aging, and issues of adaptation for elders with chronic illnesses, and the role of life-long learning for community-dwelling elders. Scott has also studied the contributions that occupations make to maintaining elders in the community with enhanced quality of life. He received a BS in occupational therapy and an MA from Tufts University, and a PhD from Boston College.

Michael J. Urban, MS, OTR/L, CEAS, MBA, CWCE, is an occupational therapist with a specialization as an ergonomic assessment specialist and has trained with the Matheson Group as a work capacity evaluator. He has experience in physical disabilities, industrial rehabilitation, and in the home care setting. Mr. Urban has consulted and overseen the development of return to work programs with an emphasis on the emergency professions. He currently works for the Department of Veteran Affairs treating clients in the polytrauma, ALS, and general outpatient clinics. He also privately consults in the areas of functional capacity evaluations, return to work programs, ADA requirements, and pediatrics. He has lectured and consulted with Yale University's Occupational and Environmental Medicine Department and assisted with research on firefighter health with Yale University's School of Medicine, Section of Emergency Medicine. Michael is serving as the current President for the Connecticut Occupational Therapy Association and previously served AOTA as a member of the Commission on Practice and as the Alternative Representative for the state of Connecticut to the AOTA Representative Assembly. Michael was recently elected as a member of the AOTF Inaugural Leaders and Legacy Society.

Lisa van Gorder, OTR/L, CEIS, is the owner and clinical director of Integrated Children's Therapies, Inc. in Hudson, Massachusetts. Her widely acclaimed lectures often draw from her experience extensive working in outpatient clinics, schools, and with early intervention programs to facilitate and obtain functional goals for children with a variety of diagnoses. In addition to her clinical experience, Lisa is certified in sensory integration, a provider for The Listening Program, and is a Certified Early Intervention Specialist from the state of Massachusetts. Furthermore, Lisa's passion and expertise with working with children with feeding issues has encouraged her to create and coordinated a variety of feeding groups for children with multiple needs.

Debra Young, MEd, OTR/L, SCEM, ATP, CAPS, owner of EmpowerAbility LLC, is a certified specialist in environmental modifications, aging in place, and assistive technology. She is a registered and licensed occupational therapist with an M.A. with specialization in Assistive Technology (AT) from Bowling Green State University, a graduate certificate in AT from Johns Hopkins University, and a Bachelor of Science degree in occupational therapy from Elizabethtown College. A Rehabilitation Engineering and Assistive Technology Society of North America–certified Assistive Technology Professional and National Association of Home Builders (NAHB) Certified Aging-in-Place Specialist (CAPS), Debra is the recipient of the 2013 NAHB CAPS of the Year Award and is an approved NAHB instructor for the Universal Design/Build and CAPS designation courses. Debra has earned the Specialty Certification in Environmental Modifications from the American Occupational Therapy Association (AOTA)—a distinction accomplished by less than 1% of occupational therapists nationally. She is the 2014 recipient of the AOTA Recognition of Achievement Award for notable contributions to the profession and its consumers in environmental modifications specialty practice. Debra has published and presented on local, state, and national levels on environmental modifications, assistive technology, universal design, and livable communities. She is currently serving on the Board of Directors of the AOTA.

Preface

Foundations of Theory and Practice for the Occupational Therapy Assistant is written specifically with the OTA student in mind. The text is divided into seven units arranged in a bottom–up hierarchy, providing students a foundation to proceed to each successive unit. The culmination of this building on process is a compilation of 13 case studies designed to put theory into practice and to encourage students to engage in high-level critical thinking skills. This comprehensive classroom-to-clinic text is designed to serve as an important resource for students as they go forward in their educational and professional OTA careers.

I set out to prepare this book to provide students and instructors with a resource that aligns with the American Occupational Therapy Association's *Centennial Vision*, which recognizes occupational therapy as a "science-driven and evidence-based profession whose role in society is to meet people's occupational needs" (AOTA, 2007, p. 613). I also wanted to bring together a diverse community of professionals whose common voice is unwavering in its conviction for the worth and value of occupational therapy. You will find that our distinguished contributors fill managerial, entrepreneurial, clinical, academic, military, research, and innovative business owner roles. The value of this organizational structure is that you will be getting real-world perspectives on all arms of the profession. All experts in the field, our contributors provide the first-hand knowledge you will need to develop the theoretical and practical skills to become a successful and well-rounded occupational therapy assistant.

You will note some features in this textbook that you may have never encountered in other textbooks. Many chapters will invite you to explore what we have named *From the Field.* They are designed as an aside within the chapter to give you a different perspective to think about, a spark of inspiration, if you will. We have created a unique icon CS to let you know that wherever it appears in a chapter, you will be certain to see the concept explored again in a case study in Unit Seven. Same or similar concepts may be explained in multiple chapters. The reason for doing this is to ensure that if you do not have the opportunity to read all of the chapters during the course(s) you are using this book for, by virtue of repetition, you will, by reading some or most chapters, be provided with what you need to know to lay the foundation for becoming an occupational therapy assistant.

In Unit One, *Our Roots, Our Future*, we begin our journey by first looking at where we began and how we have evolved and continue to evolve as a profession. Our illustrious roots are a source of pride for contemporary occupational therapy practitioners. We also explore the unique re-evolution of the occupational therapy assistant role and how today, more than ever, occupational therapy assistants are a vital and integral part of the health care and educational team. Our core values and philosophy shape the cornerstone of occupational therapy, which of course are occupations. We live in a society that constantly seeks answers and validation. Through evidence-based research of the role of occupations as a therapeutic tool, occupational therapy continues to be recognized as a leader in client care.

In Unit Two, *Theory and Guiding Principles*, build on Unit One by exploring the *Framework* (AOTA, 2014) that guides our profession and the theories that explain why and how occupations and occupational therapy is the unique and exciting profession that it is. Because our work involves direct contact with people of all ages and ability, a life span exploration of human development is important. Knowing what came before and what comes next with regard to our developmental progression, allows us to provide optimal treatment for our clients. We conclude Unit Two with a shining star and jewel of occupational therapy—the activity—and occupational analysis, a unique way in which occupational therapy practitioners prepare and tailor our interventions to ensure that they are client-centered.

Unit Three, *Scope of Practice*, begins with a look at the occupational therapy assistant's commitment to ethical practice. We then explore staying current and updated with practice issues and techniques, and expectations for documentation, management, supervisory, and team-based practice.

As we continue to lay the foundation for practice, Unit Four, *Therapeutic Techniques and Processes*, presents specific treatment techniques and processes that are unique to occupational therapy and your role as an occupational therapy assistant in carrying them out with your clients and their families.

Building on the information you have thus far been provided, Unit Five, *Common Conditions*, takes you into the actual world of treatment. We explore a wide range of issues and conditions that you as an occupational therapy assistant will encounter in your work with clients, no matter the practice area. This unit also includes reimbursement of occupational therapy services by third-party payers.

Unit Six, *Practice Settings: Traditional and Emerging*, covers the eight contexts that the American Occupational

Therapy Association has identified as areas where occupational therapy practitioners are employed and may in the future look to be employed. These chapters will prepare you for a realistic entry into practice by providing a deeper understanding of what is involved with the practice setting and the important role that an occupational therapy assistant plays in ensuring quality client care.

In Unit Seven, *The Occupational Therapy Assistant in Action: Putting Theory into Action*, we apply all that has been presented in the book to case studies. In other words, we are making the move from contextual to realistic. The 13 case studies cover life span issues and practice settings that occupational therapy assistants are likely to encounter in their work with clients. The case studies are organized and follow the Domain and Process of the *Occupational Therapy Practice Framework: Domain and Process, Third Edition* (AOTA, 2014). This organization provides you with a clear understanding of how the occupational therapy process unfolds and is implemented with our clients.

Finally, the Appendix contains a glossary of medical and professional abbreviations that could be accessed online.

Online Resources

To enhance the learning experience and reinforce the concepts presented in this text, the following resources are provided for students and instructors:

Students:

- **A Quiz Bank with NBCOT type questions** provides unlimited review and practice and is ideal for board prep.
- The Glossary of Medical and Professional Abbreviations provides a useful listing of terms that you may encounter throughout your educational and professional career.

Instructors:

- **An Instructor Manual** provides a wide range of resources to enhance teaching.
- **A robust test generator with NBCOT type questions** helps you put together tests that assess your students' understanding of the material.
- **PowerPoint Presentations** make it easy for you to integrate the textbook with your students' classroom experience, via either handouts or slide shows.

A Note on Language

Please be aware that the abbreviation OTA will be used throughout this book to describe the occupational therapy assistant role. The abbreviation OT will be used to describe the occupational therapist role. When discussing the inclusive roles that both occupational therapists and occupational therapy assistants fulfill, the term OT practitioner will be used. When describing the profession or the actual service provision, the term occupational therapy will be used. This is in alignment with the American Occupational Therapy Association.

A Final Note

In my more than a quarter of a century as an occupational therapist, I have worn many hats, including clinician, academic, manager, researcher, author, consultant, and innovator. No matter which role I have found myself in, all have significantly influenced the way I think about and participate in the world. I wish for all of you the incredible joys and riches in your journey that I have experienced as an occupational therapy practitioner.

Amy Wagenfeld

References

American Occupational Therapy Association. AOTA's centennial vision and executive summary. *Am J Occup Ther* 2007;61:613–614.

American Occupational Therapy Association. Occupational therapy practice framework: domain and process (3rd ed.). *Am J Occup Ther* 2014;68(Suppl. 1):S1–S48. http://dx.doi.org/10.5014/ajot.2014.682006

Special Note: In addition to the Student and Instructor Resources that accompany this text, readers can access a series of videos at http://thePoint.lww.com. These videos are from the highly acclaimed library of International Clinical Educators, Inc (http://icelearningcenter.com) and were chosen to supplement this text. Video clips are listed by their titles below.

Acute Care Part 5: Bed to Chair Transfers
Arranging Flowers While Standing
Dressing in Acute Care Part One
Dressing in Acute Care Part Two
Pediatric Behavior Management
Pediatrics: Fine Motor Skills Letter Formation with Play-Doh
Pediatrics: Sensory Integration and Sensory Processing: Scooterboard and Letter Recognition
Self Care: One Handed Shoe Tying
Treatment Ideas Using Objects in the Hospital Room
Upper Extremity Observations

About the Author

Amy Wagenfeld, PhD, OTR/L, SCEM, CAPS, is an assistant professor in the Department of Occupational Therapy at Western Michigan University. With over 30 years of experience as an occupational therapist, she began her teaching career in an OTA program. When not writing, researching, or teaching, Amy collaborates with landscape designers to create, program, and evaluate therapeutic gardens for children and adults in community, health care, military, and educational settings. She is the coauthor, with Daniel Winterbottom, of the recently released *Therapeutic Gardens: Design for Healing Spaces*, published by Tinder Press.

Acknowledgments

Having the privilege of publically acknowledging those who have helped to make this book possible is truly a humbling experience. I would like to begin by thanking the founders of occupational therapy, whose vision and unwavering commitment laid the foundation for what nearly a century later is a highly respected and evidence-based profession. I would also like to thank the past, present, and future leaders of occupational therapy; those whose voice have been and will be heard, and for leaders whose voices are quieter, yet no less mighty in importance.

To the American Occupational Therapy Association, I wish to thank you for being the guiding force to propel occupational therapy well into the future. It is a privilege to have joined AOTA as a student and more than a quarter century later, to have never let my membership lapse. Being an active volunteer in the association is an important part of my life. I have a great passion for being an occupational therapist and wear the title with great pride.

For my gifted and generous chapter contributors. Without your wisdom and insight, this book would not be of the incredible caliber that it is. I extend my deepest gratitude to, Naomi Abrams, Sue Berger, Karie Carbone, Vicki Case, Ann Chapleau, Carla Chase, Margaret Christenson, Alice Gandell, Debbie Grimes, Scott Homer, DeLana Honaker, Tia Hughes, Tamera Humbert, Jennifer Kaldenberg, Kevin Kunkel, Helene Lieberman, Wanda Mahoney, Diane Maxson, Kevin Piendak, Sheri Purdy, Dawndra Sechrist, Sarah Sieradzki, Stacy Smallfield, Matthew St. Laurent, Scott Trudeau, Michael Urban, Lisa Van Gorder, Sandra Weaver, and Debra Young.

Many thanks to Ellen Wagenfeld-Heintz for developing the PowerPoint slides, and to Mary Kay Arvin for writing the Test Generator and Quiz Bank questions that accompany this text.

A huge thank you to my editorial and marketing crew at Wolters Kluwer Health: Michael Nobel, Linda Francis, Priscilla Crater, and Shauna Kelley.

Thank you to my teachers and friends at Bindu for the opportunity to practice yoga and remain focused, centered, and balanced throughout writing this book. To Mauricio Rubio, thank you for helping me with typing when my fingers could not possibly do anymore work. You are the best Met son ever. To Naomi Sachs, Founding Director of the Therapeutic Landscapes Network, my deepest gratitude for your friendship, wisdom, and guidance. For my niece Ajna Wagenfeld, your gifts as a photo wizard are simply awe inspiring. Could not have done it without you! For my beloved late graduate school advisor, Carol Harding, I extend my profound gratitude for instilling in me a sense of confidence and a strong desire to write. I miss you every day.

To my parents, Drs. Morton Wagenfeld and Jeanne Wagenfeld, I thank you for your support and nurturing guidance to always reach for the stars. For my siblings, Eric, David, and Ellen, thank you for letting me practice my managerial skills on you. Being the eldest sibling does have its advantages! To my husband Jeffrey Hsi, you are nothing short of a saint. Being my steadfast supporter throughout this writing process made it possible for me to pick up the pieces and keep going, even on those long days when I thought that I had hit the wall. I am eternally grateful and love you dearly. And for our son David Hsi, DVM, MPH (a mother is entitled to brag!), you are without a doubt, the joy and light of our lives. We could not be more proud of and love you more.

And now to you, our readers. It is my sincere hope that you not only learn the important theoretical and foundational information necessary to guide you through your educational and fieldwork process, and in your professional role as an occupational therapy assistant, but that the process of reading the book is enjoyable and even inspirational. It has been a joy to write and edit this book. My best wishes to you.

Amy Wagenfeld, PhD, OTR/L, SCEM, CAPS

Contents

UNIT

I

Our Roots Our Future

The profession needs to embrace the fact that occupational therapy has different levels of practitioners and celebrate the unique contributions made by OTAs.

—Robin Jones

CHAPTER 1

Historical Perspectives of Occupational Therapy

Amy Wagenfeld, PhD, OTR/L SCEM, CAPs

Key Terms

Americans with Disabilities Act (ADA)—The 1990 landmark federal legislation that provides civil rights to people with disabilities.

American Occupational Therapy Association (AOTA)—The national organization that represents the interests and concerns of occupational therapy practitioners and students and seeks to improve the quality of occupational therapy services.

Centennial Vision—"We envision that occupational therapy is a powerful, widely recognized, science-driven, and evidence-based profession with a globally connected and diverse workforce meeting society's occupational needs" (American Occupational Therapy Association, 2007).

Founding Vision—The 1917 founding document of the profession, which states "The particular objects for which the corporation is formed are as follows: The advancement of occupation as a therapeutic measure for the study of the effect of occupation upon the human being for the scientific dispensation of this knowledge" (National Society for the Promotion of Occupational Therapy, 1917).

Individuals with Disabilities Education Act (IDEA)—A federal law requiring that all students with disabilities be educated in the least restrictive environment possible, mandating that students with disabilities be educated alongside those without disability.

Moral treatment—A 19th-century reform movement focused on curing rather than confining people with mental illness to asylums.

National Society for the Promotion of Occupational Therapy (NSPOT)—The predecessor organization of the American Occupational Therapy Association.

Occupation—A meaningful and purposeful activity; the cornerstone of our profession.

Occupational therapy—A profession that helps people do what they need and want to do through the use of therapeutic daily activities.

Learning Objectives

After studying this chapter, readers should be able to:

- Summarize the role that history plays in the current status of the profession of occupational therapy.
- Identify the roots of occupational therapy originating from multiple disciplines and state the impact on the current profession as we know it.
- Discuss the connections between the *Founding Vision* and the *Centennial Vision* of occupational therapy.
- Describe what the profession of occupational therapy "is."

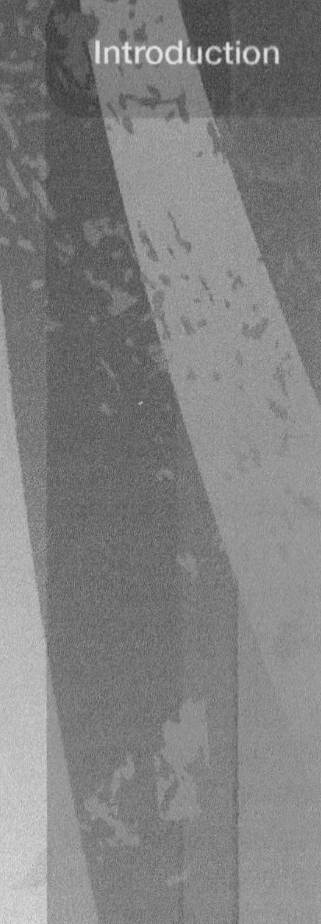

Introduction

The profession and practice of occupational therapy is richly steeped in history. In fact, the idea of occupations being curative is documented in ancient Egyptian records, when court physicians might recommend a walk in the garden to cure sadness and melancholy. As the profession evolves over time, so too does the scope of practice. While occupational therapy services have always been important, in our ever changing and complex society, the need for occupational therapy practitioners has never been greater.

The modern day definition of **occupation therapy** is

> "the therapeutic use of everyday activities (occupations) with individuals or groups for the purpose of participation in roles and situations in home, school, workplace, community, and other settings. Occupational therapy services are provided for the purpose of promoting health and wellness and to those who have or are at risk for developing an illness, injury, diseases, disorder, condition, impairment, disability, activity limitation, or participation restriction. Occupational therapy addresses the physical, cognitive, psychosocial, and other aspects of performance in a variety of contexts to support engagement in everyday life activities that affect health, well-being, and quality of life" (AOTA, 2011a, p. 1).

The AOTA also describes occupational therapy as "... helping people across the lifespan participate in the things they want and need to do through the therapeutic use of everyday activities (occupations)" (AOTA, n.d.c). To better understand these current definitions of the field, starting at the beginning and tracing the roots of the profession and looking for common threads that connect and continue to shape and define it are important.

The Moral Treatment and Reform Movement

Placing occupational therapy's history within the context of concurrent world events is important in order to appreciate that the evolution of the profession did not happen in a vacuum. Rather, world events significantly shaped and still shape occupational therapy (Hagedorn, 2001).

At the end of the 18th century and into the first half of the 19th century, due in large part to the wisdom of Philippe Pinel, a philosopher and physician, and William Tuke, a Quaker, treatment for the mentally ill underwent a transformative change (Igiugu, 2004). Instead of being treated inhumanely as had been the societal norm to this point, reform movements in the form of **moral treatment** were underway. The purpose of moral treatment was to cure rather than simply confine patients with mental illness (Dunkel, 1983). Proponents of moral treatment determined that the mentally ill were to be treated humanely and with compassion and respect. The common belief was that engaging the mind to a state of attentiveness would lead to an integration of the mind and body, and the path to wellness (Igiugu, 2004). Treatment included a balance of work and leisure activities, as well as learning methods to cope with the stresses associated with psychological issues (Dunkel, 1983). Using **occupations**, meaningful and purposeful activities, as a therapeutic tool has its roots in moral treatment (Kielhofner, 2009). Moral treatment, and associatively, the use of occupations, allowed people with mental illnesses not only to live their lives in dignity but additionally to improve their health and well-being. As such, moral treatment was based on the premise that "participation in the various tasks and events of everyday life could restore persons to more healthy and satisfying functioning" (Kielhofner, 2009, p. 17).

Based heavily on the ideologies of moral treatment, early practitioners believed that environments were a critical part of the treatment process (Kielhofner, 2009). Environments in this context included social attitudes about participating in occupations and actual participation in occupations of daily life (Kielhofner, 2009). By structuring these multitiered environments, occupational therapists could help their patients "explore potentials and learn about effective and satisfying ways to participate in everyday life" (Kielhofner, 2009, p. 24), which continues to be a central theme of the profession.

While moral treatment certainly improved the lives of patients living in mental institutions, it lacked scientific underpinnings. Toward the end of the 19th century, the popularity of moral treatment began to fade and was replaced with an insatiable interest in scientifically based treatment methods. Interestingly, with the advent of science and scientific methods, combined to some degree with the compassionate principles associated with moral treatment, there emerged a new profession, psychotherapy. Correspondingly, the blending of science and psychotherapy gave rise to what we today know as occupational therapy.

Settlement houses were an important part of the reform movement as well as the evolution of occupational therapy. Settlement houses were located in buildings in immigrant neighborhoods of large, industrialized cities. The purpose of settlement houses was to provide social services to the large influx of immigrants arriving in the United States in the late 19th and early part of the 20th centuries (Kielhofner, 2009; Wade, 2005). Services included education, health care, lodging, and food for immigrants. Hull House, located in Chicago, was the best-known settlement house in the United States (Wade, 2005). Eleanor Clarke Slagle, a social reformer and one of the profession's most distinguished founders, worked and took courses at Hull House. It is through her work that occupational therapy was linked to these important social reform institutions, because Slagle recognized that engaging immigrants in the everyday occupations offered at Hull House was curative. Slagle acknowledged that providing these kinds of opportunities for immigrants to take care of themselves and to learn new skills were meaningful and purposeful.

The Early Twentieth Century

At the conclusion of the 19th century and into the early years of the 20th century, innovations in science, technology, and medicine significantly influenced how people lived their lives. Life was becoming, for the first time, highly mechanistic and industrialized. Machines were replacing hand craftsmanship. The pace of life was increasing and scientific inquiry was flourishing. Emerging at the end of the Victorian Era in England when industrialization was on the rise, proponents of what became known as the Arts and Crafts movement opposed this trend toward industrialization. Supporters of the Arts and Crafts movement sought to reconnect people to nature and a simpler life and to foster individuality, creativity, and craftsmanship, rather than to embrace modernity, mass production, and a machine-driven industrialized society.

In addition to the tension between mechanization and industrialization and Arts and Crafts philosophy, attitudes toward people who were ill or disabled were also beginning to change. Up until now, the collective societal belief was that a person with disability either got better or could/would not lead a productive life. No longer relegated to spend their remaining years on the sidelines, there was a prevailing shift in attitude that people with disabilities had the potential to be productive members of society (O'Brien & Hussey, 2012). With the support of a passionate group of social reformers, the tide was turning, in a positive way. These salient early 20th-century issues also helped to shape the profession of occupational therapy. Physicians began to equate healthier living with being meaningfully occupied (McColl et al., 2002). That is, keeping patients engaged in something (occupations) meaningful was the key to being healthy. Instead of a rest cure, what today, we could call bed rest; the concept of a work cure involving elements of doing and being engaged in meaningful activity was now in vogue.

Much like today, in the early part of the 20th century, issues such as immigration, war, public education, and lack of availability of adequate health care plagued the United States (Schwartz, 2009, p. 682). Despite these serious social and humanitarian issues, there was a widespread spirit of optimism during this time period, which is often called the Progressive Era. The pervasive belief was that an expanding understanding of science would be the catalyst to positively influence and initiate positive change in the social, educational, and medical issues of the time (Schwartz, 2009). Those players at the forefront of implementing social change were an eclectic group from movements such as women's suffrage, arts and crafts, science, and moral treatment (Schwartz, 2009). The collective ideals of these groups would significantly influence the profession of occupational therapy (Schwartz, 2009), as would principles of moral treatment and, with the end of World War I (WWI) approaching, the need for physical rehabilitation services (Friedland, 1998).

Influence of World War I (1914 to 1918)

Heavily influenced by moral treatment and the ideology of the Arts and Crafts movement, in the early preprofessional era, an occupational therapist's work was mainly carried out in settlement houses and mental institutions. The focus of therapeutic intervention was to bolster a patient's spirits and improve independence and productivity rather than physical function (Friedland & Silva, 2008).

With the influx of wounded soldiers returning from war, moving occupations into the context of physical rehabilitation began to be explored. As well, prior to WWI, the prevailing attitude toward recovery from illness or trauma was the rest cure (Friedland & Silva, 2008). This attitude was replaced by recognition that optimal recovery involved addressing the whole body, including rebuilding self-esteem, a quality often lost or reduced following a loss in function. Engaging in occupations was thought to be an ideal way to rebuild the mind and body.

For example, Thomas Kidner, one of the profession's founders designed manual training programs that called for hands-on, creative, and holistic activities and were the basis for wartime occupational therapy. This process began at the bedside of the wounded soldiers and progressed, as the soldier improved to off-ward curative workshops, and ultimately to vocational training programs. Occupations were the catalyst to move the soldier from bedside, to curative workshop, to vocational training, and, ultimately, to return to work (Friedland & Silva, 2008).

This radical paradigm shift that soldiers with physical injury could be rehabilitated and return to a productive life was fraught with dilemma. Both moral and pragmatic issues were at play in conventional society. Morally, society needed to help those who served their country, and likewise, it was presumed immoral for the wounded soldiers to be idle (Friedland & Silva, 2008, p. 352). Pragmatically, it was felt that soldiers should not be reliant on "the state" (Friedland & Silva, 2008, p. 352). While soldiers were due a pension for their service to the country, their contribution to society was also important, both financially and for personal self-esteem. Post injury, a wounded soldier's military duty was now to get "rehabilitated" (Friedland & Silva, 2008, p. 352). It was the duty of those charged to work with these soldiers to provide optimal physical rehabilitation in order to help them reengage in a meaningful and productive life.

Concurrent with the influx of wounded soldiers returning from WWI was a sharp rise in the incidence of tuberculosis among soldiers during the war, presumably because of poor and unhygienic conditions in the trenches. Prior to WWI, the cure for tuberculosis was complete rest, fresh air, and nourishing food (Friedland & Silva, 2008, p. 352). The new role for craft-based occupations in the tuberculosis wards was seemingly to provide a diversion. Once treating physicians understood that these craft-based occupations would cause no harm, occupational therapists were welcomed on the tuberculosis wards (Friedland & Silva, 2008). Thus, the role of occupational therapists working with people with tuberculosis was born. In one short but profoundly influential period of time, the focus of occupational therapy expanded from work with the mentally ill into the physical rehabilitation setting.

During wartime, schools were set up to provide training for the earliest members of the profession. The schools actively recruited students to meet the needs of treating the large number of soldiers returning home with combat injuries. Of the eight programs in existence during WWI, the training varied, as did the backgrounds of the practitioners. To ensure constancy among the graduates, standardization of educational training programs was soon to follow.

Following WWI, the passage of two pieces of federal legislation helped propel the occupational therapy profession forward within the world of rehabilitation. The purpose of the Soldier's Rehabilitation Act of 1918 was to provide vocational rehabilitation services for injured veterans to help them return to productive civilian life. The Civilian Vocational Rehabilitation Act of 1920 provided States with a 50-to-50 matching funds mandate to provide vocational services for nonmilitary people with physical disabilities. To be eligible for these services, an individual had to have demonstrable reason to be unable to participate in "gainful" employment (O'Brien & Hussey, 2012, p. 18). Both of these Acts were important for the growth of the profession.

The Organization of the Profession

Through a creative networking process (a phrase our founders were certainly unfamiliar with!), the profession of occupational therapy was established. A seemingly disparate group of medical professionals, social workers, teachers, craftspeople, volunteers, or anyone who had something to contribute to the belief that occupation could contribute to health and healing came together to form the **National Society for the Promotion of Occupational Therapy (NSPOT)** (Fig. 1.1) (Gordon, 2009; Hagedorn, 2001; Wolf, 2007). Interestingly, these seemingly unrelated disciplines came together to begin what today is an ever-evolving, well-established, evidence-based, science-driven profession that thrives on intra- and interdisciplinary collaborations.

- The initial 2-day meeting of NSPOT was March 15, 1917, in Clifton Springs, NY (Breines, 1990; Kielhofner, 2009; Schwartz, 2003, 2009). Present at that initial meeting was a small core of key players from varying educational and philosophical backgrounds who factored significantly into the history of the profession (Fig. 1.1). They

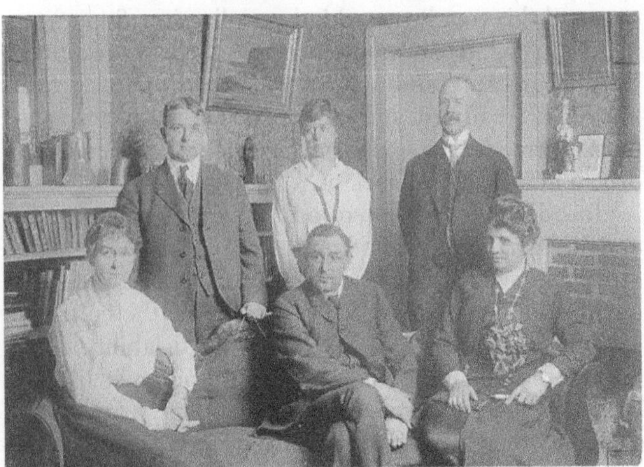

Figure 1.1 NSPOT founders.

BOX 1.1

Eleanor Clarke Slagle: Social Welfare Reformer

- Often called the mother of occupational therapy.
- Involved with NSPOT/AOTA for 20 years, she held most every role, including serving as the first vice president of the NSPOT in 1919, president of NSPOT in 1920, and executive secretary for the newly named AOTA in 1921. In addition to these roles, unlike most women of the time, she held a full-time job.
- An ardent believer in the value of therapeutic occupations and a tireless promoter for the profession of occupational therapy (Schwartz, 2009).
- Instrumental in forming the theoretical underpinnings for establishing standards of practice and treatment for the profession of occupational therapy.
- Concerns about how society of the day treated people with disabilities led Slagle to take an "invalid occupations" course at Hull House in Chicago where immigrants could receive educational and social services. She went on to study occupations and educational methods at what was the Chicago School of Civics and Philanthropy (now part of the University of Chicago) and came back to teach at Hull House (Schwartz, 2003, 2009).
- Served under Adolf Meyer as director of occupational therapy at Phipps Psychiatric Clinic in Baltimore (Bing, 1981; Schwartz, 2009). Worked with Meyer to develop a habit-training program for the patients. Expanded on Meyer's ideas of habit-training for people with mental illness, working to balance self-care, occupations, exercise, mealtime, and physical activity.
- Habit-training programs were to become a great passion for Slagle, implementing them at various other institutions she worked with and for, stating "habit-training remedially serves to overcome some habits, to modify others, and construct new ones to the end that habit reactions will be favorable to the restoration and maintenance of health" (Slagle, 1992, p. 14, in Schwartz, 2009).
- Appointed Illinois superintendent of occupational therapy and then director of occupational therapy for New York's department of mental hygiene.
- Director of the Henry B. Flavill School of Occupations.
- During World War I, she directed a 6-week training course for volunteer occupational therapists (then called reconstruction aides). In 6 months, she visited 20 hospitals, directing the training of 4,000 volunteer occupational therapists.
- Worked with the American Medical Association to establish accreditation of occupational therapy training programs and guidelines to register trained therapists.
- Wrote one book.
- In 1953, in Slagle's honor and for steadfast commitment to the profession, the AOTA created the Eleanor Clarke Slagle Lectureship, given each year at the national AOTA conference by a distinguished occupational therapist.

included Eleanor Clarke Slagle, social welfare reformer (see Box 1.1); Thomas Bessell Kidner, building tradesman/architect (see Box 1.2); William Rush Dunton, psychiatrist (see Box 1.3); George Edward Barton, architect (see Box 1.4); Susan Cox Johnson, arts and crafts teacher (see Box 1.5); Susan Tracy, occupational nurse and educator (see Box 1.6); and Herbert James Hall, psychiatrist (see Box 1.7).

- Eleanor Clarke Slagle.
- Thomas Bessell Kidner.
- Susan Cox Johnson.
- William Rush Dunton.
- George Edward Barton.
- Isabelle Newton (Barton's secretary).

What this small group of forward thinkers had in common was a commitment and belief in the effectiveness of occupations as a therapeutic tool (Schwartz, 2003). According to the AOTA, the founders were "dedicated to building a role for occupational therapy in the health care community, and to establishing an organization that would build the profession and serve its members" (AOTA, 1991). These founders wanted occupational therapy to be shaped by both the prevailing medical science and social and moral reform movements popular at the time of the establishment of the profession (Schwartz, 2003, p. 10). To the founders, occupations included "habit-training, handicrafts, graded physical exercise, and the preindustrial shop" (Schwartz, 2003, p. 8). While each founder viewed these occupations from different perspectives, the collective wisdom was that the means to good health was through engagement in meaningful occupation (Quiroga, 1995; Schwartz, 2003), or an engagement of the mind and body could positively influence a person's health and well-being (Gilfoyle, 1984). Thus, the profession of occupational therapy began in the United States. The primary objective of the NSPOT was to "study and advance curative occupations for invalids and convalescence; to gather

BOX 1.2

Thomas Bessell Kidner: Building Tradesman/Architect

- An ambassador for occupational therapy, Kidner's legacy was the development of the profession and building a "strong and accountable profession" through "standards and a registry for therapists" (Friedland & Silva, 2008, p. 354).
- President of AOTA from 1922 to 1928.
- An outspoken advocate for research–asking, how can the results of therapeutic intervention be measured and what is important to understand so as to continually challenge practitioners and the profession to achieve higher standards. *This remains the case today within the practice and profession of occupational therapy.*
- Contributions to occupations included a "method of learning for school children, a treatment for illness and injury, and as a foundation for work" (Friedland & Silva, 2008, p. 353).
- Born in England, Kidner moved to Canada as a young man. At the outset of WWI, he was awarded a governmental position as vocational secretary of the Military Hospitals Commission of Canada to ensure that wounded soldiers were either helped to return to their former assignments or retrained for other work. The process began with occupations at the bedside and progressed, as the soldier improved, to off-ward curative workshops and ultimately to vocational training programs. Kidner did not view bedside or ward occupations (generally crafts), as a carry over for job training, but as a way to instill a sense of accomplishment that would support future employment skills training (Friedland & Silva, 2008, p. 353).
- Kidner's work drew the attention of Eleanor Clarke Slagle, who visited Kidner when she was director of the Henry B. Flavill School of Occupations (Friedland & Silva, 2008).
- Kidner was secunded to the United States in 1918 where he assumed the role of advisor on rehabilitation for the Federal Board of Vocational Education. Later, Kidner worked with the National Tuberculosis Association as the head of the Advisory Service on Institutional Construction.

news of progress and occupational therapy and to use such knowledge to the common good; to encourage original research, to promote cooperation among occupational therapy societies, and with other agencies of rehabilitation" (NSPOT, 1917).

BOX 1.3

William Rush Dunton: Psychiatrist

- Frequently called the father of occupational therapy; he was a passionate supporter of occupational therapy.
- Served as a president of NSPOT in 1918.
- Began his work at Shepard Asylum, a private institution for the mentally ill. After becoming director of occupations at Shepard Asylum, spent much of his career immersed in studying the value of occupations as a therapeutic tool (Kielhofner, 2009).
- Infused moral treatment principles into the founding basis of occupational therapy.
- Wrote two books and collaborated on two occupational therapy books.
- Credited with being first to use the term occupation therapy (Bing, 1981).

Psychiatrists, who were the earliest supporters of occupational therapy, acknowledged a connection between occupation and health as a therapy (Clouston & Whitcombe, 2008). Despite this well-deserved support, at the onset of the profession, occupational therapists relied on the knowledge bases of other disciplines to guide their work, as there were no established theories of occupational therapy. What guided these pioneers were existing knowledge bases and theories from fields such as anatomy, physiology, medicine, and psychology, as well as the collective wisdom of craftspeople, architects, designers, and teachers (Hagedorn, 2001, p. 20). Due to the nature of the profession and those who practiced, adaptability prevailed, and throughout the early decades of the 20th century, practitioners began to work together and share their experiences and create a unique professional identity that continues to evolve today (Hagedorn, 2001).

The founding members of the NSPOT drafted a Founding Vision. The ***Founding Vision*** stated "the particular objects for which the corporation is formed are as follows: The advancement of occupation as a therapeutic measure; for the study of the effect of occupation upon the human being; for the scientific dispensation of this knowledge" (National Society for the Promotion of Occupational Therapy, 1917).

This vision recognized the importance of melding occupation with science. Today, we recognize the

BOX 1.4

George Edward Barton: Architect

- After contracting tuberculosis as an adult, devoted the rest of his life to service for people with physical challenges.
- Because of his ongoing health challenges, he was focused on a hospital's responsibility to its patients and to their lives after discharge.
- Established the Consolation House in Clifton Springs, NY, an early prototype of a rehabilitation center (Bing, 1981, p. 317), where after a thorough individualized in-take evaluation, patients engaged in meaningful occupations such as gardening, crafts, and woodworking to best suit their interests and needs (Fig. 1.2).
- Barton's treatment philosophy and methods fell within the realm of moral treatment for the "awakening of physical reconstruction and reeducation through the employment of occupation" (Bing, 1981, p. 317).
- He was the first to refer to the profession in the adjectival form, occupational therapy.

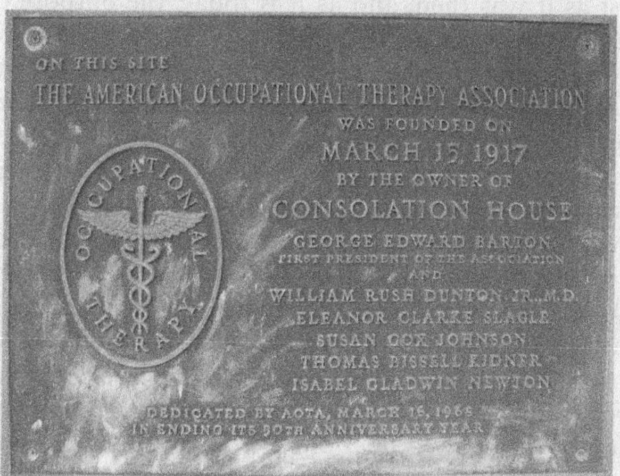
ON THIS SITE
THE AMERICAN OCCUPATIONAL THERAPY ASSOCIATION
WAS FOUNDED ON
MARCH 15, 1917
BY THE OWNER OF
CONSOLATION HOUSE
GEORGE EDWARD BARTON
FIRST PRESIDENT OF THE ASSOCIATION
AND
WILLIAM RUSH DUNTON, JR., M.D.
ELEANOR CLARKE SLAGLE
SUSAN COX JOHNSON
THOMAS BISSELL KIDNER
ISABEL GLADWIN NEWTON
DEDICATED BY AOTA, MARCH 15, 1968
IN ENDING ITS 50TH ANNIVERSARY YEAR
OCCUPATIONAL THERAPY

A

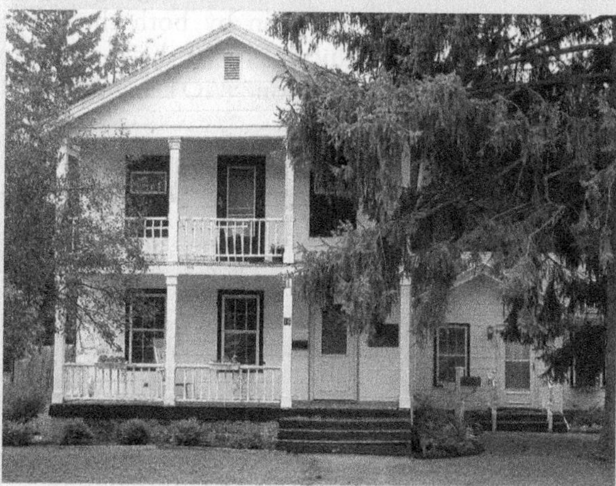

B

Figure 1.2 **A.** Historical marker, Consolation House. **B.** Consolation House today. (Photo courtesy of Natalie Pashoukos.)

BOX 1.5

Susan Cox Johnson: Arts and Crafts Teacher

- Advocate for using crafts as a therapeutic tool.
- Staff occupational therapist at Montefiore Hospital in New York.

BOX 1.6

Susan Tracy: Occupational Nurse and Educator

- The 20th century's first advocate for recognizing the benefits of using occupations with "invalids" (Bing, 1981).
- Made use of observation and experimentation to improve her practice skills and to integrate scientific principles into treatment methods.
- Tracy adopted the term occupational therapy in 1921 (it was originally proposed by George Barton) to differentiate it from vocational therapy.
- During WWI, Tracy trained nurses in occupational therapy to work with wounded soldiers.
- In Tracy's words, "The aim of occupation is to get the man well; that of vocational training is to provide him with a job. Any well man will look for a job, but the sick man is looking for health" (Bing, 1981, p. 57).

BOX 1.7

Herbert James Hall: Psychiatrist

- President of NSPOT in 1921 and was in office when the name changed to AOTA.
- A Harvard-trained psychiatrist who was interested in the multitude of problems facing individuals with mental illness.
- Started a sanatorium called the Handcraft Shops with craftsperson Jessie Luther.
- Hall's research demonstrated "physical, mental, and moral health could be restored and maintained through occupation" (Kielhofner, 2009).
- Used crafts as a therapeutic approach, as they offered the just right challenge to avoid idleness and maintain self-esteem (Kielhofner, 2009, p. 16).
- Developed a classification system for crafts. Used progressively harder occupations to grade crafts activities based on skill levels.

FROM THE FIELD 1.1

Like our founders believed, occupational therapy practitioners must have a clear understanding of what it is they do and what they can contribute to the betterment of society through melding of occupation with science. As you are beginning your OTA journey, how do you see contributing to the betterment of society through an occupational therapy profession envisioned through the AOTA *Centennial Vision* as being an evidence-based and science-focused profession?

importance of science in the advancement of our profession through occupational science and evidence-based research and practice, topics that will be discussed in upcoming chapters (From the Field 1.1).

Figure 1.3 illustrates the discussion of what this emerging profession was to be called. The early visionaries of the profession were far ahead of their time in the way they viewed the role of occupations as fostering health and well-being (Hagedorn, 2001). Their voices continue to shape the profession.

The Progression of the Profession

In 1921, following the end of WWI, the members of the NSPOT voted to change the name of the governing body of the organization to the **American Occupational Therapy Association (AOTA)**, as it is known to this day. The AOTA is the "national professional association established in 1917 to represent the interests and concerns of occupational therapy practitioners and students of occupational therapy and to improve the quality of occupational therapy services" (AOTA, n.d.b). The mission of the AOTA is "advancing the quality, availability, use, and support of occupational therapy through standard-setting, advocacy, education, and research on behalf of its members and the public" (AOTA, n.d.c). Abroad, occupational therapy was introduced in the United Kingdom in the 1930s and, following World War II (WWII), found its way to Europe and the rest of the world (Hagedorn, 2001). A call for a standardization of training was introduced, and in 1923, the AOTA adopted the *Minimum Standards for Courses of Training in Occupational Therapy* (O'Brien & Hussey, 2012). These standards included the criteria for admission to programs, the length of the program, and the course contents (From the Field 1.2).

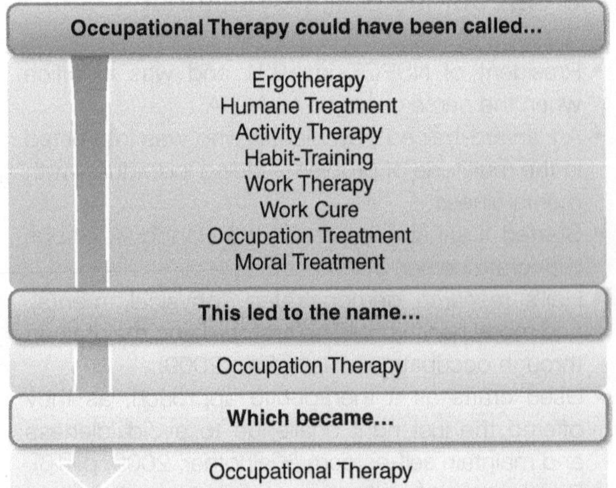

Occupational Therapy could have been called...
Ergotherapy
Humane Treatment
Activity Therapy
Habit-Training
Work Therapy
Work Cure
Occupation Treatment
Moral Treatment
This led to the name...
Occupation Therapy
Which became...
Occupational Therapy

Figure 1.3 Evolution of a name. (Bing, 1981; Friedland & Silva, 2008; Gilfoyle, 1984; Hussey et al., 2007; Schwartz, 2003, 2009).

In 1931, the AOTA created its first national registry for qualified occupational therapy practitioners, ensuring that there was now a singular and credible resource for the profession (AOTA, 1991). Just as it was then, and as it is today, the purpose of establishing standards of practice and a registry of professionals is to "protect the public, to protect the profession, and to facilitate the profession's advancement" (Friedland & Silva, 2008, p. 354). In 1935, at the request of the AOTA, the American Medical Association took on the role of inspector and accreditors for occupational therapy programs to increase the credibility of the profession (O'Brien & Hussey, 2012; Schwartz, 2003). This relationship continued until 1994, when it was determined that AOTA would function autonomously in the roles of inspector and accreditor of its programs. As it is currently known, the American Occupational Therapy Association's Accreditation Council for Occupational Therapy Education (ACOTE) is "the accrediting agency for occupational therapy education by both the United States Department of Education and the Council for Higher Education Accreditation" (AOTA, n.d).

FROM THE FIELD 1.2

The 1923 *Minimum Standards for Courses of Training in Occupational Therapy* stated that the course of study for occupational therapists was to be a minimum of 1-year long: 8 to 9 months of medical and crafts training and 3 to 4 months of clinical fieldwork in a medical setting. Compare the early standards of training to *your* curriculum. What differences do you see? What parallels can you find?

TABLE 1.1 Professional Directions: Pathways to be Taken

Status	Purpose
Remain as it was.	To improve self-esteem and sense of purpose To provide psychological support
Focus on actual return to work and skill building.	Vocational focus has little focus on physical status—nonmedical
Use occupations as part of the framework to build healthy communities.	Capacity building Teaching and social work focused
Use occupations as a means to improve physical function.	Medically focused To build strength

Friedland J, Silva J. Evolving identities: Thomas Bessell Kidner and occupational therapy in the United States. *Am J Occup Ther* 2008(May/June);62(3):349–360.

Post WWI, the profession was at a crossroad and could progress in several directions (Table 1.1). While still in its infancy, there was tension brewing between embracing the idea that occupations for occupation's sake, like gardening, crafts, and cooking, were curative (and simple) and looking at the therapeutic value of occupations through a modern and more complex scientific lens. There was a notable thirst in society for scientifically based explanations as well as scientifically based treatments. The profession of occupational therapy heeded this trend, and its treatment focus remained closely aligned with the current day medical models (Clouston & Whitcombe, 2008; Hagedorn, 2001) rather than a crafts-based focus.

Not unexpectedly, and as we will see as the century proceeds, within the profession, there was serious concern and unrest about the direction the profession was taking (Fig. 1.4).

World War II (1939 to 1945)

In terms of growth of the profession, the time between the World Wars was relatively slow, but following the onset of WWII, things once again began rolling forward. The demand for personnel to work in military hospitals was on the rise. In fact, there were not enough trained therapists to meet the needs of military hospitals, let alone anywhere else (Schwartz, 2003). To address this urgent need, 21 new training programs were established (Schwartz, 2003). Because the profession had not reached military status, and training took longer than the military could wait, emergency actions were taken, and wartime therapists were put on an extreme fast track to finish training and go to work with wounded soldiers (Hagedorn, 2001). As is the case today, with advances in medicine and technology, more soldiers were surviving their combat wounds. To meet the needs of a population that to this point had not been a focus of occupational therapy intervention, treatment shifted from crafts oriented to functional skills training (Hocking, 2007; Schwartz, 2003) (Fig. 1.5).

From a purely pragmatic perspective, during the decade of the 1930s, providing trained therapists ready to enter into professional service was urgently needed. Two additional themes directly impacting occupational therapy practice were also emerging. They were continued rapid advances in medicine and technology and the way in which people began to view people with physical disabilities in a more equitable manner (Hocking, 2007). Combined with the existing principles of occupational therapy, these three themes, an urgent need for therapists, advances in medicine and technology, and a societal shift to recognize people with disabilities, more equitably coalesced to help continue the rise of the profession (Hocking, 2007). How this information about occupational therapy practice was shared was also important; hence, from almost the beginning of the

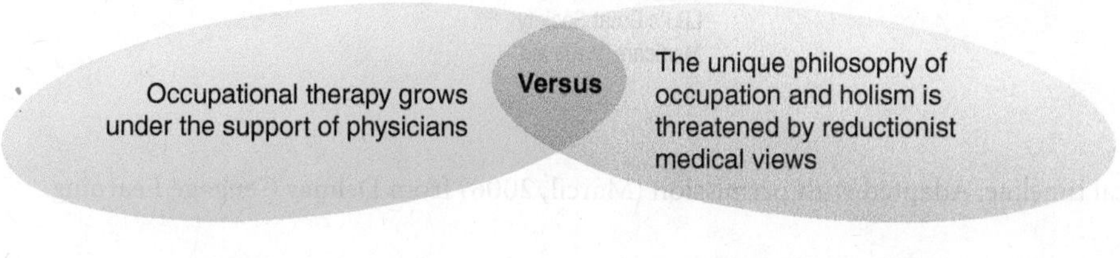

Occupational therapy grows under the support of physicians

Versus

The unique philosophy of occupation and holism is threatened by reductionist medical views

Figure 1.4 The postwar dilemma. (Hussey et al., 2007).

Archives of Occupational Therapy (1922)

↓

Occupational Therapy and Rehabilitation (1925)

↓

The American Journal of Occupational Therapy (1947)

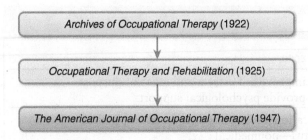

Figure 1.5 Renaming *The American Journal of Occupational Therapy* (AJOT).

profession, there was a professional journal to disseminate this information (Fig. 1.6).

Rehabilitation Movement (1942 to 1960)

The mid-20th century witnessed many rapid changes to the profession. The period of the rehabilitation movement saw a huge upswing in the need for occupational therapists that were ready and trained to work with

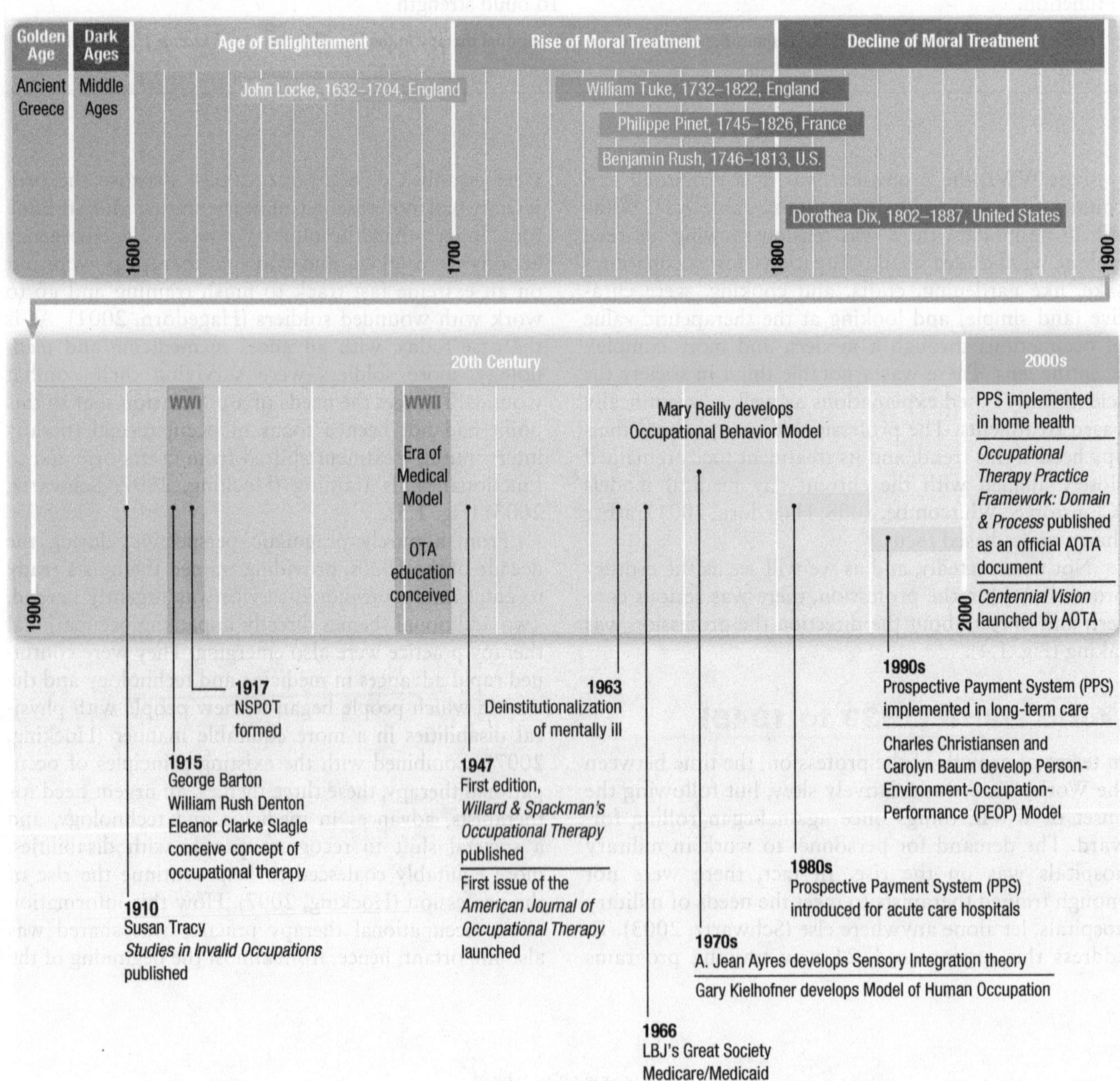

Figure 1.6 Occupational therapy historical timeline. Adapted with permission (Marcil, 2006) from Delmar Cengage Learning.

increasing numbers of soldiers with new or existing, long-term needs. With medical and pharmaceutical advances, people were living longer and often with disability. Occupational therapists trained to work with individuals with physical and psychological disabilities were highly sought after.

1945 brought on the first registration examination. Passing the examination was required to be registered as an occupational therapist. There was a move from general practitioner to specialization within physical rehabilitation (O'Brien & Hussey, 2012). To keep abreast of current trends in health care, technological advances made it necessary for occupational therapists to learn new skills, such as splinting. Consistent with the roots of the profession, the other specialty area for occupational therapists was psychosocial practice. Another specialty area of practice was just emerging, but it was not until the mid-1970s and the passage of significant federal legislation that pediatric specialty practice really came into its own.

In the late 1950s, with an increasing number of occupational therapists practicing in physical medicine and rehabilitation, there arose a serious shortage of therapists working in mental health settings, thus emerged the role of the **occupational therapy assistant**. Chapter 2 discusses the evolution and re-evolution of this position in detail.

In 1965, the Medicare program was enacted. This wide reaching federal legislation suddenly catapulted the occupational therapist's role in working with older adults in inpatient and in a more limited capacity, outpatient settings. Later, Medicare coverage was expanded to private practice. In 1988, federal legislation provided occupational therapists "the right to obtain Medicare provider numbers, thus permitting direct reimbursement for occupational therapy services" (O'Brien & Hussey, 2012, p. 20).

In 1965, the American Occupational Therapy Foundation (AOTF) was formed to promote research initiatives and occupational therapy through financial support. Today, the AOTF is a robust organization that carries out its mission to "advance research, education and public awareness for occupational therapy so that all people may participate fully in life regardless of their physical, social, mental, or developmental circumstances" (AOTF, n.d.) (From the Field 1.3).

By the 1960s, there was a recognized need for the profession to create a core to provide a reason for inclusion in the health care system and to formalize the underpinnings and body of knowledge that up to this point had been developed (Hagedorn, 2001, p. 20). It was time to create a formalized occupational science, complete with scientifically backed theories supporting the value of the profession. To this point in the history of the profession, there was an established body of knowledge that was required to become an occupational therapist. The emphasis on education was to provide information for students to be able to know what to do, without understanding the all-important *why* that comes from theories and guiding principles (Hagedorn, 2001).

> **FROM THE FIELD 1.3**
>
> The founders envisioned the future of occupational therapy as a discipline needing to stay viable in the health care system of the time. How is this any different in the 21st century?

Influenced by the scientific community, occupational therapy came under pressure to conform to a scientific biomedical practice model. It was during the 1960s and 1970s that the profession truly moved away from its roots in crafts, activities, and holism (Hagedorn, 2001, p. 20). With a continuing focus on physical rehabilitation and working with people with disabilities, the shift to specialization and more technical treatment modalities led to a decline in an occupations craft-based focus. History suggests that the founders never intended a divide to come between moral treatment and medical science (Schwartz, 2003). In the 1960s and 1970s, some leaders of the profession at the time, including Elizabeth Yerxa and Mary Reilly, spoke out against this trend that focused on physical modalities rather than occupation-based crafts in practice (O'Brien & Hussey, 2012; Schwartz, 2003) and urged the profession to "bridge the gap between the two perspectives and to practice both the art and science of occupational therapy" (Schwartz, 2003, p. 10). The end result was a concerted effort to promote research, education, and practice within the profession (Schwartz, 2003). Mary Reilly, in her 1961 Eleanor Clarke Slagle Lecture, said this about the state of the profession:

"The occupational therapy body of knowledge should include therefore, an understanding of the developmental nature of the sensory–motor systems, the patterning of aptitudes, abilities and interests, the nature of the learning process involved in the acquisition of skills. It should include also an understanding of the developmental nature of the problem-solving process and process of creativity" (Reilly, 1961, p. 89).

Late Twentieth Century

The passage of several federal laws in the 1970s and 1980s helped to further solidify the profession and open doors to new practice specialties. The Rehabilitation Act of 1973 mandated funding for and implementation of programming, service delivery, development of a set of delivery standards, research, and civil rights protections for people with disabilities. No longer were people with disabilities to be marginalized. Occupational therapy services were in great demand to help meet the mandates of the Act (O'Brien & Hussey, 2012).

Pediatric practice truly came into its own with the passage of the Education for all Handicapped Children Act (EHA) of 1975 (PL94-142). The EHA required provision of a free and appropriate education (FAPE) to all children regardless of status. Added as an amendment to PL94-142, the Handicapped Infants and Toddlers Act of 1986 extended free educational programming for preschool children aged 3 to 5 years and early interventions services for children birth to 3 years. Occupational therapy services were included in this amendment. With the passage of these laws, came a huge increase in the number occupational therapists working with children, especially in school settings (O'Brien & Hussey, 2012).

One further Act, the Technology-Related Assistance for Individuals with Disabilities Act of 1988 made provision of assistive technology and services to people with disabilities a priority. Occupational therapy practitioners have consistently provided services funded through this act (O'Brien & Hussey, 2012). Despite the passage of such groundbreaking legislation, and the rising demand for occupational therapy services, overall health care costs were on the rise, and changes to curb costs through a significant reduction in federal spending on health and welfare programs and payments to health care providers and institutions were signed into law in August of 1997. This federal law was called the Balanced Budget Act. It was designed to bring about a balanced federal budget by 2002. Some proposed spending cuts were restored in 1999 and 2000. To this day, health care costs influence the scope of service delivery for the profession.

The Professional Issues

State licensure for occupational therapy practitioners began as a controversial issue in the 1970s, but after some changes in position at the national level, it is now determined on a state-by-state basis. *Be sure to find out what legislature laws govern practice in your state.*

By the 1980s, graduate education became available, which led to a more analytical and academic approach to the theories guiding the profession. During this time, there was a move toward a social model of disability, which made holistic approaches once again more mainstream.

The 1990s brought passage of the groundbreaking **Americans with Disabilities Act** of 1990. It is commonly referred to as the ADA CS8. The ADA ensures civil rights to people with disabilities and was instrumental in further expanding the scope of practice specialties within the profession. The ADA will be explored in greater detail in Chapter 21, *Adaptive Equipment*; Chapter 22, *Assistive Technology*; and Chapter 36, *Children and Youth*. In 1991, Public Law 94–142 was renamed the **Individuals with Disabilities Education Act**. It is commonly called IDEA CS2, CS6. The IDEA requires that all students with disabilities be educated in the least restrictive environment possible, mandating that students with disabilities be educated alongside those without disability. This law also requires that local school districts provide necessary assistive technology and related services, which includes occupational therapy.

Despite the incredible advances in medicine and technology, landmark federal legislation, and a rise in the demand for occupational therapy practitioners, something had to change. Occupational therapy was being implemented in a growing number of settings, such as physical rehabilitation, mental health, and pediatric settings, yet there was a lack of theory and research to demonstrate the profession's worth. To that end, theories, such as Kielhofner and Burke's (1980) Model of Human Occupation (MOHO) and the development of an occupational science to back clinical practice, were established.

Twenty-First Century: Looking Forward

The membership body of the AOTA now exceeds 42,000 occupational therapists and occupational therapy assistants from all fifty states, the District of Columbia, Puerto Rico, and internationally (AOTA, n.d.). Throughout the world, occupational therapy continues to grow as a profession. Established in 1952, the World Federation of Occupational Therapy now contains "69 member nations around the world, an individual membership of more than 25,000 practitioners and a national organization membership that represents over 350,000 occupational therapists internationally" (WFOT, 2011). Back in the United States and as demonstrated by the forward momentum of our profession, in 2013, the Accreditation Council for Occupational Therapy Education listed 209 accredited OTA programs and 257 accredited OT programs. Compare this to 2006, when there were 129 accredited OTA programs and 148 accredited OT programs. *What does this tell you about the need and value of our profession?*

Occupational therapy began its roots as a holistic profession, in which the whole person is the focus of treatment (O'Brien & Hussey, 2012). Throughout the history of the profession, the practitioner–client/patient relationship has been critically important to the process of occupational therapy (O'Brien & Hussey, 2012).

The Centennial Vision

Because a relationship-centered model of practice was at the heart of the earliest days of the profession, it is not difficult to connect the *Founding Vision* to the *Centennial Vision* of occupational therapy. The *Founding Vision* provides today's "practitioners a sense of continuity and community with earlier generations of occupational therapists and an understanding that many of the contemporary values we currently hold were first articulated by occupational therapy's founding generation almost 100 years ago" (Schwartz, 2009, p. 681). In other words, our past guides and influences our path to the future.

The **Centennial Vision** states "We envision that occupational therapy is a powerful, widely recognized, science-driven, and evidence-based profession with a globally connected and diverse workforce meeting society's occupational needs" (AOTA, 2007, p. 613).

What connects the *Founding Vision* with the *Centennial Vision* is "a profound belief in the healing nature of occupation" (Schwartz, 2009, p. 687). What separates them is the *Centennial Vision's* expanded definition of occupational therapy that includes "preventing and overcoming obstacles to participation" (AOTA, 2007, p. 613). This clause ensures a "social justice orientation to engagement in occupations" (Schwartz, 2009, p. 867), which, while always a focus of the profession, is now clearly articulated.

When speaking of the relationship between occupational therapy and the medical model in her 2009 Eleanor Clarke Slagle Address, Kathleen Schwartz eloquently stated "occupational therapists must bend the scientific and humanistic perspectives in order to achieve occupational therapy's vision: A vision where occupation is at the heart of the intervention: not a diagnosis" (Slagle, 2009, p. 688). Take this to heart as you look forward by first looking back.

Summary

Just as our founders and early practitioners were at odds to develop a professional identity, the struggle continues today but arguably to a lesser degree in part because our well-documented historical roots guide our future and our vision is a forward looking one, firmly grounded in evidence and science. As Elnora Gilfoyle stated in her 1984 Eleanor Clarke Slagle Lecture, "Our present achievements are not a museum of finished products but an ongoing progress that is threefold: past, present, and future integrated into the upward spiral of our profession's evolution" (Gilfoyle, 1984, p. 575). Understanding how our past influences the future and the rich history we share as occupational therapy practitioners, knowing who you are and being a professional ambassador is an exciting challenge that awaits you.

Review Questions

1. Who was the first president of AOTA?
   a. Susan Tracy
   b. Eleanor Clarke Slagle
   c. Herbert Hall
   d. Adolf Meyer

2. NSPOT was formed in:
   a. March 1917
   b. June 1917
   c. March 1921
   d. July 1918

3. Which of the following was *not* proposed as a name for the profession?
   a. Ergotherapy
   b. Occupational therapy
   c. Work cure
   d. Vocational therapy

4. Who is credited as being the "father of occupational therapy?"
   a. Adolf Meyer
   b. William Dunton
   c. Thomas Kidner
   d. George Barton

5. Which of the statements below best describes moral treatment?
   a. To cure rather than confine people with mental illness in asylums
   b. A provision in federal legislature to provide elderly people with housing
   c. To insist that people attend houses of worship in order to receive pensions
   d. A belief that persons with mental illness are not equal citizens

6. The purpose of Hull House was to:
   a. Provide physical rehabilitation services for soldiers
   b. Provide habit-training programs
   c. Provide social and educational services to immigrants in Chicago
   d. Create a third-party payer system for health care during the reform movement

7. Federal legislation that requires provision of a free and appropriate education for all children is:
   a. The Education for all Handicapped Children Act (EHA)—PL94-142
   b. Soldier's Rehabilitation Act
   c. The Americans with Disabilities Act
   d. Technology-Related Assistance for Individuals with Disabilities Act

8. ________ ensures civil rights to people with disabilities.
   a. The Education for all Handicapped Children Act (EHA)—PL94-142
   b. The Americans with Disabilities Act
   c. Individuals with Disabilities Education Act
   d. Soldier's Rehabilitation Act

9. In 1923, the AOTA adopted the *Minimum Standards for Courses of Training in Occupational Therapy*. What was its purpose?
   a. To register occupational therapists
   b. To track new graduates
   c. A call for standardization of educational programs for occupational therapists
   d. To encourage occupational therapy training programs to recruit new students

10. The first occupational therapy registration exam was administered in:
   a. 1932
   b. 1988
   c. 1945
   d. 1965

11. The purpose of occupations in the TB wards, during and after WWI, was primarily for:
   a. Diversion
   b. Work
   c. Self-care
   d. Cognitive skills training

12. As part of her tireless promotion of occupational therapy, Eleanor Clarke Slagle wore many hats. Which one did she *not* wear?
   a. President of NSPOT
   b. Vice President of NSPOT
   c. Executive Secretary of AOTA
   d. Editor in Chief of the *Annals of Occupational Therapy*

13. According to Kathleen Schwartz, what do the *Founding* and *Centennial Visions* of occupational therapy share in common?
   a. They are completely disparate and have nothing in common.
   b. Both were written by people with very different professional backgrounds.
   c. A profound belief in the healing nature of occupation.
   d. A strong understanding of current world affairs.

14. What precipitated the role of the OTA?
   a. A shortage of OTs working in mental health practice settings
   b. A shortage of OTs working in pediatric practice settings
   c. The cost of malpractice insurance for OTs
   d. Medicare laws

Practice Activities

Prepare a brief script for a 2- to 4-minute synopsis of the history of occupational therapy. Choose three people: a young adult, a middle-aged adult, and an older adult. Present your synopsis to all three of these people. Ask each to relate occupational therapy to their lives. Ask them to be specific and provide concrete examples. Record the responses. Compare and contrast the responses of the young, middle-aged, and older adult, noting gender as well as age group. Share your results with your classmates. What themes do you find? Diagram the entire class' responses and present your findings at a student chapter or other OT meeting.

Select one landmark historical event in occupational therapy that is most meaningful to you. Prepare a short PowerPoint presentation linking this event to a health-related event, such as disease outbreaks, natural disasters, medical breakthrough, etc., happening in your community during this same time period. Can you find any parallels between occupational therapy and these events? Did the health-related event have any influence on the history of occupational therapy?

Research some cooking trends/recipes that were popular during a particular moment in the history of occupational therapy. Prepare a few of these recipes and share with classmates. Revisit this activity when studying Chapter 9 and prepare an activity analysis of this recipe preparation.

Thomas Kidner made no bones about expecting all occupational therapists to be ambassadors for the profession. What can you do to act as an ambassador to the profession? List 10 things and chose one to act on. How will you do it?

If you could have dinner with a founder of the profession, who would it be, and why? Write a short paper explaining your response.

References

American Occupational Therapy Association. *AOTA: a historical perspective*. 1991. Retrieved from http://www.aota.org/About/39983.aspx

American Occupational Therapy Association. AOTA's Centennial Vision and executive summary. *Am J Occup Ther* 2007;61:613–614.

American Occupational Therapy Association. *Definition of Occupational Therapy Practice for the AOTA Model Practice Act*. Bethesda, MD: American Occupational Therapy Association; 2011a. Retrieved from http://www.aota.org/Practitioners/Advocacy/State/Resources/PracticeAct/36437.aspx?FT=.pdf

American Occupational Therapy Association. Policy 5.3.1: definition of occupational therapy practice for State Regulation. *Am J Occup Ther* 2011b;58:694–695.

American Occupational Therapy Association. *About AOTA*. n.d.a. Retrieved May 3, 2012, from http://www.aota.org/About.aspx

American Occupational Therapy Association. *ACOTE Accreditation*. n.d.b. Retrieved March 3, 2012, from http://www.aota.org/educate/accredit.aspx.

American Occupational Therapy Association. *What Is Occupational Therapy?* n.d.c. Retrieved from http://www.aota.org/Consumers.aspx

American Occupational Therapy Foundation. The mission of AOTF. n.d. Retrieved from http://www.aotf.org/aboutaotf/visionmissiongoals.aspx

Bing RK. *Eleanor Clarke Slagle Lecture Occupational therapy revisited: a paraphrastic journey*. 1981. Retrieved from http://www.aota.org/Practitioners/Resources/Slagle/1981.aspx

Breines E. Genesis of occupation: a philosophical model for therapy and theory. *Aust Occup Ther J* 1990(March);37(1):45–49.

Clouston TJ, Whitcombe SW. The professionalisation of occupational therapy: a continuing challenge. *Br J Occup Ther* 2008(Aug);71(8):314–320.

Dunkel LM. Moral and humane: Patients' libraries in early nineteenth-century American mental hospitals. *Bull Am Libr Assoc* 1983; 71(3):274–281.

Friedland J. Occupational therapy and rehabilitation: an awkward alliance. *Am J Occup Ther* 1998;52(5):373–380.

Friedland J, Silva J. Evolving identities: Thomas Bessell Kidner and occupational therapy in the United States. *Am J Occup Ther* 2008(May/June);62(3):349–360.

Gilfoyle EM. 1984 Eleanor Clarke Slagle Lecture Transformation of a profession. *Am J Occup Ther* 1984;38:575–584.

Gordon DM. The history of occupational therapy. In: Crepeau EB, Cohn ES, Boyt Schell BA, eds. *Willard and Spackman's Occupational Therapy*. 11th ed. pp. 202–215. New York, NY: Lippincott Williams & Wilkins; 2009.

Hagedorn R. *Foundations for Practice in Occupational Therapy*. Edinburgh, UK: Churchill Livingstone; 2001.

Hocking C. Early perspectives of patients, practice and the profession. *Br J Occup Ther* 2007(Jul);70(7):284–291.

Igiugu MN. Instrumentalism in occupational therapy: an argument for a pragmatic conceptual model of practice. *Int J Psychosoc Rehab* 2004;8:109–117.

Kielhofner G. *Conceptual Foundations of Occupational Therapy Practice*. 4th ed. Philadelphia, PA: F.A. Davis Company; 2009.

McColl MA, et al. *Theoretical Basis of Occupational Therapy*. Thorofare, NJ: Slack, Inc; 2002.

National Society for the Promotion of Occupational Therapy. *Certificate of Incorporation*. Clifton Springs, NY: Author; 1917.

O'Brien JC, Hussey SM. *Introduction to Occupational Therapy*. 4th ed. St. Louis, MO: Mosby Elsevier; 2012.

Quiroga VA. *Occupational Therapy: The First 30 Years 1900–1930*. Bethesda, MD: American Occupational Therapy Association; 1995.

Reilly M. *Eleanor Clarke Slagle Lecture. Occupational Therapy can be One of the Great Ideas of 20th-Century Medicine*. 1961. Retrieved from http://www.aota.org/Practitioners/Resources/Slagle/1961.aspx

Schwartz KB. The history of occupational therapy. In: Crepeau EB, Cohn ES, Boyt Schell BA, eds. *Willard and Spackman's Occupational Therapy*. 10th ed., pp. 5–13. New York, NY: Lippincott Williams & Wilkins; 2003.

Schwartz KB. The 2009 Eleanor Clarke Slagle Lecture: Reclaiming our heritage: Connecting the Founding Vision to the Centennial Vision. *Am J Occup Ther* 2009(Nov-Dec);63(6): 681–690.

Slagle EC. Training aides for mental patients. *Arch Occup Ther* 2009(Nov-Dec);1(1):11–18.

Wade LC. Settlement houses. 2005. Retrieved from http://encyclopedia.chicagohistory.org/pages/1135.html

WFOT. *Member Organisations of WFOT*. 2011. Retrieved from http://www.wfot.org/Membership/MemberOrganisationsofWFOT.aspx

Wolf T. Refocusing our education efforts for the 2017 Centennial Vision. *Occup Ther Health Care* 2007;21(1/2):309–312.

CHAPTER 2

The Evolution and Re-Evolution of Occupational Therapy Assistant Training and Practice

Amy Wagenfeld, PhD, OTR/L SCEM, CAPs

Key Terms

Accreditation Council for Occupational Therapy Education (ACOTE)—The organization that accredits occupational therapy and occupational therapy assistant educational programs.

COTA Award of Excellence—Recognizes the unique role of an OTA through clinical practice, education, administrative education, publication, or presentation.

Occupational therapy assistant—A credentialed professional who works under the supervision of and in partnership with an occupational therapist to deliver safe and effective therapy services (AOTA, 2009a,b).

Representative Assembly—The body composed of representatives from identified constituencies (election areas) whose function is to legislate and establish policy for the association (AOTA, 2010).

Roster of Honor—Recognizes the contribution of an OTA to AOTA and the profession.

Terry Brittell COTA/OTR Partnership Award—Recognizes outstanding partnership and collaboration between the roles within occupational therapy.

Learning Objectives

After studying this chapter, readers should be able to:

- Explain how the role of the occupational therapy assistant began and how current practice share commonalities and is also divergent.
- State the role of the occupational therapy assistant as a vital member of the treatment team.

Introduction

The role of the occupational therapy assistant (OTA) arose out of necessity post the World War II era. The impact of the two World Wars led to a critical need for physical rehabilitation services and created a severe shortage of OTs treating people in psychiatric venues. Despite significant concern for how this role would evolve in the profession, OTAs were envisioned as being integral to direct patient care. Today with rising health care costs, an ongoing shortage of therapists, and the changing roles and responsibilities of OTs, now more than ever, the OTA is a much needed member of a treatment team. This may be in traditional practice areas or, more and more, in innovative and creative new roles. Because the future employment outlook for OTAs has never looked better, this content of this chapter focuses on the evolution of a new professional role within occupational therapy and how, with current health care trends, it continues to re-evolve.

An Overview of Professional Roles in Occupational Therapy

There are three roles that are recognized within occupational therapy, the occupational therapist (OT), the OTA, and the occupational therapy aide. All work together, yet each role has unique responsibilities and scope of practice that must be followed.

Occupational Therapist

As of 2007, OTs must complete a master's degree (in occupational therapy) in order to practice. OTs that completed their education and certification exam prior to 2007 are "grandfathered" into practice. The role of an OT is to evaluate, plan, and implement interventions, as well as to be involved with discharge planning and other communications. OTs who graduate from accredited programs are eligible to take the national certification exam (AOTA, n.d.a).

Occupational Therapy Assistant

The OTA receives an associate's degree and provides therapy services under the supervision of an OT. Based on state laws and demonstrated clinical competence, an OTA may assist with evaluations. OTAs who graduate from accredited programs are eligible to take the national certification exam (AOTA, n.d.a) (From the Field 2.1).

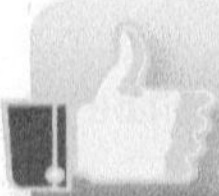

FROM THE FIELD 2.1

The American Occupational Therapy Association's accrediting agency for occupational therapy/assistant education is called the Accreditation Council for Occupational Therapy Education (ACOTE) (AOTA, 2014a,b,c). It is recognized by the U.S. Department of Education and the Council for Higher Education Accreditation (AOTA, 2014a,b,c). There are over 325 educational programs accredited by the ACOTE (AOTA, 2014a,b,c). To view the ACOTE standards that occupational therapy and OTA programs must adhere to in their curriculum design and implementation, please see http://www.aota.org/-/media/Corporate/Files/EducationCareers/Accredit/Standards/2011-Standards-and-Interpretive-Guide-August-2013.pdf.

Occupational Therapy Aide

Sometimes referred to as a restorative aide, an occupational therapy aide performs nonclinical supportive roles such as setting up occupational therapy groups and cleaning the clinic, training is typically on the job, and there is no certification process for occupational therapy aides (AOTA, n.d.a).

Defining the Role of the OTA

With the long-term job outlook for OTAs stronger than ever, before exploring the evolution and current re-evolution of the OTA role, let's begin with a question. What exactly is an **occupational therapy assistant**? According to the American Occupational Therapy Association (AOTA), "an occupational therapy assistant is responsible for providing safe and effective occupational therapy services under the supervision of and in partnership with the occupational therapist and in accordance with laws or regulations and AOTA documents" (AOTA, 2009a,b, p. 797). As set forth by the AOTA, there are formal role delineations between an OT and OTA (Table 2.1).

The OTA is supervised by an OT and carries out prescribed treatment plans (Salvatori, 2001). While the responsibility for services provided by an OTA is taken on by the supervising OT and their employer, disciplinary action for OTAs and OTs is carried out in part by the National Board for Certification in Occupational Therapy (NBCOT) (AOTA, 2010a; Salvatori, 2001). The NBCOT is a stand-alone agency that provides the initial certification of OTs and OTAs (AOTA, 2010a). Certification is important to any profession because it aligns with credibility. In terms of occupational therapy certification it "sends a message of trust and accountability to consumers about occupational therapy practitioners" (Wagenfeld & Hsi, 2003, p. 40). Occupational therapy was one of the first health care professions to initiate a credentialing and certification process (Wagenfeld & Hsi, 2003). OTAs must follow AOTA professional practice standards and adhere to a code of ethics in the delivery of services (AOTA, 2015).

Black and Eberhardt (2005) indicated about the OTA role that "its most valuable asset is to broaden occupational therapy services in all practice areas". That said, the bulk of the profession works in skilled nursing facilities and schools, but without a doubt, innovative practice is well on the rise and OTAs are now working in many unique settings, such as case management and home modification consultation. Additionally, OTAs now serve at all levels within the AOTA and are educators in OT and OTA programs, authors, and presenters.

TABLE 2.1 Role Deliniations

Service Components	Occupational Therapy Assistant	Occupational Therapist
Screening, evaluation, re-evaluation (evaluation)	Contributes to the evaluation process by implementing delegated assessments	Directs, initiates, and is responsible for all aspects of the evaluation process
	Uses up-to-date assessments and assessment procedures and follows defined protocols of standardized assessments for evaluation process	Uses up-to-date assessments and assessment procedures and follows defined protocols of standardized assessments for the evaluation process
		Analyzes and interprets data from evaluation and develops treatment plan
	Contributes to the documentation of evaluation results	Completes and documents occupational therapy evaluation results
	Communicates evaluation results while following confidentiality and privacy regulations	Communicates evaluation results while following confidentiality and privacy regulations
Implementation		Develops, documents, and implements occupational therapy intervention
	Collaborates with client to develop and implement intervention plan	Collaborates with client to develop and implement intervention plan
	Uses professional and clinical reasoning to select the most appropriate interventions	Uses professional and clinical reasoning to select the most appropriate interventions
	Documents occupational therapy services	Documents occupational therapy services
Outcomes		Selects, measures, documents, and interprets outcomes related to the client's ability to engage in occupations
		Documents changes in client's performance and capacities and for transitioning the client to other types or intensity of service or discontinuing services
	Contributes to transition or discontinuation plan by providing information and documentation to the supervising occupational therapist	Prepares and implements a transition or discontinuation plan
	Facilitates a collaborative transition or discharge process	Facilitates a collaborative transition or discharge process
	Contributes to evaluating safety and effectiveness of the occupational therapy processes and interventions	Contributes to evaluating safety and effectiveness of the occupational therapy processes and interventions

Adapted from the American Occupational Therapy Association. Standards of practice for occupational therapy. *Am J Occup Ther* 2010c;64:S106–S111.

A New Role within AOTA: The Proud History of the OTA in the Twentieth Century

It all began in March 1949 when, at the AOTA Board of Management meeting, creation of an assistant level practitioner within occupational therapy was first proposed.

The 1950s

Beginning post WWII and into the mid to late 1950s, there was increasing demand for occupational therapy services in both physical rehabilitation and psychiatric settings. However, the reality was that there were more OTs practicing in physical medicine and rehabilitation and a serious shortage of therapists working in psychiatric practice (Black & Eberhardt, 2005; Cottrell, 2000a; O'Brien & Hussey, 2012; Salvatori, 2001). This shortage of OTs made it very difficult for those needing psychiatric-based occupational therapy services to receive them. A first step to solving this problem was addressed in 1956 when the Board of Management for AOTA and the Delegate Assembly (renamed the **Representative Assembly** or RA in 1976) formed the Committee for the Recognition of Occupational Therapy Assistants (Black & Eberhardt, 2005; Yamkovenko, 2009).

At this meeting, it was proposed that a plan to develop an educational program at the assistant level be established. A committee was formed to take on this task of exploring the possibility of creating a new level of practitioner as a means of addressing the shortage of OTs (Cottrell, 2000a). In 1956, the AOTA approved a plan to recognize an additional level of practitioner within the profession, the certified occupational therapy assistant (COTA), now called OTA. Those OTs credited at the AOTA board level for leading the charge to create the role of the OTA were Ruth Brunyate Wiemer, Colonel Ruth Robinson, Marion Crampton, and Mildred Schwagmeyer (Black & Eberhardt, 2005). Robinson, who served as the AOTA president from 1955 to 1958, is associated with helping to create the scope of the OTA roles and responsibilities (Black & Eberhardt, 2005). Wiemer had a forward thinking vision for the advancement of the OTA role and felt that positive working relationships could ensue between an OTA and OT. She also believed that an OTA would, through implementation of services, positively impact clients. Weimer steadfastly believed that there was an important place for both OTAs and OTs in the entire client treatment process across a variety of practice venues, which remains true today.

In October 1957, the AOTA Board of Management accepted the committee's written document, which provided a curriculum guide and recommendations for the minimum requirements for educational standards for an OTA program. The course of study that the committee proposed covered one particular disability area, psychiatry. Consequently, completion of the earliest formal OTA training programs led to the certification in psychiatric OTA practice. It was also at this time that the designation COTA and the COTA insignia were adopted. According to official records, "the standards for the training and recognition of occupational therapy assistants in psychiatry were adopted in 1958, and were developed from guidelines which had a favorable vote of a majority of state associations in January 1956" (Black & Eberhardt, 2005, p. ix).

In 1958, a year after the committee devised a written plan for this new professional designation, it was published and distributed as an official AOTA notification regarding the training and certification of this new OTA role to governmental, mental health, and pertinent individuals (AOTA, 1958; Cottrell, 2000b). Accordingly, there have been national standards for education and an approval process for the accreditation of educational programs for OTAs since 1958. As we will explore, since the beginning, the role, education, training, and practice scope of the OTA have been the subject of, at times, intense debate.

The 1960s

In its earliest iteration, a prospective OTA attended a 3-month training program in a designated facility. The program consisted of didactic coursework and specialty skills with supervised clinical experience (Cottrell, 2000a). In 1960, the first educational psychiatric training programs were held at the Westboro State Hospital in North Grafton, Massachusetts, which today houses the Tufts Cummings School of Veterinary Medicine. The other was held at Marcy State Hospital, in Marcy, New York. Another program based on the 12-week curriculum model developed by the AOTA board was offered at a nursing home in Montgomery County, Maryland (Cottrell, 2000a). The graduates of these first formal training programs were credentialed only for psychiatric or nursing home practice. In 1965, AOTA began a pilot educational program for OTAs leading to dual certification in psychiatric and general practice (Cottrell, 2000a). By 1966, the AOTA required that all new OTA programs provide dual training in general and psychiatric practice (Cottrell, 2000a). Prior to the landmark 1958 move to formal educational standards and certification for OTAs, those working as occupational therapy aides for at least 2 years in a specialty practice area were eligible to be grandfathered at the OTA level. Doing so involved providing AOTA with three positive recommendations, including one from a current supervisor. In 1960, 2 years after commencement of formal OTA educational programs, the grandfathering clause was terminated (Cottrell, 2000a).

In 1965, two college-level associates degree programs opened their doors to the first class of OTA students. Mount Aloysius College in Pennsylvania and St. Mary's Junior College in Minnesota became the first in the country to offer an associate-degree program for OTAs. Both graduated their first class of OTAs in 1966 (Black & Eberhardt, 2005; Strezlecki, 2009). In 1986, St. Mary's Junior College merged with the College of St. Catherine. In 2009, the College changed its name to St. Catherine University, where it is 1 of 17 schools in the United States to offer both OTA and OT programs (AOTA, 2014a,b,c). Mt. Aloysius' OTA program closed in 2008.

Since 1965, an OTA is credentialed at the technical level and must complete a 2-year associate degree at 1 of nearly 300 accredited college or university programs throughout the United States (AOTA, n.d.b.). Formed in 1994, the organization that accredits occupational therapy and OTA educational programs is called the

Accreditation Council for Occupational Therapy Education (ACOTE). All OTA programs must receive initial accreditation and periodic reaccreditation by the ACOTE. The most recent version of the guiding document for this process is the *2011 Accreditation Council for Occupational Therapy Education (ACOTE) Standards and Interpretive Guide* (AOTA, 2012a,b). Recall from Chapter 1 that the AOTA has been accrediting educational programs since 1935, and at the request of the AOTA, from 1935 until 1994, the American Medical Association oversaw the process. Over the years, program length and curricula requirements have significantly changed.

By 1968, just 10 years after introducing formal AOTA endorsed educational training programs, there were more than 1,200 practicing OTAs and 20 educational programs (Cottrell, 2000a). Increasingly, more educational programs began to be located in academic settings rather than hospital or other health care venues (Cottrell, 2000a). To accommodate the significant need for OT and more OTA practitioners, today the numbers of accredited, in development stage and in applicant stage, and bridge educational programs are on the rise. The American Occupational Therapy Association URL, http://www.aota.org/en/Education-Careers/Find-School.aspx, provides up-to-date information on the status of all of the OT and OTA programs.

The 1970s and 1980s

In 1970, the AOTA approved another route to becoming an OTA. Military personnel who had worked as occupational therapy technicians for at least 12 months and were recommended by an OT were eligible for certification as an OTA (Cottrell, 2000a). By 1972, concerns about the lack of consistency in, or duration and content of OTA programs were on the rise. Programs lasted 9 to 11 months in a facilities-based institution or 2 years in an academic institution (Black & Eberhardt, 2005; Cottrell, 2000a). Not unexpectedly, the course content of these facilities-based and academic institutions varied, yet graduates of either program were equally eligible to practice as OTAs. In 1975, responding to this concern, the AOTA adopted the revised *Essentials and Guidelines for an Approved Educational Program for the Occupational Therapy Assistant*. The purpose of this document was to solidify the existing educational guidelines and to require that, by 1977, all graduates of an AOTA approved OTA programs sit for and pass a written certification exam (AOTA, 1976, 1999; Black & Eberhardt, 2005; Cottrell, 2000a). Since 1976, there have been multiple revisions to the educational standards to ensure consistency across the curriculum. *The Accreditation Standards for Educational Programs for the Occupational Therapy Assistant* replaced *The Essentials and Guidelines for an Approved Educational Program for the Occupational Therapy Assistant* in August 2006 (AOTA, 2009b).

Recognizing the desire for some OTAs to achieve upward career mobility, in 1971, the AOTA Delegate Assembly passed a resolution to determine ways in which OTAs could achieve professional advancement without further academic study. The Career Mobility Program (CMP) was established in 1973 to provide OTAs having at least two years of experience the opportunity to take the OT certification exam. But there were concerns that two years of experience were not sufficient to warrant taking the certification exam. By 1976, the criteria for CMP professional advancement was changed to "4 years of coaching practice with satisfactory delivery of direct services to clients under the supervision of an OTR, successful completion of approved therapist-level clinical fieldwork for at least 6 months, and payment of annual certification fees" (Cottrell, 2000a, p. 410). Those participating in the CMP program studied independently and received feedback from supervising OTs (Cottrell, 2000a).

This program was the focus of intense debate until its ultimate demise in 1982. Supporters of the CMP believed that skills generated from practical experiences versus academic background (and experiences) were adequate for OT level practice. They believed it was an efficient way to move OTAs into the health care system as OTs. Opponents of the CMP felt that it would undercut the value of the OT credential and, accordingly, certify as OTs those who did not, by virtue of lack of formal OT academic preparation, have the skills and knowledge necessary to provide a desired occupational therapy level of care. Noteworthy is that some OTAs also felt that the CMP program actually diminished their important role, as it possibly implied that only the OT role was of value.

While the Representative Assembly voted to continue the program, in 1982, it was discontinued because of "widespread concerns about the impact of lowering the educational standards because of and requirements for entry into the profession" (Cottrell, 2000a, p. 410). Further, many state licensure boards did not recognize OT status attained through CMP or permit CMP-certified clinicians to work in public school settings. There were also concerns about reimbursement for services implemented by CMP designates. Interestingly, in the 5 ½ years that the program was in existence, only 64 OTAs took advantage of it, but of those who did, many indicated that becoming an OT through the traditional channel would have been preferable (Cottrell, 2000a).

Although the OTA certification process was initiated in 1958, it was not until 1977 that AOTA established a certification examination for OTAs and a recertification process in the 1990s (Salvatori, 2001). To practice as an OTA, it is required to sit for and pass the national certification exam. There is much to be gained from a mandatory certification exam and national standards for education. In its earliest days, it sets and still sets OTAs apart from other assistant programs that do not necessarily require stringent standards for education and practice. According to Ruth Jones, "This provided a means to standardize and measure the knowledge and skills needed to practice as an OTA" (in Yamkovenko, 2009, p. 17). These high standards support upward career mobility (Salvatori, 2001).

OTAs who early on had trained in health care institutions or had grandfathered from occupational therapy aide to OTA had limited privileges to AOTA (Cottrell, 2000a). In 1963, the AOTA offered OTAs associate membership in the organization, with limited privileges (Black & Eberhardt, 2005; Salvatori, 2001). Continuing into the early 1970s, OTAs remained associate members but were not eligible to serve as AOTA representatives, vote in AOTA elections, vote on AOTA proposals, or receive the *American Journal of Occupational Therapy* (*AJOT*) as member benefits. A resolution to award OTAs voting rights in AOTA and the opportunity to serve on national boards was defeated in 1965 (Black & Eberhardt, 2005; Cottrell, 2000b; Yamkovenko, 2009). The resolution also recommended creation of a special division of AOTA devoted specially to OTA issues (Cottrell, 2000a; Yamkovenko, 2009). Defeat of this resolution caused a great deal of animosity and only heighted the contentious relationship that was escalating between OTs and OTAs that had existed since the inception of the assistant level role in 1958 (Cottrell, 2000a; Yamkovenko, 2009). Overcoming this division and developing a mutual sense of respect between OTAs and OTs and clear delineation of the roles and professional responsibilities of each practitioner level were the priorities. In 1972, the AOTA funded a workshop to address and quell the increasing divide (Cottrell, 2000a; Yamkovenko, 2009). A liaison between OTAs and the AOTA Council of Development was formed to help OTAs become more actively involved with the profession (Cottrell, 2000a; Yamkovenko, 2009). Efforts to transform the relationship in a more positive way were not well received by all members of the AOTA (Cottrell, 2000a; Yamkovenko, 2009). Although some resolution was achieved, there still remains a divide within the profession. Working to achieve mutual respect for the unique roles that OTAs and OTs fulfill as important members of a treatment team remains a challenge for the profession.

Despite the strife, during the 1970s, many exciting things were happening for OTAs on the national level at the AOTA. In 1975, the AOTA established the **COTA Award of Excellence** to recognize the unique role of an OTA through clinical practice, education, administrative education, publication, or presentation (Black & Eberhardt, 2005). OTAs were now eligible to receive the AOTA award of merit and to be considered to present the prestigious Eleanor Clarke Slagle Lectureship.

In 1976, OTAs were given full AOTA membership status and awarded full voting rights in AOTA. The first OTA was elected to AOTA's Executive Board in 1976 and, in 1978, saw the establishment of the COTA **Roster of Honor** for OTAs whose scholarly achievements in education, practice, and research were noteworthy (AOTA, 2011). The first recipient of the AOTA Roster of Honor was Sally E. Ryan.

In 1983, Ms. Ryan was the first OTA to be elected to the Representative Assembly, where she served as a member at large. The Representative Assembly established the COTA Advisory Committee to AOTA's Executive Board in 1986 (Cottrell, 2000a). In 1988, the COTA Forum became a permanent feature of the AOTA Annual Conference (Cottrell, 2000a). In terms of professional recognition, since its inception in the 1970s, more than 30 OTAs have received the AOTA OTA Award of Excellence, the Roster of Honor, or the **Terry Brittell OTA/OTR Partnership Award** (discussed below) (Yamkovenko, 2009, From the Field 2.2).

The 1990s

Beyond the scope of education and training, the OTA role within the AOTA continued to undergo a renaissance of sorts (Yamkovenko, 2009). The Terry Brittell COTA/OTR Partnership Award was created in 1991 to recognize outstanding partnership and collaboration between the roles within occupational therapy (Cottrell, 2000a). AOTA started an OTA networking steering committee in 1991(Cottrell, 2000a). Since the 1990s, OTAs have consistently served on the AOTA Commission on Practice, the Commission on Standards, and the Representative Assembly (Cottrell, 2000a).

Ongoing evolution from direct service provider to more expanded scope of responsibilities on a health care team helped increase awareness of the importance of OTAs in the 1990s. This increased visibility was in part due to initiation of the 1997 Advanced Practitioner program for OTAs, a self-initiated process that recognizes "achievement of an advanced level of practice within an area of occupational therapy" (Cottrell, 2000a, p. 409). The program was a catalyst for some OTAs to experience career mobility. Further, changes in health care trends have made it necessary for OTs to focus on evaluation and intervention planning, thus making it imperative that the OTA assume more responsibility for implementation of the OT's intervention plan. Health care trends and the Advanced Practitioner program have helped to increase the status of the OTA as a viable partner in health care.

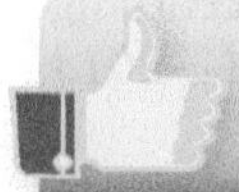

FROM THE FIELD 2.2

Kitty's Story

I became interested in OT at the age of 15 years after my niece Alison was diagnosed with spinal meningitis at 3 days old. At about 6 months old, she began home therapy with Mercedes, her OT. I was so impressed with this woman and how she could read what Alison was going to do next, but she was also able to persuade Alison to do things that we thought were impossible. Raised a country girl, I thought Mercedes' profession was too far out of my reach, but I could not stop soaking up as much as I could. When Alison was 4 years old and I was 19, I taught her to sit up without being propped against something or someone holding her upright. When my sister showed the PTs what I had taught Alison, they said I had a natural talent and to encourage me to pursue therapy. As the baby of my family, I was very naïve, protected, and basically clueless about the whole college scene. I was scared to death with the thought of going away to school, so I put occupational therapy on the proverbial back burner.

Life happened: marriage, babies, and self-employment, which is where I found out about a local private college offering an OTA program from one of our customers. I didn't have to go away to school! My husband was witness to the expressions of excitement and fear and knew he had to encourage me. I was 38 years old, married, with two children, and two businesses, could I have picked a more difficult time to go to college? Much to my surprise, I did it anyway!

I have been in this profession since 2000 and can honestly say I have never had such a satisfying job. I prefer to work in the long-term care setting. The love that is given and received is immeasurable, the wisdom that is shared is amazing, and the smallest acts are appreciated. My favorite saying to my patients is "I have to go pretend I am working," this does not feel like a job to me except that I am not at home.

Kitty Stafford, COTA/L

The Twenty-First Century

More than 50 years ago, a committee reported to the AOTA on the merits of creating a training program for OTAs for both the association and the profession as a whole (Yamkovenko, 2009). The committee envisioned that the OTA role would enhance the quality of and extend the scope of services to a greater number of people (Yamkovenko, 2009, p. 18). The increasing demands for OTA services in all sectors of practice and client care have been met with an influx of educational programs, which must undergo initial and reaccreditation processes by the ACOTE. In 1999, there were 162 accredited OTA programs (all but four culminated in an associate degree), 23 developing programs, and 13 in applicant stage (Cottrell, 2000a). In 2014, there were over 200 accredited, 20 in developing stage, and 33 OTA programs in applicant stage (AOTA, 2014a,b,c). It is safe to say that the program you are attending looks very little like what the initial three 12-week-long programs did. While the first programs addressed the immediate societal needs, today's OTA must be prepared to take on increasingly demanding and complex roles and responsibilities within an ever-changing health care system (From the Field 2.3).

Today, all OTA programs are housed in colleges or universities. The programs offer a broader range of coursework to prepare new graduates to emerge as generalists as compared to the focus on psychiatric practice. Like occupational therapy programs, the ACOTE continues to accredit OTA programs. Modern day OTA programs must follow ACOTE guidelines and curriculums so as to prepare students to be active participants in clinical, managerial, academic, and research endeavors. The current educational program is 2 years long and includes multiple fieldwork experiences (AOTA, 2011).

Today, and with regard to practice as an OTA, the AOTA *Scope of Practice* (AOTA, 2010b) states that an individual must have

FROM THE FIELD 2.3

OTA Programs

For many OTAs, the burden of additional coursework combined with work and outside responsibilities can be great (Cottrell, 2000a). To meet the needs of what are referred to as nontraditional students, many OTA and also master's of occupational therapy and doctoral programs are now offered in hybrid, weekend, or distance learning formats, although presently there are no fully online OTA programs. *What type of program do you attend? Did you choose it in part because of the structure of the program?*

- Graduated from an OTA program accredited by the ACOTE or predecessor organizations
- Successfully completed a period of supervised fieldwork experience required by the recognized educational institution where the applicant met the academic requirements of an educational program for OTAs that is accredited by the ACOTE or predecessor organizations
- Successfully passed the national certification examination for OTAs and/or met state requirements for licensure/registration (p. S76)

Because state and other regulatory agencies or boards may have their own requirements, it is your responsibility to contact the appropriate agencies to determine what specific requirements apply to practice in your geographic region (AOTA, 2010b, p. S76).

Upward Mobility

Not all OTAs have the desire to advance to the OT level. For many, there are opportunities within the traditional OTA role that are very satisfying. For others who wish to advance within the OTA role, many companies or large institutions offer career-laddering programs for OTAs to retain their professional identity while learning new skills such as leadership, management, or particular clinical skills. Those who choose to advance via career laddering tend to develop very strong collaborative relationships with their supervising OTs, which truly benefits the profession as a whole (Cottrell, 2000b, From the Field 2.4).

The Re-evolution: A Growing Profession

According to the U.S. Bureau of Labor Statistics, you have chosen wisely to pursue a career as an OTA. Not only is it a vibrant and an exciting profession, the employment outlook could not be better. According to the *Occupational Outlook Handbook, 2012–2013 Edition,*

> employment of occupational therapy assistants and aides is expected to grow by 30 percent from 2008 to 2018, much faster than the average for all occupations. Demand for occupational therapist assistants and aides will continue to rise because of the increasing number of individuals with disabilities or limited function. (Bureau of Labor Statistics, 2012)

Practically speaking, because demand for occupational therapy services continues to rise, OTs must increasingly coordinate intervention plans with OTAs. Job prospects should be *very good* for OTAs. (From the Field 2.5).

Figure 2.1 shows the projected 10-year growth of the employment outlook for OTAs. According to the 2012 Bureau of Labor Statistics, OTAs rank as the 13th most employable occupation.

What is the reason for this positive employment outlook? As our population ages, people will be more likely to develop chronic or debilitating conditions that require therapeutic intervention. Baby boomers are reaching the age where cardiac issues are more common and will require cardiac and physical rehabilitation services. With medical and technological advances, veterans returning from combat missions and other victims of trauma are surviving catastrophic wounds. They too will need ongoing physical and psychosocial therapeutic intervention. People now surviving illnesses that a generation ago may have been fatal will need therapy services. The obesity crisis is necessitating an increase in service provision for all aspects of health and wellness services implemented by OT practitioners. A rising number of students with special needs are reaching school age and, as mandated by federal law, must be provided

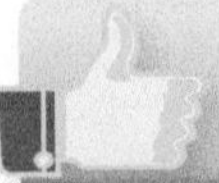

FROM THE FIELD 2.4

Educational Laddering

For those OTAs choosing to advance to OT status, there are many educational opportunities available via a process called educational laddering. This process involves transferring OTA courses to an entry-level Master's program. *Does your program offer this educational laddering opportunity? Are there any programs close to where you live that offer educational laddering?*

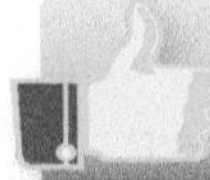

FROM THE FIELD 2.5

Local Connections

As compared to occupational therapy programs, OTA programs in particular tend to be focused on meeting the needs of a diverse group of students in their local communities. It is common for graduates of OTA programs to remain in the community where they studied to practice (Blum et al., 2008), thus strengthening local connections by having the opportunity to give back to the community. *How does this resonate with you?*

Occupational Title	SOC Code	Employment 2008	Employment 2010	Projected Employment 2018	Projected Employment 2020	Change 2008–2018	Change 2010–2020
Occupational therapy assistants	31-2001	26,600	28,500	34,600	40,800	7,900 more employed - 30% increase	12,300 more employed - 43.3% increase

Figure 2.1 Projections data from the National Employment Matrix.

a free and appropriate education in the least restrictive environment possible. This is leading to an increased need for school-based pediatric practitioners. The professional services that OTAs can provide will be in high demand in all practice areas for the foreseeable future.

There is more. Demand for therapy services may be dampened by federal legislation. From a practical and economic perspective, OTAs will be in greater demand to reduce the rising cost of occupational therapy services and to keep client costs within the federal caps on reimbursement for therapy services (Bureau of Labor Statistics, 2012). Based on the scope of practice that an OTA is qualified to implement under the supervision of an OT, addressing these issues will entail OTAs undertaking greater treatment responsibilities to help curb health care costs and make service delivery more affordable and accessible for all who require it (Yamkovenko, 2009).

Summary

The OTA designation has experienced significant challenges throughout its history. What remains indisputable is the fact that OTAs are a vital and integral part of the occupational therapy profession and, with each passing year, become more and more important for the viability of the profession. To keep occupational therapy services affordable and accessible for all who need it, the AOTA views OTAs as "collaborative partners" and integral to achieving its *Centennial Vision* (Yamkovenko, 2009, p. 17). Further, collaborating with other OT practitioners helps to ensure the scientific integrity of the profession and encourage evidence-based practice in new and traditional practice venues (Blum et al., 2008). In order to achieve the *Centennial Vision*, it is incumbent upon the profession to "ensure a workforce for multiple roles" (AOTA, 2007, p. 613). How will you meet this challenge? Remember, OTAs are important participants in education, the delivery of services, and AOTA (Yamkovenko, 2009). The future truly looks golden.

Review Questions

1. Typically an OTA does not
   a. Evaluate
   b. Treat
   c. Plan activities
   d. Adapt equipment

2. The most typical practice venues for an OTA are
   a. Work hardening centers
   b. Schools
   c. Nursing facilities
   d. B and C

3. The OTA role was established in
   a. 1917 with credentialing in 1963
   b. 1922 with credentialing in 1965
   c. 1949 with credentialing in 1965
   d. 1949 and credentialing in 1949

4. What is the main reason that the OTA role was established?
   a. Shortage of OTs practicing in pediatric settings
   b. Shortage of OTs practicing in physical rehabilitation settings
   c. Shortage of OTs practicing in psychiatric settings
   d. Shortage of OTs practicing in nursing facilities

5. The first college-level training programs for OTAs were housed at
   a. Mount Aloysius College in Pennsylvania and St. Mary's Junior College in Minnesota
   b. Mt. Ida College in Massachusetts and Western Michigan University in Michigan
   c. Tufts University in Massachusetts and Arizona State University in Arizona
   d. Lasell College in Massachusetts and St. Mary's Junior College in Minnesota

6. What was the now defunct Career Mobility Program?
   a. A means for OTAs to become members of AOTA
   b. A means to provide OTAs having at least two years of experience the opportunity to take the OT certification exam
   c. A means for OTAs to be eligible for supervisory roles
   d. A means for OTAs to serve on AOTA committees

7. The first certification exam for OTAs was established in
   a. 1999
   b. 1965
   c. 1978
   d. 1959

8. When were OTAs awarded full membership rights in AOTA?
   a. 1991
   b. 1976
   c. 1965
   d. 1959

9. Which one of the following is not an AOTA award bestowed upon an OTA?
   a. Roster of Honor
   b. Roster of Fellows
   c. Terry Brittell Award

10. Why is the role of the OTA more important than ever?
    a. Rising costs of health care
    b. Aging population
    c. Federal laws mandating services for children with special needs
    d. All of the above

Practice Activities

Make a flow chart that outlines your experiences, both personal and professional that led you to select becoming an OTA as a career path. Compare your responses with your classmates.

Make a timeline of the evolution of the OTA profession. Tie each landmark with a pertinent domestic or international historical event. What parallels can you find? Can you project into the future? What do you foresee in the ongoing re-evolution of the OTA?

Prepare a one-page flyer about what you view as the most important reasons why an OTA is an integral member of the health care team. During National Occupational Therapy month (April), make copies of this flyer and distribute it to students, faculty, and administrators at your school.

Prepare a bulletin board in your department (or, with permission, in the student union or library) that tells others about what an OTA is and does.

References

American Occupational Therapy Association. The recognition of occupational therapy assistants. *Am J Occup Ther* 1958;12:269–275.

American Occupational Therapy Association. Essentials on an approved educational program for the occupational therapy assistant. *Am J Occup Ther* 1976;30:245–263.

American Occupational Therapy Association. Standards for an accredited educational program for the occupational therapy Assistant. *Am J Occup Ther* 1999;53:583–589.

American Occupational Therapy Association. AOTA's centennial vision and executive summary. *Am J Occup Ther* 2007;61:613–614.

American Occupational Therapy Association. Guidelines for supervision, roles, and responsibilities during the delivery of occupational therapy services. *Am J Occup Ther* 2009a;63:797–803.

American Occupational Therapy Association. *History of AOTA Accreditation*. 2009b(August). Retrieved from http://www.aota.org/Educate/Accredit/Overview/38124.aspx

American Occupational Therapy Association. *Frequently asked questions about ethics*. 2010a. Retrieved from http://www.aota.org/Practitioners/Ethics/FAQs.aspx

American Occupational Therapy Association. Scope of practice. *Am J Occup Ther* 2010b;64(Suppl):S70–S77.

American Occupational Therapy Association. Standards of practice for occupational therapy. *Am J Occup Ther* 2010c;64:S106–S111.

American Occupational Therapy Association. *Occupational Therapy Code of Ethics and Ethics Standards*. Rockville, MD: American Occupational Therapy Association; 2010d.

American Occupational Therapy Association. *The Glossary of the American Occupational Therapy Association 2014*. Rockville, MD: American Occupational Therapy Association; 2014.

American Occupational Therapy Association. *2011 Accreditation Council for Occupational Therapy Education (ACOTE®) Standards and Interpretive Guide*. 2012a. Retrieved from http://aota.org/Educate/Accredit/Draft-Standards/50146.aspx?FT=.pdf

American Occupational Therapy Association. *AOTA Preconference Institute 2012*. Indianapolis, IN: American Occupational Therapy Association; 2012b.

American Occupational Therapy Association. Accreditation. 2014a. Retrieved from http://www.aota.org/education-careers/accreditation.aspx

American Occupational Therapy Association. *Educational programs for OTAs seeking OT degrees*. 2014b. Retrieved from http://www.aota.org/Education-Careers/Find-School/Bridge-Weekend/OTAs-Seeking-OT.aspx

American Occupational Therapy Association. *Find a school*. 2014c. Retrieved from http://www.aota.org/en/Education-Careers/Find-School.aspx

American Occupational Therapy Association. *Frequently asked questions about occupational therapy education*. n.d.a. Retrieved from http://www.aota.org/Educate/EdRes/StuRecruit/Education/38383.aspx?FT=.pdf

American Occupational Therapy Association. *About occupational therapy: the profession of occupational therapy*. n.d.b. Retrieved from http://www.aota.org/About/AboutOT.aspx

Black TL, Eberhardt KM. *The Occupational Therapy Assistant: Resources for Practice & Education*. Bethesda, MD: AOTA Press; 2005.

Blum JC, et al. The importance of occupational therapy assistant education to the profession. *Am J Occup Ther* 2008;62(6):705–706.

Bureau of Labor Statistics. *Occupational outlook handbook, 2010–11 edition*. 2012. Retrieved from http://www.bls.gov/oco/ocos166.htm

Cottrell RPF. COTA education and professional development: a historical review. *Am J Occup Ther* 2000a;54:407–412.

Cottrell RPF. COTA to OTR: factors influencing professional development. *Am J Occup Ther* 2000b;54:413–420.

O'Brien JC, Hussey SM. *Introduction to Occupational Therapy*. 4th ed. St. Louis, MO: Mosby Elsevier; 2012.

Salvatori P. The history of occupational therapy assistants in Canada: a comparison with the United States. *Can J Occup Ther* 2001(Oct);68(4):217–227.

Strezlecki MV. OTA program clarification. *OT Practice* 2009;14(7):5.

Wagenfeld AE, Hsi JD. Credentialing, ethics, and legalities of practice. In: Solomon A, Jacobs K, eds. *Management Skills for the OTA*. pp. 39–58. Thorofare, NJ: Slack, Inc; 2003.

Yamkovenko S. Celebrating 50 years of OTA education and practice. *OT Practice* 2009 (Feb 2);14(2):16–17.

CHAPTER 3

The Philosophical Basis of Core Values

Amy Wagenfeld, PhD, OTR/L SCEM, CAPs

Key Terms

Axiology—A philosophy that is concerned with the study of values and aesthetics.

Core values (document)—An official AOTA document originally published in 1993 whose purpose is to express the values and attitudes that are foundational to occupational therapy.

Dualism—Idea that the mind and body are separate parts or entities.

Epistemology—A philosophy that examines the nature, origin, and limits of human knowledge.

Holism—Idea that the mind and body are a single integrated system.

Humanism—In clinical work represents that clients should be treated as a person and not an object, and people are capable of change.

Metaphysical—Philosophy concerned with the mind–body relationship and whether there is a dualistic or holistic connection between the two.

Organismic—Philosophical perspective that recognizes that a person's behaviors influence the physical and social environment and, in turn, a person is impacted by changes in the environment.

Philosophy—The study of why people think and act the way that they do.

Personal philosophy—A way of life that sets the course for all thoughts and actions.

Professional philosophy—A collection of beliefs, attitudes, and thoughts that frames the way one engages in his or her work.

Values—Ideas and beliefs that an individual determines to be important.

Learning Objectives

After studying this chapter, readers should be able to

- Summarize how philosophy shapes the profession and practice of occupational therapy.
- State the importance of upholding the core values of occupational therapy in professional as well as personal conduct.
- Explain how the different branches of philosophy influence occupational therapy.
- Articulate the importance of always using person-first language.

Introduction

The philosophical base of a profession represents its core beliefs, values, ethics, and principles. This chapter explores occupational therapy's professional philosophy, core values, and your role as an ambassador to ensure that occupational therapy's highest standards are adhered to and respected, at all times.

Philosophy

It is not unreasonable to be asking yourself, what does philosophy have to do with occupational therapy and why is it being discussed in this chapter on core values? The answers to these questions should become clear as you read this chapter, but first, a basic definition. **Philosophy** refers to the study of why people think and act the way that they do. Over time, and with experience and self-reflection shaping the meaning of self and one's position in the world, each of us develops a **personal philosophy**, a way of life that sets our course for thought and action. A **professional philosophy** builds on a personal philosophy and is a collection of beliefs, attitudes, and thoughts that frames the way someone engages in his or her work. Personal and professional philosophies change with time and experience. So too do the philosophies of organizations such as occupational therapy. Our philosophies guide us to recognize the worth and value of our therapeutic goals, objectives, and interventions. From a larger-scale professional (occupational therapy) philosophical perspective, these same beliefs, attitudes, and thoughts help to provide reason for the grand design or overarching purpose of the profession. While fundamentally occupational therapy remains rooted in its original philosophy, values, and ethics systems, because times change, so too must an organization address change. To remain relevant, while maintaining true to its founding mission, our profession evaluates, responds to, and strives to consistently meet the needs of its consumers. Simply said, philosophical perspectives help to enable occupational therapy practitioners to take action and justify the reason for doing so, and on a larger scale, for the profession to evaluate and respond to change.

There are three overarching branches of philosophy that influence the foundations and practice of occupational therapy. These three branches are epistemology, axiology, and metaphysical philosophy. In discussing these philosophical perspectives, we will also explore how the concepts of **dualism** and **holism** influence epistemological and metaphysical philosophy. A dualistic perspective sees the mind and body as separate parts or entities, while a holistic perspective sees the mind and body as a single integrated system. The trend in Western medicine has moved to a holistic one, which closely aligns with the profession's *Founding* and *Centennial Visions*, and is arguably the very essence of occupational therapy (From the Field 3.1).

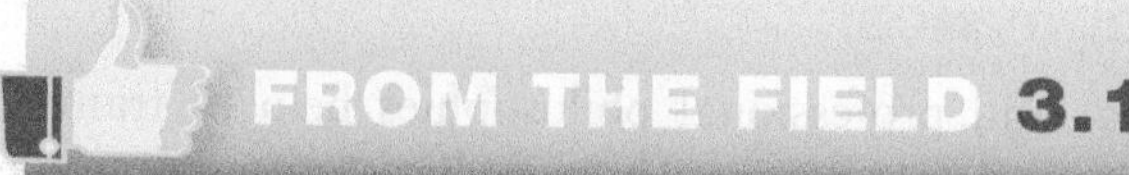

FROM THE FIELD 3.1

Person-First Language

Consider these two phrases.

"The blind person" and "Mrs. Smith, who is blind."

Which phrase more closely aligns with dualism and which with holism? Is one more deficit oriented than the other? Sensitivity to all people dictates that in written and verbal communication, we refer to the person first, rather than as a presenting disability. That is, we are people first and are not defined by our disability or challenges. To that end, "Mrs. Smith, who is blind" represents a human being who is above all a person first and who is not defined by visual challenges. Holism supports active, person-first verbal and written communication. In fact, it is incumbent upon OT practitioners, and for that matter everyone, to always use what is called person-first language. A very helpful electronic style guide on acceptable person-first language can be found at http://ncdj.org/style-guide/. It is well worth the time to download a copy of this guide for future use.

Epistemology

The component of philosophy that examines the nature, origin, and limits of human knowledge is called **epistemology**. Personal and professional philosophies are shaped by epistemological questions seeking to understand truth, namely "what is true?" We can know truth through experiences such as understanding that while a spring rain may feel refreshing on our skin, if left on long enough, wet clothing will be very uncomfortable and unwieldy. Our action plan or truth may be to choose to always carry an umbrella to avoid getting wet. In looking at epistemology from a dualistic perspective, you would attribute carrying an umbrella with you at all times to logical and rational thought; for example, the mind tells the body, "if I have an umbrella I will stay dry and not feel uncomfortable in wet clothing." A holist would arrive at the same conclusion but instead believe the mind and body are working as one to intuit that based on prior experiences of "having gotten caught in the rain without an umbrella before, having one available will keep me dry."

Axiology

The part of philosophy that is concerned with the study of values and aesthetics is called **axiology**. Aesthetics refers to an interpretation of what is beautiful or sought after, and values are the standards for determining right and wrong. As we will discuss in Chapter 12, *Ethics*, these axiological standards are the foundation of ethics, which strongly guide the occupational therapy profession.

Metaphysical

Personal and professional philosophies help to frame metaphysical questions such as "what is the meaning of life?" and "what is my purpose?" **Metaphysical** philosophy is particularly interested in the mind–body relationship and whether there is a dualistic or holistic connection between the two. A dualist will believe there is a difference between the mind and body, and a holist will say they are one in the same, working in sync with each other the mind influences the body and vice versa. For instance, a dualist may encourage a walk on the beach as a way to heal the body but does not recognize the influence of the mind on healing. On the other hand, a holistic may encourage that same walk, believing it will simultaneously and synergistically soothe the mind and strengthen the body (and soul).

Organismic and Humanistic

In addition to overarching epistemological, axiological, and metaphysical philosophies, there are also several other philosophical views that influence occupational therapy. An **organismic** perspective is one that recognizes that a person's behaviors influence the physical and social environment and in turn, a person is impacted by changes in the environment. As will be explored in Chapter 7, *Occupational Therapy Theories and How They Guide Practice*, organismic philosophy factors significantly into several occupational therapy theories. **Humanism**, one of the foundations of occupational therapy, represents that recipients of service should be treated as people and not objects. A humanistic philosophy is fluid and positively oriented in that it supports the idea that people are capable of change. Philosophies influence who we are and how we choose to behave in our personal and professional roles.

Adolf Meyer and the Philosophy of Occupational Therapy

Adolf Meyer (see Box 3.1), while not an official founding member of occupational therapy, made significant contributions to the philosophical foundation of our profession. Trained as a psychiatrist, Dr. Meyer firmly believed in and advocated for a philosophy of occupational therapy. In a seminal paper entitled *The Philosophy of Occupational Therapy* (1922) that he read at the Fifth Meeting of the National Society for the Promotion of Occupational Therapy (NSPOT) in October 1921, Dr. Meyer had a great deal to say about creation of a philosophy of occupational therapy. He believed that the concept of occupational therapy could better the lives of people with mental illness, saying, "The proper use of time in some helpful and gratifying activity [work] appeared to me a fundamental issue in the treatment of any neuropsychiatric patient" (Meyer, 1921, p. 1). Meyer noted,

> Groups of patients with raffia and basket work or with various kinds of hand work ... took the place of the bored wall flowers and of mischief makers. A pleasure in achievement, a real pleasure in the use and activity of one's hands and muscles, and a happy *appreciation of time* began to be used as incentives in the management of our patients.... The main advance of the new scheme was the blending of *work and pleasure* (emphasis added) (1922, p. 3).

Meyer spoke of this work as a compassionate substitute for physical restraint of patients with mental illness, a practice that was, if you recall from Chapter 1, *Historical Perspectives of Occupational Therapy*, commonplace prior to the moral treatment era. This conceptualization of linking activity to meaning, happiness, and fulfillment represented a milestone in the development of a philosophy of occupational therapy. Meaningful activity versus meaningless activity of ward patients was to be employed as a positive reinforcement and method for restoration.

In reading the words of Adolf Meyer, it is not hard to picture the scene at the NSPOT meeting as he presented his philosophy of occupational therapy paper, saying, "Somehow it represents to me a very important manifestation of a very general gain in human philosophy. There is in all this a development of *valuation of time and work* which is not accidental" (1922, p. 4). He went on to say,

> [man is] an organism that maintains and balances itself in the world of reality and actuality by being

BOX 3.1

Adolf Meyer: Psychiatrist and Philosopher

- Trained as a psychiatrist and though not a founder, was a major player in the development of occupational therapy and a philosophy of occupational therapy. Meyers' ideas helped to shape the professional paradigm (Kielhofner, 2009).
- Collaborated with Eleanor Clarke Slagle to develop occupational therapy services at the Henry Phipps Psychiatric Clinic in Baltimore, MD.
- Recognized a connection between the mind and body and how the environment influenced performance.
- Focused on what a patient could change—such as habits, problem solving, and negative patterns of thinking rather than on psychopathology.
- Felt that patients needed to engage in work that is meaningful to them.

in active life and active use, i.e., using and living and acting its *time* in harmony with its own nature and the nature about it. It is the use that we make of ourselves that gives the ultimate stamp to our every organ (1922, p. 5).

In essence, what is meaningful is maintaining balance through engagement in activity. In looking forward, Meyer suggested that a philosophy of occupational therapy and the implementation of meaningful work to people with mental illness would potentially,

shape for ourselves and for our patients an outlook of sound idealism, furnishing a setting in which many otherwise apparently insurmountable difficulties will be conquered and in which our new generations will find a world full of ever new opportunity and achievement in healthy harmony with human nature (1922, p. 10).

And so began the occupational therapy philosophy that to this day continues to shape the way we think about and act as occupational therapy practitioners.

Core Values

There is a strong interconnection between philosophy and values, and to say that one precedes or trumps, the other is inaccurate. **Values** are ideas and beliefs that an individual determines to be important. "Values are not rules of conduct but concepts that group together certain modes of behavior ...provide unity and become the unifying force in our philosophy" (Gilfoyle, 1984, p. 578).

TABLE 3.1 AOTA's Code of Ethics Standards and Accompanying Core Values

Core Value	Definition	Practical Example
Altruism	An individual's ability to place the needs of others before his or her own.	Participating in an occupational therapy service mission trip to create adaptive equipment for people who are underserved.
Equality	The desire to promote fairness in interactions with others.	Mr. Jones who is homosexual is provided the same level of care as Mr. Smith, who is heterosexual.
Freedom (personal choice)	Desires of the client must guide our interventions.	When working on dressing skills, allowing young Clara to select the clothes she wants to wear, even if they clash.
Justice	Occupational therapy practitioners, educators, and researchers relate in a fair and impartial manner to individuals with whom they interact and respect and adhere to the applicable laws and standards regarding their area of practice, be it direct care, education, or research.	Bob, an OTA acts within the scope of his practice and does not conduct standardized home evaluations.
Dignity	The promotion and preservation of the individuality of the client; assisting him or her to engage in occupations that are meaningful to him or her regardless of level of disability.	Mr. Johnson recently had a stroke and has limited use of his right hand. He wants to go back to his hobby of painting. The OT practitioner develops an intervention plan focusing on helping Mr. Johnson relearn how to paint.
Truth	Provision of accurate information, both in oral and written form.	Corey accurately documents his client's progress (or lack of).
Prudence	Use of clinical and ethical reasoning skills, sound judgment, and reflection to make decisions to direct practitioners in their area(s) of practice.	Julie is concerned that a child she is working with may have been abused. She immediately discusses her concerns with her supervisor and together they decide it is necessary to report their concern to the appropriate authorities and do so.

Adapted from American Occupational Therapy Association. Core values and attitudes of occupational therapy practice. *Am J Occup Ther* (1993);47:1085–1086; Peloquin SM. A reconsideration of occupational therapy's core values. *Am J Occup Ther* 2007;61(4):474–478.

A few examples of values are the concepts of loyalty, honesty, and responsibility.

Each of us has a set of implicit or explicit personal values to which we hold true and aspire to maintain. Personal values are serve as an internal barometer to determine what is right, wrong, important, and beneficial, to name a few. Ultimately, personal values can influence societal customs and rules. An organization may also have a set of explicitly stated values for its members to uphold, which is the case for occupational therapy is "key to professionalism" (Gilfoyle, 1984, p. 579). Consider what Eleanor Gilfoyle (1984) said about values,

> Our values come from our experiences, from testing what does and does not work; values are modified through the development of our profession and the environment and culture of our time. As occupational therapists, we cannot maintain our professional integrity if we let others direct our values (p. 579).

There are seven core values that define the "attitudes and values that undergird the profession of occupational therapy" (Kanney, 1993, p. 1085) and comprised the first occupational therapy **core values** document. The original document was written by Elizabeth Kanney for the Commission of Standards and Ethics (SEC). Approved by the American Occupational Therapy Association (AOTA) Representative Assembly (RA) in 1993, the core values document was then published in the *American Journal of Occupational Therapy (AJOT)*. The core values document reflected existing precedents in AOTA documents including:

- *Dictionary Definition of Occupational Therapy*; *The Philosophical Base of Occupational Therapy*;
- *Essentials and Guidelines for an Accredited Educational Program for the Occupational Therapist*;
- *Essentials and Guidelines for an Accredited Educational Program for the Occupational Therapy Assistant*;
- *Occupational Therapy Code of Ethics* (Peloquin, 2007, p. 474).

The original core values document is now incorporated into *Occupational Therapy Code of Ethics and Ethics Standards* (AOTA, 2015), which will be explored in Chapter 12, *Ethics* (Table 3.1) (From the Field 3.2).

The seven core values provide a foundation by which occupational therapy personnel guide their interactions with others, be they students, recipients of service, colleagues, research participants, or communities. These values also define the ethical principles to which the profession is committed and which the public can expect from its members (AOTA, 2015). Further, the original seven core values (below) are commitments that every OT practitioner aspires to uphold. Profound in their scope and meaning, they guide and inspire us to maintain the highest standards of practice. The seven core values are as follows:

- A commitment to altruism is manifest in caring, dedication, responsiveness, and understanding.
- A commitment to equality is conveyed through fairness and impartiality.
- A commitment to freedom leads to the enabling of choice, independence, initiative, and self-direction.
- A commitment to justice shapes the exercise of fairness, equity, truthfulness, and objectivity.
- A commitment to personal dignity is expressed through honoring the worth and uniqueness of each person, through empathy, and through respect for self and others.
- A commitment to truth is reflected in fidelity to facts and reality, in accountability and forthrightness, and in honesty and authenticity.
- The commitment to prudence is manifest through governing and disciplining the self with reason as well as with judiciousness, discretion, moderation, care, and circumspection (AOTA, 1993; Peloquin, 2007, p. 475).

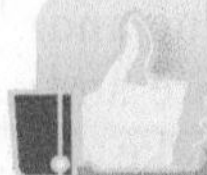

FROM THE FIELD 3.2

Values and Change

Eleanor Gilfoyle suggested that in times of organizational transitions, value systems would undoubtedly change (1984). She was emphatic in stating that external pressures not be the directional change within occupational therapy, but rather, "[we] *should change because* we *continue* to *seek the truth of our values*" (Gilfoyle, 1984, p. 579). While this directional change was in reference to large-scale philosophical and organizational change within the profession, how can this mode of thinking apply to YOU as an emerging practitioner? Consider this with regard to when you may be faced with changing roles or when you may find yourself pressured to make changes in an existing role that challenge your personal and professional values systems. *How might you respond?*

Continuing Competence

According to the AOTA (2010), the standards for continuing competence is an evolving process that tasks the OT practitioner to realistically reflect on competency and the capacity for maintaining or bettering this competency

TABLE 3.2 Standards of Continuing Competence in Occupational Therapy

Standard	Definition
Standard 1. Knowledge	Occupational therapists and occupational therapy assistants shall demonstrate understanding and comprehension of the information required for the multiple roles and responsibilities they assume.
Standard 2. Critical Reasoning	Occupational therapists and occupational therapy assistants shall use reasoning processes to make sound judgments and decisions.
Standard 3. Interpersonal Skills	Occupational therapists and occupational therapy assistants shall develop and maintain their professional relationships with others within the context of their roles and responsibilities.
Standard 4. Performance Skills	Occupational therapists and occupational therapy assistants shall demonstrate the expertise, aptitudes, proficiencies, and abilities to competently fulfill their roles and responsibilities.
Standard 5. Ethical Practice	Occupational therapists and occupational therapy assistants shall identify, analyze, and clarify ethical issues or dilemmas to make responsible decisions within the changing context of their roles and responsibilities (AOTA, 2010, p. S103–S104).

(AOTA, 2010)

going forward into the future. Continuing competence is built on a foundation of core values in that without core values, an OT practitioner is at odds to reflect on professional betterment. Continuing competency factors into "professional development and lifelong learning… [and is] a dynamic and multidimensional process in which the occupational therapist and occupational therapy assistant develop and maintain the knowledge, performance skills, interpersonal abilities, critical reasoning, and ethical reasoning skills necessary to perform current and future roles and responsibilities within the profession" (AOTA, 2010, p. S103).

The five identified standards of continuing competence for occupational therapy practitioners are knowledge, critical reasoning, interpersonal skills, performance skills, and ethical practice (AOTA, 2010). They are described briefly in Table 3.2. The full white paper is available at www.aota.org.

Our professional culture and philosophy is reflective of the fundamental concepts and beliefs associated with the therapeutic value of occupation (Gilfoyle, 1984). "Our value system emerges from our rational knowledge of occupation and our intuitive knowledge of the purposefulness of the occupational process. Values underlie our culture and form the heart of our profession" (Gilfoyle, 1984, pp. 576–577). Values are also at the center of occupational therapy's philosophy in that they guide our actions and set us apart from other health care professions (Gilfoyle, 1984). Occupational therapy's values allow us, as practitioners, to believe that through engagement in occupation, people have the capacity to change (Gilfoyle, 1984).

Summary

We are judged individually and as a profession by outcomes and behaviors (Gilfoyle, 1984), making it imperative that your professional practice reflects the core values and philosophy of occupational therapy. Committing to a lifelong process in which core values and ethical practice guide every element of your work is a commendable way to practice as an OTA.

Review Questions

1. Why are personal and professional philosophies important for all people and organizations?
   a. To enable practitioners to take action and justify the reason for doing so and on a larger scale, for the profession to evaluate and respond to change
   b. To evaluate methods of information dissemination
   c. To stay rooted in the past
   d. To avoid conflict

2. Epistemology is a philosophical orientation that focuses on:
   a. Study of values and aesthetics
   b. Dualism
   c. Making sense of what is true
   d. Seeking to understand the meaning of life

3. Humanism is a philosophical view that:
   a. Recognizes that a person's behaviors influence the physical and social environment and, in turn, a person is impacted by changes in the environment
   b. Is fluid and positively oriented in that it supports the idea that people are capable of change
   c. Addresses the basic function of human existence
   d. Posits that people are not capable of change

4. Axiology is a philosophical orientation that focuses on:
   a. Study of values and aesthetics
   b. Dualism
   c. Making sense of what is true
   d. Seeking to understand the meaning of life

5. An organismic philosophy:
   a. Recognizes that a person's behaviors influence the physical and social environment and in turn, a person is impacted by changes in the environment
   b. Is fluid and positively oriented in that it supports the idea that people are capable of change
   c. Addresses the basic function of human existence
   d. Posits that people are not capable of change

6. A dualistic philosophy views the mind and body as:
   a. A single integrated system
   b. Separate parts or entities
   c. Both integrated and separate dependent on the situation
   d. Not under conscious control

7. Metaphysical is a philosophical orientation that focuses on:
   a. Study of values and aesthetics
   b. Dualism
   c. Making sense of what is true
   d. Seeking to understand the meaning of life

8. What is the express purpose of the AOTA *Core Values*?
   a. Guide practice
   b. Define ethical principles
   c. Aspirational document to uphold a commitment to excellence in practice
   d. All of the above

9. Values are:
   a. Rules of conduct
   b. Legal tenets
   c. Ideas and beliefs one feels to be important
   d. Determined solely by society

10. Examples of values are:
    a. Dishonesty
    b. Responsibility
    c. Empathy
    d. Loyalty
    e. b, c, and d

Practice Activities

In his philosophy of occupational therapy, Adolf Meyer said, "The most important factor in [patient] progress lay *undoubtedly* in the newer conceptions of *mental problems as problems of living* and not merely diseases of a structural and toxic nature…or of a final lasting constitutional disorder on the other. The formulation in terms of habit deterioration of even those grave mental disorders presenting the serious problem of *terminal dementia* made systematic engagement of interest, and concern about the actual use of TIME and work an obligation and necessity" (1921, p. 4). What major branch(es) of philosophy best align(s) with these statements? It is dualistic or holistic? Prepare a one to two paragraph position paper that explains your thoughts.

List 10 personal values that hold true for you. Using pictures cut out from magazines, make a collage that reflects these 10 personal values. How many of the 10 align with the AOTA core values document?

Choose one of the AOTA core values listed in Table 3.1, and apply it to something you do in your daily life. Play a class-wide "Pictionary" type game in which you begin to illustrate your value (and the activity that exemplifies it) bit by bit until someone guesses what your value and activity is.

References

American Occupational Therapy Association. Core values and attitudes of occupational therapy practice. *Am J Occup Ther* (1993);47:1085–1086.

American Occupational Therapy Association. Standards for continuing competence. *Am J Occup Ther* (2010);64(Suppl):S103–S105. doi: 10.5014/ajot.2010.64S103-64S105.

Gilfoyle EM. Eleanor Clarke Slagle Lecture. Transformation of a profession. *Am J Occup Ther* 1984;38:575–584.

Kanney E. Core values and attitudes of occupational therapy practice. *Am J Occup Ther* 1993;47(12):1085–1086.

Kielhofner DO. *Conceptual Foundations of Occupational Therapy Practice*. Philadelphia, PA: F.A. Davis Company, 2009.

Meyer A. The philosophy of occupational therapy. *Arch Occup Ther* 1921;1(1):1–10.

Occupational therapy code of ethics and ethics standards. *Am J Occup Ther* 2015.

Peloquin SM. A reconsideration of occupational therapy's core values. *Am J Occup Ther* 2007;61(4):474–478.

Website of Interest

Style Guide for acceptable person-first language: http://ncdj.org/style-guide/.

CHAPTER 4

Occupations: The Cornerstone of the Profession

Amy Wagenfeld, PhD, OTR/L SCEM, CAPs

Key Terms

Activities of daily living—Self-care activities such as bathing, dressing, and toileting.

Flow—A mental process in which a person is fully immersed, absorbed, present, and focused on a task (Csikszentmihalyi, 1997).

Just Right challenge—The balance between the challenge of the activity and the skills of the person.

Meaningful—Making sense of what is being done in an occupation.

Occupation—The therapeutic application of everyday activities to improve participation in and quality of life (AOTA, 2004).

Occupation as ends—Situations when the end goal to be achieved is the occupation itself.

Occupation as means—Simple and repetitive purposeful behaviors.

Occupational adaptation—A lifelong transformation process that suggests that what we have done influences what we are to become (Nelson, 1997, pp. 535–536).

Occupational choice—The conscious decision to engage in an occupation (Kielhofner, 1992, 2009).

Occupational deprivation—Lack of participation in occupation due to factors including injury, disability, prejudice, poverty, and employment.

Occupational form—The contextual information or meaning system of occupation (Nelson, 1997).

Occupational justice—The component of occupational participation that meets individual needs and embraces social equity (Christiansen & Townsend, 2004).

Occupational participation—Engagement in work, leisure, self-care, or sleep (Christiansen & Baum, 2005, pp. 41-42).

Occupational performance and function—The doing component of occupation (Nelson, 1997).

Occupational science—The formal study of occupation.

Participation—Taking part in or involvement in life situations and activity, the act of doing a task (WHO, 2002).

Purposeful—The intention part of an occupation.

Sense of coherence—An overarching and fluid representation of confidence.

Learning Objectives

After reviewing this chapter, readers should be able to:

- Explain the concept of occupation and its application to occupational therapy practice.
- Differentiate between occupation and activity.
- Compare and contrast the dimensions of occupation and how they influence engagement in occupation.
- Apply the concepts of meaningful and purposeful when considering occupation for client treatment.
- Explain how the concepts of sense of coherence and just right challenge relate to each other.

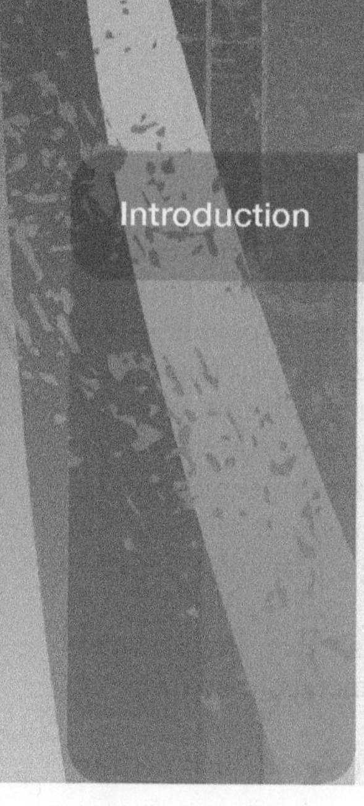

Introduction

Does it surprise you that many OT practitioners find it challenging to articulate who they are as professionals and how to explain what occupational therapy is to others outside the profession? Further, do you wonder what OT practitioners do that sets us apart from other allied health care professionals? These issues and more will be explored in this chapter, which centers on the cornerstone of our profession: occupation.

One of the most important action items you can charge yourself with doing is to develop a short and concise 30-second summary to share with others that clearly articulates what an OTA does and what exactly occupational therapy is from a historic and contemporary perspective. If you are well versed in understanding the profession's rich history, it may make you more confident about your skills and optimistic about your future as an OTA (Friedland & Silva, 2008) and better help you understand the profession's forward-looking vision.

History of Occupations

During the preoccupational therapy era, physicians recognized that a healthier lifestyle was directly connected to doing activities that were meaningful and purposeful (McColl et al., 2003). With this understanding, it was common for physicians to prescribe a balance of daily activities including meaningful work endeavors for people with mental illnesses. Supervising this new regimen was a new kind of health care professional, the occupational therapist (McColl et al., 2003). Accordingly, the term **occupation** was widely used by our profession's founders. For instance, Dunton (1919, p. 10) wrote that "occupation is as necessary to life as food and drink. ... Sick minds, sick bodies, sick souls may be healed through occupation" (Dunton, 1919, p. 10, in Bauerschmidt & Nelson, 2011). Other important figures in early occupational therapy such as Eleanor Slagle and Adolf Meyer wrote with energy and passion about the worth and value of occupation as a therapeutic tool (Bauerschmidt & Nelson, 2011). As stated in the *Articles of Incorporation of the National Society for the Promotion of Occupational Therapy* (NSPOT, 1917), the reason for this new profession was "the advancement of occupation as a therapeutic measure" (p. 1). As far back as the 1920s, the earliest occupational therapy literature sought to explore and quantify the idea of occupation as a treatment and how best to address specific patient problems using such treatment. Early on, it was suggested that to be motivating and of interest, occupation would be most therapeutic if it was designed to meet each patient's needs (McColl et al., 2003). In addition, occupation as a way to address psychological or physical issues, and looking at meaningful occupation as the conduit to providing patients with productive skills to use in preparing to return to work was also explored (McColl et al., 2003).

Three paradigms or models can be ascribed to the history of occupational therapy (Kielhofner, 2009):

- Paradigm of occupation
- Mechanistic paradigm
- Contemporary paradigm

The Paradigm of Occupation

The paradigm of occupation began in the 1940s with the rise of the scientific model in modern medicine. It led the profession to a point of philosophical and practical crisis (Kielhofner, 2009): stay with using crafts-based occupations or to explore a scientific approach to treat patients.

Mechanistic Paradigm

The outcome of the paradigm of occupation led to the mechanistic paradigm (Kielhofner, 2009). No longer only occupations based, therapeutic intervention now relied on understanding a patient's underlying biological, psychological, and physiological "inner mechanisms" or dysfunction (Kielhofner, 2009; Kielhofner & Burke, 2005). Instead of weaving or other crafts or gardening occupations, rehabilitation became more scientifically focused and relied on the use of machines and exercise. As applied to the practice of occupational therapy, inner mechanisms translated into addressing "dysfunction of treatment of components underlying occupation," which is a reductionist (vs. holistic) framework (Gray, 1998, p. 355) that put occupation more or less "on the shelf."

As with most paradigm shifts, there were benefits and detriments associated with transition to inner mechanisms. Kielhofner and Burke suggested that one benefit of shifting to inner mechanisms was the foray into a budding scientific foundation for practice (an early form of evidence gathering), but one detrimental aspect was leading the profession to a shift away from employing occupation as the central tenant of our theory and practice (in Gray, 1998, p. 355). What would prevail, a more global and holistic approach to using occupations as intervention or turning to a more scientific exercise-based approach for treatment?

Contemporary Paradigm

By the 1970s, the mechanistic paradigm was deemed ineffective and not true to the roots of occupational therapy. Yet another crisis ensued, leading to the contemporary paradigm that once again is embracing the worth and value of occupation as therapy (Kielhofner, 2009). Many well-respected contemporary OTs have clearly articulated this need for the profession to return to grounding in occupation and engagement in a purposeful activity as a means to maintain professional autonomy. It was suggested that failure to do so will only continue to fragment the profession (Fidler, 1981) and reduce professional credibility. As you will read, evidence supports the importance of engagement with a **meaningful** (CS7, CS8, CS11, CS13) and **purposeful** (CS2, CS11) task-oriented (CS5) occupational focus as a means to experience positive health outcomes. Working with clients to help them achieve what they want and need to do through the use of therapeutic occupations is what the profession began as and, once again, is revisiting.

Despite the impressive heritage that the founder's provided, they "neglect[ed] to make explicit the foundational concepts of the profession [which] created problems in understanding" and identity for future OT practitioners (Breines, 1990, p. 45): an issue that OT practitioners continue to grapple with, although to a far lesser degree than even a decade ago. Why is this? As we will explore in Chapter 5, *Evidence-Based Research Methods: Guiding the Practice*, establishment of an **occupational science**, the formal study of occupation and evidence-based practice that quantifies the worth and value of occupational therapy have propelled our profession to the forefront of the health care professions. Validating the worth of the profession rests on combining the heart of occupational therapy with research to support it. In other words, taking the best of the paradigm of occupation and the mechanistic paradigm is the foundation of the contemporary paradigm.

What Are Occupations?

According to the philosopher, Jean-Paul Sartre, doing, being, and having things are the fundamental components of human life (Sartre, 1943/1993). Occupation is a fundamental component of life. Occupations can be thought of as the therapeutic application of everyday activities to improve participation in and quality of all aspects of life such as at home, in the workplace, in school, and in the community (AOTA, 2004). They are a driving force in providing meaning to people's lives (CAOT, 2002; Hammell, 2004, p. 296). You might also like to think of occupations as mental and physical processes rather than products (Royeen, 2003, p. 610). Daily occupations define who we are as people, give us purpose, help us to structure our lives, and are "key not just to being a person, but to being a particular person" (Christiansen, 1999, p. 576).

Occupations have "dimensions" that involve performance, form, function, and choice (Christiansen & Baum, 2005).

Several dimensions of occupations are illustrated in Figure 4.1.

Nelson (1997) defined occupation as "the relationship between an occupational form and occupational performance." **Occupational form** is the "thing, or the format, that is done" (p. 533). It is the objective part of an occupation. **Occupational performance** is the actual doing. Think about stirring batter to make brownies. The occupational form includes all the movements of the hand and arm required to grasp the spoon and stir the batter and the sensory, perceptual, and cognitive skills, as well as the set up needed to move the process along. Occupational performance is the actual stirring; can the client hold the spoon without assistance, see the batter, focus, and keep the batter in the bowl? Occupational performance is influenced by occupational form. We can see and observe form and performance. There is yet another side of occupation that is subjective: meaning and purpose. Nelson (1997) described meaning as "the person's active interpretation of the occupational form" (making sense of what is done), and once meaning is found, purpose can follow, which is "the person's goal orientation... what the person wants or intends" (p. 534). If a client is uninterested in making brownies, has no one to share them with, or for dietary reasons is unable to eat them, there will likely be little or no personal meaning, purpose, or attachment associated with this task. Experiencing occupation is a dualistic process in that the internal self is influenced by external mechanisms (Kuo, 2011). Who we are is, in part, shaped by what we do. Occupations provide the experiences that enable people to become who they are and to find meaning in their lives (Christiansen, 1999). "People can change or transform themselves [and influence the quality of their lives] through a [life-long process called] **occupational adaptation**," or in Nelson's words, "as we do [or experience], so we become" (Nelson, 1997, pp. 535–536). People participate in occupations based on what they need, believe in and care about, and can do (Hockey & Wright-St. Claire, 2011).

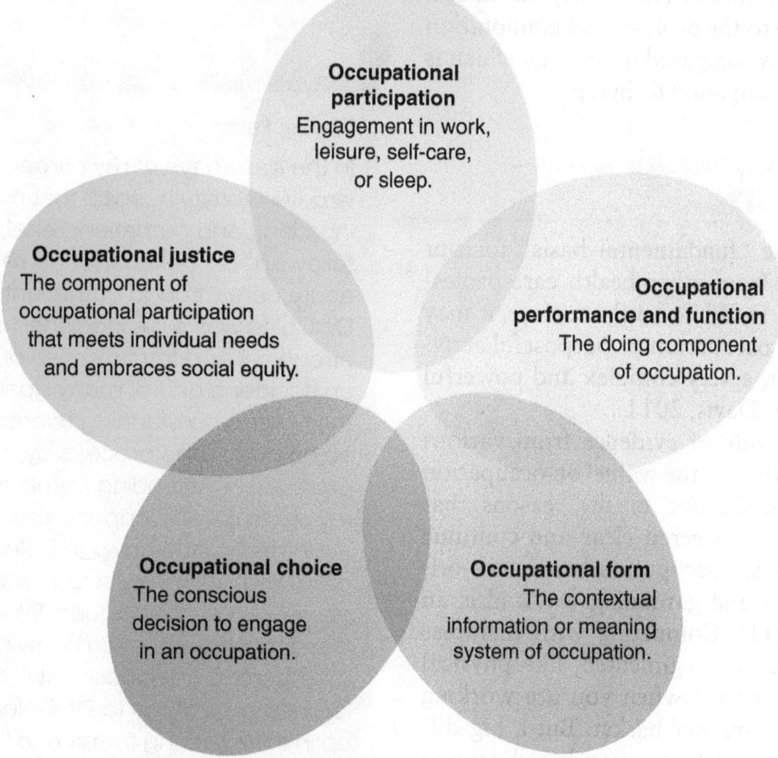

Figure 4.1 Dimensions of occupations.

While there are many definitions of occupation, the consistent characteristics are that they are and can be the following (CAOT, 2007; Christiansen & Baum 2005, p. 5):

- Human pursuits
- Directed and purposeful
- Performed in situations or contexts that influence how and with whom they are done
- Identified by the doer and others
- Give meaning to life
- An important determinant of health and well-being
- Organize behavior
- Develop and change over a lifetime
- Shape and is shaped by environments
- Have therapeutic effectiveness

Experiences are an important part of occupations of daily living (Kuo, 2011). Experiences help to organize a person's occupations and ebb and flow through time based and spatial contexts (Kuo, 2011). With respect for temporal considerations, "Occupational therapy, at its best, focuses on occupations important to each person within his or her environment" (Law, 2002, p. 646). A single occupational process evolves over time, is interrelated to other occupational processes, and almost never occurs in isolation, but is rather an interrelated processes occurring at the same, different, or overlapping times. Occupation significantly influences human development (Nelson, 1997, p. 550) and is situation specific (Royeen, 2003, p. 616).

Terminology: Occupation and Activity

Many OT practitioners use the terms occupation and activity interchangeably in the literature and within clinical practice, but arguably, they are not one in the same. John Dewey (1916), a 20th-century philosopher and educator, described occupations as ongoing activities with a set purpose. What sets occupation apart from other activities that we engage in are the "social and symbolic context[s]" that infuses them with meaning (Christiansen & Baum, 2005, p. 5). Let's think about stirring brownie batter again. If a client was given a bowl filled with water to stir, it would be an activity. The inherent movements and cognitive processes needed to stir water are the same as brownie batter, but it lacks purpose other than to move the arm and hand and to focus on keeping the water in the bowl. Stirring brownie batter is an occupation because of the symbolic contexts we associate with making this delicious treat.

In the original *Philosophical Base of Occupational Therapy* (American Occupational Therapy Association [AOTA], 1979, p. 785), the word activity was used five times and occupation only once. Comparatively, in the revised *Philosophical Base of Occupational Therapy* (American Occupational Therapy Association [AOTA], 2011, p. 607), activity appears twice and occupation and its derivatives appear 13 times. In the third edition of the *Occupational Therapy Practice Framework; Domain and Process* (AOTA, 2014), the term occupation and its derivative appears more (834 times) often than the term activity (73 times). This clearly indicates a philosophy shift relative to the professional connotation of the term occupation as compared to activity, which is a fundamental part of occupational therapy.

Why Use Occupation as a Therapeutic Tool?

Using occupation as the "fundamental basis" for our treatment sets us apart from other health care professionals (Davis, 2011, p. 1). While on the surface, it may appear that engaging in occupation or purposeful activity is simple, it is in fact, a very complex and powerful therapeutic intervention (Davis, 2011).

Despite a growing body of evidence from various disciplines clearly identifying the value of occupation and activity (WHO, 2002), one of the reasons that OT practitioners may have steered clear and continue to steer clear of traditional occupation-based task-oriented practice like crafts and gardening was and is an image issue (Davis, 2011). Competing with therapies that look very scientific and regimented, like physical therapy (Davis, 2011), is hard when you are working with a client to weave a market basket. But a big difference between a functional occupation-based activity like weaving and exercise, modalities, or nonpurposeful activity is that for the most part, clients prefer to do something that is enjoyable and purposeful like weaving a basket while still accomplishing the same goals (Davis, 2011). This brings our discussion back to the basic function of occupation: engagement in meaningful and purposeful activity to effect positive change (From the Field 4.1).

In part, the shift back to engaging clients in functional activity may be an off-shoot of third-party payers like insurance companies and Medicare requiring documentation of functional changes (Davis, 2011). This has been transformative for occupational therapy because "The importance of function and the foundation of our profession were validated" (Davis, 2011, p. 1). Described in the World Health Organization's (WHO), *International Classification of Functioning, Disability, and Health (ICF)* (2002) are 1) **participation**, which entails taking part in or involvement in life situations, and 2) activity, the act of doing a task, which is understood to positively influence health and well-being (WHO, 2002). On the other hand, disability tends to lead to reduced and less diverse occupational participation in daily life activities; including work, leisure, education, social participation, and self-care (AOTA, 2014; WHO, 2002).

While occupational participation enhances life quality, limited participation or **occupational deprivation** leads to poor health and well-being (Law, 2002; Wilcock, 1998). **Occupational justice** is a philosophical explanation for reducing or eliminating deprivation and encouraging equitable participation. According to Law (2002), "Participation in the everyday occupations of life is a vital part of human development and lived experience. Through participation, we acquire skills and competencies; connect with others and our communities, and find purpose and meaning in life"

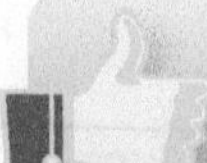

FROM THE FIELD 4.1

Playing Poker

In the early days of my career, I worked in a large university hospital that housed acute care, inpatient, and outpatient rehabilitation units. I followed "Dr. Coles" (not his real name) from acute care through outpatient rehabilitation. Dr. Coles was a distinguished professor with a strong will and terrific sense of humor. Following an accident, one of many goals for Dr. Coles was to improve his standing tolerance and balance, so he began the process by a graded standing program in a standing frame. He also needed to rebuild trunk and upper extremity control.

In getting to know Dr. Coles, I learned that one of his leisure time passions was a weekly poker game with his colleagues. Well, not being a poker player and barely even knowing how to play any card games, I decided that it was prime time to learn to play. Much to Dr. Coles' delight, I set him up in the standing frame and brought out a set of cards and chips and asked him to teach me how to play. The sessions flew by, he stood for longer periods of time every session, and to recreate the just right challenge, I would set the game up on higher surfaces and farther away from his trunk each session.

Not only was Dr. Coles standing longer, he was having fun engaging in what was meaningful and purposeful for him while increasing active range of motion in his upper extremities and developing better trunk control. And, then we added wrist weights. A simple thing—learning what mattered to Dr. Coles—changed what could have been potential drudgery, standing in a frame doing nonpurposeful activities like pinning clothespins to a vertically oriented pole, into a meaningful occupation. And, in the process, I lost an incredible amount of pretend money! I never fail to recount this story when I am lecturing to my students on the importance of engaging clients in personally meaningful occupation. It truly makes a difference and is profoundly transformative for both client and practitioner.

Amy Wagenfeld, PhD, OTR/L, SCEM, CAPs

(p. 640). Not only is working with clients to determine the appropriate occupation important, so too is focusing on enhancing the actual experience of participation, the doing of the activity. The exciting challenge in therapeutic intervention is both determining the occupation and facilitating it so that clients can actively participate and derive the maximum meaning from it. On the other hand, while research supports that our lives are enhanced through participation, it has also determined that a lack of participation or occupational deprivation leads to a decline in health and well-being (Law, 2002). Some examples of occupational deprivation are disability, unemployment, living in war zones or other marginalized areas, lack of basic resources, and racial prejudice. For instance, people living in war zones or marginalized areas such as public housing projects or other low socioeconomic housing situations often have little or no access to nature: parks, grass, or even trees. Being deprived of the opportunity to engage in outdoor occupations is equated with poorer physical and psychological health (Kuo & Sullivan, 2001; Mitchell & Popham, 2008; Park et al., 2010). Ensuring equitable opportunity for underserved people to participate in and connect with nature occurs through occupational justice. Because of the limitations they place on people, these examples prevent people from fully participating in occupation, something an OT practitioner must be sensitive to when planning for appropriate intervention. The mission of the occupational therapy profession is to engage clients in everyday meaningful and purposeful activity, and OT practitioners are uniquely positioned to align the ICF principles with our practice to develop and enhance participation for all people, no matter age, ability, or preference (From the Field 4.2).

Occupational therapy will remain pertinent for generations to come for the same reason it has flourished in the past (Nelson, 1997). Occupational therapy practitioners are the experts in implementing occupation-based practice. People have always and will always need therapeutic occupation (Nelson, 1997). Why? Humans need to be ensured of the opportunity to actively participate in life to the greatest extent possible. "The human being can attain enhanced health and quality of life by actively doing things that are personally meaningful and purposeful, in other words, through occupation" (Nelson, 1997, p. 532). For the reasons discussed, (1) third-party payers require documentation of change in function, (2) the ICF acknowledges the importance of participation and activity, and (3) evidence supports its merits (Davis, 2011); other health care professionals will be eager to use occupation, but remember, "we can dominate it with our skill and expertise" (Davis, 2011, p. 2).

FROM THE FIELD 4.2

The ICF

Familiarize yourself with a very important document prepared by a multinational panel of members of the World Health Organization called the *International Classification of Functioning, Disability, and Health (ICF)*. It can be found at http://www.who.int/classifications/icf/training/icfbeginnersguide.pdf. One of the key points of this document is recognition of the importance of participation and activity. Who better to implement meaningful and purposeful activities than OT practitioners?

Occupation as Ends versus Occupation as Means

Occupation as ends is a situation when the end goal to be achieved is the occupation itself (Trombly, 1995), such as relearning to button a shirt using a piece of adapted equipment called a button hook. Occupation as ends is a way to achieve functional goals from a bottom-up perspective, and not as a means to "[using] occupation[s] of purposeful and meaningful activity to improve performance components" (Gray, 1998, p. 357; Van Mater Stone, 2005). Occupation as ends is "the over-arching goal of all occupational therapy interventions" (in Gray, 1998, p. 357). Burke's (1983) description of occupation as ends incorporates goals and objectives to help clients regain old or learn new ways to engage in their "chosen occupational lives" (in Gray, 1998, p. 357). Looking at occupation as ends from this perspective suggests that assessment and treatment needs to be client-centered with the end goal of restoration of or recreation of "occupational lives" (Gray, 1998, p. 357). As an emerging OTA, think about how your contribution to your professional team may be influenced in the way you view occupations as ends as a bottom-up treatment approach or as the overarching goal of occupational therapy intervention or perhaps both.

Trombly (1995) suggested that **occupation as means** can be distilled down to being "limited to simple behaviors" (p. 963) that are repetitive such as doing three sets of bending and straightening the elbow 15 times in a row. Gray (1998) questioned as to whether these simple behaviors are in fact occupation or better equated with "exercise or physical modalities" that could be useful as "adjuncts to occupation...[and/or] to advance someone toward an occupational outcome" (p. 358). The AOTA (1994) position toward occupation as means as being "simple behaviors" is that they are best suited as preparation for and in conjunction with occupation, and not a substitute for occupation.

A current issue that corresponds to occupation as means is the use of physical agent modalities (PAMs). They are "procedures and interventions that are systematically applied to modify specific client factors when neurological, musculoskeletal, or skin conditions are present that may be limiting occupational performance" (AOTA, 2012, p. 1), such as heat, electrical stimulation, or massage (Bracciano, 2008). The AOTA clearly states that PAMs "may be used by occupational therapists and occupational therapy assistants [only with training and supervision and PAMs are always integrated into a broader occupational therapy program as a preparatory method for the therapeutic use of occupations or purposeful activities" (AOTA, 2008, 2012, p. 2; AOTA, 2014). Using PAMS as a substitute for occupational performance is not considered occupational therapy (AOTA, 2008; 2012; 2014).

Categorizing Occupations

Any individual's typical day is divided up into a series of occupations that can typically be categorized as work (paid and unpaid), leisure and play, self-care, and sleep.

As described by Christiansen and Baum (2005), work is an "activity required for subsistence" (p. 9), yet work such as household chores are unpaid and discretionary. A person chooses when and how to do this work. Examples of work are paid employment, volunteer jobs, and house and yard chores. Leisure and play are discretionary activities that are presumed to bring forth a sense of happiness and relaxation. Here is a paradox. For some people, yard work is actually a leisure time activity and not unpaid work. As well, a professional basketball player gets paid to do what most others do as a leisure activity. As you might be thinking, for children, play is actually a primary occupation of childhood and might even be considered work. Self-care activities (**activities of daily living** [ADLs]) are necessary for self-maintenance and include things such as bathing, dressing, and eating. Sleep is actually a self-care occupation that is necessary for survival (Christiansen & Baum, 2005). We spend approximately a third of our lives asleep. Activities of daily living are often divided into personal ADLs and instrumental ADLs, which will be discussed in the upcoming *Occupational Therapy Practice Frameworks* and *Activities of Daily Living* in Chapters 6 and 23, respectively. When working with clients, it is imperative to understand what is important for them when selecting occupation. If a client presents with limited strength and endurance or even motivation, self-care activities may not be of personal high priority, whereas a creative OT practitioner may be able to achieve the same goals and objectives focused on strength, endurance, and motivation by engaging that client in work or leisure activities that are identified as personally meaningful. Knitting is a purposeful activity that builds strength, endurance, and, for someone who enjoys it, is meaningful. When developing an intervention plan in conjunction with a supervising OT, it is very important to find out from the client, what is important to him/her. If knitting can build foundational strength and endurance, there is a reasonable chance that the client may at some point become invested in working on self-care skills due to the new found strength and endurance gained from knitting (Table 4.1).

Meaningful and Purposeful: Forming Identities

Gray (1998) suggested that for an intervention to be considered occupational, it must have meaning and purpose for the client; have a clearly defined beginning, middle,

TABLE 4.1 Categories of Occupations: The Life of a Student

Work	Leisure and Play	Self-Care	Sleep and Rest
Attend class	Sing in barbershop quartet	Shower and wash hair	Sleep on a futon
Homework	Attend daily crossfit classes	Apply makeup	Nap from 2 to 3 PM
Work full or parttime at a frozen yogurt store	Spring break in the Bahamas	Dry hair	Share a queen-sized bed with spouse or partner
Volunteer at soup kitchen	Read a novel	Make breakfast and pack lunch	Spouse or partner snores
	Go to yoga	Drive to campus	Puppy sleeps on the bed
	Paint	Clean house	
		Rake leaves	
		Deposit check at bank.	

and end; and be holistic and multidimensional in order to ensure maximal participation (p. 354). Further, in order for occupation to contain purpose, it must be done within a temporal context that imbues personal meaning (Cox & Pemberton, 2011). Failing to locate occupation into a person's routine in a realistic way may lead to learning or relearning skills in isolation. This concept can be illustrated by carefully thinking about the temporality of the occupation when working with a client on self-care skills like dressing—"Is it realistic to practice dressing at 3 PM?" (Cox's Pemberton, 2011) (Fig. 4.2).

As Wood (1995) stated, "Engagement in meaningful occupations has a kind of multiplicative impact, not merely an additive one, upon a person's state of health" (p. 47). From a psychosocial perspective, "occupation, when it is applied as activity with wholeness, purpose, and meaning to the person, can [affect people]... in ways that purposeful activity unrelated to the person cannot" (Gray, 1998, p. 356). Gray (1998) said this of OT practitioners:

> We know how to assess functional performance, how to communicate with clients to determine their interests and goals, and how to analyze activities and patterns of activity for problems and adaptive benefits. All these skills indicate occupational therapy's expertise in human engagement in purposeful and meaningful activity. Other health care team members do not possess this occupational expertise (p. 363).

How can you effectively share this information with professional colleagues and with those who are unfamiliar with occupational therapy?

Fidler (1981) suggested, "An historical tenet of occupational therapy has been that purposeful activity provides the incentive and opportunity for individuals to achieve mastery and thereby add to their sense of competence" (p. 569) in their daily lives. Hammell (2004) said that "Occupation might best be understood, not as divisible activities of self-care, productivity and leisure but as dimensions of meaning" (p. 297). Daily occupations define who we are as people (Christiansen, 1999). Defining who we are as individuals by the occupations we engage in and having the opportunity to "... express ...[our] identity in a manner that gives meaning to life" is a profoundly important part of our identity development at every stage in life (Christiansen, 1999, p. 577).

Fidler (1981) shared two assumptions relative to the underpinnings of purposeful activity. The first is that external societal influence places value on the meaning of certain tasks, such as maintaining a neat personal appearance. These types of tasks may carry greater weight and influence sense of efficacy more than tasks that have less perceived social importance. Societies' values and norms weight certain tasks and activities. Second, one's internal biology and inner drive may lead people to active mastery over certain tasks in order to experience a sense of competence and self-satisfaction. Again, the analogy

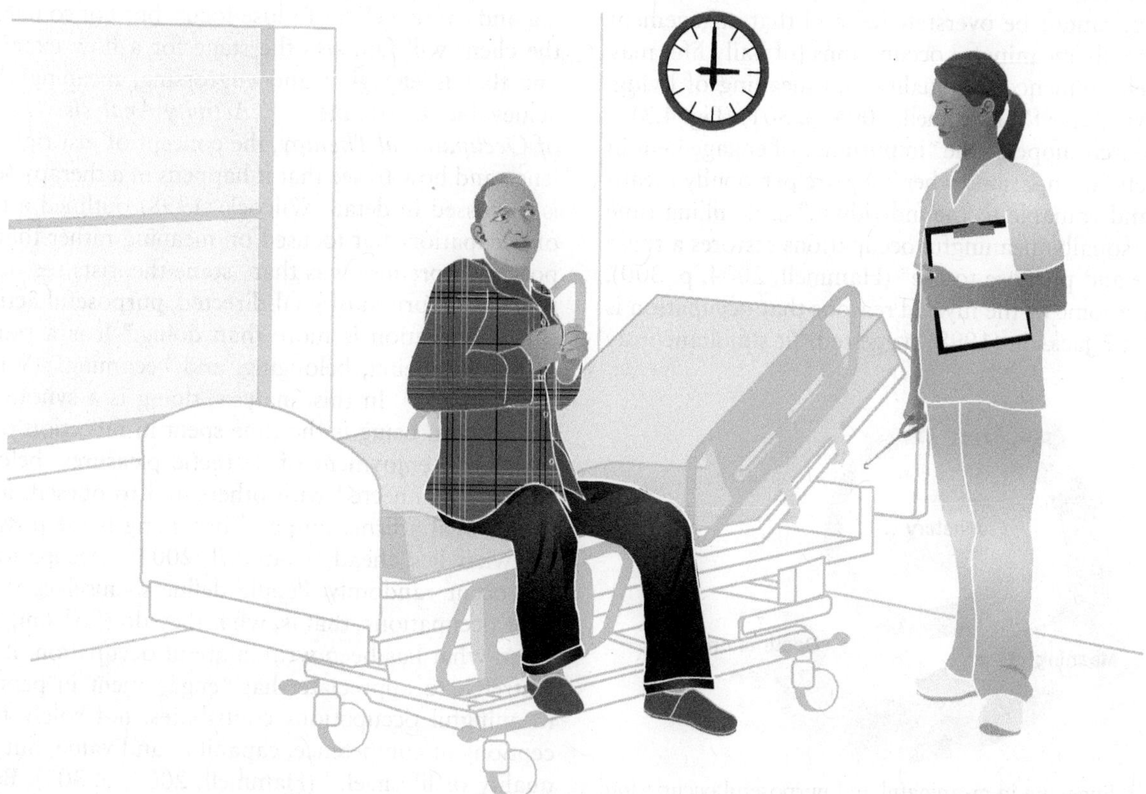

Figure 4.2 Is getting dressed for the day at 3 PM realistic therapy?

of maintaining a neat personal appearance is supported by this second assumption that we are drawn to master tasks that make us feel good about ourselves. Both external societal values and our internal processes motivate us to master meaningful and purposeful activities. Occupations that have personal meaning foster a "sense of purpose" (Hammell, 2004, p. 300). Comparatively, when people lose their ability to engage in meaningful occupation, the tendency is to devalue themselves and diminish their sense of worth and capability (Hammell, 2004). While Christiansen (1999) said this about the relationship between depression and everyday activity, "[it] can be averted when people are given an opportunity to gain personal meaning from everyday activities, when their sense of optimism is renewed, and where they believe that there is choice and control in their lives" (1999, p. 555), it is also applicable for clients with any type of challenge. **Occupational choice** gives clients a sense of empowerment, when they may feel that as a result of trauma, illness, or accident that they have little or none. It is important for OT practitioners to recognize that a client must experience a sense of competence in his/her therapeutic interventions and that mastery of skills (occupations) and doing so has the capacity to influence behaviors and actions (Fidler, 1981). Without a sense of competence or opportunity to experience mastery, there is little hope for a client to feel that he/she is capable of being an "agent of change" (Fidler, 1981, p. 571). "The importance of occupation in reconstructing a life worth living.... of filling life with meaning, cannot be overstated... and that engagement in personally meaningful occupations [of daily life] may not solely influence the quality and meaning of living, but survival itself" (Hammell, 2004, p. 301) (Fig. 4.3).

Research supports the "importance of engagement in purposeful occupations when they are personally meaningful and valuable to the individual," and "filling time with personally meaningful occupations restores a sense of value and purpose to life" (Hammell, 2004, p. 300). What are some of the myriad reasons that occupation is important? Jackson (1998) suggested, "it simultaneously and appropriately challenges the physical, cognitive, psychological, symbolic, and transcendental components of the person" (pp. 471–472).

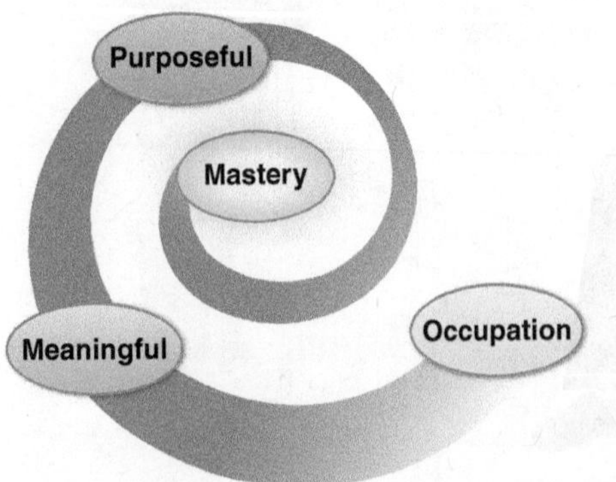

Figure 4.3 Engaging in meaningful and purposeful occupation leads to mastery of skills.

Achieving meaningfulness and participation in occupation requires a balance between the challenge of the activity and the skills of the person, which is referred to as the **just-right challenge**. Many occupational therapy practitioners often use this term to refer to a flow type of experience. The positive mental state that enables a person to be fully present and absorbed in an activity is a fluid process that Csikszentmihalyi (1997) refers to as **flow**. Flow allows people to experience a sense of balance and mastery. Flow is best experienced in structured occupations with set parameters (Law, 2002) that foster a sense of control and mastery. Occupational therapy practitioners are constantly called upon to impart the just right challenge, or flow experience, when working with clients. For example, kneading bread dough is a therapeutic activity for working on strengthening and range of motion (movement of the joints) and sensory skills. A client who dislikes baking or touching slimy things is unlikely to experience flow as he/she does not find meaning in kneading dough. The just right challenge is unlikely to occur because the activity is not a good match for the client. On the other hand, for a client who loves to bake, yet is weak or has trouble with movements in the hands and arms, kneading dough may be the ideal therapy, starting with a very light and easy to manipulate dough to a tougher and more elastic type of dough. Creating the just right challenge, not too easy to be boring and cause a client to lose focus, but not so hard that the client will fail, sets the stage for a flow experience, one that is engaging and engrossing, meaningful, and achievable. In Chapter 11, *Activity Analysis: The Jewel of Occupational Therapy*, the concept of just right challenge and how to see that it happens in a therapy session is discussed in detail. Wilcock (1998) outlined a theory of occupation that focused on meaning rather than purpose. The premise was that "some theorists see occupation as comprised of goal-directed, purposeful activities, [but] occupation is more than doing." It is a synthesis of "doing, being, belonging, and becoming" (Wilcock, 1998, p. 341). In this analysis, doing is a synonym for occupation; being is the time spent in reflection or contemplative enjoyment of aesthetic pleasures; belonging is feeling connected with others and to oneself, a sense of personal affirmation; and becoming is the possibility for what lies ahead (Hammell, 2004). Occupations do not occur randomly. People define themselves through their occupations, that is, what they do (Jackson, 1998). From what has been written about occupation, it is not a stretch to appreciate that "engagement in personally meaningful occupations contributes, not solely to perceptions of competence, capability and value, but to the quality of life itself" (Hammell, 2004, p. 303). Because our profession is grounded in engagement in meaningful activity, we are well positioned to help "meet the challenges confronting people whose identity is threatened by impairments, limitations to activity, and restrictions on their participation as social beings" (Christiansen, 1999, p. 592). We are who we are because of the daily occupations we engage in and the context, which gives them meaning (Christiansen, 1999). To that end, "[t]he central place of occupations in shaping identity and creating life meaning is so powerful that one cannot help but marvel at their implications for occupational therapy practice" (Christiansen, 1999, p. 590).

Occupations in Action: The Therapeutic Applications

Christiansen (1999) proposed that "[t]he ultimate goal of occupational therapy services is well-being, not health. Health enables people to pursue the tasks of everyday living that provide them with the life meaning necessary for their well-being" (p. 576). This systems-oriented perspective suggests that while our goal is not to heal, in order to experience well-being, clients need to be provided with opportunity to pursue occupation that will allow them to experience a sense of mastery and competence. Health depends on well-being and well-being depends on health.

The concept of occupations as a treatment modality is built on the premise that occupations are a catalyst for (1) "improving health and productivity; they could prevent secondary illness (particularly depression), help with motivation, and build self-esteem" (Friedland & Silva, 2008, p. 351), and (2) for experiencing sense of control and mastery. One of the most profound human needs is experiencing a sense of control. Depression, anxiety, and heightened sense of pain can be reduced when people experience a sense of meaning and control in their lives and achieve what Antonovsky (1987) called a **sense of coherence**. A sense of coherence helps people to cope with stress in ways that are beneficial rather than detrimental to health and well-being. There is growing evidence that many people with physical impairments, either newly acquired or of long-term duration, undergo a conceptual transformation and change the way they think about disability. If sense of coherence is strong, those with physical challenges perceive themselves to be competent and capable, choosing to minimize loss, and focus instead on ability and accomplishment (Hammell, 2004, p. 298). For most every client that you will treat, active participation in occupation depends on connecting the past (self) with the new (self) and sense of coherence. This is not to say that the focus of intervention is on disability, but rather to "blend past and present to create new and integrated occupational routines" (Jackson, 1998, p. 472).

Gray (1998) said that "Occupational [therapy practitioners] are experts in analyzing a person's ability to function in his or her environment and thus to participate in personally satisfying, organized daily routines of culturally and developmentally relevant activities: occupation" (p. 357). For maximum benefit, intervention has to mesh with an individual's needs and values and be rich in personal meaning. While doing puzzles may improve visual perception and coordination for someone who has never enjoyed puzzles, those same skills can, with a degree of creativity and patience, be addressed through engagement of personally meaningful occupation with that same client, such as perhaps, baking a cake if he/she articulates that baking is a source of positive meaning and fulfills a sense of purpose. "When therapists use occupation they are less likely to see a hand or arm; nor are they likely to simply focus on cognition, mental states, motor control, or balance. Instead, they are more apt to be synthesizers, viewing the patient as an occupational being with many strengths and needs that require integration… [into meaningful] occupational routines" (Jackson, 1998, p. 472) such as baking that cake.

Davis (2011) discussed three considerations necessary for facilitation of functional or occupation-based activities. They are task selection, environmental considerations, and therapeutic handling developing exceptional practice skills. There is a strong interrelationship between these considerations, which Davis calls "intervention with intention" (p. 3).

Although we wear many hats as OT practitioners (Fig. 4.4), what do you think is the most important skill an OT practitioner must have? Davis (2011) believes that skill is "keen observation," and the "better your observational skills are, the better a [practitioner] you will be" (p. 2). Not to mention, the more successful you will be to wear the multiple hats with competence and compassion. And further, "Strive to become a master clinician in occupation-based practice. It's what defines our profession. It's what makes us unique. And it works!" (p. 3).

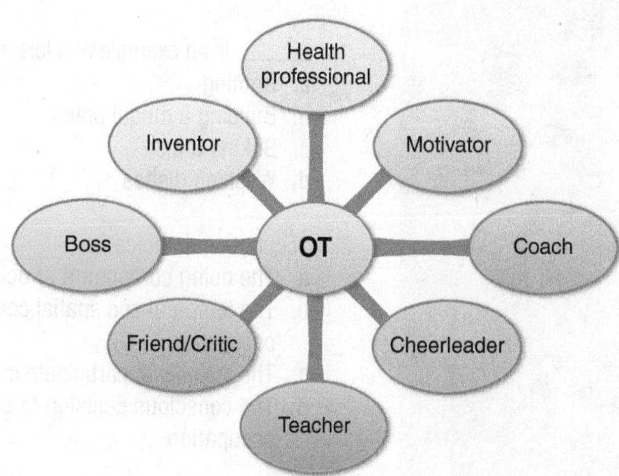

Figure 4.4 The many roles of the OT practitioner. Adapted with permission (Marcil, 2006). Delmar Cengage Learning.

Occupation in the 21st Century

With regard to the direction our profession should take, Jackson (1998) articulated that "The extent to which occupational therapists win today's tug-of-war between keeping the practice on which our profession was created—occupation—and being swept away by forces pulling us into other patterns of practice will depend on how much we value the richness and healing qualities of occupation and how able and willing we are to articulate this conviction to others" (p. 466). A decade later, a voice in occupational therapy articulates a similar concern. That is, "Today, occupational therapists struggle with the scope of their practice and voice concern over the breadth of the field" (Friedland & Silva, 2008, p. 357). Schwartz (2009) said that "Like the founders, we have a powerful tool—the use of engagement in occupation—as both a means and end to health. What we have that the founders did not is a growing body of evidence to support the efficacy of what we do, and we have the power of numbers" (p. 689). There is work to be done!

Bauerschmidt and Nelson (2011) believe that it is every OT practitioner's "personal responsibility" to have a cogent explanation to share with everyone about why we are called occupational therapists (p. 344). While it may seem like a simple task, it is anything but. Breines (1990) suggested, "[occupational] therapists can hold their heads high and articulate their identity with skill and sophistication" (p. 45). With a far better than average employment outlook, knowing who and what you are and to be able to articulate this information as you go about your professional practice as an OTA is critically important. Challenge yourself to be a true professional ambassador.

Summary

In this chapter, we reviewed the historical tenets of occupation and how our roots have supported us through three paradigms. The current paradigm represents a slow return to our founding mission: occupation as a means to foster positive health outcomes. Various definitions of occupation and different occupational categories were also discussed. As emerging OT practitioners in a society in need of the services our profession can provide, you are well poised to enter the field as an expert in understanding the profound nature of occupation. More so, you have the opportunity to apply it in meaningful and purposeful ways to the clients you will work with.

Review Questions

1. ______ is an example of a leisure occupation.
   a. Bathing
   b. Building a model plane
   c. Baking a pie
   d. Washing dishes

2. Occupational choice is:
   a. The doing component of occupation
   b. The temporal and spatial contexts of occupation
   c. The inability to participate in occupation
   d. The conscious decision to engage in occupation

3. Which one of the following is not an example of occupational deprivation?
   a. Poverty
   b. Racial bias
   c. Employment
   d. Unemployment

4. Which one of the following best describes an uncompensated work activity?
   a. Cleaning the house
   b. Trading off babysitting of your children with a friend's children
   c. Paid internship at AOTA
   d. Cleaning your yoga studio in exchange for 10 classes

5. An activity that is presented to a client that is not too hard as to insure failure but not so easy as to be boring is:
   a. The just right challenge
   b. Flow
   c. Systems theory
   d. Adaptation

6. In order for an activity to be meaningful it needs to:
   a. Make sense to the person engaging in it
   b. Last for a specific duration
   c. Be self-directed
   d. Needs to be done under controlled conditions

7. The formal study of occupation is called:
   a. Evidence-based programming
   b. Modulation review
   c. Occupational science
   d. Occupational adaptation

8. "Simple behaviors that are repetitive and purposeful" best describes:
   a. Occupation as means
   b. Occupation as ends
   c. Occupational adaptation
   d. Occupational choice

9. The *International Classification of Functioning, Disability, and Health (ICF)* recognizes the importance of:
   a. Meaning
   b. Flow and just right challenge
   c. Participation and activity
   d. Disability as reason to limit opportunities to engage in work

10. If your colleague said to you, "Mrs. Sommers refuses to get dressed today because it is 4 PM and she thinks it is a silly idea to get dressed when it is nearly time for dinner and then bed," this represents which/what components of occupation?
    a. Occupational choice and form
    b. Occupational deprivation and function/participation
    c. Occupational choice, form, and function/participation
    d. Occupational adaptation, form, choice

11. "The end goal is the occupation" itself is called:
    a. Occupation as means
    b. Occupation as ends
    c. Occupational adaptation
    d. Occupational choice

Practice Activities

As discussed in Chapter 1, Thomas Kidner, one of the founders of occupational therapy, strongly advocated for all occupational therapists to serve as ambassadors to the profession (Friedland & Silva, 2008). How do you envision using social media to get the word out about the importance of OT? Without the benefit of looking forward in the book to the units on common conditions and practice settings, think of one population or setting you might be interested in working with right now, and create the script for a video clip that you might post on the Internet that advocates for the role of an OTA in working with this population or practice area. Share this script with your classmates. When you complete the textbook, review your script, modify it, and share it with your classmates. Having the benefit of a semester plus of learning, what is different and what remains the same?

Make a list of your top fifteen most positively meaningful occupations that you engage in—work, leisure, and self-care focused. Now take this list and divide it up into the three categories listed in this chapter. Now take this list and determine what you do daily, weekly, etc. Now take this list and select your absolute favorite from each category of work, leisure, and self-care. Now take this list and determine the occupational form and performance elements involved in each of these three occupations. Repeat this activity with a family member. What did you find?

If you were to have dinner with Adolf Meyer and Eleanor Clarke Slagle tomorrow, what would you tell them about the state of occupation with regard to occupational therapy, today? Prepare a 5-minute speech and present it to your classmates.

References

American Occupational Therapy Association. *Definition of Occupational Therapy Practice for the AOTA Model Practice Act*. Bethesda, MD: American Occupational Therapy Association; 1994.

American Occupational Therapy Association. *A Guide for the Preparation of Occupational Therapy Practitioners for the Use of Physical Agent Modalities*. Rockville, MD: Author; 2004.

American Occupational Therapy Association. Physical agent modalities: a position paper. *Am J Occup Ther* 2008;62:691–693.

American Occupational Therapy Association. Physical agent modalities: a position paper (revised). *Am J Occup Ther* 2012;66(6 Suppl): S78–S80.

American Occupational Therapy Association. Occupational therapy practice framework: domain and process (3rd ed.). *Am J Occup Ther* 2014;68(Suppl 1):S1–S48. http://dx.doi.org/10.5014/ajot.2014.682006

American Occupational Therapy Association [AOTA]. The philosophical base of occupational therapy. *Am J Occup Ther* 1979;65(6):785.

American Occupational Therapy Association [AOTA]. The philosophical base of occupational therapy. *Am J Occup Ther* 2011;65(6):607.

Antonovsky A. *Unraveling the Mystery of Health: How People Manage Stress and Stay Well*. San Francisco, CA: Josey Bass; 1987.

Bauerschmidt B, Nelson DL. The terms occupation and activity over the history of official occupational therapy publications. *Am J Occup Ther* 2011;65(3):338–345.

Bracciano AG. *Physical Agent Modalities: Theory and Application for the Occupational Therapist*. 2nd ed. Thorofare, NJ: Slack; 2008.

Breines EB. Genesis of occupation: a philosophical model for therapy and theory. *Aust Occup Ther J* 1990;37:45–49.

Canadian Association of Occupational Therapists. *Enabling Occupation. An Occupational Therapy Perspective*. Rev. ed. Ottawa, ON: CAOT Publications ACE; 2002.

Canadian Occupational Therapy Association. Code of ethics. 2007. Retrieved from http://www.caot.ca/default.asp?pageid=35

Christiansen C. The 1999 Eleanor Clarke Slagle Lecture. Defining lives: occupation as identity: an essay on competence, coherence, and the creation of meaning. *Am J Occup Ther* 1999;53(6):547–558.

Christiansen CH, Baum CM. The complexity of human occupation. In: Christiansen CH, Baum CM, Bass-Haugen J, eds. *Occupational Therapy Performance, Participation, and Well-Being*. 3rd ed., pp. 2–24. Thorofare, NJ: SLACK Inc; 2005.

Christiansen CH, Townsend EA. *Introduction to Occupation: The Art and Science of Living*. Upper Saddle River, NJ: Prentice Hall; 2004.

Cox D, Pemberton S. What happened to the time? The relationship of occupational therapy to time. *Br J Occup Ther* 2011;74(2):78–89.

Csikszentmihalyi M. *Finding Flow: The Psychology of Engagement with Everyday Life*. New York, NY: Basic Books; 1997.

Davis J. The power of occupation: the key to inspired intervention. *Home Commun Health Spec Interest Sec Q* 2011;18(2):1–3.

Dewey J. *Democracy and Education*. New York, NY: MacMillan; 1916.

Dunton WR. *Reconstruction Therapy*. Philadelphia, PA: Saunders; 1919.

Fidler GS. From crafts to competence. *Am J Occup Ther* 1981;35(9):567–573.

Friedland J, Silva J. Evolving identities: Thomas Bessell Kidner and occupational therapy in the United States. *Am J Occup Ther* 2008;62(3):349–360.

Gray JM. Putting occupation into practice: occupation as ends, occupation as means. *Am J Occup Ther* 1998(May);52(5):354–364.

Hammell KW. Dimensions of meaning in the occupations of daily life. *Can J Occup Ther* 2004;5(71):296–305.

Hockey C, Wright-St Claire V. Occupational science: adding value to occupational therapy. *N Z J Occup Ther* 2011;58(1):29–38.

Jackson J. (1998). The value of occupation as the core of treatment: Sandy's experience. *Am J Occup Ther* 1998;52(6):466–473.

Kielhofner G. *Conceptual Foundations of Occupational Therapy*. 2nd ed. Philadelphia, PA: FA Davis; 1992.

Kielhofner G. *Conceptual Foundations of Occupational Therapy Practice*. 4th ed. Philadelphia, PA: F.A. Davis, Co.; 2009.

Kielhofner G, Burke J. The evolution of knowledge and practice in occupational therapy: past, present and future. In: Kielhofner G, ed. *Health Through Occupation*. pp. 3–54. Philadelphia, PA: F. A. Davis; 2005.

Kuo A. A transactional view: occupations as a means to create experiences that matter. *J Occup Sci* 2011;18(2):131–138.

Kuo FE, Sullivan WC. Environment and crime in the inner city: does vegetation reduce crime? *Environ Behav* 2001;3(3):343–367.

Law M. Participation in the occupations of everyday life. *Am J Occup Ther* 2002; 56(6):640–649.

Marcil W.M. *Occupational Therapy: What It Is and How It Works*. Clifton ParK, NY: Cengage Learning; 2006.

McColl MA, et al. *Theoretical Basis of Occupational Therapy. An Annotated Bibliography of Applied Theory in the Professional Literature*. 2nd ed. Thorofare, NJ: SLACK Inc.; 2003.

Mitchell R, Popham F. Effect of exposure to natural environment on health inequalities: an observational population study. *Lancet* 2008;372(9650):1655–1660.

National Society for the Promotion of Occupational Therapy. *Certificate of incorporation of the National Society for the Promotion of Occupational Therapy*. Bethesda, MD: Wilma L. West Library and Archives, American Occupational Therapy Association; 1917(March 15).

Nelson D. Why the profession of occupational therapy will flourish in the 21st century. *Am J Occup Ther* 1997;51:11–24.

Park BJ, et al. The physiological effects of Shinrin-yoku (taking in the forest atmosphere or forest bathing): evidence from field experiments in 24 forests across Japan. *Environ Health Prev Med* 2010;15:18–26.

Royeen CB. Chaotic occupational therapy: collective wisdom for a complex profession. *Am J Occup Ther* 2003;57:609–624.

Sartre JP. *Being and Nothingness*. New York, NY: Washington Square Press; 1943/1993.

Schwartz KB. The 2009 Eleanor Clarke Slagle Lecture: reclaiming our heritage: connecting the Founding Vision to the Centennial Vision. *Am J Occup Ther* 2009(Nov-Dec);63(6):681–690.

Trombly CA. Occupation: Purposefulness and meaningfulness as therapeutic mechanisms, 1995 Eleanor Clarke Slagle lecture. *Am J Occup Ther* 1995;49:960–972.

Van Mater Stone G. Personal and environmental influences on occupations. In: Christiansen CH, Baum CM, Bass-Huagen J, eds. *Occupational Therapy Performance, Participation, and Well-Being*. 3rd ed., pp. 93–116. Thorfare, NJ: SLACK Inc; 2005.

Wilcock AA. *An Occupational Perspective of Health*. Thorofare, NJ: Slack; 1998.

Wood W. Weaving the warp and weft of occupational therapy: an art and science for all times. *Am J Occup Ther* 1995;49:44–52.

World Health Organization. *Towards a common language for functioning, disability and health* (ICF). 2002. Retrieved from http://www.who.int/classifications/icf/training/icfbeginnersguide.pdf

CHAPTER 5

The Evidence-Based Movement: Guiding the Practice

Amy Wagenfeld, PhD, OTR/L SCEM, CAPs

Key Terms

Critically appraised papers (CAPs)—Stand-alone summaries of single studies.

Critically appraised topics (CATs)—Summarizes evidence on specific topics—less rigorous than a systematic review.

Evidence—The available facts and circumstances indicating whether or not something is true or valid.

Evidence-based medicine—Applying the best existing evidence to help make decisions about individualized patient care (Sackett et al., 1996).

Evidence-based practice—Blending the best existing evidence with clinical expertise and what is important to clients (Sackett et al., 2000).

Evidence-based research—Research standard based on evidence versus anecdotal information. There are six levels of evidence-based research.

Meta-analysis—Like a systematic review; relies on multiple methods to search and consolidate findings from multiple studies on similar topics.

PICO—A way to organize a well-written question to research and then apply the results to an evidence-based process. The acronym stands for P (patient problem or population), I (intervention), C (comparison), and O (outcome).

Qualitative research—A type of research such as case studies or findings of interviews and self-report measures that looks to gain a deeper understanding of a problem and to understand relationships rather than causation.

Quantitative research—A type of research that aims to determine causation or causal relationships; data are analyzed via statistical analyses and are reported as experimental studies.

Randomized controlled trials—Quantitative, comparative research that involves randomly assigning participants to one or more groups, one of which is a control and the others are experimental. Researchers measure and compare the outcomes or results of the different groups through statistical analyses.

Reliability—Extent to which a research tool yields the same outcomes each time it is used.

Research—Gathering or collecting information about a topic.

Sensitivity analysis—A way to predict outcomes if the results are different than what were initially predicted.

Systematic review—A research tool that consolidates and summarizes many research findings on particular topics in order to provide evidence on that topic.

Validity—Degree to which an instrument measures what it is intended to measure.

Learning Objectives

After studying this chapter, the reader should be able to:

- Describe the evidence process and articulate its importance to occupational therapy.
- Describe evidence-based research and how it influences evidence-based practice.
- Develop a plan for doing an evidence-based research review that will guide implementation of evidence-based practice.

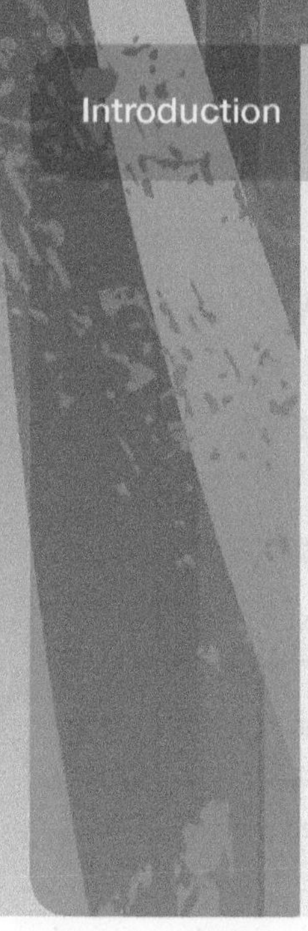

Introduction

Throughout the world and in accordance with other health professions, OT practitioners have come together to answer the challenge to globally address how to improve the quality of services by integrating research findings into clinical practice (Coster, 2005). One of the goals of the AOTA *Centennial Vision* is to see the profession recognized as "… a science-driven, and evidence-based profession" (AOTA, 2007). No matter the professional discipline, the purpose of an **evidence** process is to measure and determine the value of existing data and information (Alnervik & Linddahl, 2011). Today, the impact and influence of evidence-based practice is recognized across health care, educational, management, policy, and clinical practice settings (Bennett & Townsend, 2006). Good evidence-based practice derived from evidence-based research supports the validity of treatment interventions, which in today's health care system is critical when seeking reimbursement for services.

If one of your clients or one of their family members asked you the following question, "How do you know that what you do and how you do it really works?" (Holm, 2000, p. 575), how would you respond? In this chapter, we explore the concepts of evidence-based practice and research and its critical importance to your future work as an OTA. This will help you to be better prepared to answer this question.

Foundations of Evidence-Based Medicine

In the earliest days of occupational therapy, one of the profession's founders, Thomas Kidner, was an outspoken advocate for research. He wondered how results of therapeutic intervention could be measured and what was important to understand so as to continually challenge our profession to achieve higher standards (Friedland & Silvia, 2008). With the advent of evidence-based medicine, now more than ever, committing to use research findings as a means to support intervention and to strive for higher standards is paramount for the advancement of occupational therapy.

The concept of evidence-based medicine was first introduced in the 1980s at McMaster University medical school as a way to describe their problem-based learning approach, but the philosophical underpinnings actually date back to mid-19th century Paris and earlier. A number of recent social, political, and economic factors influenced the conceptualization of evidence-based practice including rising health care costs, shorter hospital stays, reduced number of staff, greater clinical accountability due to managed care, and client expectations (Bennett & Bennett, 2000). The Internet has also made accessing and sharing evidence information simpler for health care providers and consumers (Bennett & Townsend, 2006).

Sackett and colleagues (1996) indicated that "Evidence based medicine is the conscientious, explicit, and judicious use of current best evidence in making decisions about the care of individual patients" (p. 1). It entails "integrating individual clinical expertise with the best available external clinical evidence from systematic research" and is within the scope of every practitioner (Sackett et al., 1996, p. 1). Evidence-based medicine is, for example, administering vaccinations to children to prevent diseases such as whooping cough, hepatitis, and measles, which could lead to long-term developmental issues. It was not, and is not, the intent of evidence-based medicine to replace clinical judgment and expertise or to become formulaic, "cookie cutter" medicine. Rather, it highlights the importance of research evidence to inform clinical decision making and strengthen clinical judgment and experience and to be an integral part of clinical decision making (Bennett & Townsend, 2006; Sackett et al., 1996).

Today, evidence-based medicine, evidence-based research, evidence-based practice (EBP), and evidence-based occupational therapy practice (EBOT) are hot topics for clinicians, public health practitioners, purchasers, planners, and the public (Bennett & Townsend, 2006; Sackett et al., 1996). According to Iloh et al. (2006), "The philosophy of basing decisions on the best available research about what works is powerful and persuasive for all those with a stake in health and social care" (p. 38) including, of course, occupational therapy. In the past, our evidence was anecdotal and within each of us. It was shared or passed on from practitioner to practitioner. More recently, textbooks, journals, and the Internet have provided a forum to share expert opinions and research findings with a far-reaching global audience. While no single source of information is enough to be a definitive source of evidence, they are each an important means to disseminate information useful for evidence-based clinical practice. Throughout the world, the evidence-based movement is gaining momentum, and accordingly, to stay current and relevant, occupational therapy must remain a proactive voice in the evidence movement.

Evidence for Evidence Sake

Evidence helps to make conclusions apparent and leads to new insights for seeking other evidence (Dunn & Foreman, 2002, p. 14). Gray (1998) said, "The two ways that evidence derived from research can be used are to improve clinical practice and to improve health service management" (p. 9). Gaining evidence-based knowledge is more than an intradisciplinary process. It also entails a collaborative spirit through which knowledge from other disciplines comes together to solve problems that cannot be solved best by a single professional discipline (Dunn & Foreman, 2002, p. 19). One good example of this is universal design. It is the design of products and environments that meet the needs of the widest range of people possible without modification, regardless of age, ability, or preference (*Principles of Universal Design*, 2011). Lacking the collective knowledge of professionals in occupational and physical therapy, architecture, landscape design, environmental psychology, planning, interior, and industrial design, universal design would be unidimensional and unlikely to have the widespread positive effect on people that it does. Collaboration expands the possibilities and opens the door for creating stronger evidence (Dunn & Foreman, 2002, p. 19).

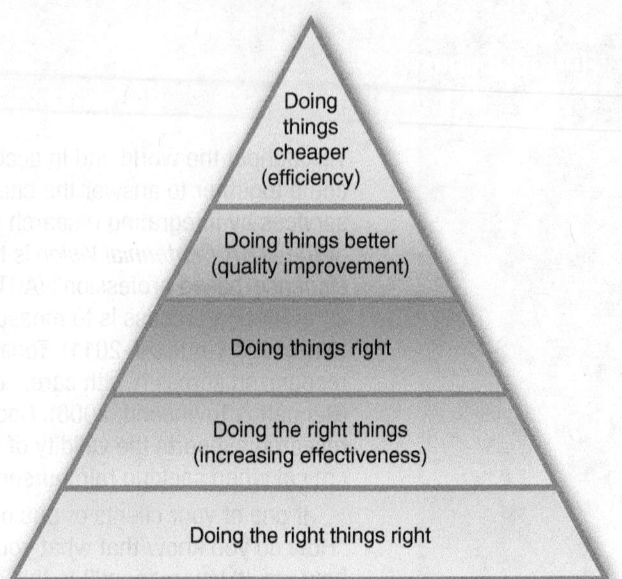
Doing things cheaper (efficiency)
Doing things better (quality improvement)
Doing things right
Doing the right things (increasing effectiveness)
Doing the right things right

Figure 5.1 The evolution of evidence-based practice.

Application to Occupational Therapy

While multiple definitions of **evidence-based practice** have guided the process within occupational therapy, the bottom line is that the purpose of any evidence-based practice is to improve clinical efficacy and provide optimal health care (Bannigan, 1997). Evidence-based practice melds clinical expertise with the best evidence available through systematic research and client values and preferences to "do the right things right" (Fig. 5.1) (Gray, 1998, p. 17, 20). It is critically important to understand that while clinical evidence can inform, it never replaces individual clinical expertise. Clinical expertise always guides whether the external evidence is applicable to the client and, if it is, how it must be woven into a clinical intervention (Sackett et al., 1996). Lacking clinical expertise, evidence has limited capacity to influence practice. Our task as OT practitioners is to reflect and take the necessary action steps to assure that clinical practice links individual clinical knowledge and skills with up-to-date evidence. This tasks OT practitioners to remain current to provide the best-quality treatment (Holm, 2000).

Implementing an evidence-based practice begins with formulating clinical questions about a client or group of clients being treated and the context or environment in which the intervention takes place. Evidence-based practice entails using good-quality research findings to find answers to these questions and inform clinical practice (Bannigan, 1997). Alnervik and Linddahl (2011) stated,

> As occupational therapists we are encouraged to reflect, discuss and have a critical approach to what we are doing. This can be the first step towards basing our work on evidence. It is by thinking through and articulating the clinical reasoning which you, often unconsciously, use on a daily basis that you can strengthen your own practice. (p. 30)

While this is a time-consuming process, the end result of ultimately implementing EBP is a win-win for clients, payers, and practitioners. Law (2002) indicated that "if done right, evidence-based practice is not a burden but a very powerful tool that helps practitioners provide a higher level of care to their clients and families" (p. 4) (Fig. 5.2).

Evidence-based practice can be distilled down to meaning that interventions are based on the strongest scientific information (Alnervik & Linddahl, 2011) so that clients can be assured of the best intervention possible and practitioners can document that interventions are effective. Occupational therapy practitioners need to employ evidence-based practice in order to do what is best (Gray, 1998, p. 20) for each client and to be methodical and be prudent in decision making (Alnervik & Linddahl, 2011). A very important component of evidence-based practice that supports making the right choices (Gray, 1998) is client-centered care. It actively involves the client in the intervention process, deliberately factoring in their wishes and expectations. As will

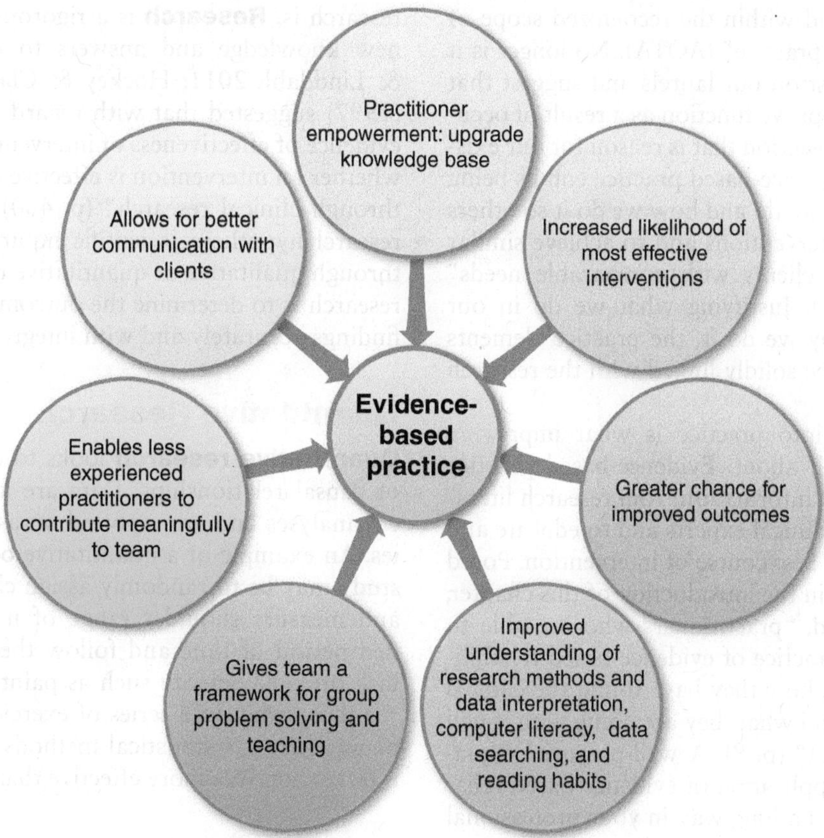
Practitioner empowerment: upgrade knowledge base
Increased likelihood of most effective interventions
Greater chance for improved outcomes
Improved understanding of research methods and data interpretation, computer literacy, data searching, and reading habits
Gives team a framework for group problem solving and teaching
Enables less experienced practitioners to contribute meaningfully to team
Allows for better communication with clients
Evidence-based practice

Figure 5.2 Positive outcomes associated with an evidence-based practice.

be stressed throughout your education and modeled in the field, client-centered care is a natural extension of the scope of occupational therapy intervention processes.

Evidence-based practice is actually a paradigm shift in that instead of implementing a same as always has been done approach, treatment is guided by up-to-date research, which allows practitioners to justify what they are doing and why it is expected to be an effective intervention (Alnervik & Linddahl, 2011, p. 9). Evidence-based practice embraces clinical skill and expertise because often it is the knowledgeable practitioners who are best positioned to implement and mentor others to implement evidence-based practice. Evidence-based practice's take-home central message is one of flexibility and open-mindedness to be able to blend the old ways with the fruits of research and new knowledge (From the Field 5.1).

FROM THE FIELD 5.1

From the Field: Expertise

Generally speaking, it takes about 10 years to become an expert in most any endeavor, including professional practice.

As a profession, we shifted away from occupation as our treatment focus. But we are returning to our core, occupation-based practice. Why? Likely, it is because evidence-based research supports the benefits associated with engagement in meaningful task-oriented occupation. For instance, Lin et al. (1997) undertook a meta-analytic study of 17 articles, including four articles on studies of patients with neurological impairments. Results of the findings of the studies designed to improve the motor performance of patients with neurological impairments showed that results were significantly better when the patients' exercises were embedded into everyday tasks than when the patients only performed rote exercises. The power of the evidence supported the efficacy of occupational therapy intervention. That is, using everyday activity in a therapeutic capacity is indeed, strong. Summarily, Taylor (1997) suggested, "the evidence-based approach does appear to be a perfect way to blend theory and practice and to demonstrate the benefits and effectiveness of occupational therapy" (p. 472). Are you ready to be part of the evidence movement?

The *Occupational Therapy Code of Ethics and Ethics Standards* (AOTA, 2015) states in clear and unequivocal terms in Principle 1C that practitioners must strive to "Use, to the extent possible, evaluation, planning, intervention techniques, and therapeutic equipment that are evidence-based and within the recognized scope of occupational therapy practice" (AOTA). No longer is it adequate for us to rest on our laurels and suggest that because our clients improve function as a result of occupational therapy intervention that is reason for our existence. Engaging in evidence-based practice entails being able to "explain what we do and how we do it so others can replicate these interventions and to achieve similar outcomes with their clients with comparable needs" (Holm, 2000, p. 576). Justifying what we do in our clinical work and why we do it, the practice elements of evidence needs to be solidly linked with the research element of evidence.

Putting evidence into practice is what improving health outcomes is all about. Evidence-based practice entails distilling down information from research literature, colleagues, and clinical experts and to educate and provide clients on the best course of intervention. Posed as a challenge to you in the introduction of this chapter, Law (2002) suggested, "practitioners who are able to adeptly explain the practice of evidence-based rehabilitation to their clients, how they have found the clinical data they are using, and what they are doing with it will be the most successful" (p. 9). A well-prepared explanation and sensible application of evidence-based rehabilitation will take you a long way in your professional career.

Evidence-Based Research

William Dunton, another occupational therapy founder, wrote

> "We are unable to present the results of research because the psychologists have not given us formulae for judging the emotional effect of pounding a copper disc into a nut dish or other occupations ... Nor have the physiological chemists given us a test whereby if we lay a bit of paper on a patient's tongue we may judge that by its turning a pale pink he is enjoying his weaving to a mild degree, whereas his neighbor shows a crimson when tested because he is having a wonderful time putting a jig saw puzzle together. In other words, we lack a quick and snappy means of measuring the emotions" (Dunton, 1934, pp. 325–326, in Schwartz, 2009). Or, in simple terms, without evidence we simply do not have the answers. How do researchers establish evidence? How can we as professional consumers know what the best evidence is so our clients can be the major beneficiaries of this research? Read on!

This section of the chapter focuses on **evidence-based research**, an inquiry process that relies on proof and facts rather than anecdotal and subjective information. Before going any further, it is helpful to establish a common ground understanding of what research is. **Research** is a rigorous process of seeking new knowledge and answers to questions (Alnervik & Linddahl, 2011; Hockey & Clair, 2011). Bannigan (1997) suggested that with regard to health care, "the evidence of effectiveness of interventions, or truth about whether an intervention is effective or not, is discovered through clinical research" (p. 480). Depending on the research hypotheses, scientific inquiry can be approached through qualitative or quantitative research. The task of research is to determine the outcomes and to report the findings accurately and with integrity.

Quantitative Research

Quantitative research looks to determine causation or causal relationships. Data are analyzed via statistical analyses and are reported on as experimental studies. An example of a quantitative occupational therapy study may be to randomly assign clients to two groups and measure shoulder range of motion over a specified period of time and follow the group who does a task-oriented activity such as painting on an easel versus those who do a series of exercises. The data would be analyzed via statistical methods to determine if one intervention was more effective than the other.

Qualitative Research

The purpose of a qualitative study is to gain a deeper understanding of a problem and to understand relationships rather than looking for causation. Using the previous conditions, a qualitative study may look at (via an interview) a client's perception of a intervention protocol such as painting at an easel to increase movement. **Qualitative research** often supplements quantitative studies and give rise to additional hypotheses, yet qualitative methods are also valued as stand-alone research. Another example of qualitative research would be a survey looking at level of client satisfaction with occupational therapy services at a rehabilitation hospital or a case study about a client who responded well to a particular intervention or who presented with an unusual situation.

Choosing the Best Sources of Evidence

The evidence arm of practice is based on clinical research evidence, whether it is derived from qualitative or quantitative studies (Sackett et al., 2000).

Bennett and Bennett (2000) suggested that "evidence for informing clinical decisions may come from various sources including clinical experience, education, textbooks, [conferences, evidence-based reports, summaries, and guidelines] discussion amongst colleagues and from clients, but evidence from well-performed research may be less prone to bias or to the tendency to believe what we want to believe" (p. 175; Alnervik & Linddahl, 2011; Bennett & Townsend, 2006). In other words, while there is an abundance of sources that help OT practitioners make intervention choices, the best choices tend to come from well-done evidence-based research studies.

It has been proposed that the "best evidence comes from studies with the strongest and most appropriate methodologies for the specific clinical question under consideration" (Bennett & Bennett, 2000, p. 176). These types of studies are the "(a) least vulnerable to bias, (b) more generalizable, and (c) more likely to yield patient outcomes that can confidently be attributed to the intervention being studied" and "...are also the studies that we must strive to plan, implement, and publish" (Holm, 2000, p. 576). Studies are most often reported on in peer-reviewed journals. A peer-reviewed journal relies on a panel of expert reviewers to weigh in on whether a study should be published in that particular journal. The hierarchy of evidence-based research ranks from one to six, with one being the most rigorous studies that are considered to produce the best evidence outcomes and six being those that produce limited evidence outcomes (Fig. 5.3). This discussion will focus on the top sources for evidence-based research: systematic reviews, meta-analysis, and randomized controlled trials.

Systematic Reviews

Systematic reviews are a consolidation and summary of the findings of many research studies that pertain to particular topics (Bannigan, 1997; Bennett & Bennett, 2000). Because individual studies may not provide enough information or are too limited in their scope, systematic reviews cull together findings from multiple studies looking at the same topic in order to improve the accuracy of findings. The intention of a systematic review is to offer an unbiased and well-argued overview of the best evidence to better inform health care practice (Bennett & Bennett, 2000).

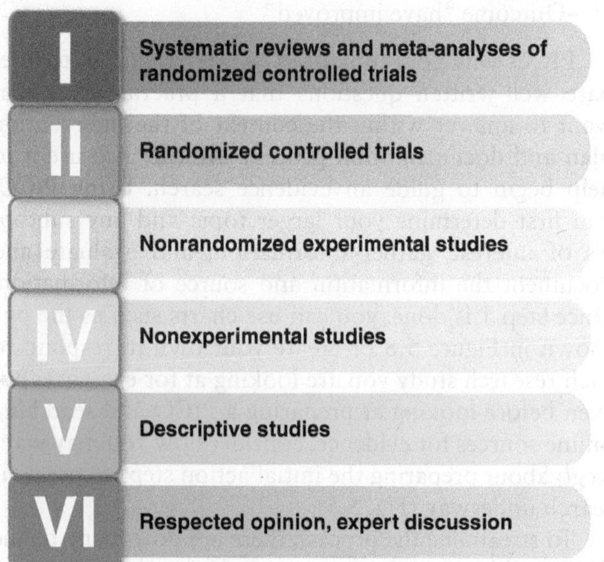

I
Systematic reviews and meta-analyses of randomized controlled trials
II
Randomized controlled trials
III
Nonrandomized experimental studies
IV
Nonexperimental studies
V
Descriptive studies
VI
Respected opinion, expert discussion

Figure 5.3 Levels of evidence as proposed by Fletcher and Sackett (1979).

Here is a good example of the value of a systematic review. In an examination of over 30 years of research on stroke rehabilitation, there was significant evidence indicating that exercise therapies did not improve upper extremity function (Teasell, 2011). Further, a systematic review of 151 studies, 123 of which were randomized controlled studies, showed greater evidence in support of a functional task approach versus impairment-focused exercise programs for stroke rehabilitation (Kwakkel et al., 2004).

Systematic reviews also point out where there are gaps in knowledge (Bannigan, 1997, p. 483) and are prepared as follows:

- Step 1. State objectives of the review and outline inclusion criteria.
- Step 2. Search for studies that seem to meet the inclusion criteria.
- Step 3. Tabulate characteristics of each study identified and assess its methodological quality.
- Step 4. Apply inclusion criteria and justify any exclusions.
- Step 5. Assemble the most complete data set feasible, with involvement of investigators, if possible.
- Step 6. Analyze results of included studies: using statistical synthesis of data (meta-analysis), if appropriate and possible.
- Step 7. Perform **sensitivity analyses** if appropriate and possible to determine if assumptions have impacted the outcomes of the systematic review.
- Step 8. Prepare a structured report of the review, stating aims, describing materials and methods, and reporting results (Watt et al., 1996; Bannigan 1997).

Critically appraised topics (CATs), which summarize evidence on specific topics, and critically appraised papers (CAPs), stand-alone summaries of single papers (Bennett & Townsend, 2006) while not as rigorous as systematic reviews, are still of significant value to researchers and practitioners. Additional resources for information about systematic reviews and CATs and CAPs include http://www.thecochranelibrary.com/view/0/AboutCochraneSystematicReviews.html and http://www.otcats.com/intro.html. The AOTA Evidence Exchange can be accessed at http://www.aota.org/en/Practice/Researchers/Evidence-Exchange.aspx.

Meta-Analysis

A meta-analysis is a statistical method that combines the results of multiple studies of similar topics. A meta-analysis should be the step that follows a systematic review.

An example of a meta-analysis is an analysis of findings of multiple studies examining the effectiveness of using a specific intervention protocol for veteran's with PTSD.

Randomized Controlled Clinical Trials

Systematic reviews, CATs and CAPs, and **meta-analyses** usually contain findings of **randomized controlled clinical trials**, a quantitative, comparative research method that involves randomly assigning participants to one or more groups, one of which is a control and the others are experimental. Using statistical analyses, researchers measure and compare the outcomes or results of the different groups. An example of a randomized control study looking at the quality of sleep for those who drink a cup of warm milk before bed (experimental) and those who do not (control).

Systematic reviews of multiple randomized controlled trials and stand-alone randomized clinical trials are most likely to "inform us and so much less likely to mislead us…[they have] become the 'gold standard' for judging whether a treatment does more good than harm" (Sackett et al., 1996, p. 2). While the gold standard of research is often equated with randomized controlled trials, they are not always appropriate for answering all types of clinical research questions.

Evidence-Based Research Implementation Process

The challenge for any OT practitioner is determining which study design best meets your evidence-based practice questions (Taylor, 2007), that is, what information will give you the best answers to your question(s). The evidence-based research implementation process (searching for related information and practice implementation) involves four steps (Fig. 5.4). Each step will be discussed in greater detail throughout this chapter.

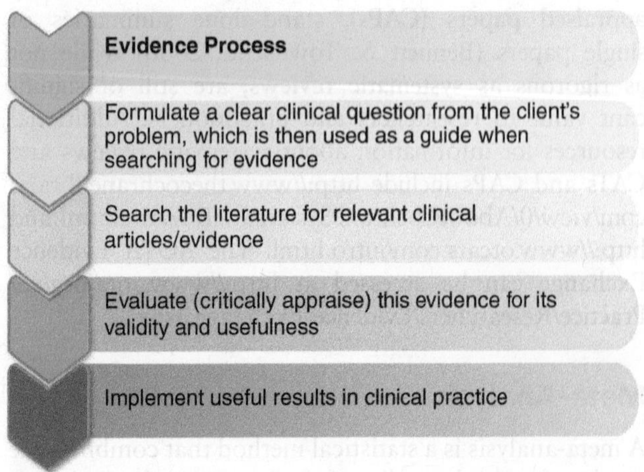

Evidence Process
Formulate a clear clinical question from the client's problem, which is then used as a guide when searching for evidence
Search the literature for relevant clinical articles/evidence
Evaluate (critically appraise) this evidence for its validity and usefulness
Implement useful results in clinical practice

Figure 5.4 Rosenberg and Donald's (1995) evidence process.

Evidence can be used to inform intervention for a single client. It can be used to change and develop departmental policies and practices. Evidence can also be used to develop clinical guidelines (Taylor, 1997, p. 472). While getting there may incur bumps along the way, the results overwhelmingly suggest it is well worth the effort. Moving to an evidence-based practice involves allotting time and infrastructure (computers and Internet access) for literature review and discussion, bringing together the collective skills of the practitioners, and a desire and commitment to work based on evidence rather than experience alone. While evidence-based practice takes time, it is not about overloading and simply building a reference base, but rather to cull out what research is relevant to the practitioner, his/her colleagues, and clients.

Search for Evidence Related to a Research Question

The optimal place to search for research evidence to answer questions is in peer-reviewed journals because they are the first line for reporting findings with enough detail so readers can come to informed conclusions about the validity and relevance of the research (Bennett & Bennett, 2000). Finding the information you need to respond to any evidence question involves doing a literature search. Today, it is easy to do so online, starting first with preparing a question and determining which key terms to use to locate the evidence. One way to organize and prepare a research question is via a **PICO** format, which stands for

P—Patient population or disease of interest
I—Intervention
C—Comparison or "compared to"
O—Outcome "have improved"

PICO was conceptualized as an organizer to prepare well-written questions that a practitioner might want to answer within the context of the intervention plan and documentation process. We can also use it to help begin to guide an evidence search. Using PICO, you first determine your larger topic and any subtopics of interest, gather information, and evaluate and document the information and source of information. Once step 1 is done, you can use charts such as the one shown in Figure 5.8 or create your own to respond to each research study you are looking at for evidence. But even before looking at preparing a PICO and searching online sources for evidence, consider how you may want to go about preparing the initial action steps to get your search underway (Fig. 5.5).

To streamline the process, there are now many online databases that contain peer-reviewed journal articles, some of which are devoted entirely to evidence and are even OT specific and, often, available at no cost (Table 5.1).

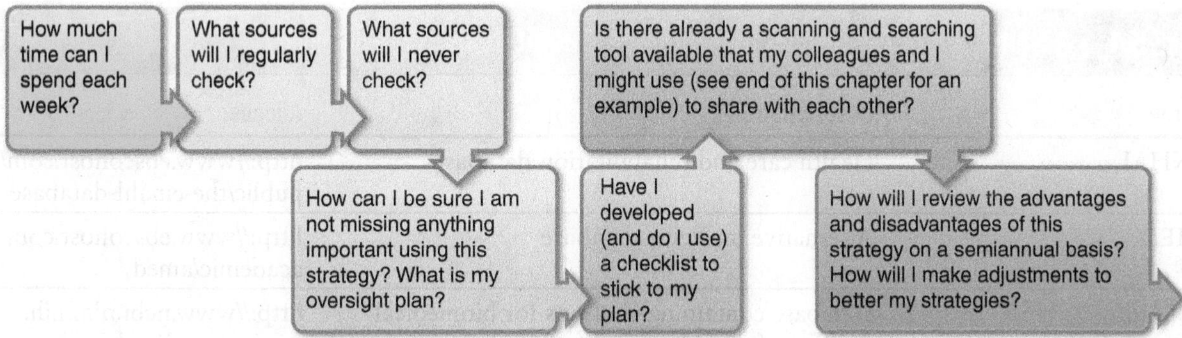

Figure 5.5 Strategies for scanning and searching the literature: what do I need to think about? (Adapted from Gray JM. *Evidence-Based Health care: How to Make Healthy Policy and Management Decisions*. London, UK: Churchill Livingstone; 1997.)

TABLE 5.1 A Sampling of Resources for Evidence-Based Research

Source	Description	Access
OTseeker	Free online database of systematic reviews and critically reviewed randomized controlled trials of OT-related research studies	http://www.otseeker.com
OTcats	Contains CATs and CAPs that focus on occupational therapy	http://www.OTcats.com
AOTA	List of systematic reviews, OT Practice Pulse, *OT Practice*, online evidence-based practice resource directory	http://www.aota.org
The Australian Occupational Therapy Journal	Devotes space for critically reviewed articles	http://www.otaus.com.au/about/australian-occupational-therapy-journal
OTevidence	Online portal provides access to EBP strategies, knowledge, and other resources.	http://www.otevidence.info/
The Cochrane Database of Systematic Reviews	Systematic reviews of primary research in human health care and health policy	http://www.cochrane.org/cochrane-reviews
Centre for Evidence-Based Medicine	Develop, teach, and promote evidence-based health care and provide support and resources to doctors and health care professionals to help maintain the highest standards of medicine.	http://cebm.jr2.ox.ac.uk/
Centre for Clinical Effectiveness	Evidence-based practice support unit that encourages and supports health professionals, managers, and policy makers to use the best available evidence to improve health care	http://www.Med.moash.edu.au/publichealth/cce/
Critical Appraisal Skills Programme (CASP)	Enables individuals to develop the skills to find and make sense of research evidence, helping them to put knowledge into practice	http://www.phru.org/casp/
McMaster Occupational Therapy Evidence-Based Practice Group	Portal for evidence-based occupational therapy research	http://www.fhs.mcmaster.ca/rehab/ebp/
University of Queensland Evidence-Based Occupational Therapy Group	Resource center for evidence-based research in occupational therapy	http://www.shrs.uq.edu.au/OT

(*continues on page 60*)

TABLE 5.1 A Sampling of Resources for Evidence-Based Research (continued)

Source	Description	Access
CINHAL	Health care and rehabilitation database	http://www.ebscohost.com/public/the-cinahl-database
AMED	Alternative medicine database	http://www.ebscohost.com/academic/amed
PubMed	Database containing citations for biomedical literature from Medline, life science journals, and online books	http://www.ncbi.nlm.nih.gov/pubmed/
Medline	Medical database containing journal citations and abstracts for biomedical literature from around the world	http://www.nlm.nih.gov/bsd/pmresources.html
PsycINFO	PsycINFO database references studies in psychology and related mental health fields	http://www.apa.org/pubs/databases/psycinfo/index.aspx
ERIC	Education literature database	http://www.eric.ed.gov/

Evaluation of Evidence

Research findings should never be taken at face value, even when published in peer-reviewed journals because despite all attempts to maintain impartiality, inherently, there are limitations of reporting on human subject research, including issues of reliability and validity (Bannigan, 1997) associated with individual studies. **Reliability** refers to the extent to which a research tool yields the same outcomes each time it is used, and **validity** is the degree to which an instrument measures what it is intended to measure. That is why systematic reviews are so important because they consolidate findings of multiple similar studies to determine their research efficacy.

Implementation in Practice

A hugely important part of the evidence-based practice process entails determining whether an intervention does more good than harm. Gray (1997) indicated that "randomized controlled trials designed to assess effectiveness often need to be complemented by cohort studies [time specific observational studies of a set group of people engaged in a specific intervention] to assess safety" so that a practitioner can determine the "balance between good and harm confirmed by a therapy" (p. 31). Evidence-based research informs questions, such as "Why does my patient need both a physical therapy exercise program and occupational therapy? What evidence do you have that cooking tasks, adapted checkers games, and those other things you do make any difference in upper-extremity motor performance?" (Holm, 2000, p. 576). In suggesting how evidence-based practice aligns with clinical expertise and evidence-based research, Holm (2000) suggested, "I would like to emphasize that if we are to practice evidence-based occupational therapy, evidence can only be used to inform clinical expertise, not replace it, and clinical expertise must be used in conjunction with the best available evidence, not substituted for it" (p. 581). To that end, OT practitioners (or any professional) must be proactive "critical consumers" (Bannigan, 1997, p. 480) in determining whether an intervention does more harm than good. Figure 5.6 illustrates the process of moving evidence from research into practice (From the Field 5.2).

Implementing evidence-based practice is important in health care provision. Changes, such as shorter hospital stays, rising costs and limited resources, fewer staff,

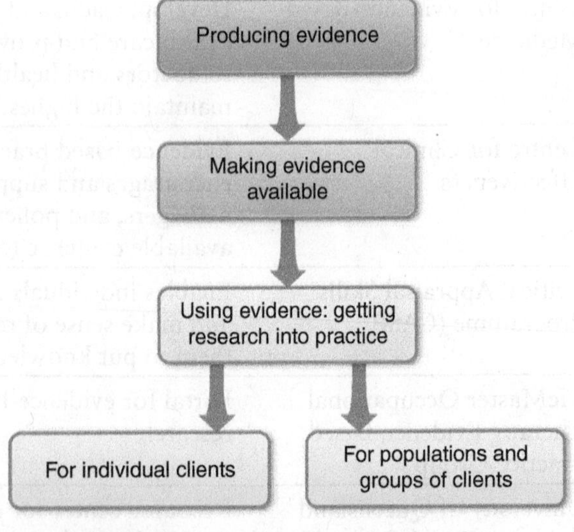

Figure 5.6 Producing evidence adapted from Gray JM. *Evidence-Based Health care: How to Make Healthy Policy and Management Decisions*. London, UK: Churchill Livingstone; 1997.

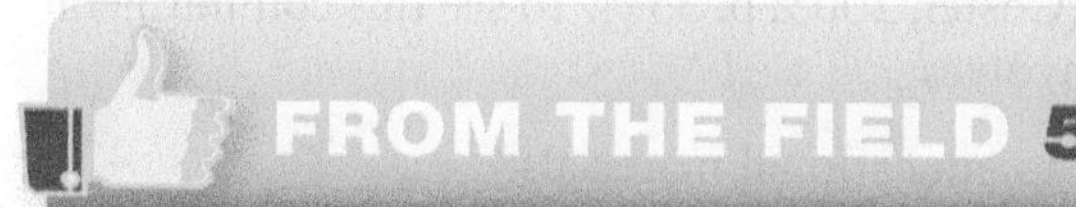

FROM THE FIELD 5.2

From the Field: Method/ology

Did you know that the terms methodology and methods are often (incorrectly) interchanged? Methodology is an idea or theory of how research on a particular topic is expected to proceed. Methods are the ways in which information is gathered and data is analyzed (Hammell, 2002).

client expectations, and managed care, have led to greater clinical accountability and justification of services and, accordingly, to implement an evidence-based practice (Bennett & Bennett, 2000; Lin et al., 2010, p. 164). While many health care professionals have identified the steps for evidence-based practice, a critical part of the process is actual implementation at the point of care. Failing to do so may negatively impact reimbursement and even the scope of practice in many settings (Lin et al., 2010). The information age has made the world a smaller place. In an effort to "spread the wealth," and serve all clients effectively and equitably, moving from a local focus to a globalized, one world approach to the provision of evidence-based occupational therapy could not be more important to our profession (Iloh et al., 2006).

Challenges to Use of Evidence-Based Practice

Despite the availability and access to evidence, there are a couple of challenges to discuss. One is that there is so much evidence that it is hard to stay current, and the other is that quantity does not necessarily equal quality with regard to evidence (Holm, 2000). There are tools to help you assess well-designed and reported research, such as Table 5.2.

Despite all good intentions, there are also a number of roadblocks to implementing evidence-based practice at individual practice and system-wide levels (Alnervik & Linddahl, 2011). While a majority of health care professionals have developed guidelines for evidence-based practice, implementation remains the overarching challenge. In fact, there is "a 17-year lag… between evidence and practice" (Lin et al., 2010, p. 164). Some of these obstacles include the following:

- Limited clinical and infrastructure resources
- Not enough time to train practitioners to locate and assess the evidence research
- Limited access to research results and relevant articles

TABLE 5.2 Evaluation Protocol—Individual Studies

Question	Yes	No	Not evident
Did the trial address a clearly focused issue?			
Was the research question(s) clearly stated?			
Were the subjects randomly assigned to control or experimental groups?			
Were all subjects accounted for at the end of the study?			
Was the literature review thorough with multiple viewpoints discussed?			
Was the study completed as a blind process?			
Was the subject group homogeneous as possible at onset of study?			
Excepting the experimental intervention, were the groups treated equally?			
How were ethical issues considered?			
Was there a robust discussion of data collection methods?			
Was the methodology appropriate and clearly stated?			
What are the key results?			
What is the statistical significance of the results?			
Can the results be generalized to my client group?			
Were all the important outcomes considered?			
Do the benefits of the invention outweigh the cost or harm?			

Adapted from Taylor MC. *Evidence-Based Practice for Occupational Therapists*. Oxford, UK: Blackwell Science; 2000.

- Relevant research is of poor quality.
- Relevant research on the patient population or problem has not been carried out (Law & Baum, 1998; Lin et al., 2010).

As with any challenge, there are also strategies available to overcome the obstacles. Cusick and McCluskey (2000) proposed several:

- Develop an evidence-based approach: keep abreast of research and collaborate in developing occupational therapy practice.
- Positively change client expectations and demands: actively involve clients in their rehabilitation and provide them with accurate information about treatment options.
- Start with local resources and requirements at the institutional level: it takes a village to make evidence-based practice a reality within a department as well as the entire institution.
- Find out what your local or state professional organizations, or others, can contribute.
- Scrutinize and make use of the national clinical guidelines available to you and your colleagues.

Despite all good intentions, challenges impeding globalization of evidence-based occupational therapy include the following: (1) a limited but growing base of research, researchers, and centers from which to disseminate what we do know about EBOT; (2) throughout the world, occupational therapy is at different stages of development, and there is not yet a level playing field from which to have a common voice; (3) English is the language of science and occupational therapy as is much of the research, which may not be translated to other languages, and, as well, evidence published in other languages is not always available in English. There needs to be a common voice from which to disseminate research; and (4) limited resources, both in terms of personnel and funding for evidence-based research (Iloh et al., 2006, p. 39). While by no means are these insurmountable challenges, they are realities that our global occupational therapy community must address in a timely manner. Be it on a local, national, or a global level, there is work to be done.

Thinking into the future, what additional strategies can you suggest for overcoming potential obstacles and roadblocks to implementing evidence-based practice at your future place of employment? Think about starting to develop strategies now to stay abreast of current evidence and in turn to integrate this knowledge into your future clinical practice.

The Future of Evidenced-Based Practice

Committing to "use the best available evidence in clinical decision making is a fundamental element of ethical practice" (Coster, 2005, p. 357). To see this commitment through involves

1. Access to educational materials.
2. Creation of an international EBP education center and a director to oversee it.
3. Arrangements to share information and access to publications on a global scale.
4. Implementation of creative strategies to close the gap between those programs and institutions with adequate evidence-based practice and evidence-based research resources and those in the developing world without.

In other words, availability of these resources must be made accessible to all OTAs (Coster, 2005). As you prepare for a career as an OTA and to meet the needs of an ever-changing and complex health care and educational system and be part of the global community, it is incumbent upon you to become well versed in evidence-based practice. Below is a self-assessment that will be useful to you going forward in your studies and ultimately into practice (Fig. 5.7).

Question 1:
Do I examine what I do by asking clinical questions?

Identify your client population and the interventions you most commonly use. Based on evidence, are you doing the right things right?

Question 2:
Do I take time to track down the best evidence to guide what I do?

Put aside time to find the answers, review the research.

Question 3:
Do I appraise the evidence or take it at face value?

While this can be difficult and time consuming, study the statistics. Do not take what an author says at face value. Be a good research consumer.

Question 4:
Do I use the evidence to do the "Right Things Right?"

Use the evidence you have gathered to develop your own clinical guideline that asks,

- Who is the right person to implement the intervention?
- What is the right thing to do?
- What is the right way to implement the intervention?
- What is the right place to implement the intervention?
- What is the right time to provide the intervention?
- What is the right result?

Figure 5.7 Evidence-based practice—a self-assessment. (Adapted from Holm MB. Our mandate for the new millennium: evidence-based practice, 2000 Eleanor Clarke Slagle lecture. *Am J Occup Ther* 2000;54:575–585.)

Summary

The forward momentum of evidence-based practice is now supported through the availability of many online resources for accessing evidence for research, professional conferences and training on occupational evidence-based practice, and, increasingly, opportunities for inter- and intradisciplinary collaboration on research projects (Lin et al., 2010) throughout the world. At its best, occupational therapy is evidence based and client-centered. Evidence indicates that a client-centered approach to occupational therapy practice leads to greater satisfaction with services and improved outcomes for clients and their families (Law & Baum, 1998). Looking at evidence from a profession-specific perspective, Iloh et al. (2006) suggested, "Evidence-based occupational therapy (EBOT) has become part of our professional psyche" (p. 38). As an emerging OTA, the importance of embracing the evidence-based movement cannot be underestimated.

Review Questions

1. The gold standard of research is considered to be:
   a. Case studies
   b. Quantitative analyses
   c. Qualitative analyses
   d. Randomized controlled trials

2. A critically appraised topic is:
   a. An appraisal of one research study
   b. An appraisal of multiple studies focused on the same topic
   c. A rigorous intervention focused on a single issue in occupational therapy
   d. A research method that attempts to find relationships

3. Causation is associated with which type of research?
   a. Quantitative
   b. Qualitative
   c. Systems
   d. Case studies

4. Which of the following is *not* an outcome associated with evidence-based practice?
   a. Improved communication with clients
   b. Practitioner empowerment
   c. Opportunity to learn and expand knowledge base
   d. Increased caseload

5. Which of the following is true?
   a. Clinical expertise trumps evidence
   b. Informal discussions with colleagues about a specific treatment intervention is an example of strong evidence
   c. Clinical expertise is needed to support evidence-based practice
   d. Clinical expertise is not needed to support evidence-based practice

6. Examples of evidence do *not* include:
   a. Systematic reviews
   b. Evidence-based clinical guidelines
   c. Critically appraised papers
   d. Critically appraised interventions

7. A research tool that consolidates and summarizes many research findings on particular topics and provides evidence on these topics best describes a(n):
   a. Meta-analysis
   b. Systematic review
   c. Survey
   d. Critically appraised topic

8. Statistical analyses are associated with:
   a. Methods
   b. Methodology
   c. Theory
   d. Conjecture

9. Which of the following evidence tools is considered to be the most rigorous?
   a. Critically appraised topics
   b. Systematic review
   c. Critically appraised papers
   d. Self-reports

10. Which of the following is NOT considered to be a roadblock to implementing an evidence-based practice with a client or group of similar clients?
    a. Time
    b. Limited access to online resources
    c. Limited available research on a particular question
    d. Client resistance

11. Which of the following does not apply as to why the evidence movement began?
    a. Burgeoning economy
    b. Rising cost of health care
    c. Staff shortages
    d. Greater accountability to clients

12. An evidence-based practice is:
    a. Client-centered
    b. Based on science
    c. Doing things the way it was always done
    d. A and B

Practice Activities

Design a PICO worksheet you can use to address the following scenarios. Be sure to tailor it to fit your unique learning style. This might include using a large sans serif font, different colored fonts for different sections of the PICO, etc.

Prepare one research question pertaining to occupational therapy that interests you, such as pediatric splinting, workplace ergonomics, or feeding techniques for adults with dysphagia (swallowing difficulties). Identify two to three key terms you will use to help you find examples of evidence. Using an evidence database (Table 5.1) of your choice, do an initial search for evidence studies. Share with your class, your question, key terms, number of studies you located, and their classification according to the levels of evidence chart (Fig. 5.1).

As a class, write one occupational therapy research question that you will all find evidence about. Individually, select one evidence database from Table 5.1 that you would like to use to research this question. Using the *Evaluation Protocol for Assessing Research Studies* (Table 5.2) or *Organizer for Database Searching* (Fig. 5.8), respond to as many of the questions as possible. Use your PICO worksheet to organize your findings in preparation for sharing them with the class.

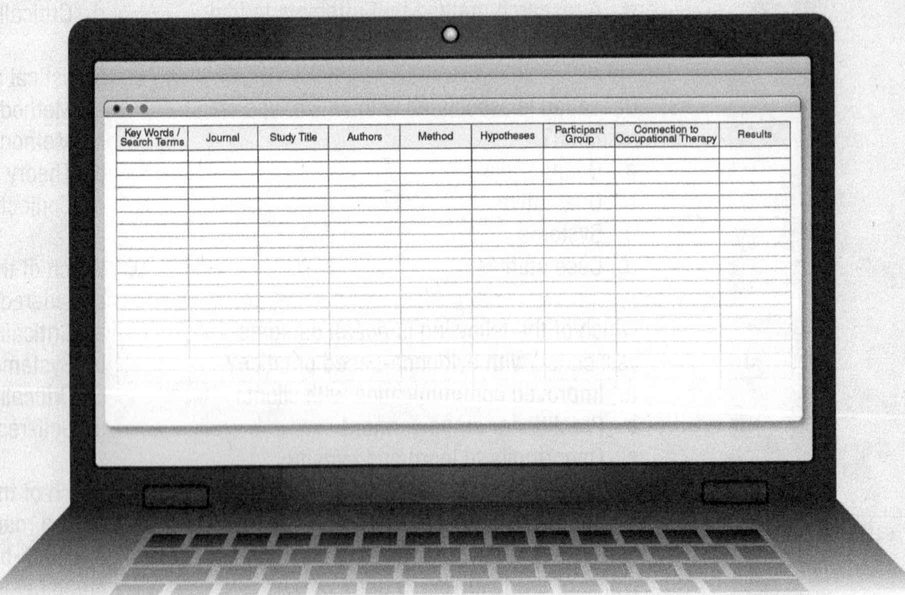

Key Words / Search Terms	Journal	Study Title	Authors	Method	Hypotheses	Participant Group	Connection to Occupational Therapy	Results

Figure 5.8 Action organizer for database searching. Create a table and type in the headings as shown on the screen. (Adapted from Alnervik A, Linddahl I. *Value of Occupational Therapy. About Evidence-Based Occupational Therapy*. Swedish Association of Occupational Therapists; 2011.)

References

Alnervik A, Linddahl I. *Value of Occupational Therapy. About Evidence-Based Occupational Therapy*. Swedish Association of Occupational Therapists; 2011.

American Occupational Therapy Association.

Bannigan K. Clinical effectiveness: systematic reviews and evidence-based practice in occupational & therapy. *Br J Occup Ther* 1997;60(11):479–483.

Bennett S, Bennett JW. The process of evidence-based practice in occupational therapy: informing clinical decisions. *Aust Occup Ther J* 2000;47:171–180.

Bennett S, Townsend L. Evidence-based practice in occupational therapy: international initiatives. *WFOT Bull* 2006;53:6–11.

Coster W. International conference on evidence-based practice: a collaborative effort of the American Occupational Therapy Association, the American Occupational Therapy Foundation, and the Agency for Healthcare Research and Quality. *Am J Occup Ther* 2005; 59(3):356–358.

Cusick A, McCluskey A. Becoming an evidence-based practitioner through professional development. *Aust Occup Ther J* 2000;47:159–170.

Dunn W, Foreman J. Development of evidence-based knowledge. In: Law M, ed. *Evidence-Based Rehabilitation—A Guide to Practice*. Thorofore, NJ: SLACK, Inc.; 2002:13–30.

Fletcher S, Sackett D. The periodic health examination: Canadian task force on the periodic health examination. *Can Med Assoc J* 1979;121:1193–1254.

Friedland J, Silva J. Evolving identities: Thomas Bessell Kidner and occupational therapy in the United States, *Am J Occup Ther* 2008, May/June;62(3):349–360.

Gray JM. *Evidence-Based Health care: How to Make Healthy Policy and Management Decisions*. London, UK: Churchill Livingstone;1997.

Gray JM. Putting occupation into practice: occupation as ends, occupation as means. *Am J Occup Ther* 1998, May;52(5):354–364.

Hammell KW. Informing client-centered practice through qualitative inquiry: evaluating the quality of qualitative research. *Br J Occup Ther* 2002;4(65):175–182.

Hockey C, Clair VW-St. Occupational science: adding value to occupational therapy. *N Zeal J Occup Ther* 2011;58(1):29–38.

Holm MB. Our mandate for the new millennium: evidence-based practice, 2000 Eleanor Clarke Slagle lecture. *Am J Occup Ther* 2000;54:575–585.

Iloh I, Taylor MC, Bolanos C. Evidence-based occupational therapy: it's time to take a global approach. *Br J Occup Ther* 2006;69(1):38–41.

Kwakkel G, van Peppen Rx, Wagenaar RC, et al. Effects of augmented exercise therapy time after stroke: a meta-analysis. *Stroke* 2004;35(11):2529–2539.

Law M. Introduction to evidence-based practice. In: Law M, ed. *Evidence-Based Rehabilitation—A Guide to Practice*. Thorofore, NJ: SLACK, Inc.; 2002:3–12.

Law M, Baum C. Evidence-based occupational therapy. *Can J Occup Ther* 1998; 65:131–135.

Lin K, Wu C, Tickle-Degnen L, et al. Enhancing occupational performance through occupationally embedded exercise: a meta-analytic review. *Occup Ther J Res* 1997;17:25–47.

Lin SH, Murphy SL, Robinson JC. Facilitating evidence-based practice: process, strategies and resources. *Am J Occup Ther* 2010;64(1):164–171.

Principles of Universal Design. Center for Universal Design, NCSU; 2011.

Rosenberg W, Donald A. Evidence based medicine: an approach to clinical problem-solving. *Br Med J* 1995;310:1122–1126.

Sackett DL, Rosenberg WMC, Gray JAM, et al. Evidence-based medicine: what it is and what it isn't. *Br Med J* 1996;312:71–72.

Sackett DL Strauss SE, Richardson WS, et al. Evidence-Based medicine: how to practice and teach EBM. 2nd ed. Edinburgh: Churchill Livingstone; 2000.

Schwartz KB. The 2009 Eleanor Clarke Slagle Lecture: reclaiming our heritage: connecting the Founding Vision to the Centennial Vision. *Am J Occup Ther* 2009, November–December;63(6):681–690.

Straus SE, Richardson WS, Glasziou P, et al. *Evidence-Based Medicine*. 3rd ed. London, UK: Churchill Livingstone; 2005.

Taylor MC. What is evidence-based practice? *Br J Occup Ther* 1997;60(11):470–474.

Taylor MC. *Evidence-Based Practice for Occupational Therapists*. Oxford, UK: Blackwell Publishing; 2007.

Teasell R. Holistic care for stroke in the context of the current health care bureaucracy and economic reality. *Top Stroke Rehabil* 2011;18(1):66–69.

Watt I, Droogan J, Wilson P. The NHS Centre for reviews and dissemination: a resource for clinical audit. *Audit Trends* 1996;4:155–157.

Retrieved from http://www.ncsu.edu/project/design-projects/udi/2011/05/09/newprinciplesposters/

UNIT

II

Theory and Guiding Principles

What makes us unique is not that we document functional outcomes but that we use occupation as the method to achieve positive outcomes.

—David L. Nelson

CHAPTER 6

The Occupational Therapy Practice Framework: Domain Process

Amy Wagenfeld, PhD, OTR/L SCEM, CAPs

Key Terms

Domain—A concept that explains the purpose of occupational therapy and the areas in which occupational therapy helps clients.

***Occupational Therapy Practice Framework: Domain and Process* (I, II, III)**—An official AOTA document that articulates "occupational therapy's contribution to promoting the health and participation of people, organizations, and populations through engagement in occupation" (AOTA, 2014, p. S2).

Process—Dynamic methods used to implement occupational therapy services.

Taxonomy—Classification into ordered categories (*dictionary.com Unabridged*, 2015).

Uniform Terminology—Predecessor document to the *Framework* whose purpose was to set forth a uniform reporting system to be used for reimbursement of occupational therapy services.

Learning Objectives

After studying this chapter, the reader should be able to:

- Explain the rationale behind development of the *Occupational Therapy Practice Framework: Domain and Process III.*
- State the importance of the *Occupational Therapy Practice Framework: Domain and Process III* to future clinical practice.
- Interpret the interconnectedness of the two parts of the *Occupational Therapy Practice Framework: Domain and Process III.*

Introduction

The philosophical and practical beliefs of the collective membership of a profession are reflected in its official documents and provide the underpinnings for decision making that impacts the meaning and transformation of the profession (Gutman et al., 2007). An example is the *Occupational Therapy Practice Framework: Domain and Process III*, which is an official document of the American Occupational Therapy Association (AOTA, 2014). It is a document meant to be read by OT practitioners and any others who want to better understand the profession.

In its original form as well as its most current iteration, the *Occupational Therapy Practice Framework III* was originally developed to "articulate occupational therapy's contribution to promoting the health and participation of people, organizations, and populations through engagement in occupation" (AOTA, 2014, p. S2). It remains a document whose purpose is to explain the domain and process of occupational therapy and builds upon the founding values of the profession (AOTA, 2014). From its inception, the *Occupational Therapy Practice Framework* did something very important; it placed focus on occupation and client-centered outcomes, which collectively are the foundation of occupational therapy practice (Gutman et al., 2007).

History of the Occupational Therapy Practice Framework: Domain and Process III

Published in 1979, the *Occupational Therapy Product Output Reporting System and Uniform Terminology System for Reporting Occupational Therapy Services* represents the first document to organize the conceptual concepts of occupational therapy (AOTA, 2014). This document was commonly referred to as ***Uniform Terminology*** or *UT (I, II, II)*. The original purpose of the *Uniform Terminology* was to develop a uniform reporting system to be used for reimbursement of occupational therapy services. There were two revisions of *Uniform Terminology* (1989 and 1994). In addition to the original concepts, the final version of *Uniform Terminology III* also provided common language for use in "clinical practice, policy-making, and education" (Butts & Nelson, 2007, p. 512).

With an expansion of existing and new practice venues, as well as an increased understanding of therapeutic efficacy of occupation on daily life functioning, the profession advanced and transformed (Youngstrom, 2002). It was widely recognized that we had outgrown the *Uniform Terminology III,* as it did not speak to expanding practice venues or to the therapeutic value of everyday occupations (Gutman et al., 2007, p. 119; Youngstrom, 2002). Reflective of contemporary practice, the *Uniform Terminology III* offered a limited scope on the use of occupation, categorization challenges of certain terms, missing terminology, and terminology that was unfamiliar to audiences beyond occupational therapy practitioners (Gutman et al., 2007, p. 119; Youngstrom, 2002). Beginning in 1999, with an understanding that the *Uniform Terminology III* was no longer meeting the needs of the profession, the AOTA Commission on Practice began to review the *Uniform Terminology III* and seek feedback from practitioners, scholars, and leaders to determine next steps. While the consensus was that there still needed to be some sort of document that put forth the constructs associated with occupational therapy's domain, it needed to be something new. Why? Practice in traditional health care settings was changing due to changing reimbursement patterns, and accordingly, practitioners had to change the way they practiced. Occupational therapy practitioners were venturing into new practice areas and seeking support for doing so. The occupation-based practice focus was taking on steam, and there was an identified need to define and articulate the meaning of occupational therapy.

This document had to clearly explain how occupation factored into the occupational therapy process and how the two were interconnected. It needed to link all practice areas together and clearly show how, collectively, all areas of practice were focused on helping people to do what occupational therapy is about: helping clients engage and participate in everyday activities that are of meaning to them (Youngstrom, 2002). A few of the countless examples of these activities are shown in Figure 6.1.

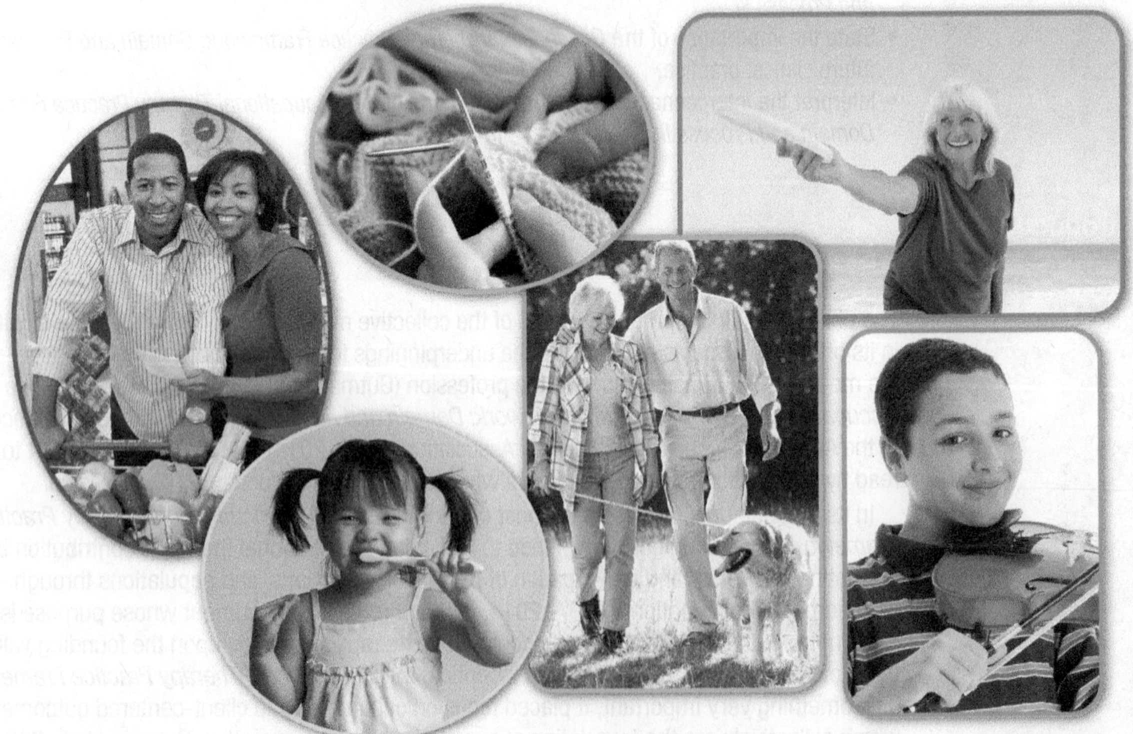

Figure 6.1 Examples of everyday occupations.

In 2002, the AOTA Representative Assembly approved the ***Occupational Therapy Practice Framework: Domain and Process*** as an official document. To make it relevant to the spectrum of health care and all other areas of practice, the *Occupational Therapy Practice Framework* had to include terminology consistent with current knowledge and also be aligned with the WHO *International Classification of Functioning, Disability, and Health (ICF)* (WHO, 2001). See also Chapter 4, *Occupations: The Cornerstone of the Profession* for a discussion about the *ICF*. The *Occupational Therapy Practice Framework* also had to explain the contribution of occupational therapy to health and make occupational therapy practitioners aware of their role within a larger societal and health context in order to stay relevant and clearly focused on client-centered outcomes regardless of whether they are individual, group, organizational, or community contexts (Youngstrom, 2002) (From the Field 6.1).

The purpose of the original *Occupational Therapy Practice Framework* was to "(1) describe the profession's philosophical assumptions, (2) define the profession's domain of concern, (3) offer direction for evaluation and intervention, and (4) help external audiences to better understand the profession's unique contribution to healthcare" (Gutman et al., 2007, p. 119). Then and now, the importance of the *Occupational Therapy Practice Framework* to the profession cannot be underestimated. Each successive edition of the *Occupational Therapy Practice Framework* has become inextricably woven into official AOTA documents, is more visible in occupational therapy education (Accreditation Council for Occupational Therapy Education, 2013; Gutman et al., 2007), and is also used by the National Board for Certification in Occupational Therapy [NBCOT] (Gutman et al., 2007; NBCOT, 2003) to generate examination questions. No matter the edition, the broad implications of the *Occupational Therapy Practice Framework* are applicable to "practice, education, research, and communications with organizations and individual persons outside the profession of occupational therapy" (Nelson, 2006, p. 512). Glomstad described the *Occupational Therapy Practice Framework* as "the 'hub' around which all other AOTA documents should revolve" (Nelson, 2006, p. 512).

FROM THE FIELD 6.1

Who Are Our Clients?

According to the *Occupational Therapy Practice Framework III*, clients are

- Persons, including families, caregivers, teachers, employers, and relevant others
- Groups, such as businesses, industries, or agencies
- Populations within a community, such as refugees, veterans who are homeless, and people with chronic health disabling conditions (AOTA, 2014)

The Occupational Therapy Practice Framework: Domain and Process III Today

The American Occupational Therapy Association is clear in stating that the *Occupational Therapy Practice Framework III* (as well as all other editions) is not a **taxonomy** (a classification system) or a theory or practice model. Rather, it is a foundational document that should be used alongside the evidence and knowledge that inform occupational therapy (AOTA, 2014). Schwartz (2010) described the *Occupational Therapy Practice Framework (II)* as a "guiding instrument for occupational therapy practitioners by helping outline the course of client-centered occupational therapy evaluation and treatment" (p. 22). This remains true with the *Occupational Therapy Practice Framework III* (AOTA, 2014). A client-centered focus posits that "All people need to be able or enabled to engage in the occupations of their need and choice, to grow through what they do, and to experience independence or interdependence, equality, participation, security, health, and well-being" (Wilcock & Townsend, 2008, p. 198).

As the title indicates, the *Occupational Therapy Practice Framework III* is divided into two parts, Domain and Process (AOTA, 2014). **Domain** is our professional scope and established body of knowledge and expertise. **Process** is the means through which we deliver occupational therapy services (AOTA, 2014). The Domain explains the purpose of occupational therapy and the areas in which we help clients (Butts & Nelson, 2007). Think of Domain as the foundation of a building, the scaffolding upon which occupational therapy practitioners develop the activities needed for treatment interventions (Youngstrom, 2002). The other part of the *Occupational Therapy Practice Framework III* is the dynamic occupational and client-centered Process and methods used to implement occupational therapy services (AOTA, 2014). Youngstrom (2002) linked Process to the structure of a building, the walls, roof, etc. as it derives from the Domain and the considerations of activities that are facilitated during Process. Collectively, Domain and Process guide occupational therapy practitioners to focus on the occupational performance that ensues from the interplay between the client, his/her context and environment, and occupations (AOTA, 2014). While Domain and Process are described as two terms, they truly are interconnected.

There are five main categories that comprise and are defined in the Domain portion of the *Occupational*

Therapy Practice Framework III (AOTA, 2014). They are areas of occupation, client factors, performance skills, performance patterns, and context and environment (AOTA, 2014, p. S1). Each of the Domains are further subdivided into subcategories and beyond. The particular value of categorizing areas of occupation, performance patterns, contexts, and activity demands is enhanced understanding of the intervention and evaluation Process by OT practitioners (Gutman et al., 2007). The five Domains of practice are carefully balanced so that one does not take precedence over another and all are equally important to occupational therapy. Three main categories comprise the Process portion of the *Occupational Therapy Practice Framework III* and are evaluation, intervention, and outcomes (AOTA, 2014). Like the Domain, each of these categories is subdivided into other applicable categories and includes explanations of each.

Summary

The *Occupational Therapy Practice Framework III* (AOTA, 2014) is the foundational guide for occupational therapy intervention because it provides the rationale for our theory and practice frames of reference and models. You may want to think of the *Occupational Therapy Practice Framework III* (AOTA, 2014) as the common ground from which OT practitioners develop and implement treatment, develop educational paradigms, and administrate. Because it is foundational, the *Occupational Therapy Practice Framework III* (AOTA, 2014) also provides the base from which to provide an individualized, holistic, and client-centered service delivery approach that our profession embraces (Dixon et al., 2011). The content of the *Occupational Therapy Practice Framework III* (AOTA, 2014) is very important for OT practitioners to understand and use, be it in educational, practice, or research endeavors.

Review Questions

1. The original AOTA document that attempted to organize the conceptual concepts of occupational therapy was the:
   a. *Occupational Therapy Practice Framework*
   b. *Core Values*
   c. *Standards of Ethical Practice*
   d. *Uniform Terminology I*

2. The original purpose of the *Uniform Terminology* was to:
   a. Document the history of the profession
   b. Develop a uniform reporting system to be used for reimbursement of occupational therapy services
   c. Organize the fee structure for occupational therapy services at every health care facility
   d. Document where occupational services could be offered

3. Which one of the below statements is *not* true with regard to the reasons why the *Uniform Terminology* was replaced by the *Occupational Therapy Practice Framework*?
   a. It no longer spoke to expanding practice venues or the therapeutic value of everyday occupations.
   b. It only provided a limited scope on the use of occupation.
   c. Was too similar to physical therapy's core documentation and was repetitive
   d. Contained terminology that was unfamiliar to audiences beyond occupational therapy practitioners

4. In what year was the first edition of the *Occupational Therapy Practice Framework* approved by the AOTA Representative Assembly?
   a. 1979
   b. 2002
   c. 2003
   d. 2013

5. The language of the *Occupational Therapy Practice Framework* had to align to which classification system?
   a. International Classification of Functioning, Disability, and Health
   b. International Classification of Health and Welfare
   c. International Classification of Functional Purpose and Meaning
   d. International Classification of Functioning, Disability, and Outcomes Measures

6. Which statement best describes the purpose of the *original Occupational Therapy Practice Framework*?
   a. (1) Describe the profession's philosophical assumptions, (2) define the profession's domain of concern, (3) offer direction for evaluation and intervention, and (4) help external audiences to better understand the profession's unique contribution to health care.
   b. (1) Describe the profession's ethical standards, (2) define the profession's domain of concern, (3) offer direction for evaluation and intervention, and (4) help external audiences to better understand the profession's unique contribution to health care.
   c. (1) Describe the profession's philosophical assumptions, (2) define the profession's domain of concern, (3) standardize all evaluation and intervention, and (4) help external audiences to better understand the profession's unique contribution to health care.
   d. (1) Describe the profession's philosophical assumptions, (2) define the profession's limitations, (3) offer direction for evaluation and intervention, and (4) help external audiences to better understand the profession's unique contribution to health care.

7. The *Occupational Therapy Practice Framework III* (AOTA, 2014) (and all previous editions) is a:
   a. Foundational theory document that should be used alongside the evidence and knowledge that inform occupational therapy
   b. Practice document that should be used alongside the evidence and knowledge that inform occupational therapy
   c. Taxonomy that should be used alongside the evidence and knowledge that inform occupational therapy
   d. Foundational document that should be used alongside the evidence and knowledge that inform occupational therapy

8. The *Occupational Therapy Practice Framework III* (AOTA, 2014) is divided into two parts, which are:
   a. Domain and Procedure
   b. Process and Practice
   c. Procedure and Practice
   d. Domain and Process

9. The five main categories of the Domain of the *Occupational Therapy Practice Framework III* (AOTA, 2014) are:
   a. Areas of occupation, client factors, performance skills, performance patterns, and context and environment occupation, practice skills, performance patterns, context, activity demand and client factors
   b. Occupation, performance skills, performance patterns, context, activity analysis and client factors
   c. Occupation, performance skills, means as ends focus, context, activity demand and client factors

10. What is the Domain of the *Occupational Therapy Practice Framework III* (AOTA, 2014)?
    a. What AOTA owns with regard to intellectual property
    b. Dynamic methods used to implement occupational therapy services
    c. Professional scope and established body of knowledge and expertise and process
    d. Dynamic methods used to discontinue occupational therapy services

11. What is meant by the Process of the *Occupational Therapy Practice Framework III* (AOTA, 2014)?
    a. Dynamic methods used to implement occupational therapy services
    b. Professional scope and established body of knowledge and expertise and process unique to occupational therapy
    c. Professional scope and established body of knowledge and expertise and process for all health care professionals
    d. Dynamic methods used to discontinue occupational therapy services

Practice Activities

Select one occupation that is meaningful to you. Gather magazine photos that represent this occupation. Using only the photos (no words), graphically illustrate how the Process of the *Occupational Therapy Practice Framework III* (AOTA, 2014) occupational therapy would focus on this occupation for a pediatric client with physical disabilities. Refer to the *Occupational Therapy Practice Framework III* (AOTA, 2014).

Use the same occupation from the above activity. Gather magazine photos that represent this occupation. Using only the photos (no words), graphically illustrate how the Process of the *Occupational Therapy Practice Framework III* (AOTA, 2014) of occupational therapy would focus on this occupation with an adult client with mental health issues. Refer to the copy of *Occupational Therapy Practice Framework III* (AOTA, 2014) included in this book.

Take a photograph of a street scene. Print the photo. Select one person from the photo and based on the five categories (occupation, performance skills, performance patterns, context, activity demand, and client factors) of the Domain of the *Occupational Therapy Practice Framework III* (AOTA, 2014), and create a fictitious profile of this person engaged in the occupation of preparing to go grocery shopping. Be creative in how you organize this profile and be prepared to share it with your classmates. Refer to the *Occupational Therapy Practice Framework III.*

References

Accreditation Council for Occupational Therapy Education. *2011 Accreditation Council for Occupational Therapy Education (ACOTE®) Standards and interpretive guide*. 2013. Retrieved from http://www.aota.org/Educate/Accredit/Draft-Standards/50146.aspx?FT=.pdf

American Occupational Therapy Association. *Occupational Therapy Product Output Reporting System and Uniform Terminology for Reporting Occupational Therapy Services*. Bethesda, MD: American Occupational Therapy Association; 1979. Retrieved from http://www.pracdept@aota.org

American Occupational Therapy Association. Occupational therapy practice framework: Domain and process (3rd ed.). *Am J Occup Ther* 2014;68(Suppl 1):S1–S48. http://www.dx.doi.org/10 .5014/ajot.2014.682006

Butts DS, Nelson DL. Agreement between Occupational Therapy Practice Framework classifications and occupational therapists' classifications. *Am J Occup Ther* 2007;61: 512–518.

dictionary.com Unabridged. Retrieved from: http://dictionary.reference.com/browse/taxonomy

Dixon M, et al. Learning the Framework as an occupational therapy assistant student. *OT Practice* 2011;16(1):15.

Gutman SA, et al. Revision of the Occupational Therapy Framework. *Am J Occup Ther* 2007;61(1):119–126.

National Board for Certification in Occupational Therapy. NBCOT homepage. 2003. Retrieved from http://www.nbcot.org

Nelson DL. Critiquing the logic of the domain section of the Occupational Therapy Practice Framework: domain and process. *Am J Occup Ther* 2006;60(5):511–523.

Schwartz DA. My turn at applying the Occupational Therapy Practice Framework. *OT Practice* 2010;l(6):22–23.

WHO. International classification of functioning, disability and health (ICF). 2001. Retrieved from http://www.who.int/classifications/icf/en/

Wilcock AA, Townsend EA. Occupational justice. In: Crepeau EB, Cohn ES, Schell BB, eds. *Willard and Spackman's Occupational Therapy*. 11th ed. Baltimore, MD: Lippincott Williams & Wilkins; 2008:192–199.

Youngstrom MJ. The Occupational Therapy Practice Framework: the evolution of our professional language. *Am J Occup Ther* 2002; 56(6):607–608.

CHAPTER 7

An Overview of Occupational Therapy Theory, Practice Models, and Frames of Reference: Guiding the Practice

Amy Wagenfeld, PhD, OTR/L SCEM, CAPs

Key Terms

Frame of reference—An organizer that provides overarching direction on how to provide treatment (Mosey).

Habituation—To become accustomed or acclimated to something.

Model—A means to organize thinking and intervention around the philosophical basis of a profession.

Theory—More than an educated guess; a group of related ideas that have been verified through analysis.

Volition—The act of willing or choosing—making choices.

Learning Objectives

After studying this chapter, the reader should be able to:

- Explain the foundational underpinnings of occupational therapy frames and practice models of references.
- Compare and contrast the frames of references and practice models described in this chapter.
- State the importance of frames of reference and practice models for the practice of occupational therapy.

Introduction

Occupational therapy theory, frameworks, and practice models provide the profession with a foundation to structure and implement treatment plans with clients. They also help to inform research and to generate new ideas. Collectively, theories, practice models, and frames of reference direct us through the actual work that we do with clients and their families. In this chapter, we explore the several theories, practice models, and frames of reference that have and continue to guide our practice.

Theory

Our knowledge of theories, whether they are simple or complex, guides our work with clients. Simply stated, a **theory** is a way to explain something. More than an educated guess, a theory is a group of related ideas that have been verified through analysis. According to Pollock and Rochon (2002), theories are developed to "explain one's observations, to enhance understanding of relationships, and to predict future events" (p. 34). In occupational therapy, theories are the foundation for models of practice and frames of reference. Beginning in the 1970s, there was a tremendous upsurge in theory in occupational therapy. The 1970s and 1980s saw the rise of sensory integration theory, neurodevelopmental theory, and psychoanalytical theory (Pollock & Rochon, 2002) and their practical applications to therapeutic intervention. Today, we continue to write about theory, to develop new theories, and to apply existing theory from other disciplines such as human ecology, psychology, business, and technology in new ways to fit within the occupational therapy framework. Some examples of current theories that are guiding our professional frames of reference include systems theory, motor learning theories, and meta-cognitive theories, which in turn inform our actions as practitioners (Pollock & Rochon, 2002, p. 35). The way we practice and implement occupational therapy intervention is based on theories. Theories are translated into practical application through models and frames of reference.

Models of Practice

A **model** helps an OT practitioner to organize his/her thinking and intervention around the philosophical basis of the profession, which in our case is occupation. Occupational therapy has two types of models, conceptual and practice. A conceptual model (also referred to as an occupation-based model) provides theoretical validation for occupational therapy by explaining why it works. A conceptual model is generic and does not deal with specific practice areas. An example of a conceptual, occupation-based model is the Lifestyle Performance Model (Fidler, 1996). By explaining how occupational therapy works, practice models provide overarching ideas for implementing practice (Cole & Tufano, 2008). An example of a practice model is the Person–Environment–Occupation Performance Model (Christiansen & Baum, 2005). We will be discussing these and other conceptual and practice models in greater detail shortly.

Frames of Reference

A frame of reference builds on theory and practice models and is a guide or "map" to treat clients (Fig. 7.1). Mosey described a **frame of reference** as "a set of interrelated internally consistent concepts, definitions, and postulates that provide a systematic description of and prescription for a practitioner's interactions with a particular aspect of a profession's domain of concern"

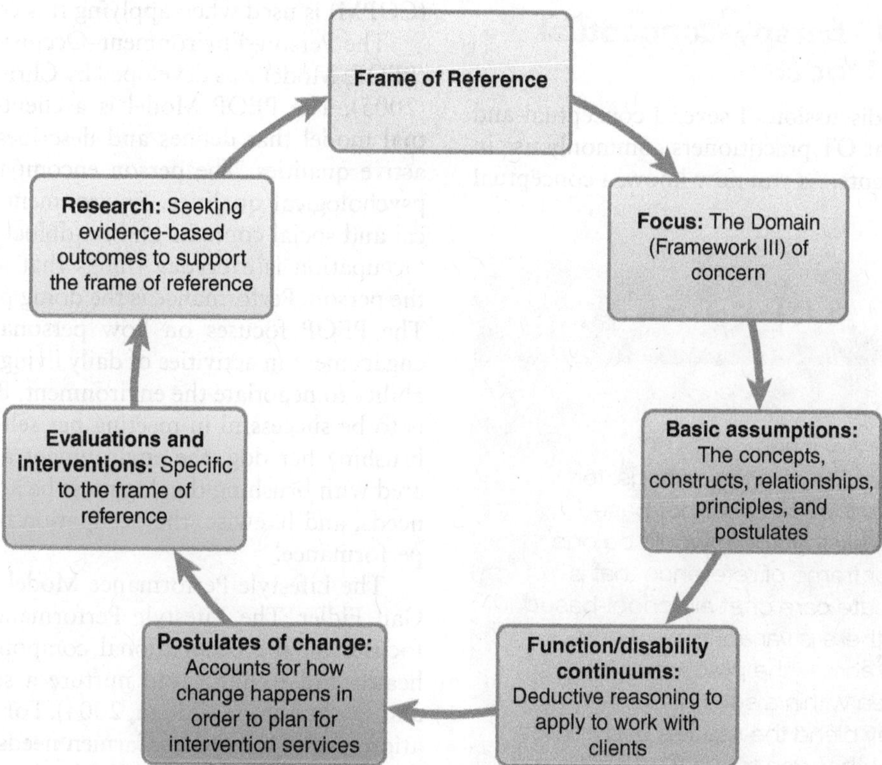

Figure 7.1 Components of an occupational therapy frame of reference. (Adapted from Cole M, Tufano R. *Applied Theories in Occupational Therapy: A Practical Approach*. Thorofare, NJ: Slack, Inc.; 2008.)

1986, (p. 129). Models may align with frames of reference. Unlike conceptual and practice models, frames of reference provide guidelines for evaluation and intervention (Cole & Tufano, 2008).

Why Understanding Theory Is Important for an Occupational Therapy Assistant

As an OTA, it is important to understand theories, practice models, and frames of reference to be prepared to help with treatment planning and other aspects of the intervention process. As well, understanding the reasoning behind treatment protocols enables you to clearly articulate to clients, families, other health care professionals, and payers why you, as an active member of the treatment team, are doing what you are doing (Jirikowic et al., 2001).

While each of our discipline-specific frames of reference addresses human occupation in different ways, they all help to guide evaluation, treatment planning, and implementation (Ikiugu, 2004). The frame of reference that is applied is based on many factors, including facility compatibility and personal frames of reference (Storch & Goldrich Eskow, 1996). In order to implement client-centered practice, OT practitioners tend to weave together different frames of reference and models in their practice to meet the specific needs of their clients (Lawlor & Henderson, 1989) (From the Field 7.1).

Occupational Therapy Conceptual and Practice Models

What follows is a discussion of several conceptual and practice models that OT practitioners commonly use in their work with clients. As you now know, a conceptual model is more theoretical, and a practice model provides overarching ideas for planning and carrying out treatment. We begin by looking at occupational therapy performance conceptual models and then discuss practice models.

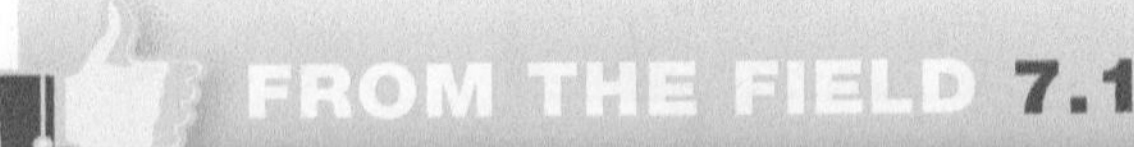

Frames of Reference

If you were to survey a number of OT practitioners at similar practice settings, for example, in acute care or at school-based settings, it is unlikely that there would be one singular model or frame of reference that is followed at all acute care or at all school-based settings. Often, there is variability between OT practitioners across the practice setting and possibly even within a setting. Some OT practitioners may blend the models and frames of reference that they use to work with clients.

The Canadian Model of Occupational Performance (CMOP) was developed by Mary Law and colleagues. It is systems based and recognizes the connections between a person, his/her environment, and occupations (Ikiugu, 2004). In this client-centered model, environment refers to how things occurring outside the body (external factors) that lead to responses (the person) influence how and why people find meaning and purpose in life (Law et al., 1996). At the core of this client-centered model is spirituality that which is self-motivating or inspirational. In this application, spirituality is "a pervasive life force, manifestation of a higher self, source of will and self-determination, and a sense of meaning, purpose, and connectedness that people experience in the context of their environment" (CAOT, 1997, p. 182).

The CMOP is well suited for many types of clients in equally as many practice settings. When applying the CMOP model, OT practitioners develop treatment plans that address goals that are important to their clients. For instance, if Mr. Walker wants to return to work as a welder (and it is realistic to do so), intervention will address how to help him achieve this goal by examining how the environment can be adapted to meet his desire to return to his role as a welder. A measurement tool called the Canadian Occupational Performance Measure (COPM) is used when applying this conceptual model.

The Person–Environment–Occupation–Performance (PEOP) Model was developed by Christiansen and Baum (2005). The PEOP Model is a client-centered conceptual model that defines and describes a person's interactive qualities. The person encompasses physical and psychological qualities. Environment represents physical and social contexts and roadblocks to performance. Occupation is everyday things that are of meaning to the person. Performance is the doing part of occupation. The PEOP focuses on how personal motivation and engagement in activities of daily living impact a person's ability to negotiate the environment. By example, if Jodi is to be successful in meeting her self-identified goal of brushing her dog, the environment and factors associated with brushing the dog must be adapted to meet her needs, and likewise, the occupation of brushing fosters performance.

The Lifestyle Performance Model was developed by Gail Fidler. The Lifestyle Performance practice model focuses on the occupational components that support health and wellness and nurture a sense of coherence and quality of life (Ikiugu, 2004). For example, if evaluation results show that Carmen needs to connect better with his peers, but issues with obesity make him feel reluctant to interact with others, an intervention plan may focus on an occupation-based healthier lifestyle choice plan. It conceptualizes the connections between a person, environment and contexts, activity profile, and perceived quality of life to improve intrinsic motivation and lead to increased self-satisfaction and an evolving lifestyle (Fidler, 1996).

The occupational adaptation model was developed by Janet Schkade and Sally Schultz. The occupational adaptation model views the person as a system comprised of three subsystems, sensorimotor, psychosocial, and cognitive. People are presumed to be active agents of change and can interact and adapt to their environments through occupational engagement using the three subsystems (Ikiugu, 2004). The model has two parts: an organizer to explain "adaptation and [also] a framework to enable occupational therapy practitioners to plan, guide, and implement interventions" (Schkade & McClung, 2001 in Cole & Tufano, 2008, p. 107).

The occupational adaptation frame of reference is holistic and supports client-centered intervention. It focuses on the dynamic interplay between a person and his/her occupational environment (Cole & Tufano, 2008, p. 107). For example, an OTA is working with Jason on adapting his workspace to make it ergonomically sound so that he can continue to do his work as a web designer, something he is passionate about. With Jason as an eager partner in the process, his OTA thinks in a holistic way about factors such as how the workspace can be designed so Jason can look at his monitor without harming his eyes, without harming his ears due to noise levels from surrounding colleagues, and without affecting his ability to focus on his work and how he will be able to do his work safely and feel productive.

The Model of Human Occupation (MOHO) was developed by Gary Kielhofner and Janice Burke (1980). The MOHO is a systems-based practice model that recognizes a person as a dynamic system who constantly interacts with and is affected by the environment via a process of input (taking in information), throughput (processing of the information), output (response to information), and feedback. The environment refers to physical contexts, objects, occupations, groups, and social–cultural situations in which performance occurs. Occupation provides meaning and purpose and enhances development at all stages of life.

Restoration involves intervention at the throughput level of the human system that addresses **volition**: making choices, **habituation**, becoming used to something, and performance within the environment. As applied to treatment, the OT practitioner directs the client to be the agent of change to accomplish goals. For example, Mrs. Liebowitz is relearning how to brush her teeth following a stroke. Her OTA will provide the necessary setup to get Mrs. Liebowitz ready to brush her teeth, but it is Mrs. Liebowitz who draws onto her personal motivation and makes the choice to relearn the activity of brushing her teeth.

Occupational Therapy Theories and Frames of Reference

Occupational therapy frames of reference provide a framework to plan and implement treatment. While not an exhaustive list, there are a number of frames of reference that OT practitioners base their work with clients on. The frameworks discussed here are categorized as occupational science, psychospiritual, psychosocial, cognitive behavioral, multicontextual, developmental, sensory integration, biomechanical and rehabilitative, and motor control.

Occupational Science

Occupational science takes into account complex relationships involving people interacting with the environment.

Occupational science is both a theory and frame of reference. It was developed by Elizabeth Yerxa. Occupational science views people as complex systems interacting with the environment. Obstacles such as disease, disability, trauma, or other life-interrupting experiences impede active engagement in occupation and participation in the environment (Yerxa, 1990). Through re-engagement in meaningful occupation, a person is able to reconnect and experience an enhanced sense of self-worth and competency (Yerxa, 2000). For example, Lisette is a 16-year-old Cuban American who has juvenile rheumatoid arthritis. She loves to knit, make jewelry, and tap dance. Her family is very close knit, and she enjoys listening to her grandma tell her stories about life in Cuba. One of her client-centered goals is to learn techniques and new ways to knit and make jewelry that will protect her joints. Because her grandma also has arthritis, Lisette is eager to share what she has learned from her OT practitioner with her grandma.

Psychosocial and Psychospiritual

These types of frames of reference provide a foundation for understanding the human psyche and how it influences engagement in occupation.

Psychospiritual Integration Frame of Reference

The psychospiritual integration (PSI) frame of reference was developed by Chris Kang. The PSI was developed largely in response to a profession-wide acknowledgment of the spiritual dimension of occupational therapy practice (please also refer to Chapter 19, *Spirituality*). The PSI has four purposes, "(i) to explore the construct of spirituality in depth; (ii) to propose a way of viewing spirituality, occupation, and therapy; (iii) to provide a link between theory and practice of enabling spirituality through occupations; and (iv), to provide suitable technology for assessment and enablement of spirituality" (Kang, 2003, p. 94). The PSI focuses on "(i) the nature of spirituality; (ii) the expressions of spirituality in everyday behaviour; (iii) the nature of spiritual occupation; and (iv) the influence of spirituality and spiritual occupations on health and well-being" (Kang, 2003, pp. 94–95). Kang (2003) describes the PSI as both a frame of reference and a conceptual practice model useful for most all clients who receive occupational therapy intervention. The purpose is to be used by OT practitioners working with individuals or groups of people whose spiritual connections are limited because of or are resulting in occupational-related issues or for those who wish to explore a spiritual connection (Kang, 2003). For example, 19-year-old Glenn was recently in an auto accident and is now a quadriplegic. Through journaling via voice-activated software on a tablet that the OT practitioner has set up for Glenn to use on his own, Glenn is able to articulate questioning his purpose in life now that he finds himself in a new and unexpected life space.

The doing and meaning psychosocial frame of reference was developed by Gail and Jay Fidler. The impact of including occupation in mental health treatment protocols can be enhanced by interactions between practitioner and client, between clients, and also the overarching influence of the occupational therapy intervention on the rest of the client's treatment regimen (Fidler & Fidler, 1954). In the doing and meaning psychosocial frame of reference, it is not the activity itself that matters, but rather the activity is the conduit to make intervention effective (Fidler & Fidler, 1954). This is a process rather than an end product-focused frame of reference. The inherent benefits of treatment are achieved through the process of participating in occupation. The act of participating leads to improved mental health, level of independent functioning, self-satisfaction, and quality of life. For instance, engaging a client to participate in baking a cake will lead to positive mental health outcomes.

Cognitive Behavioral Frame of Reference

The cognitive behavioral frame of reference is based on the premise that thought influences behavior and changes in cognitive status occur through alteration of brain chemistry or physiology.

The Cognitive Disability Model was developed by Claudia Allen. This model provides guidelines for OT practitioners to help clients adapt to chronic conditions. There are six levels of cognitive function associated with the Cognitive Disability Model (Allen, 1991; Earhart, 2008). Cognitive function ranges from less than 1, indicating a basically comatose state, to the 4.6 range, which is the minimal cognitive range associated with the ability to live independently, and the 6 and above range, which indicates normal cognitive functioning. The assessment tool associated with the Cognitive Disability Model is the *Allen Cognitive Level Screen* (ACLS-5). The fifth version of the assessment tool was published in 2007 (Allen et al., 2007).

The end goal of employing the Cognitive Disability Model in treatment is to assist clients to self-regulate. This is accomplished by helping them change thought patterns, behaviors, and environmental issues that negatively impact function (Ikiugu, 2004). It involves training to learn new habits and routine, assistance via cueing, environmental adaptations to augment upgraded occupational performance and cognitive status, and adaptation of task demands to improve function. For instance, Bella is nonverbal and can inconsistently communicate with a tabletop electronic communication system. Her OT practitioner is working with Bella to consistently touch the icon for restroom, when she needs to toilet. The OTA must be creative in finding the best way to adapt the communication system as well as Bella's methods to use the system for her to be successful in communicating when she needs to toilet. In time, the OTA plans to work with Bella on using the system to communicate other needs.

Multicontextual Frame of Reference

The multicontextual frame of reference is oriented from a cognitive–perceptual perspective.

The multicontextual approach was developed by Joan Toglia. It equates learning to the interaction between personal tasks and environmental factors. Personal variables include processing strategies and awareness of cognitive thought processes. External or environmental factors include the demands of the occupation, the task itself, and the contexts in which they occur. This is a task-oriented frame of reference; detailed task analyses are developed by the OT practitioner to help clients learn task-specific skills and also to transfer these skills to different conditions or environments, to self-monitor, and to self-motivate in order to increase cognitive capacities. For example, Mr. Clark has indicated that growing hot peppers is his favorite hobby. In order to help Mr. Clark be able to continue this hobby, his OT practitioner analyzes all the steps involved in growing hot peppers as he did prior to his injury (in an in ground garden) and determines that an alternative method of growing would be better for Mr. Clark. They discuss this plan and he is agreeable, so the OT practitioner analyzes the same activity, but now to be done in a series of pots placed on a table. This is determined to be the better option and becomes the focus of treatment. Mr. Clark intends to expand his growing repertoire by growing other vegetables and herbs in pots.

Developmental Frames of Reference

Developmental frames of reference are based on understanding that development occurs on a continuum or in a sequential fashion. Learning new skills depends on building on existing skills.

The developmental theory was developed by Lela Llorens. Developmental theory identifies the highest level of motor, social, and cognitive skills in which a client can engage and facilitates improvement in function from the outset of treatment. The OT practitioner's role is to grade activities so that the client can achieve them but is still slightly challenged to do the tasks. The purpose is to help "close the gap" in the areas in which the client is unable to perform. For example, Tanner is learning to put on his socks by himself. The OTA uses a backwards chaining approach with Tanner. The OTA does all the steps necessary to put on socks, except to pull them up over the ankles, which Tanner does by himself. When Tanner masters this, the OTA does all the steps except for pulling the socks over the heel and up over the ankles. The OTA continues this backwards chaining process until Tanner can independently put on his socks.

Sensory Integration Frame of Reference

The sensory integration frame of reference is based on the premise that a well-organized sensory system is necessary for optimal participation in daily life. This frame of reference is grounded in neuroscience.

Sensory Integration

The sensory integration frame of reference was developed by A. Jean Ayres.

The sensory integration frame of reference takes into account the whole person in many situations "from remediation of foundational neuromechanisms, to habilitation and development of skills, to prevention of problems in daily life, while promoting engagement in occupations at all ages" (May-Benson & Koomar, 2008, p. 1). This means that when working within the sensory integration frame of reference the occupational therapy practitioner addresses underlying neural structures in the brain by facilitating highly selective and specific sensory-based activities at all stages of life in order to help clients achieve maximal levels of function. This is very important because skill acquisition, learning, and overall life function depend on a well-integrated sensory system. Conversely, sensory processing issues negatively impact learning, behavior, and function. Providing meaningful client-directed sensory experiences requires an adaptive response, which leads to skill acquisition, learning, and behavioral changes (Ayres, 1994; Bundy & Murray, 2002). Based on its multifaceted orientation, the sensory integration frame of reference forms a bridge between a medical focus and occupation-based goals (May-Benson & Koomar, 2008, p. 1). For example, Miranda is seven years old and, among other things, cannot sit on her chair in school without falling off. She is given the choice of blowing bubbles or tossing rings onto a pole while lying on her belly on a rocking platform swing. She chooses bubbles. The adaptive response, an action that will lead to meeting an environmental demand that the OT practitioner is seeking while having Miranda swing on the platform swing and blow bubbles, is improved hip, trunk, and shoulder control. This will help Miranda be more aware of where her body is in space and to be able to sit in her chair without falling off (please also refer to Chapter 28, *Sensory Processing*).

Biomechanical and Rehabilitative Frames of Reference

These types of frames of reference are based on a remediation and adaptation approach to therapy. While both the biomechanical and rehabilitative frames originally focused only on physical rehabilitation, contemporary OT theorists and practitioners recognize that occupational performance is a combination of physical and mental skills. These frames are currently viewed more holistically and are recognized as being applicable to multiple practice settings.

The biomechanical frames of reference was developed by Catherine Trombly. The theoretical basis of the biomechanical frame of reference is that given an appropriate assessment and treatment program, clients will acquire the voluntary motor skills necessary to perform their desired human occupations. It is focused on remediation but also encompasses adaptation. Cole and Tufano (2008) indicate that the biomechanical frame of reference utilizes "principles of physics to movement and posture to the forces of gravity" (p. 165). It is also derived from theories in kinetics and kinematics, a science that studies the effects of forces and motion on material bodies. It embraces the concept of endurance, defined as exertion over time (Cox & Pemberton, 2011, p. 79).

The biomechanical frame of reference is the most commonly used frame of reference by OT practitioners (NBCOT, 2004). While many health care professionals apply principles of biomechanics to their intervention, OT practitioners are unique in applying these principles (i.e., motion, strength, endurance) to the occupations of daily life (Cole & Tufano, 2008). For example, the purposeful and repetitive activity of having Mrs. O'Malley string beads to make a necklace for her grandchild will strengthen and improve active range of motion of the hand and fingers.

Rehabilitative Frame of Reference

The rehabilitative frame of reference was developed by the founding members of occupational therapy, including Eleanor Slagle, Thomas Kidner, George Barton, Susan Cox Johnson, and William Dunton. The goal of this frame of reference is facilitating the greatest level of independence possible despite disease or disability processes. Enabling active participation in all domains of occupation entails working with clients on learning compensatory methods, assistive devices, and environmental modifications.

Functional restoration occurs through appropriate application of self-care and leisure activities, adaptive equipment training, use of assistive technology, environmental modifications, and ergonomic and workplace safety techniques.

The rehabilitative frame of reference is focused on improving function to the greatest degree possible, despite any limitations (Trombly, 2002). For example, in order for Mr. Jackson to shower independently, he needs to sit on a shower chair and use a long-handled sponge and soap on a rope, which is tied to the side of the shower chair to wash his feet and back (please also refer to Chapter 21, *Adaptive Equipment*; Chapter 22, *Assistive Technology*; Chapter 26, *Workplace Safety*; and Chapter 38, *Work and Industry*).

Motor Control and Learning Frames of Reference

Neurodevelopmental Therapy Frame of Reference

The neurodevelopmental therapy frame of reference was developed by Karel and Berta Bobath. Originally conceptualized as a treatment method for those with hemiplegia secondary to a cerebral vascular accident (CVA or stroke), neurodevelopmental therapy (NDT) was also later applied to children with cerebral palsy. Today, it is used in a broader sense for clients with motor control issues (Cole & Tufano, 2008). It is a preparatory method because it lays the foundation for re-establishing sensorimotor performance components that are prerequisites for occupational performance (Cole & Tufano, 2008, p. 245). For example, Sally had a stroke and cannot bend her left arm on her own. Her OT practitioner takes her arm through a series of repetitive movements that involve bending and straightening so that she can experience what normal movement feels like.

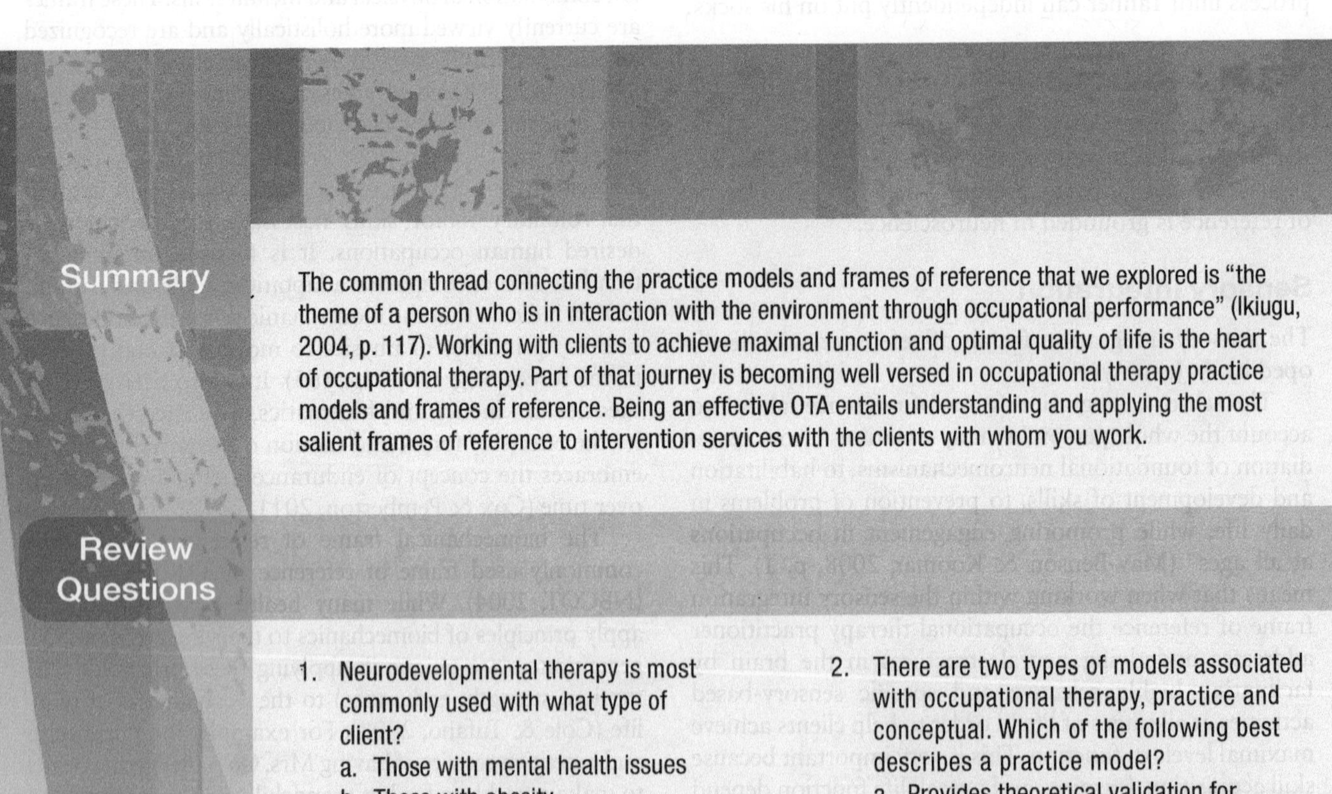

Summary

The common thread connecting the practice models and frames of reference that we explored is "the theme of a person who is in interaction with the environment through occupational performance" (Ikiugu, 2004, p. 117). Working with clients to achieve maximal function and optimal quality of life is the heart of occupational therapy. Part of that journey is becoming well versed in occupational therapy practice models and frames of reference. Being an effective OTA entails understanding and applying the most salient frames of reference to intervention services with the clients with whom you work.

Review Questions

1. Neurodevelopmental therapy is most commonly used with what type of client?
   a. Those with mental health issues
   b. Those with obesity
   c. Those with neurological dysfunction
   d. Those with arthritis

2. There are two types of models associated with occupational therapy, practice and conceptual. Which of the following best describes a practice model?
   a. Provides theoretical validation for occupational therapy by explaining why it works
   b. Generic and does not deal with specific practice areas
   c. Explanation for why a phenomenon occurs
   d. Guide for treating clients

3. The biomechanical practice model is based on:
   a. Remediation and repetition
   b. Remediation and innovation
   c. Remediation and psychosocial intervention
   d. Remediation and adaptation

4. The sensory integration frame of reference is based in *large* part on:
   a. Physiology
   b. Kinematics
   c. Neurology
   d. Anatomy

5. There are two types of models associated with occupational therapy, practice and conceptual. Which of the following best describes a conceptual model?
   a. Provides theoretical validation for occupational therapy by explaining why it works
   b. Generic and does not deal with specific practice areas
   c. Explanation for why a phenomenon occurs
   d. Guide for treating clients

6. Builds on theory and practice models and is a guide or "map" to treat clients best described as a:
   a. Conceptual model
   b. Practice model
   c. Hypothesis
   d. Frame of reference

7. The occupational adaptation model is a systems-based model based on the promise that a person is which of the three following subsystems?
   a. Sensorimotor, psychosocial, and cognitive
   b. Neurological, physiological, and cognitive
   c. Physiological, psychosocial, and cognitive
   d. Sensorimotor, psychosocial, and neurological

8. Which frame of reference is expressly stated as being process rather than product focused?
   a. Psychosocial doing and meaning
   b. Occupational adaptation
   c. Cognitive behavioral
   d. Multicontextual

9. The psychosocial integration frame of reference/model is applicable to:
   a. Clients with mental health issues
   b. Children
   c. Clients with neurological issues
   d. All clients

10. The terms input, throughput, output, and feedback apply to the:
    a. Canadian Model of Occupational Performance
    b. The Model of Human Occupation
    c. Person–Environment–Occupation–Performance Model
    d. Biomechanical frame of reference

11. Despite being recognized as outdated, which model or frame of reference continues to be widely used?
    a. Neurodevelopmental therapy
    b. Sensory integration
    c. MOHO
    d. Occupational adaptation

Practice Activities

Select a frame of reference or practice model that most appeals to you. Write a short essay that explains why it speaks to you. Try to relate your essay to a personal life experience that closely aligns to the frame of reference or practice model you selected.

Make a chart that lists all of the frames of reference and practice models discussed in this chapter. Using a different colored marker to represent each, highlight the frame of reference or practice model with its unique color. Link frames/models to each other on the basis of commonalities to another using the color-coding system you developed. What do you see? What does your color web tell you?

Select one frame of reference and design an activity based on your frame of reference.

References

Allen CK. Cognitive disability and reimbursement for rehabilitation and psychiatry. *J Insur Med* 1991;23(4):245–247.

Allen CK, et al. *Manual for the Allen Cognitive Level Screen-5 (ACLS-5) and Large Allen Cognitive Level Screen-5 (LACLS-5)*. Camarillo, CA: ACLS and LACLS Committee; 2007.

Ayres AJ. *Sensory Integration and the Child*. Los Angeles, CA: Western Psychological Services; 1994.

Bundy A, Murray E. Sensory integration: A. Jean Ayres theory revisited. In: Bundy A, Murray E, eds. *Sensory Integration Theory and Practice*. 2nd ed. Philadelphia, PA: F.A. Davis; 2002.

Canadian Occupational Therapy Association. *Canadian Occupational Performance Measure*. 3rd ed. Ottawa, CA: Author; 1997.

Christiansen CH, Baum CM. *Occupational Therapy: Performance, Participation, and Well-Being*. Thorofare, NJ: Slack Incorporated; 2005.

Cole M, Tufano R. *Applied Theories in Occupational Therapy: A Practical Approach*. Thorofare, NJ: Slack, Incorporated; 2008.

Cox D, Pemberton S. What happened to the time? The relationship of occupational therapy to time. *Br J Occup Ther* 2011;74(2):78–89.

Earhart CA. Brief history of the Cognitive Disabilities Model and Assessments. 2008. Retrieved from http://www.allen-cognitive-network.org/index.php/allen-cognitive-model/brief-history

Fidler GS. Life-style performance: from profile to conceptual model. *Am J Occup Ther* 1996;50(2):139–147.

Fidler G, Fidler J. *Introduction to Psychiatric Occupational Therapy*. New York, NY: The MacMillan Company; 1954.

Ikiugu MN. Instrumentalism in occupational therapy: an argument for a pragmatic conceptual model of practice. *Int J Psychosoc Rehab* 2004;8:109–117.

Jirikowic T, et al. Contemporary trends and practice strategies in pediatric occupational and physical therapy. *Phys Occup Ther Pediatr* 2001;20(4):45–62.

Kang C. A psychospiritual integration frame of reference for occupational therapy. Part 1: Conceptual foundations. *Aust Occup Ther J* 2003;50:92–103.

Kielhofner G, Burke JP. A Model of Human Occupation, Part 1. Conceptual Framework and Content. *Am J Occup Ther* 1980;34: 572–581.

Law M, et al. The Person-Environment-Occupation Model: a transactive approach to occupational performance. *Can J Occup Ther* 1996;63(1):9–23.

Lawlor MC, Henderson A. A descriptive study of the clinical practice patterns of occupational therapists working with infants and young children. *Am J Occup Ther* 1989;43(11):755–764.

May-Benson TA, Koomar JA. AOTA's Centennial Vision and the sensory integration frame of reference. *Sens Integration Spec Interest Sect Q* 2008;31(1):1–4.

Mosey AC. Occupational therapy: Configuration of a profession. New York: *Rawen Press;* 1986.

National Board for Certification in Occupational Therapy. A practice analysis of entry-level occupational therapist registered and certified occupational therapy assistant practice, *OTJR-Occup Participation Health* 2004;24(Suppl 1):S1–S31.

Nelson D. Why the profession of occupational therapy will flourish in the 21st century. *Am J Occup Ther* 1997;51:11–24.

Pollock N, Rochon S. Becoming an evidence-based practitioner. In: Law M, ed. *Evidence-Based Rehabilitation—A Guide to Practice*, pp. 31–45. Thorofore, NJ: Slack, Incorporated; 2002.

Storch B, Goldrich Eskow K. Theory application by school-based occupational therapists. *Am J Occup Ther* 1996;50(8):662–668.

Trombly C. Conceptual foundations for practice. In: Trombly C, Radomski MV, eds. *Occupational Therapy for Physical Dysfunction*. 5th ed., pp. 1–35. Philadelphia, PA: Lippincott Williams & Wilkins; 2002.

Yerxa E. An introduction to occupational Science, a foundation for occupational therapy in the 21st century. *Occup Ther Health Care* 1990;6(4):1–17.

Yerxa E. Occupational science: a renaissance of service to humankind through knowledge. *Occup Ther Int* 2000;7(2):87–98.

CHAPTER 8

An Overview of Human Development: Framing Who We Are

Amy Wagenfeld, PhD, OTR/L SCEM, CAPs

Key Terms

Active—Through experiences, people are active participants in shaping their course of development.
Cephalocaudal—Physical development pattern that proceeds from head down toward toes.
Cognitive development—Thinking and language development.
Continuity—Development proceeds as a gradual and ongoing process.
Discontinuity—Development occurs in distinct steps or stages.
Distal—With regard to the human body, that which is furthest from the center of the body (i.e., fingers and toes).
Fine motor skills—Tasks that rely primarily on the small muscles and joints of the wrists and hands.
Gross motor skills—Tasks that rely primarily on the larger muscles and joints in the body.
Hypothesis—Testable assumptions or predictions.
Motor development—Movement, reflex, and sensory development.
Nature—Development proceeds because of internal, biological factors.
Nurture—Development proceeds because of external, environmental factors.
Passive—The environment shapes people "doing" is not the explanation for development.
Proximal—With regard to the human body—that which is closest to the center of the body (i.e., shoulders and thighs).
Psychosocial development—Psychological and emotional development.
Resilience—The ability to adapt to change.
Sense of coherence—An overarching and fluid representation of confidence.
Spiritual development—Overarching worldview development seeking answers to questions such as "who am I" and "what is my purpose."
Teratogens—Any disease, drug, or other environmental agents that can harm a developing embryo or fetus.
Theory—A set of related ideas that describe and explain specific concepts.

Learning Objectives

After studying this chapter, readers should be able to:

- Explain the influence of human development on engagement in occupation throughout the lifespan.
- Compare and contrast developmental theories and their application to occupational therapy.
- Discuss the interconnectedness of different facets of development and how they influence human function.

Introduction

One of the most exciting things about lifespan human development is that we all experience it. While much of human development follows (for most) a typical course, we are first and foremost individuals. Embracing the individuality and uniqueness that makes our clients who they are is a really important part of our job. In fact, it is a critical piece of client-centered intervention.

What then is typical development? First of all, development is actually all about change. We are constantly changing. While it is seldom evident, you are different than you were when you began to read this chapter just moments ago. Typical development entails acquiring new skills at more or less predetermined times throughout life, such as the skills that lead up to an infant's first steps. The elegant work of theorists from disciplines such as psychology, medicine, occupational therapy, and education has helped to quantify typical developmental milestones, the range of time in which they usually happen, as well as their quality. When deviation from the normal predicted patterns of development warrants further evaluation, practitioners from many disciplines including occupational therapy, physical therapy, speech and language therapy, medical professionals, and mental health may intervene, assess, and treat. Although we continue to develop and change throughout our entire lives, assessment and intervention for developmental issues typically occurs from birth to young adulthood.

Today, many societal issues challenge what is considered the course of normal development. One example is the increased survival rates of premature babies with very complex birth complications and atypical developmental patterns. Many of these babies will require intense and long-term occupational therapy services. Another example is obesity. The obesity epidemic is threatening the physical and psychosocial health and normal development of children, not to mention altering the life course of adults as well. The role of the OTA in working to combat the effects of obesity as it impacts every facet of development is very important (AOTA, 2010). Simply said, development influences function and function influences development.

Themes Associated with Development

There are several realms of development that practitioners, researchers, and scholars concern themselves with. Although not an inclusive list, they include motor development, social–emotional development, cognitive development, and spiritual development, which primarily represent what OT practitioners concern themselves with. **Motor development** refers to postural control, reflex integration, sensory skills, and **gross** (large) and **fine** (small) **motor skills** and the way they shape movement skills. In humans, motor development proceeds in a **cephalocaudal** (head to toe) and **proximal–distal** (midline outward) manner. Large motor skills like reaching occur before grasping and release. Gross motor skills lay the foundation for precise fine motor skill work like writing, using utensils, typing, and tying shoes.

Psychosocial development begins with early attachment relationships and encompasses the ways that children learn to engage in and interpret inter- and intrapersonal relationships. Early attachment relationships often shape the way in which children approach and engage in all future relationships. Typically, the first attachment relationship a baby develops is with a parent and most often with a mother. Children who, for whatever reason (e.g., parent is ill, infant is in an orphanage), do not have the opportunity to develop a secure attachment relationship very early in life may be at risk for reactive attachment disorder, which impacts a child's ability to develop healthy relationships with family and friends.

Cognitive development refers to how thinking and language skills unfold. The process begins in utero. A fetus can hear. Studies have shown that if a fetus hears a particular song repeatedly while in the womb, he/she will recognize the song when played at birth and shortly after by turning his/her head to the source of that particular song. Reading to and talking to infants and children and reinforcing and repeating and expanding upon the sounds they make and words they form is a very important way to nurture cognitive and language development.

Spiritual development is a bit harder to quantify, but refers defining who we are and what our purpose in life is (please also refer to Chapter 19, *Spirituality*). Factors such as **resilience**, the ability to adapt to change, and **sense of coherence**, an overarching and fluid representation of confidence in one's ability to carry out life's activities (Antonovsky, 1987), are associated with spiritual development.

Motor development depends on cognitive development, which depends on psychosocial development, which depends on spiritual development, and so on. It is safe to say that a lag or disruption of development in one area ultimately impacts another (Fig. 8.1).

One of the most heated debates in the development community is whether development proceeds due to the influence of nature or of nurture. The **nature** position is that our inner biology (e.g., genetics and physiology) determines who we are and are to become. The **nurture** side of the debate argues that external environmental factors (e.g., the quality of caregiving a child receives and nutrition) determine our course of development. The debate has actually resolved to a more middle ground position, in that it is now generally accepted that we are products of both our inner biology (nature) and our environments (nurture). The relationship between factors of nature and nurture shapes our individuality. While OT practitioners cannot reverse or

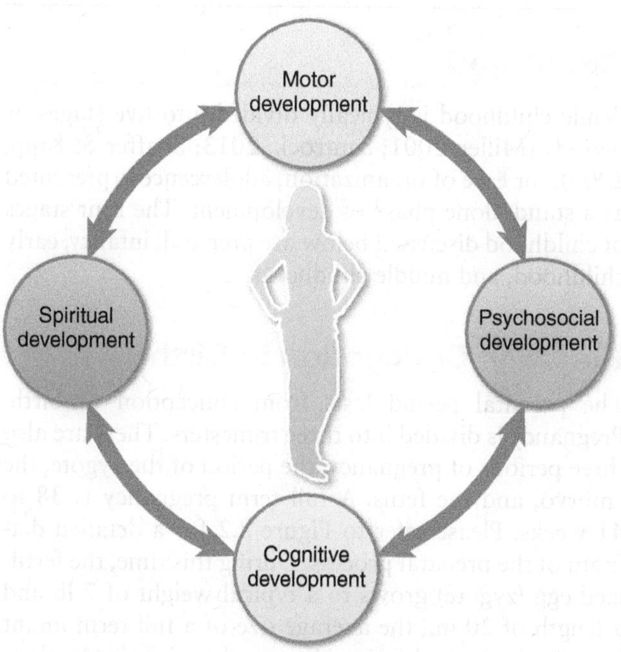

Figure 8.1 The interconnectedness of development.

alter a person's genetics or inner biology, we can and do strongly adapt or modify the environment and how clients engage with and participate in it. In fact, one of the tenets of occupational therapy is adapting environmental contexts to meet the client's need(s) (AOTA, 2014).

The active–passive debate also shapes what we know about human development. The **active** orientation suggests that through experiences, people are active participants in shaping their course of development. Think of the active orientation as being in charge of your destiny. The **passive** orientation suggests that the environment shapes people, and "doing" is not a primary factor in development. The more widely held view is the active orientation, that is, our active participation in life shapes who and what we are.

We now know that physical, cognitive, psychosocial, and spiritual development occurs throughout life and does not stop at an arbitrary age. The means by which people acquire the developmental skills necessary to participate in life are looked at through a lens of continuity or discontinuity. One who believes that development occurs in an orderly, stepwise progression following a set timetable would be considered a **discontinuity** theorist. Think of discontinuity as climbing a developmental staircase to adulthood. On the other hand, **continuity** theorists believe that development occurs in a gradual ongoing manner. Rather than steps, development proceeds in degrees. Think of continuity as a train chugging slowly along a straight track. The common ground between continuity and discontinuity is that with each new developmental skill, we are better prepared to function in the moment and to be ready to take on more new and challenging experiences.

Human Development and the Occupational Therapy Practice Framework III

As you likely now appreciate, development does not occur in a vacuum. We are a combination of nature and nurture and are active creatures that to the greatest degree possible shape our life course through occupation conducted in various environmental contexts. According to the AOTA (2014), environments or contexts are factors within and around people that significantly influence performance. The domain of occupational therapy as described in *Occupational Therapy Practice Framework III* (AOTA, 2014) includes a discussion of six contexts, cultural, personal, temporal, virtual, physical, and social. Table 8.1 outlines the contexts and their connection to performance and development (AOTA, 2014).

TABLE 8.1 **Contexts and Development**

Context	Defined	Developmental Areas Impacted by Context
Cultural	"Customs, beliefs, activity patterns, behavior standards, and expectations accepted by the society of which the client is a member" (p. S9)	Psychosocial Spiritual
Personal	"Age, gender, socioeconomic status, and educational status that are not part of a health condition" (p. S9)	Motor Cognitive Psychosocial Spiritual
Temporal	"Life stage, time of day or year, duration of the activity… and history" (p. S9)	Motor Cognitive Psychosocial Spiritual
Virtual	"Interactions occurring in real or near-time situations in the absence of physical contact" (p. S9)	Motor Cognitive Psychosocial
Physical	"The natural and built environments in which occupations occur" (p. S8)	Motor Cognitive Psychosocial Spiritual
Social	"Presence, relationships, and expectations of persons, organizations, populations with whom people have contact with" (p. S9)	Cognitive Psychosocial Spiritual

American Occupational Therapy Association. Occupational therapy practice framework: Domain and process (3rd ed.). *Am J Occup Ther* 2014;68(Suppl 1):S8–S9. http://www.dx.doi.org/10.5014/ajot.2014.682006

Developmental Theory

Much of the way we understand and explain development is based on theories. Researchers test theories by developing hypotheses, which are testable assumptions or predictions (Wagenfeld, 2005). There are several occupational therapy frames of reference and practice models that are based on developmental theory. While they are not categorized as developmental theory, occupational therapy models, or frames of references, the Canadian Model of Occupational Performance (Law et al., 1996), the Model of Human Occupational (Kielhofner, 2007), Neuro-Developmental Treatment (D'Ambrogio & Roth, 1997), and Sensory Integration (Ayres, 1994) all incorporate developmental theory into their structure. Please refer to Chapter 7, An Overview of Occupational Therapy *Theory, Practice Models, and Frames of Reference: Guiding the Practice,* for further information about these models and frames of reference. Table 8.2 provides a brief discussion of various theories of development, the theorists who proposed them, and their overarching application to occupational therapy practitioners.

Childhood

While childhood is typically divided into five stages or periods (Miller, 2001; Santrock, 2013; Shaffer & Kipp, 2009), for ease of organization, adolescence is presented as a stand-alone phase of development. The four stages of childhood discussed below are prenatal, infancy, early childhood, and middle childhood.

Prenatal: Conception to Birth

The prenatal period lasts from conception to birth. Pregnancy is divided into three trimesters. There are also three periods of pregnancy, the period of the zygote, the embryo, and the fetus. A full term pregnancy is 38 to 41 weeks. Please refer to Figure 8.2 for a detailed diagram of the prenatal process. During this time, the fertilized egg (zygote) grows to a typical weight of 7 lb and a length of 20 in., the average size of a full term infant born in the United States. At no other time in development does growth occur at such a breathtaking rate as during the prenatal stage of development. As well, at no other time in development is there as great a sensitivity

TABLE 8.2 Developmental Theorists and Developmental Concepts

Theorist	Theoretical Orientation	Continuity or Discontinuity?	Basic Premise	Application to the OT Practitioner
Jean Piaget (1896–1980)	Social Cognition (construction)	Discontinuity	Thinking and development in general are a result of internal processes. Children are at their best to develop when provided with many hands-on and observational experiences (Kamii, 1973; Piaget & Inhelder, 1969).	The OTA provides children with hands-on experiences as a means to optimize performance and function.
Lev Vygotsky (1896–1934)	Social Construction	Continuity	Children learn through social experiences. In most cases, given time and support, a child will achieve a desired skill or action (Vygotsky, 1978).	The OTA acts as a capable guide to provide mediation and support for development of more functional and increasingly complex skills.
Robert Siegler (1949–)	Information Processing	Continuity	Proposes that the mind is like a computer, the brain is the hardware and cognition is the software. Thinking skills such as memory, coding, and encoding are equated with information processing (Shaffer & Kipp, 2009).	The OTA works to improve cognitive skills through enhancing learning strategies.
Sigmund Freud (1856–1939)	Psychoanalytic (psychosexual)	Discontinuity	Personality development is, for the most part, an unconscious process that is influenced by emotions (Santrock, 2012).	The OTA may use projective and creative techniques such as art activities and journal writing to support personality development (Cole, 1998).
Erik Erikson (1902–1994)	Psychoanalytic (psychosocial)	Discontinuity	A psychosocial explanation for sequential, lifelong development of personality. Each stage has specific tasks that must be accomplished to achieve a well-adjusted or maladjusted sense of self (Erikson, 1982; Erikson, 1963).	To insure future healthy growth and development, and through specific tasks associated with each life stage, the OTA helps foster a positive sense of meaning in a child's life.
Abraham Maslow (1908–1979)	Humanistic	Discontinuity	Progressing through the hierarchy of needs, every person is motivated to mature and develop to his or her greatest potential, and ultimately, the most self-fulfilled person possible (Maslow, 1970; Maslow, 1968).	The most basic needs must be met prior to moving up the hierarchy, and like the principles and practice of occupational therapy, until fundamental skills are integrated, further progress toward goal acquisition may be impeded.

(*continues on page 90*)

TABLE 8.2 Developmental Theorists and Developmental Concepts (continued)

Theorist	Theoretical Orientation	Continuity or Discontinuity?	Basic Premise	Application to the OT Practitioner
Urie Bronfenbrenner (1917–2005)	Human Ecology, Social Systems	Continuity	A systems based theory proposing that a child develops as a result of the interactions of all parts of the ecosystem (environment) (Bronfenbrenner, 1986; Bronfenbrenner, 1979)	The OTA provides intervention at all levels of a child's environments to adapt, modify, and facilitate functional abilities.
B.F. Skinner (1904–1990)	Classical Learning	Continuity	Learning is a change in behavior that results from experiences. Humans are capable of being "shaped" by predictable patterns of learning known as reinforcement and punishment techniques (Skinner, 1974).	Reinforcement schedules are frequently used by the OTA to support and encourage learning of new and desired skills and behaviors or to extinguish undesired skills or behaviors.
Albert Bandura (1925–)	Classical Learning	Continuity	Learning or cognition develops through observation or modeling, rather than direct reinforcement (Santrock, 2012).	When working with children, modeling and observation are useful tools for the OTA. Modeling might also be used to support abstract concepts, such as modeling a kind action.
Konrad Lorenz (1903–1989)	Ethology	Continuity	Looks at the biological relationship between critical or sensitive periods in development and the importance they play in later growth. Attachment theory is based on ethology (Miller, 2001).	The OTA supports the facilitation of critical periods of development as well as helps to foster nurturing relationships between child and primary caregiver.

Adapted with permission from SLACK Incorporated: Wagenfeld A, Kaldenberg J. *Foundations of Pediatric Practice for the Occupational Therapy Assistant.* Thorofare, NJ: SLACK Incorporated; 2005.

to negative outside influences, such as exposure to maternal alcohol consumption, tobacco, radiation, and chemicals. Collectively referred to as **teratogens**, the impact of exposure to these negative influences may lead to harmful, sometimes lifetime, effects.

Infancy: Birth to 18 Months

Infancy is the period from birth to 18 months. During the first 18 months of life, typically developing infants more than triple their birth weight and grow at a very rapid rate (Table 8.3). During the first 18 months of life, typically developing children learn to walk; use their hands purposefully; begin to use language; communicate with others, to play; and develop their first and most profound attachment relationship (often with a mother). Infants learn about their world through sensorimotor experiences (Piaget & Inhelder, 1969), but cultural and psychosocial influences also guide early development.

Early Childhood: 18 Months to 5 to 6 Years

Beginning at 18 months and continuing until about age 6, early childhood is a time for children to develop peer relationships and begin to explore a first taste of independence from primary caregivers, be they at

Trimester	Period	Weeks	Size	Major developments
First	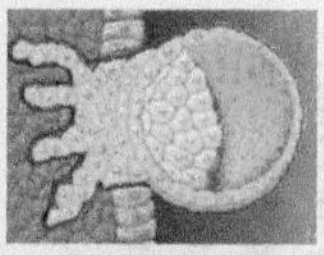 Zygote	1		One-celled zygote divides and becomes a blastocyst.
		2		Blastocyst implants into uterine wall; structures that nourish and protect the organism—amnion, chorion, yolk sac, placenta, umbilical cord—begin to form.
	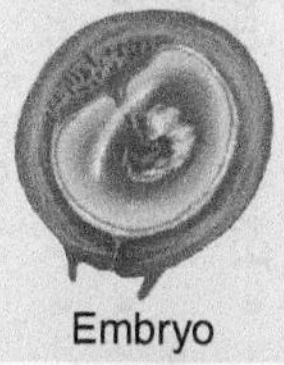 Embryo	3–4	1/4 in.	Brain, spinal cord, and heart form, as do the rudimentary structures that will become the eyes, ears, nose, mouth, and limbs.
		5–8	1 in., 1.4 oz	External body structures (eyes, ears, limbs) and internal organs form; embryo produces its own blood and can now move.
	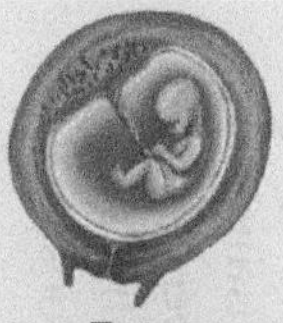 Fetus	9–12	3 in., 1 oz	Rapid growth and interconnections of all organ systems permit such new competencies as body and limb movements, swallowing, digestion of nutrients, and urination; external genitalia form.
Second	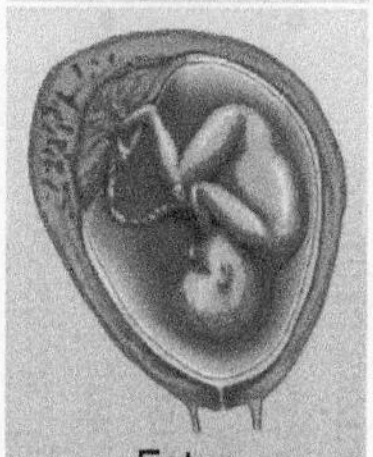 Fetus	13–24	14–15 in., 2 lb	The fetus grows rapidly. Fetal movements are felt by the mother, and fetal heartbeat can be heard. The fetus is covered by vernix to prevent chapping; it also reacts to bright lights and loud sounds.
Third	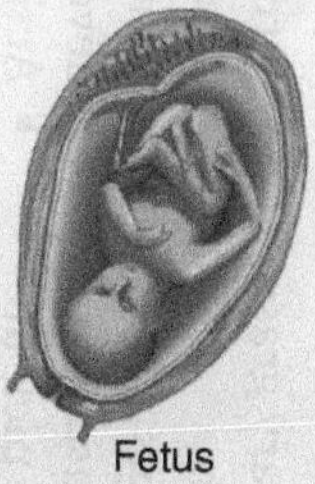 Fetus	25–38	19–21 in., 7–8 lb	Growth continues, and all organ systems mature in preparation for birth. Fetus reaches the age of viability and becomes more regular and predictable in its sleep cycles and motor activity. A layer of fat develops under the skin. Activity becomes less frequent and sleep more frequent during the last 2 weeks before birth.

Figure 8.2 A brief overview of prenatal development. (Adapted with permission from Shaffer D, Kipp K. *Developmental Psychology: Childhood and Adolescence*. 8th ed. Clifton Park, NY: Cengage Learning; 2009.)

childcare, preschool, or elementary school (Table 8.4). Associated with independence, one of the important developmental tasks of early childhood is to experience a sense of autonomy. Think about the "terrible twos." Tantrums are really a child's way of asserting him-/herself. The caregiver's job is to set limits, while respecting the child's desire to make choices, a first step toward independence.

During early childhood, engaging in the occupation of play is a very important means to nurture development (please also refer to Chapter 37, *Children and Youth*). Figure 8.3 illustrates the myriad reasons why play is so important for healthy development.

During early childhood, cognitive and language skills are also expanding at an incredible pace, as are gross and fine motor skills. By the time a child enters kindergarten, most are able to do fine motor skills such as tie shoes, hold a pencil with a mature grasp pattern, cut with scissors, and do complex gross motor skills like kick a ball, jump, navigate through obstacle courses, and have a spoken vocabulary of over 10,000 spoken words.

Middle Childhood: 6 to 10 Years

The time period between ages 6 and 10 is called middle childhood (Table 8.5). This period of development is focused on tasks relating to school and academic skills and developing close peer relationships. For children receiving special education and related services, by as early as 8th grade, initial discussion about transitioning out of public education (age 21) and what the child may do after publication education and related services terminate may begin. To master the skills of middle childhood, motor, cognitive, psychosocial, and spiritual development continues to undergo significant refinement during this time. If a child enters puberty during middle childhood, physical growth is fast and furious.

TABLE 8.3 Lifespan Developmental Milestones: Birth to 18 Months

Self-Care	Gross Motor	Fine Motor	Social/Emotional	Cognitive/Language	Sensory Motor/play
Birth to 1 month: Rapid height and weight gain; if within visual range (18 in.), eyes fix on another's face					
• Strong reflexive suck-swallow reflex allows baby to feed • Lack of established feeding schedule, feeds on demand	• Random movements with flexor withdrawal • Thoracic extension emerges • Lifts and turns head in supportive sitting • Stepping and swimming reflexes present	• Reflexive ulnar grasp	• All primary emotions are present • Reciprocal communication developing; learning that crying leads to being picked up • Makes eye contact	• Piagetian Sensorimotor stage of development (birth to 2 y) • Remembers object that reappears after 2 s • Random vocalizations	• Startles spontaneously • Alerts to and beginning to localize to sounds • Soothed by music • State modulation present, ability to be awake or to block out all stimuli and sleep • Alert 1 of every 10 h
2 months: Rapid height and weight gain					
• Rudimentary sleep-wake cycle develops	• Lifts head 45 degrees when prone on belly • Holds head fairly erect yet wobbly quality persists • Turns from side to back	• Begins to bat at hanging objects • Involuntary release • Attempts to bring hand to mouth	• Responds with interest to people • Smiles when sees human faces • Studies own movements and can repeat them	• Starting to discriminate sounds	• Self-regulation emerges • Quiets self by sucking • Studies hands • Slowly tracks objects with eyes
3 months: Rapid height and weight gain					
• Feeding schedule with longer intervals between is establishing	• Holds head up with control when prone on belly • Raises head and chest when prone on belly • Rolls from front to back • Kicks and straightens legs • Sits with support	• Ulnar grasp reflex disappearing • Voluntary grasp emerges • Attempts to reach and grasp, but cannot pick up objects	• Watches people • Recognizes primary caregivers • Primary attachment relationships developing • Actively seeks out attention of caregivers • Temperament styles and activity levels emerge • Social smile established	• Memory developing • Distinguishes speech from other sounds • Coos	• Exploratory and interactive play begins • Explores face, eyes, and mouth with hands • Localizes to sound • Visually seeks out source of sounds • Visual tracking improves; eyes now track in 180-degree plane

4 months: Rapid height and weight gain					
• Recognizes bottle • May begin to take pureed food • Feeding equated with play	• Lifts head up 90 degrees when prone on belly • Pulls to sit with assistance • Hands and arms come to midline	• Voluntary ulnar grasp continues to develop • Reaches for and grasps objects • Holds rattle with one or both hands • Shakes rattle • Brings hands together at midline	• Responds to familiar people • Starts to smile at self in mirror, but does not understand it is them • Social laughter	• Vocalization increases • Begins to imitate sounds	• Responsive for more than an hour at a time • Explores objects with mouth • Pulls dangling toy to mouth to explore • Focuses at different distances and sees in full color • Follows moving object with eyes
5 months: Rapid height and weight gain					
• May begin to teethe	• Rolls from back to front • Pulls to sit with no head lag • Balances head steadily and holds it erect in supported sitting • Begins locomotion by rocking, rolling, and twisting • Brings feet to mouth to suck on toes	• Grasps object with entire hand and explores it • Begins to release and transfer objects from hand to hand	• Smiles at mirror image of self • Clearly recognizes parents and siblings • Tries to make contact with others via smiles and vocalizations • Expresses displeasure • Matches adults emotional expressions during face-to-face interactions		• Orients self to sounds • Depth perception emerging • Sensory exploration increases
6 months: Rapid height and weight gain; reflexes integrate					
• Enjoys playing with food • Begins to finger feed • May begin to use spoon with assist	• Rolls in all directions • Balances well in ring sitting • Crawls by pulling stomach with legs and steering with arms • Primitive reflexes declining • Pulls objects towards self	• Radial palmar grasp emerges • Transfers objects from hand to hand • Reaches for toys with one or both hands	• Begins to focus away from interactions with attachment figures to the external environment • Mental representations developing, baby able to keep parent "in mind" even when not in sight • Developing subjective sense of self	• Beginning of Piagetian schemas (action plans) • Studies objects for a long time, very attentive • Turns to source when name is called • Starts to entertain self for short periods of time	• Follows path of falling objects • Depth perception developed • Pattern perception emerging • Sleep patterns emerging day and night • Hearing is more accurate • Attuned to sounds of native language

(continues on page 94)

TABLE 8.3 Lifespan Developmental Milestones: Birth to 18 Months (continued)

Self-Care	Gross Motor	Fine Motor	Social/Emotional	Cognitive/Language	Sensory Motor/play
			• Sense of humor emerges • Understands "no"	• Attention becomes more efficient • Recognition memory for people, places, and objects improves • Forms perceptual categories based on objects and similar features • Establishes joint attention with caregiver, who labels objects and events • Coos or hums to music • Makes v, th, f, s, sh, m, n, sounds	
6–8 months					
• Drinks from a cup with assist • Holds bottle independently	• Primitive reflexes integrated • Pushes up on hands and knees and rocks • Begins to creep on all fours • Bounces when held in standing • Sits independently • Assists in pull to stand from sitting • Creeps on hands and knees forward and backwards • Creeps with object in hand	• Attempts to grasp objects using raking motion • Holds two objects simultaneously • When holding objects in each hand, may hit them together • Lateral pinch developing • Can pick up a string	• Primary emotions of anger, fear, and sadness become more evident and increase in frequency and intensity • Shows interest in being part of social interactions • Wary of strangers • Firmly attached to primary caregiver (usually mother) • Objects to confinement • Sense of humor developing • Shouts for attentions	• Improved concentration • Imitates a wide variety of sounds and noises • Imitates hand movements • Points and follows what others point to • Recalls past events • Beginning to do simple problem solving • Engages in intentional, or goal-directed, behavior	• Explores body with mouth and hands • Enjoys reciprocal social games like peek-a-boo • Plays vigorously with noisy toys • Claps • Can hold an object in one hand and play with a different toy in the other hand

9–11 months					
• Grasps handle of lidded cup and drinks • Self feeds finger foods • Eats mashed table foods • Swallows with mouth closed • Developing greater skill with utensil use	• Creeps quickly and efficiently • Equilibrium/righting reflexes emerge • Beginning to take steps with hands held • Stand with hands placed on furniture • Half-kneeling emerges • Pulls up to stand • Cruises along furniture • Squats and stoops • Walks with one hand held • Crawls upstairs	• Inferior pincer grasp emerges; able to pick up small objects with flattened thumb and finger • Voluntary releases objects • Bangs objects together or singularly • Three-jaw chuck grasp developing • Removes objects from containers in one hand • Tip pinch emerging • Picks up tiny objects • Lifts lids from boxes • Turns pages of book (not exactly one at a time)	• Pushes away undesirable things (like food!) • Attachment behavior and separation anxiety is evident • Empathy emerges; may cry when another baby cries in their presence • Performs for attention • Seeks out attention and companionship • Sexual identity emerging • Not always cooperative	• Explores features of familiar people • Object permanence (ability to understand even when something is out of sight, it still exists) emerges and is well established by 11 months • Simple imitative motor behaviors improving • Imitates non-speech sounds • Imitates consonant/vowel combinations • Beginning to use gestural language • Understands and obeys some words and commands • Waves bye-bye • Memory skills improving • Working on figuring out simple relationships (such as how a button turns a toy on)	• Beginning to actively explore the world beyond the door- becoming an explorer • Deliberately chooses special toys to play with • Fears heights, afraid of vertical surfaces • Able to focus for about 5 minutes to play alone or with another adult • Enjoys water play • Uses fingers to poke and touch objects in play

(*continues on page 96*)

TABLE 8.3 Lifespan Developmental Milestones: Birth to 18 Months (continued)

Self-Care	Gross Motor	Fine Motor	Social/Emotional	Cognitive/Language	Sensory Motor/play
12–15 months					
• Feeds self with spillage • May refuse to try new foods • Assists with dressing; pulls off (doffs) socks, hats, mittens	• Stands alone • Lowers self to sitting from stand • Takes first steps using wide based gait • Crawls up and down stairs • Rolls ball in imitation	• Mature tip pincer grasp established • Puts objects into and removes them from containers and boxes • Stacks rings • Opens and closes things	• Beginning of social referencing; looking to parent to gauge own emotional response • Begins to care for dolls or stuffed toys • Starts to identify body parts • Imitates gestures and facial expressions • Resists napping and may throw tantrums	• Looks at familiar objects and persons when named • First meaningful words • Memory improves • Responds to simple 1-step directions • Identifies animals in pictures • 2 to 3 word vocabulary (12 mo) • Completes simple foam board puzzles	• Representational play, i.e. uses a spoon to feed a baby doll • Likes to squeeze, twist, and pull different kinds of textured objects
15–18 months					
• Extends arms and legs to help with dressing	• Walks forward and backwards • Walks with stable stops and starts • Walks up and down steps by holding a railing or with assist from an adult • Begins to run • Climbs on furniture	• Uses and reaches with preferred hand (dominance not yet established) • Builds a 4 block tower • Puts small objects into and removes them from a narrow necked bottle • Makes spontaneous marks with crayons	• Becomes interested in mirror image of self • Separation anxiety may persist	• Follows 1-step commands • Points to body parts upon request • 10–12 word vocabulary and accompanying gestures to communicate thoughts • Holographic speech emerges; one word conveys an entire thought	• May use objects in play in symbolic ways, such as a rectangular block becomes a train.

TABLE 8.4 Lifespan Developmental Milestones: Early Childhood: 18 Months to 6 Years

Self-Care	Gross Motor	Fine Motor	Social/Emotional	Cognitive/Language	Sensory Motor/Play
18–24 months					
• Independently spoon feeds • Removes all clothing • Drinks from cup proficiently • May show interest in toilet training	• Walks with stable gait • Sits by self in small chair • Throws ball	• Moves small objects from fingers to palm of same hand • Places pegs in holes • Puts objects into small cups or containers • Makes scribbles using a primitive grasp	• Sense of self emerges • Displays greater range of emotions • Recognizes self in mirror consistently • Shows attachment and nurturance towards a stuffed toy	• Knows most if not all body parts • Follows 2-step commands • Functional use of objects well-established • Hums	• Begins to accept wider types of touch, such as roughhousing • Tolerates different textures of clothing • Symbolic play (substituting one thing for another) • Parallel play (playing next to other children) begins • Plays alone or with others for 15 minutes
2–2.5 years: Slower height and weight gains than in infancy; walking becomes better coordinated as balance improves; running, jumping, hopping, throwing, and catching skills emerge					
• Puts shoes on and takes them off (no fasteners) • Turns door knob • Uses spoon proficiently	• Walks up and down stairs independently • Runs proficiently • Catches large ball with hands and arms	• Moves small objects from palm to fingers of same hand • Builds 6-block tower • Able to open loose jar lids • Beginning scissor skills • Imitates vertical lines on paper • Draws circles	• Coping mechanisms developing (limited) • Seeks parental approval • Self-concept and self-esteem improving • Cooperation and instrumental aggression appear • Understands causes, consequences, and behavioral signs of basic emotions • Empathy increases	• Piagetian Preoperational Stage of Development (2–7 years) • 220 word vocabulary • Utters 3-word sentences • Uses personal pronoun "I" • Refers to self by name • Begins to ask questions • Begins to sort objects by shape and color • Able to find hidden objects • Simple perspective taking emerges • Rapid acquisition of new words • Sentences start to follow basic word order of native language; grammatical markers are added • Displays effective conversational skills, such as turn taking and topic maintenance	• Independently selects toys • Parallel play • Plays house, imitates domestic tasks • Make-believe play is emerging and less dependent on realistic toys, less self-centered, and more complex.

(continues on page 98)

TABLE 8.4 Lifespan Developmental Milestones: Early Childhood: 18 Months to 6 Years (continued)

Self-Care	Gross Motor	Fine Motor	Social/Emotional	Cognitive/Language	Sensory Motor/Play
2–2.5 years: Slower height and weight gains than in infancy; walking becomes better coordinated as balance improves; running, jumping, hopping, throwing, and catching skills emerge					
• Puts shoes on and takes them off (no fasteners) • Turns door knob • Uses spoon proficiently	• Walks up and down stairs independently • Runs proficiently • Catches large ball with hands and arms	• Moves small objects from palm to fingers of same hand • Builds 6-block tower • Able to open loose jar lids • Beginning scissor skills • Imitates vertical lines on paper • Draws circles	• Coping mechanisms developing (limited) • Seeks parental approval • Self-concept and self-esteem improving • Cooperation and instrumental aggression appear • Understands causes, consequences, and behavioral signs of basic emotions • Empathy increase	• Piagetian Preoperational Stage of Development (2–7 years) • 220 word vocabulary • Utters 3-word sentences • Uses personal pronoun "I" • Refers to self by name • Begins to ask questions • Begins to sort objects by shape and color • Able to find hidden objects • Simple perspective taking emerges • Rapid acquisition of new words • Sentences start to follow basic word order of native language; grammatical markers are added • Displays effective conversational skills, such as turn taking and topic maintenance	• Independently selects toys • Parallel play • Plays house, imitates domestic tasks • Make-believe play is emerging and less dependent on realistic toys, less self-centered, and more complex.
2.5–3 years					
• Starts to brush teeth and hair • Independently dons simple clothes	• Throws ball • Walks up stairs with alternating feet • Tip toes • Walks backward • Kicks ball	• Builds 8-block tower • Can screw and unscrew 3-in. lids from jars • Strings 1-in. beads • Establishes hand dominance	• Frequently imitates caregiver behavior • Gender identity emerges • Recognizes self in a photo	• Telegraphic speech emerges- short sentences that contain only essential words "boy cookie" may mean "I want a cookie" • Increases use of pronouns • Asks "why" • Understands simple questions • Names objects in a picture • Matches and discriminates colors • Completes simple 2-piece puzzles	• Engages in more complex pretend play

3–4 years					
• Requires little help to dress and undress • Uses fork and spoon with ease • Stays dry at night	• Stands on one foot • Jumps in place • Pedals tricycle • Running, hopping, throwing and catching are more coordinated • One-foot skipping and galloping emerge	• Builds 10-block tower • Constructs a 3 to 4 block train • Strings half-inch beads • Folds piece of paper • Makes snips with scissors • Static tripod pencil grasp (3.5 to 5 years) • Copies vertical and horizontal lines, circles, square, and cross. • Draws first picture of a person • Drawing of a person consists of a head with legs	• Begins to understand different emotional responses • Becomes better at regulating emotions • Emotional self-regulation improves • Self-conscious emotions become more common • Displays humorous and mischievous behaviors • Negative and oppositional at times • Oedipal issues may emerge (romantic attachment to opposite sex parent) • Instrumental aggression declines and hostile aggression increase • Forms first friendships • Distinguishes moral rules from conventions • Preference for same sex playmates strengthens	• Puts together a 8 to 10 piece puzzle • 900 to 1,000 word vocabulary • Speaks in short sentences (4 plus words) • Uses plurals and tenses (not always correctly) • Masters increasingly complex grammatical structures • Occasionally overextends grammatical rules to exceptions • Uses private speech to guide behavior in challenging tasks • Can count to 10 by rote with no one-to-one correspondence • Tells simple stories • Language supersedes actions in communication • Follows 2-step directions • Recognizes simple shapes • Attention becomes more sustained and planned • Aware of some meaningful features of written language • Counts small number of objects and grasps • cardinality • Can tell the difference between writing and nonwriting	• Beginning to participate in more complex exploratory and imitative play • Imaginative and creative play emerges • Begins turn take in play

(*continues on page 100*)

TABLE 8.4 Lifespan Developmental Milestones: Early Childhood: 18 Months to 6 Years (continued)

Self-Care	Gross Motor	Fine Motor	Social/Emotional	Cognitive/Language	Sensory Motor/Play
• Buttons and unbuttons large buttons • Independently dresses and undresses • Ties shoes (5 years)	• Descends steps wit reciprocal gait pattern • Balances on one foot • Hops and skips • Catches ball using hands	• Able to cut straight and simple curved lines with 25% accuracy • Begins to use tools such as hammers	• Begins to mask emotions • Morality is not rule-based; focused on rewards and punishments	• Repeats a 5 to 10 word sentence • Repeats 5 to 7 numbers • Carries on a reciprocal conversation	• Pretend play is more logical • Cooperative play becomes more evident
	• Bounces a ball • Throws overhands	• Performs rapid alternating forearm movements • Copies triangle, simple words, and name with little awareness of spacing or size • Draws more elaborate, writes names	• Resolves conflicts with peers with greater ease • Guilt emerges • Peer interaction increases • Ability to interpret, predict, and influence others' emotional reactions improves • Relies more on language to express empathy • Has acquired many morally relevant rules and behaviors • Racial identity emerges • Gender-stereotyped beliefs and behavior continue to increase • Grasps the genital basis of sex differences and shows gender constancy	• Begins to be a more logical thinker • Cause and effect thinking emerges • Understands "why" questions • Begins to understand opposites such as big and little • Understands differences such as circle and square • 1 to 1 correspondence with counting 3 objects emerges • Vocabulary increases to about 10,000 words • Mastered many complex grammatical forms	

TABLE 8.5 Lifespan Developmental Milestones: Late Childhood: Age 6–10 Years

Physical	Self-Care	Gross Motor	Fine Motor	Social/Emotional	Cognitive/Language	Sensory Motor/ play
• Slower gains in weight and height continue until adolescent growth spurt • Gradual replacement of primary teeth by permanent ones throughout middle childhood • Adolescent growth spurt begins 2 y earlier in girls than in boys • Reaction time improves contributing to motor skill development • Representation of depth in drawings expands	• Uses knife to spread jelly or butter (6 y) • Uses brush or comb in functional manner • Engages a zipper • Begins to participate in instrumental activities of daily living (IADL)	• Masters ball skills • Masters bike riding (6–7 y) • Learns to swim • Learns to skate • Running, jumping, throwing, catching, kicking, batting, and dribbling are executed faster and with improved coordination	• Becomes adept at the use of school tools • Learns and masters manuscript writing • Writing becomes smaller and more legible. • Letter reversals decline • Learns and masters cursive writing • Drawing becomes increasingly more representational • Drawings become more organized and detailed; include some depth cues	• Attachment needs are also met by peers, and not only parents • Social perspective taking, understanding other's views emerges • Compliance with display rules of emotions improving • Improved sense of self • Self-esteem further develops • Self-efficacy (recognizing strengths and limits) emerges • Uses psychological traits to define self • Begins to engage in more like-gender social relationships • Self-concept begins to include personality traits and social comparisons • Self-conscious emotions of pride and guilt are governed by personal responsibility • Recognizes that people may experience amore than one emotion at a time • Increasingly more responsible and independent • Peer interaction becomes more pro-social, physical aggression declines • Self-esteem tends to rise • Adaptive set of strategies for regulating emotion present • Can "step into another's shoes" and view the self from the other person's perspective • Peer groups emerge • Becomes aware of more gender stereotypes, including personality traits and school subjects, but has a more flexible appreciation of what males and females can do	• Piagetian Concrete Operational Stage of Development (7–12 y) • Reverse thinking emerges; analyze from end, then back to beginning • Improved perception of reality • Understanding of cause and effect well established • Improved memory • Executive processes emerging; improved problem solving, better focus and attention to task • Applies logic to thinking • Pragmatics of language develop • Piagetian Formal Operational Stage of Development (12 y) • Vocabulary increases rapidly throughout middle childhood • Thought becomes more logical, as shown by the ability to pass Piagetian conservation, class inclusion, and problems • Understanding of spatial concept improves, can give clear, well-organized directions • Attention is more selective, adaptable, and planful • Uses memory strategies of rehearsal and organization • Word definitions are concrete, referring to functions and appearance • Memory strategies of rehearsal and organization become more effective. Begins to use elaboration • Use of complex grammatical construction improves • Applies multiple memory strategies simultaneously	• Fantasy play becomes more ritualized • Play takes on a work orientation in the form of formal games • Becomes interested in collections and hobbies • Organized games with rules become common

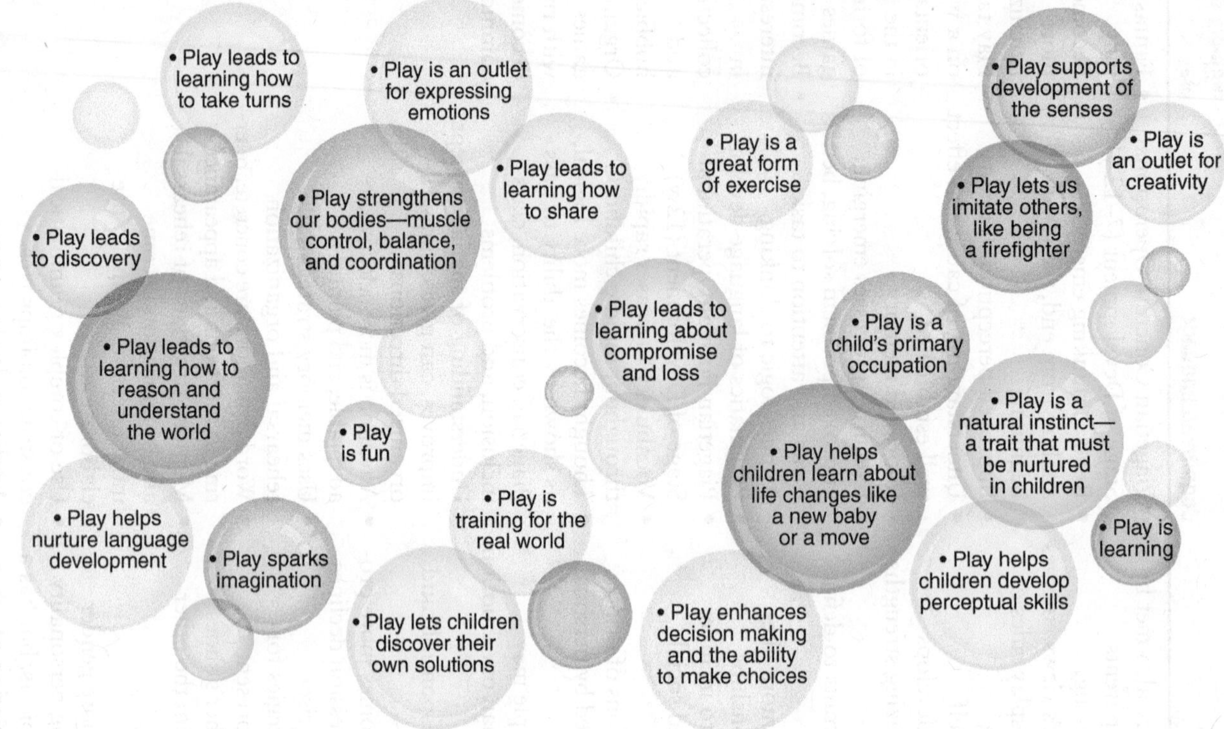

Figure 8.3 Why play is important for children.

For others, physical growth tends to slow down during middle childhood, yet for them, major changes are just around the corner.

Adolescence: 11 to 19 Years

Adolescence is a time in life that is often associated with turbulence and angst. In part, this turbulence is attributed to the significant hormonal and emotional changes that adolescents experience as they prepare to enter adulthood (Table 8.6). Many people go through puberty during adolescence (or the end of middle childhood) and, like infancy, experience rapid physical growth. Becoming comfortable and accustomed to an adult body is a challenge for many adolescents. The major tasks of adolescence are developing self-identity and autonomy, which are closely associated with psychosocial and spiritual development (From the Field 8.1).

Adulthood

Adulthood is typically divided into three periods, early adulthood, middle adulthood, and older adulthood. The themes of adulthood focus less on motor and cognitive development and more on psychosocial and spiritual development. What we do know about adulthood is that in addition to genetic predisposition to a long life, longevity is associated with daily exercise of the body (motor) by staying active by walking, swimming, and yoga. It is also known that exercising the mind (cognitive) is equally as important by doing daily mental challenges such as crossword puzzles, computations, or memorization activities. Another quality associated with longevity is a sense of belonging to a group, a family, work colleagues, social networks, friends, etc.

Early Adulthood: 20 to 40 Years

From ages 20 to 40, young adults experience peak and optimal performance within all areas of development (Table 8.7). Physical functioning is at its best and intellectual skills are sharp (Shaw & Cronin, 2005). For most young adults, the first wave of mature self-identity is experienced, leading to monumental psychosocial and spiritual developmental changes. During the early adulthood years, most people enter into committed relationships and career paths (first careers!) are determined and embarked upon.

Middle Adulthood: 40 to 65 Years

During middle adulthood, a time period from 40 to 65 years, many people begin to experience age-related physical challenges that may manifest later in life

TABLE 8.6 Lifespan Developmental Milestones: Adolescence: Age 11–18 Years

Self-Care	Gross Motor	Fine Motor	Social/Emotional	Cognitive/Language	Sensory Motor/Play
• Independent with self-care • Begins to help with meal preparation and take on other household responsibilities (IADL tasks) • Learns to manage money • Learns to navigate in the community	• Becomes proficient with all gross motor tasks	• Becomes proficient at all fine motor skills and applies this ability to all aspects of life including school work, self-care, and leisure pursuits	• Sibling rivalry tends to increase • Defining identity is important task • Self-concept becomes refined and based on other people's perspectives • Quest for autonomy may bring strife into parent-child relationship • Issues of sexuality emerge • Dating begins • Moodiness and parent-child conflict increase • Spends less time with parents and siblings • Spends more time with peers • Friendships are based on intimacy and loyalty • Peer groups become organized around cliques • Cliques with similar values unite forming crowds • Conformity to peer pressure increases • Self-esteem tends to rise • Is likely to be searching for an identity • Importance of cliques and crowd declines • Has probably started dating • Conforms to peer pressure may decline	• Conversational strategies becomes more refined • Abstract thought is cornerstone • Thinks hypothetically • Verbal and mathematical skills improve • Sense of invulnerability ("it cannot happen to me") may be problematic and danger-provoking • Becomes capable of formal operational reasoning • Becomes better at coordinating theory with evidence • Can argue more effectively • Becomes more self-conscious and self-focused • Becomes more idealistic and critical • Becomes less conscious and self-focused • Becomes better at everyday planning and decision-making	• Participates in competitive team sports

Physical milestones: If female, reaches peak of growth spurt; if male, reaches peak then completes growth spurt, voice deepens, adds muscle while body fat declines; motor performances increase dramatically; may have had sexual intercourse.

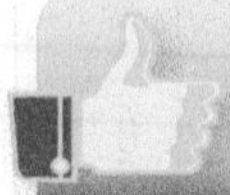

FROM THE FIELD 8.1

Considering Adolescence

Like their typically developing peers, adolescent clients struggle with developing self-identity. No matter whether it is based on physical, intellectual, or psychological challenges, it is important to provide interventions directed toward developing developmentally appropriate levels of autonomy. This approach aligns closely with client-centered intervention.

as chronic conditions (Shaw & Cronin, 2005; Table 8.8). Intellectual functioning remains sharp. In terms of psychosocial development, for most middle-aged adults, the way in which they view the world is now more sophisticated, in large part due to life experiences. Family dynamics often undergo significant change during this time. Children may leave home and live on their own, while some, due to myriad financial or social reasons, remain at home. Many middle-aged adults find themselves caring for grown children as well as their aging parents, a phenomenon known as the sandwich generation (Shaw & Cronin, 2005). Facing one's own mortality and desiring to make sure that life goals have or are going to be fulfilled are themes common to middle adulthood (Shaw & Cronin, 2005).

TABLE 8.7 Lifespan Developmental Milestones: Early Adulthood: Age 20–40 Years

Physical	Gross Motor	Social/Emotional	Cognitive/ Language
20–30 years			
• Declines in touch sensitivity; respiratory, cardiovascular, and immune system functioning; and elasticity of the skin begins and continues throughout adulthood • With decline of BMR, gradual weight gain begins in the middle of the decade and continues through middle adulthood	• Athletic skills requiring speed of limb movement, explosive strength, and gross body coordination peak early in this decade and then decline • Athletic skills that depend on endurance, arm—hand steadiness, and aiming peak at the end of this decade and then decline	• Leaves home permanently • Strives to make a permanent commitment to an intimate partner • Usually constructs a dream, an image of the self in the adult world that guides decision-making • Begins to develop mutually gratifying adult friendships and work ties • May cohabit, marry, and bear children • Sibling relationships become more companionable • With movement in and out of relationships, loneliness peaks early in this decade and then declines steadily throughout adulthood	
30–40 years			
• Declines in vision, hearing, and the skeletal system begin and continue throughout adulthood • In women, fertility problems increase sharply in the middle of this decade • Hair begins to gray and thin in the middle of this decade • Sexual activity declines, probably due to demands of daily life		• Reevaluates life structure and attempts to change components that are inadequate • Establishes a more stable niche within society through family, occupational, and community activities (for women, career consolidation may be delayed)	• As family and lives expand, the cognitive capacity to balance myriad responsibilities simultaneously improves • Creativity often peaks

TABLE 8.8 Lifespan Developmental Milestones: Ages 40–65 Years

Physical	Social/Emotional	Cognitive/Language
40–50 years		
• Accommodative ability of the lens of the eye and color discrimination declines; sensitivity to glare increases • Sharp hearing loss at high frequency occurs • Hair continues to gray and thin • Lines on the face become more pronounced, and skin loses elasticity • Weight gain continues, accompanied by a rise in fatty deposits in the torso, whereas fat beneath the skin declines • Loss of lean body mass occurs • In women, production of estrogen drops, leading to short, ending of, irregularity in the menstrual cycle • For men, quantity of semen and sperm declines, intensity of sexual response declines, but sexual activity drops only slightly; stability is more typical than dramatic change • Rates of cancer and cardiovascular disease increase, at a higher rate for women	• Modifies components of life structure, focusing on personally meaningful living • Possible selves decline and are more modest and concrete • Self-acceptance, autonomy, and environmental mastery increases • Coping strategies become more effective • Gender identity becomes more androgynous: "masculine" traits increase in women, and "feminine" traits increase in men • May launch children • May enlarge the family network to include in-laws • May care for parent with illness or disability • Sibling bonds may strengthen • Number of friends typically declines • Job satisfaction increases	• Consciousness of aging increases • Processing speed, assessed on reaction time tasks declines; compensation happens by taking large chunks of information into working memory and throughout practice and experience • Amount of information that can be retained in working memory diminishes due to decline in use of memory • Retrieving information from long-term memory becomes more difficult • General factual knowledge, procedural knowledge related to one's occupation remain unchanged or increases • Gains in practical problem solving and expertise occur
50–65 years		
• Lens of the eye loses its accommodative ability entirely • Hearing loss extends to all frequencies but remains greatest for highest tones • Skin continues to wrinkle and sag; age spots appear • Menopause occurs, usually between 50 and 55 • Continued loss of bone mass, accelerates for women after menopause. Leads to high rate of diagnosis of osteoporosis • Due to collapse of disks in the spinal column, height may drop by as much as 1 in.	• Re-evaluates life's structure and tries to change components that are inadequate • Becomes concerned with "passing the torch" • May become a grandparent • Parent-to-child child help-giving declines, and child-to-parent help-giving increases • May retire	

TABLE 8.9 Lifespan Developmental Milestones: Ages 65+

Physical	Social/Emotional	Cognitive/Language	Sensory Motor/Play
60–70 years			
• Neurons die at a faster rate, but the brain compensates through growth of new synapses • Autonomic nervous system performs less well, impairing adaptation to hot and cold weather conditions • Declines in vision continue. In terms of increased sensitivity to glare and impaired color decimation, dark adaptation, depth perception, and visual acuity • Declines in hearing continue throughout the frequency of the range • Taste and odor sensitivity may decline • Declines in cardiovascular and respiratory functions leading to greater physical stress during exercise • Aging of the immune system increases risk for a variety of illnesses • Sleep difficulties increase, especially for men • Graying and thinning of the hair continue; the skin wrinkles further and becomes more transparent as it loses its fatty layer of support • Height loss (due to loss of bone mass) continues, leading to rising rates of osteoporosis	• May become a great-grandparent • May retire	• Amount of information that can be retained in working memory diminishes further; memory problems are greatest on complex tasks requiring deliberate processing • Modest forgetting of remote memories occurs. Use of external aids for prospective memories occurs • Retrieving words from long-term memory and planning what to say become more difficult • Traditional problem solving declines; everyday problem solving remains adaptive • May excel at wisdom • Can improve a wide range of cognitive skills through training	• Touch sensitivity declines on the hands, particularly on the fingertips, less so on the arms
70 to 80+ years			
• Mobility diminishes due to loss of muscle and bone strength and joint flexibility	• As relatives and friends die, may develop friendships with younger individuals • Relationships with adult children become more important • Frequency and variety of leisure activities decline	• Cognitive changes continue	

TABLE **8.10** Sources for the Lifespan Developmental Milestones Tables (Tables 8.3–8.9)

Bergen D. *Human Development: Traditional and Contemporary Theories*. Upper Saddle River, NJ: Pearson Prentice Hall; 2008.
Berger KS. *The Developing Person Through the Life Span*. 7th ed. New York, NY: Worth Publishers; 2008.
Berk L. *Child Development*. 9th ed. Upper Saddle River, NJ: Pearson; 2012.
Bowlby J. *A Secure Base*. New York, NY: Basic Books; 1988.
Cavanaugh JC, Blanchard-Fields F. *Adult Development and Aging*. Clifton Park, NY: Cengage Learning; 2010.
Dacey JS, et al. *Human Development Across the Lifespan*. 7th ed.. New York, NY: McGraw Hill; 2008.
Denver II Online Developmental Screening. http://denverii.com/denverii/
Developmental Milestones. http://www.cdc.gov/ncbddd/actearly/pdf/checklists/all_checklists.pdf
Erhardt R. *Developmental Prehension Assessment*. Laurel, MD: Ramsco Publishing; 1982.
Feldman RS. *Development Across the Lifespan*. 7th ed. Upper Saddle River, NJ: Prentice Hall; 2013.
Frost J, et al. *Play and Child Development*. 4th ed. Upper Saddle River, NJ: Pearson; 2011.
Hawaii Early Learning Profile. http://www.vort.com/HELP-0-3-years-Hawaii-Early-Learning-Profile/
Hawaii Early Learning Profile 3–6 years. 2nd ed. http://www.vort.com/HELP-3-6-years-complements-HELP-0-3/
Hoyer W, Roodin P. *Adult Development and Aging*. New York, NY: McGraw Hill; 2008.
Krauss Whitbourne S, Whitbourne S. *Adult Development and Aging: Biopsychosocial Perspectives*. Hoboken, NJ: Wiley; 2014.
Kees DB, Schrauf RW. *Language Development Over the Lifespan*. New York, NY: Routledge; 2009.
Martin NA. *Test of Visual Motor Skills-3*. http://www.therapro.com/Test-of-Visual-Motor-Skills-3-TVMS-3-P321966C7662.aspx
McDevitt TM, Ormrod JE. *Child Development and Education*. 5th ed. Upper Saddle River, NJ: Pearson; 2012.
Piaget J, Inhelder B. *The Psychology of the Child*. 6th ed. Upper Saddle River, NJ: Pearson; 1969.
Santrock JW. *Children*. 12th ed. New York, NY: McGraw Hill; 2012.
Schaefer CE, Foy DiGeronimo T. *Ages and Stages: A Parent's Guide to Normal Childhood Development*. Hoboken, NJ: Wiley; 2008.
Shaffer DR. *Developmental Psychology: Childhood and Adolescence*. 9th ed. Belmont, CA: Wadsworth; 2013.
Steinberg L, et al. *Lifespan Development: Infancy Through Adulthood*. Clifton Park, NY: Cengage Learning; 2010.

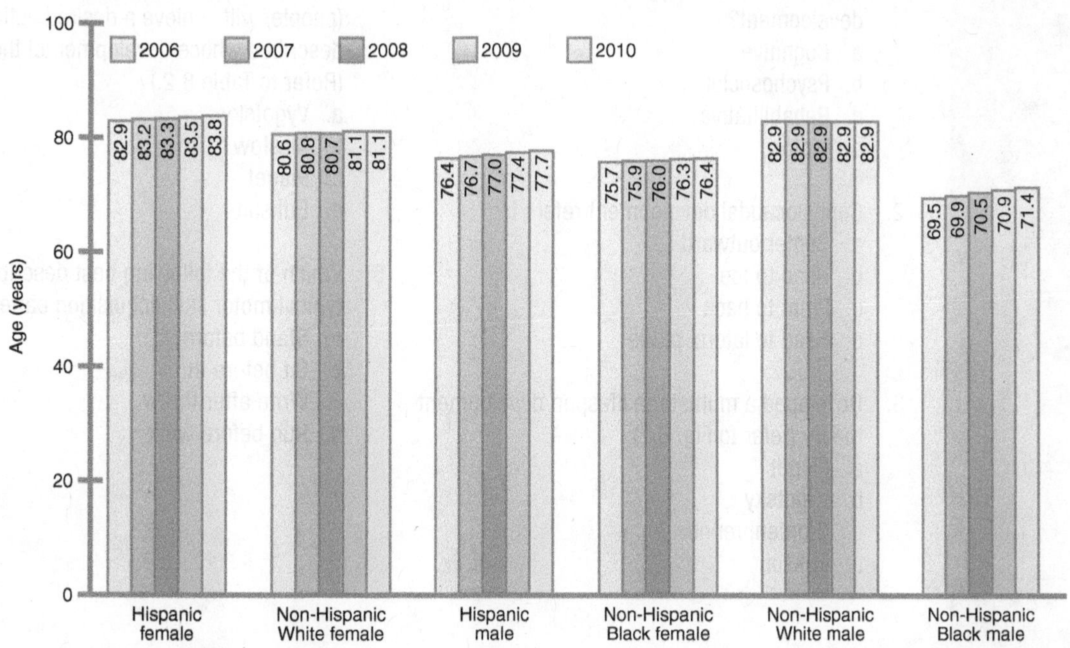

Figure 8.4 2007 CDC life expectancy statistics.

Older Adulthood: 65+ Years

The final period of life, older adult begins at age 65 (Table 8.9). The average lifespan in the United States has increased from 53 years in early part of the 20th century to 76 years in 2009 for men and from 54 to 80.9 years for women (Arias, 2014; U.S. Department of Health and Human Services, n.d.).

See Figure 8.4 for a more detailed analysis of life expectancy statistics.

Compounded in part by chronic disease and illness, normal age-related physical concerns that were just beginning to impact middle-aged adults might become problematic in older adults (Shaw & Cronin, 2005). Although not by any means inevitable, for some, cognitive function may decline and ultimately manifest as dementia. Psychosocial issues such as loss of a spouse or friends, changes in family structure, and retirement inevitably impact an older adult's life in some way (Shaw & Cronin, 2005). This is a reflective time in life, a period often associated with looking back at one's life accomplishments, but also looking forward to new challenges and experiences (Table 8.10).

Summary

There is much to be said about having a solid working knowledge of lifespan human development. While not absolutes, for most, acquisition of developmental skills occurs in an orderly fashion. Understanding the major themes of each developmental period helps you better appreciate the individuality and diversity of your clients. This knowledge helps you be prepared to develop and carry out occupational therapy intervention that is, to the greatest extent possible, client-centered and meaningful and purposeful. While the goal of development is to acquire the skills necessary to flourish and be prepared to move on to the next stage, for some, getting there is the challenge. And, these individuals will need help to do so. This is why OTAs are so important to help facilitate the process.

Review Questions

1. Which of the following is not an area of development?
   a. Cognitive
   b. Psychosocial
   c. Rehabilitative
   d. Motor

2. Cephalocaudal development refers to:
   a. Center outward
   b. Head to toe
   c. Front to back
   d. Head to lateral plane

3. Developed a multistage lifespan development theory (refer to Fig. 8.2):
   a. Piaget
   b. Vygotsky
   c. Bronfenbrenner
   d. Erikson

4. "Given time and support, most children (people) will achieve a desired action" best describes whose developmental theory? (Refer to Table 8.2.)
   a. Vygotsky
   b. Maslow
   c. Piaget
   d. Erikson

5. Which of the following best describes a typical motor skill acquisition pattern?
   a. Stand before sit
   b. Sit before throw
   c. Write after throw
   d. Run before walk

6. Which of the following best describes a proximal–distal development pattern?
   a. Raise arms upward before finger feeding
   b. Write before throw
   c. Grasp pencil before finger paint
   d. Kick before stand

7. Examples of teratogens do not include
   a. Radiation
   b. Alcohol or drugs
   c. Perfume
   d. Smoke

8. Which of the following is a developmental task associated with infancy?
   a. Jump
   b. Achieve autonomy
   c. Develop attachment relationships
   d. Complex sentence construction

9. While all of the below hold true, which of the following are the overarching major tasks of adolescence?
   a. Improve fine and gross motor skills
   b. Focus on self-identity and autonomy
   c. Improve language and mathematical skills
   d. Learn to drive and apply for college or a job

10. Peak intellectual and physical functioning occurs during:
    a. Infancy
    b. Adolescence
    c. Middle adulthood
    d. Young adulthood

11. The most recent Centers for Disease Control and Prevention 2007 statistics for all populations shows a(n) ____________ in life expectancy as compared to 2006.
    a. Increase
    b. Decrease
    c. Mixed findings
    d. No change

Practice Activities

Select one developmental theory that most appeals to you and lead a simple activity with your classmates that shows how the theory is put into action.

Interview a classmate and find out what his/her favorite leisure activity is. Write it down and then identify the gross motor, fine motor, sensory, psychosocial, and cognitive elements of the activity as well as which of the six AOTA *Occupational Therapy Practice Framework III* contexts influence it.

Interview a young adult, a middle-aged adult, and an older adult by first explaining the difference between nature and nurture and then ask them whether they believe that the obesity epidemic is the product of nature or nurture (or both). As an entire class, compile your findings and analyze your results. What trends do you see? As future OTAs, how can you positively impact this issue and be a catalyst for positive change?

References

American Occupational Therapy Association. *AOTA's Societal Statement on Obesity*. 2010. Retrieved from http://www.aota.org/.../Health-and-Wellness/Official-Docs/39432.aspx?FT=.pdfhttp://www.aota.org/Practitioners/Official.aspx

American Occupational Therapy Association. Occupational therapy practice framework: domain and process. 3rd ed. *Am J Occup Ther* 2014;68(Suppl 1):S1–S48. http://www.dx .doi.org/10.5014/ajot.2014.682006

Antonovsky A. *Unraveling the Mystery of Health: How People Manage Stress and Stay Well*. San Francisco, CA: Jossey-Bass; 1987.

Arias E. United States life tables, 2009. *Natl Vital Stat Rep* 2014;62(7):1–63.

Ayres AJ. *Sensory Integration and the Child*. Los Angeles, CA: Western Psychological Services; 1994.

Bronfenbrenner U. *Ecology of Human Development*. Cambridge, MA: Harvard University Press; 1979.

Bronfenbrenner U. Ecology of the family as a context for human development: Research perspectives. *Dev Psychol* 1986;22(6):723–742.

D'Ambrogio KJ, Roth GB. *Positional Release Therapy: Assessment and Treatment of Musculoskeletal Dysfunction*. St Louis, MO: Mosby; 1997.

Erikson E. *Childhood and Society*. New York, NY: W.W. Norton Company; 1963.

Erikson E. *The Lifestyle Completed*. New York, NY: W.W. Norton Company; 1982.

Kamii C. Pedagogical principles derived from Piaget's theory: relevance for educational practice. In: Schwebel M, Raph J, eds. *Piaget in the Classroom*. New York, NY: Basic Books; 1973:192–215.

Kielhofner G. *A Model of Human Development: Theory and Application*. 4th ed. New York, NY: Lippincott Williams & Wilkins; 2007.

Law M, et al. The Person-Environment-Occupation Model: a transactive approach to occupational performance. *Can J Occup Ther* 1996;63(1):9–23.

Maslow A. *Toward a Psychology of Being*. 2nd ed. New York, NY: van Nostrand Reinhold; 1968.

Maslow A. *Motivation and Personality*. 2nd ed. New York, NY: Harper and Row; 1970.

Miller PH. *Theories of Developmental Psychology*. 4th ed. New York, NY: Worth Publishers; 2001.

Piaget J, Inhelder B. *The Psychology of the Child*. New York, NY: Basic Books; 1969.

Santrock JW. *Child Development*. 14th ed. New York, NY: McGraw Hill; 2013.

Shaffer D, Kipp K. *Developmental Psychology: Childhood and Adolescence*. 8th ed. Clifton Park, NY: Cengage Learning; 2009.

Shaw K, Cronin A. Adulthood. In: Cronin A, Mandich M, eds. *Human Development and Performance Throughout the Lifespan*. pp. 284–305. Clifton Park, NY: Cengage Learning; 2005.

Skinner BF. *About Behaviorism*. New York, NY: Alfred A. Knopf; 1974.

U.S. Department of Health and Human Services. *The great pandemic. The United States in 1918–1919*. n.d. Retrieved from: http://www.flu.gov/pandemic/history/1918/life_in_1918/health/

Vygotsky L. *Mind in Society*. Cambridge, MA: Harvard University Press; 1978.

Wagenfeld AE. An overview of early development. In: Wagenfeld A, Kaldenberg J, eds. *Developmental Foundations of Pediatric Practice for the Occupational Therapy Assistant*. pp. 53–62. Thorofare, NJ: Slack, Inc.; 2005.

CHAPTER

9 Learning Theory

Amy Wagenfeld, PhD, OTR/L SCEM, CAPs

Key Terms

Extinction—Occurs when a behavior diminishes because there is no positive response or a negative response is stopped.

Learning—The process of transforming experience into knowledge (Kolb, 1984).

Learning styles—The myriad ways humans adapt and manage life events.

Negative reinforcement—A strategy for strengthening a desired behavior by causing a negative condition to be stopped or avoided as a consequence of the desired behavior.

Positive reinforcement—A strategy for strengthening a desired behavior through experiences that are pleasant and appealing.

Punishment—Weakens a behavior because negative conditions are imposed on a behavior.

Learning Objectives

After studying this chapter, readers should be able to:

- Compare and contrast the various theories of learning and learning styles in order to best understand how people learn.
- Explain how learning theory influences occupational therapy education and practice.
- Evaluate your personal learning style.

Introduction

Reading about learning may seem ill placed in an OTA textbook. To the contrary! Understanding how theorists interpret the learning process and how to best facilitate and nurture the processes directly correlates with successful practice. What and how you learn from your professors, supervising OTs, and other colleagues and, in turn, apply to your work with clients has a direct relationship to learning theories. Understanding the foundations of learning allows you to better able to appreciate the varied learning process clients go through along their journey to wellness. It allows you to be a better communicator and educator, whether it be with and for clients, families, and/or colleagues. Accordingly, as a future OTA, you will be helping your clients learn new skills or new and novel ways to relearn old skills. Learning does matter to our profession in terms of how we work with our clients and conduct research.

Theories of Learning

Before moving into a discussion of specific learning theories and styles, the base concept of **learning** is important to understand. According to Kolb, "Learning is the process whereby knowledge is created through the transformation of experience" (1984, p. 38). Burns' definition of learning is a "relatively permanent change in behaviour ... including observable activity and internal processes such as thinking, attitudes, and emotions" (1995, p. 99). Learning helps give meaning to our lives. There are many theories that offer explanations about how people learn. As you read about some of these theories, begin to think about how you learn and how you may effect change with the clients you work with and who, more than likely, will not learn the same way that you do.

Models of Learning Theory and Styles

We all apply learning to help us function and manage our lives, yet because we do so in different ways, theories offer explanations about different **learning styles**, or the ways in which people obtain and process information. There are several learning theories and learning styles applicable to health care professions that we will explore. Four major levels of learning styles are listed below in diminishing order of stability (Brown et al., 2008; Katz & Heimann, 1990). These are personality traits, information processing, social interaction, and instructional preference (Fig. 9.1).

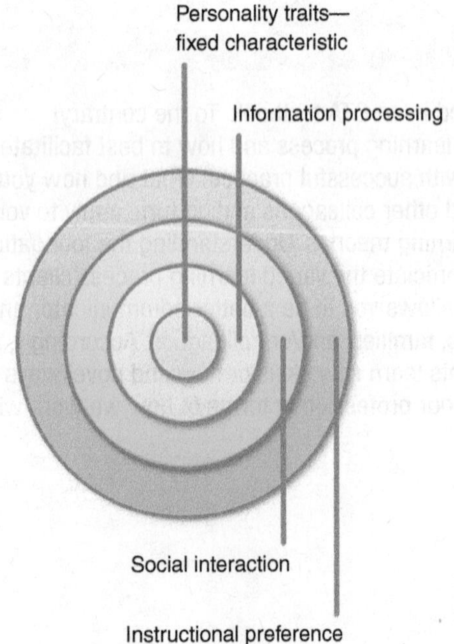

Figure 9.1 Levels of learning.

Personality Traits

You might like to visualize information processing, social interaction, or instructional preference learning theories like the layers of an onion, with personality traits as the inner core (Fig. 9.1). Personality traits, like being shy or outgoing, conscientious, and agreeable, are the constant from which the three "layers" (information processing, social interaction, and instructional preference) influence individual learning style. Each layer is less stable than the one before it; hence the outermost layer, instructional preference learning style, is considered the most unstable, yet still relevant in terms of a discussion of learning style. From these three levels of learning come three major theories of learning.

Information Processing

Developed by Lewin, the information processing theory most closely aligns with allied health research (Brown et al., 2008). It is based heavily on personality theory, out of which the concept of personality traits emerged. Personality theory is a type of psychology that attempts to quantify human nature. The four stages of Lewin's learning process are concrete experience, the actual hands-on doing part of a task. This is followed by personal reflection of the experience, which entails a retrospective look back at what was done during the concrete experience. Moving ahead, the next step is abstract conceptualization, which brings in the influence of previous experience to the learning, and finally, the last step is active experimentation, which entails finding the right fit for this new experience. Finding the right fit involves taking risks and trying out new activities and the behaviors that are associated with this active experimentation (Brown et al., 2008). By example, Tara just went downhill skiing for the first time. While sitting in the ski lodge after several runs down the gentlest slope, she thought about this fun day and how she was pleased with herself for trying something new. She then thought about how she might progress to a harder slope next time she went skiing and came up with an action plan to do so. She put her plan into action and began to work out in the gym to get stronger, to take weekly lessons, and to practice on the slopes in between lessons. In 2 months, she had advanced to a more difficult slope and was continuing to enjoy skiing.

Social Interaction

Kolb's experiential learning cycle is based on Lewin's information processing learning theory. It is commonly applied to health care practice. Similar to information processing, the root of experiential learning is personality theory. Like information processing, Kolb's experiential learning process has stages or steps (McGill & Beatty, 1995). Unlike Lewin, whose model is more linear, Kolb's model of learning suggests that the learning process can begin at any point because the process is continuous. If the concrete experience stage is preferred, it will result in "learning from specific experiences or from relating to people" (Brown et al., 2008, p. 2) (e.g., learning to count by placing objects into a box one at a time and then removing them one at a time). If the preference is reflective observation, a person will focus on keen observation and searching for meaning (e.g., watching someone knit and then trying it out), and a preference for abstract conceptualization leads to "logical analysis and systematic planning" (Brown et al., 2008, p. 2) (e.g., thinking about a new practice area for occupational therapy and then doing thorough due diligence to begin to put the idea into practice).

Kolb takes Lewin's theory a step further and defines four specific learning styles based on the direction a person takes in the processes of concrete experience, personal reflection, abstract conceptualization, and active experimentation. Kolb's four learning styles are illustrated in Figure 9.2.

Previous research found that OT practitioners generally fell in the realm of what is called accommodators or converger (see Fig. 9.2), those whose learning styles favor practical problem solving over logic and tend toward hands-on experiences (Katz & Heimann, 1990; Titiloye & Scott, 2001). Yet a more recent study of students in occupational therapy, physiotherapy, and speech pathology programs found that occupational therapy students scored lowest in the accommodator learning style domain (Brown et al., 2008). To that end, for many OT practitioners, keen observational skills, perspective taking, and our commitment to team-based work are the qualities associated with the diverger learning style (see Fig. 9.2); team players who tend to be keenly observant and look at situations as having multiple perspectives may in fact be a closer match.

Instructional Preference

Neil Fleming is associated with developing the instructional preference learning theory. Like information processing and social interaction, the instructional preference learning theory also has four categories, but unlike information processing and social interaction, they are not actual stages.

Instructional preference is considered to be the most unstable of the learning styles (Brown et al., 2008, p. 2). Developed by Fleming, an example of instructional preference learning style is VARK theory. This theory looks at instructional preference and identifies four learning styles, visual, those who learn best from looking at information; aural, those who learn best from listening to information; read/write, those who learn best from a combination of looking and doing (e.g., the physical and tactile experience of writing); and kinesthetic, those who learn best from hands-on learning (Fleming, 2001). This model acknowledges that some people do not fall

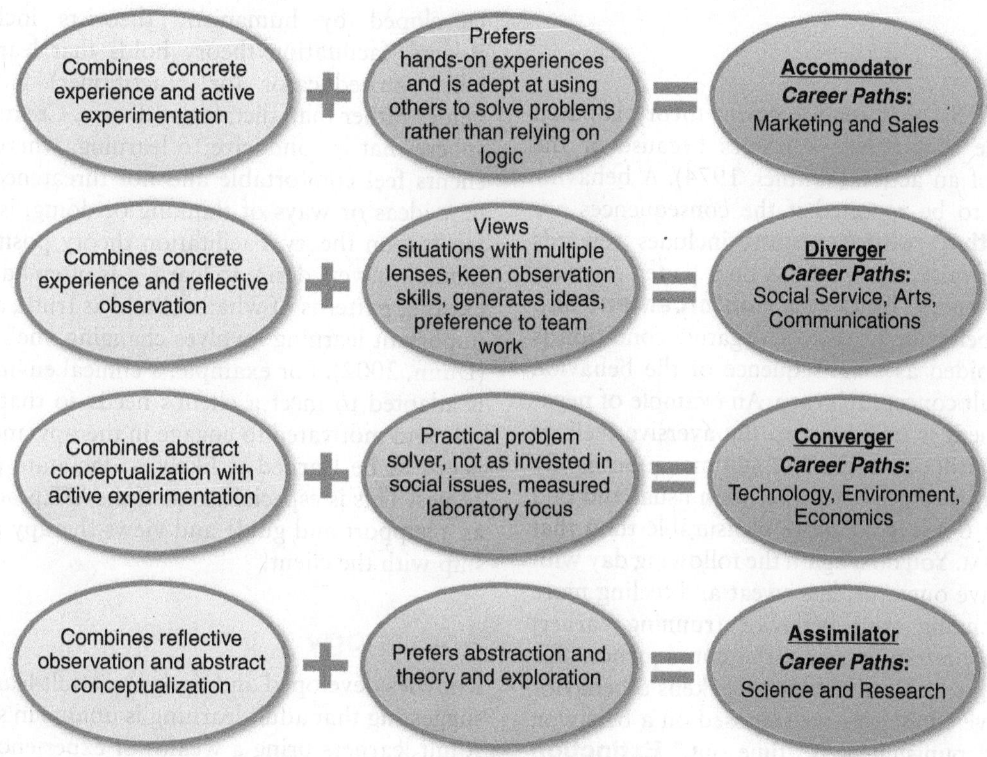

Figure 9.2 Kolb's four learning styles.

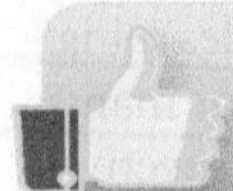

FROM THE FIELD 9.1

VARK

The VARK learning style model proposes four types of learning styles: visual, aural, read/write, and kinesthetic or a combination of the four. According to Brown and colleagues, OT practitioners tend to be kinesthetic or multimodal hands-on learners. *How does this align with the way that you best learn? Do you respond positively to practice and simulation work? Do you learn best when information is presented in a number of ways?*

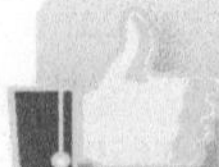

FROM THE FIELD 9.2

ABA

A common therapy approach used with people with autism spectrum disorder is called applied behavioral analysis (ABA). It is based on reinforcement theory.

neatly into one of the four categories and as such are considered to be multimodal learners (Fleming, 2001) (From the Field 9.1).

Other Theories of Learning

There are other theories of learning that do not directly align with personality traits, information processing, social interaction, and instructional preference. They are an important part of the conversation about learning theory and include, but are not limited to, reinforcement theory, holistic learning theory, facilitation theory, and andragogy.

Reinforcement Theory

Proposed by BF Skinner, reinforcement theory is based on the premise that behavior ensues because of the consequences of an action (Skinner, 1974). A behavior is more likely to be repeated if the consequences are positive. **Positive reinforcement** includes rewards such as verbal praise, a prize, an A on a paper, or other pleasant experiences. **Negative reinforcement** also strengthens a behavior because a negative condition is stopped or avoided as a consequence of the behavior. This is a difficult concept to grasp. An example of negative reinforcement is dealing with the aversive feelings of exercising outdoors in the hot summer months. By chance, one day, you get out earlier than usual and find that jogging at 6 AM is far more pleasurable than that same run at 8 AM. You do it again the following day with the same positive outcome, less sweat and feeling more refreshed. Changing your behavior (running earlier) is strengthened or reinforced by the consequence of a more refreshing run. **Punishment** weakens a behavior because negative conditions are imposed on a behavior. An example of punishment is "time out." **Extinction** occurs when a behavior diminishes because there is no positive response or a negative response is stopped. An example of extinction is ignoring someone else's behavior that is deemed inappropriate (From the Field 9.2).

Holistic Learning Theory

This theory of learning focuses on the many facets of personality that each of us manifest. These facets include the "intellect, emotions, body impulse intuition and imagination" (Laird, 1985, p. 121). In order for learning to be effective, the holistic learning theory requires that each element of our personality be working in concert with the others. For example, in order to learn the material from this chapter, a student must be able to understand it and to determine that it is important to learn for future application in practice or for an exam.

Facilitation Theory

Developed by humanistic theorists including Carl Rogers, facilitation theory holds that learning occurs when an educator (or practitioner) facilitates and guides rather than dictates or directs. Creating an atmosphere that is conducive to learning, where learners or clients feel comfortable and not threatened to explore new ideas or ways of thinking or doing, is the crux of facilitation theory. Facilitation theory posits that while humans have a desire to learn, it is often hard to change existing patterns of what we hold as truth, and the most important learning involves changing one's self-concept (Dunn, 2002). For example, a clinical environment that is adapted to meet a client's needs so that he/she feels safe and motivated to engage in therapy and learn what needs to be learned is likely to facilitate positive outcomes. This is especially true if the OT practitioner acts as a support and guide and views therapy as a partnership with the client.

Andragogy

Knowles developed andragogy or adult learning theory, suggesting that adult learning is unique in several ways. Adult learners bring a wealth of experience to a learning environment (Knowles et al., 2011). They must recognize new applications for learning and influence how learning is to be evaluated and expect that what they contribute to a learning environment when asked to do so will be acted upon (Knowles et al., 2011). For example, in this year's OTA class, Joan, a mature learner, and Zoe, a traditional learner, were paired up to research and present on multiple sclerosis to the class. While Joan, a former nurse, has a great deal of firsthand knowledge about multiple sclerosis from her time on a rehab unit, she is rather limited in her computer skills beyond basic word processing. Zoe is a whiz at preparing catchy PowerPoint presentations, but has limited clinical experience. Both are good at doing online research. Blending each of their skills, they put together a wonderful presentation that is well received by their classmates.

Summary

In this chapter, we have explored several theories of learning and learning styles that apply not only to you as a student but also to you as an emerging OTA. While none of these theories are occupational therapy specific, they provide important insight into understanding how people learn and go about learning in many different ways or styles. Looking at learning as a fluid and dynamic process goes a long way in explaining our individuality and uniqueness. Providing optimal client-centered care embraces the idea that people learn differently. Accordingly, you as an emerging OTA have the opportunity to rise to the challenge of implementing meaningful client-centered intervention services that reflect your client's learning styles. Embracing what is necessary to support individual learning differences makes for exciting practice.

Review Questions

1. Your 2-year-old daughter is misbehaving and you want to try to stop the behavior by putting her in time out. This is a classic example of:
   a. Punishment
   b. Positive reinforcement
   c. Negative reinforcement
   d. Extinction

2. Andragogy posits that:
   a. There are four levels of learning styles unique to men.
   b. Learning only occurs in a comfortable environment.
   c. Adults learn in unique ways.
   d. Learning happens as a result of the integration of mind and body.

3. Creating an atmosphere that is conducive to learning, where learners or clients feel comfortable and not threatened to explore new ideas or ways of thinking, best describes:
   a. Holistic learning theory
   b. Facilitation theory
   c. Information processing theory
   d. Instruction performance theory

4. Your client seems to learn and adapt most easily when you talk through how to do a task. This describes what kind of learner?
   a. Aural
   b. Visual
   c. Kinesthetic
   d. Linguistic

5. Learning by doing best describes a ________ style.
   a. Kinesthetic
   b. Visual
   c. Aural
   d. Read/write

6. Taking risks and trying out new activities and the behaviors pertains to which of Lewin's information processing levels of learning?
   a. Active experimentation
   b. Adaptation reconditioning
   c. Concrete experimentation
   d. Adaptive responses

7. Which of Kolb's four learning styles best describes a marketer or sales person?
   a. Converger
   b. Diverger
   c. Acquisitor
   d. Accommodator

8. Technology, environment, and economics are typically the career paths that what type of learner undertakes?
   a. Converger
   b. Diverger
   c. Assimilator
   d. Accommodator

9. "Great job!" is an example of:
   a. Negative reinforcement
   b. Punishment
   c. Extinction
   d. Positive reinforcement

10. Which of the following is considered to be the fixed characteristic of learning theory?
    a. Personality
    b. Information processing
    c. Experiential learning
    d. Instructional preference

11. Kolb's model of learning styles is:
    a. Continuous and always begins and ends at exactly the same place along the continuum
    b. Fractured and has only random patterns
    c. Continuous and begins and ends at difference places
    d. Linear and orderly

Practice Activities

Research three additional learning theories and write a short case study about a 21-year-old man with quadriplegia whose goal is to comb his hair. Integrate the premise of one of these theories into your intervention approach.

Select a learning style that best describes the way you learn. Why does this style best suit you? Compare your response with your classmates. Are there any interesting trends to report? Poll your family members. What do you find?

Layer information processing learning theory on top of the model of human occupation (refer back to Chapter 7, *An Overview of Occupational Therapy Theory, Practice Models, and Frames of Reference: Guiding the Practice*). How do the two intersect and how are they different?

Prepare a photo montage that shows people in roles associated with what Kolb identified as accommodators, divergers, convergers, and assimilators. Ask your classmates to identify who represents each of the four learning styles.

References

Brown T, et al. Learning style preferences of occupational therapy, physiotherapy and speech pathology students: a comparative study. *Internet J Allied Health Sci Pract* 2008; 6(3):1–12.

Burns RB. *The Adult Learner at Work: A Comprehensive Guide to the Context, Psychology and Methods of Learning for the Workplace*. Chatswood, NSW, Australia: Business and Professional Publishing; 1995.

Dunn L. *Theories of Learning*. Oxford Centre for Staff and Learning Development; 2002. Retrieved from http://www.brookes.ac.uk/services/ocsd/

Fleming N. *Teaching and Learning Styles: VARK Strategies*. Christchurch, New Zealand; VARK Learn Limited; 2001.

Katz N, Heimann N. Learning styles of students and practitioners in five health professions. *Occup Ther J Res* 1990;11(4):239–245.

Knowles MS, et al. *The Adult Learner: The Definitive Classic in Adult Education and Human Resource Development*. 7th ed. New York, NY: Taylor & Francis; 2011.

Kolb DA. *Experiential Learning: Experience as the Course of Learning and Development*. Englewood Cliffs, NJ: Prentice Hall; 1984.

Laird D. *Approaches to Training and Development*. Reading, MA: Addison-Wesley; 1985.

McGill L, Beatty L. *Action Learning: A Guide for Professional, Management, and Educational Development*. 2nd ed. London: Kogan Page; 1995.

Skinner BF. *About Behaviorism*. New York, NY: Alfred A. Knopf; 1974.

Titiloye VM, Scott AH. Occupational therapy students' learning styles and application to professional academic training. *Occup Ther Healthcare* 2001;15(1/2):145–155.

CHAPTER 10

The Occupational Therapy Treatment Process

Amy Wagenfeld, PhD, OTR/L SCEM, CAPs

Key Terms

Activity analysis—A way to look at the typical methods of performing an activity, the range of skills required for the performance of the activity, and the various cultural meanings that may be ascribed to the activity.

Analysis of occupational performance—The end result of a client being able to complete an occupation based on the relationship between him/her, the environment and contexts, and the activity itself AOTA, 2014, p. S13).

Client-centered approach—Service delivery that acknowledges, respects, and incorporates client wishes into the therapy plan (AOTA, 2014).

Intervention implementation—Putting the intervention plan into action (AOTA, 2014).

Intervention plan—The action plan for the occupational therapist and occupational therapy assistant to follow to provide intervention.

Intervention review—Ongoing means of reassessing the intervention plan, how it is being implemented, whether it is working, and how the client is making progress toward meeting his/her goals (AOTA, 2014).

Occupational profile—Summation of a client's occupational history and experiences, patterns of daily living, interests, values, and needs (AOTA, 2014, p. S13).

Process—The ways in which client-centered occupational therapy intervention is implemented in occupational therapy services (AOTA, 2014).

Learning Objectives

After studying this chapter, readers should be able to:

- Explain the three steps of the occupational therapy process.
- Discuss the relationship of the occupational profile and the analysis of occupational performance to the evaluation process.
- Articulate the importance of a client-centered approach to occupational therapy intervention.
- State the role of the occupational therapy assistant in the occupational therapy process.

Introduction

This chapter explores the occupational therapy process. From our previous discussion of the *Occupational Therapy Practice Framework III* (AOTA, 2014), you may recall that it is divided into two overarching areas, domain and process. This chapter provides an overview of the process area and its application to client-centered service delivery. For further detailed information, you are encouraged to refer to the *Occupational Therapy Practice Framework III* (AOTA, 2014).

The Occupational Therapy Process

As described in the *Occupational Therapy Practice Framework III*, the **process** is a means for "occupational therapy practitioners [to] operationalize their expertise to provide service to clients" via a process that involves, "evaluation, intervention, and outcome monitoring; occurs within the purview of the domain; and involves collaboration among the occupational therapist, occupational therapy assistant, and the client" (AOTA, 2014, pp. S44–S45).

While many professions organize their process into evaluation, intervention, and outcomes, occupational therapy is unique in that the process is focused on engaging in the therapeutic application of occupations as a means and method to optimize health and participation (AOTA, 2014). As discussed in Chapter 4, *Occupations: The Cornerstone of the Profession*, part of our professional uniqueness is applying the use of occupations as both means and end to the therapeutic process.

While you may be thinking that the occupational therapy process is sequential, it really is not. Instead, to accommodate for any change in client status, it is flexible (AOTA, 2014). A critically important piece of this process is establishing client-centered relationships. Recall that client can refer to a person, organization, or population (AOTA, 2014). Why is this relationship so important to the process? According to Mattingly and Fleming, the best way forward to develop a trusting relationship and correspondingly optimal therapy outcomes is through dynamic collaboration between the client and the OT practitioner (Mattingly & Fleming, 1993). Active collaboration and a trust-based relationship factor into client-centered care. Tickle-Degnen (1995) proposed three factors that nurture a collaborative and trusting practitioner–client relationship. They are:

a. The therapist's ability to listen carefully and create environments in which patients are not anxious or embarrassed to share their needs
b. The patient and therapist's ability to achieve interactional synchrony in verbal and nonverbal behavior as well as in the therapeutic activity
c. The patient's ability to find deep satisfaction in the experience (in Jackson, 1998, p. 469)

This collaborative relationship helps OT practitioners to better understand what is important in terms of intervention and what he/she and the client each brings to the table in terms of treatment. A client-centered focus validates what the client and OT practitioner each brings to the treatment process (AOTA, 2014). Figure 10.1 illustrates the importance of the client-centered process to occupational therapy intervention.

The process involves continual application and reapplication of clinical reasoning, so that an OT practitioner can "identify the multiple demands, skills, and potential meanings of the activities and occupations, and gain a deeper understanding of the interrelationships between aspects of the domain [of occupational therapy] that affect performance and those that will support client-centered interventions and outcomes" (AOTA, 2014, p. S11). The three parts of the process as described in the *Occupational Therapy Practice Framework III* (AOTA, 2014), evaluation, intervention, and outcomes, are briefly discussed below. How each part is interconnected and driven by clinical reasoning and a collaborative client-centered approach are also explored. You are encouraged to refer to the complete *Occupational Therapy Practice Framework III* (AOTA, 2014) for further information about evaluation, intervention, and outcomes.

Evaluation

An evaluation begins with an OT determining a client's needs and wants, what the client can do now, and what he/she did in the past and identifying barriers to health

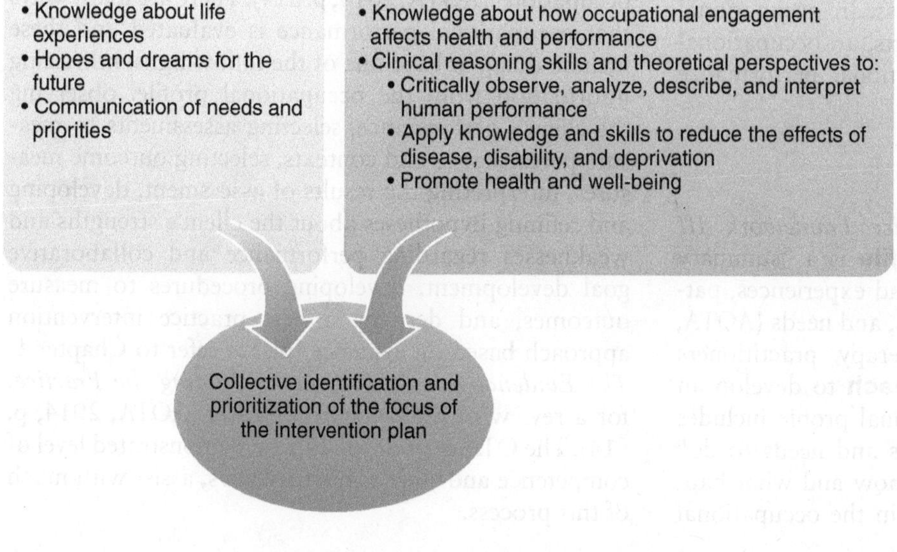

Client brings:
- Knowledge about life experiences
- Hopes and dreams for the future
- Communication of needs and priorities

Occupational therapy practitioners bring:
- Knowledge about how occupational engagement affects health and performance
- Clinical reasoning skills and theoretical perspectives to:
  - Critically observe, analyze, describe, and interpret human performance
  - Apply knowledge and skills to reduce the effects of disease, disability, and deprivation
  - Promote health and well-being

Collective identification and prioritization of the focus of the intervention plan

Figure 10.1 The client-centered occupational therapy intervention process.

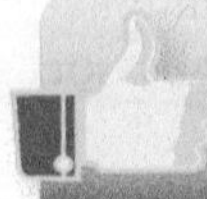

FROM THE FIELD 10.1

What's in a Word?

It really is all in the words. Did you know that there is a distinct difference between the terms disability and handicap? In their recently revised book, *Clinical Research in Occupational Therapy*, Stein et al. (2013) discuss this issue in terms of professional report and note writing. A disability is something a person is not able to do, the loss of a body part, or some type of physical or psychological impairment. A person who is unable to walk or drive a car because of a bilateral above-the-knee amputation has a disability. A handicap is a limiting factor imposed on a person by environmental conditions or another individual's actions. For example, a disability such as being unable to walk can become a handicap if there are steps or no wheelchair ramp into a friend's home or if the ramp is too steep to roll up or down safely at a favorite movie theater or if this individual has no way to get to appointments. Just because someone has a disability does not mean that he/she is handicapped. In professional writing, it is critically important to make this distinction and to not use the terms incorrectly or interchangeably.

and participation (AOTA, 2014). There is no single one-size-fits-all evaluation that OTs use; the type and focus vary from setting to setting and on client needs. Both formal and informal evaluations frequently occur throughout all phases of the process. The OT conducts the evaluation. Based on demonstrated competency and working under the supervision of an OT, an OTA may contribute to the evaluation process. In occupational therapy, the evaluation has two parts, an occupational profile and an analysis of occupational performance (From the Field 10.1).

Occupational Profile

The *Occupational Therapy Practice Framework III* states that the **occupational profile** is a "summary of a client's occupational history and experiences, patterns of daily living, interests, values, and needs (AOTA, 2014, p. S13). Occupational therapy practitioners employ a **client-centered approach** to develop an occupational profile. The occupational profile includes determining what the client "wants and needs to do" now and later, and understanding how and what happened prior to becoming involved in the occupational therapy process influences present and future occupations (AOTA, 2014). Information gathering for the occupational profile is important for the client-centered approach because it lays out client priorities and desires that will "lead to the client's engagement in occupations that support participation in life" (AOTA, 2014, p. S13). This is a very empowering part of the process as it values and respects the client as an important part of the team. What OT practitioners strive to see happen from the outset is development of a client-centered approach in order to guide the evaluation, intervention planning, and intervention and implementation process (AOTA, 2014). This is what client-centered intervention is all about.

The information gathered through the occupational profile is useful for the OT to "develop a working hypothesis regarding possible reasons for the identified problems and concerns" to determine why identified problems and concerns are present (AOTA, 2014, p. S13). While always adhering to Federal privacy laws such as HIPAA (Health Insurance Portability and Accountability Act), the OTA contributes to this process by reviewing the client's medical record and speaking with the client and his/her family and then reporting this information to the supervising OT. The findings of the occupational profile often guide in establishing client-centered outcome measures (AOTA, 2014, p. S13).

Based on the *Occupational Therapy Practice Framework III* (AOTA, 2014), an example of an occupational profile for an adult client will contain the information in Figure 10.2.

Analysis of Occupational Performance

The *Occupational Therapy Practice Framework III* describes the **analysis of occupational performance** as the "accomplishment of the selected occupation resulting from the dynamic transaction among the clients, the context and environment, and the activity or occupation" (AOTA, 2014, p. S14). There are many ways that occupational performance is evaluated and these include doing at least one of the following: synthesizing information from the occupational profile, observing the client's performance, selecting assessments to measure performance and contexts, selecting outcome measures, interpreting the results of assessment, developing and refining hypotheses about the client's strengths and weaknesses regarding performance and collaborative goal development, developing procedures to measure outcomes, and deriving a best practice intervention approach based on evidence (please refer to Chapter 5, *The Evidence-Based Movement: Guiding the Practice*, for a review of the evidence process) (AOTA, 2014, p. S14). The OTA may, depending on demonstrated level of competence and state regulatory laws, assist with much of this process.

Occupational Profile: Adult Client

Client Name: ______________________

Spouse or Significant Other: ______________________

Other Family Members: ______________________

Additional Caregiver (if applicable): ______________________

Reason for Referral: ______________________

Occupational History: Values, Interests, Life experiences; Prior pattern of participation in occupations and meanings that are associated with each.

Client Priorities and Goals:

Client Strengths General:

Client Strengths Areas of Occupation (circle all that apply): Self-Care Work Play/Leisure Rest and Sleep

Client Challenges General:

Client Challenges Areas of Occupation (circle all that apply): Self-Care Work Play/Leisure Rest and Sleep

Current contexts and environments that support participation in client centered occupation:

Current contexts and environments that limit participation in client centered occupation:

Figure 10.2 Occupational profile for an adult client.

Assessment of the client, the environment or context, the occupation or activity, and performance may be accomplished through a client interview (or with a significant other), observation of performance and context, record review, and direct assessment using formal and informal assessment tools (AOTA, 2014, p. S14). Recall from Chapter 5, *The Evidence-Based Movement: Guiding the Practice*, that the most objective client data are derived from using standardized assessment tools, which is done by an OT.

One of the best methods that OT practitioners have to understand the demands of an activity on a client is called the **activity analysis**. The activity analysis "addresses the typical demands of an activity, the range of skills involved in it is performance, and the various cultural meanings that might be ascribed to it" (Crepeau, 2003, p. 192 in AOTA, 2014, p. S41). Please refer to Chapter 11, *Activity Analysis—The Jewel of Occupational Therapy*, for a detailed discussion of the activity analysis.

Analyzing occupational performance is a complex process. It entails understanding the dynamic relationships between "the client, the context and environment, and the activity or occupation" (AOTA, 2014, p. S14). Occupational therapy practitioners weave and interconnect these factors in order to understand how they contribute to developing interventions that support occupational performance (AOTA, 2014).

Intervention

Intervention is the "skilled action(s) taken by OT practitioners in collaboration with the client to facilitate engagement in occupation related to health, well-being, and participation" (AOTA, 2014, p. S14). The information gathered during the evaluation and in conjunction with theoretical principles guides the occupation-centered intervention process (AOTA, 2014, p. 2014). The purpose of intervention is to "assist clients in reaching a state of physical, mental, and social well-being; identifying and realizing aspirations; satisfying needs; and changing or coping with the environment" (AOTA, 2014, p. S14). Please refer to Table 6 in the *Occupational Therapy Practice Framework III* (AOTA, 2014) for a list of a variety of occupational therapy interventions that are carried out with clients.

Not surprisingly, occupational therapy interventions are intended to promote health and well-being, and participation (AOTA, 2014, p. S14) and depending on for whom/what it is intended (person, organization, or population) varies. So too does the terminology used to describe for whom the OT practitioner is directing the intervention. For instance, in a health care setting, the client may be referred to as a patient and in a school setting as student, parent, teacher, or administrator (AOTA, 2014). When occupational therapy services are directed toward an organization, the members may be called consumers, such as people served by a sheltered workshop or outpatient mental health center (AOTA, 2014).

The Three Steps of the Intervention Process

There are three steps involved in the intervention process: the intervention plan, the intervention implementation, and the intervention review. The three-step intervention process integrates the findings of the evaluation process with theory, practice models, frames of references, and evidence (AOTA, 2014, p. S15). Why? Collectively, these steps guide the clinical reasoning that is necessary for occupational therapy practitioners to provide optimal intervention services.

The **intervention plan** is the action plan that OT practitioners follow. Through a description of occupational therapy approaches and specific interventions, the intervention plan describes how delivery of services will guide the process to achieve the client's identified outcomes (AOTA, 2014, p. S15). The intervention plan is client centered; it is developed in collaboration with the client (or proxies) and reflects his/her goals and priorities (AOTA, 2014, p. S15). The intervention plan is guided by the client's goals, values, occupational needs, and beliefs, health and well-being, performance skills and patterns, collective influence of the context, environment, activity demands, and client factors, context of service delivery, and best available evidence (AOTA, 2014, p. S15). Please refer to Table 8 in the *Occupational Therapy Practice Framework III* for a description of occupational therapy intervention approaches. The four steps associated with intervention planning include:

1. Development of the plan
2. Consideration of potential discharge needs and plans
3. Making recommendations for referrals to other disciplines as needed (AOTA, 2014, p. S15)

Intervention implementation involves "putting the plan into action" (AOTA, 2014, p. S15). It entails altering the context or environment, client factors, and activity in order to effect positive changes. Interventions may focus on one or more domains (AOTA, 2014, p. S15). Because life does not occur in a vacuum, nor are skills used in isolation, the expected outcome is that skills learned or relearned through intervention will be transferrable or applicable to other contexts in a client's life. There are two steps associated with intervention implementation: (1) determining and carrying out the type of occupational therapy intervention(s) selected and (2) monitoring the client's responses to interventions through ongoing assessment and reassessment of the client's progress toward meeting his/her goals (AOTA, 2014, p. S15).

The final step of occupational therapy intervention is called **intervention review**. As described in the *Occupational Therapy Practice Framework III*, it is the "continuous process of reevaluating and reviewing the intervention plan, the effectiveness of its delivery, and the progress towards outcomes" (AOTA, 2014, p. S16). Like all other parts of occupational therapy intervention, it is client centered and involves a collaborative process. Re-evaluation may call for changes in the intervention plan (AOTA, 2014, p. S16). There are three steps associated with the dynamic intervention review. They are:

1. Re-evaluating the plan and implementation methods to determine its effectiveness
2. Modifying the plan as needed
3. Determining whether occupational therapy services are to be continued or discontinued and whether alternative referral to other services are needed (AOTA, 2014, p. S16).

Outcomes

The overarching goal or outcome of occupational therapy intervention is "achieving health, well-being, and participation in life through engagement in occupation" (AOTA, 2014, p. S4). Note that there are four parts to this desired outcome: health, well-being, participation, and engagement in occupation. "Health", as defined by the WHO (2006, p. 1 in AOTA, 2014, p. S4), is "a state of complete physical, mental, and social well-being, and not merely the absence of disease or infirmity." "Well-being encompasses the total universe of human life domains, including physical, mental, and social aspects" (WHO, 2006, p. 211 in AOTA, 2014 p. S4). Participation is the "involvement in a life situation" (WHO, 2006, p. 10 in AOTA, 2014 p. S4) and Engagement in Occupation is a "performance of occupations as the result of choice, motivation, and meaning within a supportive context and environment" (AOTA, 2014, p. S4). Several of the positive and valuable multifaceted outcomes of occupational therapy intervention include "improved performance skills...improved transactional relationship[s] among the areas of the domain...[resulting in]...ability to engage in desired occupations... [and subjective (client) outcomes such as] ... improved outlook,, perceived well-being and self-efficacy" (AOTA, 2014, p. S4). Through a detailed assessment process and using well-established, and reliable, valid evaluation tools and subjective report, the OT with input from the OTA and client measures the efficacy of occupational therapy intervention to determine outcomes. Exhibit 3 in the *Occupational Therapy Practice Framework III* (AOTA, 2014) illustrates several types of occupational therapy outcomes and how they are operationalized.

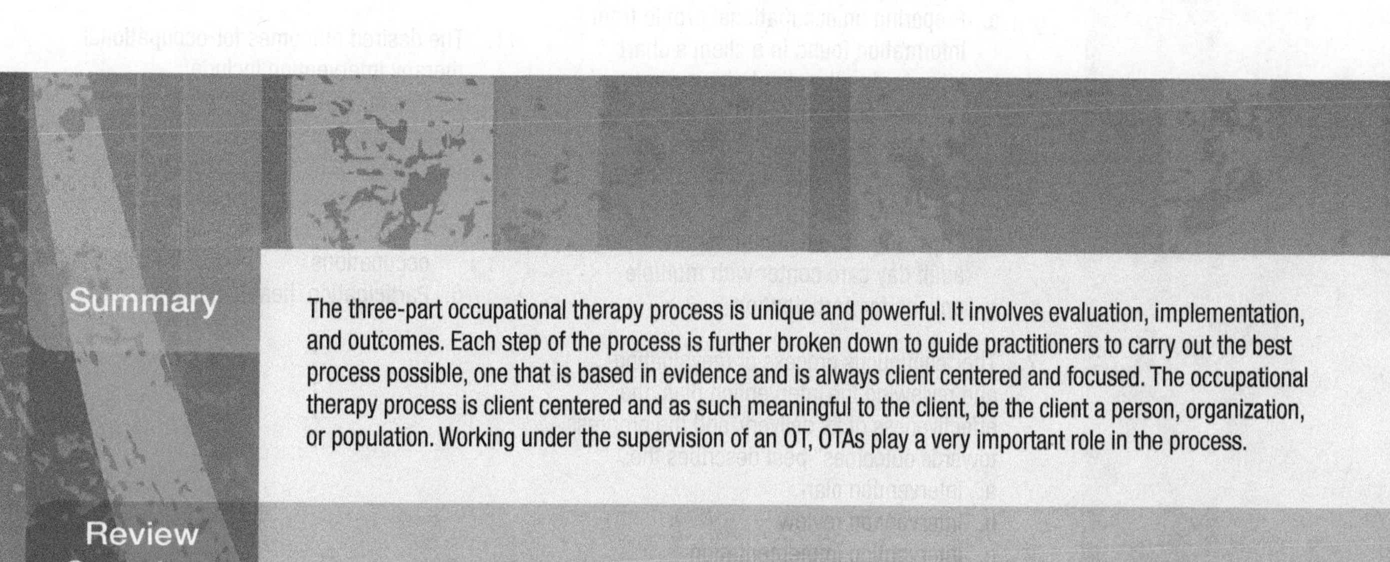

Summary

The three-part occupational therapy process is unique and powerful. It involves evaluation, implementation, and outcomes. Each step of the process is further broken down to guide practitioners to carry out the best process possible, one that is based in evidence and is always client centered and focused. The occupational therapy process is client centered and as such meaningful to the client, be the client a person, organization, or population. Working under the supervision of an OT, OTAs play a very important role in the process.

Review Questions

1. "Accomplishment of the selected occupation resulting from the dynamic transaction among the clients, the context and environment, and the activity" best describes:
   a. Activity analysis
   b. Activity performance
   c. Analysis of occupational performance
   d. Activity engagement

2. The three parts of the occupational process are:
   a. Evaluation, assessment, outcomes
   b. Assessment, plan, intervention
   c. Evaluation, intervention, outcomes
   d. Intervention, plan, outcomes

3. Which of the following best describes the role of the OTA in the evaluation process?
   a. Total autonomy with evaluation
   b. No involvement
   c. Can complete the entire evaluation with an occupational therapist on-site providing indirect supervision
   d. Depending upon competency level, may assist the OT while under his/her direct supervision

4. An example of participation or "involvement in a life situation" is:
   a. Deadheading flowers
   b. Refusing to get out of bed
   c. Bathing with assistance
   d. A, B, and C

5. The following is an example of a context or environment:
   a. Home
   b. Sewing
   c. Watching a movie
   d. Reading a book

6. Which of the following does not align with a client-centered approach?
   a. Preparing an occupational profile from information found in a client's chart
   b. Interviewing the client about what his/her life was like prior to receiving occupational therapy services
   c. Speaking with family members about the client
   d. Preparing an activity for clients at an adult day care center with multiple options for participation

7. The "continuous process of reevaluating and reviewing the intervention plan, the effectiveness of its delivery, and the progress towards outcomes" best describes the:
   a. Intervention plan
   b. Intervention review
   c. Intervention implementation
   d. Evaluation

8. Analyzing the dynamic relationships between "performance skills and patterns, contexts and environments, activity demands, and client factors" refers to which part of the evaluation process?
   a. Occupational performance outcomes
   b. Occupational profile
   c. Analysis of occupational performance
   d. Activity analysis

9. The implementation process is carried out by:
   a. The OTA under the supervision of the OT
   b. The OT and the OTA
   c. Only the OT
   d. A and B

10. The three steps of the occupational therapy intervention process are:
    a. Intervention, discussion implementation, and review
    b. Intervention plan, implementation, and assessment
    c. Intervention evaluation, implementation, and review
    d. Intervention plan, implementation, and review

11. The desired outcomes for occupational therapy intervention include:
    a. Health, participation, engagement in occupations
    b. Engagement in occupations, performance, participation
    c. Health, participation, engagement in occupations
    d. Participation, health, performance

Practice Activities

The *Occupational Therapy Practice Framework III* states that the overarching goal or outcome of occupational therapy intervention is "achieving health, well-being, and participation in life through engagement in occupation" (AOTA, 2014, p. S2). Find a photograph of an older female in a magazine and bring it to class. Based on the context in which the photo is set, discuss how in your mind, health, participation, and engagement in occupations apply to what this woman is doing.

Prepare a document that illustrates how terms other than "client" are appropriate for those we work with—as people, groups, organizations, and populations. Be creative and use pictures, charts, etc. Use specific examples. Show overlap between groups as it applies.

Your work with an OT entails helping to prepare an occupational profile for a 7-year-old boy with autism. Create a mock profile using the information about the occupational profile contained in this chapter as well as referring to the *Occupational Therapy Practice Framework III* (AOTA, 2014). Convert your occupational profile to a PowerPoint presentation and share with your classmates.

References

American Occupational Therapy Association. Occupational therapy practice framework: Domain and process (3rd ed.). *Am J Occup Ther* 2014;68(Suppl 1):S1–S48. http://www.dx.doi.org/10.5014/ajot.2014.682006

Crepeau E. Analyzing occupation and activity: a way of thinking about occupational performance. In: Crepeau E, Cohn E, Schell B, eds. *Willard and Spackman's Occupational Therapy*. 10th ed. Philadelphia, PA: Lippincott Williams & Wilkins; 2003:189–198.

Jackson J. The value of occupation as the core of treatment: Sandy's experience. *Am J Occup Ther* 1998;52(6):466–473.

Mattingly C, Fleming M, eds. *Clinical Reasoning: Forms of Inquiry in a Therapeutic Practice. Philadelphia*, PA: F.A. Davis; 1993.

Stein MS, et al. *Clinical Research in Occupational Therapy*. 5th ed. Clifton Park, NY: Cengage Learning; 2013.

Tickle-Degnen L. Therapeutic rapport. In: Trombley CA, ed. *Occupational Therapy for Physical Dysfunction*. 5th ed. Baltimore, MD: Williams & Wilkins; 1995:277–285.

CHAPTER 11

Activity Analysis: The Jewel of Occupational Therapy

Alice Gandell, MSMSP, OTR/L and Helene Lieberman, MA, OTR/L

Key Terms

Activity—A specific deed, action, or function.

Activity analysis—The process of looking at the typical methods of performing an activity, the range of skills required for the performance of the activity, and the various cultural meanings that may be ascribed to the activity. Activities are also analyzed for their therapeutic potential.

Adaptation/Adapting—Any alteration or modification in the structure or function of something or any of its parts by which that "thing" or "activity" becomes better fitted to suit the needs of the client.

Collaboration—A process of working cooperatively to achieve a goal.

Evaluation (occupational therapy)—The process of establishing a profile of the client and analysis of client's occupational performance.

Grading—Degree of change in an activity demand that occurs on a continuum from simple to complex. The change can be in one or all aspects of the activity.

Health—"State of complete physical, mental and social weel-being and not merely the absence of disease or infirmity." (WHO, 1948, p. 100).

Involvement—Taking part, being included or engaged in an area of life, being accepted, or having access to needed resources and gauged through performance (AOTA, 2014; WHO, 2001).

Meaningful activity—Activities that have an intrinsic value to an individual.

Occupation—An activity in which a person is engaged, usually indicating a purpose that is goal directed, extends over time, is composed of multiple tasks, and has meaning to their performer. Often described as the activities people engage in throughout their daily lives to fulfill their time and give life meaning.

Occupational performance—A dynamic of occupation through which a person can literally change his or her own nature by engaging in occupation.

Occupational performance analysis—The observational evaluation of a person's task performance to identify discrepancies between the demands of a task and the skill of the person (Fisher, 1998).

Occupational role—The occupations that a person ascribes to a role—they are individual and situational specific (Crepeau & Boyt Schell, 2009).

Purposeful activity—An activity that has significance to the client; tends to be goal directed.

Task—The smaller components, parts, or steps of an activity or occupation (Thomas, 2012).

Task analysis—Evaluation of the minute details involved in the steps of a task and how they relate to the activity as a whole.

Learning Objectives

After studying this chapter, readers should be able to:

- Describe the contribution of occupational therapy to health and wellness.
- Articulate the profession's focus on engagement in occupation and participation in contexts and to define and compare the terms purposeful activity, occupation, and occupational performance.
- Explain and illustrate the concept of "fit" among persons, environments, and occupations.
- Demonstrate logical thinking, critical analysis, problem solving, and creativity to the purpose of developing a "just-right fit" for clients.
- Analyze, grade, and adapt activity demands and context of purposeful activities to meet client's needs.

Introduction

In Chapter 4, *Occupations: The Cornerstone of the Profession*, we learned what occupation is and perhaps a little bit about what it is not. We must always remember that the term occupation can be misunderstood. We, as OT practitioners have adopted a specific definition, "the everyday life activities [of] individuals, groups, populations, or organizations to support participation, performance, and function in roles and situations in home, school, workplace, community, and other settings" (AOTA, 2011). Occupations are far more than just activities. **Occupations** are the activities that give our life meaning.

The way we do every **activity** is influenced by our family, community, peers, education, habit, and even personal preference and/or tastes. For example, how do you brush your teeth? Does everyone brush their teeth exactly the same way you do? Do you brush up and down or side to side? Where do you begin? Do you use mouthwash? Do you swish or gargle? What kind of toothbrush, manual or electric? Do you brush in the shower or at the sink? Do you walk around and do other things while you brush or do you stay still? Do you look in the mirror while you brush? In what ways and how much did family, community, the dentist, or others shape the way you brush?

Of course, there is a general way of brushing teeth. We need a brush, toothpaste, water, a sink, mouthwash, and perhaps few other things to brush our teeth. Toothpaste is put on the brush and brought to the mouth. Some type of motion is used to move the brush against the teeth. Then the toothpaste is ejected from the mouth by spitting, or it may be swallowed. There can be any number of steps to this activity, but this is the typical sequence of brushing teeth. As soon as we look at exactly how you or I or one of our clients do it, tooth brushing becomes one of our personal occupations, and as part of the activity analysis process, we analyze the ways in which each of us brush differently.

How do we accomplish all that we do, including working with clients to learn or relearn the task of tooth bushing? We do it in part through activity analysis. The activity analysis tool, along with our professional insights, guides OT practitioners to determine the potential value of an activity as a therapeutic agent. Through this method, we determine whether an activity is meaningful, motivates, and meets a client's needs and if it can be used to help the client develop or restore skills and abilities. Activity analysis also allows us to select, design, and grade an activity to treat a disability or functional limitation (Trombly, 1995). It is our unique professional method of determining the restorative value of an activity (From the Field 11.1).

As OT practitioners, we use activities and occupations not only to achieve our end goal but as the means by which to meet that goal (Thomas, 2012, p. 5). Occupational therapy practitioners recognize that the activities used in therapy should be within the range of a just-right challenge between client skills, interests, and abilities, which involves **grading** and **adapting** the activities to assure challenge and change. Our most valid outcome measure is the effect the activity has on the client, its value for the client, and the value it has for the client's familial, social, and cultural systems. These standards are "occupational therapy's legacy of humanistic ways, occupational justice, and timeless truths" (Royeen, 2003, p. 651).

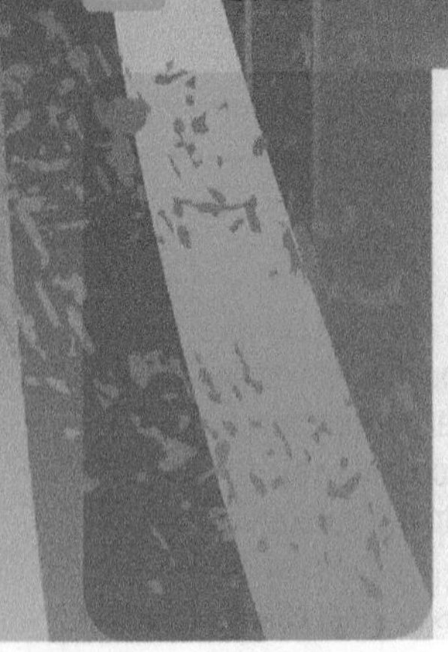

Activity analysis focuses our analysis and professional insights, thus assisting us to determine the value of an activity as a therapeutic agent. Through **activity analysis**, we determine whether an activity is meaningful, motivates, and meets a client's needs and if it can be used to help the client develop or restore skills and abilities. Activity analysis allows us to select, design, and grade an activity to treat a disability or functional limitation (Trombly, 1995). It is our profession's way of determining the restorative value of an activity. Activity analysis is a critical piece of this goal-oriented process. Thus, these unique occupational therapy "tools of our trade" are the very same occupations and activities as the goals we hope for our clients to achieve. A brief look at our rich history will verify and help frame the jewel of occupational therapy, the activity analysis.

Historical Overview of Activity Analysis

Early OT practitioners acknowledged the unity among mind, body, and spirit. They saw the connections between engagement, self-fulfillment, and **health** and used terms like work treatment, work therapy, and work cure to describe goal-directed activities in order to encourage craftsmanship, skills for the workplace, and as diversions. Practitioners as far back as during World War I incorporated activity analysis into their practice and taught activity analysis in educational and training programs (Creighton, 1992). Through analysis of activities, early OT practitioners were able to identify the skills required to engage clients in a specific activity. The first rating system for activity analysis was suggested in 1922 (Creighton, 1992). Using this system, activities were organized according to physical and emotional requirements and social properties (Creighton, 1992). This system continued through the 1960s.

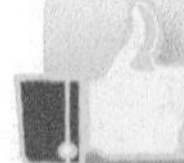

FROM THE FIELD 11.1

Analyzing an Activity

Think of an activity you did as a child. Answer the following questions.

- What is the activity?
- What materials did you need to do the activity?
- How did you do the activity—describe the steps in the correct sequence.
- Where did you do the activity?
- When did you do the activity?
- With whom did you do the activity?
- Why did you do the activity?

This exercise is a warmup for learning about the details of the activity analysis process.

Beginning in the 1970s, a number of occupational therapy frames of reference were developed and significantly influenced methods of activity analysis (please also refer to Chapter 7, *Occupational Therapy Theories and How They Guide Practice*). In part, these frames of reference guided practitioners to recognize the sensorimotor, affective, cognitive, biomechanical, volitional, contextual, and spiritual components of an activity (Creighton, 1992; Law et al., 1997).

Activity Analysis

Activity analysis or **task analysis**, which is which? These are key components of the occupational therapy treatment process. In this chapter, we will use the term activity to refer to the entire procedure or occupation associated with doing the activity. **Tasks** then become the multiple parts within the activity, which can be important to analyze, but for the scope of this chapter, we focus on the larger activity analysis process CS9. Activities and the tasks that they are composed of are the general "how and what" of anything that is done. On the other hand, occupation, as understood by OT practitioners, is the personalized "how and what" for a specific individual. We can think of this occupational personalization by the term **occupational role** (Crepeau & Boyt Schell, 2009). Within the term activity, OT practitioners also include all the values, habits, contexts, and meanings that the client ascribes to the activity.

Occupation is the combined total of the client's interaction with the environment, selected activities, and tasks. Activity analysis is the means by which practitioners design OT interventions to achieve an optimal fit between the client, the environment, and an activity. We also use **occupational performance analysis**, which is an observational **evaluation** of a person's task performance to identify discrepancies between the demands of a task and the skill of the person (Fisher, 1998) CS1-13. These are among the most important tools that we, as OT practitioners, have. We must know how to analyze activities in order to help clients function in their occupational routines and daily lives.

An Art and a Science

Activity analysis is an art and a science. It is an art because OT practitioners engage their ingenuity to offer "just-right" challenges to their clients in a multitude of occupations, activities, and tasks. We use it to support and give direction to client **involvement** in selected tasks. This support is the key to engagement in activities that can then become engagement in occupations and **participation** in life's contexts. Activity analysis is a science because we apply all the theories we have learned to accurately offer appropriate interventions to our clients. In this respect, activity analysis is employed as a clinical reasoning tool that we use to analyze **occupational performance** and to design interventions targeted at people, environments, and/or occupations.

Activity analysis lies somewhere in the middle of knowing how to perform the activity and how to use the activity therapeutically. It looks at every step, every action, and every aspect of what is needed to accomplish the activity. A detailed activity analysis helps the OT practitioner choose appropriate activities that challenge and interest the client. The presentation of the activity is structured to bring about change for the client. A thorough analysis of an activity prior to beginning it with a client helps to ensure that the activity will go smoothly.

Activity analysis is at the core of occupational therapy. The Accreditation Council of Occupational Therapy Education (ACOTE) requires that students be able to "exhibit the ability to analyze tasks relative to areas of occupation, performance skills, performance patterns, activity demands, context(s) and client factors to implement the intervention plan" (ACOTE, 2007, p. 666). Occupational therapy practitioners are skilled at considering the transactional relationship between a client's abilities, the environment, and the occupation or activity to maximize outcomes (Law et al., 1996). A change in the person, environment, or occupation leads to a change in occupational performance.

An activity analysis template that can be found near the end of this chapter has been developed for you to use as an important classroom to clinic tool. It includes aspects of the occupational therapy domain as outlined in the *Occupational Therapy Practice Framework III* (AOTA, 2014). Either turn to the template or make a copy of it and follow along with it as you read this chapter. You will also be using this activity analysis template to respond to the case studies in this chapter as well as in *Unit Seven* of this textbook.

Activity Selection

An OT practitioner may plan what he/she feels is the "perfect" treatment activity. However, if the client has no interest in the activity, it will be meaningless. If a client is unable to communicate, take the time to interview a family member or friend to discover the client's interests. Does the activity provide the opportunity to express the client's values? Every client has values or principles they stand for or oppose. An activity that supports the client's values will typically be more meaningful. Does the activity interest the client? **Meaningful activities** interest and motivate people to participate. Meaningfulness is important as it provides a source of motivation for performance (Trombly, 1995). "We can also think about our client's need to occupy time, not in the sense of 'being busy,' but also in a sense that connotes the action of doing a mental, physical, or social task that is meaningful to the person" (Fisher, 1998, p. 511). A **purposeful activity** has personal significance and tends to be goal directed.

Is the client motivated to participate in this activity? Client motivation plays a large part in encouraging the client to challenge him/herself. If the client is motivated to participate in the activity, she/he will put more effort into it. Does the activity have any spiritual meaning? This is not only the client's connection to religion or a higher power but to any personal source of connectedness in the world.

Identifying the Activity

When preparing an activity analysis, the first thing you need to do is know what the activity is so you know what is to be analyzed. You will want to categorize the activity you have chosen according to one of the eight areas of occupation as outlined in the *Occupational Therapy Practice Framework III* (AOTA, 2014) (see Activity Analysis Template). It is important to know the area of occupation the client considers this chosen activity to correspond with, as it may be one area of occupation for one person and a different area of occupation for another. For example, a person who enjoys weekend gardening would consider this activity leisure. A landscaper would consider gardening work. Gardening is a broad occupation with myriad activities associated with it. Gardening may include watering plants, planting seeds, mowing the lawn, replanting, weeding, and laying mulch. Choosing one of these smaller activities associated with gardening, like planting seeds, is more manageable for activity analysis than analyzing gardening.

Steps of the Activity

Before even starting to complete an activity analysis template, begin by writing a brief activity description describing the activity in general terms and the desired outcome of the activity. This overview summarizes the activity. Some activities will be familiar to you and others will not. Become familiar with the activity before working with your client. If your client or the client's family chooses an activity that you are unfamiliar with, ask them to explain the activity and its steps. That said, do not be caught off guard, as it is your responsibility to do back research on the activity in order to be prepared to facilitate it with your client. Good preparation and understanding of the activity will better ensure that it runs safely and smoothly. Let's consider the example of analyzing the steps of hand washing. Write out the steps to washing your hands. Make sure you include all objects and time factors needed. Now wash your hands following the steps you just wrote.

- Did you correctly sequence the steps?
- Did you forget any parts of the activity?
- If so, rewrite the steps, adding in those details and wash your hands again.

A simple activity you perform several times a day may not be so simple after all.

As you are seeing, you have to focus your thoughts on the initial step of the activity and think about how the activity unfolds. This involves carefully looking at each step or task of the activity in an orderly manner and listing all objects needed for each step. The steps should be clearly broken down so they can be easily understood and followed. An analysis also includes any time factors such as performing (or waiting for) the step for a specific amount of time.

For example, when eating cereal, one must hold the spoon functionally, steady the bowl, scoop the cereal, bring the cereal to the mouth, clear the food from the spoon with the mouth, chew, and swallow. The spoon needs to remain in the hand in order to be brought to the bowl again so the steps can be repeated until the cereal is gone. In this analysis, there are eight steps to successfully and independently eat a bowl of cereal.

How much time will the activity take? Knowing this is important for treatment planning purposes. Some activities or tasks can be completed in one treatment session. Others are done over a period of time. Can a longer activity be broken down and done over shorter periods of time? Does the activity have to be done in a specific sequence in order for it to be accomplished? Activities done in a specific sequence are most helpful to those who like things organized or need assistance organizing things in an orderly manner. Do certain parts of the activity need to be done within a specific time frame? If so, can the client attend for that long or at that time? Does the activity require any planning on the part of the client? You will want to involve clients in some level of planning even if it is a small part such as choosing a particular color of socks to don if the activity is to put on socks and shoes. Some clients function better at different times of the day than at other times. Can therapy be scheduled to take advantage of a client's optimal performance times? (From the Field 11.2).

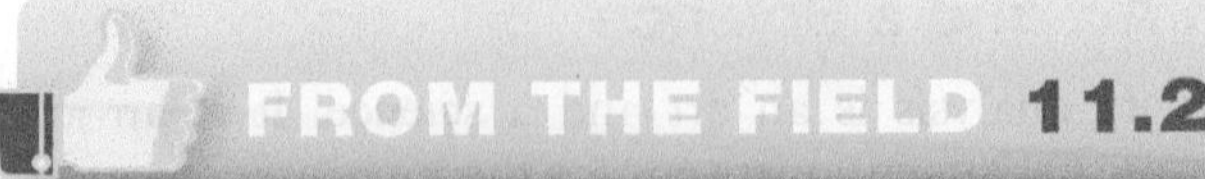

FROM THE FIELD 11.2

Activity Analysis in Daily Life

Think about this. Pay careful attention the next time you fold and put away laundry. Then watch someone else fold and put away his/her laundry. Note the differences and similarities between you and the other person's method of folding and putting away laundry. The end result is that laundry is clean and put away, yet each person has a specific manner of doing the activity.

Instructional Methods

The activity itself as well as the client's cognitive, emotional, and performance abilities must be taken into consideration when planning how to implement it. A flexible or practitioner understands that most every activity can be presented in a variety of ways. While verbal instruction is the standard method of instruction, not everyone learns best this way. Some clients will need visual instructions: step-by-step pictures of the activity, diagrams, or written instructions. Some clients need both pictures and written words. Other clients need to observe another person, usually the OT practitioner or other competent peer, do the activity. Today, we are a generation of people who are familiar with television and video, so some clients may take instruction better from a video. If none are appropriate or available, consider making one. Along with the previously discussed methods, some clients will need hand-over-hand assistance to do all or part of the activity (Fig. 11.1). Will the activity be taught individually or in a group setting? Many activities can be taught both ways. The client's performance skills and the chosen activity will determine the best method of instruction. Usually, it takes a combination of instructional methods to teach an activity.

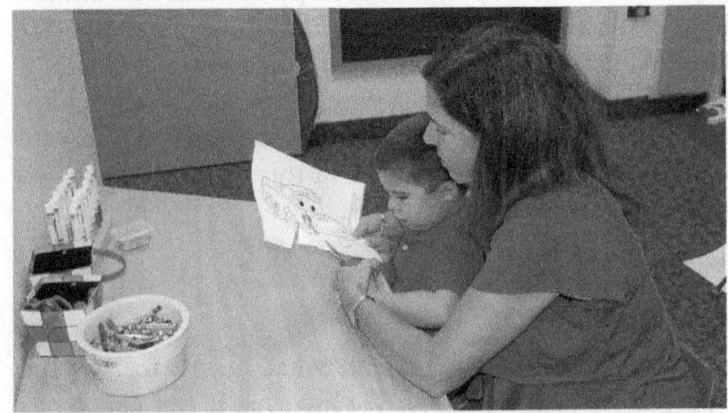

Figure 11.1 An OTA provides hand-over-hand assistance to help a child with a cutting activity. Photo provided by Lisa Van Gorder.

Activity Demands—Objects and Properties

After detailing the steps necessary to complete an activity and the methods of instruction, the OT practitioner must analyze the materials and their properties necessary for the activity. The objects include all equipment, supplies, and tools. This means everything from the salt in a recipe to the drill used in a woodworking activity. It is incumbent upon you to determine where the objects can be obtained: whether they are easily found in the home or clinic or have to be purchased. Consider the cost. Are the materials expensive or not? Are they easily found in a local store or do they need to be special ordered? Does the client already have what is needed?

Whether expensive or not, all materials and equipment have specific properties. The properties describe the objects in the activity. Properties include anything from the texture of a material or object to its safety features. The properties of the objects may prevent the client from engaging in specific activities. For example, because they are sharp, using scissors in an activity may not be appropriate for young clients or for clients who might be dangerous to themselves or others. Using flour as a cooking or baking ingredient may not be appropriate for those with asthma or food allergies.

Qualities of the Activity

When selecting an activity for a client, consider whether the activity allows creativity and self-expression. Does the client consider this a necessary activity to achieve independence in their daily life or do they wish to express themselves in some creative manner? Some clients need a great deal of structure to guide them through the activity, and other clients perform better when given more freedom within the activity. Some activities like sewing and various kinds of needlework repeat the same motion. Repetition can be beneficial for clients with limited cognition, clients that need to practice certain movements, or clients who are working to increase strength in specific muscle groups.

Environmental Demands

The type of activity and objects and their properties help determine the space or environmental requirements. Some activities can be done anywhere and others require special equipment and locations. For example, tooth brushing is most appropriate to be done in the bathroom. If the client uses a wheelchair and the bathroom is too small for the chair, it may need to be done elsewhere, like using a basin placed on a bedside table. Does the activity require open space with proper ventilation? Can it be done indoors or outdoors or both? Does the activity need to begin in a small space and then move to a larger space, as is the case with some building activities. Will the activity require a table? What size will the table be? Will the participants need to sit throughout or at some point during the activity? If so, what type of seating does the client need? Is any other furniture needed, such as a bench, cabinet, or drying rack? If the activity is messy or if it could cause staining, will a specific table surface be needed or can the surface be covered? Is a specific floor surface needed? Is the floor bumpy or smooth? A client using a walker needs to maneuver on a smooth, flat surface.

In addition to the physical layout of the room, the sensory properties of the activity must be analyzed. Lighting is an important consideration for many activities. Some activities and some clients require additional lighting. Is there glare from the sun or lighting that may interfere with the client's performance of the activity? For activities that include items that need to dry or set at specific temperatures, does the room have temperature control? Is the temperature appropriate for the client? Is it too hot, too cold, too sunny, or too dark? Is the noise level appropriate for the client? Some clients work better in a quiet environment and others prefer to work with some auditory distraction. Noise level can be manipulated to meet the client's need. A client who is returning to school needs to learn how to focus in a noisier environment. Visual input is another sensory consideration. Is there a great deal of visual stimuli such as many pictures on the wall and clutter on the counters in the treatment area? Does the client work better in a less visually distracting space or is some visual stimuli needed so the client can accommodate to it and learn to work in a visually busy environment?

Social and Cognitive Demands

Social demands may influence participation in an activity. Matching the social demands of the activity to the performance skills of your client requires careful consideration. The chronological and developmental age of the client must be addressed. For example, a 45-year-old female client with physical challenges and a developmental level of 6 months should not be given an infant rattle. A colorful bracelet may provide the same visual input the client enjoys and is more socially appropriate. What age and gender is your selected activity geared toward? Many activities are unisex and thus useful for people of all ages.

Does the activity require a great deal of money? Golf is a great activity to improve focus and visual attention, but if the client has limited financial resources, it is not an appropriate activity choice. Consider any social group memberships that the client may need to belong to or join in order to participate in this activity. Are social supports needed for activity participation? Can the activity be done alone or will assistance from others be needed to participate in the activity? Is the activity done in a group or as a parallel activity? A parallel activity is one in which people are near each other but are not communicating or working cooperatively. They may be doing the same or different activities.

Does the activity require a higher level of education or can anyone with a basic education complete the activity? What language is the client most comfortable using? If reading instructions is required, can the client read? Is the client a visual learner?

Safety Precautions

When preparing your activity analysis, carefully review every step of the activity, noting the objects to be used, the space requirements, and sensory qualities that are necessary to do the activity. Ask yourself again, does any part of the activity or objects used in the activity pose a safety risk that could potentially harm the client or others? Consider any sharp items used and any supplies that may be toxic. Does the client have any allergies or special dietary needs? Some clients may pose a flight risk so it may not be appropriate for them to engage in outdoor activities. We cannot emphasize enough the importance of being vigilant about client safety and also to know your client, including being well aware of his/her history. As OT practitioners, we are ethically obliged to do no harm.

Required Actions—Performance Skills

After analyzing the steps of the activity and the activity demands, the OT practitioner determines each action and function the body must perform when the activity is done in a typical manner. For example, when analyzing kite flying, standing for upward of 10 minutes is the norm. The *Occupational Therapy Practice Framework III* (AOTA, 2014) organizes body functions and structures under client factors. Analyzing the client's body actions and functions identifies any discrepancies between the demands of the activity and the client's abilities. In the kite flying example, imagine treating a client interested in resuming this favorite occupation who can only briefly stand with limited balance. The activity demands of kite flying are greater than the client's current abilities, so the OT practitioner must think of how to adapt the activity so the client can build the skills needed to resume kite flying.

The activity analysis template contains a column to note the performance skills and required body actions and functions for the activity that is located next to the client's performance skill–body functions and structures column. The purpose of this is to have side-by-side comparison of those actions required for the activity and the performance skills of the client to determine if the activity is feasible without adaptation. Table 11.1 analyzes the one aspect of the performance skills associated with the activity of kite flying. It immediately becomes clear that in order for the client to participate, adaptations must be made in the manner in which the activity is done.

The remainder of this chapter guides you through the many performance skills and body actions that need to be analyzed as part of activity selection. This thorough analysis of the activity is invaluable to the OT practitioner in determining how and if the client can participate. Choosing the right activity at the just-right challenge level can enhance specific performance skills and go a long way toward client goal achievement.

Motor and Praxis Skills

Motor and praxis skills are the movements and physical actions one must do to perform an activity. This includes but is not inclusive of bending, reaching, and grasping. It also includes the planning of and carrying out of physical movement(s). Some of these plans may be internally directed, and some follow the directions given from another person (Ayres, 1995).

Body Functions

The term body function refers to the "physiological functions of body systems" (WHO, 2001, p. 12). Body functions need to be considered when analyzing an activity since the activity could impact body functions. The client's body functions determine whether or not or in which way the client will be able to engage in the activity. These functions do not work in isolation and one function and/or system can influence another.

TABLE 11.1 Analyzing Kite Flying

Performance Skill—Required Body Actions and Functions for Activity	Client Performance Skill—Body Function/Structure	Client Precautions	Adaptations/Grading
Activity is done in standing for 10 min.	The client is able to stand for 2 min.	The client has poor endurance and standing balance.	Have the client sit every 2 min of the activity with support as needed and alternate between standing and sitting to fly a kite. Increase standing time as endurance increases.

Neuromusculoskeletal and Movement-Related Functions

Neuromusculoskeletal and movement-related functions include joint mobility and stability, muscular strength, endurance, and tone (AOTA, 2014). Table 11.2 briefly analyzes one body function/structure movement and performance skill for a right-handed client recovering from left elbow surgery who must remain in a splint stabilizing the left elbow at 45 degrees for 8 weeks post-surgery and is unable to stabilize food while cutting.

Body Systems

The cardiovascular/hematological system includes the heart, veins, arteries, and blood. Dysfunction of these systems may lead to hypertension, hypotension, and postural hypotension. If a client has heart disease and uses an external oxygen supply, there is significant precaution to be followed.

The respiratory system includes the nose, mouth, pharynx, epiglottis, larynx, and lungs. Its function is "inhaling air into the lungs, the exchange of gases between air and blood, and exhaling air" (WHO, 2001, p. 87). The OT practitioner must be aware of a client's respiration rate and any possible hindrances to airflow such as chronic obstructive pulmonary disease or emphysema.

The immune system fights off infection and protects us from diseases. There are many disorders that negatively affect the immune system such as lupus, rheumatoid arthritis, and HIV/AIDS. Allergic reactions are autoimmune responses. An OT practitioner must be aware of any client immune system deficiencies and the necessary precautions to be taken.

The digestive system includes the esophagus, stomach, large intestine, small intestine, colon, and anus. Dysphagia and aspiration are included in the area of digestion. Clients with digestive disorders may need to engage in activities in proximity to a restroom. Participation in food-related and cooking activities may be limited for the client with problems in this area.

The excretory system includes the kidneys, bladder, ureters, and urethra. Does the client need the restroom frequently? Is the client incontinent or have a catheter? Is a restroom nearby?

The dermatological system includes functions of the skin, hair, and nails. Is the client sensitive to certain textures or products? Does the client have thin skin or bruise easily? Is the client prone to skin breakdown? A client undergoing certain forms of chemotherapy may experience tenderness and cracking of the skin around the fingernails and fingertips.

Sensory and Perceptual Functions

Sensory and perceptual information is necessary to engage in activity. This includes detecting the sensation, processing the information, and responding appropriately to the incoming information (Ayres, 1995). The senses help distinguish between sensations that require responses and those that can be ignored (please also refer to Chapter 28, *Sensory Issues*). When the systems are performing optimally, sensory and perceptual information keeps us safe.

Visual functions include acuity and how we use vision. Diseases of the eyes such as cataracts or macular degeneration can make things appear blurred or hazy and significantly affect performance. Visual–perceptual functions combine the reception and cognition of visual stimuli (Schenk, 2005). What is seen with the eye must be interpreted by the brain. These skills include visual attention, visual memory, matching, figure ground, depth perception, position in space, form constancy, and visual closure (please also refer to Chapter 31, *Vision*). Auditory functions include acuity, or how well a person can hear, and auditory discrimination, the ability to differentiate between sounds. Vestibular functions provide the body with information on the speed and direction of movement. The vestibular system responds to changes in the body's position (Ayres, 1995). Taste functions enable people to discriminate between edible and nonedible material, hot and cold, sweet, sour, salty, and bitter. Smell function enables people to identify dangerous odors as well as pleasant ones. Smell function is often altered as a result of chemotherapy and aging.

Proprioceptive functions allow people to understand where their position in space is. Touch functions enable people to identify objects without seeing them and to differentiate between sharp and dull, rough and

TABLE 11.2 Analyzing Cutting Food Post-Surgery

Movement and Structure	Required Body Action and Functions/Performance Skill for Activity	Client's Body Functions/ Structure/Performance skill	Client Precautions in this Area	Adaptations/Grading
Elbow movement	Elbow held at about 80 degrees of flexion holding fork to stabilize food.	Elbow stabilized in a splint at 45 degrees of flexion.	Unable to flex or extend elbow. Elbow stabilized at 45 degrees.	Use a rocker knife.

smooth, etc. Temperature functions enable people to distinguish between hot and cold. Pain functions enable the person to recognize that something is amiss in the body. Understanding a person's pain level is important in treatment. We often informally assess pain on a scale of 1 to 10, with 10 being a very high level of pain and 1 being no or very little pain.

Emotional Control and Regulation

Emotional control and regulation are behaviors clients use to identify, manage, and express feelings (AOTA, 2014). We express our feelings through words, actions, facial expressions, and body language. Emotional regulation skills are those behaviors needed to express feelings. Some activities can evoke feelings of sadness or happiness. Some activities can elicit aggression. Engagement in well-thought-out activities may also help a client develop coping mechanisms and build frustration tolerance.

Does the activity contribute to the client's self-esteem? Self-esteem is a feeling of personal pride and respect for oneself (*Merriam Webster Online Dictionary*, 2015). Self-esteem is demonstrated by assertiveness and assurance in competence (WHO, 2001). Does the activity provide an opportunity for the client to test reality? Sometimes, clients' perceptions of what they are able or unable to do are inaccurate. Engaging in a meaningful therapeutic activity may help a client recognize his/her abilities. Clients are often pleasantly surprised by what they can do when engaged in a motivating activity.

Communication and Social Skills

Communication includes receptive communication, the ability to understand what is said or read, and expressive communication, the ability to verbally express one's needs and wants. Although the most familiar manner of communication is verbal, some clients may communicate with pictures or gestures or use sign language. Some clients use a combination of systems to communicate. Expressive communication may be affected by oral motor control issues. It is important to consult with a speech pathologist or OT knowledgeable in oral motor control if you suspect oral motor control issues.

Cognitive skills include executive functioning such as higher-level thinking, decision making, memory, judgment, abstract thinking, problem solving, and planning. A client's ability to demonstrate appropriate judgment and safety awareness helps the OT practitioner determine if an activity is appropriate and what level of supervision is required.

Organizational skills may be necessary for some activities. Organizational skills include the ability to put like items together, arrange items or events in an orderly manner, and/or correctly carry out a sequence of steps. Multitasking is the ability to do more than one thing at a time. The ability to focus on several events at once such as paying the bills while talking on the phone is an example of multitasking.

The above description of required body actions, functions, and performance skills is not an exhaustive list. Although the activity itself may be the constant factor, every person performs it differently. The OT practitioner takes on the challenge of adjusting the manner in which the activity is performed to ensure optimal outcomes.

Performance Patterns

Performance patterns are developed and established over time. Performance patterns are influenced by many factors in the client's life. Once established, it is difficult to change some of these performance patterns. Performance patterns include habits, routines, roles, and rituals (AOTA, 2014).

Habits are automatic behaviors that are typically done on a day-to-day or regular basis. Some of these habits are very useful and help support performance. Some habits or automatic behaviors can be harmful and/or interfere with occupational performance. A client who smoked a cigarette after dinner for 30 years may find this a hard habit to break even after having a heart attack.

Does the performance of the activity utilize, reinforce, or help create routines? Routines are established sequences of occupations or activities that provide a structure for daily life (AOTA, 2014, p. S21). For example, awakening at 6 AM every morning, doing 10 push-ups, 20 situps, putting on running gear, and going for a 2-mile run before breakfast is a routine. Routines are observable and repetitive. They are embedded into culture (Fiese et al., 2002, Segal, 2004). Routines can help to organize one's time in order to be productive.

Does the activity reinforce a client's customary role? Roles are those behaviors shaped by a culture or society. Ideally, an individual determines if a role is acceptable. For example, some women accept the role of caretaker in the home and do the laundry and house cleaning and others do not. Some clients need to develop new roles. This is especially true after an injury that limits or prevents the client from performing previous roles. Children learn new roles as they go through the many stages of the developmental process.

Rituals are symbolic actions with spiritual, cultural, or social meaning that contribute to the client's identity and reinforce the client's values and beliefs (Fiese et al., 2002). Rituals do not have to be religious in nature. Going swimming every morning is a ritual for someone linked to a belief in a healthy lifestyle.

Context and Environment

Every activity is done within a specific context or environment. There are a variety of contexts to consider. One is the physical context. This includes the place in which the activity is done. The social context involves who is present when doing an activity. Is the person alone, with the OT practitioner, with other clients, with family members? How many people are in the room? Are the people familiar or strangers? What are the others doing? Cultural context includes the customs, beliefs, and expectations of the society of which the client is a member (AOTA, 2014). Personal context refers to demographic factors. This includes the client's age, gender, educational level, and socioeconomic status (WHO, 2001). The virtual context refers to those interactions absent of physical contact. This includes using the phone, emailing, using Skype, texting, and online chat rooms. Temporal contextual factors have to do with time: the time of day, the day of the week, the time of the year, and the season, as well as time allotted for the activity. All contexts influence the client's performance in some way.

Knowing your client's current performance skills, patterns, and goals as well as the relationship between the client's, environment, and occupation is critically important to ensure **client-centered** intervention, which embraces the concept that the client's wishes and desires with regard to therapy are the focus of the intervention process. It also lays the foundation for a **collaborative** client–practitioner working relationship. Part of client-centered intervention involves thorough activity analysis. Having this information paves the way to provide a good fit and a just-right challenge based on the selected intervention process. It lays the foundation for a process of working cooperatively to achieve a goal.

Grading and Adapting Activity

Grading and **adapting** an activity are core functions of occupational therapy. It is the ability to make small and subtle changes to an activity or any of its parts, thus enabling a client to successfully engage in the activity. Grading can increase or decrease the demands of an activity or change the way the activity is done. Grading can and should be altered continuously during a treatment session as the client meets or falls short of meeting the challenges of the activity. Grading requires that an OT practitioner be alert and flexible and always ready to change the course of the activity during a treatment session. Incremental modifications are made in response to the individual's dynamic changes and provide opportunity for gradual development of skill and related therapeutic benefits (Hinojosa et al., 1993). Grading can be continued at the same rate or changed during a treatment session or from one treatment session to the next on an as-needed basis. Grading activities need to challenge the client's abilities by progressively changing the process, tools, materials, or environment of a given activity to gradually increase or decrease the performance demands (Hinojosa et al., 1993). This position reflects the changes that are presumed to occur in a client's performance skills or needs.

The role of the OTA in grading activities to meet client needs is unequivocal. According to the *ACOTE Standards for Occupational Therapy Assistants*, "the occupational therapy assistant will be able to grade and adapt the environment, tools, materials, occupations, and interventions to reflect the changing needs of the client and the sociocultural context" (ACOTE, 2007, p. 668). The OTA should also be able to "teach compensatory strategies, such as use of technology, adaptations to the environment, and involvement of humans and nonhumans in the completion of tasks" (AOTA, 2007, p. 668). The client's current performance skills and goals dictate the type of grading necessary. There are many ways to grade an activity to increase or decrease the activity demands. The OT practitioner uses careful judgment to determine whether the activity demands should be increased or decreased.

Grading an Activity

The following suggestions are ideas to grade an activity. They are not intended to be comprehensive lists as the ways in which nearly every activity can be graded must be based on the client's performance skills, body structures, and goals, and not be proscribed. Instead, these lists can and should be expanded to be as long and detailed as the OT practitioner's creativity allows (Table 11.3).

Activity Adaptation

Adaptation is directed at "changing the demands of the occupation so they are congruent with the person's ability level" (Crepeau & Boyt Schell, 2009, p. 370). Adaptation is a process that actually changes an aspect of the activity or the environment to enable successful performance. The adaptation may remain in place for the long term and/or can be removed when no longer needed. Although some adaptations may follow the same techniques used for grading, the purpose of grading is to increase or decrease the activity demands, whereas adaptation allows the client to participate in the activity. For example, following shoulder surgery, a client returns home and to cooking in his kitchen. He needs to have the items from the pantry shelves placed on the counter because he cannot reach high enough to retrieve items from the shelves. As his range of motion improves, the activity is graded and the items are placed on the first shelf, thereby challenging the client to reach higher. As time progresses, the surgeon determines that the client's range of motion will not increase any further. What was initially a technique to grade the activity by placing the items on a higher shelf has now become a permanent adaptation as the client will be able to reach to the first shelf and no higher.

TABLE 11.3 How to Grade an Activity

Structuring an activity	Select a familiar or new activity Do the activity in a familiar or new way Select the activity for the client or let the client choose it Structure the activity or allow it to be unstructured Increase or decrease the duration of the activity Keep the activity simple Add additional steps to the activity to increase the complexity Alter the cognitive demands of the activity Increase or decrease the repetitions for part or all of the activity Structure predictable or unpredictable outcomes Increase or decrease some weight to the activity (if strengthening is a goal)
Tool selection	Object selection can be larger or smaller to accommodate hand grasp goals Shape of the tool can change to accommodate hand grasp goals Select heavier or lighter tools Textural changes to accommodate sensory needs Assistive devices to make the activity easier
Environmental contexts	Have the client stand or sit Select different types of seating options—therapy balls, stools, chairs, etc. Place parts of activity in different areas of the treatment space so client must access components while moving about the clinic or environment Change the position of the activity to increase or decrease range of motion: higher up, lower down, a little further away
Temporal contexts	Duration of the activity; short or long or somewhere in between Time the task to measure progress Initiate the activity for the client Have the client initiate the activity Allow time for client to take breaks; it is very important to include this in the intervention plan
Instructional methods	Type of instruction/cues given—visual, verbal, physical Frequency of instruction and cueing Vary the duration between the time instruction is given and start of activity Eliminate some steps in instructions to encourage the client to problem solve
Social contexts	Engage with client more or less frequently during the activity Encourage other staff/clients/family to talk to the client during the activity Have more or fewer people in the treatment area Include familiar or unfamiliar people in the treatment area Have younger or older people in the treatment area Structure as individual or group activity Add a level of competition to the activity Have the client work cooperatively with someone

TABLE 11.3 How to Grade an Activity (continued)

Treatment environment	Work in a large or small treatment area Work in a familiar or unfamiliar treatment area Include more or fewer items in the treatment area to increase or decrease sensory distraction Select specific types of items in the environment to increase or decrease sensory distraction Adjust for more or less noise in the treatment area Increase or decrease the visual stimuli in the environment
Physical demands	Structure specific movements Increase repetitions of a specific movement Unilateral or bilateral activity Sit or stand to work
Cognitive factors	Change the memory demands Alter the problem-solving demand Ask the client to read the activity instructions (if written material apply) Have client determine how to obtain materials for an activity (use computer search, make a phone call) Remove one or several written or verbal directions to address memory skills such as sequencing
Emotional factors	Add a level of frustration to the activity (i.e., sabotage—NOTE: this needs to be done with extreme caution and insight and under the direct supervision of an OT) Encourage the client to interact with other clients including asking to share materials Provide more or less praise/feedback Alter the way feedback is provided—verbal or nonverbal or decreased to find the just-right challenge for the client.

Grading and adapting activities are an essential part of occupational therapy and a skill that with time and practice becomes instinctive to the OT practitioner. It is the incremental grading to meet the client's performance skills that help clients' achieve goals and participate in activities. The adaptations that help client's engage in occupation are as numerous and individual as the clients (From the Field 11.3).

Activity Analysis Template

We have come to a very important place in the chapter. Up to this point, you have been provided with the base information necessary to complete an all-important activity analysis. Now, it is time to look at the activity analysis template that has been designed for you and integrates what you have learned about in this chapter and apply it to future activity and occupational performance analysis. This template is going to be useful for you going from classroom to clinical practice (Fig. 11.2).

Case Studies

What follows are two case studies of clients with whom we have had the honor and privilege to work with in our private and clinical practices. Make a copy of the

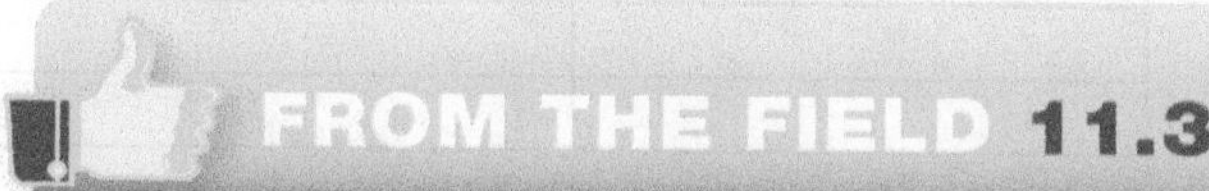

Creativity

Occupational therapy technology has its roots in the creativity of the individual practitioner who finds out what works or does not work in the real world of practice. The insightful, inventive practitioner uses his or her specialized knowledge together with skilled observation and clinical judgment to both evaluate and develop our technology (Schön, 1983).

Activity Analysis Form

Page 1

Activity ______

Area of Occupation:

_____ Activities of Daily Living
_____ Instrumental Activities of Daily Living
_____ Rest and Sleep
_____ Education
_____ Work
_____ Play
_____ Leisure
_____ Social Participation

Brief Activity Description:

______

Describe how the activity is done: (Add more space and steps if necessary.)

Step 1 ______
Step 2 ______
Step 3 ______
Step 4 ______
Step 5 ______
Step 6 ______
Step 7 ______
Step 8 ______
Step 9 ______
Step 10 ______

Sequencing and Timing:

How much time will the activity take? ______
Can it be broken down and done for short periods of time? ______ How? ______
Does activity have to be done in a specific sequence? ______ Why? ______
Do certain parts of the activity have to be done in a specific time frame? ______ If so, which ones? ______

Does this activity require the client to plan parts of the activity? ______ If so, which parts? ______

Method of Instruction:

- Verbal: __ Oral
- Visual: __ Pictures __ Written Words __ Video __ Demo __ Diagram
- Tactile Cueing: ______
- Group Instruction: ______
- Individual Instruction: ______

Activity Demands:

Objects Used	Properties	Where purchased/found	Cost

Qualities of the Activity:

Does the activity allow for creativity? ______ Which parts? ______
Is the activity structured or unstructured? Explain why. ______
Does the activity have repetitive parts? ______ What are they? ______

Figure 11.2 Activity analysis template.

Activity Analysis Form (continued)

Page 2

Environmental Requirements: _____ Indoors _____ Outdoors _____ Either

Room size ______________ Seating ______________ Furniture ______________ Lighting ______________
Ventilation ______________ Temperature ______________ Floor surface ______________
Table surface ______________ Noise level ______________ Visual Stimuli ______________

Safety Precautions: ________________________________

Social Demands:

_____ Male
_____ Female
_____ Either

_____ Group activity
_____ Individual activity

Educational level needed: ______________
Group membership needed? _____ Yes _____ No
Activity is done: _____ Alone _____ Group _____ Parallel activity
If with others, a minimum of how many people are needed? _____

Required Actions/ Performance Skills:

	Performance Skills/ Required Body Actions & Functions for Activity	Performance Skills/ Client's Body Function/ Structure	Client Precautions	Adaptations/Grading
Body position and motion				
Trunk control				
Trunk endurance				
Crossing midline				
Head movement				
Shoulder movement				
Elbow movement				
Wrist movement				
Hand skills				
Upper extremity strength				
Upper extremity endurance				
Upper extremity coordination				
Fine motor manipulation				
Unilateral task				
Bilateral task				
Hip movement				
Knee movement				
Ankle movement				
Lower extremity strength				
Lower extremity endurance				
Lower extremity coordination				
Muscle tone				

Figure 11.2 *(continued)*

Activity Analysis Form (continued)

Page 3

Required Actions/ Performance Skills (continued):

	Performance Skills/ Required Body Actions & Functions for Activity	Performance Skills/ Client's Body Function/ Structure	Client Precautions	Adaptations/Grading
Motor reflexes				
Motor planning				
Cardiovascular/hematological function				
Immunological function				
Respiratory function				
Digestive function				
Excretory function				
Dermatological function				
Visual function				
Visual-perceptual function				
Auditory function				
Taste function				
Smell function				
Proprioceptive function				
Touch function				
Pain function				
Temperature function				
Emotional control/regulation				
Impulse control				
Expressive communication				
Receptive communication				
Oral motor control				
Collaboration with others				
Judgment/safety awareness				
Executive functions				
Reading				
Calculations				
Memory				

Figure 11.2 *(continued)*

Activity Analysis Form (continued)

Page 4

Required Actions/ Performance Skills (continued):

	Performance Skills/ Required Body Actions & Functions for Activity	Performance Skills/ Client's Body Function/ Structure	Client Precautions	Adaptations/Grading
Organization skills				
Multitasking				
Others as needed:				

Additional Client Factors:

How does the activity provide the opportunity to express the client's values?

How does the activity interest the client?

How is the client motivated to participate in this activity?

How does the activity have any spiritual meanings for the client?

How could the activity positively contribute to the client's self-esteem?

How does the activity offer opportunity for affective expression?

____ Aggression ____ Sadness ____ Happiness ____ Love ____ Others

How does the activity provide an opportunity for the client to test reality?

Performance Patterns:

How does the performance of this activity reinforce useful habits?

How does the performance of this activity reinforce poor habits?

How does the performance of the activity utilize, reinforce or help create routines?

How does the activity reinforce a customary role for the client?

How does the activity help establish a new role for the client?

How does the activity reinforce rituals performed by the client?

Context and Environment (describe):

Physical

Social

Temporal

Cultural

Personal

Virtual

Additional Information:

Figure 11.2 *(continued)*

activity analysis template to keep near you as you read the case studies. Challenge yourself to complete all, if not most, of the information as it applies to each case study you are about to read.

Meet Kimmy

Kimmy is a bright, curious, social 5-year-old. Evaluations indicated that she was a highly intelligent child. In some ways, she is a "typical" child, curious about everything, wanting to assert her independence, play with friends, go to school, and communicate. She was seen for OT twice weekly in her home from the time she was 6 months old until the family moved when she was 7 or 8 years old.

Kimmy was born with congenital nemaline myopathy, a rare condition that left her weak to the point of initially being unable to sit independently, eat "real" food, play outside, go to school, even roll over in bed, and talk. She was fed via a gastric tube. She had a tracheostomy and used a ventilator at night and sometimes during the day when breathing was a challenge. The relationship between Kimmy and the OT was a close one. Relationships with her parents and the other therapists who worked with her were collaborative and inventive in order to meet Kimmy's goals.

At age 5, Kimmy's broad goals for herself, as she communicated them to us through gestures, pictures, and simply with her expressive eyes, aligned with the goals of her parents and therapists. They included the following:

1. Find ways to provide typical developmentally appropriate life experiences for Kimmy.
2. Help her maintain or increase what muscle strength and range of motion she has.
3. Improve her means of communication, especially with peers and others outside her family and therapists' networks.
4. Improve back muscles and balance reactions to the point that Kimmy can sit unsupported for up to 30 minutes at a time 3 to 5 times a day for meals, play, and therapy in order to meet insurance company criteria for obtaining a power wheelchair.
5. Provide alternate means where necessary, to accomplish these goals.

As soon as Kimmy was able to sit upright for up to 30 minutes supported, she was brought to the table for meals with her parents. She "ate" from her gastric tube while they ate their meal. After receiving clearance from her pediatrician, Kimmy was given "tastes" of what her parents ate. She especially loved sweet and salty things like French fries with catsup and ice cream. During occupational therapy, Kimmy was challenged to sit independently while we baked simple cookies and various soft foods such as pudding that she could lick off a spoon or let melt in her mouth. These activities were graded by Kimmy; she began by simply watching the activity and allowing the spoon to be brought to her lips and in time progressed to being able to reach above table height to add ingredients to the bowl and stir the mixture. Eventually, she was able to independently dip a spoon into a low-sided bowl and bring foods like pudding to her mouth.

Kimmy enjoyed board games and other age-appropriate games. This was made possible with adaptations such as larger game pieces and placing a magnetized sheet under the board and on game pieces so they would not move or fall over as easily. She had to reach for, grasp, and move the pieces that the OT gradually made heavier as Kimmy became stronger.

Kimmy was not initially eligible for a power chair. She had to be able to sit for extended periods of time and operate the chair safely. What 5-year-old child wants to be pushed by their parent while playing with other children? The solution to this dilemma came in the form of a battery-operated play car that she could use when playing outside with other children. Initially, Kimmy had to work hard to sit upright with only a seat belt and some cushions for support. She quickly learned how to sit in the car for up to an hour with little or no support, exceeding our goal for her. She did not have the strength to operate the car's "gas" pedal with one foot, so she taught herself how to get both feet on the pedal and push to go. This self-determined innovation had the added value of strengthening her legs. Her upper extremities also became stronger simply because of their position when steering the car. The social component of connecting with friends was solved by Kimmy herself. If no one was out playing, she would go to their homes, drive up to the front door, bump against it with her front bumper, and then wait. When the door was finally opened, Kimmy would back away slightly and gesture for her friend to come out and play (Fig. 11.3).

Kimmy and her parents loved Mickey Mouse and went to Disneyland whenever they could. After seeing her steer her car, the insurance company agreed to a power chair. The family purchased a wheelchair-fitted van and began spending time with Mickey.

Kimmy worked at using a marker or piece of chalk to write and draw. She could even tell a joke with this creative system and would cover her mouth with her hand, shake her head up and down, and indicate that she was laughing. She eventually learned to use a battery-operated communication board mounted on her chair. From there, she began using a computer. Later, when she learned to read, she wrote short stories and poems on her computer (Fig. 11.4).

Meet Les

We met Les in an inpatient rehabilitation facility, where he had been for the past 5 weeks. Les is a single, 45-year-old male. Three months ago, Les had a stroke, which affected his speech and the right side of his body. He is right handed.

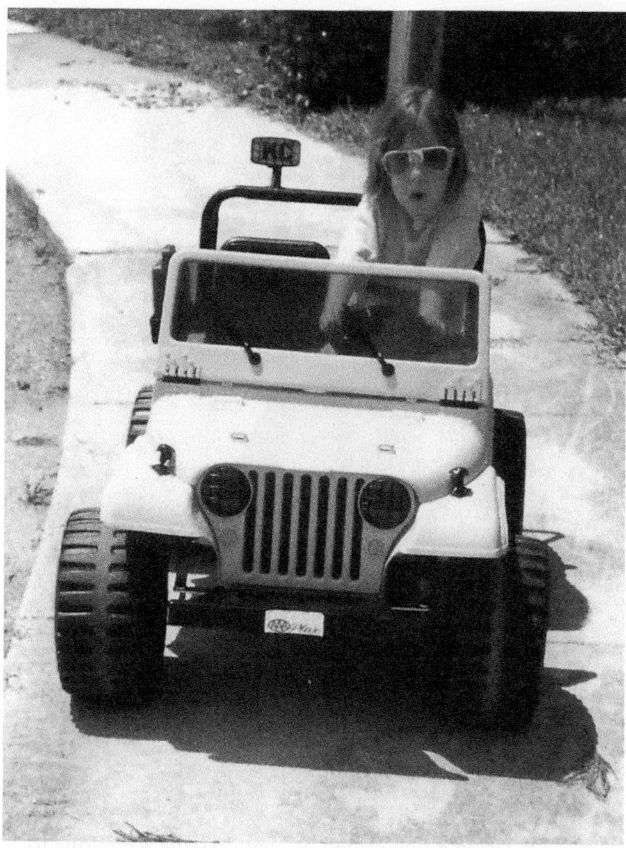

Figure 11.3 Kimmy driving to a friend's home to play.

Prior to the stroke, Les worked in a very physically challenging job, installing and repairing satellite receiving dishes and their circuitry. He frequently had to climb high ladders atop buildings and power towers. He was adept at climbing and working in high places. He also demonstrated excellent dexterity and problem-solving skills while working with electrical currents. Les is an outdoorsman. He is an avid fisherman and managed to go fly fishing and hiking at least once every few months.

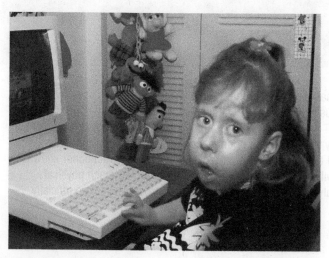

Figure 11.4 Kimmy drawing on the computer and playing educational games.

In his various therapies, Les is currently learning to walk with a cane. This was graded up only last week from a walker. He is working on oral speech as well as learning to use an iPad communication program. He is able to clumsily raise his right arm and has enough gross grasp in his right hand to hold a drinking glass but is not yet strong enough to lift the glass and bring it to his mouth. Les will soon be transitioning to outpatient therapy.

Les has managed to communicate to his OTA that he knows he will not be returning to his former job. His boss has reassured him that he will have a job when he returns to work although it will probably be in the office or warehouse. Les is motivated to work toward this goal.

Les lived alone in a small, one-story home for many years and wishes to return to doing so. Family members live close by and are in agreement with this arrangement. They have promised to look in on him and help in any way they can such as with transportation, shopping, meal preparation, and so forth. Les would ultimately like to be able to do these things for himself. He also wishes to return to his outdoor interests of fishing and hiking.

The most immediate goal agreed upon between the evaluating OT and Les is to increase right upper extremity functional grasp, strength, and range of motion (ROM) at shoulder, elbow, wrist, and hand for all activities of daily living (ADL) skills. These include dressing, hygiene, and eating. The independent activities of daily living (IADL) skills of simple meal preparation and light shopping are included in the goals as Les' status improves. Les will also work on learning one-handed adaptations to his typical daily activities and tasks. He is trying very hard to reach his goals and is willing to make adaptations if they mean his ticket to independence. These adaptations may be temporary, in which case they will serve as graded activities for the present time, as was the walker, and will hopefully give way to decreased reliance on adaptations as time goes on.

In terms of self-care, one-handed eating skills are addressed during meals, and dressing techniques are being addressed during therapy sessions and practiced in his room at appropriate times each morning and evening. The OTA provides suggestions about how to incorporate his right hand more for daily activities as he progresses. Working on various activities to increase functional right-hand grasp and active right-arm use in therapy has led to Les being able to steady his plate by lifting his right arm and placing his forearm around it. Les now holds the fork in his left hand and is able to scoop up soft food without spilling and spear cut-up meat. Les's self-identified long-term goal is to eat right

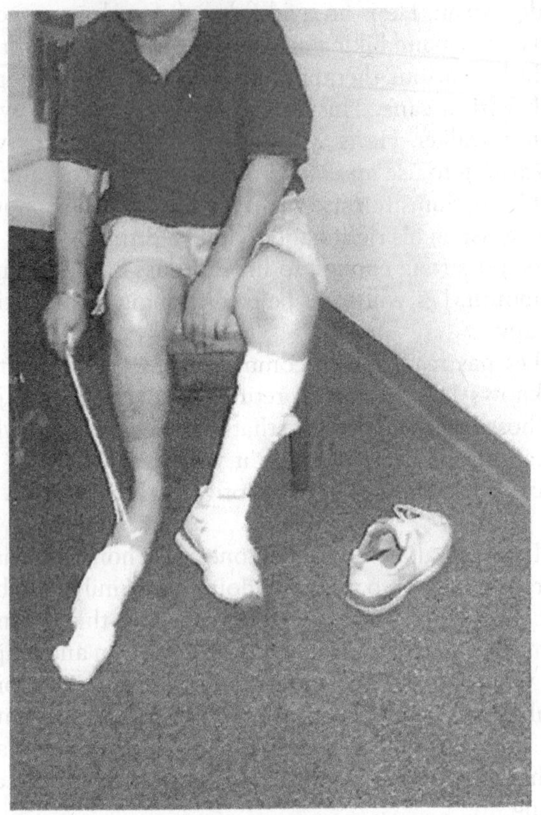

Figure 11.5 Using a sock aid to don socks.

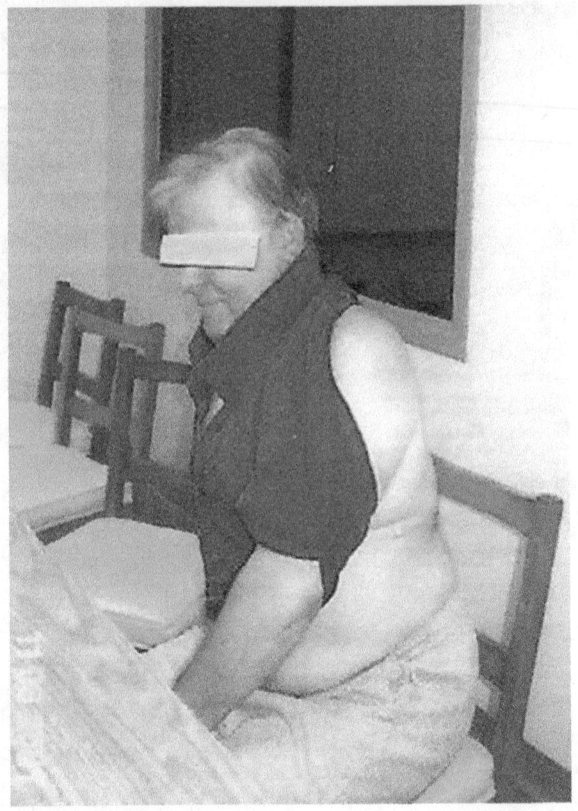

Figure 11.6 Using a one-armed or hemidressing technique to don a T-shirt.

handed as he did before having a stroke. For now, Les is wearing drawstring pants and loose-fitting T-shirts that are easier for him to put on and are more comfortable for his therapy sessions. Dressing goals include using snap-front pants with progression to button-front pants. Putting a shirt on and taking it off is being addressed as is putting on and removing shoes and socks (Figs. 11.5 and 11.6). For the present, he wears slip-on or Velcro closure shoes. These may remain as an adaptation if he is unable to do one or two hand shoe tying.

Summary

The process of preparing an activity analysis shows us that even a simple activity has many complex parts. Activity analysis can be a rigorous but extremely rewarding endeavor. Despite the challenge, activity analysis unequivocally helps OT practitioners engage our clients in occupation and participation to match the just-right fit of the activity to the client's performance skills. Contrary to what makes those who do understand occupational therapy think it is off the cuff play, the OT practitioner knows that each activity has a purpose that will help the client overcome challenges and reach physical or emotional goals. When you start analyzing every activity you do and/or observe, you are officially thinking like an OTA.

Review Questions

1. An activity is:
   a. A specific deed, action, or function as it is done by a specific individual
   b. A general or universal outline of how anyone might do a certain activity
   c. Usually but not necessarily goal directed
   d. Always goal directed
   e. Both b and c

2. The terms occupation, activity, and task may be used interchangeably in the context of an activity analysis.
   a. True
   b. False

3. OT practitioners seek to personalize the goals, contexts, environments, and techniques of a selected activity to achieve:
   a. Competence in the activity
   b. Adaptation of the activity
   c. An exercise in activity analysis
   d. An optimal fit between the client and all the component parts of the activity

4. Activity analysis is an art and a science because:
   a. The practitioners attempt to challenge their client in a variety of occupations, activities, and tasks
   b. It is used in order to support and give direction to a client's involvement in selected tasks
   c. We use it to analyze occupational performance and to design appropriate interventions for our clients
   d. We apply all the theories we have learned to accurately offer appropriate interventions to our clients
   e. *All of the above*

5. "Occupational therapy's legacy of humanistic ways, occupational justice, and timeless truths" are based on:
   a. The effect the activity has on the client
   b. The value it has for the client's familial, social, and cultural systems
   c. Our standard instructions for each activity and the way we present it to the client
   d. A and B

6. Grading can:
   a. Increase or decrease the demands of an activity or change the way the activity is done
   b. Be done continuously during an intervention session as the client meets or is not able to meet the challenges of the activity
   c. Can be continued at the same level or changed from one intervention session to the next
   d. All of the above

7. Adaptation and grading differ how?
   a. Adaptation challenges the client's abilities by progressively changing the process, tools, materials, or environment of a given activity.
   b. The purpose of grading is to increase or decrease the activity demands, and adaptation allows the client to participate in the activity at their current level.
   c. Grading is the process that actually changes an aspect of an activity or the environment to enable successful performance in that activity.

8. Les's current inability to use his right upper extremity to put his T-shirt on is:
   a. A required body function
   b. A client body function
   c. A client precaution
   d. An adaptation or grading

9. The occupational therapy assistant:
   a. Does only what the OT tells him or her to do regarding the activities to use with a client.
   b. Is on the front lines to interpret the goals established by the OT and interpret them into activities that are meaningful for the client.
   c. Works independently to decide which activities to do with the client.

10. In terms of communication and social skills, expressive and receptive communication refers to:
    a. Verbal/written and understanding
    b. Written and sign language
    c. Verbal/written and augmentative communication
    d. Verbal/written and computer skills

Practice Activities

Revisit "Meet Kimmy" in this chapter. Look at her pictures. Create a goal and write an activity analysis for it and a performance analysis for Kimmy. Include any adaptations needed. Your plan and goals will not be the same as those described by the OT who worked with Kimmy. Apply your personality, your imagined relationship with Kimmy and her family, and your individual way of thinking and problem solving. That is the way it should be.

If you were Les's OTA, how would you respond to each one of his goals? As Les makes progress in using his right upper extremity, how could you grade up the activities? What adaptations in other occupations of his life might be of help later if he is unable to increase use of his right upper extremity?

Les's home is a short walk away from the grocery store. If he walks to the store, how might he get his parcels home? How would he retrieve groceries from the shelves in the store? What could be done to help him prepare a simple frozen meal or cut food? Are there task-oriented, meaningful activities related to fly fishing that Les could participate in that might increase right upper extremity use at the same time? What activities could Les participate in that would use some of the tools with which he is familiar, such as wire cutter, long-nose pliers, and screwdriver? What time(s) of day seem most appropriate for working on the goals Les and his therapist have established? As well, think of some activities that might interest Les that would work on his problem-solving skills and right-handed dexterity.

Practice interviewing another person to learn what occupations, activities, and tasks are important to them. Use this information to construct an occupational profile. An example of an occupational profile can be found in Chapter 10, *The Occupational Therapy Treatment Process*.

Describe the cultural and personal contexts of baking a cake from the standpoint of a baker who bakes for a livelihood and a woman who enjoys baking a cake for her family. How does context influence meaning and purpose? What tasks are needed for this activity as a work occupation and as a leisure occupation? How do they compare and/or contrast? Select one task in the activity of baking a cake as a work and leisure occupation. What are the demands of the task (required actions body functions, body structures) and how do they compare?

References

American Occupational Therapy Association. Occupational therapy practice framework: domain and process (3rd ed.). *Am J Occup Ther* 2014;68(Suppl 1):S1–S48. http://dx.doi.org/10.5014/ajot.2014.682006

AOTA. *Definition of Occupational Therapy Practice for the AOTA Model Practice Act*. 2011. Retrieved from http://www.aota.org/Practitioners/Advocacy/State/Resources/PracticeAct/36437.aspx?FT=.pdf

ACOTE. Accreditation standards for an educational program for the occupational therapy assistant. *Am J Occup Ther* 2007;61:662–671.

Author. *Scholastic Pocket Dictionary*. New York, NY: Scholastic Reference; 2005.

Ayres AJ. *Sensory Integration and the Child*. Los Angeles, LA: Western Psychological Services; 1995.

Creigton C. The origin and evolution of activity analysis. *Am J Occup Ther* 1992;46:45–48. http://dx.doi.org/10.5014/ajot.46.1.45

Crepeau EB, Boyt Schell BA. *Analyzing Occupations and Activity*. In: Creapeu EB, Cohn ES, Boyt Schell BA, eds. *Willard and Spackman's Occupational Therapy*. 11th ed. Baltimore, MD: Lippincott Williams & Wilkins; 2009:359–374.

Fiese BH, Tomcho TJ, Douglas M, et al. A review of 50 years of research on naturally occurring family routines and rituals: cause for celebration? *J Fam Psychol* 2002;16: 381–390.

Fisher AG. Uniting practice and theory in an occupational framework. 1998 Eleanor Clarke Slagle Lecture. *Am J Occup Ther* 1998;52(7):509–521.

Hinojosa J, Sabari J, Pedretti L. Position paper: purposeful activity. *Am J Occup Ther* 1993;47(12):1081–1082.

Law M, Cooper B, Strong S, et al. The person–environment–occupation model: a transactive approach to occupational performance. *Can J Occup Ther* 1996;63:9–23.

Law M. Distinguished scholar lecture: participation in everyday life. *Am J Occup Ther* 2002;56:640–649.

Law M, Polatajko H, Baptiste W, et al. Core concepts of occupational therapy. In: Townsend E, ed. *Enabling Occupation: An Occupational Therapy Perspective*. Ottawa, ON: Canadian Association of Occupational Therapists; 1997: 25–56.

Merriam Webster online dictionary. Self-estem; 2015. Retrieved from www.merriam webster.com/dictionary.self-esteem

Preamble to the Constitution of the World Health Organization as adopted by the International Health Conference. New York, 19-22 June, 1946, signed on July 1946 by the representatives of 61 States. (Official Records of the World Health Organization, no. 2, p. 100 and entered into force on 7 April, 1948).

Royeen CB. Chaotic occupational therapy: collective wisdom for a complex profession. *Am J Occup Ther* 2003;57:609–624.

Schenk CM. Visual perception. In: Case-Smith J, ed. *Occupational Therapy for Children*. 5th ed. Philadelphia, PA: Elsevier Mosby; 2005:412–446.

Schön DA. *The Reflective Practitioner*. New York: Basic Books; 1983.

Thomas H. *Occupation-Based Activity Analysis*. Thorofare, NJ: Slack, Inc.; 2012.

Trombly CA. Occupation: purposefulness and meaningfulness as therapeutic mechanisms. 1995 Eleanor Clarke Slagle Lecture. *Am J Occup Ther* 1995;49(10):960–972.

World Health Organization. *International Classification of Functioning, Disability, and Health, Short Version*. Geneva, Switzerland: World Health Organization; 2001.

UNIT

III

Scope of Practice

The ethos of occupational therapy restores our clear-sightedness so that we see what is essential: We are pathfinders. We enable occupations that heal. We cocreate daily lives. We reach for hearts as well as hands. We are artists and scientists at once.

—Suzanne M. Peloquin

CHAPTER 12

Ethics

Amy Wagenfeld, PhD, OTR/L, SCEM, CAPs

Key Terms

Autonomy—To respect the right of the individual to self-determination, privacy, confidentialy, and consent." (AOTA, 2015, p. 4, paragraph 2).

Beneficence—"Demonstration of" a concern for the well-being and safety of the recipients of their services" (AOTA, 2015, p. 2, paragraph 5).

Deontological—The action is right unto itself.

Ethical actions—"A manifestation of moral character and mindful reflection… a commitment to benefit others, to virtuous practice of artistry and science, to genuinely good behaviors, and to noble acts of courage" (AOTA, 2015, p. 1, paragraph 3).

Ethical behavior—Involves several concepts including universalism, disinterestedness, and cooperation.

Ethical practice—Identify, analyze, and clarify ethical issues or dilemmas to make responsible decisions" (AOTA, 2010d standards for continuing competence document).

Ethical reasoning—An internal debate about right and wrong conduct.

Ethics—"The study of standards of conduct and moral judgment" (Guralnik, 1986, p. 481).

Fidelity—"Treat clients, colleagues and other professionals with respect, fairness, discretion, and integrity" (AOTA, 2015, p. 8, paragraph 1).

Nonmaleficence—"To refrain from actions that cause harm" (AOTA, 2015, p. 3, paragraph 2).

Justice—"Promote fairness and objectivity in the provision of occupational therapy services." (AOTA, 2015, p. 5, paragraph 2).

State Regulatory Boards—Entity that has legal jurisdiction over occupational therapy practitioners.

Teleological—The consequences of actions.

Veracity—"Provision of comprehensive, accurate, and objective information when representing the profession" (AOTA, 2015, p. 6–7, paragraph 2 (p.6), paragraph 1 (p. 7)).

Learning Objectives

After studying this chapter, readers will be able to:

- Explain the meaning and purpose of the AOTA *Occupational Therapy Code of Ethics* (AOTA, 2015) and how it impacts your role as an occupational therapy assistant.
- Understand the differences and similarities between ethical reasoning, actions, and behaviors and how they influence the profession.
- Become familiar with the six principles of the *Occupational Therapy Code of Ethics* (AOTA, 2015) and articulate the meaning of each as it applies to clinical practice as an occupational therapy assistant.

Introduction

Take a moment to think about how you feel when you are acting at your best. What comes to mind? What physical sensations do you feel right now? Contrast this to thinking about how you feel when you are at your worst. What emotions and physical sensations do you experience? Can you apply this line of thinking to what you envision as representative of an ethical community, business, government, and society? The standards of behavior we ascribe to ourselves, to others, and to groups are what ethics are all about. Velasquez et al. (2009) at the Markkula Center for Applied Ethics at Santa Clara University describe not only what ethics are but also what they are not. Ethics are not feelings. Feeling contribute to the ethical choices we make. Ethics are not religion. Not everyone is religious, but ethics apply to everybody regardless of religious preference. Ethics is not following the law. While a good legal system incorporates ethical standards, laws can veer away from what is ethical. Think about totalitarian regimes. Are their laws ethical? Ethics are not following culturally accepted norms. Sometimes, culturally accepted norms are terribly unethical, like slavery was in the United States pre–Civil War. Just because everyone is doing something does not make it ethical. Ethics is not science. While science can provide information to guide ethical thinking, reasoning, and action, it is not ethics. You may be starting to wonder, if ethics are not based on feelings, law, religion, accepted social practice, or science (Velasquez et al., 2009), just what are they? In this chapter, we explore the concept of ethics and how they apply to occupational therapy and to you, as an emerging OTA.

Ethics

As defined by the *Webster's New World Dictionary*, **ethics** are "the study of standards of conduct and moral judgment" (Guralnik, 1986, p. 481). The study of ethics looks at concepts such as "right versus wrong, justice, equality, free will, and responsibility" (Bloom, 1994, p. 52). Ethical theories can be **teleological**, focusing on the consequences of actions, or **deontological**, in which the action is right unto itself—in essence it is doing the right thing (Cummings, 1993). Ethical principles encompass four standards, "(a) prudence- choosing the right means, (b) temperateness—acting in moderation, (c) courage—being willing to do what is right, and (d) justice—treating others with respect and honor" (Wagenfeld & Hsi, 2003, p. 47).

According to Cummings (1993), **ethical behaviors** specific to occupational therapy practice include universalism, being nonbiased in the ways we treat and interact with others; disinterestedness, not being solely driven by money while always providing the best possible treatment (note: this does *not* mean working for free); and cooperation, being collaborative and engaged in working with and sharing information with others.

Ethical action is "a manifestation of moral character and mindful reflection. It is a commitment to benefit others, to virtuous practice of artistry and science, to genuinely good behaviors, and to noble acts of courage" (AOTA, 2015, p. 1, paragraph 3). When we act in an ethical manner as OT practitioners, we uphold the high standards to which our profession calls for.

Ethical reasoning is an internal debate about right and wrong conduct. According to the Association of American Colleges and Universities, ethical reasoning involves a self-assessment of "ethical values and the social context of problems, ...[of] ethical issues in a variety of settings, [and] think[ing] about how different ethical perspectives might be applied to ethical dilemmas and consider[ation of] the ramifications of alternative actions" (*assessment.aas.duke.edu/documents/ethicalreasoning.pdf*).

Velasquez et al. (2009) suggest that people undertake a specific process to making **ethical decisions**. This sequence is illustrated in Figure 12.1.

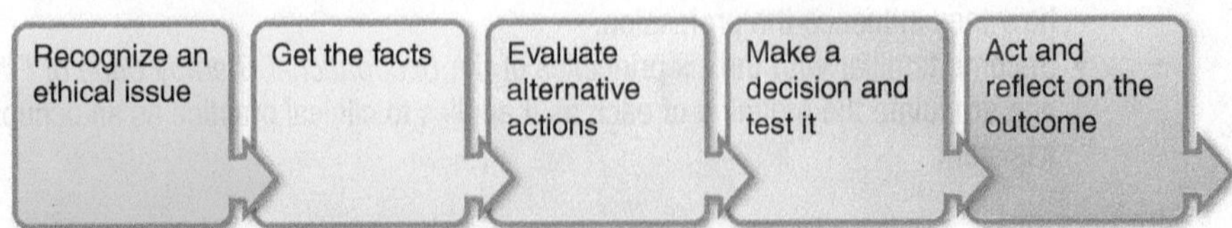

Figure 12.1 The sequence of ethical decision making. (Adapted from Velasquez M, et al. A framework for thinking ethically. 2009. Retrieved from http://www.scu.edu/ethics/practicing/decision/framework.html)

The AOTA *Standards for Continuing Competence* (AOTA, 2010c) contains five standards, one of which is **ethical practice**. According to this standard,

> Occupational therapists and occupational therapy assistants shall identify, analyze, and clarify ethical issues or dilemmas to make responsible decisions within the changing context of their roles and responsibilities.
>
> The individual must demonstrate in practice the following:
>
> - Understanding and adherence to the profession's *Code of Ethics Standards* (AOTA, 2010a; 2015), other relevant codes of ethics, and applicable laws and regulations
> - The use of ethical principles and the profession's core values to understand complex situations
> - The integrity to make and defend decisions based on ethical reasoning
> - Integration of varying perspectives in the ethics of clinical practice (p. S105)

Ethical Dilemmas: Where to Go for Help

If you have concerns about professional ethical issues, it is important to know where to turn for assistance. The AOTA is a first-line resource for help in terms of providing resources on how to approach dealing with ethical issues. As we will discuss in greater detail shortly, the Commission on Ethics (EC) is an important resource to become familiar with as they are tasked to review ethics complaints that involve occupational therapy. Other sources of assistance that you may turn to for help with ethical issues are your supervisor, the human resource department at your place of employment, the National Board for Certification of Occupational Therapy (NBCOT), and your local and **state licensing or regulatory boards**. It is incumbent upon you to vet ethical concerns when they arise, rather than simply waiting to see if they resolve on their own. As you will soon read, the six principles of the *Occupational Therapy Code of Ethics* (AOTA, 2015) explicitly state that as OT practitioners, we must aspire to hold ourselves to the highest standards in our professional and personal conduct. This includes facing ethical issues head on and reporting them to the appropriate personnel for their immediate attention From the Field 12.1.

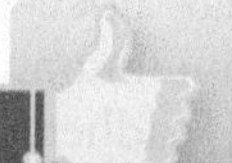

FROM THE FIELD 12.1

Hints for Negotiating

Negotiating a professional contract (or any contract) is an important skill to master. There are some things for you to think about in order to make the process and outcomes work best for you, including addressing head on, how potential ethical concerns you have may be addressed by your future employer.

1. Before you are even offered a contract, make a list of things that are important to you such as vacation, salary, billing expectations, location, payback, and noncompete clauses.
2. Make a list of ethical concerns that you want to vet with any prospective employer such as supervisory roles and responsibilities, billing, confidentiality issues, and equitable intervention services for all.
3. Prepare a statement that you request be put into your contract stating that an employer will not violate the AOTA's *Occupational Therapy Code of Ethics* (AOTA, 2015), your state licensure law, Medicare regulations, or any other state or federal law with regard to practice standards or payback clauses for sign on bonuses or scholarships.
4. Read your contract several times *before* you sign it.
5. The time between receiving a contract and signing it is the *only* time you can negotiate points two and three above. During contract negotiation is when you have the most leverage.
6. There is little or nothing you can do after you sign to try to change the terms of a contract.
7. Of course, there are no guarantees that all or some of your requests will be granted, but unless you speak up, nothing will change.
8. If you find that the terms of the contract are not palatable and the employer is not willing to amend the contract, you must decide if you wish to proceed with accepting the job.

Adapted from Kornblau B. How to avoid some ethical dilemmas. *Adv Occup Ther Pract* Retrieved from http://occupational-therapy.advanceweb.com/Article/How-to-Avoid-Some-Ethical-Dilemmas.aspx

Code of Ethics

Originally drafted in 1998 as the *Occupational Therapy Code of Ethics*, and revised in 2005, the current *Occupational Therapy Code of Ethics Standards*

(AOTA, 2015) is an important aspirational document that every OT practitioner should, at minimum, be familiar with and, optimally, consistently adhere to in professional practice. The most recent version, *Occupational Therapy Code of Ethics Standards* was published in 2015 (AOTA, 2015). The *Occupational Therapy Code of Ethics Standards* (AOTA, 2015) is as follows:

> "… an AOTA official document and a public statement tailored to address the most prevalent ethical concerns of the occupational therapy profession. It should be applied to all areas of occupational therapy and shared with relevant stakeholders to promote ethical conduct. (AOTA, 2015, p. 1, paragraph 2). "It is a commitment to benefit others, to virtuous practice of artistry and science, to genuinely good behaviors, and to noble acts of courage" (AOTA 2015, p. 1, paragraph 3). Further, "Occupational therapy personnel, including students in occupational therapy programs, are expected to abide by the Principles and Standards of Conduct within this Code" (AOTA, 2015, p. 1, paragraph 3)."

The revised *Occupational Therapy Code of Ethics Standards* integrates four previous ethics documents, the *Occupational Therapy Code of Ethics* (2010a; 2005), the *Guidelines to the Code of Ethics* (AOTA, 2006), and the *Core Values and Attitudes of Occupational Therapy Practice* (AOTA, 1993). The *Occupational Therapy Code of Ethics* (AOTA, 2015) clearly acknowledges that occupational therapy remains firmly grounded in seven core concepts, as identified in the seminal *Core Values and Attitudes of Occupational Therapy Practice* document (AOTA, 1993). They are altruism, equality, freedom, justice, dignity, truth, and prudence. (Please refer to Chapter 3, *Core Values and Philosophy*, for a more detailed discussion of these seven concepts). The *Code of Ethics Standards* "provides aspirational Core Values that guide members toward ethical courses of action in professional and volunteer roles, and delineates enforceable Principles and Standards of Conduct that apply to AOTA members" (AOTA 2015, p. 1, paragraph 2).

The historical foundation of the *Occupational Therapy Code of Ethics* is derived from "ethical reasoning surrounding practice and professional issues, and empathic reflection regarding these interactions with others" (AOTA, 2005; 2006; 2010b, p. S17). The *Occupational Therapy Code of Ethics* is deeply rooted in ethical action, "a manifestation of moral character and mindful reflection. It is a commitment to benefit others, to virtuous practice of artistry and science, to genuinely good behaviors, and to noble acts of courage" (AOTA, 2015, p. 1, paragraph 3).

Because it is aspirational and not legal in intent, the *Occupational Therapy Code of Ethics* (AOTA, 2015) is designed to protect the public and to reinforce its confidence in the occupational therapy profession. It is not intended to resolve private business, legal, or other disputes for which AOTA believes are better suited for other avenues of resolution (AOTA, 2015).

As you have just read, the *Occupational Therapy Code of Ethics* (AOTA, 2015) is an aspirational rather than legal document. Remember, ethics are not laws, but shape the development of them. With regard to occupational therapy, what agency is responsible for what when ethical violations are identified? Figure 12.2 illustrates that because AOTA is a voluntary membership agency, it has no legal authority over its members. The NBCOT regulates practice, credentialing, and a practitioner's eligibility or ineligibility to practice. The legal authorities for occupational therapy are the state, regional, and territorial boards who are ultimately responsible for the investigation and prosecution of ethical misconduct.

The *Occupational Therapy Code of Ethics* (AOTA, 2015) is based on six moral principles and standards: beneficence, nonmaleficence, autonomy, justice, veracity, and fidelity. What follows is a brief description of these principles and standards associated with occupational therapy. The *Code and Ethics Standards* (AOTA, 2015) can be found in its entirety online at http://www.aota.org/media/-/Corporate/Files/AboutAOTA/Officialdocs/Ethics/CodeofEthics.pdf

Beneficence

Principle 1. "Occupational therapy personnel shall demonstrate a concern for the well-being and safety of the recipients of their services" (AOTA 2015, p. 2, paragraph 5).

The concept of **beneficence** encompasses all types of action that are intended to help others, including preventing and removing harm (AOTA, 2015). To help clients make informed choices, it is incumbent upon OT practitioners to thoroughly understand and articulate the benefits and risks of treatment procedures (Wagenfeld & Hsi, 2003). There are 10 identified actions of beneficence in the *Occupational Therapy Code of Ethics* (AOTA, 2015) that occupational therapy practitioners are strongly urged to adhere to in their scope of practice.

Nonmaleficence

Principle 2. "Occupational therapy personnel shall refrain from actions that cause harm" (AOTA, 2015, p. 3, paragraph 2).

Nonmaleficence means to do no harm under any circumstances. An OT practitioner must maintain an ongoing internal dialogue of what constitutes nonmaleficence. This principle often is examined under the context of

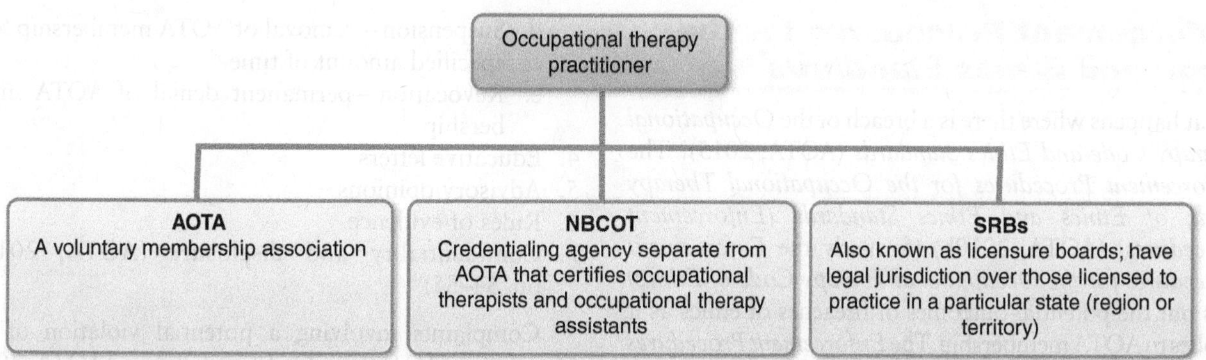

Figure 12.2 Who does what: AOTA, National Board for Certification in Occupational Therapy, and state (regional or territorial) regulatory boards. (Adapted from American Occupational Therapy Association. Frequently asked questions about ethics. 2010b. Retrieved from http://www.aota.org/Practitioners/Ethics/FAQs.aspx)

due care (AOTA, 2015). There are 10 identified actions of nonmaleficence in the *Code of Ethics Standards* (AOTA, 2015) that OT practitioners must refrain from in their scope of practice.

Autonomy

Principle 3. "Occupational therapy personnel shall respect the right of the individual to self-determination privacy, confidentiality, and consent" (AOTA, 2015, p. 4, paragraph 2).

Autonomy posit that OT practitioners must follow a client's wishes within the accepted standards of care and to always maintain and protect client confidentiality. Autonomy factors prominently into health care ethics. It does so particularly with regard to respecting and carrying out a client's wishes in terms of the direction of their care. Autonomy and confidentiality extend to students, research subjects, and all who seek information about occupational therapy services. There are 10 identified actions of autonomy in the *Occupational Therapy Code and Ethics* (AOTA, 2015) that OT practitioners must follow to in their scope of practice.

Justice

Principle 4. "Occupational therapy personnel shall promote fairness and objectivity in the provision of occupational therapy services" (AOTA, 2015, p. 5, paragraph 2).

Justice goes beyond simply following the law. It embraces justice and impartiality on any number of social and cultural levels. It levels the playing field and calls for following the rules and for equitable treatment and benefits for all people regardless of any challenges they face. Prioritizing services in a just and moral manner is a challenge that all OT practitioners must address head on. There are 16 identified actions of justice in the *Occupational Therapy Code of Ethics* (AOTA, 2015) that OT practitioners must provide to in their scope of practice.

Veracity

Principle 5. "Occupational therapy personnel shall provide comprehensive, accurate, and objective information when representing the profession" (AOTA, 2015, p. 7, paragraph 1).

Truthfulness, candor, and honesty comprise the principle of **veracity**. In health care systems, veracity encompasses "comprehensive, accurate, and objective transmission of information and includes fostering the client's understanding of such information" (Beauchamp & Childress, 2013, in AOTA, 2015, p. 7, paragraph 1). We pay due respect to others when exercising veracity. We apply veracity to establish trust relationships. Being transparent and avoiding deception with clients and research participants is a necessary part of veracity. Veracity is balanced with other ethical principles and cultural sensitivity and organizational policies and procedures. There are 10 identified actions of veracity in the *Occupational Therapy Code of Ethics* (AOTA, 2015) that OT practitioners must provide in their scope of practice.

Fidelity

Principle 6. "Occupational therapy personnel shall treat colleagues and other professionals with respect, fairness, discretion, and integrity" (AOTA, 2015, p. 8, paragraph 1).

The principle of **fidelity** derives from the Latin root fidelis meaning loyal. In the health professions, fidelity refers to maintaining good faith relationships between various service providers and recipients. In the context of this principle, fidelity applies most to maintaining collegial and organizational relationships as well as balancing "duties to service recipients, students, research participants, and other professionals as well as to organizations that may influence decision-making and professional practice" (AOTA, 2015, p. 8, paragraph 2). There are 13 identified actions of fidelity in the *Occupational Therapy Code of Ethics* (AOTA, 2015) that OT practitioners should adhere and aspire to in their scope of practice.

Enforcement Procedures for the Code and Ethics Standards

What happens where there is a breach of the *Occupational Therapy Code and Ethics Standards* (AOTA, 2015)? The *Enforcement Procedures for the Occupational Therapy Code of Ethics and Ethics Standards (Enforcement Procedures)* (AOTA, 2010b) (formerly the *Enforcement Procedures for the Occupational Therapy Code of Ethics)* lays out the potential outcomes of breaches of ethics as it applies to AOTA membership. The *Enforcement Procedures* (AOTA, 2010a) recently underwent series of revisions by the AOTA's Commission on Ethics (AOTA, 2010a, p. S4). The *Enforcement Procedures* (AOTA, 2010a) are applied to maintain compliance with the *Occupational Therapy Code of Ethics* (AOTA 2015). The primary purpose of the *Enforcement Procedures* is to "ensure objectivity and fundamental fairness to all individuals who may be parties in an ethics complaint" (AOTA, 2010a, p. S4). Acceptance of AOTA membership commits individuals to adherence to the *Occupational Therapy Code of Ethics Standards* and cooperation with its *Enforcement Procedures* (AOTA, 2015, p. S4). There are seven issues that the AOTA EC focus on when dealing with a potential ethical issue. The seven issues are as follows:

1. Professional responsibility and other processes
2. Jurisdiction
3. Disciplinary actions/ sanctions (pursuing a complaint)
   a. Reprimand—a formal expression of disapproval of conduct communicated privately by letter from the EC Chairperson that is nondisclosable and noncommunicative to other bodies (e.g., state regulatory boards [SRBs], National Board for Certification in Occupational Therapy [NBCOT]).
   b. Censure—a public expression of formal disapproval
   c. Probation of Membership Subject to Terms—failure to meet terms will subject an AOTA member to any of the disciplinary actions or sanctions.
   d. Suspension—removal of AOTA membership for a specified amount of time
   e. Revocation—permanent denial of AOTA membership
4. Educative letters
5. Advisory opinions
6. Rules of evidence
7. Confidentiality and disclosure (AOTA, 2010b, pp. S4–S5)

Complaints involving a potential violation of the *Occupational Therapy Code and Ethics* (AOTA 2015) may be initiated by any person, group, or entity within or outside AOTA (AOTA, 2010a, p. S6). Following a period of up to 90 days, the EC reviews and investigates the complaint and determines whether further action is to be taken and notifies involved parties. This investigation phase is followed by a review and decision process. Respondents (those who are under review for an ethical violation) may come before a disciplinary council to respond to or refute charges or sanctions. An appeals process follows the review and decision process. Notification of final decisions is put in writing and sent via certified delivery service to all parties. Records and reports are kept in the AOTA Ethics Office for 5 years. Decisions regarding sanctions and other disciplinary action are publicized only after the appeals process has been completed.

Because neither AOTA nor its EC is a legal entity, actions taken by the Commission do not impact an occupational therapy practitioner's right to practice, but do impact membership in the AOTA. The NBCOT that *does* have authority to revoke an occupational therapy practitioner's credentials, making him/her ineligible to practice. To that end, the goals of the NBCOT are to "promote public health, safety, and welfare by establishing maintaining, and administering standards, policies, and programs" of occupational therapy practitioners at all levels of practice (NBCOT, 2005; Rose, 1996, p. 613).

Summary

In large part, engaging in ethical practice with clients, research participants, and colleagues is a key to success in practice. While ethics are not laws, they are principles to which all practitioners should aspire to uphold in their scope of practice as well as how they live their lives. How do you aspire to fill these large shoes that past, current, and future OT practitioners have walked in and will continue to walk in?

Review Questions

1. The *Occupational Therapy Code of Ethics Standards* principle of fidelity is:
   a. Treating colleagues and other professionals with respect, fairness, discretion, and integrity
   b. Transparency with regard to treatment and research protocol
   c. Maintaining confidentiality and respecting a client's wishes with regard to the direction of treatment
   d. Doing no harm

2. Which of the following is not an intended purpose of the *Occupational Therapy Code of Ethics Standards*?
   a. Educate the general public and members regarding established principles to which occupational therapy personnel are accountable
   b. Socialize occupational therapy personnel to expected standards of conduct
   c. Describe the means by which investigation of ethical violations are implemented
   d. Assist occupational therapy personnel in recognition and resolution of ethical dilemmas

3. Which of the following entities oversees credentialing for occupational therapy practitioners?
   a. AOTA
   b. SRBs
   c. IRBs
   d. NBCOT

4. What is the most serious disciplinary action the AOTA Ethics Commission can take against a member of AOTA?
   a. Reprimand
   b. Censure
   c. Revocation
   d. Probation

5. A deontological ethical theory focuses on:
   a. Doing the right thing
   b. Finding a balance between perception and effect of an action
   c. Focusing on the consequences of the action
   d. Presumptive action

6. An internal debate about right and wrong action best describes:
   a. Ethical theory
   b. Ethical behavior
   c. Ethical reasoning
   d. Ethical action

7. Which of the following best describes beneficence?
   a. A concern for the well-being and safety of the recipients of their services
   b. To respect the right of the individual to self-determination
   c. To refrain from action that may cause harm
   d. To provide services in a fair and equitable manner

8. Which of the following entities is responsible for handling legal issues with regard to occupational therapy?
   a. AOTA
   b. SRBs
   c. IRBs
   d. NBCOT

9. To intentionally refrain from actions that cause harm best describes which of the *Occupational Therapy Code of Ethics Standard* principles?
   a. Nonmaleficence
   b. Beneficence
   c. Justice
   d. Fidelity

10. To comply with institutional rules, local, state, federal, and international laws and AOTA documents applicable to the profession of occupational therapy best describes which of the *Occupational Therapy Code of Ethics Standard* principles?
   a. Nonmaleficence
   b. Beneficence
   c. Autonomy
   d. Justice

11. A teleological ethical theory focuses on:
   a. Doing the right thing
   b. Finding a balance between perception and effect of an action
   c. Focusing on the consequences of the action
   d. Presumptive action

Practice Activities

Choose one of the ethical dilemmas below. Applying ethical theory, reasoning, actions, and behaviors, work with a classmate to prepare a short skit with two different outcomes for the ethical dilemma you choose. Poll your class to determine which outcome is interpreted as most ethical. Expand this activity by creating a longer list of dilemmas and acting them out.

1. Your supervising therapist has asked you to evaluate Mrs. Smith and fill her in on the results.
2. You are on a home visit to see an 18-month-old client. When you begin your session, you notice that the client has a series of round burns on her forearm.
3. You are working on a per diem basis at a skilled nursing facility. You have been instructed that you must bill a minimum of the equivalent of 10 hours per day and are being paid for 8 hours a day.

Identify 10 ethical acts that you observe in 20 to 25 people that you know and also strangers doing in a span of 24 hours. Place a check mark next to all that you do on a daily basis. Place a star next to all you do on a weekly or monthly basis. Place a hash mark next to those you never do. Share you results with your classmates. What ethical behaviors did you observe the most? Least?

You are on your first fieldwork placement in a rehabilitation facility. One of your patients is recovering from a self-inflicted gunshot wound to the head that resulted in left hemiparesis and very limited use of his left upper extremity. He is left-handed. Because you know that client-centered practice is the best way to implement the therapy process, you are pleased to observe that your supervising OT is following the principle of autonomy and confidentiality by asking the client to share what his goals are for therapy. The client replies that he wants to regain enough control of his left hand to be able to hold a gun and try to finish what he started (suicide). How do you view this scenario through the lens of ethics and occupational therapy?

References

American Occupational Therapy Association. Core values and attitudes of occupational therapy practice. *Am J Occup Ther* 1993;47:1085–1086.

American Occupational Therapy Association (2014). Enforcement Procedures for the Occupational Therapy Code of Ethics Standards. *Am J Occup Ther*, 2014;68(Suppl.):S3–S15. doi: 10.5014/ajot.2010.64S4-686S02

American Occupational Therapy Association. (In Press). Occupational therapy code of ethics. *Am J Occup Ther* 69(Suppl.3). Retrieved from from http://www.aota.org/-/media/Corporate/Files/AboutAOTA/OfficialDocs/Ethics/Code-of-Ethics.pdf

American Occupational Therapy Association. Occupational therapy code of ethics. *Am J Occup Ther* 2005;59:639–642.

American Occupational Therapy Association. Guidelines to the occupational therapy code of ethics. *Am J Occup Ther* 2006;60:652–658.

American Occupational Therapy Association. Enforcement procedures for the Occupational Therapy Code of Ethics and Ethics Standards. *Am J Occup Ther,* 2010a;64(Suppl.):S4–S16. doi: 10.5014/ajot.2010.64S4–64S16

American Occupational Therapy Association. Occupational therapy code of ethics and ethics standards. *Am J Occup Ther* 2010b;64(Suppl.):S17–S26. doi: 10.5014/ajot.2010.64S17–64S26

American Occupational Therapy Association. Standards for continuing competence. *Am J Occup Ther* 2010c;64(Suppl.):S103–S105. doi: 10.5014/ajot.2010.64S10–64S105.

Association of American Colleges and Universities. *Ethical reasoning value rubric*. n.d.. Retrieved from http://www.assessment.aas.duke.edu/documents/ethicalreasoning.pdf

Beauchamp TL, Childress JF. *Principles of Biomedical Ethics*. 6th ed. New York, NY: Oxford University Press; 2009.

Bloom GM. Ethical issues in occupational therapy. In: Jacobs K, Logigian MK, eds. *Functions of a Manager in Occupational Therapy* (rev. ed.), Thorofare, NJ: SLACK, Inc.; 1994:52–66.

Braveman B, Bass-Haugen JD. Social justice and health disparities: an evolving discourse in occupational therapy research and intervention. *Am J Occup Ther* 2009;63:7–12.

Cummings G Sr. Principles of occupational therapy ethics. In: Ryan SE, ed. *Practice Issues in Occupational Therapy: Intraprofessional Team Building*. Thorofare, NJ: SLACK, Inc.; 1993:307–314.

Guralnik DB (Editor in Chief). *Webster's New World Dictionary*. New York, NY: Simon and Schuster; 1986.

National Board for Certification in Occupational Therapy. *NBCOT organizational principles*. 2005. Retrieved from http://www.nbcot.org/index.php?option=com_content&view=article&id=90%3Aprinciples-and-mission&catid=17&Itemid=14

Rose BW. In: Cox JB, et al. ed., *State Regulation and Specialty Certification of Practitioners*. 1996. *The occupational therapy manager*. pp.603–625. Bethesda, MD: AOTA.

Velasquez M, et al. *A framework for thinking ethically*. 2009. Retrieved from http://www.scu.edu/ethics/practicing/decision/framework.html

Wagenfeld AE, Hsi JD. Credentialing, ethics, and legalities of practice. In: Solomon A, Jacobs K, eds. *Management Skills for the OTA*. Thorofare, NJ: SLACK, Inc.; 2003:39–58.

CHAPTER 13

Supervision in Occupational Therapy

Tia Hughes, DrOT, MBA, OTR/L

Key Terms

Aide (technician)—A therapy personnel member who is trained by an occupational therapist or an occupational therapy assistant to perform specifically delegated tasks. These nonskilled and nonbillable tasks are to be performed only after competency has been determined.

Competency—An individual's actual performance in a specific situation refers to one's capacity to perform job responsibilities.

Cosignature—A signature on a document that indicates that more than one individual was responsible for the information in the document. In the field of occupational therapy, the term is often used when a supervisor signs a document to identify that there was oversight by him or her in the work done.

Interrater reliability—The level at which two or more individuals arrive at the same results following the administration of the same process.

Licensure—Within occupational therapy, recognition from a state or territory that a practitioner has met the requirements to practice in the field of occupational therapy for the time indicated by the license. Each state or territory determines these criteria as well as disciplinary action for those individuals not meeting the required standards.

Malpractice—The breach by a member of a profession of either a standard of care or a standard of conduct usually results in damage to a client.

Manager—The process of governing, directing, and controlling.

Occupational therapist—Initially certified practitioner who is responsible for all aspects of occupational therapy service delivery and who is accountable for the safety and effectiveness of the occupational therapy service delivery process.

Occupational therapy assistant—Initially certified practitioner who delivers occupational therapy services under the supervision of and in partnership with occupational therapists.

Practitioner—An occupational therapist or an occupational therapy assistant.

Scope of practice—The range of professional duties and abilities as defined by the profession's guidelines, regulatory bodies, and licensure statues and rules.

Staff evaluation—Review of staff performance usually completed during a predetermined time frame and including informal and formal assessment strategies. The goal of staff evaluation is to identify staff strengths, areas for improvement, and professional development plans.

Supervision—The process of overseeing the work of others. This often includes the acknowledgement of responsibility for those individuals who are under one's care.

Learning Objectives

After studying this chapter, readers will be able to:

- Recognize the various roles of the occupational therapy assistant with regard to supervision.
- Identify common dilemmas occupational therapy assistants face when supervising others.
- Identify skills needed to become an effective supervisor in occupational therapy settings.

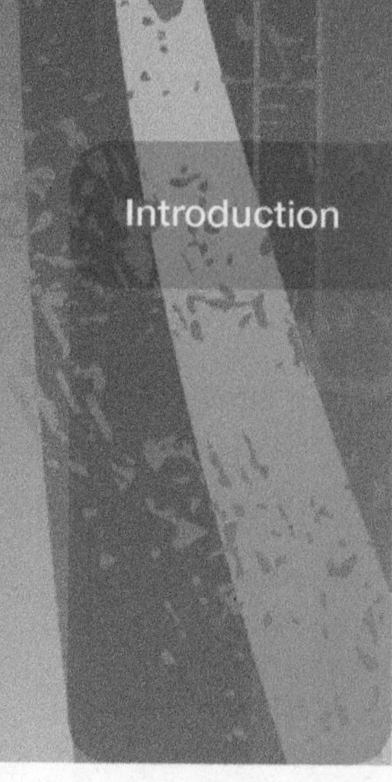

Introduction

Jane is an occupational therapy assistant who has been working as a staff OTA in a public school system for 2 years. After a move to a new part of the state, she found an opportunity working for a large private pediatric practice. During her interview, she was asked about her ability to supervise others. Working in any occupational therapy setting will require **supervision** skills at some point. For Jane, she was asked to consider supervision from the initial interview. What does she know about supervision when she was not a manager for her former employer? What did the interviewer mean when she asked about supervising others? It is helpful to understand the roles that may be associated with supervision in an occupational therapy practice setting.

Roles in Supervision

In the field of occupational therapy, there are three personnel members: occupational therapists, occupational therapy assistants, and **occupational therapy aides (sometimes referred to as rehabilitation technicians)**. OT and OTA personnel are considered **practitioners** whereas an **aide** or technician is not. Why does this clarification matter? These labels are important in legislative and practice documents. You may find that an insurance provider or a state **licensure** act clarifies who may do the various responsibilities in a therapy setting. If you read that a "therapist" must be responsible for a task, it must be an occupational therapist, but if you read that a "practitioner" is responsible, the task may be performed by either an occupational therapist or an occupational therapy assistant. Jane may be asked to supervise other assistants or aides or volunteers. Depending upon her role within the site, she may even find herself supervising occupational therapists. She will never supervise the provision of care that an OT provides a client since that contradicts the occupational therapy assistant **scope of practice** (AOTA, 2014a,b; 2005). This would be considered **malpractice**. She may, however, perform as a **manager** in her department or clinic to supervise workloads, document flow, and budgets. For the purpose of this chapter, the term supervision will relate to the oversight of the occupational therapy process. Please refer to Chapter 15, Management, to learn more about the role of the manager.

For Jane, her credential as an OTA offers her supervision rights as determined by many regulators. The scope of practice as outlined by her state will assist her as she clarifies her rights and roles in the therapeutic process. Note: What are the regulations for practice in your State? Although she may have had a certain level of autonomy in her school system, she may not within her new work environment. Why would that be? It may have to do with things other than state regulations.

Jane's pediatric clinic will likely receive reimbursement from a number of insurance sources, private pay, and Medicaid intermediaries. This will have an impact on the level of supervision she will need from the OT. Some payment providers have clear guidelines related to the provision of therapy providers. Some ask for **cosignatures**, some require a distinct amount of face-to-face supervision, some require the OT to see the child at a certain visit, and some have no specifications. Because of the volume of reimbursement policy, some organizations choose to provide supervision considering the lowest common denominator. In other words, they offer OT supervision at the level of the most stringent of the payers. In that way, there is little to no chance that the supervision will be compromised. Still, other companies choose to have payer identifiers so that the supervision is provided as to meet the specific regulations. Not following regulations may result in lack of reimbursement, charges of negligence or fraudulent billing, or state censure. One cannot use ignorance as an excuse for oversight (AOTA, 2010). The law expects professionals to know their supervision regulations and state practice acts. Although many states have chosen to follow AOTA's model state regulations, there is a wide range of interpretation of those guidelines.

Competency and Supervision

Jane's new supervisor explained the work flow of the clinical site and told Jane that based upon her previous experience she will start with clients after her week of orientation. One of her first clients is new to the setting and has a diagnosis of cerebral palsy. She was asked to perform a pediatric assessment on the child and report to the OT with the results. Jane has performed the assessment twice while in the school setting with her former administrator. What are the concerns she should have now?

Within your academic education, you will be exposed to a number of assessment tools used in client evaluations. Based upon your state, you will likely have a role in the evaluation process under the supervision of the OT. Jane had this experience in the school system administering a particular assessment. She should, however, have concerns as she begins her new role in this outpatient pediatric setting. One of those is service **competency**. She was found to be competent in the administration of the tool with her last supervisor, but would she be considered competent by the new OT? Jane should be concerned, but more important, the OT should be concerned. There is no magic number of how many times the OT watches Jane perform the assessment. Instead, the OT's judgment must indicate whether or not Jane is able to administer the test accurately and relay the results in a manner that will allow the OT to interpret the results appropriately (From the Field 13.1).

Jane should be concerned about administering the assessment in a new setting. Is she used to administering the tool with children who have physical limitations and require adaptations during the assessment? Has she administered this having parents present? Has she used the same tools that this clinic uses for the assessment subtests? Jane should share these thoughts with her OT supervisor and request that the supervisor oversee the administration on at least one child to ensure **interrater reliability** (Bladen, 2011). Many OT practitioners would not be comfortable asking for this oversight for fear of being considered incompetent or unsure of his or her skills. It is, indeed, quite the opposite. Jane is welcoming the oversight with the intent of providing the best care with exceptional professional communication regarding the care of the client. This is an example of how the supervision process is a collaborative one; it involves the person supervising and the one being supervised. Experienced OTAs request meetings with supervising OTs often when the OT is not aware of the need to meet (From the Field 13.2).

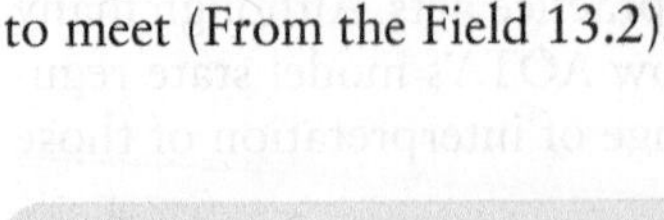

FROM THE FIELD 13.1

Document

When documenting a session in which there was supervision and OT collaboration, it is important to state such within the note even if a cosignature is not required.

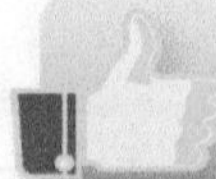

FROM THE FIELD 13.2

Supervision Defined

AOTA defines supervision as a "cooperative process in which two or more people participate in a joint effort to establish, maintain, and/or elevate a level of competence and performance. Supervision is based on mutual understanding between the supervisor and the supervisee about each other's competence, experience, education, and credentials. It fosters growth and development, promotes effective utilization of resources, encourages creativity and innovation, and provides education and support to achieve a goal (AOTA, 2005, p. 1)."

Supervision of Others

Jane is more and more comfortable at the pediatric clinic every week, and her apprehension about this new environment is slowly disappearing. She is approached by her clinic manager and asked to take a level I OTA intern student, Sarah. Jane feels like she has little choice, and she is worried about what this extra responsibility will mean.

The supervision of therapy students is both a responsibility and an honor. To be selected as a clinical fieldwork educator (CFE) means that you have been found to have exceptional clinical and personal skills that will benefit a student studying in the field of occupational therapy (From the Field 13.3).

The intern can bring many benefits to your setting, but you must remember that the intern is working as your "agent" during client care. This means that the intern is working under your license and/or certification as he or she provides care to your client. Your job as a CFE will require demonstration and teaching, but it will also include supervision. You must ensure that the intern's comments, actions, and work behaviors follow company expectations, best practice, and therapeutic interactions

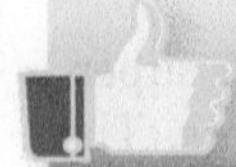

FROM THE FIELD 13.3

Clinical Fieldwork

Students who have a positive fieldwork relationship with their clinical fieldwork educator are more likely to take students after graduation.

that you approve (Hall et al., 2012). This may require regular meetings, documentation review, technique training, and even homework provision. In this way, the student will grow clinically and professionally while representing you in a safe and clinically sound way.

Student supervision is regulated by state statues and rules, by clinical settings, by corporate guidelines, by the related college, and by the Accreditation Council for Occupational Therapy Education (ACOTE). According to ACOTE, a practitioner may take on a level II student intern after one full year working in the setting that the internship will take place.

There are policies regarding how much experience the supervisor (CFE) must have, how long the internships will last, how much direct oversight the student has, and how the student will be assessed. Be sure to check with your clinical site as well as the school that sends the students to your setting to make sure that you are following all of the regulations that apply to you. In this way, you protect your clinic, your clients, the student, and yourself.

To Jane's surprise, she truly enjoyed her time with her intern, Sarah. The clinic decided to hire Sarah as a therapy aide 2 days per week while she completes her OTA program. She is excited to be at the clinic again, but Jane had new concerns.

Jane will now be supervising Sarah as a therapy aide, so she must be aware of clinic policies regarding the supervision as well as possible regulations that may impact the supervision. Most states have rules or regulations regarding the supervision of therapy aides/technicians. Some states allow the aide to do anything that the supervising practitioner allows and oversees, whereas other states will not allow the aide to touch a client who is receiving occupational therapy services. It is imperative that you become aware of the laws and rules in the state in which you work. In addition to the state rules, many settings have policies related to the use of a therapy aide. The service extender is a phenomenal way to keep OT practitioners at the side of the client while other unskilled employees cover nonessential clinic duties. Some of these activities include client transport, filing, equipment cleaning, stocking, inventory, activity setup, and general office duties. Jane will need to participate in Sarah's **staff evaluation** (Mackey & Whitfield, 2007). This review allows for a collaborative assessment of Sarah's performance at the setting. The review may take place after a probationary period, every year, or any other time frame determined by the setting (From the Field 13.4).

To assign direct client care to the aide opens several potential challenges. Will the aide follow best practice, understand evidence-based care, recognize client symptoms, or be able to document client performance using accurate observation and communication skills? Would this be acceptable to you if you were a client? Would you want to travel to a specialty occupational therapy clinic to have someone who has no occupational therapy education providing your direct care? Most likely, the answer is "no."

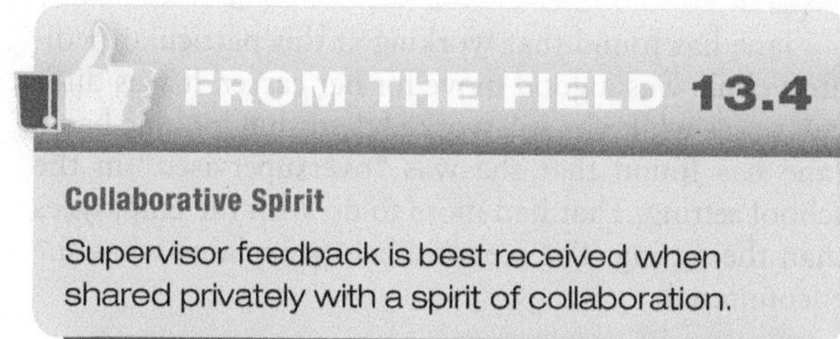

Collaborative Spirit

Supervisor feedback is best received when shared privately with a spirit of collaboration.

Continuation of Supervising Others

Two years later, Jane is enjoying her promotion to team leader for the clinic's adaptive preschool program. Sarah was hired as an OTA after completing her education, and Jane's clinic manager has given her two bonuses in the past year for her exceptional parent reports. She now supervises three OTAs, two aides, and one student every year. There are six OTs, five SLPs, and four PTs at the clinic. She has comfortably accepted this "sandwich" situation in which she supervises employees while being supervised by others.

The OTA has a unique dilemma that the OT does not with regard to supervision. The OT is able to complete the therapy process independently. The OTA cannot. Instead, the OTA provides therapy under the supervision of the OT. For Jane, this means that she could potentially have 6 OTs supervising her therapy services. Can you imagine any of the dilemmas this can produce?

Having a number of supervisors can be a bit of a juggling act. To be successful, the OTA needs a good memory, good interpersonal skills, and flexibility. Let's discuss why this is. Imagine that Jane is treating 10 children 1 day. Of these 10 children, there are 5 OTs involved as the overseeing therapists. Jane knows each child well, and she has been seeing each one for at least 4 months. As she treats each child, Jane must consider the intervention protocol desired by each of the OTs. She must utilize the documentation style requested by each OT.

In an ideal world, the setting would have standardized intervention protocols and documentation styles, but that is seldom the case. Because each OT has unique specialty skills, training, theoretical beliefs, and personal experience, the OTA working with the OT must function within those parameters. Jane remembers that when working with Monica's clients, she uses more sensory integration techniques, and when she works with Barbara's clients, she uses a more behavioral approach. How did Jane determine these approaches? She did this by meeting with the OTs on a regular basis to cotreat, to have her service competency assessed, and to work on intervention planning. In this manner, the team collaborates to ensure that the child will receive the intervention that the supervising OT has determined.

Jane has found that working at this particular pediatric clinic was a good move for her career. It was difficult to see while she still worked there, but looking back, Jane has found that she was "oversupervised" in the school setting. That had more to do with the employees than the setting. The scenario below explains what she encountered.

Supervision Scenario

In her first 2 years as an OTA, Jane worked in a county school system with several OTAs and OTs. At each school, there was a different OT who was responsible for the assessments, intervention planning, and team coordination. Some schools were more desirable than others. Some of the OTs would leave her messages telling her to deliver items to teachers, do filing, and call parents. Some schools had her treating 75% of the children, and others asked her to pick up supplies between school visits. Jane assumed that this was normal; that she needed to follow the direction and requests of the OTs she worked with. In actuality, this is far from fact. Jane was working for the school system and not for each OT. Her therapy manager, the district OT, would have been the individual who would have determined her work requirements, schedule, and duties. Once Jane changed jobs, it became clear to her that she had a manager who oversaw her work duties and she had OTs she collaborated with for intervention intervention.

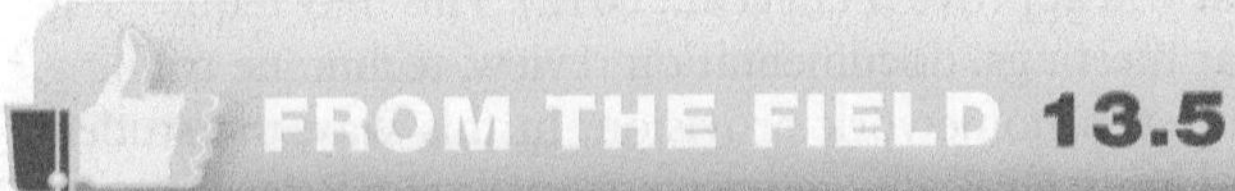

Factors Affecting Supervision

The specific frequency, methods, and content of supervision may vary by practice setting and are dependent upon the following:

1. Complexity of client needs
2. Number and diversity of clients
3. Skills of the OT and OTA
4. Type of practice setting
5. Requirements of the practice setting
6. Other regulatory requirements

More frequent supervision may be necessary when

1. The needs of the client and the occupational therapy process are complex and changing.
2. The practice setting provides occupational therapy services to a large number of clients with diverse needs.
3. The OT and OTA determine that additional supervision is necessary to ensure safe and effective delivery of occupational therapy services.

Levels of Supervision

As we have reviewed, OT supervision takes place in many forms: supervising coworkers, students, and aids. The amount, frequency, and style of supervision one needs are based upon many factors (see From the Field 13.5). Some of the common supervision levels for occupational therapy are listed in Table 13.1.

The level of supervision that is required for intervention supervision is determined by state and reimbursement regulations. Competent practitioners also follow supervision protocols based upon the severity of the client condition, secondary factors such as assistance needed, the familiarity with the situation, and experience with a certain technique (Table 13.2).

TABLE 13.1 Levels of Supervision in Occupational Therapy

Level of Supervision	Definition
General	Overseeing practitioner is available as needed, but no planned reviews are required
Monthly	Overseeing practitioner meets with the treating practitioner once monthly
Intermediate	Overseeing practitioner meets with treating practitioner several times monthly
Daily	Overseeing practitioner meets with treating practitioner every day
Telesupervision	Overseeing practitioner is available to meet with treating practitioner through electronic means (phone/video conference) as needed
Geographic	Overseeing practitioner is available to meet with treating practitioner by remaining nearby within a set geographic area
Direct	Overseeing practitioner is available to the treating practitioner within the same intervention setting during the time that treatment takes place

TABLE 13.2 Helpful Resources

Helpful Resources
AOTA position statement—Guidelines for Supervision, Roles, and Responsibilities during the Delivery of Occupational Therapy Services (2009).
AOTA State Affairs Group (2012). Occupational therapy assistant supervision requirements. http://www.aota.org/Practitioners/Licensure/StateRegs/Supervision/36455.aspx
State occupational therapy Statues and Regulations http://www.aota.org/Practitioners/Licensure/StateRegs.aspx on the AOTA Web site

When Jane began working at the pediatric clinic, she was told by her manager that the setting protocol was for her to have an OT on site at all times during her first 6 months of work due to the newness of the setting. After 6 months, the setting would reassess her skills and competency to address her supervision needs. Even after 1 year, there were still some intervention sessions that gave Jane cause for alarm. She recognized that she still required supervision when working with involved oral–motor cases and with medically fragile children. The OT would hand the case over to Jane only when she showed competency, and Jane would arrange the intervention of these children at times when the supervising OT was present. In this manner, the collaboration of supervision created the most client-centered situation; one in which the child's needs came first. For other cases, Jane was comfortable knowing that the supervising OT was available on a cell phone in the chance that a question arose during the intervention session.

Becoming an Exceptional Supervisor

Just as some individuals are better at managing and leading, some are simply better at supervising. Why is that? Why can't everyone have these skills? The answer is simple. All practitioners can be good supervisors if they wish to (Parkinson et al., 2010). Having the desire to be excellent is the key component in achieving excellence. Some of these skills include the following:

1. Observation skills—these are similar to those used with clients. Good observation skills allow the overseeing practitioner to gain insight into coworker behaviors, skills, strengths, and areas for improvement.
2. Communication skills—these are similar to those used with the client. Constructive criticism, active listening, compliments, suggestions, clinical questioning, and educating can come across as extremely helpful or terribly hurtful depending upon the tone, timing, and attitude associated with the interaction.
3. Awareness of regulations—supervision guidelines vary state to state and across payor sources. It is important to know these guidelines and to have a plan to document the compliance with them.
4. Teaching skills—much like breaking down a task for a client, the supervisor must understand how to build skills for those who are supervised. This may take place through formalized training courses, one-to-one sessions, group inservices, or directed readings.

Summary

Whether we like it or not, working in occupational therapy, practitioners will have oversight throughout our careers. This supervision can come from a number of sources. For the OTA, this may involve state regulations and licensure, payor guidelines, setting policies, therapist oversight, and professional scope of practice standards. The amount of supervision required during the provision of OT services is dependent upon many factors and is subject to change if one changes practice areas or settings. Supervision is put into place to ensure the safe, current, and efficient care of the client. Without systematic oversight, those receiving our care cannot be sure that intervention meets the expectation of the clinical setting, the payor, and the profession. As we participate in the supervisory relationship and document those activities, we can assure our stakeholders that we are taking a proactive role in intervention accountability.

Review Questions

1. Which of the following individuals is *not* an OT practitioner?
   a. Staff OT
   b. Managing OT
   c. Staff occupational therapy aide
   d. Staff OTA

2. Which one of the following groups will have supervision guidelines for occupational therapy?
   a. State occupational therapy association
   b. Medicare
   c. Internal Revenue Service
   d. National Service Associations

3. What is the recommendation of the AOTA with regard to supervision of OT personnel?
   a. The AOTA has no such recommendations.
   b. Direct supervision needs to occur during all OTA sessions.
   c. Supervision needs to take place during reevaluation sessions.
   d. Supervision is based upon several factors related to the setting and client.

4. When can an OTA supervise a level II OTA intern student?
   a. Once service competency is met
   b. After passing a fieldwork supervision course
   c. After 1 year in the intervention setting
   d. When the supervising OT deems it appropriate

5. If an OTA follows an inappropriate OT request for patient intervention, the OTA will likely be guilty of:
   a. Malpractice
   b. Fraud
   c. Forgery
   d. Unprofessionalism

6. What is sandwich supervision?
   a. Supervising several individuals with different experience levels
   b. Supervising others while being supervised
   c. Being supervised by individuals both older and younger than yourself
   d. Supervision that varies day to day based upon the supervisor mood

7. What is the appropriate response to a supervisor who is asking you to perform a task you feel uncomfortable completing?
   a. "I will get to it."
   b. "I will do the best I can."
   c. "I would prefer to have a supervisor with me for the intervention."
   d. "I am not able to comply with your request."

8. While supervising a new OTA, you notice that she stopped treatment to take a personal phone call and did not adjust charges to indicate this personal time. The best intervention in this case is:
   a. Step in while she is on the phone and instruct her to return to her client treatment
   b. Update the charge sheet to accurately reflect the intervention and discuss this observation at her next staff review
   c. Approach the patient while she is on the phone to ensure no gap in intervention during the session
   d. Address this immediately after the session in private and have her correct the charge sheet

9. While supervising a new OTA, you notice that he is transferring a patient with poor balance and is not using a transfer belt despite your previous instruction. The best intervention in this case is:
   a. Let the supervising OT know about your concerns
   b. Discuss with the OTA after the session in a low-threat environment
   c. Approach the OTA during the intervention and offer a transfer belt; discuss privately afterward
   d. Ask the OTA to step aside and use the time to educate the OTA about patient safety while you perform the transfer

10. After working as an OTA for several years, you move to another state. There may be new supervisory regulations that you must follow. Who is responsible for this new information?
   a. The supervisor is responsible to inform you as their employee.
   b. The AOTA is responsible to have this information on their Web site.
   c. The individual OTA is responsible to be informed of these regulations.
   d. The hiring company is responsible to make sure that their employees are aware of these regulations.

Practice Activities

Get into a group of four students. Each student will choose a different state. Using the Internet and helpful Web sites such as AOTA, the state's occupational therapy association, and the state occupational therapy licensure department, compare and contrast the different supervision guidelines of those three states.

Based upon what you know about the supervisory relationship, create a supervision checklist. The checklist should include each of the skills or aptitudes that the OTA should display in the provision of treatment.

According to the role of the occupational therapy aide, create two scenarios in which the aide would be able to work under the supervision of the OTA. Create two scenarios in which it would be inappropriate for the aide to perform a particular task.

References

AOTA. *Model State Regulation and Supervision, Roles, and Responsibilities During the Delivery of Occupational Therapy Services.* Bethesda, MD: AOTA; 2005.

AOTA. Guidelines for Supervision, Roles, and Responsibilities During the Delivery of Occupational Therapy Services. 2014;68, S16–22.

AOTA. Scope of practice for occupational therapy. *Am J Occup Ther* 2014; S43–40.

AOTA. AOTA code of ethics. *Am J Occup Ther* 2010;64.

Bladen A. The importance of evidence based supervision: a best practice model of supervision based on the voice and insights of occupational therapists and grounded in evidence. *Aust Occup Ther J* 2011;58:100.

Hall M, et al. Positive clinical placements: perspectives of students and clinical educators in rehabilitation medicine. *Int J Ther Rehabil* 2012;19(10):549–556.

Mackey H, Whitfield L. (2007). Supervising assistant practitioners: evaluating a reflective diary approach. *Int J Ther Rehabil* 2007;14(11): 503–511.

Parkinson S, et al. Professional development enhances the occupational therapy work environment. *Br J Occup Ther* 2010; 73(10):470–476.

CHAPTER 14

Documentation to Meet Reimbursement Guidelines

Vicki Case, OTR/L

Key Terms

Functional maintenance programs—Programs that are often developed for clients who have been discharged from therapy but will remain in a skilled nursing facility. The programs facilitate skills that are present but not utilized unless compensations or adaptations are provided.

Informed consent—A legal and ethical communication process between client (or authorized agent) and clinician that results in the client's authorization or permission to participate in evaluation and intervention (Schenker et al., 2011).

Medical necessity—The intervention or intervention is consistent with the diagnosis, and failure to provide the intervention could jeopardize or significantly compromise the client's condition or quality of medical care (NovaCare, 1996).

Negative prognostic indicators—Signs that indicate barriers inhibiting rehab potential.

Positive prognostic indicators—The indicators that the client has good rehab potential, which is essential for third-party reimbursement.

Restorative programs—Programs that facilitate the learning of new skills in an attempt to "restore" the client's previous abilities.

Screening—The process of determining if a client requires the skilled services of an occupational therapy practitioner. It helps to identify changes in functional status such as improvements or declines in physical or cognitive abilities (Author, n.d.a).

Standardized assessments—Methods used for data collection that have established reliability and validity.

Learning Objectives

After studying this chapter, readers should be able to:

- Understand the steps to, the purpose of, and the importance of the documentation process.
- Describe the occupational therapy process and characteristics for screening to determine the need for occupational therapy services.
- Describe the role of the occupational therapy assistant related to administering standardized and nonstandardized assessments and the evaluation process.
- Explain the importance of medical necessity and how to consistently document it.
- Identify the components of goal writing and progress notes.
- Accurately identify the components of SOAP and DAP notes.

Introduction

Documentation is one of the most important aspects of being an occupational therapy assistant. It showcases who we are as a profession and holds us accountable for meeting the needs of our clients. Documentation is the picture that we paint of our clients that will be looked at by third-party payers. It is the only one that the payers will see. Documentation is the key to coverage for all therapy. The reality is that if it is not documented, it has not been done. Documentation serves many other purposes. It facilitates communication between the occupational therapy team, the rehab team, and other disciplines outside of the rehab team. If another discipline reads your note, they should be able to understand what is being done by the client in therapy and what progress is being made toward goals. It facilitates continuity of intervention for our clients. Documentation also serves as a tool to advocate for our profession and provides our profession with data for evidence-based research. Documentation that instructors and supervisors provide to students and practitioners can enhance the learning process. Documentation allows OT practitioners to reflect on our reasoning skills and justify continued intervention for our clients.

Through good documentation, we can ensure that medical necessity is documented. **Medical necessity** answers the question "why does this client need and continue to need the skilled services of an OT practitioner?" Documentation is part of the unspoken contract with our clients and their families and should be viewed as equally as important as providing the best possible care through current intervention approaches. More importantly, documentation is the only concrete evidence connecting the OT practitioner's reasoning process used during the course of intervention and the client's final outcome. By documenting medical necessity, you are decreasing your risk or denial of reimbursement for services (NovaCare, 1996). In this chapter, we explore documentation procedures relevant to third-party reimbursement for clients in medical practice settings like skilled nursing, home health, and rehabilitation facilities. While reimbursement guidelines differ for other practice settings like pediatric private practice, the characteristics of good documentation is consistent across no matter where you are employed.

Why Document?

Good documentation of medical necessity answers questions like why does this client need therapy now, what happened to indicate the need for a specialized provider, and is there supporting nursing/physician documentation? If a client has had a recent hospitalization, it is usually easy to identify the specific problem/event that occurred along with the onset date. Looking at an example of a client living in a skilled nursing facility will help you begin to appreciate the methods and value of good documentation.

Mr. Wong had a recent total hip replacement and is unable to dress or bathe his lower body and transfer without assistance. If Mr. Wong can recover in the natural course of healing, then services provided will not be considered reasonable or necessary. Often for long-term care residents of nursing facilities, an evaluation is warranted when there has been a change in function documented by the physician or nursing staff and/or services are in response to an identified problem or concern voiced by the client or family. Documenting Mr. Wong's prior level of function is also important to show medical necessity. It is important to remember to be specific and to paint a clear and objective picture of this client to the reviewer to have the best chance for reimbursement for services.

Prior to the fall, Mr. Wong was ambulatory with a walker and required standby assistance for dressing, bathing, and toileting. He was active in facility activities and often attended outings with family and local faith-based groups. An OT practitioner will want to document the answer to this question, "why can't this client do what he did before?" This involves describing the diagnosis or change in function in terms of its impact on Mr. Wong's functional abilities. In doing so, the OT practitioner may note the following. After the fall, Mr. Wong suffered a pubic fracture and a right temporal contusion. He expresses fear and pain and exhibits general weakness, which limits participation in self-care and mobility. He generally requires moderate assistance with self-care and mobility.

The Documentation Process

The documentation process can be conducted electronically or with handwritten notes. This is facility dependent. Documentation also involves multiple steps and can be done in differing ways. Documentation may also include preparing incident reports, home programs, and protocols. Since every facility has differing policies, make it a point to become an expert on knowing what is expected of you regarding documentation.

Electronic Medical Records

More and more frequently, documentation is being conducted electronically, using a keyboard and computer or tablet. An electronic medical record (EMR) contains a client's entire medical history from one practice. An EMR is typically used by providers for diagnosis and intervention. You may be called upon to do electronic documentation for intervention that you provide to clients. There are plusses and minuses associated with EMRs. The plusses are that it is easier to track data and monitor progress, but the negative is that it can be difficult to share with practitioners outside of the practice (HealthIT.gov, n.d.).

Step One: Screening

A **screening** is performed to determine if an evaluation is warranted. Screenings are performed in all practice settings, just with differing procedures. A screening helps OT practitioners to identify changes in functional status such as improvements or declines in physical or cognitive abilities. The screening process is usually done quarterly in a long-term care unit or when a functional change has been identified. It may occur at any time in a school-based practice setting. A screening can be recommended by any member of the intervention or educational team.

There are four characteristics of screenings. The first characteristic is that they are brief and should be completed in less than 15 minutes. Secondly, they are to be "hands off." Data for the screening may be collected through observation, review of the medical record, and/or discussion with the team members who are recommending the screening and who have functional change and reported and disseminated in a format consistent with facility guidelines. The third characteristic of a screening is that it does not require a physician's order. Because it does not, it is not a billable service in a medical model (fourth characteristic). New OT practitioners often wonder, "What should I be looking for or asking about when I screen a client?" What follows are a few general questions to think about when preparing for or doing a screening in a nursing facility:

- Is the (potential) client in a wheelchair? If so, how does he/she look in the wheelchair (e.g., sitting posture, ability to propel it)?
- Are there observable joint contractures? Do joints appear to be stiff?
- Does the (potential) client have orthotics or positioning devices?
- Has there been in improvement or decline in function in ADL, work, or leisure skills?
- What is the (potential) client's mobility skills like? Any recent falls?
- Does the (potential) client have any pressure areas?

Step Two: Informed Consent

Informed consent is permission obtained from a potential client or other responsible party to evaluate and treat a client. We have a legal and ethical duty to obtain informed consent before starting intervention. Clients should be informed regarding intervention recommendations and consequences of refusal to participate (From the Field 14.1).

Step Three: Evaluation

Prior to the start of evaluation and intervention, a physician's order must be obtained to ensure reimbursement from third-party payers. Sometimes, a client is admitted to a facility with an order for intervention, but if not, it must be requested by the OT. It is good practice to document receipt of the physician's order for intervention in the initial progress note. This documentation is usually performed by the OT. The OT is also responsible for the evaluation process, but the OTA may assist with aspects of the evaluation. The OTA may perform interviews and observe performance with functional activities. The results of the interviews and observations will be documented by the OT.

Occupational therapy assistants may be asked to perform standardized and nonstandardized assessments once

FROM THE FIELD 14.1

Ensuring Informed Consent

If a client is unable to sign an informed consent form, it is necessary for an authorized family member or caregiver to do so prior to beginning intervention. No matter if it is a client, family member, or caregiver who signs the informed consent form, it is important for an OT practitioner to clearly explain the intent of therapy in a way that is understandable and free of jargon. If there is a language barrier, it is appropriate for an interpreter to assist with the process.

competency is established. The OT must interpret and document the results of the assessments. **Standardized assessments** are used for data collection and can be completed in a variety of formats including an interview, observation, or test. In order for the assessment to be standardized, it must have established reliability and validity. Specific procedures are followed when administering a standardized assessment in order for the results to be accurate (please also refer to Chapter 5, *The Evidence-Based Movement: Guiding the Practice*).

Step Four: Goal Writing

Components of Goals

There are a variety of methods that lay out the basic components of goal writing. The ABCD method uses the terms audience, behavior, condition, and degree (Kettenbach, 2009) as components of the goal writing process. The FEAST method breaks down goal writing into steps that include function, expectation, action, specific conditions, and timeline (Borcherding, 2000; Borcherding & Kappel, 2002). The RHUMBA (or RUMBA, as it is sometimes known) method encompasses client factors such as relevant/relates, how long, understandable, measurable, behavioral, and achievable components (College of St. Catherine [CSC], 2001; McClain, 1991) into the goal writing process. SMART is another commonly used goal writing method and includes significant, measurable, achievable, and related components (Sames, 2009).

All of the methods discussed provide the basis to develop good goal writing skills. There is another method that can be used to achieve excellence in goal writing. This method does not have an official name but could be called the "clue" method. With this method, the following questions need to be asked: "*Who* will do it? *What* do you want to happen? *How* will it happen? And *when* will it happen?"

The *who* is *always* the client, the individual who is to perform the desired behavior(s). To be client centered, your goals should always start with "the client will..." and never "the caregiver will (unless it is a specific caregiver education goal)..." Sometimes, this is challenging to do when a client is lower functioning and may not be able to speak or perform any sort of functional activities. Despite any challenge, as long as you keep your focus on the client, you will write an appropriate "who."

Examples of "who":

- The *client will* dress lower body with minimal assistance with use of adaptive equipment.
- The *client will* tolerate passive range of motion (ROM) and splinting for improved skin integrity and hygiene. (In this example, the client is not performing the ROM or applying the splint, but the goal is still written with the focus on the client.)

The *what* are the underlying body functions, client factors, and performance skills that affect the area(s) of occupation. These are the skills and abilities required for occupational performance. As you see, there must always be an area of occupation associated with preparing client-centered goals.

Some statements will only have an area of occupation. The functional outcome a.k.a. area of occupation is your "so what?"

Basic examples of "what":

- The client will dress his upper body (*area of occupation*) with minimal assistance.
- In 3 weeks, client will improve UE dressing (*area of occupation*) from moderate assistance to minimal assistance.

Based on the client, some goal will also include an underlying body function, client factor, or performance skill factors that impact function.

Complex examples of "what":

- In 2 weeks, the client will improve right-hand fine motor coordination (*body function*) to enable client to button shirt (*area of occupation*) with minimal assistance.

The *how* is the condition and/or measurement standard. The condition includes the human or nonhuman requirements necessary for optimal performance. Examples include verbal cueing, adaptive equipment, and special compensatory techniques. The measurement standard is the level of assistance or objective criterion against which performance is measured. There are not always both a measurement standard and condition included in a goal.

Example of "how":

- The client will dress the upper body with minimal assistance (*measurement standard*) and with use of button hook (*condition*).

The *when* component is the time frame in which a client is expected to complete a goal.

Example of "when":

- In 2 weeks (*when*), the client will improve lower extremity dressing from moderate assistance to minimal assistance with use of adaptive equipment.

Summary example of the *who, what, how, when* goal writing method

- In 2 weeks (*when*), the client (*who*) will improve postural control and endurance (*what*) in order to perform lower body dressing (*what*) with use of adaptive equipment (*how*) and minimal assistance (*how*).

Step Five: Progress Notes

Progress note formats, whether prepared as handwritten or electronic medical records, vary depending on facility guidelines. The three typical progress note formats are

TABLE 14.1 The SOAP Note

Subjective: What clients say, how they feel about, or react to therapy.

- Must relate to the O and A. It is not just a random statement.
- This is part of the client's response to intervention and must always be included in the note.
- May include direct or paraphrased comments by the client such as complaints, attitudes, emotions, and/or self-assessment of progress to meet goals or behavioral response to intervention (e.g., client is cooperative, lethargic). Behavioral responses are helpful to include, especially if a client is nonverbal or has poor communication skills.

Example of the *subjective* portion of the progress note:

- Client states that he is fearful of falling when sitting on the edge of the bed and when bending over.

Objective: What happened? Who did what?

- Number of visits, refusals, withheld interventions
- What the OT practitioner did and any co-intervention that occurred
- What did the client do? Compare the performance of the current week to the performance from the prior week.
- Document objective data related to body functions and client factors and also the functional status related to the short-term goals.
- Results of standardized assessments
- Barriers to intervention
- Report caregiver education and conferences attended related to your client. Give yourself credit for the things you do relative to working with a client.

In the *objective* portion of the note, indicate any **positive prognostic indicators.** These are indicators that the client has good rehab potential and are essential to document for reimbursement purposes. Positive prognostic indicators should be documented in the evaluation and re-evaluation and in weekly notes. Documentation of positive prognostic indicators helps support medical necessity.

Examples of positive prognostic indicators include a client's:

- Ability to follow directions, problem solve, and initiate activity
- Motivation
- Prior history of independence of performance areas addressed in intervention plan goals

Negative prognostic indicators are signs that indicate poor rehab potential and may indicate that intervention is not medically necessary (Author, n.d.b). Many clients will have some negative prognostic indicators but often still benefit from skilled occupational therapy services. For example, a client may be unresponsive to environmental stimuli but needs splints for positioning for improved skin integrity and hygiene. In this case, the prognosis pertains to specific goals. The prognosis is good for the client to benefit from a splinting program in order to have improved skin integrity and hygiene. Poor skin integrity and hygiene may lead to a domino effect of serious and negative medical outcomes, so a splinting program may in fact be cost-effective in the long run, not to mention be the best intervention approach for the client.

Another common situation is clients with progressive conditions like dementia. Good practice is to address head-on what third-party payers might consider to be a negative prognostic indicator. The "O" part of the note might say "the client has a progressive cognitive condition, yet is still able to follow one step verbal directives, is cooperative with caregivers, and has the potential to finger feed and perform basic grooming skills with supervision."

Examples of negative prognostic indicators:

- Poor orientation
- Inability to follow direction(s)
- Medical instability
- Absent or inadequate arousal

Example of the *objective* portion of the progress note:

Client was seen five times this week with a focus on dressing skills, perception, and balance skills. Client requires maximum assistance for donning pants and moderate assistance with upper extremity dressing. Last week, the client required maximum assistance with upper body dressing. Client has difficulty with R/L discrimination and displays poor dynamic sitting balance. Client continues to voice fears of bending forward to don/doff pants, shoes, and socks and cannot flex trunk past 90 degrees of hip flexion. The client is able

TABLE 14.1 The SOAP Note (continued)

to perform grooming with minimal assistance but required moderate assistance last week. Last week, client required moderate assistance with self-feeding and, this week, is able to self-feed with minimal assistance and use of built-up utensils and plate guard. Attended care plan meeting to discuss client's discharge plan with care team is pending.
Assessment: What does it all mean?
• The OT practitioner's professional interpretation from the *S* and the *O* part of the note • Assessment of the effectiveness of the intervention plan and changes to the intervention plan • A quick overview of the client's functional abilities and limitations • Indicate, if any, goals that were achieved and if progress is being made toward other goals including the outcome. • If no progress is being made or is slow, include an explanation or possible explanation (e.g., client was ill; had a deep vein thrombosis [DVT]). • Be cautious about how the negative prognostic indicators are documented as it will affect the determination of rehab potential. • Document any modifications that need to be made to the existing goals. • Medical necessity; why does the client continue to need the skilled services of occupational therapy? Summarize primary problems that indicate need for continued occupational therapy services. Example of *assessment* The client is making progress with upper body dressing, grooming, and self-feeding. The client has difficulty with lower body dressing skills secondary to poor balance, perceptual deficits, and fear of falling. The client continues to require the skilled services of occupational therapy to promote independence with balance and perceptual skills to improve independence with dressing, grooming, and feeding skills. Despite fear of falling, client articulates motivation about participation in therapy and desires to return home.
Plan: Now what?
• What, if any, intervention techniques and modifications are needed? • Plans for caregiver education, patient education, and family interaction • Report of communication between OT and OTA • Frequency and duration of intervention • Rehab potential Example of a *plan* Client to receive occupational therapy services 5×/week × 3 weeks with intervention to focus on UE/LE dressing, grooming, feeding, postural control, and perceptual deficits. Client has excellent rehab potential and continues to require occupational therapy services secondary to his high prior level of function, motivation, and insight into his disability.

narrative, SOAP, and DAP. SOAP and DAP notations are a way of categorizing information into specific sections. SOAP is the acronym for subjective, objective, assessment, and plan. DAP is the acronym for data, assessment, and plan. While the narrative note is written in a paragraph format and does not have specific sections, it still requires that the same information in a SOAP or DAP note be included. This section focuses on the SOAP (Table 14.1) and DAP (Table 14.2) formats, which, because of their set structure, are often a good way for the beginning OT practitioner to learn to write progress notes.

DAP notes are another common way of documenting client progress. The *data* section includes information related to your observations of behaviors related to client factors and body functions. This section also includes the client's functional status related to the short-term goals. The data section includes the information that is put in the "O" portion of a SOAP note. The *assessment* section includes the same information that is included in the "A" section of a SOAP note. The *plan* section includes the same information that in the "P" section of the SOAP note.

Documenting Functional Progress

Third-party payers look for documentation of weekly functional progress. If the client is not progressing, then third-party payers will not want to pay for the services. Progress is documented in a variety of ways. Some of the more common ways to show progress are as levels of assistance (e.g., total, maximal, moderate, minimal,

TABLE 14.2 DAP Note

Data:
Same as the objective portion of a SOAP note but may include subjective statements from the patient. Can include • Objective measurable information • What the patient did and said • Results of assessments • Levels of assistance • Caregiver training Example: The client was observed crying in her room this morning and arrived 15 minutes late to the self-esteem group. Her hair was not brushed, and she wore only a pair of sweat pants, a hospital gown, and slippers. She initially refused to answer questions, but with encouragement from other group members, the patient started to open up to the group. The patient made several negative comments about herself but was able to identify some positive qualities about herself with support from the therapist. Discussion with her nurse revealed that her mother visited the previous evening and refused to allow the patient to be released. Nursing states that the patient became very upset stating that her mother would not allow her to explain her wants and needs.
Assessment:
OT practitioner's professional interpretation of the data portion of the note. Can also include • Quick overview of the client's functional performance • Barriers to intervention and reasoning for those barriers • Goals achieved and why others were not achieved • Medical necessity Example: The patient appears to have low self-esteem as indicated by negative remarks made in group. With encouragement, she is able to identify positive qualities about herself and responds well to encouragement from others. Client appears to be poorly motivated to dress and groom herself, which may be due to frustrations related to her wanting to be discharged.
Plan:
Can include the following: • Intervention needed for the following week(s) • Any plans for caregiver education • Frequency and duration of future intervention • Rehab potential Example: Continue intervention daily with a focus on self-esteem, communication skills, and assertiveness training.

standby, independent) and improvements in performance skills, client factors, and/or body functions (e.g., ROM, muscle strength, balance). There are other ways to show progress that may be more subtle but are just as important. They include a decrease in number of refusals to participate in intervention, increased consistency, increased generalization of skills acquired in intervention, addition of a new skilled functional activity, and addition of a new skilled compensatory technique (Author, n.d.b). Occupational therapy practitioners must document medical necessity on a weekly basis by showing the progress the client has made thus far and what you expect next week and why. Remember, medical necessity needs to be a documented thread throughout weekly progress notes.

Must-Have Components of Goal Writing and Progress Notes

An easy way to ensure that you have documented important components in your goals and progress notes is to make sure that they are skilled, functional, and measurable. Using skilled terminology is a must and in simple terms means "make yourself sound smart!" Use your current *Occupational Therapy Practice Framework III* (AOTA, 2014) terminology. The second component of documentation is to make it functional. This answers the question, "so what?" As you document, it is a good practice to frequently ask yourself, "so what?" If you recall, "so what?" is the area of occupation being addressed. For a goal or statement to be functional, it must include an area of occupation (e.g., ADL, IADL, education, work, play, and leisure). Documentation of functional outcomes belongs in daily/weekly notes and in monthly intervention plans.

Examples of nonfunctional statements:

- The client has improved UE ROM ("so what?").
- The client has improved muscle strength ("so what?").

Examples of functional statements:

- The client has improved UE ROM, so he/she can now independently comb his/her hair.
- The client has improved muscle strength enabling him/her to dress the upper body with minimal assistance.

The measurable portion of documentation answers the questions, from where, to where, and, sometimes, by when?

Example of a nonmeasurable statement/goal:

- Client will increase bilateral shoulder ROM.
- The client has improved muscle strength.

Example of a measurable statement/goal:

- In 2 weeks (by when), the client will increase bilateral shoulder ROM from 60 degrees (from where) to 90 degrees (to where) of shoulder flexion to enable client to independently comb hair.
- The client demonstrated fair + (from where) upper extremity muscle strength last week. This week, the client demonstrates good – (to where) muscle strength, enabling him to transfer with minimal assistance to and from the toilet.

Step Six: Discontinuation Summary

The plan for discontinuation should be determined at the time of initial evaluation and reassessed as the client progresses through therapy. The OT writes the summary, but the OTA may provide input to the process. The OTA is often responsible for developing functional maintenance programs (FMPs) and restorative and home programs for their clients in cooperation with the OT. **FMPs** are often prepared for clients who have been discharged from therapy but will be remaining in a skilled nursing facility. The programs facilitate skills a client has but are not functional unless compensations or adaptations are provided (Author, n.d.a). Developing an FMP and the time spent educating nursing staff is a skilled and billable service. Implementing an ongoing FMP is a nonskilled service that should be delivered by facility nursing staff and not OT practitioners. The FMP identifies and enhances residual functional abilities during skilled intervention by rehabilitation professionals. The FMP serves three main purposes, one of which is to include helping a client maintain the ability to function at his/her optimal level within the given environment. An FMP also helps the client access skills he/she has not been able to access previously/recently such as designing a (self) finger feeding program, and thirdly, they help to reduce the burden of care for caregivers within the client's current environment. Remember that an FMP is a routine program to maintain current level of functioning and prevent declining functional status and not skilled therapy (Author, n.d.a). It is important to stay abreast of Centers for Medicare and Medicaid Systems guidelines to determine the current payment regulations for FMPs.

Restorative programs are typically developed for clients who are still on therapy caseload but need extra support from specially trained nursing staff or restorative aids. Restorative programs facilitate learning new skills in an attempt to restore the client's previous abilities (Author, n.d.a). Examples of restorative programs include ambulation programs and feeding programs. The goal of the restorative program is to teach, train, and reinforce a newly acquired level of function. These programs are directed and supervised by OT practitioner. Restorative programs may also begin when occupational therapy services have been discontinued and/or there are no skilled therapy needs.

Documentation Tips

All documentation needs to be completed in a timely manner and follow the guidelines provided by the AOTA, state, employer, and third-party payers. If you are late with any documentation entry, indicate the current date and the date that it is a late entry for (e.g., 1/23/99 late entry for 1/22/99). Do not make a habit of late entries. It should be the exception, and not the rule. Documentation should be written in black ink unless otherwise specified and should not include abbreviations, unless authorized by the facility or payers. Information should never be added or changed in a note. Writing data in a medical chart and then removing the information is illegal. In most situations, federal and state laws permit only the person who made the entry to correct any errors in that entry, providing that they are the ones who found it. If incorrect information is written, a single line should be drawn through the incorrect information. The OT practitioner should sign/initial and write the date above the line. You can then write the correct information following the error. Never erase, scratch out, write over, or cover errors with whiteout paint. Making a medical entry for another person and signing the same entry for that person are illegal. After you have finished your note, a straight line should be drawn from the end of the entry to the end of the line or margin of the paper. This discourages anyone from adding information at a later time. EMRs have their own set of requirements for completion, which are often facility based. Medical records must be maintained as a permanent, legal file for each client. Medical records should be organized, legible, concise, clear, accurate, complete, current, and objective.

Summary

In this chapter, we discussed the purpose of documentation, including goal development and note writing. Although many OT practitioners view documentation as drudgery, it is equally as important as providing excellent clinical intervention. Good documentation can be the difference between being reimbursed for services or not. Good documentation comes with a great deal of practice as well as sound mentoring from a colleague who is a skilled documenter. As you progress through your studies and enter the workforce, remember that you have the capacity to be a top-notch documenter.

Review Questions

Indicate if each statement is part of the subjective, objective, assessment, or plan portion of a SOAP note.

1. The client improved R shoulder ROM from 90 degrees of flexion to 110 degrees of flexion.
2. "I want to transfer by myself."
3. Client has difficulty with lower body dressing secondary to poor postural control and perceptual deficits.
4. Client performs upper extremity dressing with moderate assistance.
5. Client demonstrates improved fine motor coordination.
6. Pain limits performance with ADLs.
7. Will administer the *Motor-Free Visual Perceptual Assessment* (*MVPT*).
8. Client continues to require skilled occupational therapy services secondary to difficulties with functional transfers as well as bathing and dressing.
9. Educate family on functional transfers.
10. Client scored a 4.2 on the *Allen Cognitive Level Screen*.

Practice Activities

- Read goals below and identify the five components of each.

In 3 weeks, the client will improve fine motor coordination to enable client to button shirt independently.
Who (participant):
What (client factor/body function/performance skill):
What (area of occupation):
How (condition):
How (measurement standard):
When:

In 4 weeks, the client will improve upper extremity muscle strength and dynamic standing balance to enable client to perform toilet transfers with minimal assistance.
Who (participant):
What (client factor/body function/performance skill):
What (area of occupation):
How (condition):
How (measurement standard):
When:

- Read the case study below and identify the positive and negative prognostic indicators. Determine if this client is a good candidate for occupational therapy.
  Mr. Marks is a 73-year-old male with a diagnosis of right CVA with left hemiparesis. Prior to hospitalization, he was independent with all ADL, IADL, and mobility. Currently, Mr. Marks requires maximal assistance with all ADL, IADL, and mobility. He demonstrates left neglect and significant perceptual deficits. He is often confused and has poor judgment and problem-solving skills. Mr. Marks has a wife and three children who visit daily and are very involved in his therapy. Mr. Marks is motivated to participate in therapy and wants to return home.
  Positive prognostic indicators:
  Negative prognostic indicators:
  Is Mr. Marks a good candidate for therapy and why/not?

- Make the following statements skilled, functional, and measurable statements or goals:
  1. The client has increased ROM.
  2. The client will increase muscle strength.
  3. The client has improved fine motor coordination.
  4. The client will improve visual perceptual skill.
  5. The client has improved balance.
  6. The client will improve ability to sequence activities.
  7. The client has improved gross motor coordination.
  8. The client will improve postural control.
  9. The client has improved orientation.
  10. The client will increase activity tolerance.

References

American Occupational Therapy Association. Occupational therapy practice framework: Domain and process. 3rd ed. *Am J Occup Ther* 2014;68(Suppl 1):S1–S48. http://www.dx.doi.org/10.5014/ajot.2014.682006

Author. *Living the Values: A Clinician's Guide for the Facility Based Clinical Orientation Process*. NovaCare, Inc; n.d.a.

Author. *Self-Study Series: Documentation Training Program*. NovaCare, Inc; n.d.b.

Borcherding S. *Documentation Manual for Writing SOAP Notes in Occupational Therapy*. Throrofare, NJ: SLACK, Inc.; 2000.

Borcherding S, Kappel C. *The OTA's Guide to Writing SOAP Notes*. Throrofare, NJ: SLACK, Inc.; 2002.

College of St. Catherine. *Goal Writing: Documentation Outcomes. (Handout)*. St. Paul, MN: Author; 2001.

HealthIT.gov. *What is an Electronic Medical Record (EMR)?* n.d. Retrieved from http://www.healthit.gov/providers-professionals/electronic-medical-records-emr

Kettenbach G. *Writing Patient/Client Notes: Ensuring Accuracy in Documentation*. 4th ed. Philadelphia, PA: FA Davis, Inc.; 2009.

McClain LH. Documentation. In: Dunn W, ed. *Pediatric Occupational Therapy*. pp. 231–244). Thorofare, NJ: SLACK, Inc.; 1991.

NovaCare. Medical necessity made explicit. *Clin Adv* 1996;1:1–2.

Sames K. *Documenting Occupational Therapy Practice*. 2nd ed. Upper Saddle River, NJ: Pearson/Prentice Hall; 2009.

Schenker Y, et al. Interventions to improve patient comprehension in informed consent for medical and surgical procedures: a systematic review. *Med Decis Making* 2011(January/February);31(1):151–173.

CHAPTER 15

Management

Amy Wagenfeld, PhD, OTR/L SCEM, CAPs

Key Terms

Commission on Accreditation of Rehabilitation Facilities (CARF)—An independent, nonprofit organization focused on advancing the quality of services you use to meet your needs for the best possible outcomes. CARF provides accreditation services worldwide at the request of health and human service providers (Commission of Rehabilitation Facilities (2012), http://www.carf.org/home/).

Joint Commission on Accreditation of Healthcare Organizations (JCAHO)—Is an independent, not-for-profit organization that accredits and certifies more than 19,000 health care organizations and programs in the United States. Joint Commission accreditation and certification is recognized nationwide as a symbol of quality that reflects an organization's commitment to meeting certain performance standards (Joint Commission on Accreditation of Healthcare Organizations, 2012a, http://www.jointcommission.org/about_us/about_the_joint_commission_main.aspx).

Manager—Someone who is responsible for staff or employees and directs and supervises a business or enterprise and plans, directs, monitors, and takes corrective action of individuals or groups of people (About.com, 2012, http://management.about.com/od/policiesandprocedures/g/manager1.htm; Merriam Webster Dictionary, Online, 2012, http://www.merriam-webster.com/dictionary/manager).

Transactional leader—Leads by exception (Snodgrass et al., 2008).

Transformational leader—Inspires, energizes, and stimulates employees (Snodgrass et al., 2008).

Learning Objectives

After studying this chapter, readers should be able to:

- Identify qualities and styles associated with good management.
- Recognize the importance of the role of the OT practitioner as a middle-level manager.
- Compare and contrast transformational and transactional leadership style.
- Understand the external constraints associated with management in the health care sector.

Introduction

Management may be a topic that seems far into the future and perhaps not even in or on your mind in the early stages of your studies but nonetheless is an important topic to explore. Management issues, no matter where they occur, be they ones in which you are the recipient of an inspirational manager or one that is more challenging, directly impact your role in an organization. In fact, Gardner (1999) suggested that "Good management

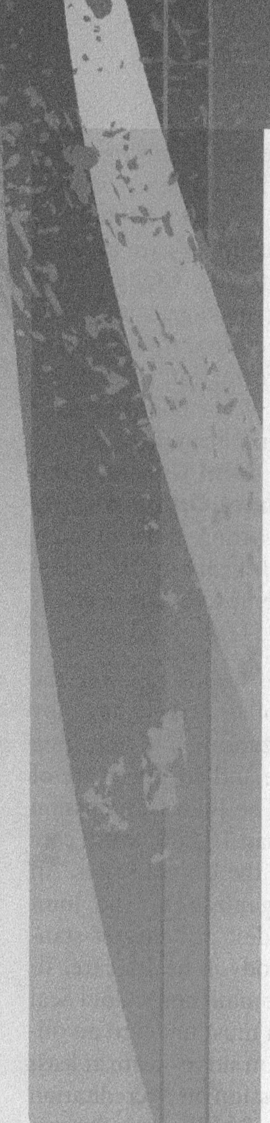

cannot create leaders. Instead, good management can create environments in which leaders and leadership qualities can incubate and evolve" (p. 15). One day, you may find yourself in a managerial role, and knowing what makes for good leadership and how to manage in the most fair and equitable manner possible can have far-reaching consequences for you, those you manage, your colleagues, the organization as a whole, and, of course, your clients (please also refer to Chapter 40, *Management and Education—Career Options for the Occupational Therapy Assistant*).

Research supports the idea that money is not everything when deciding whether to stay at a job. Issues such as management style, leadership behavior, and staff job satisfaction may actually be the deciding factors (Broadbridge, 2001; Williams et al., 2012). In fact, high levels of job satisfaction are associated with lower rates of stress and good health. A recent evaluation of leadership and health research noted that positive leadership behaviors correlated with a 27% reduction in sick leave and a 46% reduction in disability pensions (Kuoppala et al., 2008). Conversely, low levels of job satisfaction are associated with higher rates of absenteeism (Healy & McKay, 2000; Markussen et al., 2011; Rees & Smith, 1991).

Staff experiencing good leadership are 40% more likely to report high levels of psychological well-being, including lower levels of anxiety and depression (Kuoppala et al., 2008) than are their counterparts who work under leaders lacking good leadership behaviors. Williams et al. (2012) noted that

> the overall conclusions of the employee health research shows that the lack of certain leader behaviors can increase heart disease, promote musculoskeletal pain, foster sick leave, increase anxiety and depression, as well as lead to stress or even burnout. Positive leader behaviors can reduce sick leave, increase attendance and reduce anxiety, depression, stress and burnout. (http://www.boston.com/jobs/employers/hr/nehra/2011/02/the_impact_of_leader_behavior.html)

Job satisfaction is the key to employee stability and for making forward progress within a department (Broadbridge, 2001). It has been shown that OT practitioners who are satisfied with their jobs stay where they are and are more likely to remain within the profession (Moore et al., 2006). What then is a good manager? Do you have the qualities it takes to be a manager that your staff will look up to and respect?

What Is a Manager?

A **manager** or leader's duty is to be responsible for staff or employees. A manager directs and supervises a business or enterprise and plans, directs, monitors, and takes corrective action of individuals or groups of people (About.com, 2012, http://management.about.com/od/policiesandprocedures/g/manager1.htm; Merriam Webster Dictionary, Online, 2012, http://www.merriam-webster.com/dictionary/manager). Managers are formally appointed to their positions and are accountable for results (Guo & Calderon, 2007, p. 75). In the rehabilitation professions, practitioners typically rise to managerial ranks on the basis of clinical skills and ability, and not necessarily because of demonstrated leadership experiences (Atkinson, 1997; Battilana et al., 2010; Petchey et al., 2013). This lack of leadership experience and formal training often makes for a lag in getting up and running in a newfound and often foreign and perhaps ill-fitting role (Harrison, 2011). More so, many new and inexperienced managers lack the confidence needed to lead (Harrison, 2011). Because an occupational therapy manager must wear multiple hats, learning to lead well and to lead with confidence is critically important.

A manager supervises employees and ensures that proper procedures are in place and implemented in order for OT practitioners to balance role delineation with ethical and legal practice when teaming with OTAs (Bailey & Schwartzberg, 2003). The typical roles an occupational therapy manager takes on in a health care setting are, in descending order of time allocation, (1) supervision, (2) departmental representative to the larger organization, (3) staff recruitment, and (4) maintaining an active caseload (Gamble et al., 2007). Bridging the gap between no or limited leadership experience and being thrust into a role that requires a more or less 180-degree shift in professional responsibilities is a craft to be honed. Being aware of and taking on good leadership styles and qualities is no easy task. Becoming an effective manager is well worth the effort, as the end result may be a staff that is motivated and satisfied and more likely to stay. In turn, this positive climate only makes intervention that much better, and who is the ultimate beneficiary of this positive work environment? Our clients.

There are typically three tiers of leadership in a health care organization. Because there are definite similarities between organizational structure in health care and other types of corporations, parallels can be drawn in the way that managers function. As well, the skills required to be a manager are the same, regardless of the level or the venue in which management ensues. Let's start at the top. Upper-level management refers to corporate-level leadership such as a corporate executive officer (CEO), president, or vice president. The upper-level tier of management is responsible for the entire organization, including its staff and resources and, accordingly, for the higher-level decision making that impacts an entire organization.

While there are OT practitioners who are in upper-level managerial roles in a typical health care environment, most function at what is called the middle level. Middle-level managers are accountable to and report to upper-level management. In this role, OT practitioners have control over and are responsible for a segment of the organization, rather than the whole. For example, a middle-level occupational therapy manager is responsible for the occupational therapy department or perhaps, and depending on the organizational structure, the entire rehabilitation department and volunteers. Sandwiched between upper and primary management, the middle-level manager is in a unique position to view the organization from both a top-down and bottom-up perspective and is better able to maintain a finger on the pulse of the myriad trends impacting the organization (Guo & Calderon, 2007). Middle-level managers are also well positioned to "recommend changes that could be of political and financial benefit to the organization" (Guo & Calderon, 2007, p. 78).

A primary- or first-level manager in a health care system is a staff member who has supervisory responsibilities for students on fieldwork experiences or aides. First-level managers report to middle managers. An organization's survival and success depends on all levels of management and requires that they be well integrated with each other in order to accomplish its goals (Guo & Calderon, 2007).

External Issues Impacting Health Care Management

Beginning in the early 1990s, issues such as managed care, increased health care regulation, stiff economic competition, and intraorganizational conflicts began to and still overshadow management practices (Guo & Calderon, 2007, p. 76). In health care systems, quality management (QM) procedures are developed to measure whether quality of care is acceptable, including adhering to established standards of practice and achieving determined outcomes (Logigian, 1999). In other words, QM (and quality assurance) is all about accountability. Another method of determining quality of care is called continuous quality improvement (CQI). CQI involves creating environments that bring managers and staff together with the common goal of constantly striving to improve quality of care (Health Information Technology Research Center [HITRC], 2013). What does not meet acceptable health care standards must be improved upon to meet established standards. The **Joint Commission on Accreditation of Healthcare Organizations (JCAHO)** factors prominently in setting and maintaining standards for high-quality health care in the United States, including occupational therapy departments at health care centers. Founded in 1951, the JCAHO

> seeks to continuously improve health care for the public, in collaboration with other stakeholders, by evaluating health care organizations and inspiring them to excel in providing safe and effective care of the highest quality and value. The Joint Commission evaluates and accredits more than 19,000 health care organizations and programs in the United States. An independent, not-for-profit organization, The Joint Commission is the nation's oldest and largest standards-setting and accrediting body in health care. To earn and maintain The Joint Commission's Gold Seal of Approval™, an organization must undergo an on-site survey by a Joint Commission survey team at least every three years. (Joint Commission on Accreditation of Healthcare Organizations, 2012b, http://www.jointcommission.org/about_us/history.aspx)

To meet these challenges, the trend in leadership turned to "focused management teams [which] have replaced more traditional management structures" making it incumbent upon today's managers to be collaborative and measured risk takers and visionaries (Gardner, 1999; Guo & Calderon, 2007, p. 76). That is, in the spirit of success, and as compared to the past when the trend was a more authoritative and hierarchical management style, today's management structure in health care is increasingly collaborative and team focused at all levels. This collaborative spirit opens the door for middle-level managers to enact a more "participatory decision making, trust building, enthusiastic, and creative" climate for staff and to be better positioned to advocate for them (Guo & Calderon, 2007, p. 76; Moore et al., 2006).

Management and Managerial Roles

It is very important to understand that managerial skills are behaviors and not personality traits (Whetten & Cameron, 2005). While personality attributes and styles influence management, behaviors are the observable actions that managers "do." A pat on the back for a job well done is a behavior, but so too is verbal praise. A manager's personality attributes and styles may influence the behavior taken to praise an employee's good work. Management skills are controllable, that is, how a manager behaves is under his/her control (Whetten & Cameron, 2005). A manager can respond with a knee-jerk reaction to an adverse situation or be more reflective. Unlike some personality traits or IQ that are relatively consistent throughout life, management skills can be learned and improved (Whetten & Cameron, 2005). There is a great deal of overlap that is necessary to carry out good management (Whetten & Cameron, 2005). Sometimes, management skills are seen as contradictory; one size does not fit all (Whetten & Cameron, 2005). The same applies for different situations and tasks that warrant managerial oversight.

A manager is accountable for many tasks. "A manager's roles, skills and competencies are interrelated and are all necessary to be a successful manager" (Guo & Calderon, 2007, p. 80). Guo and Calderon proposed that middle-level occupational therapy managers have five overarching roles, as a planner, negotiator, coordinator, problem solver, and leader (Guo & Calderon, 2007). These roles are explained in Table 15.1 and expanded upon throughout this chapter.

Facing and dealing with the realities of financial constraints is a large part of a middle manager's job. A manager must balance high standards of client care with financial constraints and the needs and desires of the department while aligning with overarching organizational goals. Reimbursement structures are fixed, so the balancing act a middle-level manager must deal with involves determining "proper staff ratios, educational and skill levels of personnel, and scope of services"

TABLE 15.1 Typical Roles of a Middle-Level Occupational Therapy Manager

Planner	Being a planner is the most basic and bottom-line managerial function. Planning is the means by which a manager determines measurable action steps and the ways they will be accomplished (Braveman, 2006). Planning involves making decisions today that will influence future outcomes. The purpose of planning is to promote order. Planning is critical for obtaining and managing funding and reimbursement resources. Strategic planning is part of global planning. It requires balancing quality service delivery with budgetary and time constraints.
Negotiator	Being a negotiator involves bargaining and finding the simplest solutions to meet goals. Negotiating involves inter- and intraorganizational networking in order to foster change and forge new collaborative relationships. Successful negotiating involves an ongoing process of positioning, bargaining, and repositioning.
Coordinator	Setting up and designing roles and responsibilities within a department, determining lines of authority, and reporting structures and knitting all these pieces together into a well-run department (Braveman, 2006) are organizational tasks associated with coordination. Coordination entails carrying out and managing quality improvement programs and initiatives. It also involves setting and reassigning standards of performance, staff evaluation, and correction (Braveman, 2006). Quality improvement is a calculated method used to transform organizations through evaluation and improvement of exiting systems to elicit better outcomes. Quality improvement touches closely on assuring change in health care and is supported by the Joint Commission on Accreditation of Healthcare Organizations and the Commission of Rehabilitation Facilities.
Problem solver	Problem solving involves finding solutions that will result in the best outcomes with the least amount of time and effort. Problem solving involves clearly identifying goals, identifying obstacles, and obtaining upper-level management buy-in before implementing a solution.
Leader	As a leader, a manager promotes and sustains quality improvements in health care. Managers need to provide direction and consistent leadership so that the departmental objectives align with and meet set goals (Braveman, 2006). Leaders are designers and stewards of their organizations.

Adapted from Guo KL, Calderon A. Roles, skills, and competencies of middle managers in occupational therapy. *Health Care Manage* 2007;26(1):74–83.

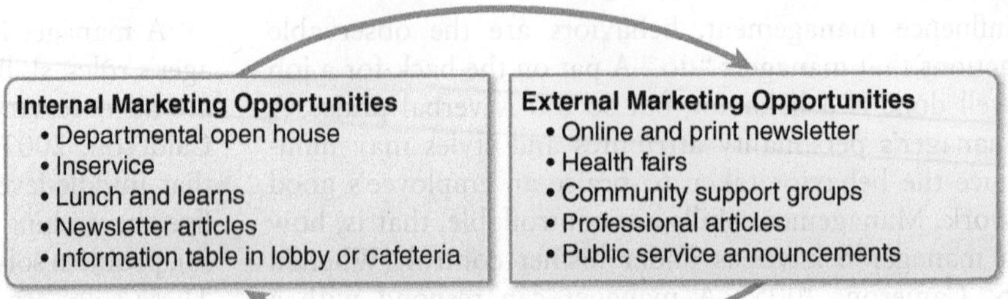

Internal Marketing Opportunities
- Departmental open house
- Inservice
- Lunch and learns
- Newsletter articles
- Information table in lobby or cafeteria

External Marketing Opportunities
- Online and print newsletter
- Health fairs
- Community support groups
- Professional articles
- Public service announcements

Figure 15.1 Marketing tips.

(Guo & Calderon, 2007, p. 77) in order to determine which staff is most competent to perform each of the necessary functions of the department in an ethically and fiscally responsible manner. Cost containing while not encroaching on meeting client needs and maintaining ethical boundaries is an ethical dilemma all middle-level occupational therapy managers face.

In a climate of intense competition and shrinking funding for services, a manager is well served to think about and write down what makes the department he/she leads unique and to create a branding that identifies its uniqueness (Stahl, 2007). This short paragraph is the key for how and to whom a manager will market the department and the services it provides (Fig. 15.1). The message should be short, clear, understandable, and concise so that it positively resonates with potential clients and the general public. Optimally, it will contain the department's (and umbrella organization's) mission, vision, and philosophical statements. This exercise could be considered a mini–business plan, which we will discuss shortly. Stahl (2007) suggests three angles to consider when marketing, (a) the services the department performs, (b) how these services help clients function better, and (c) how these services will impact physical and emotional health and well-being. Summed up, a manager is well served to think of all that the department offers as potential solutions for clients.

Managerial Challenges

Intertwined with an ever changing and complex health care system are myriad other challenges that organizations must face in order to not only survive but to also grow. These challenges include but are not limited to market competition, cost containment, ethical issues, and quality assurance (Guo & Calderon, 2007). In order for an organization to survive, managers at all levels must recognize and respond to external (such as fiscal) and internal (such as staff supervision) challenges (Guo & Calderon, 2007). Faced with these challenges, managers have a unique opportunity to bring about positive change. According to Guo and Calderon (2007), middle-level managers are uniquely positioned to balance optimization of the organization with individual employee goals so that staff can be positioned to perform at their best.

Managerial Styles

Snodgrass and colleagues suggest that one of the most widely recognized and researched theories of leadership is called the full-range leadership theory (FRLT) (Snodgrass et al., 2008). The FRLT posits "three categories of leadership outcomes; extra effort, effectiveness, and satisfaction" (Snodgrass et al., 2008, p. 39). Extra effort simply means that because of their manager's leadership style, employees are willing to work harder. Effectiveness is the perception that a manager is effective and satisfaction refers to the extent to which employees are satisfied with their manager (Snodgrass et al., 2008). Because research indicates that leadership styles are correlated with leadership outcomes, two particular components of the FRLT are noteworthy, transformational leadership (TL) and transactional leadership (TR) (Snodgrass et al., 2008). What is particularly interesting about TR and TL leadership styles is that they have been studied in diverse organizations such as the military, education, and politics, but scant research exists on the implications of these leadership styles in health care organizations, particularly with occupational therapy.

Transformational leaders are inspirational and energize and stimulate their employees (Snodgrass et al., 2008). Their vision and mission are readily apparent to those they manage (Moore et al., 2006). Transformational leaders inspire staff to look beyond themselves and focus on the greater good of the group (Snodgrass et al., 2008). Transformational leaders are able to inspire and excite their employees to recognize that extra effort pays off. And intellectually, a TL leader helps staff understand that through problem-solving rational solutions to problems can be resolved (Snodgrass et al., 2008).

A **transactional leader** is "often a prescription for mediocrity in the absence of TL" (Snodgrass et al., 2008, p. 39). Transactional leadership is leadership by exception, meaning that this type of manager establishes standards and intervenes only if they are not met. A TR leader uses contingent rewards. Employees are aware of what the expectations are and what will happen if they are not met (Moore et al., 2006). Transactional leadership is rewards and punishment focused. There are two forms of TR leadership, constructive and corrective. In the constructive form, TR leadership involves individual and group work, setting up contracts for work objectives, determining capabilities of staff, and setting up a compensation and rewards system (Snodgrass et al., 2008, p. 39). In the corrective form, TR is passive, waiting for mistakes to happen, and also active by monitoring for errors to occur (Snodgrass et al., 2008, p. 39). Research findings suggest that TL styles are more positively associated with leadership than TR, with the exception of the TR leadership contingency rewards contract (Snodgrass et al., 2008). Combining TL leadership with TR leadership contingent rewards appears to be the most effective way to manage (Snodgrass et al., 2008) leadership outcomes. With increasing numbers of occupational therapy assistants entering the workforce who may someday assume managerial roles, it is important to understand how leadership styles can positively or negatively influence the shape and direction of any therapy department, regardless of the venue.

Managerial Skills

A therapy program or clinical practice, or for that matter any business, succeeds or fails because of the people who are involved with it (Broadbridge, 2001), including staff and managers. A manager should be a visionary (Guo & Calderon, 2007; Stahl, 2007), which means having short- and long-range visions for a department. A good manager is a marketer and passionate champion for the department, both within and outside the organization. An occupational therapy manager is best able to fulfill the five roles (planner, negotiator, coordinator, problem solver, and leader) just discussed because of their skills. There are many skills that correlate with these five roles and are associated with good management.

The Manager as Planner

Good planning entails "identify[ing] and prioritize[ing] issues" (Guo & Calderon, 2007, p. 80). A manager can determine the effectiveness of strategic planning efforts through a SWOT analysis (Braveman, 2006). SWOT stands for

- Strengths—what strengths can be identified as a result of the strategic planning process
- Weaknesses—weaknesses can be identified as a result of the strategic planning process
- Opportunities—ideas and ways to move forward
- Threats—obstacles that threaten or block forward momentum

It goes without saying that a manager must be honest on all levels from budgeting, to staff management, to communicating, and more. Think about the original AOTA *Core Values* (AOTA, 1993). Among them were values such as truth, dignity, equality, and prudence. According to Broadbridge (2001), managers who possess core values such as these are better able to retain (happy) employees. Managers need to be big picture people but also to be acutely aware of and attend to details (Fig. 15.2).

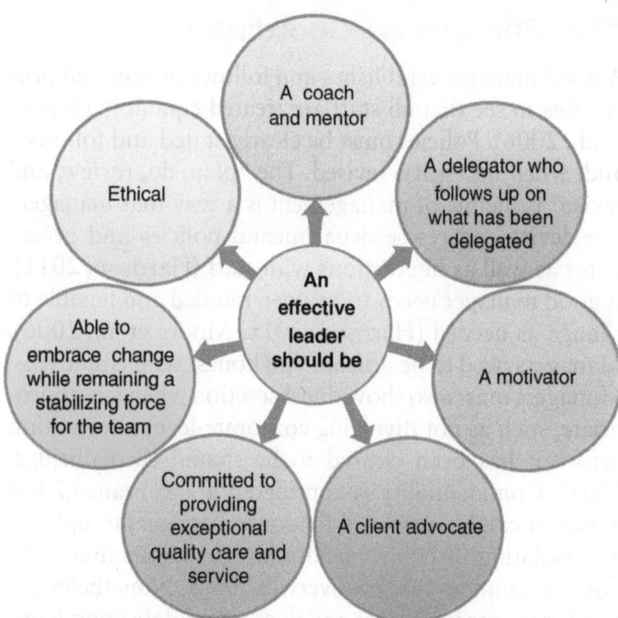
A coach and mentor
A delegator who follows up on what has been delegated
A motivator
A client advocate
Committed to providing exceptional quality care and service
Able to embrace change while remaining a stabilizing force for the team
Ethical
An effective leader should be

Figure 15.2 What effective managers need to remember to do. Adapted from Broadbridge B. Leadership and staff management. In: Prabst-Hunt W, ed. *Occupational Therapy Administration Manual*. pp. 63–80. Clifton Park, NY: Delmar, Cengage Learning; 2001.

The Manager as Negotiator

Managers should be approachable and not feared (Moore et al., 2006). Good managers respect and encourage diversity and demonstrate doing so by their actions (Broadbridge, 2001). A good manager advocates for the needs of the staff (Moore et al., 2006). Successful managers are rooted in the belief that all employees are worthy of their respect. While a manager may not agree with everything an employee says or does, each employee deserves to be treated with respect. Trust building is an important part of successful management (Gardner, 1999). Rebuilding lost trust is very difficult to accomplish (Broadbridge, 2001). Doesn't it just make sense that a staff member who feels respected is going to do a better job than is one who feels slighted or marginalized? Managers should strive to inspire their staff to feel that they are capable of reaching higher and to aspire to higher standards and professional goals (Moore et al., 2006).

The Manager as Coordinator

A good manager establishes and follows polices and procedures to see that all staff are treated equitably (Moore et al., 2006). Policies must be clearly stated and followed and, when necessary, revised. The "plan, do, review, and revise" principle of management is a way that managers can devise and revise departmental policies and procedures as well as interactions with staff (Harrison, 2011). A good manager needs to be open minded and flexible to change as needed (Harrison, 2011; Moore et al., 2006). Managers need to be upfront and honest with employees. Managers must also show due discretion when it is appropriate, such as not divulging corporate-level information before it has been cleared to be shared (Broadbridge, 2001). Confidentiality is considered a "no-brainer," but in fact, it can be very hard for some managers to uphold. It is isolating to be in a leadership role. Sometimes, the urge to confide can be overwhelming. Nonetheless, a good manager is discreet and does not violate confidentiality (Broadbridge, 2001). As an employee, you have the right to tell a nondiscreet manager that you feel uncomfortable being the recipient of confidential information that you should not be privy to knowing.

A manager needs to balance correcting an employee who has erred with keeping the positive spark and excitement alive. A good manager will shape and modify employee behavior in order to gain the necessary skills to perform tasks in compliance with organizational policies and procedures (Guo & Calderon, 2007). A good manager never criticizes an employee in front of other employees or certainly never in earshot of clients; exercising discretion is critically important. Constructive feedback is far better received than is harsh and judgmental criticism. When offering constructive feedback, it is important to be timely and specific and follow it up with constructive suggestions for how to better performance. Generalizations are not helpful. Positive feedback should be sincere and provided on a regular basis. Maybe you are familiar with the adage, "catch someone in the act of doing something right." This means that for positive feedback to stick, praise someone in the moment they are doing something right because it is then more likely to happen again (Broadbridge, 2001). And finally, a good manager schedules regular "office hours" to meet with employees and also shares tokens of appreciation with the staff (Broadbridge, 2001).

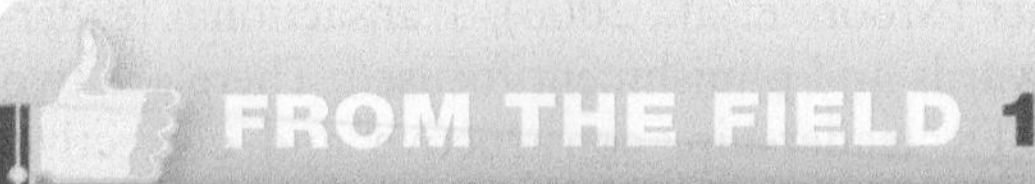

Take a Moment

Managing stress is no easy task for managers or those they manage. Three simple but effective ways to manage stress follow.

1. Close your eyes and take three, slow and deep breaths. Start from your belly and slowly inflate your chest to the count of 5. When you feel you cannot take any more air, take one additional tiny sip. Slowly release all of the air to the count of 7. When you feel as if all the air in your body is gone, repeat this exercise two more times.
2. Make a fist with your dominant hand. Feel the tension all the way up to your shoulder. Do not hold your breath! Beginning with the uppermost point on your shoulder, begin to slowly, very slowly, release the muscle tension as you slowly, but evenly inhale and exhale.
3. Stand against a wall with arms along your side and hands and fingers relaxed. While gently breathing, inhaling and exhaling, from your belly up to your chest and back down again, point the index finger of your right hand toward the floor. You will find that if you coordinate exhalation with stretch, there is more of a release. Feel the stretch and release of tension throughout your neck, shoulder, arm, and hand. Repeat with the left arm. Repeat on both sides as needed.

The Manager as Problem Solver

An astute manager understands that it is okay to disagree and that a climate that allows for such discourse to take place is necessary to create a positive working environment (Broadbridge, 2001; Guo & Calderon, 2007). It is not, though, acceptable to foster a climate in which there is behind-the-scenes dialogue that marginalizes any employee. It is unethical and very detrimental to the health of the department, not to mention its employees. Good management involves adopting a "fix it and move on" attitude to ensure that the mission of the department is realized (Broadbridge, 2001). A good manager keeps a close pulse on stress levels within the department and takes steps to, when possible, reduce it. One way to do so is to incorporate stress reduction breaks for staff during the workday (From the Field 15.1).

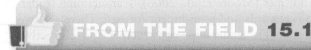

A component of problem solving is quality improvement. Part of quality improvement at the departmental level is preparing and sharing performance reviews with staff. It is understood that the best way for an employee to change a behavior is if he or she is apprised of what needs to be done. Second-guessing never accomplishes anything positive. A performance review allows a manager to sit down with an employee to discuss his/her strengths and areas of challenge and strategies to improve performance skills. A performance review generally looks at an employee's

- Written and communication skills
- Teaching skills
- Teamwork
- Customer service
- Patient advocacy
- Flexibility time management and productivity
- Organizational skills
- Clinical problem skills
- Ability to optimize the functional abilities of clients
- Clinical competencies specific to the job

The Manager as Leader

A prime indicator of a health care organization's success is to retain employees. The best way to retain employees is to create an environment in which employees experience a high level of job satisfaction. Broadbridge (2001) likens an employee to an "internal customer" and as such needs to be treated with "respect and dignity" (p. 63). Motivating employees and offering challenges and sincere opportunities to contribute to the department's betterment all help to account for employee retention and job satisfaction (Broadbridge, 2001). Moore et al. (2006) identified five qualities that managers would do well to implement to positively contribute to staff job satisfaction. They are "effective communication, approachability, consideration, advocacy, and appropriate application of policies" (p. 317). A manager's leadership style factors significantly into creating a healthy and desirable work environment for employees. In fact, a good manager considers and treats internal customers (staff) as well as they treat external customers (clients) (Broadbridge, 2001). According to Broadbridge (2001), "good leadership skills are essential to maintain a high level of staff satisfaction, productivity, and cohesiveness" (p. 63). A good manager can be the deciding factor for whether an employee stays or leaves a job. When strategizing how to best retain employees, and to avoid staff burnout, creative thinking is necessary (Fig. 15.3).

Remember money is not usually the deciding factor for whether an employee stays or goes. Options such as flextime and increased departmental responsibilities can positively enhance the working environment (Broadbridge, 2001). Although it is easy to say and harder to do, a successful manager is able to motivate staff so that they want to stay with the organization (Broadbridge, 2001; Guo & Calderon, 2007). When staff demonstrate competency, a good manager recognizes and rewards this through provision of increased autonomy (Moore et al., 2006). The following list contains additional ideas for ways a manager can motivate and improve job satisfaction and in turn increase staff retention.

- Staff reinforcement—noting a job well done.
- Employee appraisals—annual evaluations or at as needed as greater frequencies.
- Involving an employee in his/her evaluation is an empowering experience.
- Wage increases—this is always welcomed.
- Benefits—exploring fringe benefits that may be increased if salary cannot.
- Flexible hours—can actually improve staff productivity.
- Part-time options—job sharing or part-time positions help people who need or want to more easily balance personal and professional roles.
- Opportunity for advancement—for those who seek it, providing opportunities to explore different roles within the organization is very meaningful.

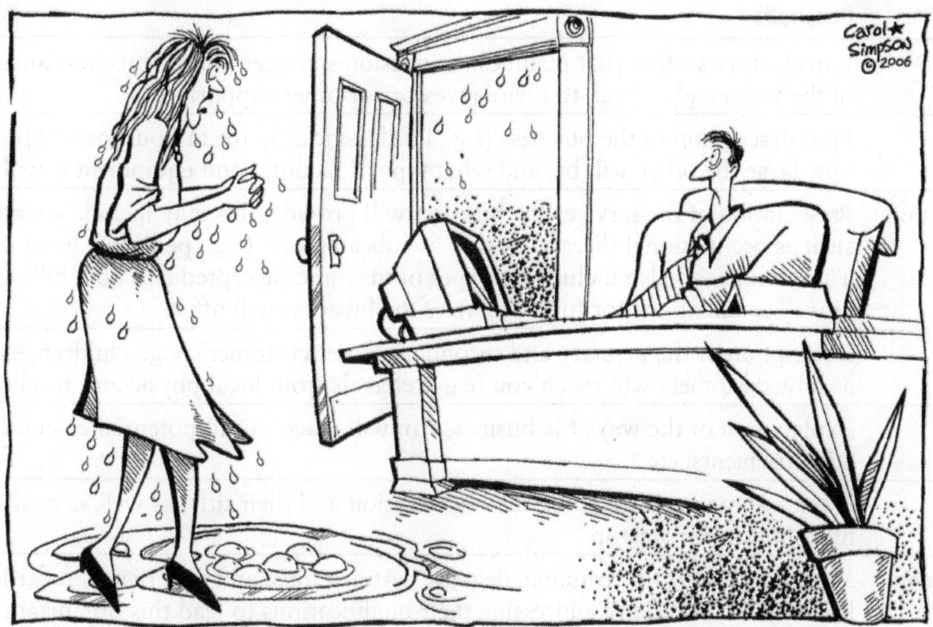

"It's the sprinkler system, sir... employee burnout keeps setting it off."

Figure 15.3 © Carol Simpson, 2006. Reprinted with permission.

- Cohesive work environment—stays positive and does not tolerate destructive communication in the department.
- Professionally challenging position—to avoid burnout or to recharge employees' batteries, offer enrichment opportunities to learn new skills and to strive for excellence.
- Job security—as best as possible, ensure that employees understand that their job is safe.
- Ability to be involved in political issues regarding occupational therapy—encourage employees to serve on local, regional, and national occupational therapy committees. It is good press for the department as well.
- Memberships in community service organizations—provide time off for employees to attend social service group meetings or events, as well as pay for memberships in these groups. It is good for morale, good for all involved, and of course good press for the department (adapted from Broadbridge [2001] and Guo and Calderon [2007]).

Good communication and good management go hand in hand. A good manager communicates all the time, and not just when problems arise (Guo & Calderon, 2007; Harrison, 2011). A good manager provides the tools needed for employees to provide the best level of care possible. Doing so requires a manager with excellent communication skills so employees know exactly what is expected of them (Harrison, 2011). Even when there is nothing much to say, a good manager is visible and around and about in the department (Broadbridge, 2001). Managers who are predictable, are consistent, and are able to admit to mistakes are more likely to be trusted than are ones who are erratic and unwilling to concede to having been wrong (Gardner, 1999; Guo & Calderon, 2007; Moore et al., 2006).

A good manager is a teacher and a mentor (Guo & Calderon, 2007). To that end, a good manager should also have demonstrably good clinical skills, so that staff feels that their leader is also a capable clinician (Moore et al., 2006). Taking this idea further, managers who are willing to step in and take on a caseload when staffing issues demand is held in higher regard than is one who does not "join the team" in times of need.

Business Plan

Whether in the future you aspire to be an entrepreneur and use your skills as an OTA in new and unique ways, want to expand your role at a facility where you will work, become a manager at an organization, or need to envision how to move a department in new ways, the tool to help you think and organize your ideas is called a business plan (Fig. 15.4). Preparing a business plan is both challenging and, hopefully, fun. Like the visionary statement we discussed, a business plan involves clear-headed thinking about future goals and ways in which you can work toward making them happen. During your career as an OTA, you may prepare several business plans as your interests change and evolve. There are many samples and templates available online and in business books. Components of a sample business plan are shown in Table 15.2.

TABLE 15.2 Components of a Sample Business Plan

Component	Description
Executive summary	Introductory section that includes the mission statement of the business and the objectives of the written plan (e.g., to invite investors or other supporters)
Company summary	Brief description of the business (e.g., its classification for tax purposes, where it is located, how large the office will be, and what type of facilities and equipment it will have)
Service description	Presentation of the services the business will provide; this may include a major category such as occupational therapy as well as subcategories (e.g., pediatric, hand therapy, etc.). This section can also include the types of insurance accepted and how billing takes place, as well as intentions for future services the business will offer.
Customer description	Description of the primary and secondary target customers (e.g., children, elderly), as well as how customers will reach you (e.g., referrals from local physicians, teachers, and others)
Marketing	Explanation of the ways the business can/will reach out to potential customers (referrals, advertisements, etc.)
Management summary	Names of the people leading the organization and their title, as well as positions to be filled in time for startup
Management team	More specific details (training, degrees, certifications, and experience) regarding the leaders listed above, especially addressing their qualifications to lead this organization
Financial plan	Detailed presentation of costs for starting up the business, projected profit/loss statements, and projected balance sheets

Summary

By now, you are aware that being a manager is more than being a "nice person." There are numerous roles a manager must take on and, in the spirit of doing so, possess unique qualities that enable him or her to lead with levelheadedness, fairness, dignity, enthusiasm, grace, a collaborative spirit, and honesty and integrity. Good managers have a vision for the future to move a department in a positive direction that aligns with organizational policies and procedures yet, at the same time, meets the needs of the staff for whom they are responsible. For many, managerial roles are unpalatable, yet for equally as many, this is a role that others actively seek out and thrive in doing.

Review Questions

1. Which of the following is not typically a primary reason for leaving a job?
   a. Management style
   b. Salary
   c. Leadership behavior
   d. Job satisfaction

2. How are many occupational therapy managers appointed to leadership roles?
   a. Consensus
   b. Seniority in department
   c. Proven clinical skills
   d. Proven leadership abilities

3. A transformative manager:
   a. Leads by exception
   b. Closely monitors and watches for errors
   c. Offers contingent rewards
   d. Inspires and motivates

4. A typical occupational therapy manager functions at what level in a health care organization?
   a. Upper level
   b. Primary level
   c. Middle level
   d. First level

5. An example of leading by exception is which of the following?
   a. "You know what you were supposed to do, and you failed to follow procedures,"
   b. "Read my mind,"
   c. "I know you can do it; next time will be easier,"
   d. "Great job, can you share what you learned with the rest of the staff?"

6. A first- or primary-level occupational therapy manager might be responsible for:
   a. Student and aide supervision
   b. Supervising students
   c. Budgeting and in-service education
   d. Hiring staff and practitioner staff performance reviews

7. A good manager provides staff with constructive feedback. Which of the following is not an example of constructive feedback?
   a. I noticed you seemed to be struggling to transfer Mr. Jones to the shower chair today. Let's figure out how we can make this easier and safer for both of you.
   b. I like how you maintained really nice eye contact with Mrs. Austin today. Because she cannot speak, you were "reading" her response to therapy by looking at her eyes to give you an indication of how things were going. That inspired a lot of trust.
   c. You seemed to be nervous about presenting in the staff meeting today. Would you like to talk about it?
   d. You were obviously nervous about how to engage Kayla today. Is this always the case? What should I know about this?

8. A type of leadership in which employees are aware of what the expectations are and what will happen if they are not met is called:
   a. Transformational
   b. Transdisciplinary
   c. Transactional
   d. Translational

9. The typical order of time spent doing occupational therapy managerial tasks is in descending order.
   a. Supervision, departmental representative to the larger organization, staff recruitment, and maintaining an active caseload
   b. Staff recruitment, supervision, departmental representative to the larger organization, and maintaining an active caseload
   c. Departmental representative to the larger organization, supervision, staff recruitment, and maintaining an active caseload
   d. Maintaining an active caseload, supervision, departmental representative to the larger organization, and staff recruitment

10. Which are qualities associated with good managerial style?
   a. Approachable, motivating, judgmental, flexible
   b. Fair, inflexible, does not carry a caseload, present
   c. Approachable, fair, inspirational, open minded
   d. Approachable, fair, nondiscretionary, open minded

Practice Activities

Respond to each of the following scenarios with an example of constructive feedback and an example of harsh criticism. While you are doing this exercise, make note of how you feel when preparing examples for each scenario. This is important to internalize as you prepare to be an employee and perhaps one day a manager.

1. Bob has come in late 5 of the past 8 workdays. He arrives out of breath and somewhat in disarray.

2. Carolyn and Jamie were hired at the same time and are both new graduates. Carolyn relies on Jamie to help her organize her treatment plans for her pediatric clients. Jamie is always eager to help.

3. Melissa has been working in the department as an OTA for 12 years. She has seen many colleagues come and go, yet she remains a loyal employee, never asking for anything or seemingly never expecting anything. She has never asked to go to conferences, yet when offered, she accepts the invitation. She does what is asked of her, but does not initiate anything.

4. Justin is a new graduate who is the proverbial "know-it-all." He does not hesitate to tell others what he thinks is the correct way to implement treatments or to construct adapted equipment, or for that matter anything. The other staff members are showing signs of anger and frustration.

5. No matter how many times Tara is instructed in departmental policy on using task-oriented purposeful activity versus exercise modalities, she continues to select exercise activities that lack meaning and purpose to use with her client.

Based on TR/TL managerial styles as well as other good managerial qualities discussed in this chapter, work through this exercise. Your department has four OTs and three OTAs. Registration is open for the national AOTA conference, and two OTs and two OTAs would like to attend. The manager would also like to attend. How would you solve this dilemma?

Make a list of qualities that best describe a favorite professor. Make another list of qualities that best describes a favorite boss. Make a list of qualities that best describe you. Make two more lists of qualities that best describe a professor and a boss that you do not care for. Take all the data, and make a graph of your findings. Compare your graph to the qualities of good management described in this chapter.

References

About.com. A New York Times Company. *Management*. 2012. Retrieved July, from http://management.about.com/od/policiesandprocedures/g/manager1.htm

American Occupational Therapy Association. Core values and attitudes of occupational therapy practice. *Am J Occup Ther* 1993;47: 1085–1086.

Anderson B. Sample business plan. In: Prabst-Hunt W, ed. *Occupational Therapy Administration Manual*. pp. 185–193. Clifton Park, NY: Cengage Learning; 2001.

Atkinson DE. Rehabilitation management and leadership competencies. *J Rehabil Adm* 1997;21(4), 249–260.

Bailey DM, Schwartzberg SL. *Ethical and Legal Dilemmas in Occupational Therapy*. Philadelphia, PA: FA Davis Co; 2003.

Battilana J, et al. Leadership competencies for implementing planned organizational change. *Leadersh Q* 2010;21(3):422–438.

Braveman B. *Leading and Managing Occupational Therapy Services: An Evidence-Based Approach*. Philadelphia, PA: FA Davis Co; 2006.

Broadbridge B. Leadership and staff management. In: Prabst-Hunt W, ed. *Occupational Therapy Administration Manual*. pp. 63–80. Clifton Park, NY: Delmar, Cengage Learning; 2001.

Commission of Rehabilitation Facilities. *About CARF*. 2012. http://www.carf.org/home/

Gamble JE, et al. A case study of occupational therapy managers in NSW: roles, responsibilities and work satisfaction. *Aust Occup Ther J* 2007;56:122–131.

Gardner JF. Leadership and organizational behavior. In: Jacobs K, Logigian MK, eds. *Functions of a Manager in Occupational Therapy*. 3rd ed., pp. 11–24. Thorofare, NJ: SLACK, Inc.; 1999.

Guo KL, Calderon A. Roles, skills, and competencies of middle managers in occupational therapy. *Health Care Manag*, 2007;26(1):74–83.

Harrison L. *Top Tips: People Management Skills*. Haymarket Business Publications; 2011. Retrieved from http://www.printweek.com/Business/article/1050307/business-inspection-supervisors-front-line/

Health Information Technology Research Center (HITRC). *Continuous Quality Improvement (CQI) Strategies to Optimize Your Practice*. National Learning Consortium; 2013. Retrieved from http://www.healthit.gov/sites/default/files/tools/nlc_continuousqualityimprovementprimer.pdf

Healy CM, McKay MF. Nursing stress: the effects of coping strategies and job satisfaction in a sample of Australian nurses. *J Adv Nurs* 2000;22(4), 11–14.

Joint Commission on Accreditation of Healthcare Organizations. *About the Joint Commission*. 2012a. Retrieved from http://www.jointcommission.org/about_us/about_the_joint_commission_main.aspx

Joint Commission on Accreditation of Healthcare Organizations. *History of the Joint Commission*. 2012b. Retrieved from http://www.jointcommission.org/about_us/history.aspx

Kuoppala J, et al. Leadership, job well being, and health effects—a systematic review and a meta-analysis. *J Occup Environ Med* 2008;50:904–915.

Logigian MK. Quality management. In: Jacobs K, Logigian MK, eds. *Functions of a Manager in Occupational Therapy*. 3rd ed., pp. 119–127. Thorofare, NJ: SLACK, Inc.; 1999.

Markussen S, et al. The anatomy of absenteeism. *J Health Econ* 2011;30(2):277–292.

Merriam Webster Dictionary, Online. *Manager*. 2012. Retrieved from http://www.merriam-webster.com/dictionary/manager

Moore K, et al. The influence of managers on job satisfaction in occupational therapy. *Br J Occup Ther* 2006;69(7):312–318.

Petchey R, et al. *Allied Health Professionals and Management: an Ethnographic Study. Service Delivery and Organisation Programme*. National Institute for Health Research. 2013. Retrieved from http://www.nets.nihr.ac.uk/__data/assets/pdf_file/0006/85056/FR-08-1808-237.pdf.

Rees DW, Smith SD. Work stress in occupational therapists assessed by the Occupational Stress Indicator. *Br J Occup Ther* 1991;54(8):289–294.

Snodgrass J, et al. Occupational therapy practitioners' perceptions of rehabilitation managers' leadership styles and the outcomes of leadership. *J Allied Health* 2008;37(1): 38–44.

Stahl J. *The 7 Fundamental Management Skills for Leaders at All Levels*. New York, NY: Kaplan; 2007.

Whetten DA, Cameron KS. *Developing Management Skills*. 6th ed. Upper Saddle River, NJ: Pearson Learning, Inc; 2005.

Williams R, et al. *The impact of leader behavior on employee health: lessons for leadership development*. 2012. Retrieved from http://www.boston.com/jobs/employers/hr/nehra/2011/02/the_impact_of_leader_behavior.html?s_campaign=8315.

CHAPTER 16

Working Together: Clinical Reasoning and Collaboration

Tamera Keiter Humbert, DEd, OTR/L

Key Terms

Activity analysis—Considering the components of activities or modalities used in the therapy sessions or general activities.

Clinical reasoning—The comprehensive cognitive process that practitioners use to make decisions about intervention based on the judgments made about the person receiving the therapy.

Conditional reasoning—Understanding the whole condition of the client including the family, social, and physical contexts that the client is engaged and imaging future possibilities for the client.

Culturally responsive care—Understanding and appreciating cultural differences between people and its application to intervention.

Ethical reasoning—Understanding and making decisions about intervention approaches when there are resulting ethical considerations and conflicts.

Evidence-based practice—Using theory and research to substantiate the approaches used in practice.

Interactive reasoning—Understanding the client as an individual or demonstrating connected knowledge.

Intuitive reasoning—A way of thinking and being with clients that entailed sensitivity to the practitioner's own emotions and those of the clients.

Narrative reasoning—The use of storytelling and story creation in order to share the client's story.

Occupational performance analysis—Assessing various aspects of the client and his/her contexts.

Pragmatic reasoning—Understanding the practical limitations in the delivery of therapy.

Procedural reasoning—Understanding the client's underlying problem and then setting goals and planning intervention accordingly.

Learning Objectives

After studying this chapter, readers should be able to:

- Describe the collaborative relationship between occupational therapists and occupational therapy assistants in the context of describing the supporting documents from AOTA.
- Discuss the evolution within the profession with the use of activity analysis, occupational performance analysis, and evidence-based practice.
- Explain the types of clinical reasoning and identify the use when given select intervention scenarios.
- Articulate the understanding of clinical reasoning with the OTA practitioner and the considerations of the OT/OTA supervisory relationship.

Introduction

This chapter was created out of a desire to assist students in understanding how OT practitioners think about and make sense of their professional world. As a former clinician and fieldwork supervisor and now more recently as an academic educator, I have come to appreciate the complexity in which exceptional students and practitioners think about and respond to therapeutic issues. This underlying thinking process utilized by OT practitioners is referred to as **clinical reasoning** and the development of such through education and clinical practice is highly regarded in the field. Additionally, the collaborative relationship between the OT and OTA further enhances clinical reasoning and is further supported by the profession (Lyons & Crepeau, 2001). To that end, the primary focus of this chapter is twofold: first, to highlight the OT/OTA collaborative relationship and, second, to assist students in comprehending the constructs of clinical reasoning and in understanding how OT practitioners think while engaged in practice. The term clinical reasoning is being used in this chapter, reflecting the historical representation of this concept as it relates to the OTA. It should be noted that the term professional reasoning is also currently being promoted, a more contemporary term that reflects the diverse nature of occupational therapy practice.

As recognized by the American Occupational Therapy Association (AOTA, 2009), and by authors Tryssenaar and Perkins (2001) and Boyt Schell and Schell (2008), the development of clinical reasoning takes years to fully develop and mature; however, it is my belief that as we make the thinking process as explicit as we can, the process moves from a nebulous, vague skill to one that can be logical and systematic. This is not to say that there is much about clinical reasoning that is still considered an art that needs to be experienced and intuitively developed (Chaffey et al., 2012; Toth-Cohen, 2008). Clinical reasoning is not a cookbook approach or flow chart approach when thinking about intervention. As OT practitioners, we need to be aware of the multiple aspects of someone's life as well as consider the best therapeutic approaches in order to provide appropriate intervention. We need to take into consideration many aspects when thinking about occupational therapy practice.

While there is a difference in the academic preparation, facilitation, and focus of clinical reasoning between OTs and OTAs, there can be and should be fundamental and basic levels of clinical reasoning and analysis present for all practitioners. Despite using the inclusive term OT practitioner throughout this chapter, I have also used the designation OT and OTA when it is relevant to past research and when describing the collaboration process.

Also, this chapter is full of stories from real-life events. These stories have come from my personal and work experiences, student's shared experiences, and other OT practitioners' narratives and explanations of their clinical reasoning. They have shared their unique perspectives related to this topic, but the names and logistics have not always been presented or may have been changed in order to insure privacy and confidentiality. The stories or images presented are offered as examples to the materials. I wish to thank all of the individuals who have supplied stories or shared their perspectives with me. It is in the dialogue and deeper understanding of one another that clinical reasoning and sensitivity is fully developed.

Collaboration and Working in a Team Model

The OTA has a great opportunity to work collaboratively with a variety of other practitioners within potential career choices. Whether you are working in a traditional medical model, a psychiatric model, a social milieu approach, a school system, or other nontraditional avenues of consultation and entrepreneurial efforts, you most likely will be working with others. According to AOTA, the OTA practitioner is required to work in collaboration with and under the supervision of an OT when the role is clearly identified with occupational therapy (AOTA, 2009). As an OTA, you would be responsible to understand and follow the supervisory expectations according to AOTA and any applicable state licensure bodies (AOTA, 2009, 2012). See Table 16.1 for the applicable documents of AOTA

TABLE 16.1 American Occupational Therapy Association Documents Related to the OTA Practitioner

Title	Date of Publication	Purpose
Guidelines for Supervision, Roles, and Responsibilities During the Delivery of Occupational Therapy Services	Original document 2004; updated version 2014	This document contains four sections: 1. General Supervision 2. Supervision of Occupational Therapists and Occupational Therapy Assistants 3. Roles and Responsibilities of Occupational Therapists and Occupational Therapy Assistants During the Delivery of Occupational Therapy Services 4. Supervision of Occupational Therapy Aides
Jurisdictions Regulating Occupational Therapy Assistants (OTAs)	May 2011	Listing of states that license or certify the practice of OTAs and the dates when the legislative process was enacted
Occupational Therapy Assistant Supervision Requirements	January 2012	Listing of all state regulations for OTA practitioners according to specific state licensure/certification laws
Occupational Therapy Profession: Continuing Competencies Requirements	January 2012	Competency requirements for OT and OTA practitioners' renewal of license/certification according to specific state standards
Scope of Practice	Original document 2004; revised version 2014	Outlines the educational and certification requirements/qualifications to become an OTA
Standards of Practice	Revised document 2010	This document outlines the requirements for OTs and OTAs for the delivery of occupational therapy services.

regarding certification and supervisory and continuing competency expectations.

There are several key considerations related to the supervisory relationship between the OT and OTA. First, the expectation is that you will need to have supervision when working in the context of occupational therapy. Secondly, the amount and frequency of that supervision varies from state to state by the established licensure and certification laws. You are responsible to understand and follow those requirements. Thirdly, there is another expectation that you continue to develop your skills, knowledge, and clinical reasoning through continuing education opportunities. The state in which you work may have specific standards that need to be met and documented to maintain your license or certification.

The role of the OTA has dramatically changed over the past sixty years, and the current understanding from AOTA (2009) is that the OTA does use clinical reasoning within and supported by the collaborative relationship with the OT. Throughout this chapter, I will be describing the term clinical reasoning, or the way practitioners think in practice, and will be integrating the concept of supervision and collaboration within that discussion.

The Background to Clinical Reasoning

The concept of clinical reasoning can be looked at from multiple angles, all of which help to explain its importance to the practice of occupational therapy.

Historical Background

As a profession, occupational therapy has gone through various periods of growth and different levels of understanding and focus. There has been an evolution related to how OT practitioners think about therapy, and this evolution can be identified through the professional literature. In the early inception of the profession, the concepts expressed about occupational therapy included the value of occupation or the value of doing and being (Quiroga, 1995). Over the years, the occupational therapy literature supported the application of these concepts to various groups of individuals and those with specific diagnoses. If you look through the *American Journal of Occupational Therapy* (*AJOT*) in the first decades of its inception, you will find articles related to "doing" therapy. Table 16.2 has a sampling of the various article titles.

TABLE 16.2 Sample of *AJOT* Articles from the Early Decades Reflecting Therapy Practice

Hurt SP. Occupational therapy in the rehabilitation of the poliomyelitis. *Am J Occup Ther* 1948;2(2):83–87
Wellerson TL. Occupational therapy program for eye patients. *Am J Occup Ther* 1951;5(4):146–148, 175
Lucci JA. Daily living achievements of the adult traumatic quadriplegic. *Am J Occup Ther* 1958;12(3):144–147, 160
Morris AG, Vignos P. A self-care program for the child with progressive muscular dystrophy. *Am J Occup Ther* 1960;14(6):301–305
Runge M. Self-dressing techniques for patients with spinal cord injury. *Am J Occup Ther* 1967;21(6):367–375

As time went on, particular theories and specific therapeutic approaches were also explained and promoted. Theory applied to practice became more explicit, and authors began to provide a rationale or theoretical principles to support the practice of occupational therapy. In addition to the expanse of theories and understanding of different diagnoses, the field of occupational therapy continued to develop into new practice arenas as funding increased, and the profession responded to the needs and demands of society. How occupational therapy addressed these new areas were also described in the literature. Table 16.3 lists examples of articles from *AJOT* that highlight theory and advanced practice.

Most recently, the focus of the professional literature has moved to a research-based approach, challenging OT practitioners to utilize the best practice methods available and to have a greater appreciation and understanding of how the therapy we provide has impacted someone's life, the community, and society. It is no longer important to just apply the concepts of theory or to understand what approaches are available; it is an expectation that OT practitioners understand various approaches used in therapy, understand the research supporting such approaches, and challenge their own understanding about the outcomes of the therapy they provide. See Table 16.4 for examples of these articles.

Activity Analysis, Occupational Performance Analysis, and Evidence-Based Practice

As the occupational therapy profession has evolved, so has the appreciation for how one thinks about therapy. Understanding the different thinking processes of practitioners has become more explicit and comprehensive over the past several decades. It has also shaped how educators teach this thinking process to students. For years, students were taught how to analyze the various activities used in the therapy sessions (Lamport, 2001). The belief being if students and practitioners could analyze the properties of specific activities used in therapy, they could choose the correct activity to give to the client or modify the activity if needed CS-5. For example, if an OT practitioner knew the inherent differences between making a cake from scratch versus using a box mix, they could choose which of one of these two baking activities would best match the goals and needs of the client. This form of analysis is referred to as **activity analysis** and continues to be used in some form today (see Chapter 11, *Activity Analysis, The Jewel of Occupational Therapy*).

In the mid-1990s, a greater understanding of the thinking processes used by practitioners was realized by the seminal research of Mattingly and Fleming (1994). This thinking process is known as clinical reasoning, and

TABLE 16.3 Sample of *AJOT* Articles that Incorporate Theory and Expanded Practice Arenas

Girls GM, Clark-Wilson J. The use of behavioral techniques in functional skills training after severe brain injury. *Am J Occup Ther* 1988;42(10):658–665
Bunning ME, Hanzlik JR. Adaptive computer use for a person with visual impairments. *Am J Occup Ther* 1993;47(11):998–1008
McAnanama EP, Joffe RT, Kelner M, et al. Discharge planning in mental health: the relevance of cognition to community living. *Am J Occup Ther* 1999;53(2):129–135
Bedell G. Daily life for eight urban gay men with HIV/AIDS. *Am J Occup Ther* 2000;54(2):197–206
White BP, Mulligan SE. Behavioral and physiologic response measures of occupational task performance: a preliminary comparison between typical children and children with attention disorder. *Am J Occup Ther* 2005;59(4):426–436

TABLE 16.4 Sample of *AJOT* Articles that Highlight Evidence-Based Practice

Hammon-Kellegrew D. Constructing daily routines: a qualitative examination of mothers with young children with disabilities. *Am J Occup Ther* 2000;54(3):252–259
VanLeit B, Crowe TK. Outcomes of an occupational therapy program for mothers of children with disabilities: impact on satisfaction with time use and occupational performance. *Am J Occup Ther* 2002;56(4):402–410
Baker NA, Cidboy EL. The effect of three alternative keyboard designs on forearm pronation, wrist extension, and ulnar deviation: a meta-analysis. *Am J Occup Ther* 2006;60(1):40–49
Dudgeon BJ, Tyler EJ, Rhodes LA, et al. Managing usual and unexpected pain with physical disability: a qualitative analysis. *Am J Occup Ther* 2006;60(1):92–103
Arbesman M, Pellerito JM Jr. Evidence-based perspective on the effect of automobile-related modifications on the driving ability, performance, and safety of older adults. *Am J Occup Ther* 2008;62(2):173–186

it moves beyond the focus of the activities used in therapy to how a practitioner interacts with clients and to how we understand and engage the individual receiving therapy services. This additional level of thinking allows OT practitioners to make decisions about the intervention session based on the judgments made about the client receiving the therapy (Boyt Schell & Schell, 2008).

With an increased understanding that therapy is not only about the activities used in therapy but more importantly the person(s) receiving therapy, the thinking process or analysis taught in educational programs moved to an **occupational performance** perspective (Thomas, 2011). If OT practitioners need to understand and appreciate the person receiving therapy intervention, they also need to analyze various aspects of the person and their contexts as well as the context in which the therapy is provided. This perspective is referred to **occupational performance analysis** (Thomas, 2011).

It is also important to note that another level of analysis or critical thinking process is being promoted in the profession and being taught in occupational therapy-related education. It entails using theory and research to substantiate what approaches should be used in practice and is called **evidence-based practice** (see Chapter 5, *Evidence-Based Practice Methods: Guiding the Practice*). This thinking process is valuable and challenges practitioners to be critical of the ways therapy is provided and to evaluate which activities and approaches are considered to be the best and most effective (Tickle-Degnen, 2000) (From the Field 16.1).

Mattingly and Fleming's Clinical Reasoning Model

Mattingly and Fleming (1994) described a conceptual model detailing how OTs think and perceive in the midst of practice. Their significant work and resulting book *Clinical Reasoning: Forms of Inquiry in the Therapeutic Process* (1994) is grounded by their research of fourteen experienced OTs. They asked the OTs to review videotapes of their own evaluation and intervention sessions, as well as other OT's sessions, periodically over a two-year period of time. The researchers asked the OTs to reflect on the process and to describe their approach and responses to the client situations through narrative storytelling. The intent of the study was to bring the tacit or semiconscious awareness and knowledge of the OTs to a conscious level in order for them to articulate and examine their practice. Mattingly and Fleming (1994) recognized the role that tacit knowledge plays in clinical practice and the need to have this knowledge become explicit in order to promote professional recognition and growth.

Mattingly and Fleming (1994) assert that clinical reasoning, a form of phenomenological thinking or meaning making, goes beyond scientific reasoning and evidence-based practice associated with critical thinking to determine the "good" for each particular client. Instead of discovering universal solutions to client scenarios and then anticipate, predict, and control the end results when providing intervention, the experienced OT utilizes a process of inquiry to understand a particular phenomenon in order to make meaning of the perceived client problem. Mattingly and Fleming (1994) promote a practical, *results-in-action*, approach that suggests OTs improvise from general theoretical ideas and rules of thumb to the specific requirements of a particular situation. Mattingly and Fleming (1994) state,

FROM THE FIELD 16.1

Research

In accordance with building a strong evidence-based practice base, the American Occupational Therapy Association has identified translational, intervention, and health services research as a high priority for the profession. (AOTA/AOTF, 2011)

> Central to the occupational therapy approach to reasoning was the notion that treatment success was very dependent upon a process that the therapists referred to as 'individualization'...[which] runs counter to the assumption that true knowledge is generalizable and that scientific knowledge can be converted into law [general] statements. (p. 338)

Mattingly and Fleming (1994) describe clinical reasoning as a dynamic, fluid process in which values, norms, and symbolic meaning are utilized to guide, gauge, frame, and formulate thought. They suggest that the clinical reasoning used during intervention relies on a large number of cues from a variety of sources including the client, the environment, past experiences, and one's knowledge. However, the OT also utilizes a more conscious, analytical process when they run into conflicts and problems during practice.

While Mattingly and Fleming focused their research on OTs, both OTs and OTAs (within the collaborative OT/OTA relationship) use tacit and habituated thought processes when paying attention to various relevant cues in the intervention environment and then unconsciously shift therapeutic interventions in response to the cues (Lyons & Crepeau, 2001; Mattingly & Fleming, 1994). Tacit knowledge is gained primarily from experience. This experience, as well as reflection about the intervention sessions, enables OT practitioners to make meaning of the therapeutic situation. Mattingly and Fleming (1994) and Lyons and Crepeau (2001) suggest that the more reflective the OT practitioner is, the more competent he or she becomes in the use of technical skills and client interaction.

Types of Clinical Reasoning

Mattingly and Fleming (1994) identified three primary forms of thinking and perceiving within the clinical reasoning process along with one underlying form of reasoning, narrative reasoning. According to Mattingly and Fleming (1994), this underlying form of reasoning or **narrative reasoning** that OT practitioners use includes storytelling and story creation in order to share the client's story, understand the client's perspective of the illness or disability, make meaning of and explain what they saw in practice, investigate the motives of the client, make sense of the client's experience, link the client's actions with the internal motivation and goals of the client, and determine how to approach the client in therapy.

Case Example: When OT practitioners are trying to think through a client case with a supervisor or colleague, they frequently share the client's story as part of the discussion. In my supervision of students and practitioners, I remember them saying things like "Mrs. Jones is a 46 year old mother. She really wants to do what is best for her kids but is struggling to understand how to deal with Billy, her youngest son. Billy seems to be having the greatest problem interacting with his peers. He gets upset quickly when there is conflict and leaves the room without any explanation." Beyond narrative reasoning, the clinical reasoning process evolves to encompass three distinct cognitive processes: procedural, interactive, and conditional reasoning.

Procedural reasoning includes the components of problem identification and definition, goal setting, and intervention selection and planning (Mattingly & Fleming, 1994). This critical thinking process is often utilized as a starting point when the OT initiates therapy. For example, when the OT receives a referral for services, he/she will complete a thorough initial assessment including gathering information regarding the client's age, diagnosis, environment, and any other pertinent, objective information in order to determine the needs of the client and to begin formulating goals for the client. The OT will use this information to begin to think about the underlying concern or issue to be addressed in therapy.

Case Example: While completing an initial assessment, I read in the chart that the client has had a stroke or cerebral vascular accident (CVA). My past knowledge and experiences alerts me to what that means from a pathological and functional standpoint. I understand the possibilities of what the client might be dealing with and then go about the actual physical, cognitive, and psychosocial assessment with the client, keeping this in mind. As I perform the assessment, I make mental notes as to how the stroke has actually affected the client and begin to make some decisions as to what is the most significant issues or primary concerns that need to be addressed. I should further understand what the current research and theory is in understanding how to best address these concerns.

It is important to note that procedural reasoning is also used throughout the intervention sessions when determining how the client is responding to the therapy activities and what areas of concern need to be furthered addressed. Within the collaborative relationship with the OT, the OTA utilizes procedural reasoning to understand the underlying concerns and reasons for the intervention plan (Lyons & Crepeau, 2001).

According to Mattingly and Fleming (1994), **interactive reasoning** is related to understanding the client as an individual or demonstrating connected knowledge, understanding the disability from the client's perspective, understanding the person as an individual within a culturally constricted point of view, and intuitively individualizing intervention. The term client-centered care has been around for some time and takes into perspective interactive reasoning. It suggests that through conversation and interaction, we get to know the client (and family when applicable) to understand what is most valued and important for them in the therapy process. We need to not only be respectful of what they value and believe but integrate our approach to address their concerns, strengths, values, and needs. This may lead to conflict and a need to resolve any differences between client, family, and practitioner, but the ideal is to always consider the client's desires when developing goals and intervention. Interactive reasoning requires active judgment related to the OT practitioner's own values and their ethical and moral decision-making skills.

Case Example: As I am completing an initial assessment with Mr. Smith, a 56-year-old gentleman with a diagnosis of a CVA, I found out that he is the president of a small company. Though it is hard to understand what he is saying because the stroke has affected his speech (procedural reasoning), he tells me that he needs to get home and back to work as soon as possible. I found out that he is married with three adult children. As we discuss his physical challenges at the moment (poor balance, not able to use of his right arm and hand, and not able to stand, walk, or sit independently—all from my procedural reasoning), I became aware that he is not interested in doing his own self-care. He believes his wife can assist with that. He is most interested in being able to get up on his own and to "get around" again. My own knowledge and experience suggests that addressing his daily activities of self-feeding and dressing to be important occupations to address after a stroke (procedural reasoning, occupational performance analysis, and evidence-based practice). Also, after a brief chat with Mrs. Smith, I learned that she works fulltime and desires her husband to "do as much for himself" as possible. Now I need to take all of this information and work with both Mr. and Mrs. Smith on identifying realistic goals for the intervention sessions.

Conditional reasoning is considered a projective mode in which the OT practitioner understands the whole condition of the client including the family, social, and physical contexts that the client is engaged, imagines how the condition could change, and engages the client in the construction of a new conditional image (Mattingly & Fleming, 1994). The OT practitioner reflects on the success or failure of the clinical encounter from a procedural and interactive standpoint, imagines the client in future contexts based on past and current roles, and engages the client to participate in the therapy session while assisting the client and family in understanding possibilities for the future. The OT and OTA, in collaboration with the OT, make meaning of the therapy sessions and interpret the successes as progression to future potential images for the client (Mattingly & Fleming, 1994). The OT practitioner's engagement with the client in forming new concepts and images of the future is performed through the narrative, storytelling process.

Case Example: From my previous work experience and knowledge, as well as evidence in the literature, I understand that the recovery from a stroke is quite variable and can be very lengthy in terms of how much recovery is expected and how long it might take. I need to be realistic as well as hopeful for both Mr. and Mrs. Smith as we move ahead in the intervention planning and delivery of services. For many people who have not had direct experience dealing with the aftermath of a stroke, most people struggle to imagine what the future will look like. As I begin and work through the therapy sessions, I "show" both Mr. Smith and his wife what is possible. I might begin the therapy session, teaching Mr. Smith to roll onto his side and then push up to sit at the edge of the bed (activity analysis). I might use the controls on his bed to help make the activity easier for him (activity analysis). I might have him experience what it is like to sit at the edge of the bed, providing just the right amount of support so that he is safe and feeling secure. Our conversation during that time would include giving him some idea as to what we will be working on in the next few days so that he might begin to practice with the nursing staff the art of "getting around" (occupational performance analysis).

Additional Types of Clinical Reasoning

Additional types of clinical reasoning, beyond what Matting and Fleming initially identified, have been described in the occupational therapy literature. The two most notable and reported supplementary types of reasoning include pragmatic reasoning and ethical reasoning. **Pragmatic reasoning** is related to the specific characteristics of the treatment setting, such as length of stay, insurance reimbursement, and institutional policies (Schell & Cervero, 1993). It recognizes that there are practical and everyday limitations that need to be understood and integrated into intervention planning and the delivery of therapeutic services.

Case Example: I am working with Mr. Smith in an acute care, hospital setting. The average length of stay at this hospital for someone with private insurance and with a diagnosis of a CVA is 5 days with one occupational therapy session provided per day. Considering this realistic limitation, I need to decide what is most practical and realistic to address during the intervention sessions that would have the greatest impact and meet the desires and needs of Mr. and Mrs. Smith within five sessions. I would need to understand not only what time I have but what the policies and procedures of the therapy department, nursing department, and hospital are. Am I permitted to see Mr. Smith alone in his hospital room versus having him transported to the therapy gym? What role do I have as an OT practitioner and what role does physical therapy have in addressing the goals of functional mobility and "getting around"? I need to be very cognizant of these issues while I am planning and delivering therapeutic intervention.

TABLE 16.5 Ethical Principles according to AOTA

Principle	Description
Beneficence	Occupational therapy personnel shall demonstrate a concern for the well-being and safety of the recipients of their services.
Nonmaleficence	Occupational therapy personnel shall intentionally refrain from actions that cause harm.
Autonomy and confidentiality	Occupational therapy personnel shall respect the right of the individual to self-determination, privacy, confidentiality, and consent.
Justice	Occupational therapy personnel promote fairness and objectivity in the provision of occupational therapy services.
Procedural justice	Occupational therapy personnel shall comply with institutional rules, local, state, federal, and international laws and AOTA documents applicable to the profession of occupational therapy.
Veracity	Occupational therapy personnel shall provide comprehensive, accurate, and objective information when representing the profession.
Fidelity	Occupational therapy personnel shall treat clients, colleagues and other professionals with respect, fairness, discretion, and integrity.

AOTA. *Occupational Therapy Code of Ethics and Ethical Standards*; 2015. www.AOTA.org

Ethical reasoning is the awareness and cognitive process of understanding and making decisions about intervention approaches when there are resulting ethical considerations and conflicts. Ethical reasoning takes place when the OT practitioner considers the various ethical principles that are involved in a case, identifies any inherent conflict between the principles, determines the value and significance of the principles to the case, and understands the dynamics of the various constituents' stake in the dilemma. Decisions are made by a process of assessing the significance of the principles, the people involved, and the potential outcomes. Table 16.5 lists specific ethical principles.

A detailed discussion of these principles is presented in the AOTA *Occupational Therapy Code of Ethics and Ethics Standards* (2015). Please also refer to Chapter 12, *Ethics*.

Case Example: I wish to honor Mr. Smith's primary desire to "get around" (autonomy). I also understand that presently he requires moderate assistance from a knowledgeable and experienced person to safely get from a lying to a sitting position. Mr. Smith should not be attempting to perform this task on his own or he will suffer significant injury. I instruct both Mr. and Mrs. Smith to wait for nursing staff or therapy staff to assist when getting up to prevent any potential harm (nonmaleficence). However, Mr. Smith states that to get better, he needs to practice and do it on his own. The conflict is between Mr. Smith's desires and wishes (autonomy) and his safety (nonmaleficence). A third ethical principle may also be at stake. I know from my discussions with Mr. and Mrs. Smith, my personal experiences with past clients, and evidence in the literature that allowing Mr. Smith opportunities to get up and practice this skill will be beneficial for his overall physical and mental health (veracity). I need to consider what is best for his health and would be most beneficial in his recovery (beneficence). However, doing what is best in this case could very well put Mr. Smith in danger of falling and possibly breaking a hip. There is a conflict between what is best (beneficence), what Mr. Smith desires (autonomy), and keeping Mr. Smith safe (nonmaleficence). I would need to consider all of these aspects when making a final determination as to what information and instructions I provide to both Mr. and Mrs. Smith in the therapy session regarding his ability to practice getting around.

Culturally Responsive Care Analysis and Intuitive Reasoning

In addition to Mattingly and Fleming's (1994) clinical reasoning types and pragmatic and ethical reasoning, several ways of knowing or understanding have also been identified in contemporary occupational therapy literature. While these have been identified as important, the concepts are still being investigated and understood with some attempts to integrate them into practice and in education settings. The first such consideration is the understanding and appreciation of cultural differences between people (Dickie, 2004). The term cultural sensitivity or **culturally responsive care** (Muñoz, 2007) has been not only suggested but highly supported as part of all of clinical reasoning and cultural analysis. Occupational therapy practitioners must be aware of how culture is part of a client's life and how to best support the beliefs and assumptions about care (Kondo, 2004; Toth-Cohen, 2008). In addition, the OT practitioner must be aware of one's own culture and how our beliefs and assumptions about health, disability, wellness, and intervention impact what we do in practice and how that practice is based on and influenced by our world views (Unsworth, 2004).

The other contemporary consideration is termed **intuitive reasoning**. Chaffey et al. (2010) conducted a preliminary study with OTs in mental health practice to understand how they utilized clinical reasoning in therapy. They identified a way of thinking and being with clients that entailed sensitivity to their own emotions and those of the clients. Chaffey et al. (2012) then conducted a second study to determine the correlation between emotional intelligence and the use of an intuitive cognitive thinking style with OTs employed in mental health practice. Experienced OTs tended to report use and preference for emotional competencies during practice more than novice OTs.

Research on the Use of Clinical Reasoning within Occupational Therapy Practice and Education

Initial research studies related to Mattingly and Fleming's clinical reasoning model were conducted with OTs and indicated that the OTs utilized a variety of clinical reasoning skills in practice (Alnervik & Sviden, 1996; Case-Smith, 1997; Fossey, 1996). While there is limited research from which to draw conclusions, there is some indication that the use of various forms of clinical reasoning may be related to the particular activities in which the OTs were engaged. In addition, there were noted differences in the use of clinical reasoning between experienced and novice OTs (McKay & Ryan, 1995; Strong et al., 1995).

The research also suggests that clinical reasoning is evident in occupational therapy practice arenas within and outside the medical model or hospital practice setting, where the initial Mattingly and Fleming (1994) study was conducted. Various articles have been written to support how therapists think about intervention with clients with strokes (Kristensen et al., 2011), brain injury (Kulpers & Grice, 2009; Kulpers & McKenna, 2009), cancer (Purcell et al., 2009), and dementia (Toth-Cohen, 2008). In addition, articles have been written to highlight particular practice areas including community-based practice (Taylor et al., 2007), pediatric intervention (Kramer et al., 2009), and driving programs (Unsworth, 2011). These articles highlight important and significant factors to consider in practice and, at times, provide protocols articulating applicable approaches based on the most effective intervention.

More recently, the research has been directed to the various ways clinical reasoning may be further enhanced in the therapy clinic and within education. The assumption behind this research is that when the clinical reasoning process is made explicit and one can articulate his or her thinking methods, clinical reasoning will become stronger. The methods or approaches to facilitate and enhance clinical reasoning are reviewed in Table 16.6.

Clinical Reasoning Skills and the Occupational Therapy Assistant

To date, there has only been one published study in the *American Journal of Occupational Therapy* related to the understanding of clinical reasoning and OTAs (Lyons & Crepeau, 2001). Lyons completed a phenomenological case study with an experienced OTA, exploring the working partnership of the OTA with two supervising OTs as it related to promoting efficacious clinical reasoning (Lyons & Crepeau, 2001). Lyons first conducted an initial interview with the experienced OTA in order to gain background history. For 3 days, she then observed the OTA throughout her workday. She took notes related to the interaction between the OTA and the OT supervisors. In order to determine the accuracy of interpretations of these observations and for further clarification from the participant and the supervising OTs, she conducted follow-up interviews. Multiple themes emerged in the study. First, clear examples of interactive, pragmatic, procedural, conditional, and narrative reasoning were employed throughout the supervisory relationship. Lyons (1999) describes this process metaphorically as being in tandem, much like riding a tandem bicycle. At times, the OT would initiate or lead the clinical reasoning process, while the OTA would contribute information. Other times, the OTA would initiate or lead the clinical reasoning process, and still on other occasions, they would mutually share information and hypothesize options for problematic situations or to better understand the therapy process.

Lyons (1999) further identified the complexities and responsibilities of clinical reasoning within this tandem supervisory process. Lyons (1999) espoused that both the OT and the OTA need to take responsibility for their contributions to the supervisory dialogue and demonstrate a mutual level of trust and respect for each other's level of skill and judgment. Lyons (1999) also suggested that there may be various factors that interfere with any tandem supervisory relationship. These factors may include blindly trusting the OTA's clinical reasoning skills, having limited information by the OT due to not being actively engaged with clients, having limited to no time for problem solving, dealing with an apathetic or uninvested OT,

TABLE 16.6 Examples of Educational Approaches in the Facilitation of Clinical Reasoning

Utilizing head-mounted video cameras to capture therapy sessions that can be reviewed and discussed at a later time	Unsworth (2005)
Using computer-aided cases to stimulate problem solving	Taylor et al. (2007)
Explicitly applying theory to practice cases	Lee et al. (2009)
Using developed conceptual and mapping strategies to better articulate thinking patterns	Greber et al. (2007); Greber et al. (2011); Parkinson et al. (2011)
Integrating the use of evidence-based practice with clinical reasoning	Cameron et al. (2005); Janes and Metzger (2011); Tickle-Degnen (2000); Tomlin and Borgetto (2011)
Reviewing and critiquing clinical reasoning through peer audits, case reports, and case studies	Aas and Alexanderson (2012); Torcivia and Gupta (2008)
Completing reflective journals	Hansen et al. (2011)
Supporting fieldwork education including online discussions during fieldwork	Scanlan and Hancock (2010)
Incorporating classroom-as-clinic activities into the curriculum	Benson and Hansen (2007); Neidstadt (1996)
Problem-based teaching/learning approach and activities	Scaffa and Wooster (2004)
Teaching a professional thinking approach curriculum	Bannington and Moores (2009)
Teaching an occupational science curriculum	Wood et al. (2000)
Active learning activities in the classroom	Kramer et al. (2007)

working with inexperienced or naïve practitioners, or not valuing the OTA's judgment. In her research, Lyons (1999) asserts that the key to the promotion of clinical reasoning within the supervisory relationship is effective communication skills. She states "Communicating with the OTR and conveying clinical reasoning is a critical aspect of the COTA [role]" (p. 92). Lyons (1999) began her study by stating her assumption that the OTA does utilize clinical reasoning in practice. However, she states

> Thus, there are many complex factors that affect the supervision and service competency of COTAs. If the literature reflects current clinical practice, OTR and COTA teams are not openly discussing these complexities. It is tacitly assumed that COTAs will somehow develop clinical reasoning skills to guide their intervention sessions by the time they make the transition to an intermediate level of practice. There has been no dissemination of techniques that OTRs can use to enable COTAs to reason more effectively or to assess their ability to clinically reason. Also, if clinical reasoning happens primarily in supervisory sessions, there has been no model for the supervision that describes how this may best be achieved. (1999, p. 95)

Lyons and Crepeau (2001) described the use of clinical reasoning with an experienced OTA as it is facilitated or initiated within the supervisory relationship. While this study is based on one case study, there is some additional evidence in the literature that clinical reasoning may be present and utilized by the experienced OTA. De La O (2008a) describes her work through a home health agency and the clinical reasoning needed for that particular practice. In a follow-up article, De La O provides opportunity for a supervising OT to share his perspective about the OTA role with such work (De La O, 2008b). The literature also provides examples of academic faculty supporting and facilitating clinical reasoning with OTA students. Greenburg and Plotnick (2011) describe a teaching/learning project between OT and OTA students where ethical reasoning scenarios are discussed and challenged. Additionally, Gonzalez et al. (2010) provide an example of OT and OTA student collaboration in carrying out an exercise program with community adults experiencing developmental challenges. While the literature and evidence is limited, there is some recognition and support of OTA students and practitioners gaining and using clinical reasoning skills within the OT/OTA collaborative relationship.

Summary

The use of clinical reasoning skills is complex and multidimensional. The development of such skills comes through an active learning approach and a dedication to articulating and challenging our own thinking processes. The OTA along with supervising therapists needs to spend time developing relationships where communication and problem-solving skills are acknowledged and supported.

Review Questions

Mrs. Smith is a 76-year-old woman with the admitting diagnosis of Alzheimer disease. She was found by a neighbor as she was wandering in the street and taken to the emergency department. Mrs. Smith was evaluated by the emergency room physician and admitted to the Behavioral Health Unit for further evaluation and intervention. The OT completes the initial evaluation and begins the intervention plan. She asks the OTA to include Mrs. Smith in the morning exercise group.

1. The OTA brings Mrs. Smith to the exercise group where they perform simple stretching exercises. As the group is progressing, the OTA notices that Mrs. Smith is having a significant amount of difficulty following the directions. The OTA provides some additional directions and modifies the exercises by slowing the routine down in order for Mrs. Smith to better participate in the group. The analysis that helped the OTA downgrade the activity is defined as
   a. Occupational performance analysis
   b. Evidence-based practice
   c. Activity analysis
   d. Conditional reasoning

2. After the group, the OTA begins to consider the reasons for Mrs. Smith's challenges, in particular what aspects of her cognitive skills are most challenged. This type of reflection is referred to as
   a. Narrative reasoning
   b. Procedural reasoning
   c. Interactive reasoning
   d. Conditional reasoning

3. Later in the day, the OTA reads through the social history found in the chart. She finds out that Mrs. Smith is a widow and has two grown children who do not live in the area. In addition, Mrs. Smith was an elementary school teacher for forty years. This information would be used to help formulate which type of clinical reasoning?
   a. Narrative reasoning
   b. Pragmatic reasoning
   c. Interactive reasoning
   d. Ethical reasoning

4. The OTA then shares with the OT what she found as being the most effective way to engage Mrs. Smith in the therapy session. The OTA states "when you give Mrs. Smith two choices, she is able to respond well." This is which reasoning type?
   a. Narrative reasoning
   b. Procedural reasoning
   c. Conditional reasoning
   d. Interactive reasoning

5. The following day, there is conversation at the nursing station as to whether or not Mrs. Smith might be able to go on a walk outdoors with the staff. There is concern that she might wonder off if there is not enough staff to provide oversight and supervision. However, there is also concern expressed about Mrs. Smith getting some exercise and fresh air. These concerns are related to which reasoning type?
   a. Pragmatic reasoning
   b. Interactive reasoning
   c. Ethical reasoning
   d. Procedural reasoning

6. As the nursing staff and the OTA discuss this situation further, the OTA states that the OT is off sick today and that will leave the unit short of additional help for the walk. This concern is related to which clinical reasoning type?
   a. Pragmatic reasoning
   b. Ethical reasoning
   c. Conditional reasoning
   d. Procedural reasoning

7. Later in the day, the OTA attends the intervention team meeting. Based on the discussion with the OT the previous day, the OTA states that the occupational therapy department is recommending that Mrs. Smith need additional support at home after discharge. The OTA further states that Mrs. Smith should be able to complete all of her basic ADLs with minimal support from a caregiver. This comment comes for which clinical reasoning type?
   a. Pragmatic reasoning
   b. Conditional reasoning
   c. Ethical reasoning
   d. Procedural reasoning
8. As the OTA completes her end-of-the-day responsibilities, she receives a phone call from the OT stating that she has been diagnosed with gallbladder disease and needs to have surgery next week. She will be away from the unit for two additional weeks. The OTA considers the issue of supervision and the need to make sure she has adequate supervision from a qualified OT. The OTA wishes to make sure to understand the exact requirements for supervision before going to the department administrator with her requests for supervision. The OTA would look at which document to understand these considerations?
   a. Guidelines for Supervision, Roles, and Responsibilities During the Delivery of Occupational Therapy Services
   b. Jurisdictions Regulating Occupational Therapy Assistants
   c. Occupational Therapy Assistant Supervision Requirements
   d. Standards of Practice
9. The OT and OTA collaborate over the phone in regard to the supervisory requirements and the coverage needed for the OT's absence. As the OT puts together a plan to present to the department administrator, the OT uses the following AOTA document to support her request for additional OT coverage during her absence:
   a. Scope of Practice
   b. Jurisdictions Regulating Occupational Therapy Assistants
   c. Occupational Therapy Profession: Continuing Competencies Requirements
   d. Guidelines for Supervision, Roles, and Responsibilities During the Delivery of Occupational Therapy Services
10. As the OTA continues to provide group sessions on the Behavioral Health Unit, she feels competent to continue with the sessions but is concerned about the need for new clients to be evaluated by a qualified OT. This concern would be applicable to which of the following ethical principles:
   a. Beneficence
   b. Veracity
   c. Social justice
   d. Procedural justice

Practice Activities

Pull the AOTA documents described in Table 16.1 and review the specific requirements for OT/OTA supervision according to state regulations. Discuss the similarities and differences between state regulations.

Discuss ethical principles and how one might make a decision when an ethical dilemma is involved (in the case example from the chapter).

Share and discuss how OT and OTAs best collaborate within a supervisory relationship.

Read/share articles or biographies of client's perspectives about therapy or the rehabilitation process and discuss ways in which to better develop an understanding of the long-term needs of clients.

References

Aas RW, Alexanderson K. Challenging evidence decision-making: a hypothetical case study about return to work. *Occup Ther Int* 2012;19(1):28–44.

Alnervik A, Sviden G. On clinical reasoning: patterns of reflection on practice. *Occup Ther J Res* 1996;16(2):98–111.

American Occupational Therapy Association and American Occupational Therapy Foundation. Occupational therapy research agenda. *Am J Occup Ther* 2011;65(6 Suppl.):S4–S7. doi:10.5014/ajot.65S4

AOTA. *Occupational Therapy Code of Ethics and Ethical Standards*; 2015. www.AOTA.org

AOTA, Commission on Practice. *Guidelines for Supervision, Roles, and Responsibilities During the Delivery of Occupational Therapy Services. Am J Occup Ther* 2014;65:S4–S22.

AOTA, Scope of Practice for Occupational Therapy. *Am J Occup Ther* 2014:S39–S40.

AOTA, State Affairs Group. *Occupational Therapy Assistant Supervision Requirements*; 2012. www.AOTA.org

Bannington K, Moores A. A model of professional thinking: integrating reflective practice and evidence based practice. *Can J Occup Ther* 2009;76(5):342–350.

Benson JD, Hansen AMW. Moving the classroom to the clinic: the experiences of occupational therapy students during the "living lab". *Occup Ther Health Care* 2007;21(3):79–91.

Boyt Schell BA, Schell J. *Clinical and Professional Reasoning in Occupational Therapy*. Philadelphia, PA: Lippincott Williams & Wilkins; 2008.

Cameron KA, Ballantyne S, Kulbitsky A, et al. Utilization of evidence-based practice by registered occupational therapists. *Occup Ther Int* 2005;12(3):123–126.

Case-Smith J. Variables related to successful school-based practice. *Occup Ther J Res* 1997;17(2):133–153.

Chaffey L, Unsworth CA, Fossey E. Relationship between intuition and emotional intelligence in occupational therapists in mental health practice. *Am J Occup Ther* 2012; 66(1):88–96.

Chaffey L, Unsworth CA, Fossey E. A grounded theory of intuition among occupational therapists in mental health practice. *Br J Occup Ther* 2010;73(7):300–308.

De La O TO. Home health from the occupational therapy assistant perspective. *Home Community Spec Interest Sect Q* 2008a;15(4):1–3.

De La O TO. Insights from an occupational therapist and home health agency owner. *Home Community Spec Interest Sect Q* 2008b; 15(4):3–4.

Dickie V. Culture is tricky: a commentary on culture emergent in occupation. *Am J Occup Ther* 2004;58(2):169–173.

Fossey E. Using the Occupational Performance History Interview (OPHI): therapists' reflections. *Br J Occup Ther* 1996;59(5):223–228.

Gonzalez TR, Carrasco SC, Sparkman L. Helping OTAs exercise their intervention skills. *OT Pract* 2010, September 27;15(17):17–19.

Greenburg NS, Plotnick HD. Professional ethics collaboration between community college and graduate occupational therapy programs. *Educ Spec Interest Sect Q* 2011;21(2):1, 2.

Greber C, Ziviana J, Rodgers S. Clinical Utility of the four-quadrant model of facilitated learning: perspectives of experienced occupational therapists. *Aust Occup Ther J* 2011;58(3):187–194.

Greber C, Ziviani J, Rodger S. The Four-Quadrant Model of Facilitated Learning: using teaching learning approaches in occupational therapy. *Aust Occup Ther J* 2007;54(1): S31–S39.

Hansen D, Larsen JK, Nielson S. Reflective writing in level II fieldwork: a tool to promote clinical reasoning. *OT Pract* 2011;16(7):11–15.

Janes WE, Metzger L. Evidence perks: introducing…the Journal Club Toolkit. *OT Pract* 2011;16(22):9, 20.

Kondo T. Cultural tensions in occupational therapy practice: considerations from a Japanese vantage point. *Am J Occup Ther* 2004; 58(2):174–184.

Kramer J, Bowyer P, O'Brien J, et al. How interdisciplinary pediatric practitioners choose assessments. *Can J Occup Ther* 2009; 76(1):56–65.

Kramer P, Ideishi RI, Kearney PJ, et al. Achieving curricular themes through learner-centered teaching. *Occup Ther Health Care* 2007;21(1/2):185–198.

Kristensen HK, Borg T, Hounsgaard L. Facilitation of research-based evidence within occupational therapy in stroke rehabilitation. *Br J Occup Ther* 2011;74(10):473–483.

Kulpers K, Grice JW. The structure of novice and expert occupational therapists' clinical reasoning before and after exposure to a domain-specific protocol. *Aust Occup Ther J* 2009;56(6):418–427.

Kulpers K, McKenna K. Upper limb rehabilitation following brain injury: complex, multifaceted and challenging. *Br J Occup Ther* 2009;72(1):20–28.

Lamport NK. *Activity Analysis and Application*. 4th ed. Thorofare, NJ: Slack, Inc.; 2001.

Lee SW, Taylor R, Kielhofner G. Choice, knowledge, and utilization of a practice theory: a national study of occupational therapists who use the Model of Human Occupation. *Occup Ther Health Care* 2009;23(1):60–71.

Lyons KD. *Clinical reasoning in tandem with the occupational therapists: a case study of the clinical reasoning of an occupational therapy assistant*. Unpublished Master's Thesis. University of New Hampshire; 1999.

Lyons KD, Crepeau EB. Case report: the clinical reasoning of an occupational therapy assistant. *Am J Occup Ther* 2001;55(5):577–581.

Mattingly C, Fleming M. *Clinical Reasoning: Forms of Inquiry in a Therapeutic Practice*. Philadelphia, PA: F.A. Davis; 1994.

Neidstadt M. Teaching strategies for the development of clinical reasoning. *Am J Occup Ther* 1996;50(8):676–684.

McKay EA, Ryan S. Clinical reasoning through storytelling: examining a student's case story on a fieldwork placement. *Br J Occup Ther* 1995;58(6):234–238.

Muñoz J. Culturally responsive caring in occupational therapy. *Occup Ther Int* 2007;14(4): 256–280. doi:10.1002/oti.238

Parkinson S, Shenfield M, Reece K, et al. Enhancing professional reasoning through the use of evidence-based assessments, robust case formulations and measurable goals. *Br J Occup Ther* 2011;74(3):148–152.

Purcell A, Fleming J, Haines T, et al. Cancer-related fatigue: a review and conceptual framework to guide therapist' understanding. *Br J Occup Ther* 2009;72(2):79–86.

Quiroga V. *Occupational Therapy: The First 30 Years*. Bethesda, MD: The American Occupational Therapy Association; 1995.

Scaffa ME, Wooster DM. Brief report—effects of problem-based learning on clinical reasoning in occupational therapy. *Am J Occup Ther* 2004;58(3):333–336.

Scanlan JN, Hancock N. Online discussions developing student's clinical reasoning skills during fieldwork. *Aust Occup Ther J* 2010;57(6):402–408.

Schell BA, Cervero RM. Clinical reasoning in occupational therapy: an integrative review. *Am J Occup Ther* 1993;47(7):605–610.

Strong J, Gilbert J, Cassidy S, et al. Expert clinicians and students' views on clinical reasoning in occupational therapy. *Br J Occup Ther* 1995;58(3):119–123.

Taylor B, Robertson D, Wiratunga N, et al. Using computer-aided case based reasoning to support clinical reasoning in community occupational therapy. *Comput Methods Programs Biomed* 2007;87(2):170–179.

Thomas H. *Occupation-Based Activity Analysis*. Thorofare, NJ: Slack, Inc.; 2011.

Tickle-Degnen L. Gathering current research evidence to enhance clinical reasoning. *Am J Occup Ther* 2000;54(1):102–105.

Tomlin G, Borgetto B. Research pyramid: a new evidence-based practice model for occupational therapy. *Am J Occup Ther* 2011;65(2):189–196.

Torcivia EM, Gupta J. Designing learning experiences that lead to critical thinking and enhanced clinical reasoning. *OT Pract* 2008;13(15):CE1–CE8.

Toth-Cohen S. Using cultural-historical activity theory to study clinical reasoning in context. *Scand J Occup Ther* 2008;15(2): 82–94.

Tryssenaar J, Perkins J. From student to therapist: exploring the first year of practice. *Am J Occup Ther* 2001;55(1):19–27.

Unsworth CA. Gaining insights to the clinical reasoning that supports an on-road driver assessment. *Can J Occup Ther* 2011; 78(2):97–102.

Unsworth CA. Using a head-mounted video camera to explore current conceptualizations of clinical reasoning in occupational therapy. *Am J Occup Ther* 2005;59(1):31–40.

Unsworth CA. Clinical reasoning: how do pragmatic reasoning, worldview and client-centredness fit? *Br J Occup Ther* 2004;67(1): 10–19.

Wood W, Nielson C, Humphrey R, et al. A curricular renaissance: graduate education centered on occupation. *Am J Occup Ther* 2000;54(6):586–596.

CHAPTER 17

Staying Current

Amy Wagenfeld, PhD, OTR/L, SCEM, CAPs

Key Terms

AOTF—American Occupational Therapy Foundation; "serves the public interest by supporting occupational therapy research [education], and increasing public understanding of the important relationship between everyday activities (occupations) and health. It accomplishes its aims primarily through grants and scholarships, through programs, and through publications" (American Occupational Therapy Foundation, n.d.b. http://www.aotf.org/aboutaotf.aspx).

AOTA—American Occupational Therapy Association; "the national professional association established in 1917 to represent the interests and concerns of occupational therapy practitioners and students of occupational therapy and to improve the quality of occupational therapy services" (American Occupational Therapy Foundation, n.d.a., http://www.aota.org/About.aspx).

NBCOT—National Board for Certification in Occupational Therapy; "a not-for-profit credentialing agency that provides certification for the occupational therapy profession" (NBCOT.org).

OT Connections—AOTA's online community.

Resume—A document intended to construct a professional identity in order to get a job interview.

WFOT—World Federation of Occupational Therapists (WFOT) is an international organization that promotes "occupational therapy as an art and science internationally" (wfot.org) (World Federation of Occupational Therapists, 2011).

Learning Objectives

After studying this chapter, readers should be able to:

- Understand why staying current in occupational therapy is important.
- Know where and how to access information in order to stay current.
- Develop an action plan to stay current in occupational therapy as a student and also going forward as an occupational therapy assistant.

Introduction

It is always good practice to stay current about your profession, no matter what it is. Staying current enables you to maintain a pulse on new, emerging, and pertinent issues and on issues related to reimbursement for services and to be better connected with your profession. Staying current helps you to know what the current trends are in practice and reimbursement regulations and, in turn, to apply them to the work you do with clients, in research, or in education. Staying current also demonstrates your commitment to learning

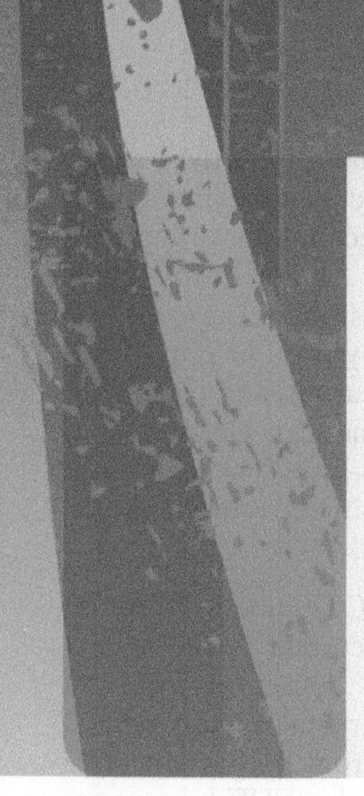

and using your knowledge to become a steward of any profession. Starting now, in the early stages of your educational career, is the perfect time to make a pact with yourself to stay current, interested, and committed to occupational therapy.

It is increasingly easy to stay current and knowledgeable about pretty much anything. Undeniably, it is also overwhelming. The Internet has made connecting to others as well as accessing information simple. With simplicity does come pitfalls, as much of the information available electronically is not always credible or reliable. For instance, when doing electronic searching for information to keep you current about occupational therapy, it is important to remember that many .com URLs are not as well vetted or reliable as .org or .edu URLs. The accuracy of information that is on the Internet varies widely, from quackery to highly respectable. In this chapter, we explore ways to stay current about occupational therapy and to do so as a discerning consumer. We will also explore how staying current also includes preparing a resume and cover letter and keeping it updated and ready to submit when applying for your first professional OTA job.

Home Base for Occupational Therapy: AOTA

The first place to look for information about current issues associated with occupational therapy is the **American Occupational Therapy Association** (**AOTA**). The URL for the AOTA is www.aota.org. The AOTA is a voluntary agency boasting a membership of over 50,000 OT practitioners. The AOTA website provides links for students, practitioners, educator–researchers, and those wanting to know more about occupational therapy. The home page contains headline information about issues pertinent to the profession. Because the site is updated constantly, it is important to check in on a very regular basis. Readers can access an abundance of other information, including some AOTA documents and white papers, publications, academic program information, and downloadable information for the general public from the home page. You can also find out about conferences that are either occupational therapy specific or of interest to OT practitioners. Attending conferences is an ideal way to stay current on specific topics as well as to network with colleagues.

Membership in AOTA allows you to access far more information than as a nonmember, including access to AOTA publications, official AOTA documents, the *Evidence-Based Practice Resource Director* and Critically Appraised Topics and Papers (CATs and CAPs), and a discount on AOTA's evidence-based practice guidelines (AOTA.org). While membership is voluntary, it is an investment well worth the money, as member-only benefits provide access to current information about occupational therapy that is unavailable anywhere else. Not only that, membership provides connections to fellow occupational therapy colleagues. Students are entitled to a reduced membership rate.

AOTA publications are available to members only. There are several, including the *American Journal of Occupational Therapy*, which is an official publication of the AOTA. Published seven times per year, it is a peer-reviewed journal that focuses on practice, research, and health care issues impacting occupational therapy (http://www.aota.org/Pubs/AJOT_1.aspx). It is available in print and online, and members have electronic access to back issues. The AOTA *Evidence Exchange* is a great tool to access evidence-based information on occupational therapy. *OT Practice,* published in print and electronic formats, "covers professional information on all aspects of occupational therapy practice today" (http://www.aota.org/Pubs/OTP.aspx). Back issues are available online to members. The AOTA publishes eleven different *Special Interest Section Quarterly Newsletters (SIS)*. Each SIS focuses on a specific practice area. AOTA members have access to all of the 11 e-newsletters and, depending on membership type, receive one *SIS Quarterly* in print form (http://www.aota.org/Pubs/SISQs.aspx). Members can also sign up to receive the AOTA *1-Minute Update* every other week in their inbox. Collectively, these AOTA resources keep members updated, current, and in the know about occupational therapy.

How about getting actively involved with AOTA as a means to stay current? There is an entire section of the AOTA website devoted just to students. It is easily accessed from the home page of AOTA and lists many ways to connect with the profession. A program that AOTA developed for its members is called the Coordinated Online Opportunities for Leadership (COOL) database (Yamkovenko, 2010). It links AOTA members with volunteer projects within the association.

Another way to stay current and be engaged with fellow occupational therapy practitioners is through a portal called **OT Connections** that is open to AOTA and non-AOTA members. It is an online community that enables OT practitioners, students, and consumers to interact, connect, and share on professional topics of interest to them. And last, but hardly least, participate or check out any of the AOTA special interest section forums within OT Connections to read about what members are saying and thinking. AOTA is truly your home for updated information about the profession.

For our colleagues in other parts of the world, your national and state or province associations are also the first place to search for current information about issues impacting occupational therapy in your country.

Affiliate Occupational Therapy Resources

There are a number of affiliate resources for occupational therapy practitioners that are discussed below.

The American Occupational Therapy Foundation

Becoming familiar with the **American Occupational Therapy Foundation (AOTF)** is another way to stay current about occupational therapy. The AOTF was founded in 1965 and "serves the public interest by supporting occupational therapy research [education], and increasing public understanding of the important relationship between everyday activities (occupations) and health. It accomplishes its aims primarily through grants and scholarships, through programs, and through publications" (http://www.aotf.org/aboutaotf.aspx). The goals of the AOTF are to support and facilitate the following:

Leadership development—facilitate the development of current and potential leaders in occupational therapy.

Financial stability—grow the foundation's capacity to pursue its mission.

Public awareness—increase public and professional knowledge and understanding of the following:

- The health benefits of participation in everyday activities
- The unique contribution of occupational therapy to health and quality of life

Research—support research initiatives that grow capacity and advance best practices in occupational therapy.

Education—support educational initiatives that strengthen the profession of occupational therapy.

Technology—foster the use of technology to improve practice and enhance quality of life (http://www.aotf.org/aboutaotf/visionmissiongoals.aspx). The AOTF and AOTA work closely to offer opportunities to further "research, education, and leadership in occupational therapy" (American Occupational Therapy Foundation, n.d.c., http://www.aotf.org/programspartnerships/jointinitiativeswithaota.aspx).

Jointly supported by the AOTF and AOTA, an important resource for staying current is the Wilma L. West (WLW) Library, which houses a large and invaluable compilation of occupational therapy-related materials. With materials dating from 1910 to the present, the information contained in the WLW Library are occupational therapy specific as well as pertain to topics relating to occupational therapy such as psychology, rehabilitation, and health care. The contents of the WLW Library are indexed in OT Search, which is an online bibliographic database. In the future, there are plans to include full text resources when possible, but for now, OT Search is an invaluable resource for OT practitioners looking to review the profession's past as well as to stay current. Anyone can sign up for a membership to OT Search, but AOTA members receive a discount. And yes, there is a student membership rate for OT Search. Some colleges and university libraries subscribe to OT Search, so be sure to check and see whether yours is a member.

National Board for Certification in Occupational Therapy

The National Board for Certification in Occupational Therapy, Inc. (NBCOT) is the not-for-profit agency that oversees the certification process for the profession (nbcot.org). The mission of the NBCOT is "serving the public interest by advancing client care and professional practice through evidence-based certification standards and the validation of knowledge essential for effective practice in occupational therapy" (nbcot.org). The NBCOT coordinates with state regulatory and licensing agencies to share information about practitioner credentialing, conduct, and issues pertaining to certification (nbcot.org). The vision of the NBCOT is "Certified occupational therapy professionals providing effective evidence-based services across all areas of practice worldwide" (nbcot.org). The NBCOT is an important organization to be familiar with to learn about current credentialing and regulatory issues impacting the profession on national and state/territorial levels (From the Field 17.1).

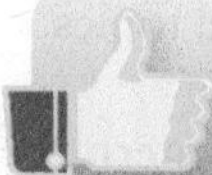

FROM THE FIELD 17.1

Keep Learning!

Not only is it required to maintain certification (and often, state licensure), one of the best ways to increase your knowledge base and improve your service delivery is to take continuing education (CE), professional courses. It can lead to some unexpected outcomes: discovering a new skill, networking, or even leads for new jobs.

International Home Base for Occupational Therapy: WFOT

The mission of the **World Federation of Occupational Therapists (WFOT)** is promotion of "occupational therapy as an art and science internationally (WFOT)." The URL for WFOT is www.wfot.org. The Federation supports the development, use, and practice of occupational therapy worldwide, demonstrating its relevance and contribution to society (http://www.wfot.org/AboutUs/FundamentalBeliefs.aspx). There are 73 member nations linked to the WFOT. The group is comprised of over 25,000 individual OT practitioners and a national organizational level membership comprising more that 350,000 practitioners throughout the world (http://www.wfot.org/Membership/MemberOrganisationsofWFOT.aspx). The WFOT home page (wfot.org) is internationally focused and provides an abundance of current information about conferences, programs, research, and news pertaining to the international occupational therapy community. The WFOT has an online resource center to enable members to stay current. The WFOT has established collaborative working relationships with the World Health Organization and the United Nations. AOTA members are eligible to join the WFOT.

State Associations

Every state, the District of Columbia, and Puerto Rico have occupational therapy associations. To easily locate a particular association, the AOTA website home page has a link to state and US territorial organization Internet sites. Many state occupational therapy organizations publish online or print newsletters that are available only to members. In case you might be wondering, state licensure does not require membership in a state occupational therapy association. Remember that state regulatory agencies control the legal aspects of occupational therapy practice, whereas national and state occupational therapy associations are completely separate organizations in which membership is voluntary.

That said, and like membership in AOTA, it is always a good idea to belong to your state organization. And like AOTA, state occupational therapy associations offer reduced student membership rates. Membership gains you access to an online and in-person community of colleagues, access to up-to-date practice and regulatory issues that are specific to your state or region, and access to publications that are unavailable to nonmembers.

State occupational therapy associations are volunteer run. Existing officers and committee chairs are always delighted to bring new volunteers into the fold. Consider being a volunteer starting now; it is a great way to share your talents, to learn more about the profession, to gain leadership and participatory experiences, to connect with colleagues, to give back to your profession, and to have a lot of fun.

Local Associations

Some, but not all regions of the United States, have formed local occupational therapy associations. These groups tend to be less formal than state organizations. They are typically formed to meet a specific need. For instance, in the Boston area, there is a sensory integration group that meets on a regular basis to talk about issues relevant to OT practitioners who use sensory integration techniques in their practice. Student OT and OTA chapters run through a local college or university could also be considered a local association. Getting involved on the local level is a grassroots means to getting involved with the profession. If you have ideas for a special study or practice group, starting on a local level may be a sensible way to begin.

Reading, Reading, Reading

As we discussed in Chapter 5, *Evidence-Based Research Methods: Guiding the Practice*, staying current with regard to evidence and occupational therapy involves a serious commitment to frequently accessing online evidence databases. While a list of several of these databases and what they include were provided in that chapter, several of these online links are also provided below in the section called Resources. Please refer to Chapter 5, *Evidence-Based Research Methods: Guiding the Practice* for the complete descriptive list. The best and most rewarding way to stay current with evidence is to do so as part of a journal club. A shared minds experience allows for discussion and sharing of ideas that would not happen if you are searching and learning in isolation. If distance and time is an issue, consider holding your journal club as a Skype meeting or online chat.

Conferences and Continuing Education

Attending conferences is a great way to stay current. Many occupational therapy conferences offer discounted rates for students. The AOTA holds an annual conference that attracts thousands of attendees from the United States and abroad. "Conference," as it is affectionately known, is an unprecedented opportunity to get current on most everything about occupational therapy. In addition to hundreds of workshops, short courses, and institutes, there are formal and informal networking events. All educational sessions at AOTA meet the standards for CE credits (CE), which are required for NBCOT renewal and, in differing amounts on a state-by-state basis, for licensure renewal. There are also stand-alone student professional and social events (in addition to full access to all other educational forums) at the annual AOTA conference. As a student or looking into the future, consider submitting a proposal to present at Conference. You can share what is current in your world of occupational therapy with your colleagues (From the Field 17.2).

State occupational therapy associations typically present annual conferences, which is another closer to home, ideal way to network and stay current on practice and research issues in the field. CE credits are offered at state conferences. Since state conferences are smaller than the AOTA national conference, you may encounter less competition to have a proposal accepted to present. Student rates for state conference are usually available, and sometimes, you may even attend on a work in exchange for admission basis. Local associations may also offer seminars and workshops on specialized topics. Often, there is CE credit available for attendees.

Every four years, the WFOT convenes an international conference that celebrates current practice and research trends in occupational therapy throughout the world. It is a large-scale event that brings together a global community. Attending a WFOT conference is truly an amazing way to connect face to face with other OT practitioners. CE credit is available for attendees.

Staying current by attending conferences and workshops to earn required CE credits to maintain certification and licensure is important. Other ways to stay current and earn CE credits are through online webinars, online or written courses, and face-to-face seminars sponsored by various organizations. Be sure to check that any course you are considering taking has been authorized as a provider for CE credit by your state association. In most states, CE providers are required to include a stock statement provided by the association on their course brochure indicating approval by the state association to offer the course for credit. Of note, not all states accept credit for courses that have AOTA CE credit approval. Be sure to look carefully and be aware of your state's status.

On AOTA's home page, there is a tab for CE that directs you to detailed information about CE requirements. As well, your state association is also a resource for determining the CE requirements for licensure renewal.

> **FROM THE FIELD 17.2**
>
> **PDU Handbook**
>
> The NBCOT requires that all certificants (OTR and OTAs) receive 36 professional development units (PDU) within a set three-year certification period. The NBCOT website (www.nbcot.org) provides access to the *PDU Handbook*, which clearly outlines the requirements and process for tracking and self-reporting these units for initial OTA and OTR certification and recertification.

Online Communities

In addition to *OT Connections*, the AOTA online community, sites such as LinkedIn and Facebook offer numerous opportunities to connect with OT practitioners throughout the world. These communities are yet another way to stay current and up to date on issues relevant to occupational therapy.

The First Job Application: Resume and Cover Letter

Being familiar with and making good use of resources that provide you with information such as the AOTA, AOTF, NBCOT, and WFOT and attending conferences and seminars are crucial for staying current with occupational therapy. Staying current also includes preparing a resume and cover letter and keeping it updated and ready to use when applying for your first professional OTA job. In this section, we explore how to compose a cover letter and resume and why both are such important precursors to a job interview.

The Cover Letter

Most every word processing program contains templates for creating a cover letter. Look at the options carefully and determine which template matches the position for which you are applying. Because a cover letter is often the first thing a potential employer sees about you, it must be well written with professional language and contain no slang or abbreviations, it should be organized, and it should say what needs to be said in a clear and concise manner. Check carefully for typos and grammatical errors, as they tend to send a message of carelessness, which you certainly want to avoid. In a cover letter, it is important to focus on the positive and the skills you have that make you the ideal candidate for the job. For instance, if a job requires one year of experience and you are a new graduate, talk about internship and fieldwork experiences and other hands-on learning experiences that are relevant for the job. But—and this goes for any position at any point in your career—never, ever be dishonest about your experiences or qualifications. It is unethical.

The first paragraph of a well-written cover letter talks about the advertised position you are applying for and how you learned about it. Without repeating your resume, the second paragraph discusses how your skills and experiences, educational background, and credentials are relevant to the position. Your final paragraph thanks the potential employer for considering you for the position and discusses how you can be reached and will follow up. Your cover letter should not be more than a single page. Double space the body of the letter and hand sign it. If the application process is online only, an electronic signature should appear as, /Your Name, Credentials/. Below is an example of a well-written cover letter for an OTA position at a local acute care hospital (Fig. 17.1). Be sure to tailor your cover letter to best match a job description.

The Resume

The purpose of a **resume** is to construct a professional identity in order to get a job interview (Fig. 17.2). Like cover letters, there are an abundance of resume template options available from your word processing program or the Internet. Your resume should be neat, concise, and free of spelling and grammatical errors. It should summarize your professional and volunteer work history as well as accomplishments. A resume should be formatted to fit a job description. That is, information may need to be rearranged to highlight information that is particularly relevant to a job description. However, as with the cover letter, it should only contain information that is true (From the Field 17.3).

Staying Current in Collaboration with Others

Ideally, your first job as an OTA is one in which you are hired as part of a medium to large department staffed with OTs and OTAs. Working with other staff provides you with built-in mentoring opportunities. A mentor–mentee relationship can be built around sharing and learning about current practice techniques. There is much to be gained from an inspirational mentor. Sources for identifying and finding a mentor include approaching a professor or fieldwork educator who motivates you, reaching out to a presenter at a conference you attended, and/or contacting the author of an article, book, or blog whose work is of interest to you.

Consider asking some upfront questions in your interview. During your job interview, ask your interviewer whether the practitioners in the department provide evidence-based intervention and how they derive the knowledge to do so. Knowing that they are committed to this model of practice tells you that they are abreast of current trends within occupational therapy.

When appropriate, another way to stay current and to learn from others is to engage in collaborative inter- and transdisciplinary models of intervention. An interdisciplinary model means that practitioners from different disciplines work as an integrated team while maintaining their professional roles. In a school-based setting when the OT, PT, and speech and language practitioners and teachers are meeting regularly to coordinate, implement, and discuss the outcomes of, for instance, a child's seating system, a sensory diet, or communication system, they are engaging in interdisciplinary practice. Interdisciplinary practice is not to be confused with multidisciplinary practice. In multidisciplinary practice, team members do not collaborate but work individually as team members, while an interdisciplinary team collaborates. A transdisciplinary model means that practitioners from different disciplines are competent enough in their roles to switch "hats" and function in a different capacity. Interdisciplinary and more so transdisciplinary practices are closely associated with early intervention work. Based on the team composition and leadership structure, an OT practitioner may find him/herself fulfilling roles traditionally associated with a speech and language pathologist or physical therapist. For instance, an OT practitioner may focus on complex positioning and swallowing with an infant with severe spasticity associated with cerebral palsy. Or the speech and language pathologist may be integrating fine motor activities into his/her language-based intervention plans. Newly graduated practitioners are usually not well suited for transdisciplinary practice. But it is very enriching work and

1234 Home Address
City, State 12345
222-333-4444
job.applicant@email.com

July 12, 2015

Ms. Lauren Evans*
Human Resources Manager
Acute Care Hospital
54321 Healthcare Road
Get Well, CA 12345

Dear Ms. Evans,

I read with great interest on Job Finder, the advertisement for an occupational therapy assistant position at Acute Care Hospital. My skills, professional and volunteer experiences, and educational background make me an ideal candidate for this position. I am fully certified and licensed in the state of XX as an occupational therapy assistant.

As a 2014 honors graduate of the (School Name) occupational therapy assistant program, I am well trained to work in an acute care setting. My fieldwork experiences as well as community service experiences have prepared me well to work with children and adults with physical disabilities. Before starting the occupational therapy assistant program I worked for a year as a skilled nursing assistant in a residential care facility for adults with developmental disabilities. It was during this time that I realized that I wanted to become an occupational therapy assistant, as the scope of work that occupational therapy assistants perform aligns with my professional interests. Since graduating I have spent the past two years working as an occupational therapy assistant in a skilled nursing facility, where I work closely with occupational therapists to provide high quality care to our patients. I am deeply committed to working with adults with physical disabilities and feel that I would be a value asset to your occupational therapy department.

A resume is enclosed with this cover letter. If I can provide you with any additional information regarding my qualifications for the occupational therapy assistant position, please do not hesitate to contact me. Thank you for your consideration of my application, Ms. Evans. I look forward to hearing from you.

Sincerely Yours,

[Signature]

Job Applicant, OTA/L

* If there is no contact name provided in the job posting, address the cover letter to "Search Committee" or omit a salutation entirely

Figure 17.1 Sample cover letter.

Job Applicant
2468 Street Avenue
Somewhere, State 12345
resume@email.com
222-333-4444

OBJECTIVE

To obtain an occupational therapy assistant position in (setting) and work as part of a team to provide high quality occupational therapy services.

EDUCATION

2011 AA with Honors, Your College/University, City, State

AWARDS

Varsity Letter Women's Swim Team, Your College
Team Captain 2010 Women's Swim Team, Your College
Martin County Special Olympics Volunteer of the Year 2008

OCCUPATIONAL THERAPY ASSISTANT CERTIFICATION AND LICENSURE

NBCOT Certification
State (name) Licensure(s)

WORK EXPERIENCE

2014-present Staff occupational therapy assistant, Kind Care Skilled Nursing Facility, Anywhere, MI, USA.
Under the supervision of an occupational therapist, treated patients using a task-oriented approach, trained and educated families in patient care, and developed an IADL cooking group for patients and their families.

2011-2014 Staff Occupational Therapy Assistant, John Doe Center, Someplace, TX, USA
Worked with a team of seven occupational therapists and occupational therapy assistants to provide care for adults with developmental disabilities. Educated nursing staff on proper lifting techniques and worked with clients on prevocational skills.

2008-2009 Certified Nurse Aide, Happy Assisted Living Facility, Here, AL, USA.
Provided direct patient care, including assistance with feeding and bathing, and light housekeeping. Taught a weekly chair yoga class as a volunteer.

VOLUNTEER EXPERIENCE

2009-2011 Treasurer, Your College Occupational Therapy Assistant Student Service Club
2007- present Swim Coach, Martin County Special Olympics

SPECIALIZED SKILLS

Proficient with word processing and other computer skills
Certified yoga instructor
Fluent English and Spanish speaker

Figure 17.2 Sample resume.

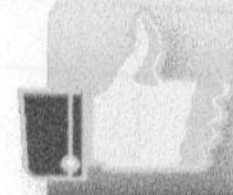

FROM THE FIELD 17.3

Update Your Resume

A brief word to the wise from one who has been there: Make it a habit to update your resume on a regular basis. It is really hard to remember professional experiences, awards, conference presentations, publications, or anything else relevant to add to your resume long after they occurred. It will take you longer and cause more aggravation to try to update a resume while you are applying for a job. Set your calendar or some type of reminder system to update your resume on a monthly basis. Even if there is nothing to add, spend a few moments tweaking your resume. Speaking from experience, it will make your life far easier!

something to look forward to as clinical skills and confidence levels improve with experience and ongoing learning.

Resources

The following list of Internet resources will be helpful to keep you current throughout your educational and professional career.

American Occupational Therapy Foundation—AOTF.org
American Occupational Therapy Association—AOTA.org
National Board for Certification in Occupational Therapy—NBCOT.org
AOTA OT Connections—http://otconnections.aota.org/
AOTA *Evidence Exchange*—http://www.aota.org/Educate/Research/Evidence-Exchange.aspx
American Journal of Occupational Therapy—http://www.aota.org/Pubs/AJOT_1.aspx
OT Practice—http://www.aota.org/Pubs/OTP.aspx, http://www.aota.org/Pubs/Enews/1MinUpdate.aspx
Wilma L. West Library—American Occupational Therapy Foundation, n.d.d. http://www.aotf.org/resourceswlwlibrary/otsearch.aspx
The Cochrane Database of Systematic Reviews—http://www.cochrane.org/cochrane-reviews
Medline—http://www.nlm.nih.gov/bsd/pmresources.html
PubMed—http://www.ncbi.nlm.nih.gov/pubmed/
CINHAL—http://www.ebscohost.com/public/the-cinahl-database
OTcats—OTcats.com
OTseekervotseeker.com

Summary

Staying current involves making a conscious effort to stay engaged with the profession. The advantages of doing so far outweigh the negatives. Staying current enables you to be knowledge about the profession, which in turn, can be applied to your practical work, making you better positioned to provide your clients the highest quality of care possible. Staying current links you to current colleagues and invites you to reach out and connect with new ones. Staying current takes you out of your comfort zone and entices you to join local, state, and national and even international occupational therapy organizations and to actively engage in the myriad opportunities they offer. Staying current in occupational therapy entails reaping many rewards.

Review Questions

1. Where would you go to find out current information about occupational therapy credentialing?
   a. AOTA
   b. NBCOT
   c. AOTF
   d. NBCOT
2. The AOTA online community, OT Connections is
   a. A member-only benefit
   b. Available to OTs exclusively
   c. Open to all
   d. Available to members at a reduced rate
3. Membership in state occupational therapy associations is
   a. Mandated on a state-by-state basis
   b. Overseen by state regulatory agencies
   c. Mandatory
   d. Voluntary
4. A member-only benefit of AOTA is
   a. Access to the Wilma L West Library
   b. Online access to *AJOT* and *OT Practice*
   c. Reduced rate access to *AJOT* and *OT Practice*
   d. Free state association membership
5. A cover letter should *not*
   a. Be concise and free of spelling and grammatical errors
   b. Be lengthy and restate all that is in the resume
   c. Be one size fits all and used as is for all job applications
   d. B and C
6. The Wilma L West Library database is called OT Search. The database currently contains
   a. Full text materials
   b. Information from the last 25 years only
   c. Only occupational therapy-specific information
   d. Bibliographic citations only
7. The purpose of a resume is to
   a. Outline a person's professional identity in order to get a job interview.
   b. Provide in-depth information about a person's employment history.
   c. Substitute for a job interview.
   d. Call attention to a person's deficiencies in their employment history.
8. A cover letter and resume should
   a. Never change
   b. Be tailored to fit the job description
   c. Contain mistruths and misleading information to ensure an interview
   d. Be lengthy and verbose
9. Sources for current information about occupational therapy can be found at
   a. AOTA, AOTF, NBCOT, WFOT, state associations, evidence-based databases
   b. AOTA, AOTF, all Internet sites ending in .com, WFOT, state associations, evidence-based databases
   c. AOTA, AOTF, NBCOT, WFOT, state associations, evidence-based databases
   d. AOTG, AOTF, NBCOT, WFOT, state associations, evidence-based databases
10. The World Federation of Occupational Therapy, whose mission is promotion of "occupational therapy as an art and science internationally," is an important source for current information because
    a. It has a large member nation and keeps a pulse on international issues pertinent to occupational therapy practitioners throughout the world.
    b. It derives its information from the AOTA.
    c. It is evidence based.
    d. It's exclusive community of members controls the information that is disseminated.

Practice Activities

Contact your state occupational therapy association to learn what volunteer opportunities are available to you. Choose one and write a brief description about why you are an ideal candidate to fill this role.

Explore various resume templates and choose one that serves you best. Prepare a resume, being sure to include as much detail as you can while still being concise and to the point. Share your resumes with classmates for constructive feedback.

Write a cover letter for the following job posting. Keep in mind that you are to write it as if you were a new graduate with no professional job experience (yet).

The Easter Seals Foundation of Harbor City is seeking a full-time occupational therapy assistant with two years of experience to work in our preschool classroom with children with multiple physical and mental disabilities. The candidate must be self-starting, creative, and team focused. Serious applicants only should apply. The closing date for applications is September 30.

Make a list of ten ways and the frequency with which you will stay current about occupational therapy. Note when you will begin the process. Track your ability to stay on task for the duration of your educational program. If you have been diligent about staying current, it is highly likely that this will become a good habit that stays with you throughout your career.

Work with a partner and plan an evidence-based journal club. How will you organize it? Advertise it? What format will it take? Plan on the meeting lasting 15 minutes. Each partner group can host one meeting. After each group has hosted a meeting, evaluate what worked best and what could be improved upon.

References

American Occupational Therapy Foundation. *About AOTA*. n.d.a. Retrieved from http://www.aota.org/About.aspx

American Occupational Therapy Foundation. *About AOTF*. n.d.b. Retrieved from http://www.aotf.org/aboutaotf.aspx

American Occupational Therapy Foundation. *Joint Initiatives with AOTA*. n.d.c. Retrieved from http://www.aotf.org/programspartnerships/jointinitiativeswithaota.aspx

American Occupational Therapy Foundation. *OT Search*. n.d.d. Retrieved from http://www.aotf.org/resourceswlwlibrary/otsearch.aspx

The Linux Information Project. Peer-review Definition. 2005. Retrieved from http://www.linfo.org/peer_review.html

World Federation of Occupational Therapists About Us. Retrieved from www.wfot.org

World Federation of Occupational Therapists. *Member Organisations of WFOT*. 2011. Retrieved from http://www.wfot.org/Membership/MemberOrganisationsofWFOT.aspx

Yamkovenko S. Participation in your Association is COOL: Volunteering made Easier. 2010. Retrieved from http://www.aota.org/News/Announcements/COOL.aspx

UNIT

IV

Therapeutic Techniques and Processes

Occupation is so much more than just activity!

—Charlotte Brasic Royeen

CHAPTER 18

Ensuring Purposeful and Meaningful Interventions

Scott L. Homer, MS, OTR/L

Key Terms

Activity analysis—An analysis of what is required of the client to participate in a chosen activity, and the relationship of the activity's requirements to engagement in occupation.

Intervention—The process and skilled actions taken by OT practitioners in collaboration with the client to facilitate engagement in occupation related to health and participation.

Intervention approaches—Specific strategies selected to direct the process of interventions that are based on the client's desired outcome, evaluation data, and evidence.

Meaning—The sense that a person makes of a situation.

Occupational profile—A summary of a client's occupational history, patterns of daily living, interests, values, and needs.

Purpose—The desire to do something about a situation.

Learning Objectives

After studying this chapter, readers will be able to:

- Define key terms related to the occupational therapy processes of evaluation and intervention.
- Recognize the unique approach that occupational therapy practitioners utilize to help clients achieve their goals.
- Describe the process of gathering pertinent information in an occupational profile and activity analysis to guide decision making in planning interventions.
- Explore the qualities of selected intervention choices to ensure that they are purposeful and meaningful to the client.

Introduction

Through the use of case examples and with the *Occupational Therapy Practice Framework: Domain and Process (3rd Edition)* (AOTA, 2014) as a guide, this chapter introduces the reader to the importance of choosing meaningful and purposeful interventions. Occupational therapy's unique philosophy and perspective are examined with a series of stories that illustrate effective interventions. Key terms are defined within the context of the narrative, as each section builds upon the previous information to culminate in an appreciation for occupational therapy intervention.

What Is the Point?

Dylan was not amused. The last thing he wanted to do today was to be dragged to see yet another "specialist" for his arm. For the whole year leading up to the surgery that stopped his seizures, he had been poked and prodded by neurologists, therapists, and surgeons. Now that his hair was finally growing back the way he liked it, and he had been seizure free for months, his mom was insisting he get his left hand evaluated. Again. He already went through this at school after the surgery and did all of the tests and writing they wanted him to, and now, it was supposed to be his summer break.

As they sat in the waiting room at the clinic, Dylan grumbled to his mom, "I'm tired of being an experiment!" He didn't see the point. He was getting along just fine with one hand. Slumped over his smartphone, Dylan didn't notice the occupational therapist come in to the waiting area to call him in. He was surprised to see her looking over his shoulder at the adventure game he was engrossed in. "So, you like knights and dragons?" she asked, causing Dylan's character to lose the battle because of her distraction. As he put the phone away and entered the therapy room, he fully expected another round of measuring and exercising as he had grown accustomed to.

When the occupational therapist picked up a pair of long foam tubes and walked with Dylan toward a hanging bolster, he finally cracked a smile. "Let's attack this dragon!" she suggested, giving the bolster a firm whack with a tube (Fig. 18.1). Of course Dylan reached for his weapon with his right hand, but when she offered him the use of two swords, he couldn't help but use his weaker hand too. In the flurry of blows that followed, Dylan was too engaged slaying his dragon to notice the tear of joy in his mother's eye.

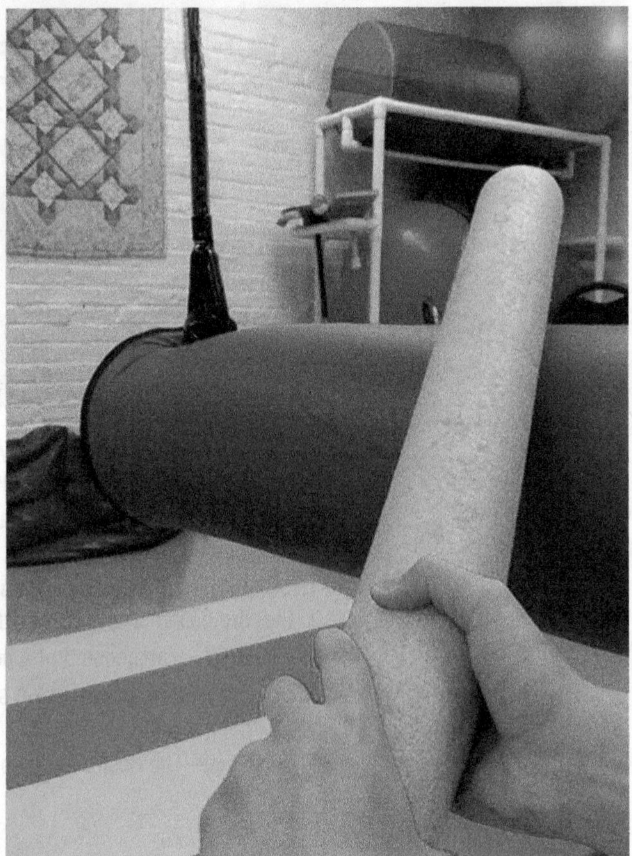

Figure 18.1 Let's attack this dragon!

Occupational therapy is different. Students entering the field sense this and feel a spark of interest in learning what that difference is. Clients and family members who experience occupational therapy know this and develop their own idea of what the difference is. Other professionals acknowledge this and debate what qualities of OT practitioners separate them from other allied health disciplines. Those who work in the profession, OTs and OTAs, create that difference in their use of purposeful and meaningful interventions for the clients they serve.

You are entering the exciting world of occupational therapy, eager to complete your studies and enter the practice arena to help clients achieve their goals. Perhaps reading this chapter holds neither purpose nor meaning to you yet. This is merely another assignment to complete and check off an ever-growing list: another barrier slowing you on your path to graduation. Is your attitude toward this reading similar to Dylan's frustration with yet another therapy appointment? Are you having trouble finding "the point" of this assignment? Consider this: your purpose drives you to succeed, just as it motivated you through the application process to enter this program. The meaning that these words will provide is a glimpse into your future. Each writer in this textbook, indeed in all writings of our profession, has been in your situation. Each of us had to begin somewhere, and that path begins with learning about what has come before. The key to absorbing and making this knowledge meaningful is to relate it to your present role as a student and your eventual future as an OT practitioner.

Authors need to provide definitions to ensure the reader can follow the intent and relate to what is being discussed. In his article entitled, *Therapeutic Occupation: A Definition*, David Nelson defines the terms "purpose" and "meaning" in words that serve this chapter well. "**Meaning** is the sense that the person makes of a situation" (Nelson, 1996, p. 776). Thus, meaning is a personal assessment that each of us makes based upon many factors; certainly, prior experience and cultural traditions play major roles. Purpose is defined as evolving from meaning; "after a person finds meaning in a situation, he or she experiences **purpose**, or the desire to do something about the situation" (Nelson, 1996, p. 777). In a scholarly paper such as Professor Nelson's, it is refreshing to read a phrase as simple as "do something." For all of the lengthy debates and myriad definitions of what our profession's specialty is, it seems that the way we help people could be summed up in a two-letter action word: *do*.

How do OT practitioners "do?" It surely can't be as simple as it sounds. The intuitive nature of an occupational therapy intervention may lead the casual observer to jump to the conclusion that we are "just winging it" when we work with our clients. Perhaps you have already observed this phenomenon in your exploration of the field or in guided observations as part of your education. This illusion of natural ease of interaction between practitioner and client comes from careful analysis of occupations, deep study of all aspects of human nature, and genuine empathy CS9. Despite outward appearances, OT practitioners are not making it up as they go along. Our profession is guided by an official document entitled the *Occupational Therapy Practice Framework: Domain and Process, 3rd Edition,* published by the American Occupational Therapy Association (AOTA, 2014) (please also refer to Chapter 8, *The Occupational Therapy Practice Framework: Domain and Process*).

The beauty of an occupational therapy session is that it capitalizes on the client's interests, motivations, strengths, and, sometimes, weaknesses. The time that practitioner and client spend together, and even the time that we spend preparing for this session, is known as an occupational therapy **intervention**. The *Occupational Therapy Practice Framework III* (AOTA, 2014) describes many types of **intervention approaches** and supplies the following definitions of these terms:

Intervention: The process and skilled actions taken by occupational therapy practitioners in collaboration with the client to facilitate engagement in occupation related to health and participation. The intervention process includes the plan, implementation, and review (p. S15).

Intervention approaches: Specific strategies selected to direct the process of interventions that are based on the client's desired outcome, evaluation data, and evidence (p. S15).

These definitions begin to unravel the essence of what OT practitioners do. Foremost in the description is the inclusion of the client's desires through collaboration between practitioner and client. We do not create our interventions in isolation. We include the client in the planning of the interventions and that makes all of the difference in the doing. Whatever we chose to employ as an intervention, we ensure purpose and meaning by listening to our clients and helping them determine what they need.

However, to arbitrarily assign a purpose without meaning does not meet the needs of our clients and can be seen as "pointless." In the case of Dylan, the well-intentioned OT practitioners at his school pushed for him to utilize his left hand for writing or keyboarding, but, perhaps unbeknownst to the practitioners, he had swiftly found compensatory strategies for interacting with his smartphone one-handed. The goal of two-handed typing may have had a great purpose but was absent meaning for this young client. These words of caution should guide us in choosing interventions: "we must not confuse or assume that occupations that have an added purpose are also meaningful" (Ferguson & Trombly, 1997, p. 514).

In essence, it takes purpose *with* meaning to provide "the point" of a given task, occupation, or activity. Each person individually assigns meaning, as a sum of his or her experiences and culture. Purpose occurs when motivation has been provided to entice the person to *do something*, or engage in the occupation presented. But the client must be an active, willing participant. The OT practitioner's ability to provide a motivating and challenging intervention harnesses an inherent human desire to *do something*. This empowers our clients to truly have a hand in their own well-being. According to Trombly (1995), our behavior and time is organized by our sense of purpose, but it is the personal meaning that motivates our participation in occupation.

In the opening vignette, the OT practitioner had Dylan engaging in imaginative play as a purposeful and meaningful intervention. His delight at this fun and unexpected tactic underscores what makes OT practitioners so effective in motivating our clients. One needs only to look briefly at the *Areas of Occupation* in Table 1 of the *Practice Framework III* (AOTA, 2014) to see that the occupational therapy profession values and promotes play as an occupation. Play is a therapeutic intervention. Take a moment and really think about that. Occupational therapy *is* different!

Analyze, then Personalize

Jim cursed his bad luck. All of his years on horseback working for the railroad patrol, he had never had a fall. Now here he was, laid up in the nursing home after a tumble in his own bathroom. And what a tumble it was. The doctor said he had fractured his hip and it would be months before he could move his leg like he used to. He wasn't moving much of anything like he used to, it seemed; everything hurt. He hadn't felt his eighty-five years of age so acutely before that fall, and now, it took all he had just to sit up on the edge of his bed.

When the young man came in and announced that he was from "occupational therapy," Jim curtly informed him that he had probably been retired for as long as the boy had been out of diapers. The young man laughed but then pulled up a chair next to Jim and started explaining what he meant by "occupation." Jim was not much interested in the conversation until the young man did what nobody else had taken the time to do since he had been whisked away from his home by ambulance in the dead of night. He asked Jim about himself—about his life.

Jim was not sure what made him share so much about himself, but soon, he had revealed his feelings after his wife's death, detailed some of his old hobbies, and lamented about the distance he felt from his son. By the time Jim found himself in the occupational therapy room, the young man had set him up with some tools that he had never expected to find in a place like this. Sure they were not as nice as the ones in his workshop, but the leatherworking tools felt natural in his hands. He could have selected a better piece of leather if he could get to the Western store, but the scraps in the therapy cupboard were not half bad.

Jim took the young therapist's advice and started crafting a belt for his son. As his fingers found their way along familiar paths, he slowly stopped noticing the ache in his surgical site (Fig. 18.2). In a few days, when the belt was complete, Jim had all but forgotten the pain. He had stood at the workbench while completing much of the project, with the young man patiently by his side. Jim even took the opportunity to teach him a few things about leatherworking tools and techniques as he worked. He felt more and more like himself as they worked in this way; a quiet partnership that helped Jim in more ways than he could express.

What is it about engagement in a purposeful task that transports us from the very worries that threatened to immobilize us? One might conjecture that busying one's hands and mind allows an escape from present concerns. Perhaps instead, we should acknowledge that we are never more in the moment than when we are truly focused on a purpose that has personal meaning to us. Our motor patterns and senses remember the past learning that has brought us to a level of skill at the task. Our hopes to complete a project allow us a goal-driven sense of purpose with an eye to the achievable future. Our present efforts are focused at accomplishing the task at hand. Thus, engagement in an occupation that has purpose and meaning allows functioning in the present, past, and future simultaneously.

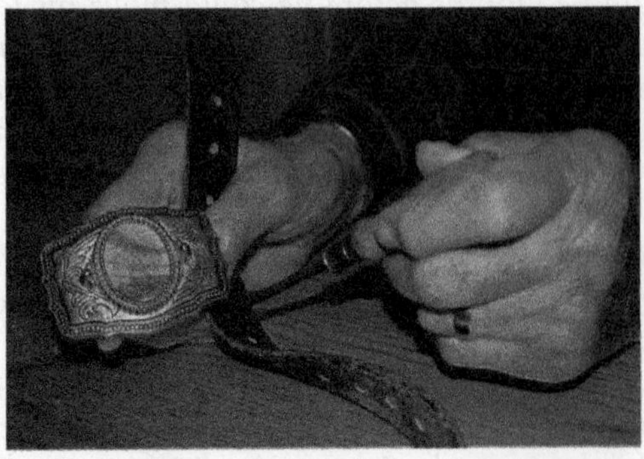

Figure 18.2 His fingers found their way along familiar paths.

How do OT practitioners discover what has purpose and meaning to our clients? Is it written in their medical charts or individualized education plans for us to look up? Once again, our *Occupational Therapy Practice Framework III* guides us. An essential part of the occupational therapy evaluation is the **occupational profile**, defined as "information about the client's needs, problems, and concerns about performance in occupations" (AOTA, 2014, p. S13). Occupational therapy assistants play a vital role in the evaluation process by helping to collect valuable information that fills in this profile. In Jim's story, the conversation that took place at his bedside was a description of this process. Interviewing our clients about their daily living patterns and values can be done during an intervention or whenever the opportunity presents itself. The key to a good interview is asking open-ended questions and employing active listening (please also refer to Chapter 10, *Principles of Therapeutic Intervention*, and Chapter 16, *Working Together: Clinical Reasoning and Collaboration*). Armed with this essential information about *who* our clients are and *what* they do, OT practitioners are in a unique position to provide purposeful and meaningful interventions.

A thorough occupational profile provides the tools to ensure motivation and help the client meet his or her needs. However, choosing the best intervention approach—one that meets these needs, yet provides a challenge to the client—requires an additional skill. At the heart of the occupational therapy, intervention is the **activity analysis** (please also refer to Chapter 11, *Activity Analysis: The Jewel of Occupational Therapy*). The *Occupational Therapy Practice Framework* (AOTA, 2014) uses Table 3 to illustrate the components of a given activity that require careful analysis. In summary, OT practitioners systematically breakdown and "analyze the demands of an activity to understand the specific body structures, body functions, performance skills and performance patterns that are required and to determine the generic demands the activity or occupation makes on the client" (AOTA, 2014, p. S12). Looking to Jim's case example, the OT practitioner determined from the occupational profile that Jim had work history with and a continued interest in horses, identified himself with Western culture, and had been a leatherworker in his spare time. Analyzing the steps of this activity helped the OT practitioner pair the task of making a leather belt with Jim's values and interests. An added benefit was that Jim was motivated to fashion the belt as a gift for his estranged son. While performing the work, Jim experienced a lifting of his burdens, both the physical pain from his surgery and some lightening of his emotional load. What happened in those occupational therapy sessions that facilitated this change?

A founder of our profession, Adolf Meyer, wrote a paper entitled *The Philosophy of Occupational Therapy* in 1922 that first articulated many of the beliefs that form our profession's philosophy to this day. He saw firsthand through his work as a psychiatrist that the active engagement in occupations had remarkable health benefits to his patients. When discussing the types of occupations that he had witnessed to be most therapeutic, he gave future generations of OT practitioners a plan for their interventions. He stated, "I am convinced that a premium should be put on the production of things that are finished in one or a few sittings and yet have an independent emotional value. They must give the satisfaction of completion and achievement, and that in the eye of the maker and of those for whom he has tried to work" (Meyer, 1922, p. 641).

For Jim, the satisfaction of completion, of achievement, and of doing something that held meaning and purpose for him was achieved in a few occupational therapy sessions. His helpless frustration melted away as he had an opportunity to demonstrate his worth to himself, despite his recent misfortunes. Jim already had the potential to get back to the life he was accustomed to before his fall, but something was holding him back. Indeed, his fractured hip was repaired by his surgical team and rendered better than new with prosthetic components. However, his pride, confidence, and sense of self-worth had been damaged beyond the reach of diagnostic equipment or orthopedic surgeons. The psychological impact of his condition was keeping Jim from his potential through his self-doubt and despair. With the right guidance in occupational therapy, Jim was able to find his self-confidence again through engagement in the leatherworking activity selected for him after gathering information on his occupational profile and a careful activity analysis. When you are instrumental in this process, from learning about a client's life to selecting an appropriate intervention to seeing it through completion, you will experience the great satisfaction that comes from helping others help themselves.

We Are What We Do

Connie's stroke had left her weak, confused, and scared. Thoughts swirled in her head, but her voice betrayed her and she could not express what she wanted to say. She felt trapped in the wheelchair, trapped in her own body. When the aide came to her room to wheel her to a therapy session, she closed her eyes in silent frustration. A homemaker and caregiver for her seven children and thirteen grandchildren, she was not accustomed to having others wait on her. A kind woman approached her at their destination and introduced herself as an occupational therapy assistant. Connie was not sure what this meant, but could only muster a nod of her head as a greeting.

Over the days that followed, Connie began to look forward to the occupational therapy sessions. Her favorite part of the visits were when the two women looked through magazines and pictures together as Connie gestured to things that drew her attention. Soon, her new friend had discerned that Connie liked to cook. Indeed, it was her passion. Visits from her children during these therapy sessions confirmed what Connie had struggled to express. Before long, Connie's daughter had brought in her recipe book and some cookware from home. To her surprise, there was a kitchen at the hospital right next door to the therapy department.

Given the opportunity to reignite her passion, Connie became a force to be reckoned with. Her words still had trouble forming, but her gestures and facial expressions made it clear who was in charge in the kitchen. As the delicious dishes increased in complexity over time, the hospital staff began to linger around the kitchen during and after Connie's sessions. The pride Connie had in her work was evident as she served her baked delicacies to the nurses and therapists who had helped her. She felt alive again, and found that her expressions of gratitude through her occupation of cooking were even more poignant than any words of thanks she would have said (Fig. 18.3).

Motivation and opportunity are central themes of Connie's story, and they resonate within the narratives of Jim and Dylan as well. It is important to realize that in many cases, occupational therapy practitioners are not *teaching* clients how to perform a task; the client is often the expert. We use our skills to tap into the intrinsic motivation of our clients and give them *opportunities* to perform the occupations that they desire.

Influential OT researchers and authors have supplied us with qualitative narratives and quantitative data that put these nebulous concepts into definable terms. Suzanne Peloquin eloquently described an OT practitioner's role as that of a pathfinder who cocreates daily lives by helping clients discover novel ways to perform

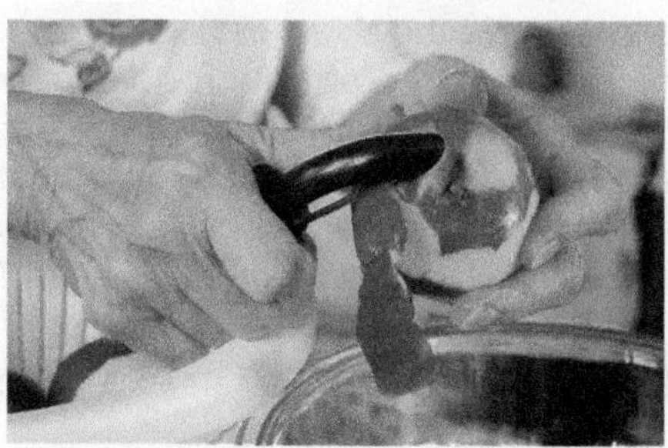

Figure 18.3 She felt alive again.

familiar tasks within their new limitations (Peloquin, 2005). Gary Kielhofner wrote prolifically on the subject of human volition, habituation, and performance capacity in developing his *Model of Human Occupation* (Kielhofner, 2002) (please also refer to Chapter 7, *Occupational Therapy Theories and How They Guide Practice*).

The opportunities that occupational therapy provides are invaluable in allowing the motivation within our clients to blossom. It is vital to recognize that each of us has our own sense of values and meaning, and therefore, we are each motivated differently. An unfortunate scenario is when new OT practitioners experience frustration in the field by finding that some clinics prescribe the same activities for each client, in a "cookie cutter" fashion (see from the Field 18.1). This is not what occupational therapy was intended to provide. Again looking to Adolf Meyer's philosophy for guidance, we find that nearly a century ago, he affirmed that "our role consists in giving opportunities rather than prescriptions" (Meyer, 1977, p. 641). Each client's intervention should be as unique as his or her occupational profile, as our lives are ultimately defined by what we *do*. Hold true to this ideal in your own practice, and occupational therapy will continue to distinguish itself as a field that is holistic, humanistic, and *different*.

FROM THE FIELD 18.1

Therapeutic Use of Self

A recent graduate sent the following e-mail:

"I am working in an adult setting and am trying to find some valuable resources for treatments. The majority of clients are LTC [long term care], with limited ROM [range of motion], some form of dementia, amputees, TBI [traumatic brain injury], stroke, fractures, you name it. I do the same things repeatedly and would love to find some other treatments that address their limitations and support the goals. Many are very weak and not weight bearing, so transfers are always a big deal. Also, for some older folks they really do not want to participate because they do not see the benefit in therapy. All in all, it is a big challenge to get them up and motivated!"

My response, in part, was as follows:

"You describe a common issue facing health care professionals, and the immediate answer I have to motivate your clients is for you to employ your therapeutic use of self. The best tool you possess to help others is your own enthusiasm, energy and caring. The long-term care population often have multiple comorbidities and can be rather frail, depressed, and some have lost hope. This is a major challenge in our healthcare system, but I believe that we as OT practitioners have the skills needed to make a difference. Find out who your residents are and what makes them tick—then remind them how good it feels to be alive and doing what motivates them! Give them choices in a situation where they may feel that they have lost all. The benefits of active participation are inherent in participation! The mind is engaged, the body is active…and we heal."

A Final Note

Three case examples were woven throughout this chapter to put faces on the concepts discussed therein. In each case, the story wrapped up with a successful intervention that helped the client improve. Not every client story has a "happily ever after" ending. There are many challenges in this profession—some may even seem insurmountable. It is very difficult to act as a pathfinder for some clients, as they may be lost in their own despair far beyond a recognizable trail. Others will try as hard as they are able and still fall short of their desired outcomes. Remember this as you practice the art and science of occupational therapy. You are in a unique position to help others help themselves live life to its fullest (Fig. 18.4). You have chosen a wonderful profession with innumerable rewards. Even though some days may be rough, the benefits will far outweigh the difficulties.

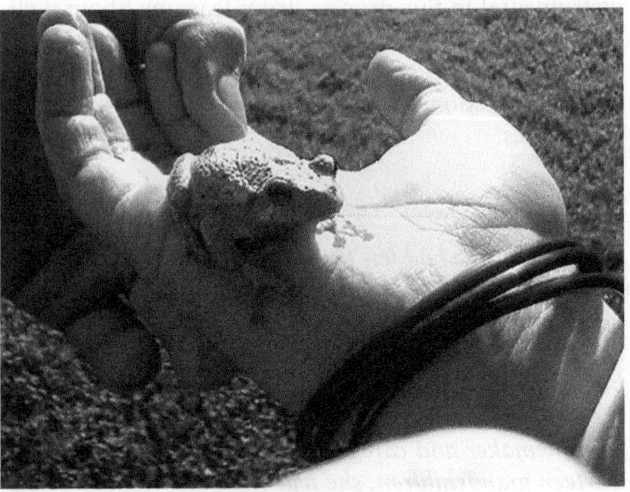

Figure 18.4 Living life to its fullest.

Summary

In this chapter, we explored the ways in which OT practitioners ensure purposeful and meaningful interventions. Through several threaded case studies, the foundational components of occupational therapy practice were isolated, examined, and then reintegrated to illustrate the process of intervention. The occupational profile and activity analysis are essential tools in this process, and as future OTAs, you will find that assessing these becomes intuitive as you practice. If we simplify the essential definition of occupation to the verb "do," then we can see the value of our profession in these words: "doing is so important that it is impossible to envisage the world of humans without it" (Wilcock, 1998, p. 249).

Review Questions

1. The sense that a person makes of a situation is defined as:
   a. Purpose
   b. Meaning
   c. Sensation
   d. Cognition

2. An occupational profile consists of:
   a. Occupational history
   b. Patterns of daily living
   c. Interests, values, and needs
   d. All of the above

3. The activity analysis is useful to
   a. Determine the properties of a chosen activity
   b. Prescribe the best activity for all clients
   c. Assign a task based on cognitive levels
   d. Evaluate a client's level of independence

4. The intervention plan, implementation, and review are all parts of:
   a. The intervention method
   b. The intervention strategy
   c. The intervention process
   d. The intervention outcome

5. According to Adolf Meyer, the OT provides:
   a. Prescriptions
   b. Opportunities
   c. Structured work
   d. Respite

6. Which author described an OT practitioner's role as that of a pathfinder?
   a. Suzanne Peloquin
   b. Gary Kielhofner
   c. David Nelson
   d. Adolf Meyer

7. In Jim's story, what was the most likely reason for his depressed mood in the long-term care facility?
   a. Pain from his fracture
   b. Loss of his sense of self-identity
   c. Frustration with discharge planning
   d. Confusion over his hip precautions

8. According to Ferguson and Trombly, we cannot assume that occupations with an added purpose are also:
   a. Therapeutic
   b. Relevant
   c. Meaningful
   d. Goal directed

9. The Model of Human Occupation, as authored by Gary Kielhofner, is concerned with human:
   a. Volition
   b. Habituation
   c. Performance capacity
   d. All of the above

10. What was a common theme to all of the OT interventions in the case study stories presented in this chapter?
    a. They were all elderly clients.
    b. All of the practitioners were OTAs.
    c. The interventions were personalized and occupation based.
    d. The OT practitioners had established intervention ideas prior to meeting the clients.

Practice Activities

Have a classmate send you an e-mail about a particularly frustrating aspect of your program of study. Put yourself in a therapeutic role, and craft a thoughtful response that helps illustrate the purpose and meaning as you understand it.

Dylan, Jim, and Connie were provided as examples from the author's own clinical experiences. Think of someone that you know who has been through a difficult situation. Create a brief narrative from his or her point of view. Work with a classmate to brainstorm a good therapeutic use of self that you could employ to help with the difficult situation.

Look at your next activity analysis assignment as an opportunity to tap into the power of occupational therapy. Challenge yourself to look at everyday tasks as therapeutic tools that you will soon employ to help others. How do you choose the best interventions? Analyze, then personalize!

References

American Occupational Therapy Association. Occupational therapy practice framework: domain and process. 3rd ed. *Am J Occup Ther* 2014;68(Suppl 1):S1–S48. http://dx.doi.org/10.5014/ajot.2014.682006

Ferguson JM, Trombly CA. Effect of added-purpose and meaningful occupation on motor learning. *Am J Occup Ther* 1997;51(7):508–515.

Kielhofner G. *Model of Human Occupation: Theory and Application*. 3rd ed. Philadelphia, PA: Lippincott Williams & Wilkins; 2002.

Meyer A. The philosophy of occupational therapy. *Am J Occup Ther* 1977;31(10):639–649. (Originally published in 1922.)

Nelson DL. Therapeutic occupation: a definition. *Am J Occup Ther* 1996;50:775–782.

Peloquin SM. The 2005 Eleanor Clark Slagle Lecture—embracing our ethos, reclaiming our heart. *Am J Occup Ther* 2005;59(6), 611–625.

Trombly CA. The 1995 Eleanor Clark Slagle Lecture—occupation, purposefulness and meaningfulness as therapeutic mechanisms. *Am J Occup Ther* 1995;49(10):960–972.

Wilcock AA. Reflections on doing, being, and becoming. *Can J Occup Ther* 1998;65(5): 248–256.

CHAPTER 19

Spirituality and Occupational Therapy: A Beginning Conversation

Tamera Keiter Humbert, DEd, OTR/L

Key Terms

Beliefs and practices—Center on trusting in a higher power to cope with an illness or crisis and/or connecting with something greater than ourselves.

Cultural sensitivity—Considering specific behaviors and beliefs related to practice and the client.

Flow—A state of being when an activity becomes so gratifying that it becomes spontaneous and automatic.

Life meaning—The underlying beliefs and assumptions about the reason(s) for our existence, the reason(s) we are living and part of this world.

Occupational integrity—Integrating into one's occupational choices what matters most.

Occupational value—The selection of and engagement in occupations that hold importance.

Occupations of spirit—Select activities that may specifically elicit spiritual awareness and practice.

Resilience—The ability of a person to persevere in extreme situations.

Spirituality—Personal quest for understanding answers to ultimate questions about life, meaning, and the sacred or transcendent; a pervasive life force, manifestation of a higher self, source of will and self-determination; sensitivity to the presence of spirit; gives meaning to occupations.

Learning Objectives

After studying this chapter, students should be able to:

- Articulate the definitions of spirituality as defined in key documents of the American Occupational Therapy Association and the Canadian Association of Occupational Therapy.
- State and describe the constructs of spirituality as found in the OT literature.
- Describe the consideration when incorporating spirituality into occupational therapy practice.

Introduction

For this chapter on spirituality, I will take you on a journey that will not only provide some considerations but also, I hope, enrich your understanding of spirituality as it relates to the practice of occupational therapy. I will first provide an introduction to several key documents that support the understanding of spirituality. Next, I will review constructs that relate to spirituality as represented in the OT literature. The intent of this chapter is to provide a cursory review of the subject, allowing the readers to consider some fundamental ideas about spirituality that have been written within the field of occupational therapy.

I love this quote: "Pinning jelly to the wall takes the right equipment and dedication to conquer the task" (author unknown). In many respects, talking about spirituality is

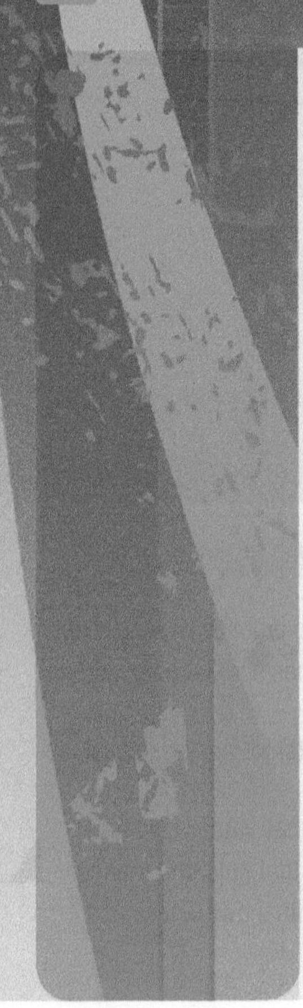

like pinning jelly to the wall. My experience has been that when anyone uses the word "spirituality" in conversation, one of several responses usually happens. Sometimes, people light up with excitement and often add their own curiosity and insights to the dialogue. Others look apprehensive and reluctant to engage the topic, and others seem to roll their eyes, literally or figuratively, giving the sender of the comment the notion that they are not interested in or tired by the whole conversation. Wherever you find yourself in these scenarios, or possibly in another one altogether, everyone is welcome to this conversation.

Let me start with some brief considerations. First, you might ask, "Why should we study spirituality anyway?" Not only is this topic becoming more common in mainline culture today, clients are interested in incorporating spirituality into their daily lives, including and especially after a major life crisis (Heinz et al., 2010; Hilbers et al., 2010; Kang, 2003). As practitioners, we need to be aware of that desire, especially if we proclaim that we are trying to be culturally responsive and that we provide client-centered care.

We also know from the limited research conducted with OT students and practitioners that many of us are uncertain as to how to respond to this topic. Reasons cited for this reluctance include not wanting to impose our own views on others, not wanting to confuse spirituality with religious beliefs and practices, not understanding how occupational therapy should incorporate spirituality into practice, and not being sure how to even document or get reimbursed for such discussions with clients and families (Kirsh et al., 2001; Thompson & MacNeil, 2006). You might then ask, "Should we just leave this to the 'spiritual' professionals like ministers, rabbis, priests, mullahs, shamans, humanist counselors, spiritual directors, and chaplains?" According to the research, while most of us are uncertain how to respond to the topic of spirituality, OT practitioners do recognize its value and importance in our personal and professional lives (Collins et al., 2001; Taylor et al., 2000).

The Official Word about Spirituality and Occupational Therapy

The American Occupational Therapy Association (AOTA) has begun to consider this topic and publish statements about such in official documents. The first contemporary and endorsed public nod to **spirituality** came through the first edition of the *Occupational Therapy Practice Framework: Domain and Process* (*OTPF*) published in 2002. In this document, spirituality was considered a context in which people engaged. However, in the next version of the *OTPF (OTPF-II)*, the understanding of spirituality took a major shift in focus. The definition for spirituality given in the *OTPF-II* was "The personal quest for understanding answers to ultimate questions about life, meaning, and the sacred or transcendent, which may (or may not) lead to or arise from the development of religious rituals and the formation of community" (AOTA, 2008, p. 634; Moreira-Almeida & Koenig, 2006, p. 844). The *OTPF-II* provided direct references to spirituality as well as references implicit to spirituality that included religious practice. I would like to take a side note here to say that most practitioners would consider religious and faith-based practices as spiritual but spirituality does not need to be religious or faith based.

The definition for spirituality given in the most recent edition of Occupational *Therapy Practice Framework III* is "the aspect of humanity that refers to the way individuals seek and express meaning and purpose and the way they experience their connectedness to the moment, to self, to others, to nature, and to the significant or sacred" (Puchalski et al., 2009, p. 887 in AOTA, 2014, p. S7). This shift moves from a more rational or inquisitive approach in understanding the mysteries and questions of life to seeking and expressing meaning and purpose. Spirituality is now considered to have influence, motivating individuals to engage in occupations and finding meaning or purpose in life (p. S7). Spirituality and ritual are now also more explicitly related to the IADL occupation of religious and spiritual activities and expressions (Fig. 19.1).

What is important to note with these major documents is that there has been a change in the past twelve years as to how AOTA, the official organization of OT practitioners in the United States, is talking about spirituality. While many in the field (inside as well as outside the United States) have written about the topic for at least the past 20 years, it has been only recently that AOTA has attended to the concepts in any endorsed capacity. What is also important to understand is that other OT practitioners and organizations beyond AOTA have formally spoken about spirituality for a much longer time.

We now turn to the Canadian Association of Occupational Therapy (CAOT) to find additional

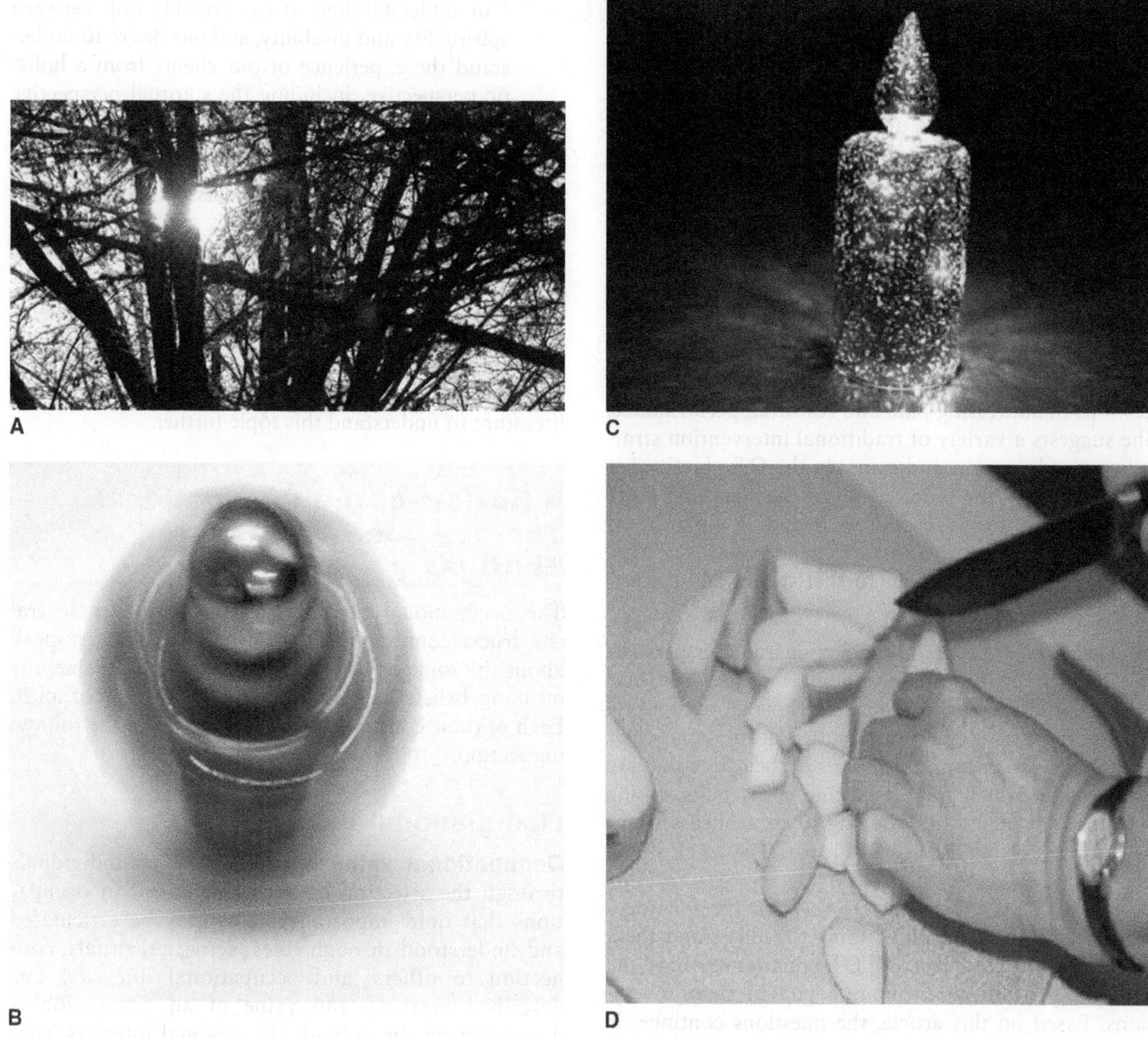

Figure 19.1 Some images and items that can be related to spirituality.

perspectives about spirituality. The Canadian occupational therapists point to 1919 as a landmark time when the understanding of the integration of mind–body–spirit was conveyed in the association's emblem and badge worn they wore (CAOT, 2002). This publically supported identification of spirituality has a long history with Canadians. In accordance with that history, the CAOT unveiled the *Canadian Model of Occupational Performance (CMOP)* in 1997 (Fearing et al., 1997) and in 2002 revised the model again (CAOT, 2002). Both documents provided a model for practice that endorses spirituality. Within this model, spirituality was defined as "a pervasive life force, manifestation of a higher self, source of will and self-determination, and a sense of meaning, purpose and connectedness that people experience in the context of their environment" (CAOT, p. 182). Spirituality was identified as the central core of the individual. In 2007, the model was further revised. The latest, and most current, revision of the model, the *Canadian Model of Occupational Performance and Engagement (CMOP-E)*, has maintained the original definition of spirituality with the addition of the phrases "spirituality is sensitivity to the presence of spirit" and "spirituality resides in persons, is shaped by the environment, and gives meaning to occupations" (CAOT, 2007, p. 374).

The question may be asked, "Is spirituality primarily about an aspect of an individual?" Is it what practitioners are to pay attention to and recognize and whenever applicable incorporate the client's perspectives about spirituality into assessment and intervention? Bouthot et al. (2011) provide suggestions as to how to understand an individual's spirituality through the use of the *Faith and Belief, Importance, Community, and*

Address in Care (FICA) Spiritual History Assessment. The authors promoted the understanding and support of OT practitioners, at least in a medical health care environment, to ask questions of clients to better understand their beliefs and faith practices. However, directly following this article in the same *OT Practice* publication was an article entitled "Physical, Mental, and Spiritual Approaches to Managing Pain in Older Clients" by Shelia Haines Szafran (2011). In this article, Szafran speaks about pain and the implication it has in the performance of occupations. (Whatever age you may be, if you have suffered serious or long-standing pain, you understand this concept.) Szafran goes on to provide specific assessment and intervention suggestions in addressing pain and restoring performance. She suggests a variety of traditional intervention strategies to reduce pain and cautions the OT practitioner in approaching the older client when suggesting more contemporary forms of practice including mindfulness training, meditation, and movement-based activities like tai chi and qigong. She further speaks about spirituality as

> ...an area of occupation affecting an older person's ability to manage pain. Finding meaning and purpose in defining the quality of life is an occupation that may cause relief from suffering for some older people who encounter changes in their lives that are unplanned, including acquiring a disability, losing support systems, and moving to controlled settings such as nursing homes. (2011, p. CE-6)

Szafran (2011) continues to say that the therapeutic relationship is vital in helping to understand these perspectives of the client and OT practitioners have the ability to provide and facilitate hope with those discussions. Based on this article, the questions continue. Is spirituality more than understanding and respecting clients' beliefs and practices, but also about the therapeutic relationship and the process of providing hope through the discovery of meaning and purpose in life? Could it also be considered an occupation?

In the first published book entirely and specifically related to spirituality in occupational therapy, Mary Ann McColl (2003) wrote what assumptions or motivations guided that text. Along with the historical understanding and value of spirituality as described by the CAOT, she also acknowledged the following assumptions by the collective authors in this edited text:

- Our natural human drive to understand what lies beyond the known realm of our earthly experience and our senses;
- The impetus provided by our work as health care professionals to better understand existential questions about death, pain, and suffering;
- Our understanding of the possible link between spirituality and disability, and our desire to understand the experience of our clients from a holistic perspective, including the spiritual perspective (McColl, 2003, p. 208).

The focus of spirituality with those words just got even larger, expanding the understanding to something beyond what we can tangibly experience, to also include larger questions as to the meaning of life and how one makes meaning of life circumstances and disability. (With such diverse understandings of spiritually, it is getting harder to pin that jelly to the wall.) We need additional "tools" to make sense of this topic. We need to look at the larger collection of occupational therapy literature to understand this topic further.

A Review of the Occupational Therapy Literature Related to Spirituality

The occupational therapy literature provides several constructs connected with spirituality. Authors speak about the topic as it relates to occupational value, life meaning, beliefs and practices, and occupations of spirit. Each of these constructs will be discussed in the following section.

Occupational Value

Occupational value is experienced by individuals through the selection of and engagement in occupations that hold importance. This may be articulated and understood through roles, activities, rituals, connection to others, and occupational integrity. The described meaning and value of an occupation is dependent on the individual's personal interests, routines, and values related to choosing, performing, and engaging select occupations ($). Various occupational therapy authors have shared stories depicting clients finding meaning through specific occupational activities such as baking, playing card games, writing in a journal, giving manicures, caring for hair, doing laundry, singing, making jewelry, and washing dishes (Leslie, 2006; Mathis, 2006; Strzlecki, 2009; Whitney, 2010).

In one example, Bowen (2006) shared a story of an 87-year-old woman who found particular meaning through structured occupations, routines, and habits when the activities brought her "loving support, the expression and demonstration of caring, interaction, gentle humor and quiet guidance" (p. 48). Whitney (2010) also found by personally engaging in the occupation of writing, "her spirit was touched" (p. 33). She states, "For me, writing is an action of my spirit.

I have rituals, habits and a writer's lens through which rich moments of life filter into my brain and fall into imaged pages or possible novels or essays or poems" (p. 33). Thibeault (2012d) also spoke about the beauty and intensity of such activities that become rituals and "ceremonies of life," particularly as they are aligned with grief and loss (p. 218).

In another example, Ramugondo (2005), an African OT, shared her perspective of mothers living with a diagnosis of HIV/AIDS. The mothers often saw their child who also had HIV/AIDS as a "dying being" and experienced challenges identifying and connecting with their mother role. However, during the meaningful occupational activity of play, mothers were then able to reconnect with their children and themselves. Ramugondo states through the use of play, the mother "reconnects with her own spirit since spirituality is related to one's understanding of one's role in life" (2005, p. 319).

While OT practitioners embrace the concept of engagement in occupations and promote that concept through therapeutic tasks, there is also an acknowledgment that individuals personally discover, choose, and engage in occupations that specifically reflect values and beliefs, that give life meaning, and that allow the expression of the essence of who were are (Pentland & McColl, 2012, p. 142). According to Pentland and McColl, **occupational integrity** means "integrating into one's occupational choices what matters most" (p. 142). It is an intentional act to make those choices. Furthermore, it is understood that occupational values are not stagnant. They are dynamic and often make significant shifts when we are faced with a new disability, injury, or illness or when dealing with a long-term crisis (McColl, 2012). The simple act of making and enjoying a cup of coffee may move from a mundane daily task that required very little effort or thought prior to a devastating accident to one that now brings a sense of peace and enjoyment when accomplishing the task and through the gratitude in being able to do so.

Utilizing valued occupations within occupational therapy intervention suggests one of several things. First, it implies that the therapeutic activities utilized in the therapy sessions should reflect the valued occupations and roles of the client. For example, Leslie (2006) chose to include select activities with an 18-year-old adolescent with an intellectual disability who had been in a catatonic state. These activities were chosen to complete during intervention because of the meaning they had for the client before she entered the catatonic state. In another example, Mathis (2006) incorporated baking pecan pies with her client. "The purpose of the activity was to work on standing balance, endurance, upper extremity strengthening and reach"; however, the OT practitioner made these goals meaningful to the client through the use of a former valued occupation and role (Mathis, 2006, p. 16). The implicit understanding behind the use of meaningful activities is that we might tap into the fundamental essence of the person through that activity.

Secondly, utilizing valued occupations within intervention may also suggest that the practitioner appreciates the meaning of a therapeutic activity beyond its common understanding. Activities may actually be symbolic or be representative of something greater or grander than the commonly held perception of the task. Occupational therapy practitioners should not only consider what the client holds as valuable and helpful in restoring or maximizing function but may also consider what additional activities might be introduced in therapy that will spark a spiritual or meaningful connection for the client. Peloquin (1997) introduced the idea that self-care activities, such as hair care and grooming, can be meaningful to a client beyond just a daily or routine task. Such tasks may be valued and used in therapy because of the impact that activity has on making oneself presentable and attractive. In addition, Rosenfeld (2001) and Urbanowski (1997) identified daily tasks such as brushing teeth, toileting, dressing, grooming, and cooking activities as having a spiritual component. Beyond just the completion of a valued role, the use of these daily activities may be utilized as a way of fostering an inspired or spiritual state of discovery or being.

Thirdly, Thibeault (2012b) provides a glimpse as to how we as OT practitioners may recognize, bring to light, and support meaningful and valued occupations as clients shift focus and readjust to life experiences. Thibeault shares the story of her own father who was dealing with the ravages of dementia and how he moved from his past beloved roles and occupations of reading the latest government reforms and following the stock exchange to appreciating the time spent with grandchildren in completing homework. Readjusting and leaving go of past and insignificant activities in order to take on different occupations may be realized by clients and families and encouraged by and supported in therapy.

Life Meaning

Life meaning reflects the underlying beliefs and assumptions about the reason(s) for our existence, the reason(s) we are living and part of this world. For some, these thoughts may not be conscious, attended to, articulated, or even considered until a crisis occurs (McColl, 2012). Thibeault (2012a) provides several stories of individuals she met throughout her work internationally. Men and women who have had to deal with epidemics, extreme poverty, political injustice, violence, and the stigma and rejection related to disability. The meaning that these individuals gave to their suffering and life provided a deeper understanding of the person's

FROM THE FIELD 19.1

Attention Restoration Theory

Developed by environmental psychologists Rachel and Stephen Kaplan, attention restoration theory suggests that people experience relief from mental stress and fatigue through access to nature, being in it or even viewing it through a window. For some in a state of unrest, nature imbues a spiritual quality and fosters a sense of peace and meaning.

mission in life and the value that his/her life still held in light of the extreme challenges (From the Field 19.1).

After the tsunami devastated South Thailand, many affected by the destruction felt unmotivated and were subsequently not engaged in any occupations due to a lack of physical and emotional resources. A group of OT students intervened by providing group activities, individual occupations, and social interactions. "Through the use of dancing, which resulted in relaxation; the participants focused on meaningful occupations consequently relieving boredom and depression" (Pongsakri, 2007, p. 32). According to the author, these meaningful occupations served to provide the participants with a spiritual experience through feelings of "excitement, discovery, competence, satisfaction, pride, and awareness of an increase of self-esteem" (Pongsakri, 2007, p. 32). Thibeault (2012c) also highlights the concept of **resilience**, or the ability of a person in extreme situations to persevere and to utilize volition repeatedly and steadily through a process of transformation CS-5.7.

Select activities may be provided therapeutically to explicitly discover and make sense of current suffering, trauma, pain, and even the death process (McColl, 2012). For example, Trump (2001), working within a hospice setting, was able to engage a client in the meaningful occupation of writing letters to her daughter in order to facilitate reflections about her life. As an active participant in this process, the client "had a sense of accomplishment when the task was completed and a sense of peace from knowing that her daughter would read her words" after she passed on (Trump, 2001, p. 10). According to Trump, the OT practitioner can play a crucial role in facilitating one's life meaning in this type of setting.

Occupational therapy practitioners have and continue to play diverse roles in facilitating participation in valued occupations as well as shaping new life meaning (Dawson & Stern, 2007; Jung et al., 1999). Occupational therapy practitioners are able to recognize the "goal is not that [clients] are merely performing disjointed activities but that they are doing personally meaningful occupations that will in turn define the person" (Dawson & Stern, 2007, p. 4).

According to Reid (2010), "Participation in meaningful occupations helps organize, give meaning and a sense of presence in clients, a requirement for being in the world" (p. 24). Vrkljan (2000) further states that clients must engage in activities that are meaningful and functional in order to assist them in a successful transition from past to future occupational performance. In this transition, we help create new meaning for the client. Occupational therapy intervention may incorporate different activities and occupations into therapy in order to restore a sense of continuity and consequently enhance or reaffirm life meaning (Rosenfeld, 2004).

Billock (2009) specifically discusses ways for OT practitioners to facilitate meaningful occupations in the home environment through the use of special objects such as pictures, items from ones travels, and treasured gifts. The use of these objects may be used to "support the potential for experiencing spirituality" by furthering the life narrative of the client and reassuring or reaffirming life meaning (Billock, 2009, p. 3). The use of discussion and conversations, engaging in storytelling, and offering activities that support grieving all may contribute to a new or reinforced sense of life meaning (McColl, 2012).

Beliefs and Practices

Beliefs and practices center on trusting in a higher power to cope with an illness or crisis and/or connecting with something greater than ourselves. Spencer (2007) wrote about a 54-year-old woman who had a stroke. Through the woman's grieving process, she sought out a higher power and declared that she did not want to be confined to a wheelchair the rest of her life. As time progressed, she was able to become thankful for her blessings and the small incremental improvements made in therapy. Another client with spastic paralysis found similar comfort in communicating with and having a relational understanding of a higher power (Doughton, 1996). Two OTs discussed personal experiences resulting from a crisis where they had a sense of another presence or realm beyond the physical one (Forhan, 2010; Hatchard & Missiuna, 2003). The authors expressed an appreciation of their beliefs and the spiritual experiences that helped them to find comfort and hope for the future.

As expressed earlier, religious expressions may be part of the spiritual experience for the individual, but it is not an expectation for all individuals. According to Rosenfeld (2000), "spirituality does not necessarily imply a belief in [a higher power] ...recovery frequently requires finding one's spiritual center ...a connection with the human spirit, one's inner voice, the spirit of love, or valued group" (p. 17). There is an indication that spirituality surrounds more than the doing of occupations and is part of a larger conceptualization, appreciation, and understanding of life. Pentland and McColl (2012) state:

> For some, spiritual meaning is associated with the concept of higher being and may conform to religions or faith traditions. For others, spiritual meaning derives from a sense of connection—with others, with nature, with the past, present, and future (p. 147).

Supporting beliefs and practices of clients, families, and communities entails practitioners to utilize knowledge and skills about such practices in order to facilitate client's engagement in any desired routines. Billock (2009) notes, "Religion often influences spiritual experience by providing its practitioners with occupations such as reading theological books, praying, meditating and attending religious services" (p. 3). As well, Feeney and Toth-Cohen (2008) emphasize the importance of listening to our client's comments and observing objects in the client's rooms in order to best serve the clients routines and practices during therapy. Swedberg (2001) also suggests that OT practitioners should promote roles within faith communities if and only if the client expresses this as a meaningful occupation.

Occupations of Spirit

The use of the term **occupations of spirit** is not a common phrase but has been used in the OT literature. It entails recognition of select activities that may specifically elicit spiritual awareness and practice. Gourley (2001) notes:

> [there is] virtually no difference between occupational therapy and spirituality ... the spiritual realm is purpose and meaning and we are access to it because we operate in there all the time. As OT's, we facilitate the purpose and meaning of life, and that's what heals patients. (pp. 13–14)

Similarly, Christiansen (1997) states "Activities of spirit can create opportunities for meaning making, which is necessary for establishing an identity, gaining a sense of control, and connecting one's personal story or narrative to something greater than self" (pp. 170–171).

Occupational therapy was also seen as relevant in the use of occupations of the spirit to guide intervention. Rosenfeld (2001) articulates:

> Occupations of the spirit can foster an inspired state of spiritual function by including charitable projects, offering forgiveness, preparing traditional foods, crafting religious objects, celebrating holidays, singing hymns, practicing tai chi and yoga, meditating, studying, having contact with nature, and performing tasks with clarity and purpose. (p. 20)

Creative occupations are one specific medium that may be used to facilitate spiritual awareness, have a positive influence on a client's health and well-being, and provide transformational opportunities (McColl, 2012). Sadlo (2004) espouses that humans seem to have an intrinsic drive to purposefully utilize creative occupations to relieve symptoms such as depression. "The growing discontent and spiritual disconnection may be linked with a lack of experience in making beautiful things in this age of passive occupations such as watching television" (Sadlo, 2004, p. 95).

Clients can use creative activities to promote well-being. "Creativity is a synthesis of intellectual, emotional and spiritual intelligence, and requires integration of the performance sub-systems" (Sadlo, 2004, p. 95). According to Sadlo (2004), OT practitioners should recognize and value the creative nature of occupations. Toomey (2012) further suggests that we need to recognize the inherent risk involved in creative expression. Creative activities often elicit feelings of vulnerability. The client as well as the creative task needs to be honored and the client supported through the process.

While the term occupations of spirit is not a common one found throughout the literature, it does present an image that some of the activities that OT practitioners utilize (based on the client's valued goals and meaningful routines) may produce a spiritual connection with the client. Activities such as deep relaxation, meditation, imagery, chanting, and restorative yoga may support or facilitate wellness practices but may as well promote spiritual experiences and personal growth (Dickenson, 2012). Engaging in nature and creating spaces for reflection and renewal may restore health and provide spiritual grounding (Unruh, 2012). While some OT practitioners may purposefully introduce select activities into the therapy session that are inherently spiritual to the client, clinicians have the responsibility to recognize when therapy approaches this state and respect the perimeters in using such. McColl (2012, p. 195) suggests four questions to consider before utilizing such activities as direct intervention tools:

- Is the client's problem spiritual in nature?
- Would the client be receptive to a direct spiritual intervention?
- Is the therapist equipped to offer spiritual intervention?
- Would the workplace support it?

Additional Constructs

States of being may also be associated with spirituality as mentioned in the occupational therapy literature. While not predominant in the literature, there are some articles that equate an emotional or affective response of the person with the engagement of a valued activity or in the completion of a therapeutic goal. This was seen through the expression of joy and through flow. In one article, a child displayed extreme happiness while independently completing activities of daily living. After struggling for some time to be able to put his shirt on by himself, he finally accomplished the task. The therapist stated he began to dance, calling it the "Indepen-dance" conveying tremendous joy after his success. The OT stated, "The word independence will now be associated with a dance that expresses the spirit of the person, not just a task" (Gavacs, 2009, p. 32).

On the other hand, when an activity becomes so gratifying that it is done for personal reasons, and when one becomes so involved in what she is doing that she becomes spontaneous and almost automatic, that is called **flow**. Nesbit (2006) described her personal journey through breast cancer treatment and recovery. During this process, she reflected on her experiences and the coping mechanisms that she utilized to endure and persevere through her treatments and recovery. She used valued occupational activities such as walking, engaging in music and nature, swimming, and painting. She connected with others through periods of socialization, and she found life meaning through humor, by having attitudes of gratitude and grace, and in times of solitude. The activities she engaged in frequently elicited "flow" for her, a state of being that provided the author with ways to enrich her life during a time of grief and loss. With flow, the author found ordinary, everyday experiences to be spiritual, and through this, she found meaning in her life.

Application and Considerations in Practice

While the authors mentioned in the previous section may have advocated an understanding of spirituality in terms of one or more of the constructs described, the implication is that all of these constructs might be aspects of or part of the larger construct of spirituality. The client that we may be working with comes to the therapy sessions with elements of his or her "being" and spirituality. To recognize these aspects of a person and to attend to them within the therapy process is not only suggested by the authors but reinforced as a way that clients may find new meaning in their lives and hope for the future.

It is also important to understand that these constructs provide descriptions of various aspects of spirituality associated with an individual but may not be representative of/for all individuals. For example, someone might not acknowledge nor desire to give credence to a higher power or spiritual belief system. Someone may never experience a state of flow, while others may not engage in select spiritual activities. The aspects noted are recognized but not required to be in existence or accepted by the person in order for the person to consider him/ her as spiritual. Just as we are taught to be client centered in therapy as it relates to the person's desires and goals for life, we acknowledge the need for a client-centered approach in understanding spirituality with those we collaborate with and provide therapy services.

Therapeutic use of self supports the OT practitioner's understanding of his or her own belief system and values as well as taking initiative to further develop **cultural sensitivity** and responsive care when working with clients. In order to facilitate meaningful occupational therapy, OT practitioners need to spend time researching and gaining knowledge about the specific culture related to his or her area of practice, setting, and client practices. According to Fox (2009), cultural sensitivity allows an OT practitioner to provide the best intervention possible because the intervention is based on the client's belief and value system. As we become culturally sensitive to the values and beliefs of clients, we are better able as practitioners to respect any differences between the client's beliefs and our own. Through the development of cultural sensitivity, the OT practitioner is then able to maintain appropriate boundaries when working with clients.

Australian authors Swarbrick and Burkhardt (2000) emphasize the importance of "being aware of one's personal spiritual beliefs that affect a client's occupations, behaviors...and coping strategies in relation to loss, injury, and illness" (p. 2). These authors describe their understanding as to how that therapeutic relationship is created. The relationship is first supported by recognizing the OT practitioner's own belief system and values in order to maintain perspective within the occupational therapy process. Additionally, it is the "therapist's caring, intentional presence [that] fosters sharing of [client's] spiritual concerns" (Swarbrick & Burkhardt, 2002, p. 2). Gabriel (2005) also espouses "to fully understand spirituality as it guides our interactions with others, we must first understand and nurture spirituality in ourselves" (p. 207).

McColl (2012) further challenges OT practitioners to honestly assess their personal comfort level with this topic and understand personal–professional boundaries. Notwithstanding, she also encourages us to "adapt a willingness to learn from the experiences of patients and accept our own limited understanding" (McColl, 2012, p. 274). Developing attitudes of courage, justice, compassion, agency, and awareness strengthens the therapeutic use of self (McColl, 2012, p. 278), and integrating our own transformative experiences and personal growth helps to develop authenticity.

Summary

My clinical experience as both an OTA and OT as well as my involvement as a fieldwork supervisor, an administrator, and an educator and researcher is that most OT students and practitioners are most comfortable in understanding and utilizing the constructs related to valued occupations within therapy. We make it a point to try to understand what holds significance for the individual receiving therapy and do what we can to incorporate those activities into the practice setting in which we work. We also need to be aware that some of the activities that we introduce to the therapy session may or may not have any relevance for the person and may not touch the spiritual or essence of the person. The question may then be asked: "Is this still therapy or not?" In other words, does a therapeutic activity need to hold significant relevance for it to be therapeutic? Does every therapeutic activity need to be one that is considered meaningful? And are all meaningful activities spiritual ones? Is the ultimate goal in therapy to have a "spiritual" experience or is it that we need to be aware that our therapy activities and approaches might evoke a spiritual response from the client?

As seasoned OT practitioners, we often pull from our own professional and personal knowledge gained throughout the years and are able to offer hope and motivation and new life meaning by providing new images of possibility and adding to the life narratives of clients, families, and communities. Mattingly and Fleming (1994) describe this clinical reasoning process as reframing narratives for clients. Even though we can provide these insights and new images to clients during the therapy process, what can become a challenge at times is how to respond to clients and families who are questioning the meaning of life, suffering, pain, and death in a more philosophical or faith-based perspective. It will not be uncommon to work with clients, families, and communities who will question out loud why such devastating life events and circumstances are occurring and wonder how to make sense of those traumatic events. We, as OT practitioners, usually do not have the language or the professional background to adequately address these global questions and in many respects are not totally cognizant of how we personally make sense of these issues either. In the times when clients and families are explicitly articulating life meaning questions and wish to discuss the concerns openly, we should rely on other professionals, such as chaplains, to engage these conversations further.

The other challenge for OT students and practitioners at times is the understanding of different religious traditions and faith-based beliefs and practices. In order to best support clients, families, and potentially communities in the resumption of valued occupations that encompass these faith or spiritual practices, we must have some understanding of what those beliefs, rituals, and activities include. As mentioned earlier, this takes an openness and willingness to expand our therapeutic use of self and the willingness to discover and ask pertinent questions to be better informed and culturally responsive and sensitive.

Lastly, while we can envision and support spirituality as part of the process of engaging clients in meaningful roles and activities, in finding new life meaning, and engaging in select practices, what might be more challenging for a student or practitioner is the idea of "occupations of spirit." According to the official documents of AOTA, we engage in a host of activities or occupations including activities of daily living, instrumental activities of daily living, rest and sleep, work, education, play, leisure, and social participation. All of these occupations entail "doing" or performing, and therapy subsequently tends to focus on such. However, we do not have a category, as of yet, specifically related to spiritual occupations. That is where I think the conversation sometimes gets uncomfortable. Are there really occupations particularly related to spirituality, or is spirituality embedded in the other already stated occupations? Are occupations of spirit about "being" and not so much about the "doing?" Could it be both possibilities? We just added some more jelly to the wall!

What does this mean for you as students? I think it means several things. First, we must know what we are speaking about when discussing spirituality. What does it actually mean? Throughout this chapter, I have tried to provide ways in which spirituality has been understood by many clinicians and researchers in the field of occupational therapy. Various perspectives and aspects of spirituality were presented. To further converse about this topic beyond this chapter, I think you need to know how to begin the conversation and appreciate where it might be going.

It also means that we need to be self-reflective, understanding our own biases and appreciations about the topic and the aspects that we are comfortable with and the ones that we may not be as comfortable with. We can start by pondering and thinking about our own understanding about life meaning and purpose. Beyond that, we also need to develop our therapeutic use of self and challenge ourselves to become more knowledgeable about other's beliefs and practices.

As professionals, we also need to further the dialogue about such matters as we do with other topics and subjects and continue to collect the evidence that supports the use of meaningful occupations. Most of the research related to spirituality and occupational therapy completed at this point in our history is related to students' and practitioners' perspectives (comfort and use) regarding spirituality. We have some qualitative research that provides insights into what is most meaningful to recovery from the client's perspective, but we need even more. There are also beginning conversations in the global occupational therapy community as to how spirituality ties into occupational justice concerns and as a profession, we need to be inclusive in letting all parties and all cultures be part of that dialogue.

Lastly, as professionals, we need to also be attentive to our own personal self-care and nurture. We often do not openly speak about this in the field but recognize the importance with clients. We need to attend to our physical, emotional, and spiritual self-care so that we have the energy and stamina to attend to the needs of others.

Special Acknowledgments

I wish to thank Lauren Rossi, MS, OTR/L, and Amanda Sedlak, MS, OTR/L, for all of their work on this topic and continued support over the years. Their inspiration and excitement provided much energy in getting the original comprehensive literature review completed. I also thank Ellen Wascou for her photography and her gift of seeing beauty in the world. Special thanks to the Pendle Hill community, a Quaker retreat center that provided me many hours of respite and a spiritual place to write.

Review Questions

1. Which institution has the longest history of supporting the concept of spirituality in occupational therapy through the publication of professional texts and documents?

2. Name the four primary constructs of spirituality as outlined in the chapter.

3. Describe the four primary constructs of spirituality as outlined in the chapter.

4. An occupational therapy practitioner elects to use tai chi as an intervention strategy to improve balance because she understands the client engages in physical activities on a regular basis and finds great meaning in such activities. Which spirituality construct would support this approach?

5. An occupational therapy practitioner elects to use tai chi as an intervention strategy to facilitate a sense of calm and well-being because she understands the client engaged in similar practices before his injury and his goal for therapy is to continue to deal with the pain that is impeding his daily routines and to find healing through personal self-discovery. Which spirituality construct would support this approach?

6. An occupational therapy practitioner elects to use tai chi as an intervention strategy to promote occupational performance. She understands that prior to the client's accident, he engaged in regular tai chi sessions held at the local Buddhist community. Which spirituality construct would support this approach?

7. Describe three considerations in the professional development and use of spirituality in occupational therapy practice.

8. An occupational therapy practitioner elects to use the activity of making a collage with a resident in Hospice to facilitate a discussion regarding end-of-life concerns. Which spirituality construct would support this approach?
9. An occupational therapy practitioner elects to use the activity of making a collage with a resident in Hospice to facilitate a discussion regarding what activities the client wishes to engage in during the next several weeks. Which spirituality construct would support this approach?
10. An occupational therapy practitioner elects to use the activity of making a collage with a resident in Hospice to facilitate a discussion regarding coping through life crisis. Which spirituality construct would support this approach?

Practice Activities

Before reading the chapter, define and describe your personal definitions of spirituality and share any ideas of how occupational therapy and spirituality might be connected.

Using the pictures in the chapter, have a discussion as to any reactions of these pictures to spirituality. Do they fit or not?

Share and discuss personal spiritual practices and benefits if you are comfortable doing so. If you are comfortable, share your narrative/story regarding your recovery through a personal challenge or life event.

References

American Occupational Therapy Association. Occupational therapy practice framework: domain and process. *Am J Occup Ther* 2002;56(6):609–639. doi:10.5014/ajot.56.6.609

American Occupational Therapy Association. Occupational therapy practice framework: domain and process (2nd ed.). *Am J Occup Ther* 2008;62(6):625–683. doi:10.5014/ajot.62.6.625

American Occupational Therapy Association. Occupational therapy practice framework: domain and process (3rd ed.). *Am J Occup Ther* 2014;68(Suppl. 1):S1–S48. http://dx.doi.org/10.5014/ajot.2014.682006

Billock C. Integrating spirituality into home health occupational therapy practice. *Home Community Health Spec Interest Sect Q* 2009, March;16(1):1–4. Retrieved from http://www.aota.org

Bouthot J, Wells T, Black RM. Spirituality in practice: using the FICA spiritual history assessment. *OT Pract* 2011;16(3):13–16.

Bowen JE. Reflections from the heart: the healing- within relationship. *OT Pract* (2006, January);11(1):48. Retrieved from http://www.aota.org

Canadian Association of Occupational Therapy. *Enabling Occupation: An Occupational Therapy Perspective, revised edition*. Ottowa, ON: Canadian Association of Occupational Therapists, CTTC; 2002.

Canadian Association of Occupational Therapy. *Enabling Occupation II: Advancing an Occupational Therapy Vision for Health, Well-Being & Justice Through Occupation*. Ottowa, ON: Canadian Association of Occupational Therapists, CTTC; 2007.

Christiansen C. Nationally speaking: acknowledging a spiritual dimension in occupational therapy practice. *Am J Occup Ther* 1997, March;51(3):169–172. Retrieved from http://www.aota.org

Collins JS, Paul S, West-Frasier J. The utilization of spirituality in occupational therapy:

beliefs, practices, and perceived barriers. *Occup Ther Health Care* 2001;14(3–4):73–92. Retrieved from http://informahealthcare.com/loi/ohc

Dawson DR, Stern B. Reflections on facilitating older adult's participation in valued occupations. *OT NOW* 2007, September/October;9(5):3–5. Retrieved from OT Search.

Dickenson J. A spiritual journey—a personal perspective. In: McColl MA, ed. *Spirituality and Occupational Therapy*. 2nd ed. Ottawa, Ontario: CAOT Publications; 2012:259–268.

Doughton KJ. Unlocking your client's hidden talents. *OT Week* 1996, June;10(26):18–19. Retrieved from OT Search.

Fearing VG, Law M, Clark J. An occupational performance process model: fostering client and therapist alliances. *Can J Occup Ther* 1997;64(1):7–15.

Feeney L, Toth-Cohen S. Addressing spiritually for clients with physical disabilities. *OT Pract* 2008, March;13(4):16–20. Retrieved from http://www.aota.org

Forhan M. Doing, being, and becoming: a family's journey through perinatal loss. *Am J Occup Ther* 2010;64(1):142–151. Retrieved from http://www.aota.org

Fox L. Native American spirituality: a truly holistic perspective. *Home Community Health Spec Interest Sect Q* 2009, March;16(1):1–4. Retrieved from http://www.aota.org

Gabriel L. Reflections on spirituality: implications for ethics education. In: Purtilo R, Jensen G, Royeen C, eds. *Educating for Moral Action: A Sourcebook in Health and Rehabilitation Ethics*. Philadelphia, PA: F.A. Davis; 2005:203–214.

Gavacs M. Reflections from the heart: the dance of independence. *OT Pract* 2009, June;15(10):32. Retrieved from http://www.aota.org

Gourley M. The spiritual realm of occupational therapy. *OT Pract* 2001, April;6(8):13–14. Retrieved from http://www.aota.org

Hatchard K, Missiuna C. An occupational therapist's journey through bipolar affective disorder. *Occup Ther Mental Health* 2003;19(2):1–17. doi:10.1300/J004v19n02_01

Heinz AJ, Disney ER, Epstein DH, et al. Pilot study on spirituality: a focus-group study on spirituality and substance-user treatment. *Subst Use Misuse* 2010;45(1–2):134–153. doi:10.3109/10826080903035130

Hilbers J, Haynes AS, Kivikko JG. Spirituality and health: an exploratory study of hospital patients' perspectives. *Aust Health Rev* 2010;34(1):3–10. doi:10.1071/AH09655

Jung B, Salvatori P, Missiuna C, et al. The McMaster lens for occupational therapists: bringing theory and practice into focus. *OT NOW* 1999, March/April;10(2):16–19. Retrieved from OT Search.

Kang C. A psychospiritual integration frame of reference of occupational therapy. Part 1: Conceptual foundations. *Aust Occup Ther J* 2003;50(2):92–103. doi:10.1046/j.1440-1630.2003.00358.x

Kirsh B, Dawson D, Antolikova S, et al. Developing awareness of spirituality in occupational therapy students: are our curricula up to the task? *Occup Ther Int* 2001;8(2):119–125. Retrieved from http://onlinelibrary.wiley.com/journal/10.1002/(ISSN)1557-0703

Leslie CA. Reflections from the heart: life's lessons. *OT Pract* 2006, April;11(6):44. Retrieved from http://www.aota.org

Mathis TK. The magic in a pecan pie. *OT Week* 1996, June;10(25):16. Retrieved from OT Search.

Mattingly C, Fleming M. *Clinical Reasoning: Forms of Inquiry in a Therapeutic Practice*. Philadelphia, PA: F.A. Davis; 1994.

McColl MA. *Spirituality and Occupational Therapy*. Ottawa, Ontario: CAOT Publications; 2003.

McColl MA. *Spirituality and Occupational Therapy. 2nd ed*. Ottawa, Ontario: CAOT Publications; 2012.

Moreira-Almeida A, Koenig HG. Retaining the meaning of the words religiousness and spirituality: a commentary on the WHOQOL SRPB group's "A cross-cultural study of spirituality, religion, and personal beliefs as components of quality of life". *Social Sci Med* 2006;63:843–845.

Nesbit SG. Using creativity to experience flow on my journey with breast cancer. *Occup Ther Mental Health* 2006;22(2):61–79. doi:10.1300/J004b22n02_03

Peloquin SM. Nationally speaking: the spiritual depth of occupation: making worlds and making lives. *Am J Occup Ther* 1997, March;51(3):167–168. Retrieved from http://www.aota.org

Pentland W, McColl MA. Occupational Choice. In: McColl MA, ed. *Spirituality and occupational therapy. 2nd ed*. Ottawa, Ontario: CAOT Publications; 2012:141–149.

Pongsakri M. Occupational therapy eases the suffering of tsunami victims. *WFOT Bull* 2007, May;55:30–33. Retrieved from Cinhal.

Ramugondo EL. Unlocking spirituality: play as a health-promoting occupation in the context of HIV/AIDS. In: Kronenberg F, ed. *Occupational Therapy Without Borders: Learning from the Spirit of Survivors*. New York, NY: Elsevier/Churchill Livingstone; 2005:313–325.

Reid D. Mundane occupations: providing opportunity for engagement and being-in-the-world. *OT NOW* 2010, March/April;12(2):24–26. Retrieved from OT Search.

Rosenfeld MS. Spiritual agent modalities for occupational therapy practice. *OT Pract* 2000,

January;5(2):17–21. Retrieved from http://www.aota.org

Rosenfeld MS. Exploring spiritual contexts for care. *OT Pract* 2001;6(11):18–25. Retrieved from http://www.aota.org

Rosenfeld MS. Motivating elders with depression in SNFs. *OT Pract* 2004, June:21–28. Retrieved from http://www.aota.org

Sadlo G. Creativity and occupation. In: Molineux M, ed. *Occupation for Occupational Therapists*. 1st ed. Malden, MA: Blackwell Publishing; 2004:90–100.

Spencer K. A whole new world. *Top Stroke Rehabil* 2007;14(4):93–96. doi:10.1310/tsr1404-93

Strzlecki MV. Careers: luck of the draw. *OT Pract* 2009, January;14(1):7–8. Retrieved from http://www.aota.org

Swarbrick P, Burkhardt A. Spiritual health: implications for the occupational therapy process. *Mental Health Spec Interest Sect Q* 2000, June;23(2):1–3. Retrieved from http://www.aota.org

Swedberg L. Facilitating accessibility and participation in faith communities. *OT Pract* 2001, May;6(9):CE1–CE8. Retrieved from http://www.aota.org

Szafran SH. Physical, mental and spiritual approaches to managing pain in older clients. *OT Pract* 2011;16(3), CE-1–CE-8.

Taylor E, Mitchell JE, Kenan S, et al. Attitudes of occupational therapists toward spirituality in practice. *Am J Occup Ther* 2000;54(4):421–427. Retrieved from http://www.aota.org

Thibeault R. Occupational gifts. In: McColl MA, ed. *Spirituality and Occupational Therapy*. 2nd ed. Ottawa, Ontario: CAOT Publications; 2012a:111–120.

Thibeault R. Occupational therapy values. In: McColl MA, ed. *Spirituality and Occupational Therapy*. 2nd ed. Ottawa, Ontario: CAOT Publications; 2012b:103–110.

Thibeault R. Resilience and maturity. In: McColl MA, ed. *Spirituality and Occupational Therapy*. 2nd ed. Ottawa, Ontario: CAOT Publications; 2012c:121–130.

Thibeault R.Ritual: ceremonies of life. In: M. A. McColl, *Spirituality and Occupational Therapy*. 2nd ed. Ottawa, Ontario: CAOT Publications; 2012d:217–222.

Thompson BE, MacNeil C. A phenomenological study exploring the meaning of a seminar on spirituality for occupational therapy students. *Am J Occup Ther* 2006;60(5):531–539. Retrieved from http://www.aota.org

Toomey M. Creativity: spirituality through the visual arts. In: McColl MA, ed. *Spirituality and Occupational Therapy*. 2nd ed. Ottawa, Ontario: CAOT Publications; 2012:233–240.

Trump SM. Occupational therapy and hospice: a natural fit. *OT Pract* 2001, November;6(20):7–8, 10–11. Retrieved from http://www.aota.org

Unruh A. Appreciation of nature: restorative occupations. In: McColl MA, ed. *Spirituality and Occupational Therapy*. 2nd ed. Ottawa, Ontario: CAOT Publications; 2012:249–256.

Urbanowski R. Spirituality in everyday practice. *OT Pract* 1997, December;2(12):18–23. Retrieved from http://www.aota.org

Vrkljan BH. The role of spirituality in occupational therapy practice. *OT NOW* 2000, March;2:1–5. Retrieved from OT Search.

Whitney R. Reflections from the heart: the spirit catches me and I write it down. *OT Pract* 2010, September;15(16):33. Retrieved from http://www.aota.org

CHAPTER 20

Crafts in Occupational Therapy

DeLana Honaker, PhD, OTR and Debbie Grimes, COTA

Key Terms

Arts and Crafts movement—Emerged as a reaction to the industrial revolution and mass production of products. Reed (1989) posited in her Slagle Lecture that the Arts and Crafts movement revitalized the tenets of moral treatment into a new rationale, which the founders and early leaders of occupational therapy were quick to understand and embrace.

Craft—An activity involving skill in making things by hand.

Moral treatment—"Respect for human individuality and a fundamental perception of the individual's need to engage in creative activity…" (Bockoven, 1971, p. 223).

Learning Objectives

After studying this chapter, readers should be able to:

- Explain the origins of crafts in occupational therapy.
- Identify at least three crafts that can be used with clients with varying needs and goals.

Introduction

Review occupational therapy's past, and the role of crafts in the profession becomes a golden thread woven throughout our history and within the tapestries of the lives of our clients. Two primary philosophies guided the evolution of occupational therapy: an ideology of pragmatism called moral treatment and the Arts and Crafts movement. "Both philosophies were concerned with creating a healthy society by addressing the meaning of activity in human lives" (Breines, 1989, p. 462).

Moral Treatment

In essence, **moral treatment** was "respect for human individuality and a fundamental perception of the individual's need to engage in creative activity..." (Bockoven, 1971, p. 223). The age of moral treatment largely occurred during the 1800s and was a revolutionary perspective in the treatment of persons with mental health issues from mild depression to mental retardation to extreme psychosis and even chronic physical health conditions (Peloquin, 1989) such as cerebral palsy or "weak chests." Prior to advancement of moral treatment, these individuals were often placed in poor houses, madhouses, "insane asylums," or sanatoriums, many of which operated under abysmal conditions such as limited and poor-quality food and water, lack of hygienic facilities, shackling, or keeping residents behind bars, abuse, filth, etc. Moral treatment tenets included understanding the patient's life circumstances and how these contributed to the patient's mental health rather than to assume that the patients were subhuman and had lost their reason (Peloquin, 1989). Another was recognizing the critical link between the patient's activities and activity patterns and his or her physical and mental health. Patients were encouraged to engage in purposeful work in the facility such as maintenance, gardening, cooking, and sewing, and maintenance of their personal spaces and selves (Breines, 1989; Peloquin, 1989; Peloquin, 1994). However, moral treatment lost favor in the latter part of the 1800s until the emergence of occupational therapy in the early 1900s (Peloquin, 1989; Reed, 1986). Bockoven (1971), a psychiatrist, stated that "the history of moral treatment in America is not only synonymous with, but *is* the history of occupational therapy before it acquired its 20th century name of 'occupational therapy'" (p. 225).

Arts and Crafts Movement

The **Arts and Crafts movement** emerged in reaction to the industrial revolution with the automation and factory production of many goods originally created by craftsmen. In the 1800s, Europe and America evolved from "... an agrarian to a manufacturing economy; from a cottage industry to a mass production society; from a consumer-driven marketplace to a producer-driven marketplace; from a patronage system to an industrial wealth system; from pride in workmanship to concern for profit..." (Reed, 1986, p. 599). Reed (1986) further posited that these factors all played a role in the demise of moral treatment in the late 1800s. The emergence of the Arts and Crafts movement revitalized the tenets of moral treatment into a new rationale, which the founders and early leaders of occupational therapy were quick to understand and embrace (Reed, 1986). Arts and crafts in occupational therapy were used as a way of promoting health through "doing" and provided an outlet for creative energy and purposeful activity for both mental illness and for long-term physical conditions such as tuberculosis and, later, physical rehabilitation (Reed, 1986). In his *Philosophy of Occupation Therapy* (1922), Adolf Meyer, a psychiatrist and ardent supporter of occupational therapy, stated:

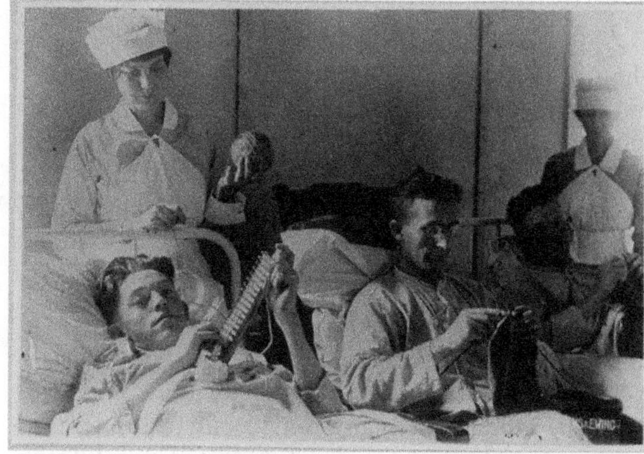

Figure 20.1 Occupational therapy during WWI bedridden wounded is knitting. Otis Historical Archives, National Museum of Health and Medicine.

> Groups with raffia and basketwork or with various kinds of handwork and weaving and bookbinding and metal and leatherwork took the place of wall flowers and mischief makers. A pleasure in achievement, a real pleasure in the use of activity of one's hands and muscles and a happy appreciation of time began to be used as incentives in the management of our patients. (p. 2)

With the advent of World War I, reconstruction aides (predecessors to occupational and physical therapists) began working with injured veterans using exercise programs and crafts; "the concept of occupational therapy's role in rehabilitation [during and after WWI] was one of using crafts to reactivate the minds and motivations of the mentally ill and the limbs of the veterans starting them on their way to vocational training" (Woodside, 1971, p. 227) (Figs. 20.1 and 20.2).

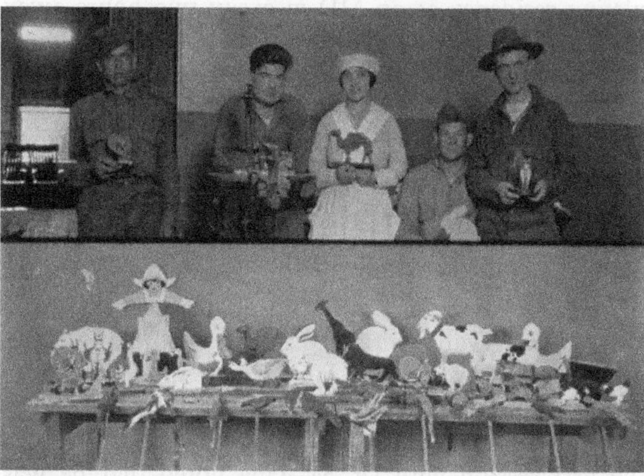

Figure 20.2 Occupational therapy. Toy making in psychiatric hospital. World War I era. Otis Historical Archives, National Museum of Health and Medicine.

Using Crafts in Therapy Today

The use of crafts in occupational therapy has waxed and waned as the profession attempted to further define itself and provide a unique service to a variety of clients (Bissell & Mailloux, 1981; Reed, 1986). Do crafts still have a role in occupational therapy today? Most emphatically, yes! As Reed noted, our founders believed crafts serve multiple purposes including the following:

- The treatment should, in each case, be specifically directed to the individual's needs.
- The production of a well-made, useful, and attractive article, or the accomplishment of a useful task, requires health exercise of mind and body, gives the greatest satisfaction, and thus produces the most beneficial effects.
- Novelty, variety, individuality, and utility of the products enhance the value of an occupation as a treatment measure.
- Quality, quantity, and salability of the products may prove beneficial by satisfying and stimulating the patient but should never be permitted to obscure the main purpose (Reed, 2006, p. 24).

Crafts, as opposed to exercise programs or games, serve as a means of eliciting desired performance as opposed to being just an activity to stave off boredom. Critical to using crafts as a treatment modality is the understanding that any craft used with the client is individualized to his or her needs and leads to a meaningful and valued *end product* rather than simply "something to do." For many clients, one of the unique aspects of crafts is that it is viewed as nonthreatening, and mastery of the craft can lead to mastery of other occupations as in the case of Dr. M.

Dr. M

Dr. M was pursuing a postdoc in neurology after completing residency as an MD in a city two hours away from his family; he regularly drove back to be with them most weekends. On one of these trips, his car was hit by a drunk driver who crossed the median late at night and hit Dr. M head on. Dr. M was rushed by helicopter to a trauma hospital and eventually required an amputation of his left arm at the shoulder. He also experienced right knee damage that required surgery and use of a one-handed walker for 2 months. Upon his transfer to the rehabilitation wing of the hospital 2 weeks post-op, Dr. M was evaluated for occupational therapy and physical therapy services. Jana, a new grad OTA, was assigned to work with Dr. M and noted that his goals included learning ADLs and IADLs one-handed. In the first session with Dr. M, Jana noted that he was depressed and seemed apathetic. While demonstrating scar massage on Dr. M's amputation site, Jana engaged Dr. M in conversation and he shared that at the time of his accident, he was finishing up his dissertation research in which he used a cryostat and ultramicrotome to examine some minute differences in thin slices of diseased brain tissue. He sighed and stated that he did not think he would be able to continue that work with only one hand now. Jana, in her effort to be positive and helpful, stated that she was sure he would be able to do his research again, but Dr. M was clearly dejected and repeated that he would not be able to continue his research. Jana respected his perspective but in her mind, she became determined to show Dr. M that he could go on to finish his postdoc in neurology and then pursue his goal to work as a neurologist. Jana discussed her treatment plan with her OT, Lisa, who agreed with Jana's plan to help Dr. M continue in achieving his lifelong dreams. Typically, Jana would help a client in a similar situation as Dr. M select a nail clipper board from a medical supply catalogue, but this time, she decided that they would make the nail clipper board as part of therapy. Although Dr. M had woodworking experience from working as a child with his dad in the garage workshop, he was not too sure that he would be able to make the nail clipper board now that he just had a right hand, but Jana assured him that it would be possible and that she would help. They began by asking the hospital maintenance staff for a board piece that was 2 inches wide by 4 inches long and half an inch thick. Using clamps and sanding boards (thin boards that Jana had glued various grit sandpaper onto), the first session was spent sanding the board smooth. Next, Dr. M used a slightly damp cloth to clean the dust from the bottom surface of the board. Then, he and Jana problem solved how he could cut out a piece of nonskid drawer liner fabric; she suggested that he stabilize it by placing the hammer on the fabric, which worked. Next, Dr. M and Jana problem solved how he could open the rubber cement jar one-handed; he decided to wrap excess nonskid fabric around the jar, press it between his chest and table edge, and then open the jar lid with his right hand. Next, Dr. M applied a layer of rubber cement on the bottom of the block and then applied the fabric piece and set the block aside to dry overnight. In the next session, Jana and Dr. M problem solved how he would attach the clippers Jana bought at the local drug store. Dr. M figured out that the clipper could be attached using a screw inserted in the hole at the end of the clippers and then two penny nails to each side of the clippers to anchor it. To do this, he put the board in a clamp, using some poster gum, and marked with a felt-tip pen where the screw and nails would go. Once that was done, he removed the clipper and poster gum, and then, he and Jana problem solved how he would use the screwdriver and the hammer. To hold the nails, he used the poster gum again by pushing a penny nail in a ball of gum and then placing the point of the nail on the marked dot, and then pressing the gum down on the wood to stabilize the nail. He then used the nail to hammer it into the wood block. Doing the same process with the other nail and for the mark for the screw hole, he hammered the nail enough to make a hole to start the screw hole. He removed that nail and the poster gum. Next, he slid the clippers in so that the hole in the clippers aligned with the hole he had made for the screw, and then molded the poster gum to the sides of the clipper to further stabilize it. He then screwed in the screw until it was flush with the clipper. He finished the board by applying a layer of tung oil to the board. Just as Dr. M finished the clipper board, he said to Jana, "I guess if I can do this, I could continue with my research...." Jana smiled and said she would try to see if there was a cryostat or ultramicrotome in the research wing of the hospital. Luckily, she found exactly that, and the next day's therapy session was spent in the lab with Dr. M and Jana problem solving how he would use this equipment with just one hand.

While one would not necessarily see a connection between a craft project and using sophisticated medical research equipment, Jana's purpose in using craft as a therapy modality for Dr. M was simply to use techniques he was already familiar with from working with his dad in his woodworking shop and then problem solving how he would still use those same skills one-handed. It was the nonthreatening craft project and the process that allowed Dr. M to realize that he could apply the same problem-solving skills in achieving his dissertation research.

Crafts beyond the Clinic

Prior to Social Security disability benefits, which were not available until 1956 (United States, 2012), learning a craft as a client in the early days of occupational therapy often served as means of support for earning money despite having a mental or physical disability. Craftsmanship is still a highly valued skill, just take a look at the popularity of craft shows and fairs as well as craft consignment shops. Learning a craft today certainly has value as a means of partial or full financial support for a client receiving occupational therapy services. In addition, creating a home business as a craftsperson can also provide a much valued worker identity role (Dickie, 2003) that may have been previously eliminated due to an illness or disability as in the case of Mary Sue.

Mary Sue

Mary Sue, a 47-year-old woman diagnosed with schizophrenia and depression, is back in the psychiatric hospital as she had stopped taking her medications again and was a danger to herself. Judy, the OT for the facility, and Maria, the OTA, had noticed that several clients often demonstrated this type of "bounce back" pattern; the clients would leave the hospital stable on his or her medications and then return in a few months, having stopped the medication and requiring hospitalization again. Over time, they asked clients probing but gentle and nonjudgmental questions to determine what caused this pattern. It appeared that all the clients were living on some type of public assistance or benefits, which was meager at best, and it often came down to buying food or cigarettes, paying rent, or paying for medication (From the Field 20.1). In some situations, the problem was limited public transportation or limited funds to pay a driver or taxi to get the medications. Judy and Maria realized that there were several issues at stake and made a concerted effort to collaborate with the unit's social worker to help with some of the issues. But Maria also believed that if the clients had some way to make "pocket change" to supplement their disability support, they would also better able to ensure they had access to their medications. Maria and Judy discussed this issue at length and agreed that these patients were unable to consistently hold typical or regular jobs due to the nature of their disabilities but that a flexible way to earn money when they were able would be very helpful. Maria thought that if she taught clients some simple craft skills along with skills on how to maintain a small home craft business, they might be successful. With Judy's approval, Maria decided to try her plan with Mary Sue. Maria taught Mary Sue how to make simple but elegant serving sets such as a cake plate or a chip and dip set (the steps below), and once Mary Sue had made several serving sets on her own with beautiful results, Maria began to problem solve with Mary Sue about how to create a small business making and selling her wares. First, they created a simple business plan, which included a supplies list and then did an Internet search and a field trip to a local box store to determine the best prices for the supplies. Next, Maria showed Mary Sue how to track her supplies' expenses, inventory, and income, using a simple bookkeeping booklet downloaded from a source online. Next, Maria

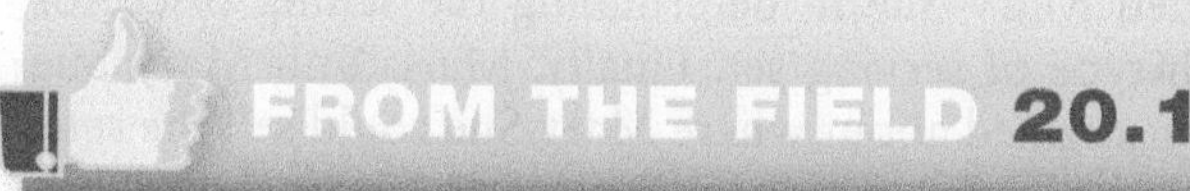

Smoking

Although you may have personal views about using limited funds to buy cigarettes, please note that smoking IS a significant addiction that is often beyond the client's abilities to overcome.

guided Mary Sue in determining the selling price for each type of serving set. Finally, Maria and Mary Sue brainstormed about where Mary Sue could sell the sets. They discussed renting a table at local craft shows, but Mary Sue was not sure that she would be comfortable talking with that many people or if she would have reliable transportation to the shows. They eventually decided that selling her sets at a local craft consignment store and possibly a local gift shop would be a better option for Mary Sue. Maria made contact with a local gift shop manager who agreed to sell the sets for Maria for a 20% commission on the sale price. With these details settled, Mary Sue needed to determine how she would finance the first set of supplies for her venture; she only needed $54 to get started and she decided to ask her sister for help. Mary Sue's sister was impressed with the mini–business plan Mary Sue presented to her and agreed to buy the supplies for Mary Sue. Maria kept in touch with Mary Sue's social worker and once visited the local craft consignment store where she saw Mary Sue's serving sets on display; Maria was also thrilled to see that Mary Sue had come up with additional designs for her serving sets. The social worker reported that Mary Sue was not always able to make the sets but when she was, she did make another $100 to $200 a month, which was very helpful on her limited income. Judy and Maria also noticed that Mary Sue had not "bounced back" into the facility since starting her small craft business and discussed Mary Sue's success and decided to implement similar programming with other clients for whom this might be a successful endeavor (Fig. 20.3).

Materials and Supplies

- 2 dinner plates
- 2 matching bowls
- 1 candle holder
- Loctite Glass Glue
- Dishwashing soap, water, and lint-free towel

Tools Needed

- 12-inch ruler
- Washable marker

Instructions for All Pieces

- Wash plates, bowls, and candle holder in warm sudsy water.
- Be sure to remove price stickers and other marks.
- Thoroughly dry pieces using the lint-free towel.

Cake Plate Instructions

1. Put a thin line of glue along the bottom edge of bowl.
2. Carefully and quickly (you have less than a minute before the glue begins to harden) place the bowl on the center of the plate bottom.
3. Let the cake plate dry for 1 hour upside down. Then, turn right side up.
4. The cake plate is safe to put in the dishwasher after glue has cured for 1 week.

Chip and Dip Set Instructions

1. Put a thin line of glue along the bottom edge of the bowl.
2. Carefully and quickly (you have less than a minute before the glue begins to harden) place the bowl on the center of the iron candle stand.
3. Let the bowl dry on the iron candle stand for one hour.
4. Apply glue to the bottom of the candle holder and place carefully in the center of the plate. Let the candle holder dry for one hour.
5. The chip and dip set is safe to put in the dishwasher after glue has cured for 1 week.

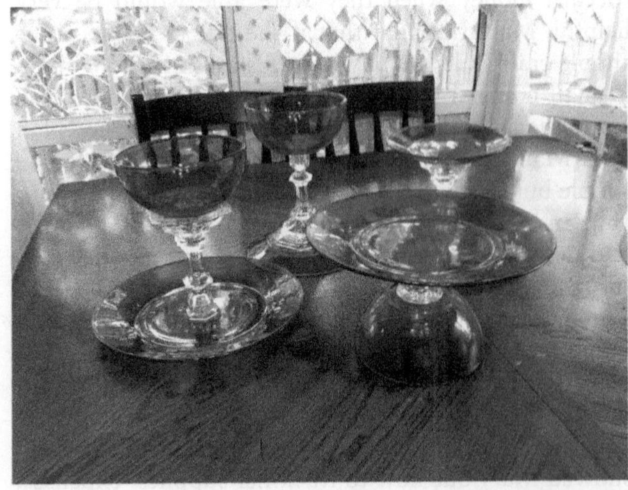

Figure 20.3 Cake plate and chip and dip sets.

Implementing Crafts in Practice

How would you incorporate the use of crafts in occupational therapy practice? The remainder of this chapter focuses on case studies in which crafts are used to meet the personal needs or goals of clients with a variety of conditions.

Charlie, Jose, Candace, and Mason

One of the key skills OT practitioners develop with time is the ability to quickly grade a craft activity to meet the needs of the client and their goal(s) or to meet the needs of several clients and their goals. Katie, a seasoned OTA who works for a public school district, had a super busy Tuesday. At one of her schools, she had four children with different needs but not a lot of time to create new craft activities for each so she decided to choose one craft activity, snowman, but to grade it to meet the needs of all four students. For Charlie, a first-grader who functions at a developmental age of 13 months and who had a goal to tolerate various textures, she drew an outline of a snowman on a piece of blue construction paper. Then, she and Charlie smeared glue on the construction paper; Katie cued Charlie to stay within the lines. After washing his hands, Katie had Charlie scoop and pour little handfuls of sugar on the glue, making sure to cover all the glue areas and then they set it aside to dry. The next time Katie saw Charlie's mom, she was thrilled that she had some "refrigerator art" from Charlie and put it up with that of his two brothers (Fig. 20.4).

Next, Katie saw Jose in his prekindergarten classroom during small group time; Jose had goals to address fine motor delays. Although Jose was the only child in the classroom who received occupational therapy services, in the spirit of inclusion, Katie set up a small group activity center that Jose and several of his classmates would circulate to. She pulled out several other predrawn snowmen on blue papers. In this activity, the children, including Jose, put equal dollops of white glue and shaving cream in the middle of the snowman shape and then smeared it while staying within the lines. Jose loved that the mixture had a foamy texture. Next, Katie had the children make snowflakes by putting fingerprints of the mixture all around the paper. Finally, the children put raisins on the snowman to make buttons and facial features and then added cotton swabs for the arms. In this part of the activity, Katie provided some minimum assistance to Jose's his raisins in the right places (Fig. 20.5).

Katie saw both Candace (a first-grader with hemiplegic cerebral palsy and goals to address bilateral coordination) and Mason (a third-grader who had sensory processing disorder and had goals for improving constructional praxis) together for her next session. Katie had Candace staple a dinner-sized paper plate to a dessert-sized paper plate and then cut out a black hat (Katie had predrawn this using a white crayon on black construction paper) and a strip of colorful tissue paper. Next, Candace drew the facial features and the buttons on the paper plate snowman and then glued the hat on.

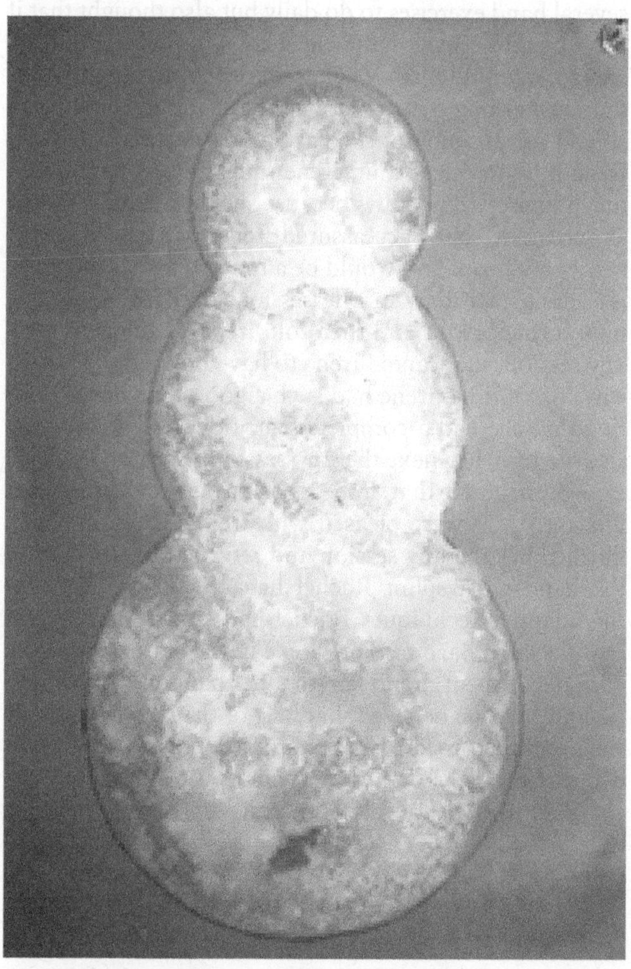

Figure 20.4 Charlie's snowman.

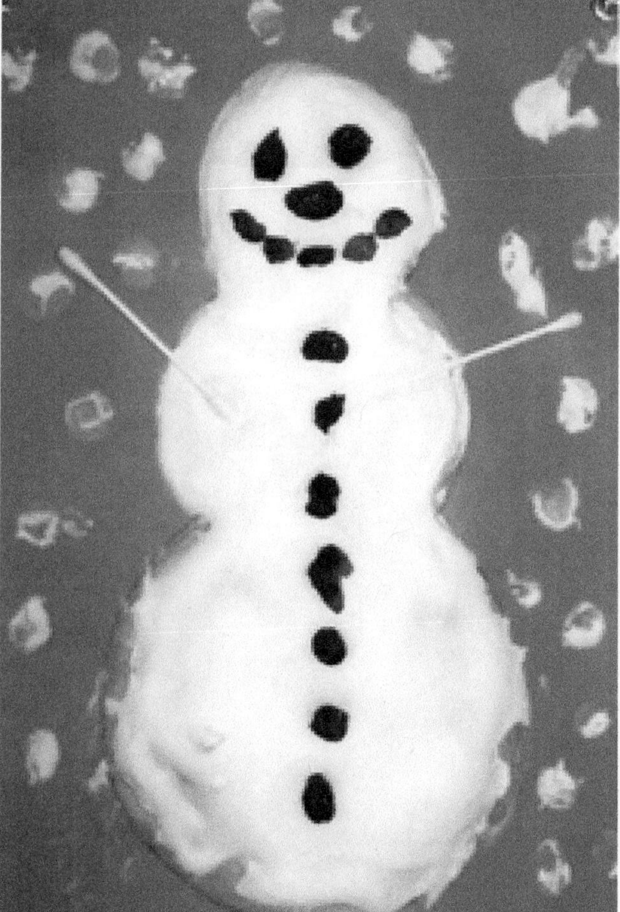

Figure 20.5 Jose's snowman.

Finally, Candace tied the tissue like a scarf around the neck. Meanwhile, Mason followed Katie's demonstration in folding a piece of white paper accordion style. Next, Mason traced a paper doll snowman template on the folded paper, ensuring the "hands" were on the folds with verbal cues from Katie. Then, he cut out the snowman out with verbal cues and then decorated his snowman using markers (Figs. 20.6 and 20.7).

Irene

Irene experienced significant carpal tunnel pains in her right hand; she noticed that this pain was particularly worse when she did repetitive tasks at her factory job on the assembly line. The pain was getting to the point that she was having difficulty doing her job, and she reported it to her supervisor. Irene consulted a hand surgeon as required by her worker's comp insurance provider, and the surgeon recommended occupational therapy as Irene's carpal tunnel syndrome was not severe as to require surgery at this time. Irene was assessed by Rachel, an OT and certified hand therapist, and Rachel determined that several therapy sessions were needed to reduce swelling of the carpal tunnel area and to develop adaptations to the way that Irene did her job on the assembly line. While Rachel did an on-site visit to Irene's work to observe the adaptations that could be made so that Irene could do her job, Barb, an OTA, worked with Irene in the clinic to reduce the swelling in her right hand. Barb showed Irene several hand exercises to do daily but also thought that if Irene could keep her hand elevated with the hand/fingers spread, it would further help reduce the swelling. Rather than just asking Irene to sit with her hand up and fingers spread for 10 minutes several times a day, Barb showed Irene how to finger knit. Irene said she had never been much interested in crafts because she didn't think herself as "creative," but Barb assured Irene that this craft was nearly fail proof and would be a fun way to get this exercise done each day. In one session, Barb showed Irene how to finger knit and then told Irene by the next therapy session, she wanted Irene to have finished at least 40 rows of knitting. Irene had such a good time finger knitting that she had a complete scarf done by the time she returned for her next therapy session! Barb and Rachel also both noted that Irene's edema had decreased significantly and were pleased with Irene's progress. Irene finished her therapy session and returned to work using the hand glove/splint Rachel had created for her and the adaptive techniques Rachel had shown her. Several months later, Barb ran into Irene in the craft store in the yarn department; Irene said that her hand was much better and that she believed that part of the reason was that she continued to do hand knitting almost daily during her coffee breaks or in the evenings after her shift; she also said that she loved being "crafty" (Fig. 20.8).

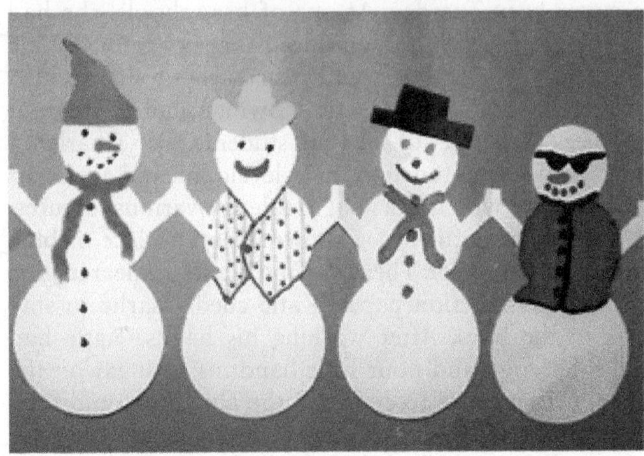

Figure 20.7 Mason's snowmen.

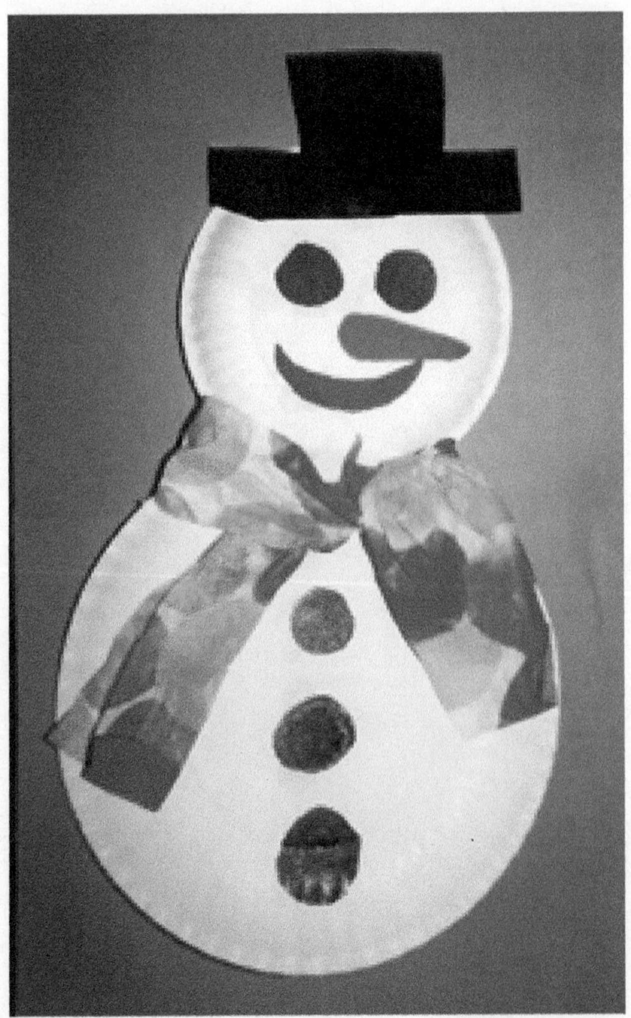

Figure 20.6 Candace's snowman.

List of Supplies

- One to two skeins of yarn depending on desired length of scarf

Note: "Chunky" or "fluffy" yarn makes a thicker scarf.

- Two hands

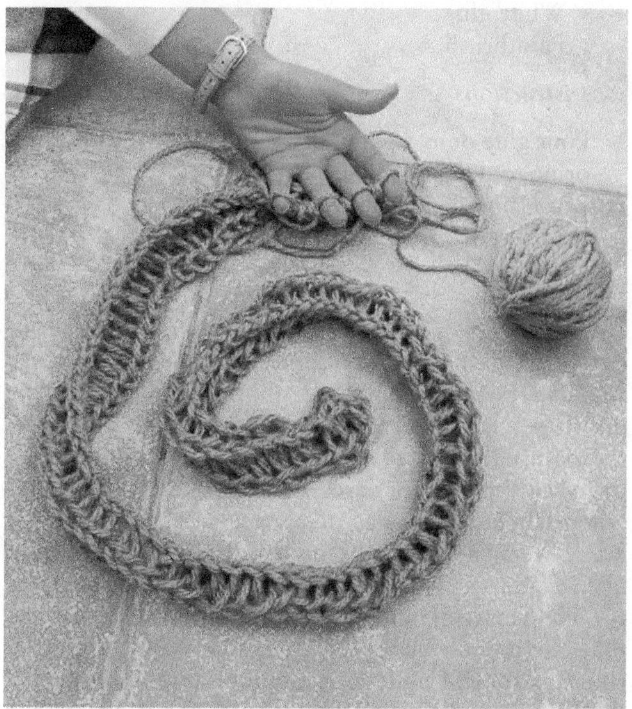

Figure 20.8 Irene's finger knitting.

Instructions

1. Use your nondominant hand as your frame. Put the ball of yarn behind your hand, with a 6" tail in front of your hand.
2. Using the yarn attached to the ball, weave it behind your index finger, in front of your middle finger, behind your ring finger, and in front of your pinkie. Make sure that you do not pull the yarn too tightly.
3. Continue to weave the yarn—all the way around your pinkie in front of your middle finger and in front of your index finger.
4. Repeat steps two and three working from your index finger to your pinkie and back again. Hold the yarn end with your thumb to your palm so it does not get in your way. You now have two loops on your finger.
5. Lift the lower loop on each finger over the top loop and off your finger, letting the loop down the back. There is now a loop on each finger.
6. Repeat steps two, three, and five until your knitting is desired length.
7. To finish your piece, take the loop from your pinkie and place it on your ring finger, above the loop already there. Lift the lower loop over the top loop and off your finger, letting it drop down the back. Place the remaining loop from your ring finger on your middle finger, and repeat lifting off/moving over until you have one loop left on your index finger.
8. Cut the yarn attached to the ball, leaving a 6" tail, and then pull the tail through the last loop.
9. If desired, make three strands of the same length and then braid the strands into one scarf by pulling a six-inch yarn piece through each stitch of the last row of each strand and then tied in a knot to tie all three strands together while making a fringe.

Mildred

Mildred, a 72-year-old woman with Alzheimer's, was living at home with her husband who tended to her until his recent fatal coronary. Initially, Mildred went to live with her only daughter and her family, but Mildred steadily declined and her Alzheimer's worsened to the point that she was often forgetful, would wander the house during the night, and one night even wandered out of the house only to be found by the police a few hours later. Her physician believes that the loss of her husband was a significant event that accelerated Mildred's Alzheimer's and he recommended that Mildred move to the memory care unit at the local skilled nursing facility. Mildred is physically mobile and physically able to complete most of her ADLs with verbal cues, but she is beginning to demonstrate agitated behaviors when she is confused and these behaviors are occurring several times each day. Mildred was evaluated by the facility OT and goals included independence in ADLs and decreasing Mildred's agitation. Cheryl, the OTA, spends most of her day in the unit and initially works with Mildred on using laminated picture sequence boards in completing all the steps of each ADL task. Cheryl also tries several calming techniques with Mildred, but nothing seems to be particularly effective. Over time, Cheryl observes that Mildred seems slightly calmer when looking at old photographs in a coffee table book. She asks Mildred about these pictures in one of Mildred's more lucid moments and Mildred tells her that the pictures remind her of her picture albums "at home." Cheryl begins to think and decides to call Mildred's daughter and arranges to borrow Mildred's albums; she scans many of the pictures and then prints them. Since Cheryl has saved all the photos (in an encrypted file), she is able to print out more pictures as needed. Over the next several occupational therapy sessions, Cheryl and Mildred make collages, and on Mildred's more lucid days, they even make scrapbook pages. Overwhelmingly, the staff on the unit notice that Mildred is experiencing fewer agitated periods, down from several in a day to only three to four a week. Not only did Cheryl find the right trigger to calm Mildred effectively, she also made the collages and scrapbook pages a purposeful activity greatly treasured not only by Mildred but also by her daughter and grandchildren when Mildred passed away 2 years later (Fig. 20.9).

Nancy

Nancy has a history of diabetes that eventually led to a right leg below-knee amputation and current placement in the inpatient rehabilitation center. Nancy was an

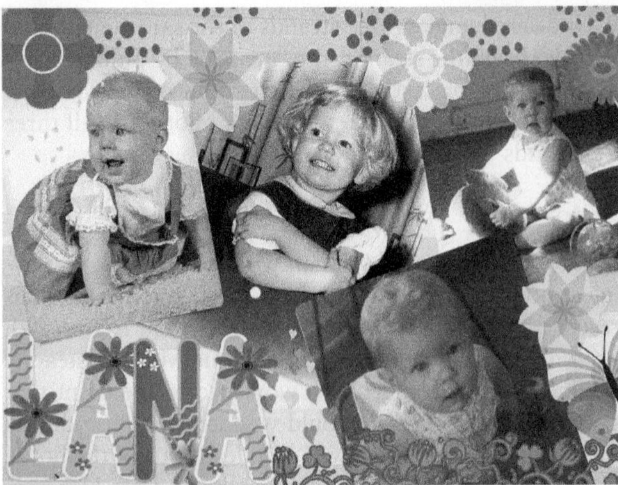

Figure 20.9 Mildred's scrapbook page.

avid gardener prior to her amputation and her husband brought her flowers every other day. There were several raised beds in the rehabilitation center and Nancy's OTA, Becky, developed a treatment plan that included gardening with adaptive strategies. For the days that they could not get out into the planting beds, Becky and Nancy made some pretty vases to set on the tables in the dining room while working on standing balance and endurance. The vases were a huge hit with the staff and residents, and in other therapy sessions, Nancy made vases for patients to have in their rooms (Fig. 20.10).

Supplies

- Different sized and shaped jars
- Food coloring

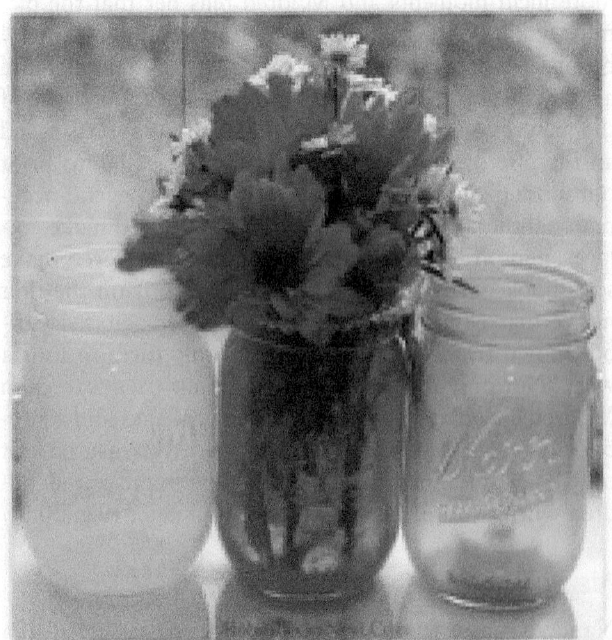

Figure 20.10 Nancy's tinted vases.

- White glue
- Paintbrush

Instructions

1. Pour glue onto a paper plate and mix with food coloring to desired tint.
2. Brush tinted glue all over the jar.
3. Let it dry for 24 hours.

Betty

Betty loved to decorate for the holidays. However, she had become depressed about her deteriorating multiple sclerosis because she and her husband made the painful choice to place her in a nursing home in order to receive the care she needed during the day when her husband was not home. He picked her up every weekend to go home and be with her family. She loved to show pictures of her house all decorated for Thanksgiving and Christmas, but it made her sad that she could not do that anymore. Lucy, the OTA, told her that of course, she could continue with her decorating activities. They would come up with a plan to make some decorations for her room, taking into account Betty's fluctuating energy levels and fine motor skills. In the first project, Betty decided to create a pinecone wreath for her door so she could put an orange-colored ribbon on the top for November and change it to a red-colored ribbon for Christmas. Eventually, Betty had four seasonal wreaths for her door that only required a small change of ribbon for the specific holidays (Fig. 20.11).

Mark

Mark was a very quiet man who had returned to the states after a military tour in the Middle East with burns from an explosion and limited shoulder range of motion and posttraumatic stress disorder (PTSD). He witnessed nine of his fellow soldiers die in that explosion. Not surprisingly, he had the nightmares and flashbacks but would not talk about them to anyone in the rehab unit of the veterans' hospital. In high school, Mark took art classes and was a very good sketch artist. Joe, a fellow soldier and OTA, decided to suggest painting as a modality that would help with the shoulder ROM and hopefully as a way for Mark to express his feelings. Mark refused at first saying he was not a painter, but Joe gently prodded him to give it a try and more as a method to "exercise the shoulder" than as an outlet for the feelings. Mark began with abstract paintings, big eruptions of black and gray. He only spoke to Joe in vague terms at first when describing his paintings, but as time progressed, he would discuss some of the meanings of the paintings and eventually his

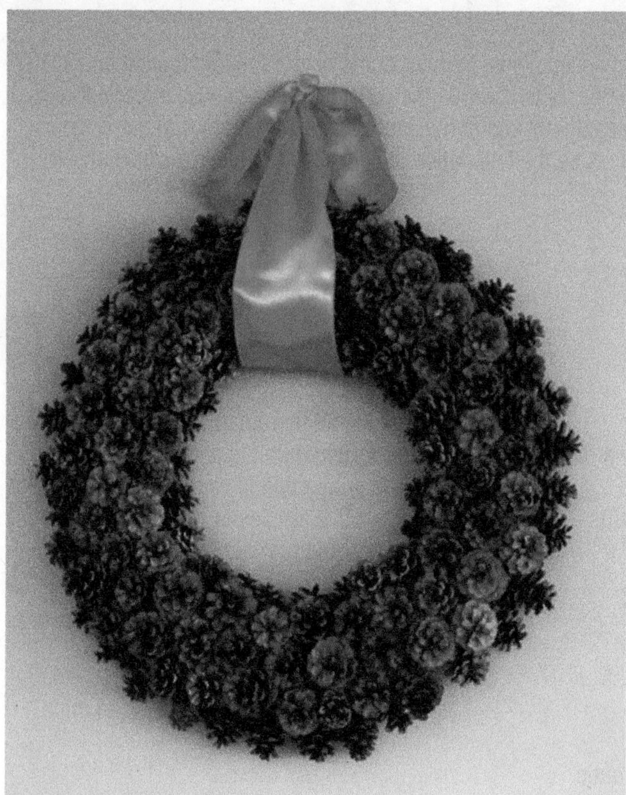

Figure 20.11 Betty's pinecone wreath.

experiences overseas. Joe and Mark kept in touch after Mark was discharged and Mark shared that whenever he was feeling some of the PTSD symptoms, he always returned to painting until he could work out what the triggers were or the feelings associated with them.

Matthew

Mathew had a typical birth, but at age 2, he was diagnosed with spinal muscular atrophy. As he grew older, all of his muscles slowly lost function. He was evaluated at age 5 by a home health OT. Due to his weakened immune system, Matthew needed home health services and home teaching from the local school district. By this age, Mathew was on a ventilator, had to be in bed as his spinal cord muscles could no longer support him in a sitting position, had lost his ability to speak but was able to blink to indicate preferences, and was only able to move his index fingers and big toes. According to his home teacher, cognitively, he was functioning at kindergarten level. Matthew's goals included activities that facilitated pincer grasp, visual–perceptual and tracking, and finger flexion and extension to indicate wants and make choices from picture cards or using his electronic communication systems. Staci, Matthew's OTA, often saw him just before the home teacher arrived for his daily lessons; Staci knew that Matthew was learning to read *The Very Hungry Caterpillar* by Eric Carle and decided to do corresponding craft activities. Today, she decided they would create paper chain caterpillars. Staci placed Mathew's hand above a paper plate with a dollop of glue and asked him to bend his finger to dip into the glue. She then placed his hand above a strip of construction paper and had him extend his finger to dot the glue onto the paper at one end. Next, Staci pulled the other end of the strip over the glue to make a loop. Then, she placed another strip through the loop and then had Matthew put more glue on the end of the strip while she pasted the loop. They continued until they had several caterpillars. Then, Staci helped Matthew place two glue dots on one loop so that she could attach squiggly eyes. Once the caterpillars had dried, Staci and the nurse placed them in different parts of the room (e.g., around his IV stand, hanging from the ceiling, on the footboard of the bed) to work on visual tracking skills. Matthew loved his caterpillars and often would try to gaze at his family members, his teacher, or the nurse and then to a caterpillar to "show" them his masterpieces (Fig. 20.12).

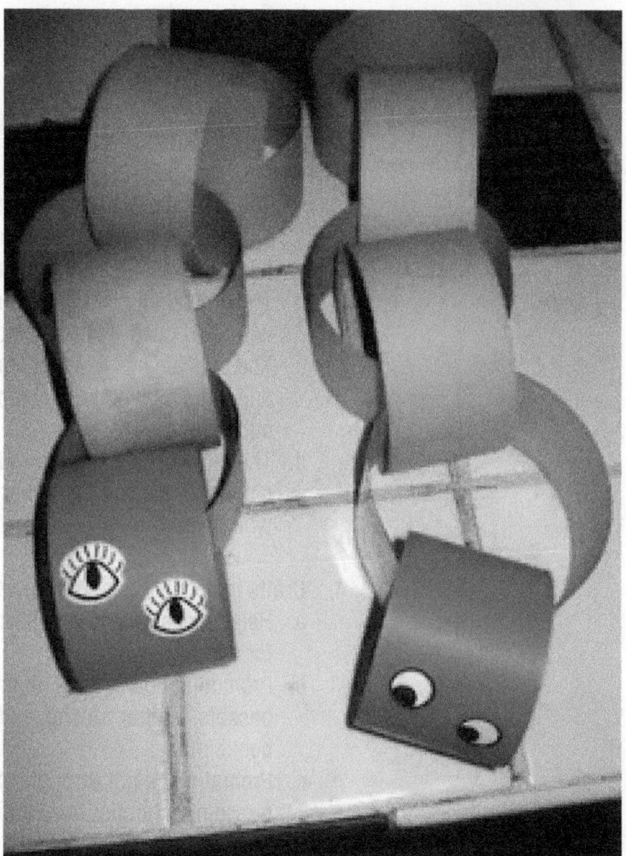

Figure 20.12 Matthew's hungry caterpillars.

Summary

Holding a significant place in the history of occupational therapy, crafts have been and remain an important treatment modality for OT practitioners to use with their clients. Crafts play an important role in most every practice setting. They are meaningful and purposeful activities for many and can open the door to new business ventures as well as be the foundation to help clients achieve a sense of self-confidence and worth.

Review Questions

1. Two major philosophies significantly influenced the practice of occupational therapy:
   a. Socratic method and Arts and Crafts movement
   b. Pragmatism and Arts and Crafts movement
   c. Moral treatment and pragmatism
   d. Moral treatment and impressionist movement

2. In the early years, crafts as a therapeutic modality was used by:
   a. Nurses
   b. Social workers
   c. Psychiatrists
   d. Reconstruction aides

3. A tenet of moral treatment is understanding:
   a. The critical link between the patient's activities and activity patterns and his or her physical and mental health
   b. The critical link between purposeful work and good mental health
   c. The critical link between crafts and patients who were deemed as subhuman
   d. The influence of a person's life circumstances on his or her health and well-being

4. Crafts in occupational therapy are about:
   a. Helping clients find an alternative means for earning money
   b. Promoting health through making baskets, leather tooling, and bookbinding
   c. Promoting health through "doing" and providing an outlet for creative energy and purposeful activity
   d. Helping clients express their deepest feelings and fears

5. Occupational therapy founders believed crafts served multiple purposes including:
   a. The production of well-made, useful, and attractive articles or the accomplishment of a useful task
   b. The pathway to link occupations and exercise
   c. The development of a healthy mind and strong body
   d. The critical connection between mind, body, and spirit

6. Crafts, as opposed to exercise programs or games, are:
   a. An activity a client does to stave off boredom
   b. Individualized to the client's needs and leads to a meaningful and valued end product
   c. Its nonthreatening nature
   d. Individualized to meet the needs of the institution by providing free labor in maintenance of the facility

7. Teaching a client a craft can:
   a. Provide a much-valued worker identity role, that of craftsperson
   b. Provide a role within the facility
   c. Lead to another form of occupation
   d. Lead to a productive and valued hobby or leisure activity

8. In the case study that involves Charlie, Jose, Candace, and Mason, the OTA:
   a. Provided each child the necessary assistance needed in order for the child to feel successful
   b. Individualized the craft activity as desired by the child
   c. Created a new activity for each child
   d. Graded one activity to meet the needs and goals for all four children

9. In the case study of Matthew, what other craft activities could the OTA have done that would have met his goals?
   a. Created a caterpillar magnetic game board that would have allowed Matthew to use his index finger to push his game piece to the next spot on the board
   b. Created a caterpillar balloon animal to hang from his IV pole
   c. Created a caterpillar sock puppet to put on Matthew's hand
   d. Created a caterpillar drawing by having Matthew choose by eye gaze which color marker to use

10. In the case study of Mildred, the OTA tries several interventions to decrease Mildred's agitation; the most effective intervention was:
    a. Using laminated picture sequence boards
    b. Calming techniques
    c. Looking at old photographs in a coffee table book
    d. Making collages and scrapbook pages using pictures from Mildred's family photo albums

Practice Activities

Complete an activity analysis of one or more of the crafts mentioned in this chapter.

How would you grade the craft activities noted in the case studies? Select one and demonstrate how you could grade it for your classmates.

Create a thematic unit for a group of clients. It should consist of a minimum of eight activities that are age and skill appropriate for the group of clients and include alternative activities in case your original idea does not work out.

Think of someone you know with special needs—what goal do or should they have and how would you address the goal using a craft activity?

References

Bissell JC, Mailloux Z. The use of crafts in occupational therapy for the physically disabled. *Am J Occup Ther* 1981;35:369–374.

Bockoven JS. Legacy of moral treatment—1800's to 1910. *Am J Occup Ther* 1971;25:223–225.

Breines EB. Media education based on the philosophy of pragmatism. *Am J Occup Ther* 1989;43:461–464.

Dickie VA. Establishing worker identity: a study of people in craft work. *Am J Occup Ther* 2003;57:250–261.

Meyer A. Philosophy of occupational therapy. *Arch Occup Ther* 1922;1:1–10.

Peloquin SM. Moral treatment: contexts considered. *Am J Occup Ther* 1989;43:537–544.

Peloquin SM. Moral treatment: how a caring practice lost its rationale. *Am J Occup Ther* 1994;48:167–173.

Reed KL. Tools of practice: heritage or baggage? 1985 Eleanor Clarke Slagle Lecture. *Am J Occup Ther* 1986;40:597–605.

Reed KL. Occupational therapy values and beliefs: the formative years: 1904–1929. *OT Pract* 2006;11(7):21–25. Reprinted in Slater DY. (2008). *Reference Guide to the Occupational Therapy Ethics Standards* (pp. 121–125). Bethesda, MD: AOTA Press.

United States Social Security Administration. (2012, November 14). *Frequently Asked Questions*. Retrieved from http://www.ssa.gov/history/hfaq.html

Woodside HH. The development of occupational therapy 1910–1929. *Am J Occup Ther* 1971;25:226–230.

CHAPTER 21

Adaptive Equipment and Adaptive Devices

Margaret Christenson, MPH, OTR/L, FAOTA

Key Terms

Adaptive equipment and/or assistive devices—Products, apparatus, and occasionally services that make it possible for a person with a disability to perform everyday activities, preferably without assistance from another person.

CANIS—A genus of carnivorous mammals, of the family Canidae, including the dogs and wolves.

Slope and rise—The steepness or angle of a slope is dependent on the length of a ramp and the height of the rise.

Universal design—Products, services, or environments that meet the needs of the widest range of users possible regardless of age, ability, or preference.

Learning Objectives

After studying this chapter, readers should be able to:

- Explain the factors that came together to impact the development of rehabilitation.
- Describe at least five assistive devices that may compensate for age-related physical changes in the bathroom of an older client.
- Discuss falls prevention and how assistive devices play an important role in reducing fall risk.

Introduction

Adaptive equipment (AE) or **assistive devices** (AD) are part of the much larger category of assistive technology (AT), which is discussed in Chapter 22. Tools or items defined as AE or AD (these terms are used interchangeably) include a wide variety of products, apparatus, and occasionally services that make it possible for a person with a disability to perform everyday activities, preferably without assistance from another person. Occupational therapy intervention plans often include AE as a long-range adaptation for a client.

The purpose of AE includes helping a person move around, see, communicate, eat, take care of toileting needs, and/or get dressed. These tasks are thoroughly delineated in Table 1 of the *Occupational Therapy Practice Framework III* (AOTA, 2014). These tasks are referred to as activities of daily living (ADLs) or instrumental activities of daily living (IADLs) (please also refer to Chapter 23, *Activities of Daily Living*). In this chapter, we will look at some of the AE or durable medical equipment used to assist people to engage in ADL/IADLs as well as the functional categories where they are applied. Durable medical equipment refers to devices that are "primarily and customarily used to serve a medical purpose, and generally are not useful to a person in the absence of illness or injury" (DRNPA, 2012, p. 7). To find out if Medicare will cover the cost of a particular piece of AE, visit www.Medicare.gov.

Because it is difficult to separate AE from assistive technology (AT), we will also briefly discuss AT and its relevance to helping clients lead productive lives. Keep in mind that like AE, "Assistive technology is any service or tool which can help an older person or a person with a disability perform activities that might otherwise be difficult or not be possible" (Eldercare Locator, 2012). There are no private insurance plans or public program that will pay for all types of AT (Christenson, 2011). However, "assistive technology may be funded under Medicare Part B as durable medical equipment, prosthetic devices, and orthotic devices. Medicare Part B pays for power wheelchairs and augmentative communication devices" (DRNPA, 2012, p. 7). Vocational rehabilitation is another federal source of funding for AT (From the Field 21.1).

"Almost anything *can* be adapted to help in a task" (amhistory.si.edu/polio/howpolio/assistive.htm, n.d.). This statement described the urgent situation of patients during the polio epidemics of the mid-20th century and is included in a display entitled "Whatever Happened to Polio?" at the Smithsonian's National Museum of American History in Washington, DC (Smithsonian, n.d.). The display tells the story of the polio epidemics of the 1950s in America. During this period, when people returned home from the hospital following the acute phase of polio, there were no devices available to help them do daily tasks. We will discuss how their needs were, in large part, the catalyst for the disability rights era, development of the field of physical rehabilitation, and adaptive equipment.

We Are People First

There has been and continues to be much discussion about the correct terminology to use when describing a person with a disability. The World Health Organization (WHO) defines disability as an umbrella term, covering impairments, activity limitations, and participation restrictions and characteristics of the natural, built, cultural, and social environments (WHO, 2012). Overcoming the difficulties faced by people with disabilities requires interventions to remove environmental and social barriers. A person is more or less disabled based on the intersection between himself/herself and the many types of environments within which he/she interacts (WHO, 2001). Such terms as differently abled and physically challenged and, most recently, handicapable have been suggested as appropriate descriptors for people with disability (Wheelchair Dancer, 2012). You may encounter some of these words when discussing disability with colleagues or clients or when you are searching for information about assistive devices. Many people feel very strongly about a term. As you have likely noted, in this textbook, we use the phrase "*person with* a disability." Remember the person comes first.

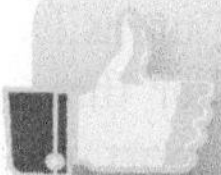

FROM THE FIELD 21.1

Funding Assistive Devices

Finding information on funding for assistive devices is always a challenge. The online booklet *Assistive Technology: How to Pay for the Device or Service that You Need* is available at www.drnpa.org. It is an excellent resource, and although it was created for the State of Pennsylvania, it may lead you to ideas for funding resources in your area.

Historical Account of Assistive Devices—from Cane to Contemporary

The first adaptive device is not identified as such, but we can speculate it was when someone needed to reach and retrieve an item and grabbed a stick or rod to assist in the task. As time passed, the humble stick began to signify authority or, when moved with force through the air, a weapon and, when it was leaned upon, a walking stick or a cane. Indeed, the stick has served many purposes throughout history (Monek, 1997). The terms cane and walking stick are used interchangeably. There are at least two explanations of how the term "cane" became part of our lexicon. The most commonly recognized explanation in the Western world is that after the 16th century, materials such as reeds, sugarcane, palms, rattans, and bamboo were used to make shafts. The term "cane" was adopted to describe these walking devices (Monek, 1997).

However, there is a second more colorful explanation for the term cane. In Roman times, packs of wild dogs infested the streets. Pedestrians had to carry a heavy stick with a short, sharp point to defend themselves against these savage animals (Monek, 1997). This club, by natural substitution of cause and effect, was called **CANI**, which meant literally "for a dog." A more befitting term could not have been chosen. The plural of CANI is CANIS (CANES), the precise designation by which they are now known (Monek, 1997, p. 20).

During the Crusades, hundreds of thousands of pilgrims traveling to the Holy Land used strong sticks about five feet long with a pointed metal spike at the bottom to dig into the earth on steep inclines and to fend off ferocious animals, much as the original users had done in Rome (Monek, 1997). The top portion was hollow and could be unscrewed to conceal religious relics and valuables. Many items were smuggled across borders in the cane (Monek, 1997). As the 19th century came to a close, so too did the routine using of canes. By the mid-20th century, canes were used primarily by hikers and climbers, or as an orthopedic aid (Monek, 1997). Other assistive devices may have had a similar history beginning as something basic and evolving into something more applicable for someone with a disability, but history most colorfully documents the evolution of the cane.

Today, we face a major issue that usually is not solvable through use of a wheelchair or a cane, although either may help. This dire public health issue is that as people age, they usually become more susceptible to falls. Understandably, as falls increase, people become fearful of repeat falls (please also refer to Chapter 35, *Health and Well-Being,* and Chapter 37, *Productive Aging*). Thus begins a downward spiral. Fear of falling may impact stability and stamina because when people are afraid, they exercise less. Reduced movement or activity causes people to be less able to do common daily tasks. When a person experiences movement issues, adaptive equipment is often the critical mediator for many to perform simple activities of daily living, such as bathing and dressing. Despite challenges and even if they have difficulties with daily tasks, most people still see themselves as active and healthy (Yeung, 2003). This is important to understand because for many older individuals, a combination of AE may make the difference between being able to ambulate and live independently or require placement in a long-term care facility (please also refer to Chapter 33, *Rehabilitation, Disability, and Participation*).

Assistive Devices or Equipment

Occupational therapy practitioners use the term "assistive" to describe items that may be prescribed to help a client do a specific task. Assistive devices vary in their complexity. Many pieces of AD are surprisingly simple, but their impact on the lives of the user can be enormous. Some are as simple as a reacher, a tool that helps you grab an object you cannot reach, a cane to make moving around easier, and a grab bar attached to an adjacent wall or on the floor to provide support to get up from a seated position. More complex AE includes both manual and motorized wheelchairs, and amplification devices for a telephone or television that make sounds easier to hear.

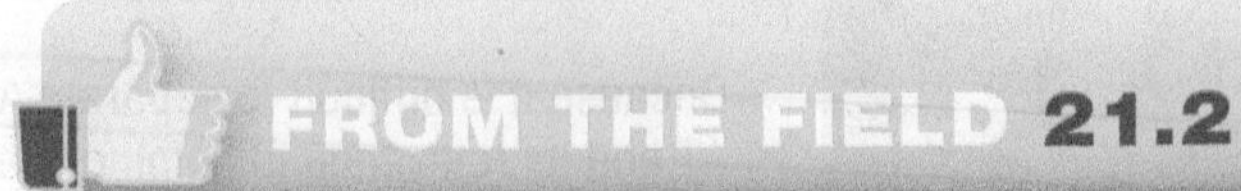

Causes of Disability

If you consider the possibility of becoming physically disabled, you may think that accidents are usually the cause. However, 73% of all disabilities are caused by illness, so fewer than one-third are the result of an accident (Principal Financial Group, 2012).

Just because someone needs a specific adaptation or adaptive product does not mean that he or she will accept and use it. How these tools or equipment are introduced and recommended is extremely important in determining whether it will be used. Part of any unwillingness to use AE may be reluctance to change. However, when you think about it, the main reason clients resist AE is all in the words. As we just discussed, "assistive" implies the "need for help," and most people want to be perceived as healthy and active. What typically happens is that people "make do" until a looming crisis becomes overwhelming and there is little choice but to seek help. An important role as an OTA is to be sensitive to a client's feelings. When introducing an "assistive device," it is important to convey that it will make doing the task easier rather than to focus on disability issues (From the Field 21.2).

Universal Design

Another way to encourage clients to use AE is to recommend products that are **universally designed.** This design approach means that a wide range of people, no matter their age or ability, can use the tool or product to make tasks easier. An example is the OXO brand of universally designed kitchen tools. Their vegetable peeler has a large, well-contoured handle that color contrasts with the blade and requires very little effort to use by right- or left-handed people. And it looks nice. Creating utensils and other tools/products that people *want* rather than something they merely *need* is an exceedingly important concept associated with universal design. Most people are inclined to want (and use) something that is attractive rather than something that looks utilitarian.

Therefore, the aesthetics of the item is an important consideration in convincing people to want the items that they need.

In addition to recognizing the importance of aesthetics, universally designed products must be developed with various users' needs in mind. The result is a product that is usable by the broadest spectrum of individuals possible. In the case of OXO, it means designing products for young and old, male and female, left- and right-handed,

FROM THE FIELD 21.3

Stephen Hawking

Without high-tech AE, the brilliant physicist and author, Stephen Hawking, would be unable to communicate. Hawking has a slowly progressing form of amyotrophic lateral sclerosis (ALS). A speech generating device has enabled Hawking to operate a computer keyboard by using small movements of his body. A voice synthesizer then speaks what he has typed. For lectures and media appearances, Hawking speaks fluently through his synthesizer. His device uses a predictive text entry system (like a Google search), which requires only the first few characters of a word in order to automatically complete the spoken output. When he prepares answers without the synthesizer, he has to enter each letter manually, and his system can only produce words at a rate of about one per minute (Stephen Hawking, n.d.).

and many with special needs (OXO, n.d.). Occupational therapy practitioners have a great deal of expertise to add to the universal design process (From the Field 21.3).

Who Benefits from Adaptive Equipment?

Individuals who benefit most from AE are those who have difficulty in one of the following:

Vision
Hearing
Mobility
Balance
Sitting
Rising
Bending
Reaching
Climbing stairs
Lifting and carrying items
Grasping
Cognitive skills such as reasoning, memory, and problem solving

Adaptive equipment and assistive devices and technologies such as wheelchairs, walkers, canes, prostheses, hearing aids, visual aids, and specialized computer software and hardware can be used to increase productivity, hearing, vision, and communication capacities. More specifically, mobility aids assist with ambulation or otherwise improve someone's ability to move about. These devices enable freedom of movement similar to, for instance, unassisted walking or the ability stand up from a chair. Reachers, kitchen utensils with built-up handles, grab bars, and bath chairs assist with doing daily living activities. There is AE designed to help people write. Examples of low-tech assistive writing devices include easy grasp pens or pen and pencil grippers (Fig. 21.1B). A high-tech innovation is the Livescribe Smartpen, which records everything you write and hear (Fig. 21.1A).

With the assistance of these devices and technologies, people experiencing loss in function are better able to enhance their abilities and are, hence, better able to live independently and participate in their home and community (WHO, 2001). Since able-bodied people usually take doing ADLs or IADLs independently for granted, they rarely stop and think about what life would be like if they were unable to walk under their own power, hear without the assistance of a hearing aid, eat, dress, or take care of toileting themself. For many people with physical, sensory, or cognitive disabilities, this is not a reality. Fortunately, modern industry has and continues

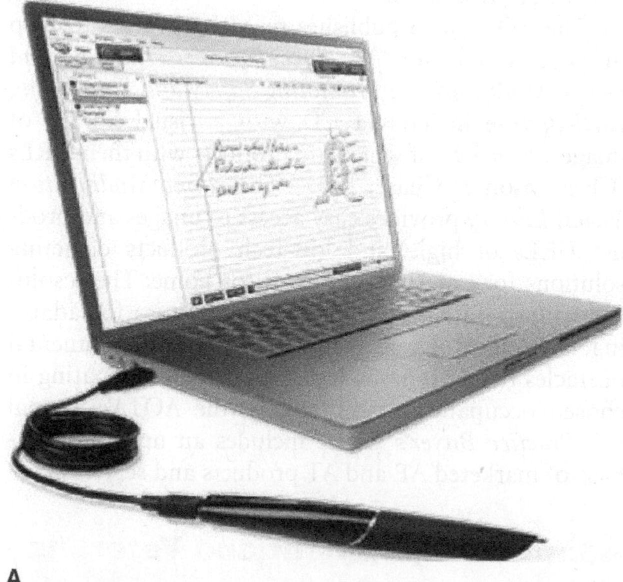

A

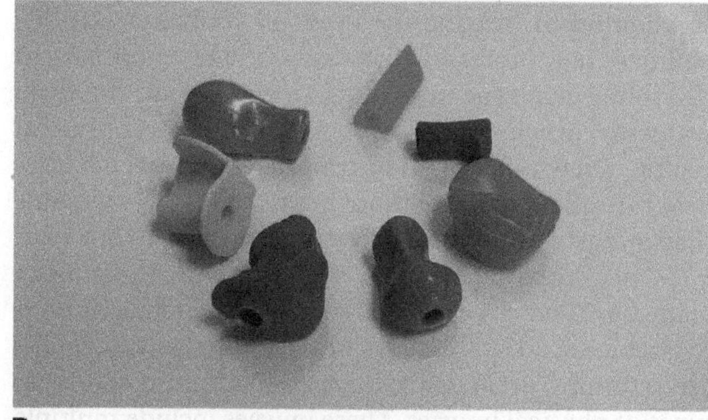

B

Figure 21.1 **A:** The Livescribe Smartpen (www.livescribe.com) **B:** Pencil grippers.

to make it possible to have different adaptations in the home and workplace to make it possible to conduct these tasks with little or no assistance.

Resources for Adaptive Equipment

Finding the appropriate product for a client may take time and research, but there are several ways to make this task easier. Consult with your colleagues. They are an important front-line resource. You can look at catalogs and talk with AE vendors at conferences. An online image search like Google Images can also be helpful, especially if you have an idea of what you are looking for and can visualize or describe it but do not know what it is called.

AbleData (www.AbleData.com) is an Internet resource that provides objective information about AE, AT, and rehabilitation equipment. Almost 40,000 product listings are included in 20 different categories in the database. AbleData is supported by the National Institute on Disability and Rehabilitation Research (NIDRR). Wheelchair Net (www.wheelchairnet.org) is another Internet resource of multiple companies that carry many AE and AT resources.

The AOTA also publishes several resources to help in your search for AE. *Occupational Therapy and Home Modifications: Promoting Safety and Supporting Participation* includes a CD with a visual library of images, over 200 of which are products with their URLs (Christenson & Chase, 2011). The *Home Modification Visual Library* provides easy access to images and product URLs of high- and low-tech products depicting solutions for potential problems for home. These solutions illustrate a wide range of possibilities for adapting, circumventing, or compensating for environmental obstacles that may impede clients from participating in chosen occupations. Additionally, the AOTA's annual *OT Practice Buyer's Guide* includes an updated database of marketed AE and AT products and services.

Adaptive Equipment and Veterans Care

In addition to meeting the needs of civilians with disabilities, our profession has always and continues to rise to the challenge of treating veterans returning from war with complex physical, cognitive, and psychological injuries. New types of body armor and improved battlefield care allow many of those injured to survive wounds that in past wars would have proved fatal. More than 95% of troops wounded in the Iraq and Afghanistan wars have survived, many with catastrophic injuries (Marchione, 2012). Because of these advances, veterans are returning home with different (and more complex) types of physical injuries. These injuries include multiple amputations, traumatic brain injury (TBI), and posttraumatic stress disorder.

A rise in survival rates, coupled with resultant often severe and complex polytrauma, has led to increased research in ways to enable these veterans to actively participate in daily living. To meet the needs of wounded veterans, the trickle-down effect of this innovation research from recent as well as past military conflicts has historically led to advances in AD and technology for veterans and, in turn, their applicability for the civilian population. For instance, the developer of Stove Guard, a reminder system that turns off a stove, personally shared with me how he had been able to make several improvements to his product through grants targeted for assistance to veterans with TBI. Although the Stove Guard was originally designed for people with dementia, due to recent product improvements, the manufacturer is now reaching out to a wider market, including veterans with TBI. Like their fellow soldiers from previous wars, product design research increased and continues to increase in response to an identified need to provide veterans with AE that is intended to improve the quality of their lives.

Poliomyelitis and the Emergence of Assistive Devices

Prior to the middle of the 20th century, poliomyelitis (polio) was referred to by several names including infantile paralysis because of its propensity to affect children (please also refer to Chapter 30, *Physical Conditions*). Infantile paralysis or polio was the first disease of epidemic proportions in US history that left those who survived with major disabilities. Because polio primarily affected children, there was tremendous public compassion for its survivors.

For the first time in US history, the combination of the return of disabled veterans of World War II and the polio epidemics of the 1950s created an influx of people with different disabilities but comparable need to live independently or with help to carry out daily living tasks. This identified need evolved into a common goal of developing organized and supported rehabilitation services. It was during this time that federal agencies led by the Department of Veterans Affairs began addressing technological issues of rehabilitation including client mobility, communication, and transportation that would forever shape the lives of those living with disabilities (Mann & Lane, 1995).

The Evolution of the Disability Rights Movement and Federal Legislation

The polio epidemics not only changed the lives of those who survived them but also facilitated profound cultural changes, spurring grassroots fund-raising campaigns that would revolutionize medical philanthropy. Along with veterans wounded in WWII, the polio epidemics gave rise to the modern field of rehabilitation. As one of the largest groups of people with a specific disability worldwide, survivors of polio helped to advance the modern disability rights movement through campaigns for social and civil rights of those with disabilities. For the most part, people who had been paralyzed by polio were fighters. As they matured (remember, a majority of people who developed polio were children), they began to demand the right to participate in mainstream society.

Prior to the mid-20th century, there was limited federal financial assistance for people with disabilities. In 1950, *Aid to the Permanently and Totally Disabled* was enacted, followed by other national programs for those with disabilities. Correspondingly, in 1961, the American National Standard Institute (ANSI) under the designation A117.1 published voluntary standards called *Making Buildings Accessible to and Usable by the Physically Disabled.* As they were voluntary standards and included minimal requirements, they were often ignored. In the mid-1960s, a federal commission found that the biggest obstacle facing persons with disability from being employed were inaccessible buildings. While the ANSI standards opened the door for recognizing the need for public accessibility, the beginning of public building accessibility came into its own in response to Congressional passage of the *Architectural Barriers Act* of 1968. It required that if federal funds were used to design, construct, alter, or prepare to lease a building, it had to be accessible.

As we now know, those who survived polio and veterans with disabilities were at the forefront of the disability rights movement that emerged out of these early volunteer standards and federal acts. They were instrumental in advocating for legislation such as the *Rehabilitation Act* of 1973, which placed even more clout on the *Architectural Barriers Act* of 1968 by protecting qualified individuals from discrimination based on their disability. The 1970s and 1980s saw additional federal acts for the education of children with "handicaps" and began the federal codes for accessible design.

The monumental and historic *Americans with Disabilities Act* (ADA) was signed into law in 1990. It has been responsible for many positive changes for persons with disabilities. The ADA extends civil rights protection to people with disabilities. The focus of the ADA is to make accessibility standardized in any portion of a building that is open to the general public. Many of its associated guidelines focus on specific public building accessibility, especially lobbies, restrooms, dining rooms, restaurants, and admissions offices (Christenson & Chase, 2011).

In case you may be wondering why we are discussing ADA and other federal accessibility legislation in this chapter on assistive devices typically used in the home, it is because there is a misperception that ADA standards apply to all situations, be they in public buildings or in a private home. They do not! Many product vendors and sometimes contractors recommend ADA standards to client for their home. For instance, ADA code states "Thresholds at doorways shall not exceed ¾" (19 mm) in height for exterior sliding doors or ½" (13 mm) for other types of doors" (ADAAG, 2002, Table 6.21). However, a ½" rise of a threshold will be difficult for someone with a shuffling gait to lift their feet over, or a person using a walker to lift the front legs or wheels over, or for a wheelchair user to roll over. Despite ADA code, a better, more universal option is a no-threshold design in a home. Understanding the profound importance of the ADA with regard to public accessibility is very important. So too is understanding that not all ADA code aligns well with what people may need in their homes to function at their greatest capacity (From the Field 21.4).

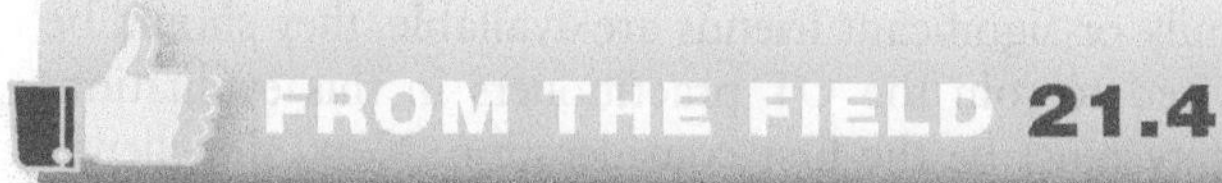

If you are working under the supervision of an OT as part of a home modifications team, consider the following. When planning the location of cabinet shelves, electrical outlets, light switches, closet rods, and other items that a client must reach, check and be sure that indeed, everything is within reach. While ADA code stipulates heights and placements of the aforementioned, a better calculation to use to determine the appropriate height or depth for cabinetry or placement of other fixtures is called the optimal reach zone (ORZ) (Wylde et al., 1994). The ORZ advocates a smaller reach area than ADA stipulates.

The *Assistive Technology Act* was originally signed into law in 1998 (US Government, 1998). Often called the Tech Act, it refers to assistive devices as "assistive technology devices" and defines them as "any item, piece of equipment, or product system that is used to increase, maintain, or improve functional capabilities of individuals with disabilities" (NECTAC, 2012). One could argue that this definition also encompasses AD, because it is difficult to neatly delineate between AD and AT. The Tech Act was amended in 2004 to "develop, support, expand, or administer alternative financing programs (AFPs) to allow individuals with disabilities and their family members, guardians, advocates, and authorized representatives to purchase AT [AD/AE] devices and services" (Federal Register, 2012).

Selecting Adaptive Equipment

The OTA, working under the supervision of the OT, may be called upon to conduct a client needs assessment by determining the functional capacity of the individual. As well, determining the desired occupation(s) of the person in his or her home is of greatest value when it is done as a team effort with the client *and* in the location (e.g., home or long-term care facility) where the AE will be used. If family or significant friends are available, they should be invited to join the OT practitioners in this evaluation. Safety must be the first consideration. Next, the client's desire and motivation to participate in a particular occupation and how AE can facilitate these desired outcomes is addressed. To enhance their use, products that are well suited to the client should be selected. When presented with options for AE, clients should be guided to plan ahead and think about how their needs may change over time. Ideally, when AE is at all complex, either with setup or use, the OT practitioner should train the client and his or her family to use it correctly.

Your clients and their caregivers may need assistance when deciding to obtain AE. Using AE may change the mix of services that a client requires or may affect the way that those personal services are provided. For instance, a client may be able to bathe independently by purchasing several pieces of equipment, including a bath bench, a long-handled soap brush, a handheld shower, and grab bars. By using this AE, the client will no longer need a home-health aide to assist with bathing. There is always more to the story, as this client has very few visitors and the family is concerned that the client will become more isolated without the aide's visit. The occupational therapy home assessment team will need to discuss the pros and cons of these arrangements and assist the family to make appropriate plans (From the Field 21.5).

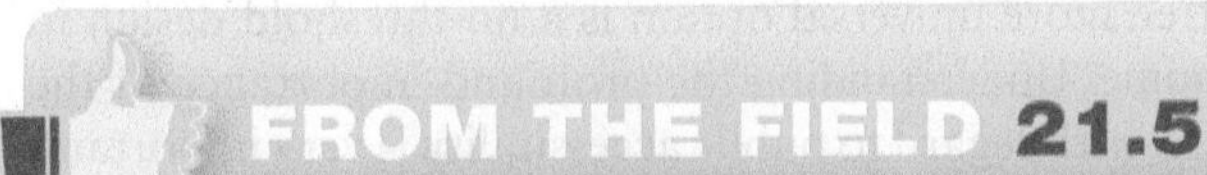

FROM THE FIELD 21.5

Fred Sammons

As groups of people with similar disability (e.g., survivors of polio) became quantifiable, there was growing interest in designing and providing helpful simple daily living tools. So too, the needs and the benefits of these products, with occasional tweaking for use with other groups of people with disability, became obvious. A small cottage industry began to develop. One of the founders of this industry was Fred Sammons, OTR/L, FAOTA. Following military service during the Korean War, Sammons began his career as an OT. A few years into his practice, he joined the staff of a clinic that treated people with amputations. It was there that he began to design and build devices to assist individuals to function better in their everyday lives. The demand for his devices grew and Sammons, Inc., was established in 1965 and has grown to a multimillion dollar business. It is now called Sammons Preston and is a part of Patterson Medical, Inc. Sammons received an Honorary Doctorate from Western Michigan University and is an Honorary Life Member of the American Occupational Foundation Board (AOTF, n.d.).

Aging in Place/Aging in Community

As they grow older, most people want to age in place in their homes, and many say they are modifying their residences to enable them to do so. As the name implies, aging in place is a concept associated with remaining in one's home until death. With an aging population and escalating health care and long-term care costs, nearly 90% of seniors indicate that they want to age in place, whether they need basic help or not (AARP, 2011; Bayer & Harper, 2000). Even if people need help with basic care or more complex medical care for loved ones or themselves, they would prefer the care to commence in current homes. With this in mind, home becomes the center of care. To foster this increased desire to receive care at home, most existing homes will require modifications, or new homes will need to be universally designed to align with successful aging in place. Along with structural changes, providing the infrastructure for life support equipment will also need to be considered during construction (or modification) so the home is equipped with, for example, adequate power. In addition to home modifications, AE will also play an active role in meeting clients' needs to safely age in their homes. Training clients and their caregivers in proper use of AE needs to be an integral part of the client's home care plan.

Assistive Equipment as a Part of Environmental (Home) Modifications

In the following section, AE solutions are presented to compensate for physical challenges typically linked to age-related changes. However, injuries or illness at any age may cause similar limitations. Although some of these limitations may be short term, a client may still require AE, but just for a shorter period of time. The younger client with foot surgery may have the same non–weight-bearing status as the older person who is unable to walk because of a chronic disease. Please note, there are also myriad solutions available to address use of AE for sensory and cognitive challenges but are beyond the scope of this chapter. Readers are encouraged to pursue further research on these topics.

Physical Changes, Physical Challenges

Physical skills are influenced by tone, strength, endurance, flexibility, balance and coordination, gait, and both voluntary and involuntary movement (AOTA, 2014). For the purposes of our discussion, they are divided into ten categories: stability, mobility, carrying items, climbing stairs, sitting, rising, bending, reaching, grasp, and pinch. Within each of these categories, we will look at various situations in the home to consider and adaptations to address the skill and help improve a client's optimal function. Like all other work involving client assessment, your role as an OTA in working with clients with home modifications will be done under the supervision of an OT.

The following information is reprinted from *PresentEase: Compensations for Age-Related Physical Changes*, M. A. Christenson, 2039 Lifease, Inc.®2002 by Lifease, Inc. Reprinted with permission.

Stability and Mobility

Stability is the ability to stand upright and move about without losing one's balance. The degree of a stability-related problem determines the kind and amount of support used or needed. The joints promote stability that allows for movement. Stability is the most important function to consider when dealing with falls prevention. Mobility is the capacity to move over a variety of surfaces whether walking or rolling, including lifting the foot up and over a rise or an obstacle. Surface resistance and degree of incline may be limiting factors associated with mobility.

Challenge: Entryway. Front entry doors should have a flat-entry zero threshold and a protected overhang. A small wood/metal, rubberized wedge-type ramp can be placed up to or over an existing threshold if it is not possible to renovate. Similar inserts exist for sliding doors. When ramps are needed because there are steps to navigate, ideally, they should have a 1:20 **slope and rise**; for every 1 foot of elevation, there should be twenty feet of extension. Please note, ADA ramp slopes between 1:16 and 1:20 are preferred with 1:20 being the easiest to use (ADAAG, 2002). At this slope and rise, no railing is required, and it allows someone using a wheelchair to move up and down the ramp with greater ease. The ability to manage an incline is related to both its slope and its length. Wheelchair users with disabilities affecting their arms or with low stamina have serious difficulty navigating long and steep inclines.

Challenge: Step edges. Many falls occur when there is a single step to navigate. Highlighting risers and edges of steps with brightly colored paint, particularly the top and bottom steps, as well as threshold steps, like those leading to a basement is important. Stair lighting or a string of LED lights along carpeted steps helps increase safety (From the Field 21.6).

Challenge: Outdoors. Ground surfaces should be kept clear and antislip whether from ice and snow or moss and wet leaves. Moss inhibitors can be applied to walkways. Ice grippers worn on shoe bottoms can reduce the possibility of slipping on ice or snow. In northern climates, slipping on black ice is often the cause of falls. Black ice is a thin coating of ice that is virtually impossible to see. It often occurs when ice melts and refreezes.

FROM THE FIELD 21.6

Front Steps

With the front steps depicted in the picture below, the minimum change needed to improve the safety factor would be to install handrails on both sides of the steps and color contrast the risers and top edge of the steps. Alternatively, a 1:20 ramp could be installed. The best change, of course, would be a no-step entrance (Fig. 21.2).

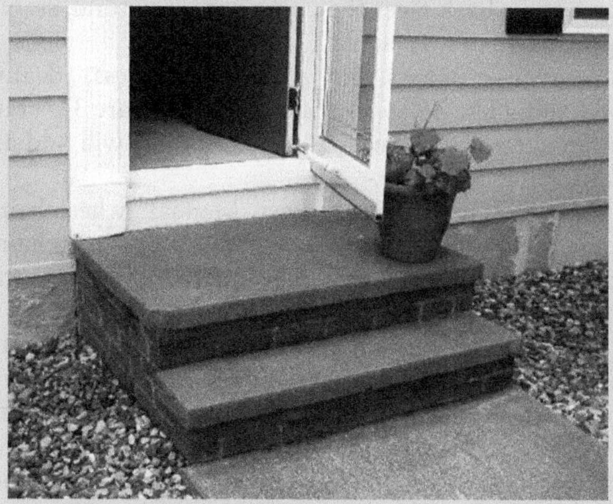

Figure 21.2 Two-step entry to a home (www.lifease.com).

Challenge: Getting the mail. For many people, the mailbox is an important link to family and friends, but making more than one trip to check if mail arrived can be tiring. Mail Alert (Fig. 21.3) is a device that fits on the mailbox door with a receiver that is kept in the house. When the mailbox door is opened, the alarm goes off in the house to alert someone that mail has arrived.

Challenge: Flooring. Remove scatter rugs on smooth floors, as they are truly a trip and fall hazard. If a client

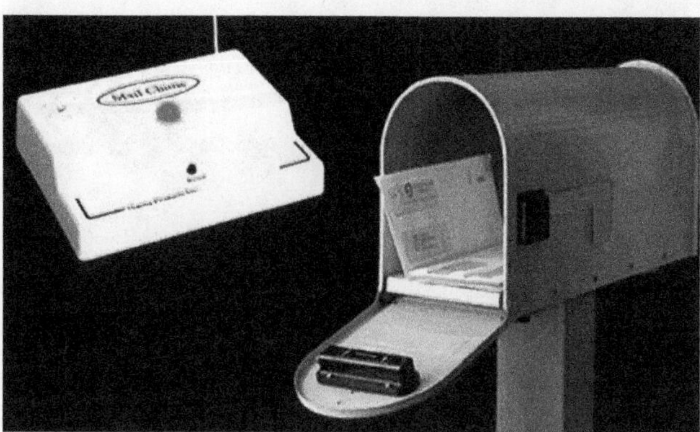

Figure 21.3 Mail Alert (www.gadgetshack.com).

is reluctant to remove them, suggest using nonslip material between the floor and rug and tuck fringes beneath the rug. Shiny surface flooring material looks wet. For someone who is fearful of falling, this misperception may produce an added layer of concern to their life. This glare can be reduced by substituting carpet, lightly buffed sheet vinyl, unbuffed tile, or wood flooring. In the bathroom and kitchen, floor covering should be laid to the back wall so someone using a wheelchair can access the sink, counter, and cooktop without having to deal with a change in flooring surface.

Challenge: Furniture arrangement. Stable furniture and handrails can be used for support. By turning furniture so its back faces the traffic path, a natural, stable support system is created.

Challenge: Doors. For wheelchair access, ideally, doors should be 36" wide. Many doorways are 32", but if more clearance is needed, an offset hinge will add an additional 2" of space.

Challenge: Turning radius. Manual wheelchairs require a turning radius of 5 feet. Most motorized chairs are wider and may require a turning radius of as much as 7 feet.

Challenge: Bathroom safety. Most people need something for support as they enter or exit a bathtub, get up from the toilet, or even move about the bathroom. They need grab bars (Fig. 21.4).

Grab bars are available at various price points and come in a variety of styles, colors, and textures. They can also be an attractive home accessory. With safety a foremost concern and if products are equal, for clients with a strong aesthetic sense, finding the more attractive option versus a standard institutional-looking grab bar (or any adaptation) may encourage and increase the likelihood that it will be used. Grab bars should be mounted vertically for entering or leaving the bathtub, horizontally on the wall opposite the tub opening, and vertically at entrance to bathtub to support getting in or out. They may also be installed on the wall by a commode and in place of towel bars around the bathroom. Grab bars need to be attached on studs or on 2" × 6" supports placed between the studs. If they are being installed on an exterior wall of brick or if the wall surface is covered with ¾" plywood, supports can be placed wherever needed. Grab bars can also be attached to walls with fasteners like WingIts, which allow grab bars or other products to be installed without structural backing (blocking). Please be aware that towel bars should never be used as grab bars, although grab bars can be used as towel bars.

Grab bar installation may become problematic if done by an "amateur carpenter." Encourage family members to seek out qualified professionals. Your local areas on aging or senior service centers may provide lists of preferred contractors.

Challenge: Showers. Although shower pans are available in up to a 3′ × 3′ size, a shower that small is impossible for anyone using a wheeled commode chair to maneuver effectively within. A "wet room" is a good alternative. It has no curb to cross to walk or roll into the shower area and has a handheld shower, a gradual slope to the drain, and an optional glass block wall (Fig. 21.5). Curbless showers should be large enough to allow full access for a shower chair. A long narrow shower built with glass blocks and a sloped floor to drain eliminates the need for a shower door. If there are doors on curbless showers, they should be installed with a tight seal on the door.

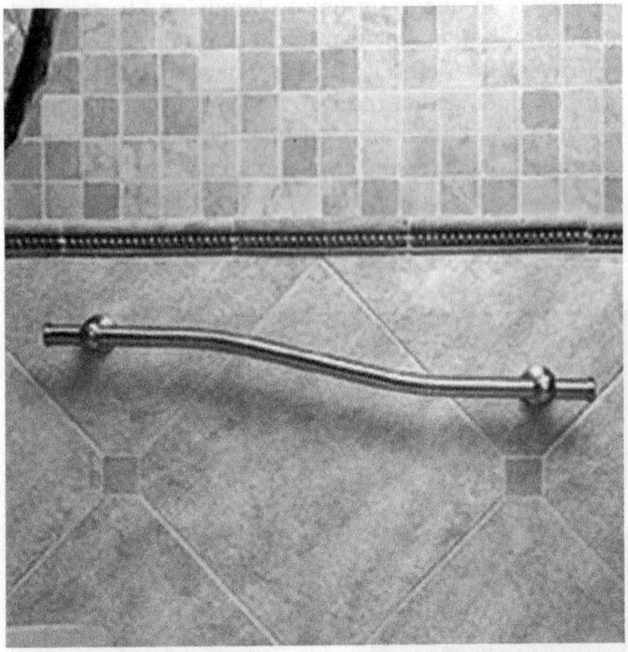

Figure 21.4 An aesthetically pleasing grab bar (www.adaptmy.com).

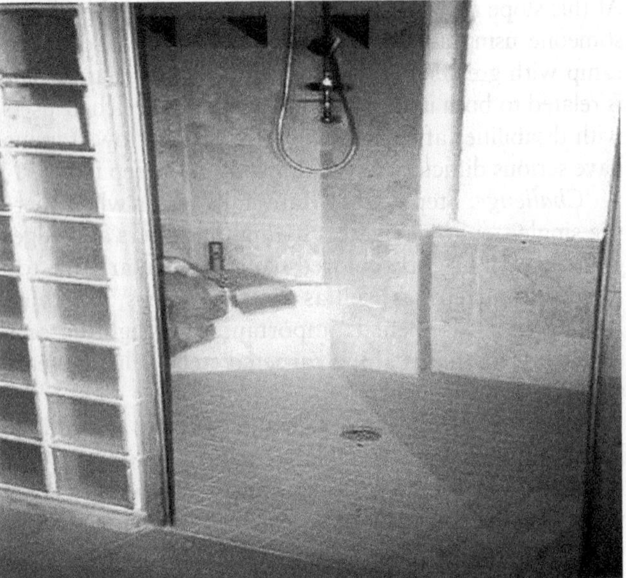

Figure 21.5 A wet room with a curbless roll-in shower (www.lifease.com). M. Christenson, (reproduced with permission).

Lifting and Carrying

Lifting is the process of moving something from below to at or above ground level. Lifting a heavy item from a lower cupboard shelf to the counter can be made easier by using an appliance lifter (Fig. 21.6).

Carrying is the process of lifting an item and moving it from one place to another. A variety of carts, trolleys, and other wheeled devices can transport items at home. A sturdy plant trolley on casters works well to move heavy trash bags or boxes from one area to another.

Climbing Stairs

Climbing stairs requires a combination of endurance, balance, leg strength, and also arm and hand strength if a handrail is used.

Challenge: Handrails. In public buildings, handrails often have a horizontal extension to provide support before or after climbing or descending stairs (Fig. 21.7). An extension is an important adaptation because it prevents shirt sleeves or purse straps from catching on the end cap of the railing, which could become a fall risk. This feature should be included on home handrails. Handrails on stairs, ramps, or other locations should contrast in color with the wall, be 1¼" to 1½" in diameter, and placed no more than 1½" from a wall.

Challenge: Ascending and descending stairs. Stair gliders allow people to get to another floor in a home. A curved chair glide has a self-leveling transport system that moves the lift carriage along a low-profile rail and around corners. A straight chair glide goes up a single flight of stairs. The seat and foot platform fold up to save space.

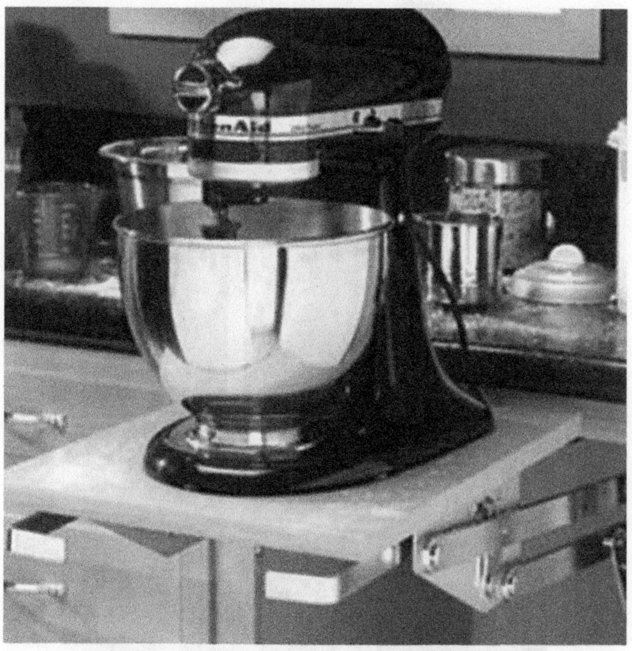

Figure 21.6 Appliance lifter (www.adaptmy.com).

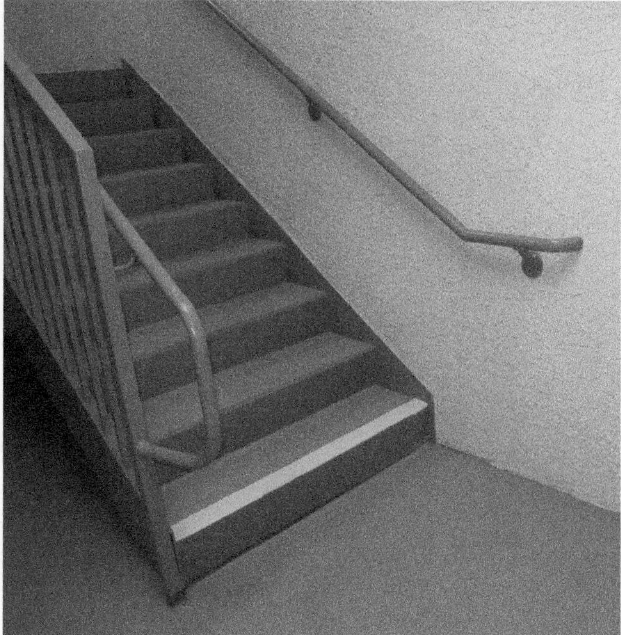

Figure 21.7 Color contrasting handrail with horizontal extension. (Amy Wagenfeld, reproduced with permission).

Challenge: Ascending and descending stairs. Plans for a home elevator can be included prior to construction of a two-story dwelling. It is done by siting identical closets one above the other on each floor, accounting for correct dimensions to accommodate the elevator and a mechanical room on the first floor. Home elevators increase the resale value of a house.

Sitting and Rising

Sitting and rising are the combined capabilities of getting up or down from a raised surface such as a bed, toilet, or couch. It also includes arising from the floor, tub bottom, and ground. The amount of support one needs to sit or rise includes handholds or anything sturdy to grasp or lean on.

Challenge: Chairs. Chairs should have wide solid arms, good neck support, and ample space underneath for a person to place the feet to allow ease in sitting and rising. A sled base chair (Fig. 21.8) is easy to get up from and easier to move, but canes or walkers can get caught on the horizontal supports (Christenson, 1990).

Challenge: Tables. A table must be high enough to allow the arms of a wheelchair to go under it. With round pedestal tables, wheelchair foot pedals often touch the pedestal, so it is hard to pull up close to the table. Tables with legs are preferred, and they happen to be more stable. But, in long-term care facilities, tables with legs are often avoided because they can get nicked from wheelchair foot pedals. Tables suited for people using wheelchairs are higher than for those

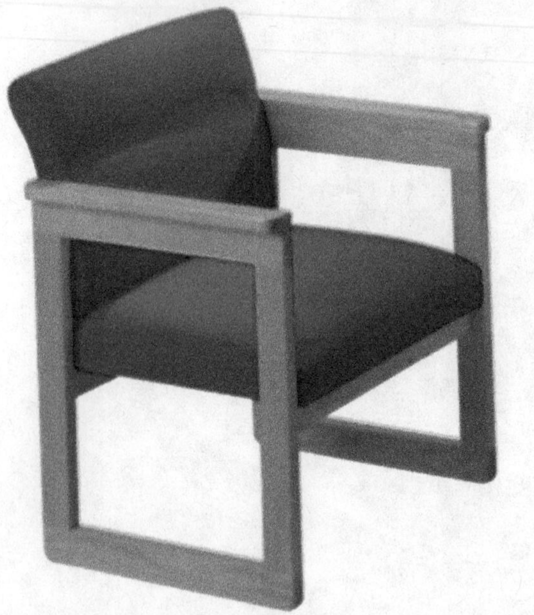

Figure 21.8 Sledbase chair (www.beyondtheofficedoor.com).

who are ambulatory and thus uncomfortable for them. Because of this design dilemma, table assignments at long-term care of senior facilities are often segregated: a sad example of how environments can separate rather than bring people together. A simple solution for the home or long-term care facility is to obtain a square table with apronless leaves. A person in a wheelchair can sit where one of these leaves has been placed. A clearance height of 29 ½″ (or more) from the floor will accommodate the arms of most wheelchairs (Fig. 21.9).

Challenge: Toilet/commode. Using a raised or regular height toilet is an individual decision. Raised toilets are referred to as comfort height, which is about 18″ from the floor. This height makes it easier for most to sit down or get up. However, if a client is unable to place both feet on the floor, a standard-height toilet, which is about 15″ from the floor may be the best solution. Installing grab bars around a standard or comfort height toilet should always be strongly recommended. If there is a wall beside the toilet, a grab bar could be installed there and a fold-down bar on the opposite side. If there is no wall, fold-down bars on both sides of the toilet can be installed. If grab bar installation is impossible, a grab pole may be installed (Fig. 21.10).

Challenge: Bathing. A "bath chair" does not automatically have a back, nor is a "bath bench" backless. Vendors and manufacturers use the terms interchangeably. A bath chair or bench is placed in a tub or shower. It has no extension on the outside of the tub. A client needs to be able to step into the tub and then sit down on the chair or bench. A bench or backless chair may be used if the client has good trunk stability. A bench is better suited for a client who requires assistance in bathing, because the caregiver can more easily reach the client's back. Of course, if the bench has no back on it, the client must have adequate trunk stability to hold him/herself erect.

If a client is unable to lift his/her feet over the edge of the bathtub, a transfer chair or bench with an extension

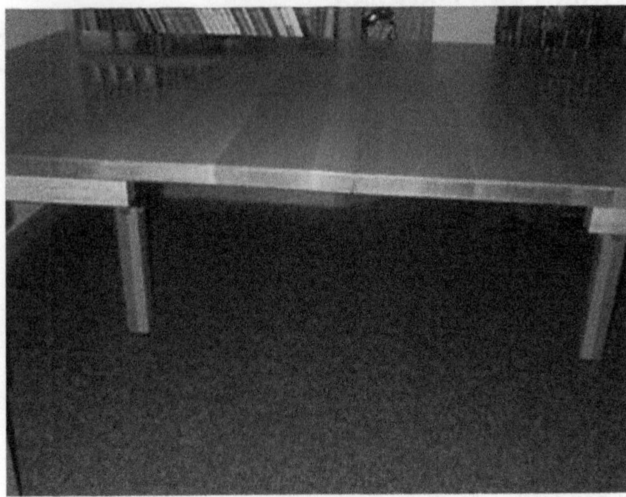

Figure 21.9 Square table with apronless leaves (www.lifease.com). (Reproduced with permission).

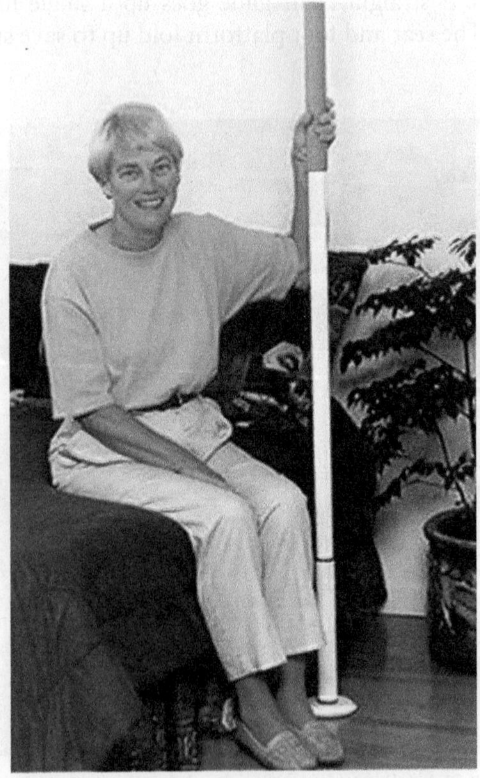

Figure 21.10 Grab pole (www.adaptmy.com).

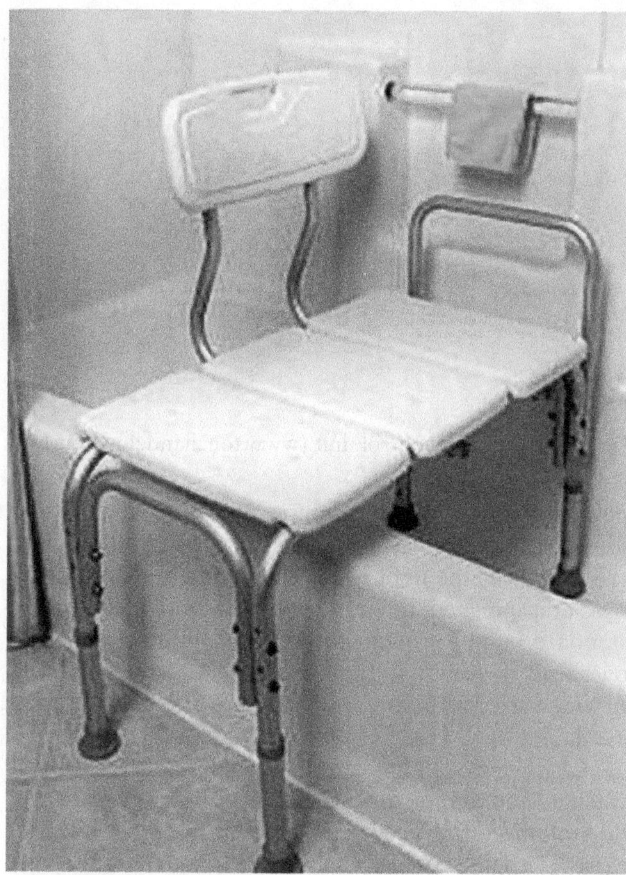

Figure 21.11 Bathtub transfer bench with extension (www.adaptmy.com).

over the side of the tub is recommended (Fig. 21.11). Shower doors should be replaced with a curtain because a shower curtain allows for more room to maneuver the body when getting in and out of the tub. To avoid water splashing onto the floor when the transfer bench or chair is being used, cut two slits in the bottom of the shower curtain, so when it is pulled closed, the flap that is created by the slits drapes over the transfer extension of the bench or chair. Measure twice and cut once. Carefully mark out exactly where and how high the slits need to be made with the shower curtain closed around the extension of the bench or chair. If desired, a handheld shower can be installed in the shower or tub to make bathing easier.

Bending and Reaching

Reaching is the action away from the body at or above shoulder level, at or below knee level, or away from body directly in front or to the side. Bending is the process of bringing the shoulders and arms down, by leaning forward to hip level when standing.

Challenge: Cupboard. Open shelves make it easier to reach items. A corner cupboard with revolving corner shelves makes accessing corners easier. Pullout shelves in place of stationary ones eliminate much reaching and bending (Fig. 21.12). Most kitchen shelves can be retrofitted. Over-counter cabinets are not useful for clients who are unable to reach them.

Challenge: Dishwasher. A raised dishwasher reduces the need to bend. A counter can be raised 6″ to 8″ to accommodate a dishwasher. This raised dishwasher/higher counter arrangement is particularly helpful if there are taller people in the household. If the dishwasher is in a cabinet, it may be able to be raised 18″. This extra height enables those in wheelchairs to reach the inside back corner of the dishwasher. It also happens to be a good height for anyone standing to load/unload the dishwasher.

Challenge: Washer and dryer. In the laundry room, washer and dryers with front controls can be placed on a platform. Platforms may be purchased that accommodate many brands of frontloading washers and dryers.

Challenge: Bedroom closets. Lowering the closet rod in a bedroom closet makes accessing clothing easier. Work with a client to determine the appropriate height to place the rod. A pull-down closet rod also makes it possible for someone who is short or uses a wheelchair to access a high closet rod (Fig. 21.13). Storing shoes on a closet shelf rather than on the floor makes them easier to retrieve.

Challenge: Dustpan and reachers. A long-handled dustpan reduces the need to bend when sweeping.

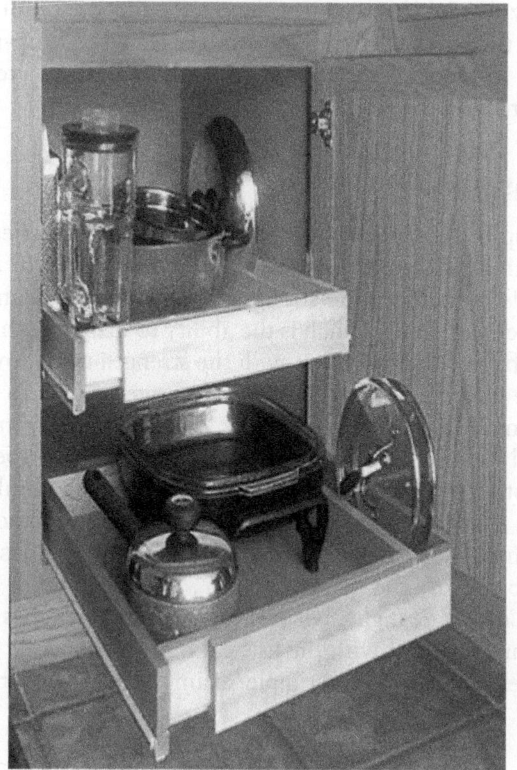

Figure 21.12 Pullout shelving (www.stacksandstacks.com).

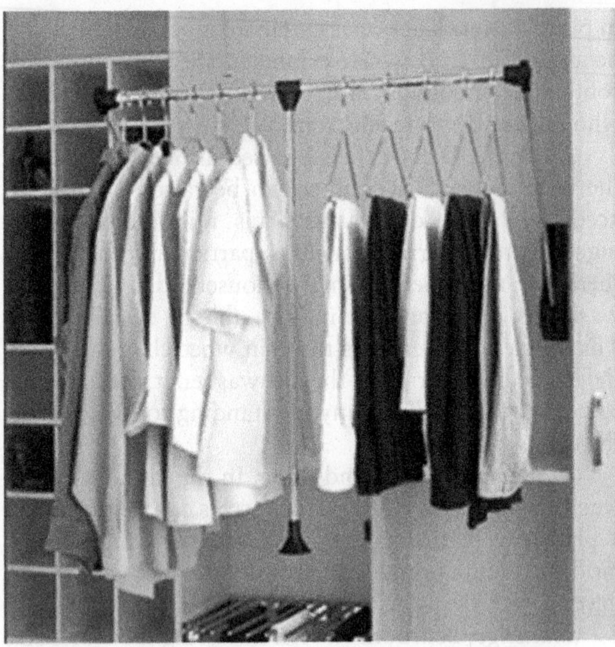

Figure 21.13 Pull-down closet rod (www.adaptmy.com).

Reachers are now available at many pharmacies and department stores and are helpful with all activities that require accessing something too far to safely reach.

Challenge: Cooktop. Reaching over burners to turn on controls that are located at the back of a stove is dangerous. Some argue against front controls, as small children can access them. A safe solution is to remove the knobs when the stove is not in use or purchase commercially available covers to place over the knobs. Stoves with the controls placed in front are usually a drop-in or slide-in model. Freestanding models typically have the controls on the rear panel.

Grasp and Pinch

Grasp is the capacity to move the hand into a variety of positions and to manipulate an object with one or both hands; it includes the strength to grasp, release, and/or squeeze an object. Pinch is the ability to bring the thumb and fingers in opposition with the strength to remove or close an object like a clothespin or tweezers or to pick up small items like paper clips. For those with limited hand function, a criterion for recommending a specific adaptive device is whether it can be easily manipulated with a closed fist without needing to grasp or pinch. If so, most individuals with hand or wrist difficulties will be able to use the item.

Challenge: Light switches. Rocker light switches may be turned on/off with the fist, palm of the hand, or even the elbow and are a simple example of a universally designed feature. Stable lamps with switches located near the base are easier to turn on/off than those with switches near the light bulb. They are also safer. A control unit plugged into an electrical outlet converts a standard lamp to touch control and eliminates reaching overhead or fumbling for the lamp switch (Fig. 21.14). A wide variety of remote switches are also commercially available.

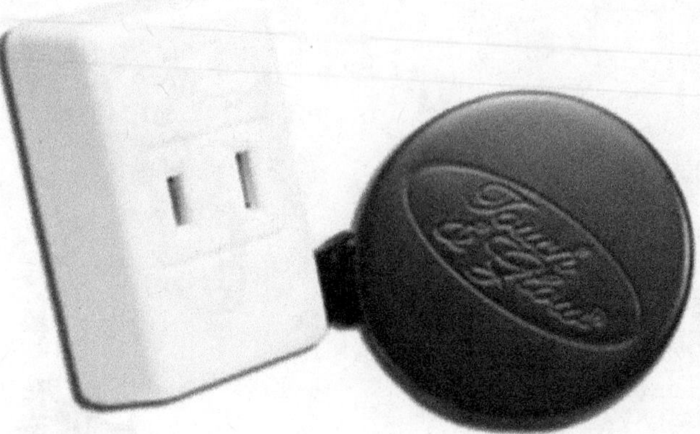

Figure 21.14 Touch control unit (www.touchandglow.com).

Challenge: Appliances. If new appliances such as washers and dryers, dishwasher, stoves, and microwaves do not meet the needs of someone with a disability, existing appliances will need to be adapted so they are safe and usable. For example, building up the buttons of appliances will make them easier to manipulate. For clients with tremors or visual disabilities, you may outline appliance buttons, especially flat ones, with glue or puffy paint to provide a distinct tactile cue as to where to turn on or depress a touch type switch or knob. Be creative and try different solutions.

Challenge: Door handles. Lever door handles are much easier to use than are doorknobs because you do not need to grasp them. They can be operated with an open hand, fist, or elbow. The side of the lever door handle facing the door should not be hollow as the surface is rough and uncomfortable and fingers could get abraded.

Challenge: Faucets. Lever faucets require less grasp to operate than do round faucet knobs. Shower controls that can preset water temperature and have a lever-type handle are easier to operate than standard knob faucets.

Challenge: Drinking glasses. Something as simple as glassware can be selected to increase hand function. A best option is to recommend textured plastic glasses that will not easily slip out of someone's hands.

Infusing AE into home modifications helps ensure that a client is better prepared and enable the client to fulfill his/her desire to age in place with dignity.

Summary

This chapter began by looking back at the evolution of AE and how those who were on the front line of experiencing disability were instrumental in bringing about change in how they and future generations of people with disability were to be accorded equal rights. We explored how adaptive tools and devices can maximize participation in daily living. In this chapter, we also discussed recommendations for adaptive equipment and home modifications to address physical capabilities. Sometimes, due to physical challenges, people need extra help in order to function and carry out daily activities. Help may come in the form of AE. Despite needing AE, there are other factors that may influence someone's decision about whether to use or not use a recommended adaptive device. These factors include values and preferences, which are very personal. As well, some older adults may be reluctant to use AE and AD due to denial that they need it, embarrassment about using it, or perceived social stigma associated with using the devices and tools (Aminzadeh & Edwards, 2001). As the aesthetics of adaptive products improves and they are, based on principles of universal design, increasingly incorporated into various mainstream settings, there may come an increase increased rate of acceptance of AE.

An OT practitioner must have detailed knowledge of AE so that he or she can search out and recommend products that go beyond meeting just a client's basic needs. Although the assistive devices you recommend may be logical solutions to help a client attain his/her goals, in the end, the final decision about using the equipment is up to the client. Your job as an OTA is to thoroughly understand what you are recommending and to be prepared to explain why you feel any adaptive equipment that you recommend will help a client be an active participant in his/her own life. It is an exciting prospect to be preparing to undertake.

Note

The author and publisher have no financial stake in the products or companies discussed in this chapter, nor do they endorse any of them.

Review Questions

1. What is the preferred slope of a ramp?
   a. 1:12
   b. 1:20
   c. 1:14
   d. 1:15

2. What is the most important function when dealing with falls prevention?
   a. Stability
   b. Mobility
   c. Strength
   d. Range of motion

3. "Primarily and customarily used to serve a medical purpose, and generally are not useful to a person in the absence of illness or injury" best describes:
   a. Assistive technology
   b. Workplace safety regulations
   c. Self-care
   d. Durable medical equipment

4. Why do people typically abandon or choose to not use adaptive equipment?
   a. Perceived social stigma
   b. OT practitioner approach to recommending it
   c. Aesthetics
   d. Do not feel it is necessary
   e. All of the above

5. Creating products that people *want* rather than something they merely *need* is an exceedingly important approach associated with:
   a. Universal design
   b. Adaptive design
   c. Home modifications
   d. Accessible design

6. Which of the following adaptive equipment may best help a client with poor balance bathe independently?
   a. Reacher, soap on a rope, long-handled sponge, handheld shower, tub seat
   b. Soap on a rope, long-handled sponge, bath bench with back and transfer extension, handheld shower
   c. Tub seat, long-handled sponge, handheld shower
   d. Tub seat with back, handheld shower

7. A wet room:
   a. Has no threshold to the shower
   b. Is useful for people with poor stability and mobility
   c. Can be universally designed
   d. All of the above

8. What two factors were the catalyst for the disability rights movement and the introduction of adaptive equipment?
   a. WWII veterans and polio epidemic
   b. HIV/AIDS and obesity
   c. Polio and CVA
   d. Vietnam veterans and obesity

9. A reliable resource for learning about adaptive equipment and assistive technology options is:
   a. Google
   b. AbleData
   c. ADAAG
   d. ADA

10. The ideal grab bar placement in the bathroom is:
    a. Vertically for entering or leaving the bathtub; vertically on the wall opposite the tub opening or on the wall by a commode and in place of towel bars around bathroom
    b. Horizontally for entering or leaving the bathtub; vertically on the wall opposite the tub opening or on the wall by a commode
    c. Vertically for entering or leaving the bathtub; horizontally on the wall opposite the tub opening or on the wall by a commode and in place of towel bars around bathroom
    d. Anywhere is fine, and towel bars are an adequate substitute for grab bars

11. Which of the following is an example of a universally designed product found in commercial and residential buildings?
    a. Pull cord–operated ceiling fan
    b. Two-handled faucet
    c. Bathtub
    d. Rocker light switch

Practice Activities

Bring your vegetable peeler to class. Because they are such a mainstream product, hopefully, someone will have an OXO peeler. Compare and contrast the features of each peeler and determine which meets the qualities associated with universal design, and why.

Prepare a 1- to 2-minute elevator speech that you could give to a client and his/her family that explains why AE is important, when it is recommended. Share your speech with your classmates.

On a piece of graph paper, sketch a bathroom layout for a wheeled mobility user who had a stroke. Refer to the many guidelines and recommendations in this chapter as well as in Chapter 22, **Assistive Technology** for additional information.

References

AARP. *Aging in Place: A State Survey of Livability Policies and Practices*; 2011. Retrieved from http://www.aarp.org/home-garden/livable-communities/info-11-2011/Aging-In-Place.html

ADAAG. ADA accessibility guidelines for buildings and facilities (ADA); 2002. Retrieved from http://www.access-board.gov/adaag/html/adaag.htm#4.8

American Occupational Therapy Association. Occupational therapy practice framework: domain and process (3rd ed.). *Am J Occup Ther* 2014;68(Suppl. 1):S1–S48. http://dx.doi.org/10.5014/ajot.2014.682006

Aminzadeh F, Edwards N. Exploring seniors' views on the use of assistive devices in fall prevention. *Public Health Nurs* 2001;15: 297–304.

AOTF. *Honorary life member of the board, Fred Sammons*; n.d. Retrieved December from http://www.aotf.org/aboutaotf/honorary-lifemembersoftheboard/fredsammons.aspx

Bayer A, Harper L. *Fixing to Say. A National Survey on Housing and Home Modification Issues*; 2000. Retrieved from http://assets.aarp.org/rgcenter/il/home_mod.pdf

Christenson M. *Aging in the Designed Environment*. Binghamton, NY: Haworth Press; 1990.

Christenson MA. *PresentEase: Compensations for Age-Related Physical Changes*. Orlando, FL: Lifease, Inc.®2002 by Lifease, Inc.; 2002.

Christenson M. Environmental adaptations: foundation for daily living. In: Christiansen C, Matuska K, eds. *Ways of Living*. 4th ed. Bethesda, MD: American Occupational Therapy Association; 2011:510–511.

Christenson M, Chase C. *Occupational Therapy and Home Modifications: Promoting Safety and Supporting Participation*. Bethesda, MD: AOTA Press; 2011a.

Christenson M, Chase C. *Visual library on CD. In Occupational Therapy and Home Modifications: Promoting Safety and Supporting Participation*. Bethesda, MD: AOTA Press; 2011b.

Disability Resources Network of Pennsylvania. *Assistive Technology: How to Pay for the Device or Service that You Need*; 2012. Retrieved from http://drnpa.org/wp-content/uploads/2012/10/assistive-technology-how-to-pay-for-the-device-or-service-that-you-need1.pdf

Eldercare Locator. *Assistive Technology*; 2012. Retrieved from http://www.eldercare.gov/Eldercare.NET/Public/Resources/Factsheets/Assistive_Technology.aspx

Federal Register. *Federal register. Volume 77, Number 153*; 2012. Retrieved from http://www.gpo.gov/fdsys/pkg/FR-2012-08-08/html/2012-19477.htm

Mann WC, Lane JP. *Assistive Technology for Persons with Disabilities*. Bethesda, MD: The American Occupational Therapy Association; 1995.

Marchione M. *U.S. Vets' Disability Filings Reach Historic Rate*; 2012, May 28. Retrieved from http://usatoday30.usatoday.com/news/health/story/2012-05-28/veteran-disability/55250092/1

Monek F. *Canes Through the Ages*. Atgle, PA: Schiffer Publishing , Ltd.; 1997.

NECTAC. *Federal Definitions of Assistive Technology*; 2012. Retrieved November from http://www.nectac.org/topics/atech/definitions.asp

OXO. *About OXO, Universal Design*; n.d. Retrieved from http://www.oxo.com/Universal-Design.aspx

Principal Financial Group. *Financial Security: A Step by Step Guide to Life Insurance*. Des Moines, IA: Principle Financial Group; 2012.

Smithsonian National Museum of American History. Assistive technology; n.d. Retrieved from www.amhistory.si.edu/polio/howpolio/assistive.htm

Stephen Hawking. *Stephen Hawking*; n.d. Retrieved from www.hawking.org.uk

U.S. Access Board. *Regulatory Assessment of the Final Revised Accessibility Guidelines for the Americans with Disabilities Act and Architectural Barriers Act*; 2004. Retrieved from http://www.access-board.gov/ada-aba/reg-assess.htm

US Government. Assistive Technology Act of 1998; 1998. Retrieved from http://www.section508.gov/508Awareness/html/at1998.html

Wheelchair Dancer. *Wheelchair Dancer*; 2012. Retrieved from: www.cripwheels.blogspot.com

World Health Organization. *Definition of Disability, Accessing Safety*; 2001. Retrieved from http://www.who.int/disabilities/world_report/2011/chapter1.pdf

World Health Organization. *Disability and Health Fact Sheet*; 2012. Retrieved from http://www.who.int/mediacentre/factsheets/fs352/en/index.html

Wylde MA, Robbins AB, Clark S. *Building for a Lifetime: The Design and Construction of Fully Accessible Homes*. London, UK: Anova Books; 1994.

Yeung Y. Educating older adults in AT. *OT Pract*, Bethesda, MD: American Occupational Therapy Association 2003;8(15):12–15.

CHAPTER 22

Assistive Technology

Debra Young, MEd, OTR/L, SCEM, ATP, CAPS

Key Terms

Assistive technology—High- or low-technology items used to increase a person's functional skills.

HAAT—Human Activity Assistive Technology.

ICF—International Classification of Functioning, Disability and Health.

MPT Model—An assessment tool that encompasses Matching Person and Technology.

MSIPT—A systematic motor access assessment that looks at movement, control site, input method, position, and targeting.

PEOM—Person–Environment–Occupation Model.

RESNA—Rehabilitation Engineering and Assistive Technology Society of North America.

SETT Framework—Student Environment Tasks Tools.

Learning Objectives

After studying this chapter, readers should be able to:

- Summarize assistive technology legislation as it relates to occupational therapy practice.
- Apply assistive technology models to occupational therapy practice to guide the use of assistive technology as a preparatory method to support occupational performance.
- Explain the assistive technology assessment process to feature match match assistive technology to client needs to support occupational performance.
- Be aware of assistive technology supports that maximize fit and support client occupational performance with the targeted outcome of client carryover of use.

Introduction

Occupational therapy practitioners have longstanding expertise in providing services to clients that incorporates assistive technology (AT) and environmental modification (AOTA, 2009). This chapter will provide an overview of AT as a preparatory method to support daily occupational performance, via assessment, selection, provision, and education, and training in use of the devices and systems (AOTA, 2014).

History of Assistive Technology

Assistive tool use is far from a new concept. Humans have used tools to complete daily tasks for thousands of years. Many of these tools dating back to the sixth or seventh century BC (Bodine, 2013) were created out of necessity, such as partial dentures, artificial legs and hands, and drinking straws.

Throughout history (and prehistory), people across myriad cultures have creatively adapted, developed, and used special tools and devices to help others with special needs in their societies (King, 1999). Many early innovations were done to meet the needs of persons with disabilities, but ultimately became mainstream tools. In fact, the earliest documented account of optical and lens technologies, eyeglasses, came from Venice around AD 1300 (King, 1999). In 1808, Pellegrino Turri built the first typewriter for a friend who was visually impaired to help his friend write legibly (A Brief History of Typewriters, n.d.; Adler, 1973). Alexander Graham Bell's lifelong work was inspired by his mother who was hearing impaired. Bell's patent for the telephone, a byproduct of his studies with persons with hearing impairments, was granted in 1876 Alexander Graham Bell Biography, n.d.). While the tools have advanced considerably, since their earliest iterations, we continue to develop, use, and integrate many assistive tools into our daily routines.

Assistive Technology Legislation

While early technological innovations were developed purely out of necessity, in modern times, AT services have been moved to the forefront through Federal legislation (Table 22.1). In 1975, the Individuals with Disabilities Education Act (IDEA) was passed, requiring public schools to provide a free and appropriate public education (FAPE) to all students with disabilities in the least restrictive environment (please also see Chapter 36, *Children and Youth*). This legislation further provided that public schools are required to develop Individualized Education Programs (IEPs) to meet each student's individualized needs (DOJ, 2009). It is within the IEP that occupational therapy services, along with any accommodations and supports, including AT, are determined and specified.

Furthering the scope of accommodations for persons with disabilities, in 1988, the Fair Housing Amendment Act was passed. This Act prohibits housing discrimination on the basis of race, color, religion, sex, disability, familial status, and nationality (DOJ, 2009). This protection extends to private housing, state and local government housing, and housing that receives Federal financial assistance (DOJ, 2009). The Act further provides for residents that landlords make reasonable accommodations to maximize the accessibility of their living space, along with any common use spaces. It is these reasonable accommodations that fall into a category of AT called architectural access AT.

In 1988, the Hearing Aid Compatibility Act (HAC) was passed in an effort to ensure that all "essential telephones are hearing aid compatible" (FCC, n.d.). In 1990, the Television Decoder Circuitry Act ensured that "to the fullest extent made possible by technology, deaf and hearing-impaired people should have equal access to the television medium" (FCC, 1990). This led to closed captioning on television, a milestone for persons who are hearing impaired that is now a widely accepted and well-integrated feature in our televisions for people with and without a hearing impairment. The benefits of this technology are universal, allowing viewers to watch television in sound-sensitive environments (e.g., library, offices) and increasing

TABLE 22.1 Brief Chronology of Federal Legislation Pertaining to People with Disabilities

1975	Individuals with Disabilities Education Act (IDEA) P.L. 94–142
1988	Fair Housing Amendment Act P.L. 100–430 [42 USC 3604]
1988	The Hearing Aid Compatibility Act (HAC) of 1988 P.L. 100–394 [47 USC 610(b)]
1990	The Television Decoder Circuitry Act, Section 3 P.L. 101–431 [47 USC 303 (u)]
1990	Americans with Disabilities Act (ADA) P.L. 101–336 [42 USC 12101]
1996	Telecommunications Act Title 1- P.L. 104–104 [47 USC 255], Title III-P.L. 104–104 [47 USC 613]
1998	Rehabilitation Act Section 508 P.L. 93–112 29 [U.S.C. § 794d]
1998	Workforce Investment Act P.L. 105–220 [29 USC 701]
1998	Carl D. Perkins Vocational and Technical Education Act Amendments of 1998 P.L. 105–332 Section 1 (b) [20 USC 2302]
1998	Assistive Technology Act P.L. 105–394 [29 USC 2201]

comprehension for dialogue that is spoken quickly and/or with unfamiliar accents or in an environment with background noise.

1990 was a landmark year, as it saw inception of the Americans with Disabilities Act (ADA). The ADA is a civil rights law that "prohibits the discrimination and ensures equal opportunity for persons with disabilities in employment, state and local government services, public accommodations, commercial facilities and transportation" (DOJ, 2009). AT is one intervention used to provide reasonable accommodations to ensure equal opportunities for persons with disabilities.

To further accessible communication and update a law created sixty two years earlier, the Telecommunications Act was amended in 1996 to require telecommunications equipment manufacturers and telecommunications service providers to ensure that such equipment and services are accessible to and usable by persons with disabilities, if readily achievable (DOJ, 2009). This includes telephone service, telephone book access, and cable programming.

The rise of the Information Age saw the passage of Section 508 of the Rehabilitation Act in 1998. In an attempt to keep up with the ever-changing technology landscape that permeates the way Americans work, live, and play, this law established requirements for electronic and information technology developed, maintained, procured, or used by the Federal government to be accessible to people with disabilities (DOJ, 2009).

1998 was a busy year for AT legislation, as it engendered three other laws. The Technology-Related Assistance for IDEA brought awareness and support for the benefit of AT for persons with disabilities. Otherwise known as the "Tech Act," this legislation provides funding to states to facilitate the development, evaluation, application, and delivery of AT devices and services (ATAP, n.d.). Two other relevant laws passed in 1998 are related to employment:

- The Workforce Investment Act, which defines technology in the vocational rehabilitation process and mandates its use in job planning and retention of people with disabilities (USDOL, n.d.).
- The Carl D. Perkins Vocational and Technical Education Act Amendment, which defines vocational technical education as organized educational programs offering sequences of courses directly related to preparing individuals for paid or unpaid employment (USDOE, n.d.).

Assistive Technology

Assistive technology was first defined in Federal law in the IDEA. The IDEA defines an AT *device* as:

> Any item, piece of equipment, or product system, whether acquired commercially off the shelf, modified, or customized, that is used to increase, maintain, or improve functional capabilities of a child with a disability.

> IDEA defines AT *services* as
>
> Any service that directly assists a child with a disability in the selection, acquisition, or use of an AT device. Such terms include the following:
>
> A. The evaluation of the needs of such child, including a functional evaluation of the child in the child's customary environment
> B. Purchasing, leasing, or otherwise providing for the acquisition of AT devices by such child
> C. Selecting, designing, fitting, customizing, adapting, applying, maintaining, repairing, or replacing of AT devices
> D. Coordinating and using other therapies, interventions, or services with AT devices, such as those associated with existing education and rehabilitation plans and programs
> E. Training or technical assistance for such child or, where appropriate, the family of such child
> F. Training or technical assistance for professionals (including individuals providing education and rehabilitation services), employers, or other individuals who provide services to, employ, or are otherwise substantially involved in the major life functions of such child (IDEA, n.d.)

In occupational therapy practice, AT is considered a preparatory method used concurrently with occupations to support daily occupational performance (AOTA, 2014). AT covers a large spectrum of low- and high-tech devices from a simple pencil grip to complex environmental systems that manage households, as it can be usable everywhere people work, live, and play. These supports fall into a variety of categories to meet the needs of occupations (Table 22.2) (From the Field 22.1).

While all categories of AT fall within the occupational therapy practitioner's scope of practice, several of the categories may benefit from a team approach for best client outcomes. One example is augmentative and alternative communication, a means to help people without or with limited verbal language communicate. Interprofessional collaboration between an OT practitioner and a speech and language pathologist brings knowledge of the client's best possible access for use of a speech device along with the setup of the device to meet the client's specific communication needs (Fig. 22.1).

Depending upon a client's needs, collaboration with, or referral to, an OT practitioner who has additional training, skills, and knowledge in an area of AT may also be warranted. Adaptive driving is one example. An OT practitioner may be working with a client who has sustained a spinal cord injury and is interested in

TABLE 22.2 Categories of Assistive Technologies

Adaptive Driving	Environmental Controls/Switches
Adaptive Sports/Recreation	Low Vision Aids
Adaptive Toys/Games	Memory/Organizational Aids
Alternative Formats/Methods	Mobility
Architectural Access: home/public	Prosthetics/Orthotics
Assistive Listening	Seating/Positioning
Augmentative/Alternative Communication	Self Care/ADLs
Computer Access	Service Animals
Computer-Based Skill Development	Vehicle Modification
Educational Access	Worksite Modification

getting back to driving. Referral to an occupational therapist with adaptive driving training and can provide preassessment driving screens and/or behind-the-wheel driver rehabilitation evaluation, recommendations, and training may be needed (Fig. 22.2).

Assistive Technology Models

There are several models of AT that are important to understand. They include the International Classification of Functioning (WHO, 2001), Disability and Health, the Person–Environment–Occupation Model (Law et al., 1996), and the Human Activity Assistive Technology Model (HAAT) (Cook & Miller Polgar, 2014). All are discussed below.

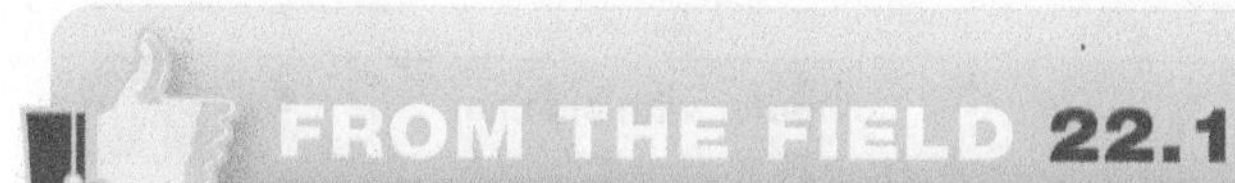

A Spectrum of Options

Within each AT category, there are spectrums of choices that run from no-tech/low-tech to high-tech options. Consider a third grade student who may have difficulty with the motor aspects of writing. A continuum of considerations for AT from simple to complex is shown in Figure 22.3, and some examples are in Figure 22.4.

Determining which device will best meet a client's needs and improve occupational performance, and subsequently if that device will be a low-tech option versus a high-tech option, is part of the AT assessment process that an OTA may be called upon to work with an OT to facilitate.

International Classification of Functioning, Disability and Health

The **International Classification of Functioning, Disability and Health (ICF)** was published by the World Health Organization (WHO) in 2001 with the overall aim "to provide a unified standard language and framework for the description of health and health related states" (p. 3). The ICF is an individual and population health measurement framework. The framework classifies individuals based on the following components:

- Body functions
- Body structures
- Activities and participation
- Environmental factors
- Personal factors

These components are organized on a checklist (WHO, 2003), which allows for analysis of an

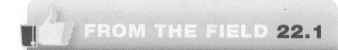

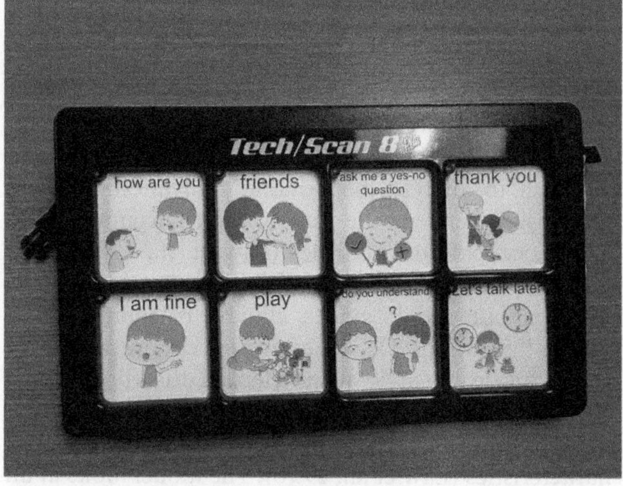

Figure 22.1 An example of an augmentative communication device.

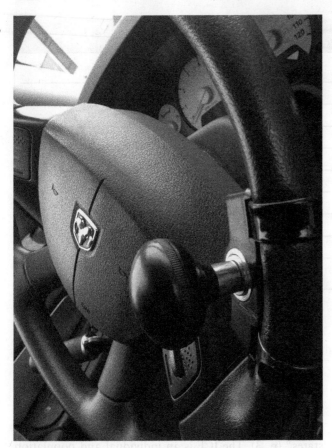

Figure 22.2 Examples of a spinner knob and hand control for adaptive driving.

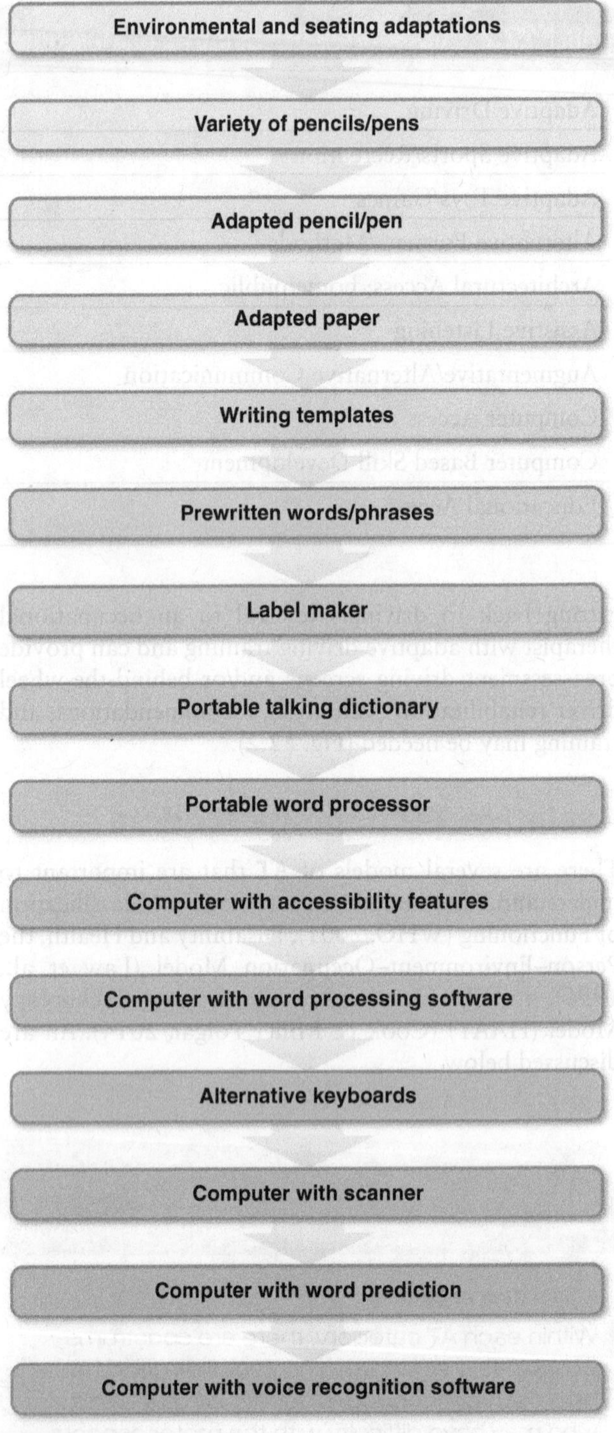

Figure 22.3 A continuum of low- to high-tech AT communication devices. Adapted from Gierach J. *Assessing Students' Needs for Assistive Technology (ASNAT)*. 5th ed. Milton, WI: Wisconsin Assistive Technology Initiative; 2009.

individual's health and the impact of the environment and how these factors may subsequently influence an individual's activity and participation.

Person–Environment–Occupation Model

As OT practitioners, we constantly look at the environments in which a person must act, the occupations they need to engage in, and the personal factors that impact their performance in these occupations in various environments. This is the **Person–Environment–Occupation Model (PEOM)** developed by Mary Law and colleagues (Law et al., 1996). It is a transactive framework and approach to analyze the dynamic and interdependent relationship between the person, the environment, and his/her occupations and roles (Law et al., 1996). This model does not prescribe specific assessments or interventions, but rather guides clinical reasoning about what interventions OT practitioners choose and why. In this approach, it is acknowledged that behavior is influenced and cannot be separated by contextual influences, temporal factors, and physical and psychological characteristics (Law et al., 1996). The model looks at an individual holistically, as all areas of a person's life may impact occupational performance.

There are four major constructs of the PEOM. The "Person" is made up of a series of intrinsic factors (e.g., psychological, cognitive, physiological, spiritual, and neurobehavioral) that compose one's set of skills and abilities (Law et al., 1996). The person brings to the context their own set of attributes, skills, knowledge, and experience.

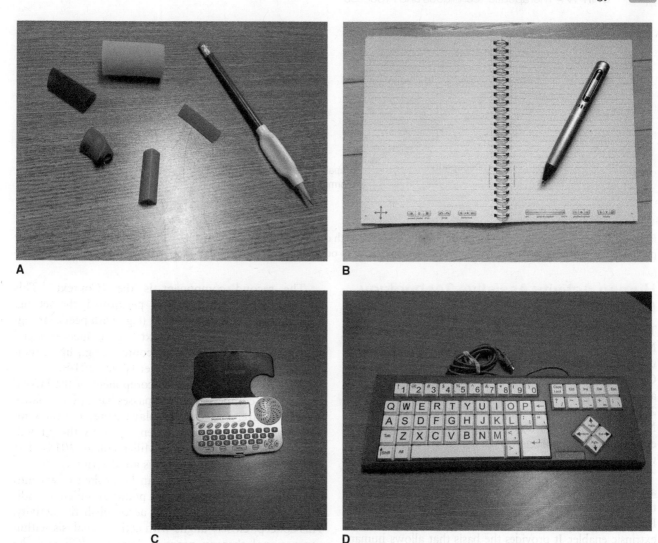

Figure 22.4 A–D. Examples of low- to high-tech AT communication devices.

Aligning with the AOTA *Occupational Therapy Practice Framework III* (AOTA, 2014), these are client factors and performance skills. The client is a unique being who assumes multiple roles and cannot be separated from contextual influences (Law et al., 1996). The basic assumptions of the model are that the person is continually developing and is intrinsically motivated (Law et al., 1996).

The second construct is the "Environment." This construct considers that participation is always impacted by extrinsic characteristics of the environment in which it occurs (Law et al., 1996). Aligning with the AOTA *Occupational Therapy Practice Framework III*, these extrinsic environmental factors are the external physical and social conditions that surround the client along with the cultural, personal, temporal, and/or virtual contexts within which occupational performance takes place (AOTA, 2014).

Construct three is "Occupation." Occupations refer to self-directed meaningful tasks and activities engaged in throughout a life span (Law et al., 1996). People engage in occupations to fulfill an intrinsic need for self-maintenance, expression, and life satisfaction and that are carried out within multiple environments and contexts to satisfy individual roles (Law et al., 1996). The temporal aspect that encompasses the occupational routines of an individual over time (e.g., day, week, life span) is an important consideration as the interaction of all three components varies (Law et al., 1996).

The fourth construct is "Occupational Performance and Participation." This is the outcome of the interaction of the person, the environment, and one's chosen occupation (Law et al., 1996).

The model constructs are represented via three concentric circles that dynamically interact with one another over time. The more the circles (constructs) overlap, the better the "fit" and subsequent maximization of occupational performance. The less the circles overlap, "fit" is minimized, which compromises occupational performance (Fig. 22.5).

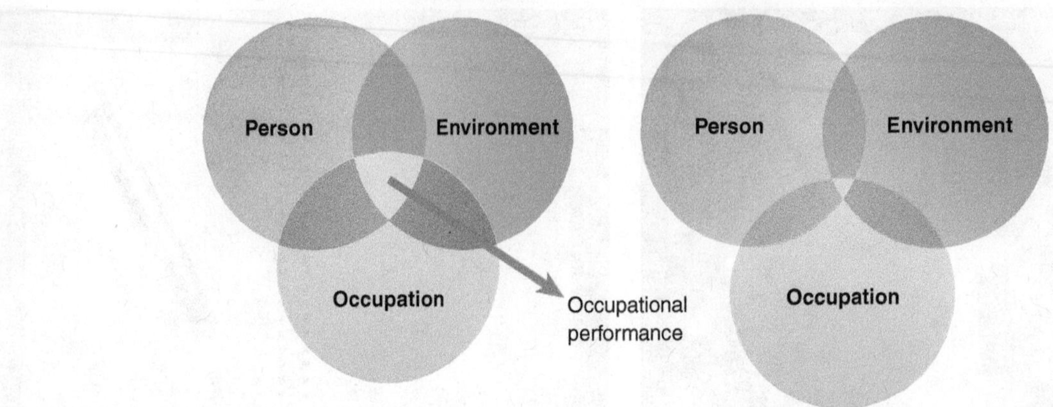

Figure 22.5 Person–Environment–Occupation Model (PEOM) with concentric circles showing "fit." (Adapted from Law M, et al. The person-environment-occupation model: a transactive approach to occupational performance. *Can J Occup Ther* 1996;63(1):9–23.)

Human Activity Assistive Technology Model

The original **Human Activity Assistive Technology (HAAT)** Model by Cook and Hussey (Fig. 22.6) was developed using the foundations of the ICF, the Canadian Model of Occupational Performance and Enablement (CMOP-E), and the PEOP (see Table 22.3) (Cook & Miller Polgar, 2014). It is also adapted from the Human Performance Model (Bailey, 1989) and often used by human factors engineers and psychologists in the design and application of technology. There are four components of this model. The "Human" is the intrinsic enabler and takes into consideration the underlying abilities, level of proficiency, and what that person brings to a new task or skill (Cook & Miller Polgar, 2014). The AT component within this model is the extrinsic enabler. It provides the basis that allows human performance to improve (Cook & Miller Polgar, 2014).

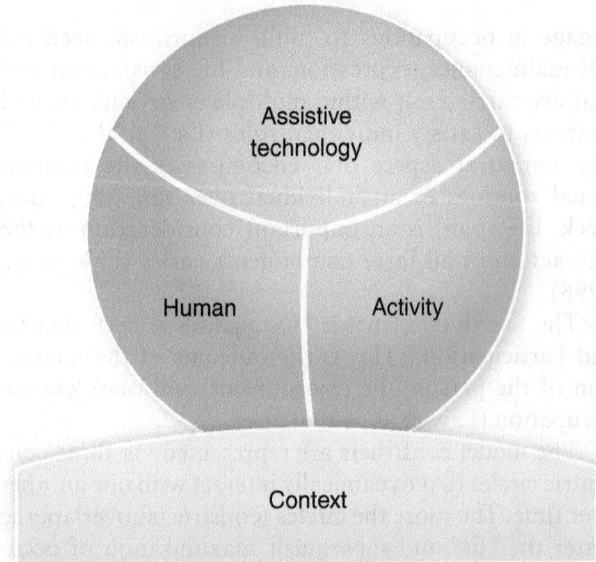

Figure 22.6 The HAAT model. Reproduced with permission. Cook AM, Miller Polgar J. *Assistive Technologies: Principles and Practice*. 4th ed. St Louis, MO: Elsevier; 2014.

The second component is the "Context." This refers to where the activity is performed, the setting/environment, the social context (e.g., with peers, strangers, family), the cultural context (e.g., influences social context), and/or the physical context (e.g., light, temperature, sound) (Cook & Miller Polgar, 2014).

The "Activity" is the third component of the HAAT Model. This component encompasses basic performance areas: self-care, work/school, play/leisure, and the temporal contexts and where, when, and how the AT will occur and be used (Cook & Miller Polgar, 2014). The activities an individual performs are determined by that person's life roles. Activities can be broken down into smaller tasks to help determine points at which an individual may need assistance to accomplish the activity. This concept closely aligns with activity analysis within occupational therapy practice. Like the ICF and the PEOP, the HAAT analyzes the fit of the person, participating in a given activity, within a specified environment. The HAAT differs in that it takes these three components and then considers AT as the extrinsic enabler. Not only is the HAAT a model, but it is also an approach to AT assessment.

Process

This section explores the use of AT within the occupational therapy process.

Assessment

The AOTA *Occupational Therapy Practice Framework III* (AOTA, 2014) places AT under preparatory methods and tasks. It is used as part of a therapy session in preparation for (or as previously discussed, as a preparatory method), or concurrently with, occupations and activities to support daily occupational performance (AOTA, 2014). Considering the use of AT is one part of the occupational therapy process: a process that starts with development of an occupational profile.

TABLE 22.3 Comparing the ICF, PEOP, and HAAT Models

ICF	PEO Model	HAAT Model
Body Functions and Structures	Person	Human
Environmental Factors	Environment	Context
Activities and Participation	Occupation	Activity
		Assistive Technology

The occupational profile is a summary of a client's occupational history and experiences, patterns of daily living, interests, values, and needs (AOTA, 2014). Frequently, information is gathered for the occupational profile through the occupational therapy process. This client-centered approach assists with identifying client priorities and subsequent targeted outcomes.

Activity analysis is another component of the occupational therapy process. Occupational therapy practitioners analyze the demands of an activity or occupation to understand the specific body structures, body functions, performance skills, and performance patterns that are required and to determine the generic demands the activity or occupation makes on the client (AOTA, 2014) (see also Chapter 11, *Activity Analysis*). This is followed by analysis of occupational performance. This systematic approach provides the evidence for the intervention process, which may include AT.

Human Factors

Human factors, also known as ergonomics, are "an applied science concerned with the characteristics of people that need to be considered in designing things that they use in order that the people and the things will interact most effectively and safely" (Merriam-Webster Online, n.d.). As OT practitioners, "characteristics of people that need to be considered" (Merriam-Webster Online, n.d.) align with client factors and performance skills included in the *AOTA Occupational Therapy Practice Framework III* (AOTA, 2014). Regarding AT, human factors such as client factors and performance skills influence the many aspects of how people (e.g., user, family, caregiver, professional) interact with devices and technologies. Client factors and performance skills have a significant impact on the success or failure of AT interventions. As much as 75% of success in AT use is attributable to human factors (King, 1999). A thorough occupational profile in combination with knowledge of technology devices aids in determining how a user may interact with a device and subsequently provides for feature-matching–appropriate AT to meet a person's needs. King describes 10 essential factors that relate to carryover of AT use or possible abandonment (King, 1999) (Table 22.4).

According to King's device continuum, when an AT device or system is easy to understand and use (transparent), there is greater likelihood the device will be used (King, 1999). AT that is less intuitive and requires a person to be taught to use (opaque) runs the highest risk for failure of adoption. Along with this continuum, King describes nine other factors that contribute to the success of a user adopting an AT device. As OT practitioners, considering the use of AT must be done as a client-centered process. A thorough occupational profile, activity analysis, and analysis of occupational performance will provide pertinent information to help with feature-matching–appropriate AT.

Baker's Basic Ergonomic Equation (BBEE), developed by Bruce Baker, is a heuristic in mathematical form that looks at AT success from a holistic perspective. Its original intent was to look at augmentative communication device use, but was later readapted by King for overall application with AT use (King, 1999). King determined a correlation between four factors associated with technology use or abandonment, including motivation to do the task (the major determiner), physical effort, cognitive effort (including linguistic effort), and time involved and their applicability to predict AT device success/use (King, 1999).

The main premise of the formula involves motivation plus four "load" factors: physical effort, cognitive effort, linguistic effort, and time efficiency. The equation relates the likelihood of a successful experience with a device (S) to a user's motivation to complete a task (M), the physical effort (P), cognitive effort (C), linguistic effort (L), and time load (T), the amount of time it takes to activate and control a device (King, 1999). This formula is represented as

$$\text{Likelihood of success (S)} = \frac{\text{M}}{(\text{P}+\text{C}+\text{L}+\text{T})}$$

If motivation is high and the other four factors are low, it would be predicted that the user would have a successful experience with an assistive device. The longer and harder it is to perform a task with the AT device, the higher the user's motivation must be if he/she will use the device to complete a task.

TABLE 22.4 Assistive Technology Makeup and Human Factors Influencing Use or Abandonment

Factor	Description
Device transparency–translucency–opacity continuum	User-friendliness and how open usage is to new users (e.g., the more complex the device, the more "opaque" its use is likely to be).
Cosmesis of devices	Aesthetic appeal of a device and the user's opinions and social acceptability toward them.
Mappings of commands and actions	The device's interface should follow expected patterns, does it map the way we think it should operate?
Affordances	Qualities afforded by the materials used in a device's design (e.g., strength, durability).
Learned helplessness	Internalization of difficulties experienced with a device as a personal failure.
Feedback from controls	Manipulation of the device should result in communicative feedback to the user.
Knowledge in the head versus knowledge in the world	Recognizing that knowledge of how to use a device may be conveyed by a device or expected as common knowledge.
Constraints on device usage	Limitations placed on the device usage due to physical, sensory, cultural, or other reasons.
Fail-safe mechanisms	Features to prevent harm or device misuse.
Error prevention	Features that prevent or limit mistakes or help insure successful usage of a device.

Adapted from King TW. *Assistive Technology: Essential Human Factors*. Boston, MA: Allyn & Bacon; 1999.

Human–Technology Interface

Occupational therapy is inherently a client-centered practice that considers the client (human) in domain and process (AOTA, 2014). When considering AT, the human–technology interface is an integral part of the equation and is the boundary between the human and the AT across which information is exchanged (Cook & Miller Polgar, 2104). The interaction between user and the AT device or system includes how the user will operate a device (input) and the feedback that the device will provide (output). Cook & Miller Polgar, 2014 discuss three elements of the human–technology interface:

- Control interface
- Selection set
- Selection methods

The control interface is the hardware that a person uses to control a device such as a switch (Fig. 22.7), mouthstick, and joystick (Cook & Miller Polgar, 2014).

The control interface may send two different types of signals (input) to a device, discrete or continuous.

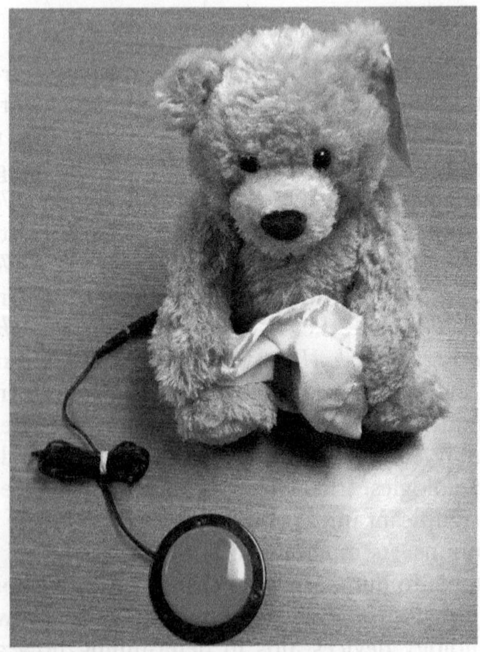

Figure 22.7 A control interface such as a switch allows a client to more easily activate a toy or other objects.

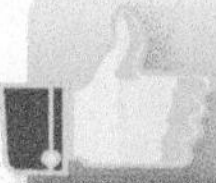

FROM THE FIELD 22.2

Control Interfaces

Examples of control interfaces:

- A light switch (control interface) sends discrete input to a light (device) to turn it on or off. Continuous input results in successively greater or smaller degrees of output.
- A dimmer switch (control interface) provides continuous input to the light allowing for a range between dim and bright versus just on and off.

A control interface with a discrete input sends a fixed signal to the device (From the Field 22.2).

The selection set are the items from which choices are made (Cook & Miller Polgar, 2014; Lee & Thomas, 1990). The selection set may have a visual or auditory representation. Examples include icons on a tablet or smartphone, letters on a keyboard, or auditory choices provided via an augmentative communication device. The size, modality, and type of selection set are determined based on user needs and abilities (Cook & Miller Polgar, 2014).

Part of the occupational therapy AT assessment process implemented by an OT for determination of a user's selection method is the means in which a user is going to access a given device to make a choice from the provided selection set. Direct selection is when the user can randomly choose any item within the selection set (Cook & Miller Polgar, 2014). The user can go directly to the target and select a choice via preferred access method. Examples of direct selection are using an index finger to access icons on a tablet or speaking to choose from a list of contacts to call via a smartphone.

Indirect selection requires the user to go through intermediate steps to make a selection (Cook & Hussey, 2008). Scanning a selection set is one form of indirect selection. The process of scanning involves providing the choices of a selection set to a user in a specified order with auditory and/or visual feedback. Consider an augmentative communication device with eight choices: if the user is unable to direct select each of the choices, use of indirect selection through scanning may provide the user access to the device. There are a variety of types of scanning approaches, including the following:

- Sequential scanning (automatic): each choice of the selection set is scanned independently with feedback provided by visual and/or auditory feedback. For example, each of the eight choices on an augmentative communication device is highlighted one at a time, in order from right to left and top to bottom with an auditory cue (beep) to denote each scanned item. A switch, an additional step/component, is connected to the device and activated by the user to make a selection.
- Directed scanning: user selects direction of the scan and then choices are sequentially scanned (Cook & Miller Polgar, 2014), for example, an augmentative communication device with two rows and four columns (eight choices within the selection set) in which the user activates a switch to initiate vertical scanning of the two rows of choices on the device. Next, the user activates the switch on the first icon in the second row, and the device begins to horizontally scan each of the four (columns) choices. The user then activates the switch a third time to make a selection from the four choices within that second row.

Transmission Methods

Transmission in AT refers to systems that require a signal for the device to be controlled (Cook & Miller Polgar, 2014). Transmission methods typically relate to and should be considered for determination and recommendation of electronic aids for daily living (EADLs). EADL are devices that enable a person to control elements within an environment (Fig. 22.8). For example, a client who sustained a C4 spinal cord injury lacks the functional ability to use a standard remote control for the television and requires an adaptation to be able to control the television. These types of devices, previously known as environmental control units (ECUs), started as stand-alone units that provided alternative access to controlling the environment. In their early form, many of these types of devices used direct wiring, X-10 house wiring, as well as infrared, ultrasound, and radio frequency to assist with transmitting a signal. With of the advent of an abundance of mainstream technologies, transmission methods have changed dramatically. We are still seeing devices that have X-10 capability, along with infrared and radio frequency, but with the trend toward mobile systems, the market is surging with devices that run on wireless technologies.

When feature-matching possible AT to meet a client's needs, the following is a list of potential considerations with regard to transmission methods:

- Can the device be used in the needed environment, or does the transmission method preclude this (e.g., with regard to a wireless technology choice, user does not have wireless capability within their home environment and/or cannot sustain the cost of having wireless technology)?
- Does the device require line of sight for the signal to be sent and received (e.g., a television remote

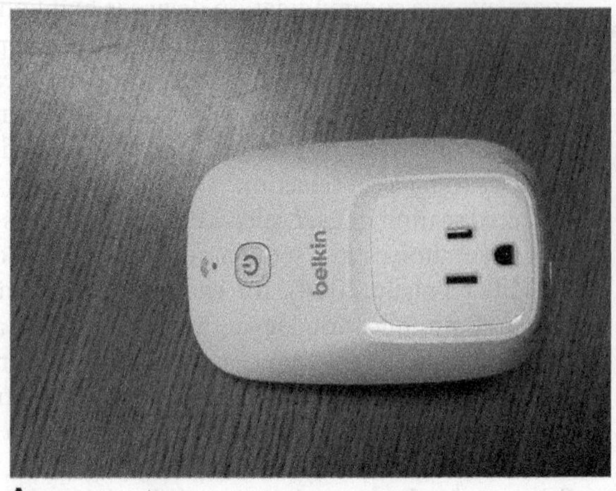

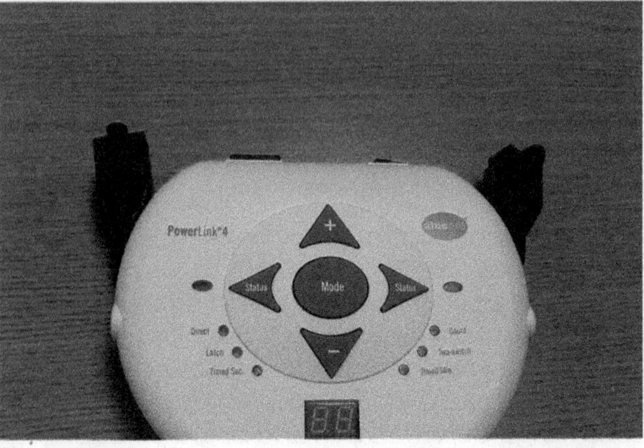

A B

Figure 22.8 **A,B.** WeMo Switch x-10 EADL and Powerlink control device.

control uses infrared transmission, signal can only be received if there is line of sight, and nothing blocking the signal between the remote and the television)?

- If the system uses direct wiring and/or X-10 house wiring, what is the backup in case of a power outage?
- What is the range the device will transmit a signal? Does this impact a client's ability to control items within an environment (e.g., turning on first floor lights when on second floor, unlocking door to home when exiting vehicle in driveway)?
- Is there any concern for signal interference (e.g., radio-frequency transmission, accidentally controlling a neighbor's garage door instead of one's own)?
- Is there limited Internet availability or transmission concern secondary to living in rural environments?

Assistive Technology Assessments

There are a variety of AT assessment approaches that OTs use. The commonalities between these assessment approaches are feature matching a device to a client's needs to maximize occupational performance and ensure successful carryover of use. Several are briefly described; however, further exploration into the multitude of available AT assessments is encouraged.

Movement, Control Site, Input Method, Position, and Targeting Assessment

The **Movement, Control Site, Input Method, Position, and Targeting Assessment (MSIPT)** is a systematic motor access assessment comprising of five major components: movement, control site, input method, position, and targeting (Glennen & DeCoste, 1997). The assessment approach is an adaptation from the Hugh MacMillan Medical Center MSIP assessment (Goosens & Crain, 1986). The five major components include the following:

- M: assess movement, available movements, and any concerns (e.g., range, reliability, accuracy, quality, speed of movements, muscle tone, spasticity, abnormal reflexes, fatigue)
- S: control site, point of contact with the input device, and actual part of the body used to access the device (e.g., left cheek to touch a switch, right index finger to touch a display screen)
- I: input method, equipment used (e.g., keyboard, joystick, touchscreen, switch) (Fig. 22.9)
- P: position of input method, actual placement of input devices and device to be controlled
- T: targeting, an individual's ability to access a device using direct selection or scanning; a measure of the accuracy of the selection (e.g., target size, number of keys/cells to activate) (Glennen & DeCoste, 1997)

The MSIPT also considers speed of overall response, accuracy of overall method, reliability, and overall quality. The goal of the MSIPT is to assess motor access options for AT use and make determinations of best possible access method/s. The assessment gathers data on at least two to three MSIPT components in an effort to show evidence to support recommendations.

Matching Person and Technology

The **Matching Person and Technology** (MPT) model was developed to provide an individualized approach to determination of appropriate AT with the outcome goal of device adoption (Institute for Matching Person and Technology, n.d.). This model considers user's expectations, preferences, background, family and environmental influences, and economic factors in the determination of appropriate AT (Institute for Matching Person and Technology, n.d.). This model attempts to

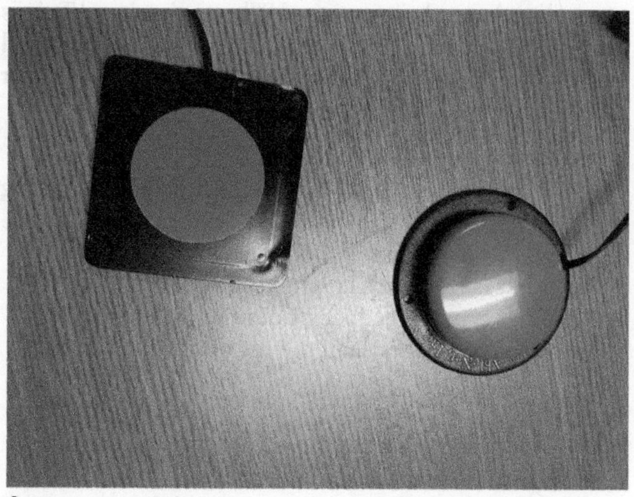
A

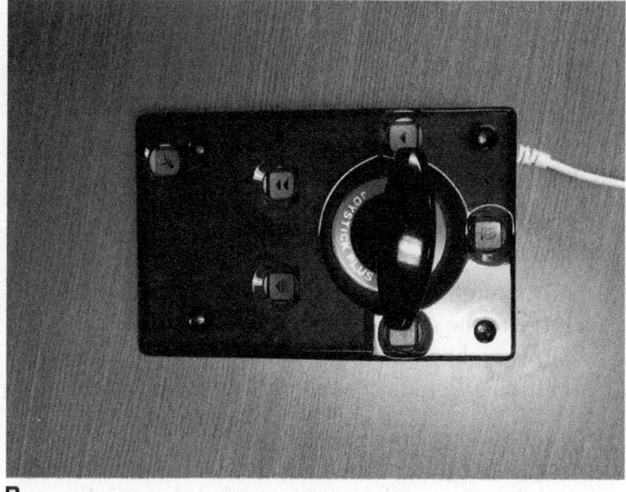

B

Figure 22.9 A. Plate switch and jelly bean switch. B. Joystick mouse.

identify characteristics including user's expectations, preferences, background, and family and environmental influences that lead to either AT device adoption or abandonment. There are three main components of the MPT model:

- Milieu: the environments in which the person uses the technology
- Person: the individual's characteristics and preferences
- Technology: the technology's functions and features (Institute for Matching Person and Technology, n.d.)

The MPT assessment process is a series of self-checklist and questionnaire assessment forms. Part of the process is choosing the appropriate forms to assess the individualized user needs, for example, using the Educational Technology Predisposition Assessment (ET PA) form for a student versus the Workplace Technology Predisposition Assessment (WT PA) for an employee. The target outcome of the assessment is the selection of an appropriate AT device that is adopted and used rather than abandoned. While the MPT model of AT assessment is targeted for adults with disabilities, a second model, Matching Assistive Technology & Child (MATCH) was developed to meet the needs of children.

Student Environment Tasks Tools Framework

The **Student Environment Tasks Tools (SETT)** Framework was created by Joy Zabala (Fig. 22.10). It was designed to aid the process of gathering, organizing, and analyzing data to inform collaborative problem solving and decision making regarding AT and appropriate educational programming for students with disabilities (Zabala, n.d.).

The "Student" factor of the framework looks at

- What does the student need to do?
- What are the student's current abilities and limitations?

The "Environment" factor analyzes all aspects of the environment needed to complete an educational task:

- What is the physical arrangement of the environment, and are there any special concerns?

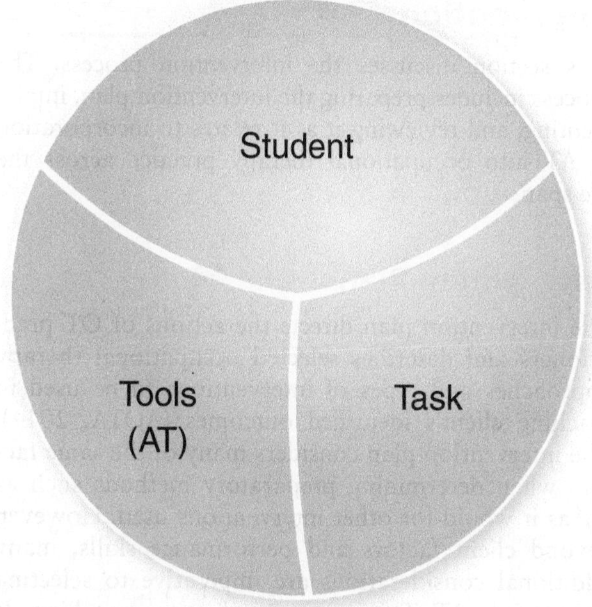

Figure 22.10 SETT Framework. (Diagram and information is based on and attributed to Dr. Joy Zabala, www.joyzabala.com and adapted with permission.)

- What materials and equipment are available to the students, and what resources are available to the people supporting the student?

The "Tasks" factor probes further into what activities take place in the environment and how difficult they may be for the student:

- What activities support the student's curriculum?
- What are the critical elements of the activities?
- How might the activities be modified to accommodate the student's special needs?
- How might technology support the student's active participation in those activities? (Zabala, n.d.)

By completing the first three areas of the SETT, the AT selection team is now ready to take this information and determine whatever is needed that might support the student's active participation in the specified activities. Once the first three factors are analyzed, the team can determine the "Tools." The specific and individualized information gathered from the first three factors assists in the feature matching of AT to meet the student's individualized needs. Questions that the AT assessment and selection team needs to ask are as follows: what strategies might be used to invite increased student performance? What no-tech, low-tech, and high-tech options should be considered when developing a system for a student with these needs and abilities doing these tasks in these environments? Also, how might these tools be trialed with the student in the natural environments in which they will be used (Zabala, n.d.)?

Intervention

This section discusses the intervention process. The process includes preparing the intervention plan, implementing, and reviewing it as it relates to incorporation of AT into occupational therapy practice across the life span.

Intervention Plan

The intervention plan directs the actions of OT practitioners and describes selected occupational therapy approaches and types of interventions to be used in reaching client's identified outcomes (AOTA, 2014). The intervention plan considers many of the same factors when determining preparatory methods such as AT as it would for other interventions used. However, beyond client factors and performance skills, many additional considerations are imperative to selecting appropriate AT. This process is feature matching. It utilizes evidence to assist with matching technology to meet a client's individualized needs and abilities. An ideal system is a flexible one, one that can adapt to a client's needs over time. When selecting AT, it is important to start the process with a client-centered approach. The information gathered about each client needs to include the following:

- What are the user's goals?
- What are the user's values and beliefs regarding AT?
- What are the user's functional capabilities?
- What is the user's cognitive status?
- What type of feedback does the user need?
- What position(s) will the user be in?

Considerations:

- Determine what the client does not want first!
- Determine what the client wants.
- Feature match to person's needs/abilities.
- The ideal system should be flexible and adaptable to client's needs and varying positions in which it is used over time. For example, a client with muscular dystrophy uses a head switch when lying in a hospital bed to call a caregiver for assistance. The system should allow for the client to be able to access the switch whether in supine and sidelying on either side, for example, constraints on device usage (King, 1999), if the client were to have a spasm or reflex as well as if the bed is positioned with the head up or down, for example, fail safe mechanisms (King, 1999) (Fig. 22.11).
- Understand and be able to explain the cost–benefit of the device.
- Remember that what works for one person does not necessarily work for another.
- Recommendations should be *individualized* to the person so that it fits his/her lifestyle and allows him/her to accomplish everyday tasks and perform daily routines.

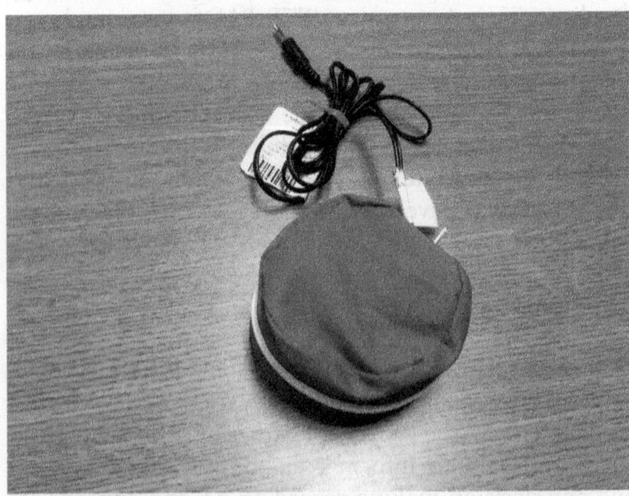

Figure 22.11 A pillow switch can be used with a client who is positioned in supine.

Also consider:

- What position will client be using AT in: seated in a wheelchair, standing, sidelying, or supine in bed.
- Is portability a factor; can it be accessible in any environment?
- Where will the device be used: in one or more rooms inside, outside, or both?
- What is the space availability in the client's home and/or work/school environment?
- Are there barriers and opportunities in environment(s) such as light/temperature/sound/radio-frequency interference?
- Think about installation, training, maintenance, and repair.
- What are the anticipated repair and maintenance issues? Is there a backup system in place should the device need repair or maintenance?
- Could existing technology be modified to meet client's needs rather than recommending new AT?
- What are the sources and availability of funding?
- Are there opportunities for training client and caregivers?

Intervention Implementation

Intervention implementation is the process of putting the intervention plan into action (AOTA, 2014). This is the time when the user has the opportunity to use the AT for the specified activity within the specified environment. Providing time for trials with AT allows for data to be collected regarding its effectiveness of use. It further allows for the OT practitioner to make modifications, as necessary, to optimize client occupational performance. Trials with AT provide for opportunity to obtain client feedback and gauge receptiveness of use, foreshadowing device adoption or abandonment. This is also a way to cost contain. Trials will determine if a device is worth purchasing or not, thus eliminating potential for spending money on a device/system that does not get used. Every State Tech Act program has an AT loan program. This is one option for obtaining loaner AT equipment for clients.

Integral to AT intervention implementation is education and training. It is recommended that all people who will come in contact with the device/system should be educated and trained on its use. This supports the client's carryover and overall success with use. For example, consider an older adult who safely uses a power scooter for functional mobility in a long-term care facility. The client has been trained on its use within the facility and has demonstrated safe carryover of use. It is important to also train the staff who work with the client, as they may need to assist with charging the device, monitoring it for maintenance and repair, as well as monitoring the client to ensure continued safe use. Clear and comprehensible documentation is imperative. Staffing changes for those who work with the client may be an ongoing challenge. Putting supports or a system in place that allow for new caregivers to be trained helps to provide continued care for the client, regarding their AT during times of transition (From the Field 22.3).

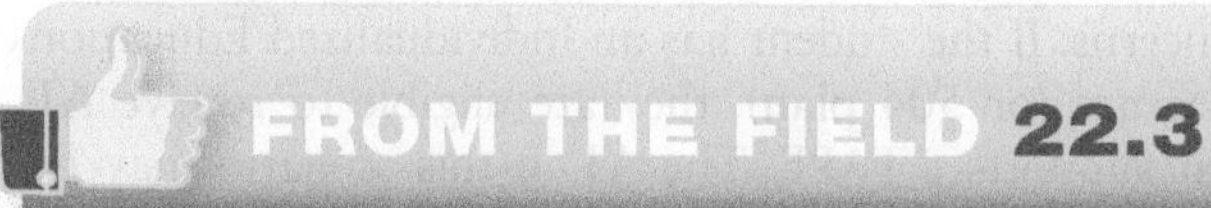

Considerations

When making an AT selection, it is important to think about the following:

- Is it difficult to install?
- Does it require multitasking to use?
- Does the recommended device interface with other AT client uses?
- What functions are needed/most appropriate?
- What transmission method will work in the environment(s)?
- Can a trial with actual device be facilitated?

Intervention Review

Intervention review as it relates to AT entails taking a closer look at the data obtained via the trials and analyzing it to determine success of use as it corresponds to the targeted outcome/outcomes. In this stage of the process, the OT practitioner is determining which of the AT devices/systems trialed best meet the client's needs. If the answer is none, determining the underlying reasons that may have impacted success is integral to selecting additional devices/systems for trial. This may require gathering more information via the occupational profile, activity analysis, analysis of occupational performance, and intervention to ensure each part of the process was thoroughly integrated into the plan. If though, an appropriate fit is found, device provision via coordinating funding and/or providing funding resources is the next step in the process of procuring AT for a client.

Funding

Funding for AT is very individualized. Funding varies based upon who the user is, where the user is receiving services, what AT is being used, and in what environment. For example, a client may be a fourth grade student with cerebral palsy who receives occupational therapy services within a public school system. This student may have seating, communication, and curricular (e.g., reading, writing) concerns. If the student has an Individualized Education Program (or 504 plan), they are eligible to receive AT that supports a FAPE. The AT in this scenario may be funded by the school district when needs are determined to be and justified as education necessary. However, this student may also be a Medicaid beneficiary. In this situation, the student is eligible to use Medicaid funding to assist with both the seating and positioning along with the communication concerns, if needs are determined to be and justified as medically necessary.

From a medical model perspective, different AT funding sources may be available to a client along the continuum of care. Consider a client who has sustained a traumatic brain injury and is currently receiving services at an inpatient rehabilitation hospital. While in inpatient rehabilitation, the client may use Medicare, Medicaid, and/or private insurance to fund AT. Once discharged from rehabilitation, that client may now be eligible to receive funding from vocational rehabilitation to assist with return to work. If the client was injured on the job, he/she may be eligible to receive workmen's compensation funding for any and all AT to return to previous life roles. For clients who may not readily have access to the abovementioned funding sources, as an OTA, having a knowledge of local and state programs is important to providing resources to your clients and their caregivers. Many states also provide low-interest loan programs to assist with obtaining AT. Clients who self-fund may be eligible to deduct the AT expenses as part of their medical deduction, work expenses, and/or miscellaneous work expenses on their taxes. In order for the AT to qualify as a deduction, the purchase must demonstrate that it not only provides assistance to the client but that it was purchased specific to meet a specific need. Table 22.5 provides an overview of AT funding sources.

TABLE 22.5 Overview of AT Funding Sources

Area Agencies on Aging
Civic and service associations (e.g., Rotary Club, Kiwanis Club, Elks Club)
Community Development Block Grant (CDBG) programs
Disability organizations (e.g., National Multiple Sclerosis Society, ALS Association)
Faith-based organizations
Health Promotion and Falls Prevention Grants
Loan programs
Long-term care insurance
Medicaid
Medicare
Schools
Self-funding and fund raisers
State Assistive Technology Projects
State agencies (e.g., Division of Vocational Rehabilitation, Division for the Visually Impaired)
Veterans Administration
Workmen's compensation

Certifications

Use of AT is within the purview of occupational therapy practice. For both OTs and OTAs, the progression from entry-level to advanced-level knowledge and skills related to technology and environmental interventions evolves through education and experience (AOTA, 2009). It is the ethical responsibility of OT practitioners to ensure that they are competent in the services they provide and routinely seek out new knowledge and techniques that apply to their practice (AOTA, 2010). Occupational therapy practitioners with an interest in technology and environmental modifications may also seek out certification within this area of practice. Currently, there are two AT-related certifications. AOTA offers the Specialty Certification in Environmental Modifications (SCEM). The application requires employment information along with evidence of a specified amount of hours of work as an OT or OTA and a minimum number of direct delivery of occupational therapy services within the environmental modifications area of practice. The application also contains a reflective portfolio section for documenting ongoing professional development or lifelong learning, continuing competence, and the ability to meet 12 identified criteria. The criteria are based on the AOTA *Standards for Continuing Competence: Knowledge, Critical Reasoning, Interpersonal Skills, Performance Skills and Ethical Practice* (AOTA, 2010). There is also an ongoing professional development section of the application, which includes a self-assessment and professional development plan.

A second certification is the Assistive Technology Professional (ATP) from the **Rehabilitation Engineering and Assistive Technology Society of North America (RESNA)**. The ATP recognizes demonstrated competence in analyzing the needs of consumers with disabilities, assisting in the selection of appropriate AT for the consumer's needs, and providing training in the use of the selected device(s) (RESNA, n.d.). Applicants are required to complete and pass a 200-item multiple-choice examination to qualify for certification.

Additional Resources

WATI free publications http://www.wati.org/?pageLoad=content/supports/free/index.php

WHO ICF Checklist: http://www.who.int/classifications/icf/training/icfchecklist.pdf

Summary

AT, from its simplest form, such as eyeglasses, and pencil grips to complex smartphones and communication systems plays an important role in our daily lives, no matter if we have disabilities or not. Occupational therapy practitioners are integral in assisting clients to select and use AT to optimize performance and participation. It is an exciting area of specialization to consider and which to obtain gain additional skills and training.

Review Questions

1. Which law provides for accommodations and supports, including AT for school-age children?
   a. The Americans with Disabilities Act
   b. The Individuals with Disabilities Education Act
   c. The Rehabilitation Act
   d. The Assistive Technology Act

2. Assistive Technology is defined as:
   a. Devices and equipment used to improve functional capabilities
   b. Evaluation of the needs of a client
   c. Training for the client, family, and caregiver
   d. All of the above

3. What are the four constructs of the Person–Environment–Occupation Model (PEOM)?
   a. Person, Environment, Occupation, Occupational Performance
   b. Person, Environment, Occupation, Occupational Justice
   c. Person, Environment, Occupation, Quality of Life
   d. Person, Environment, Occupation, Role Competence

4. Which of these clients may benefit from assistive technology?
   a. A 74-year-old woman with arthritis
   b. A 16-year-old girl with ADHD and developmental delay
   c. A 25-year-old man with high-level quadriplegia
   d. All of the above

5. What factor is least important when selecting AT that will support client adoption of use versus abandonment?
   a. Device aesthetics
   b. User-friendliness of the device
   c. Price
   d. Device durability

6. Which of the following categories of AT may require a referral to an occupational therapist with additional knowledge and skills?
   a. Low-vision aids
   b. Complex environmental modifications (CEM)—home environment
   c. Adaptive driving
   d. A and B
   e. All of the above

7. Which client might utilize indirect selection?
   a. A 65-year-old woman status post total knee replacement
   b. A 10-year-old girl with spastic quadriplegia cerebral palsy
   c. A 27-year-old man with T8 paraplegia
   d. A 53-year-old man status post right above-the-knee amputation

8. What is not a part of AT implementation?
   a. Completing trials
   b. Training the client, family, caregivers, and professionals
   c. Developing system for future trainings
   d. Provision of AT device/system

9. You are working in an outpatient setting with an 82-year-old client who has macular degeneration. She was successful with using a video magnifier to read her books, bills, and menus. She is interested in obtaining this device. Which funding sources might she be eligible to use?
   a. State Agency: Division for the Visually Impaired
   b. State assistive technology loan program
   c. Community Development Block Grant
   d. A and B
   e. All of the above

10. Choose the statement that is true.
   a. Certification is necessary for OT practitioners to utilize AT as a preparatory method.
   b. Use of assistive technology is not within the scope of OTA practice.
   c. Specialty Certification in Environmental Modifications (SCEM) is offered by the Rehabilitation Engineering and Assistive Technology Society of North America (RESNA).
   d. Assistive technology is within the purview of occupational therapy practice.

Practice Activities

Choose a device/technology that you use on a daily basis. Analyze the device for usability. What are the pros and cons of that device as it relates to human factors?

Feature Match: Review the features (pros and cons) of an AT device. Summarize the features relative to the abilities of individuals who could use this device. Give examples of how the device would be used by an individual in multiple environments.

Make a prototype of an AT device for a specific use, such as for adapted gardening, bowling, cooking, or grooming.

References

A Brief History of Typewriters. The Classic Typewriter page. n.d. Retrieved from http://site.xavier.edu/polt/typewriters/tw-history.html

Adler M. *The Writing Machine*. London: George Allen & Unwin; 1973.

Alexander Graham Bell Biography. *Encyclopedia of World Biography*. n.d. Retrieved from http://www.notablebiographies.com/Ba-Be/Bell-Alexander-Graham.html

American Occupational Therapy Association. *Specialized knowledge and skills in technology and environmental interventions for occupational therapy practice*. 2009. Retrieved from http://www.aota.org/-/media/Corporate/Files/Secure/Practice/OfficialDocs/Skills/SKS-Tech-Environmental-2010.pdf

American Occupational Therapy Association. *Standards for continuing competence*. 2010. Retrieved from http://www.aota.org/-/media/corporate/files/secure/practice/officialdocs/standards/standards%20for%20continuing%20competence%202010%20revision.pdf

American Occupational Therapy Association. *Occupational Therapy Practice Framework: Domain and Process*. 3rd ed. *Am J Occup Ther* 2014;68(Suppl. 1):S1–S48. http://dx.doi.org/10.5014/ajot.2014.682006

Association of Assistive Technology Act Programs (ATAP). Highlights of Tech Act Project Accomplishments. n.d. Retrieved from http://www.ataporg.org/highlights.html

Bailey RW. *Human Performance Engineering*. 2nd ed. Englewood Cliffs, NJ: Prentice-Hall; 1989.

Bodine C. *Disability: Key Issues and Future Directions: Assistive Technology and Science*. Thousand Oaks, CA: SAGE Publications, Inc.; 2013. doi: http://dx.doi.org/10.4135/9781452218434

Cook AM, Miller Polgar J. *Assistive Technologies: Principles and Practice*. 4th ed. St Louis, MO: Elsevier; 2014.

Department of Justice (DOJ). *A guide to disability rights laws*. 2009. Retrieved from http://www.ada.gov/cguide.htm#anchor65310

Federal Communications Commission (FCC). *Television Decoder Circuitry Act of 1990*. 1990. Retrieved from http://transition.fcc.gov/Bureaus/OSEC/library/legislative_histories/1395.pdf

Federal Communications Commission (FCC). *Hearing aid compatibility for wireline telephones*. n.d. Retrieved from http://www.fcc.gov/guides/hearing-aid-compatibility-wireline-telephones

Gierach J. *Assessing Students' Needs for Assistive Technology (ASNAT)*. 5th ed. Milton, WI: Wisconsin Assistive Technology Initiative; 2009.

Glennen S, DeCoste DC. *The Handbook of Augmentative and Alternative Communication*. San Diego, CA: Singular Pub. Group; 1997.

Goosens C, Crain SS. *Augmentative Communication Assessment Resource*. Wauconda, IL: Don Johnston Developmental Equipment; 1986.

IDEA. 20 U.S.C. Part A, Section 602. n.d. Retrieved from http://idea.ed.gov/download/statute.html

Institute for Matching Person and Technology. *Matching person and technology website*. n.d. Retrieved from http://www.matchingpersonandtechnology.com/mptdesc.html

King TW. *Assistive Technology: Essential Human Factors*. Boston, MA: Allyn & Bacon; 1999.

Law M, et al. The person-environment-occupation model: a transactive approach to occupational performance. *Can J Occup Ther* 1996;63(1):9–23.

Lee KS, Thomas DJ. *Control of Computer Based Technology For People With Physical Disabilities: An Assessment Manual*. Toronto: University of Toronto Press; 1990.

Merriam Webster Online. Ergonomics [Medical Definition]. n.d. Retrieved from http://www.merriam-webster.com/dictionary/ergonomics

Rehabilitation Engineering and Assistive Technology Society of North America (RESNA). Get Certified. n.d. Retrieved from http://www.resna.org/certification

United States Department of Education (USDOE). The Carl D. Perkins Vocational and Technical Education Act, Public Law 105–332. n.d. Retrieved from https://www2.ed.gov/offices/OVAE/CTE/perkins.html

United States Department of Labor (USDOL). Workforce Investment Act Laws and Regulations. n.d. Retrieved from http://www.doleta.gov/usworkforce/wia/act.cfm

World Health Organization. *International Classification of Functioning, Disability and Health: ICF*. Geneva, Switzerland: World Health Organization; 2001.

World Health Organization. *ICF Checklist, Version 2.1a, clinician form for international classification of functioning, disability and health*. 2003. Retrieved from: http://www.who.int/classifications/icf/training/icfchecklist.pdf

Zabala J. *The SETT Framework: Critical areas to consider when making informed assistive technology decision*. n.d. Retrieved from http://www.joyzabala.com/

CHAPTER 23

Activities of Daily Living and Instrumental Activities of Daily Living

Sheri Purdy, OTR/L, CLT and Kevin Piendak, EMBA, OTR/L

Key Terms

Activities of daily living (ADL)—Activities oriented toward taking care of one's body.

Assessment—Specific tools, instruments, or procedures used to obtain data during the evaluative process (AOTA, 2005).

Barrier—An obstacle that impedes completion of a task (Merriam-Webster.com, 2012).

Client centered—An orientation that honors the desires and priorities of clients in designing and implementing interventions.

Doff—To take off or remove.

Don—To put on.

Durable medical equipment—Equipment that can withstand repeated use, is primarily and customarily used to serve a medical purpose, and is generally not useful to a person in the absence of illness or injury (US Department of Health and Human Services, 2005).

Equipment—Devices used to promote independence including adaptive equipment (e.g., reacher, sock aide, dressing stick) or durable medical equipment (e.g., tub seat, tub bench, commode).

Instrumental activities of daily living (IADL)—Activities to support daily life within the home and community that often require more complex interactions than self-care used in ADL (AOTA, 2014).

Instrumental activities of daily living (IADL)—Activities to support daily life within the home and community that often require more complex interactions than self-care used in ADL (AOTA, 2014).

Intervention planning—Process in which activities are chosen with goals established and modified to enhance functional performance toward an outcome.

Quality of life—A client's dynamic appraisal of life satisfactions (perceptions of progress toward identified goals), self-concept (the composite of beliefs and feelings about themselves), health and functioning (including health status, self-care capabilities), and socioeconomic factors (e.g., vocation, education, income) (American Occupational Therapy Association, pp. 625–683).

Task-oriented activity—An activity that has inherent meaning and purpose for a client.

Learning Objectives

After studying this chapter, readers should be able to:

- Recognize the role of occupational therapy assistant in the training of clients with activities of daily living and instrumental activities of daily living tasks.
- Understand the value that the occupational therapy assistant and the occupational therapist roles play in the assessment and intervention planning for all clients.

- Identify assistive devices/equipment designed to enhance performance and independence within the context of activities of daily living.
- Explain how to incorporate activities of daily living components into intervention planning.
- Recognize how performance skills can impact successful completion of activities of daily living and instrumental activities of daily living.

Introduction

At the heart of occupational therapy practice is the philosophy of helping clients become independent with all of life's activities of daily living (ADL) and instrumental activities of daily living (IADL). As identified in the *Domain* of occupational therapy (AOTA, 2014), OT practitioners incorporate these skills, tasks, and functional performance components into all of our client's daily routines and intervention planning activities. Throughout this chapter, you will learn the value and importance of your role as future OTAs in the assessment and intervention planning of ADL and IADL and also to identify which daily tasks are classified as ADL versus IADL. You will also learn to distinguish between which daily tasks are classified as ADL or IADL with varied diagnoses and different levels of impairments. Occupational therapy assistants play a vital role in working with clients to improve ADL and IADL skills in order to maximize quality of life.

Overview of Activities of Daily Living

As identified by the *Occupational Therapy Occupational Therapy Practice Framework III*, **activities of daily living (ADL)** are defined as "activities that are oriented toward taking care of one's own body" (adapted from Rogers & Holm, 1994, pp. 181–202; AOTA, 2014, p. S19). ADL also are referred to as basic activities of daily living (BADLs) and personal activities of daily living (PADLs). Whether referred to as ADL, BADL, or PADL, these activities are "fundamental to living in a social world; they enable basic survival and well-being" (Christiansen & Hammecker, 2001, p. 156) CS1-13. Table 23.1 contains a summary of ADL and their definitions as stated in the *Occupational Therapy Practice Framework III* (2104).

Overview of Instrumental Activities of Daily Living

Activities to support daily life within the home and community often require more complex interactions with the self and environment than ADL and are called **instrumental activities of daily living (IADL)**. See Table 23.2 for a description of IADL as stated in the *Occupational Therapy Practice Framework III* (2104).

A person's perceived **quality of life** varies based on their current situation, life experiences, and psychological and physical status. ADL and IADL are key components to enhancing a client's quality of life. The ability to care for oneself and/or others goes to the core of our self-worth as individuals CS1-13. As OT practitioners, if we are able to work with clients to increase their ability to perform these tasks at their most proficient level possible, we have also assisted with enhancing their quality of life. In order to develop an appropriate intervention plan, it is important to be competent to assess and identify each client's strengths and limitations for core components of ADL/IADL skills work.

Assessment of ADL/IADL

At the beginning of every occupational therapy intervention session, it is important to take the time to completely and accurately assess the client's current functional status. It is incumbent upon every OT practitioner to select and use a variety of tools (activities and adaptive equipment) to effectively complete this process and make it as client centered as possible. But before even starting the intervention, the OT must complete a detailed **assessment**. Per AOTA practice guidelines, an OT must complete the initial evaluation (AOTA, 2009, pp. 175–176). Each assessment should always begin with gathering a detailed client profile. This includes prior medical history, prior level of function, current living situation, and caregiver support structure. To be **client centered**, clients need to be given the opportunity to express their desired goals and outcome, and in turn, OT practitioners must incorporate this information into the client's therapy goals and intervention plan. In a nutshell, it is simply making sure

TABLE 23.1 Domain of Activities of Daily Living

ADL Domain	Definition
Eating	The ability to keep and manipulate food or fluid in the mouth and swallow it
Feeding	The process of setting up, arranging, and bringing food [or fluid] from plate or cup to the mouth; sometimes called self-feeding
Grooming/hygiene	Obtaining and using supplies; removing body hair (e.g., use of razors, tweezers, lotions); applying and removing cosmetics; washing, drying, combing, styling, brushing, and trimming hair; caring for nails (hands and feet); caring for skin, ears, eyes, and nose; applying deodorant; cleaning mouth; brushing and flossing teeth; or removing, cleaning, and reinserting dental orthotics and prosthetics
Bathing	Obtaining and using supplies; soaping, rinsing, and drying body parts; maintaining bathing position; transferring to and from bathing positions
Dressing	Selecting clothing and accessories appropriate to time of day, weather, and occasion; obtaining clothing from storage area; dressing and undressing in a sequential fashion; fastening and adjusting clothing and shoes; and applying and removing personal devices, prostheses, or orthotics
Bowel and bladder	Completing intentional control of bowel movements and urinary bladder and, if necessary, using equipment or agents for bowel and/or bladder control
Toileting	Obtaining and using supplies; clothing management; maintaining toileting position; transferring to and from toileting position; cleaning body; and caring for menstrual and continence needs (including catheters, colostomies, and suppository management)
Functional mobility	Moving from one position or place to another (during performance of everyday activities), such as in bed mobility, wheelchair mobility, and transfers (e.g., wheelchair, bed, car, tub, toilet, tub/shower, chair, floor). Includes functional ambulation and transporting objects

American Occupational Therapy Association. Occupational therapy practice framework: domain and process (3rd ed.). *Am J Occup Ther* 2014;68(Suppl. 1):S1–S48. http://dx.doi.org/10.5014/ajot.2014.682006; Uniform Data System for Medical Rehabilitation. *The Functional Independence Measure (FIM) The IRF-PAI Training Manual*. Buffalo, NY: Author; 2012:III28–III30.

that you are factoring the needs and wishes of your client into all aspects of their intervention plan.

When gathering information for the assessment, the OT asks the client about his/her medical history. The OTA may take an active role in this process. If a client is unable to provide this information, the OT practitioner seeks the information from family members, caregivers, or medical records. As OT practitioners often seek information from client medical records, they need to be familiar with medical diagnoses and the limiting factors that may hinder the client's ability to participate in ADL/IADL activities. Because disease and past and present functioning impact every client differently, the end results are individualized barriers/limitations toward achieving independence with ADL/IADL that must be addressed in the intervention process.

To accurately determine how significant a client's present barriers/limitations are, it is essential to understand the client's prior level of function CS1-13. It is important to seek out information about the client's daily routine prior to the occupational therapy assessment. A typical day in the lives of clients varies, so it is critical to gather the relevant information about the details of their typical day, such as those described in Tables 23.1 and 23.2. As has been discussed, if a client is unable to provide an accurate synopsis of his/her daily life, you will need to gather this information from family members or caregivers. Remember, it is all about client-centered intervention.

Understandably, awareness of the client's living situation and support structure prior to the assessment is vital to establish an appropriate intervention plan that meets the client's functional goals as well as to deliver client-centered intervention. It is important to learn about the client's home setup and evaluate the contexts in which ADLS will be performed postdischarge. This includes learning about any **durable medical equipment (DME)** and assistive **equipment** that the client owns and/or uses on a daily basis. Durable medical equipment, which is equipment that can withstand repeated use, is primarily and customarily used to serve a medical purpose and is generally not useful to a person

TABLE 23.2 Domain of Instrumental Activities of Daily Living

IADL Domain	Definition
Meal preparation and cleanup	Planning, preparing, and serving well-balanced, nutritional meals, cleaning up remaining food and dishes/utensils after meals
Shopping	Preparing shopping lists (grocery and other); selecting, purchasing, and transporting items; selecting method of payment; and completing money transactions
Care of others (including selecting and supervising caregivers)	Arranging, supervising, or providing the care for others
Care of pets	Arranging, supervising, or providing the care for pets and service animals
Communication management	Sending, receiving, and interpreting information using a variety of systems and equipment including writing tools, telephones, typewriters, audiovisual recorders, computers, communication boards, call lights, emergency systems, Braille writers, telecommunication devices for the deaf, augmentative communication systems, and personal digital assistants
Child rearing	Providing the care and supervision to support the developmental needs of a child
Safety and emergency management	Knowing and performing preventive procedures to maintain a safe environment as well as recognizing sudden, unexpected hazardous situations and initiating emergency action to reduce the threat to health and safety
Community mobility	Moving around in the community using public or private transportation, walking, or biking
Financial/economic management	Using fiscal resources, including various methods of financial transaction and planning and financial planning with long-term and short-term goals
Health management and maintenance	Developing, managing, and maintaining routines for health and wellness promotion, such as physical fitness, nutrition, decreasing health risk behaviors, and medication routines
Religious observance	Participating in religion, "an organized system of beliefs, practices, rituals, and symbols designed to facilitate closeness to the sacred or transcendent"

American Occupational Therapy Association. Occupational therapy practice framework: domain and process (3rd ed.). *Am J Occup Ther* 2014;68(Suppl. 1):S1–S48. http://dx.doi.org/10.5014/ajot.2014.682006

in the absence of illness or injury (US Department of Health and Human Services, 2005), and assistive equipment both contribute to helping a client maintain an independent lifestyle (**CS8, 11**). Both will be discussed in further detail in this chapter. It is also important to know about specialized services that the client may receive including, but not limited to, meal delivery, home services like cleaning and self-care assistance, and transportation services **CS12**.

The next step in the assessment process is to thoroughly evaluate the client's current ADL/IADL functional level. Both standardized and informal assessments are used to gather this information. Administering standardized and informal assessments can be done via questionnaires, simulated performance testing, and/or observation or actual performance activities (From the Field 23.1). Please refer to Table 23.3 for a comprehensive list of various ADL/IADL assessments and corresponding information. It is important to understand the role that the OTA plays in this process. Although the OT typically completes a majority of the assessment process, there are many opportunities for the OTA to participate in the data collection based on demonstrated competence and experience. A collaborative partnership between the two practitioners is vitally important to successfully establish an appropriate intervention plan for the client.

It is important to stay up to date on assessment tools and intervention protocols. Please refer to Chapter 5, *The Evidence-Based Movement: Guiding the Practice,* for a detailed discussion about how to find evidence-based research to support the assessment selection process. Assessments are generally expensive, so OT practitioners are wise to do a thorough analysis of which assessments they will purchase. Some assessments will not be available for purchase unless an OT has been trained to administer it. Some assessments may be

TABLE 23.3 ADL/IADL Assessments

Age Group	ADL/IADL Assessments	Standardized
Newborn—24 Months	*Prefeeding Skills Checklist*	No
Adolescents—Adults	*Assessment of Occupational Function (AOF)*	Yes
	Occupational Performance History Interview (OPHI-II)	Yes
	Occupational Self-Assessment	Yes
Adult—Elderly	*A-One*	Yes
	Amps	Yes
	Barthel Index	No
	Direct Assessment of Functional Abilities (DaFa)	Yes
	Functional independence measure (FIM)	Yes
	Kitchen Task Assessment (KTA)	Yes
	Kohlman Evaluation of Living Skills (KELS)	Yes
	Milwaukee Evaluation of Daily Living Skills (MEDLS)	No
	Performance Assessment of Self-Care Skills (PASS)	No
	Routine Task Inventory (RTI-II)	No
Elderly	*Independent Living Scales (ILS)*	Yes
All Ages	*Canadian Occupational Performance Measures (COPM)*	Yes

Adapted from Burns AP. Appendix B: assessment tool grid. In: Sladyk K, Jacobs K, MacRae N, eds. *Occupational Therapy Essentials for Clinical Competence*. Thorofare, NJ: SLACK, Inc.; 2010:542–544.

purchased online and come with instructions and scoring forms, but knowing if the assessment tool is reliable and/or valid and meets the needs of what has to be assessed should factor into determining whether it should be purchased (From the Field 23.1).

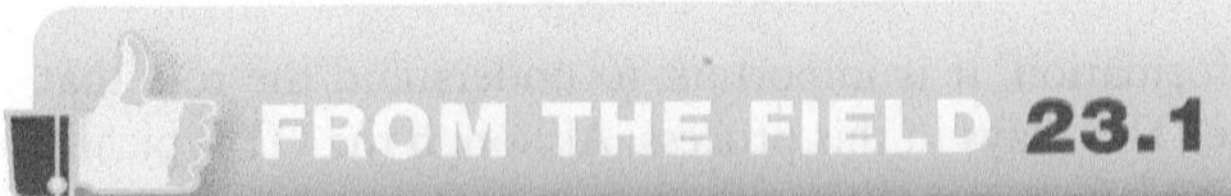

Standardized and Nonstandardized Assessments

A standardized assessment is one that has established reliability and validity; it has been determined to measure what it was intended to do. Scores on standardized assessments can be compared to others who have taken it, such as IQ tests. A nonstandardized assessment does not have established reliability and validity. Results cannot be compared to others. An example of a nonstandardized test is a checklist. Both standardized and nonstandardized assessments are important components of the evaluation process.

While Table 23.3 provides a sampling of assessment tools, the list is not inclusive. There are numerous standardized and nonstandardized assessments to measure ADL/IADL that are available to OT practitioner. It is the responsibility of every OT practitioner to research, select, and use the appropriate assessments that best meets the client's needs. All OT practitioners are encouraged to incorporate current evidenced-based research and practice into their assessment and intervention processes and be open to updating their skill set and practice tools as new best practice research and practice guides our professional decision making and actions.

Developing an Intervention Plan for ADL/IADL

Once the assessment is complete, it is the OT practitioner's responsibility to develop an appropriate intervention plan for ADL/IADL activities. This begins with identifying the client's current functional performance limitations as compared to his/her prior level of function. This includes but is not limited to those activities as identified in Tables 23.1 and 23.2.

Once functional limitations have been identified, the next step in the intervention process is for the OT practitioner to identify the barriers preventing a client from improving functional skills. The barriers may include medical precautions, physical or emotional limitations, lack of or limited support systems, or environmental challenges within the home or community. Based on occupational therapy's holistic intervention philosophy, the OT practitioner must consider all potential barriers in order to assure that the correct interventions are chosen to address the functional problem areas that the client presented during the assessment CS1-13.

Intervention activities should be chosen based on theoretical frames of reference in collaboration with client-centered goals (please also refer to Chapter 7, *Occupational Therapy Theories and How They Guide Practice*, and Chapter 14, *Documentation*). To put it another way, OT practitioners should base their intervention decisions on theoretical approaches that have been supported by evidence and that will specifically address their client's needs. Selecting appropriate intervention activities that have been validated through evidence-based research supports the success of occupational therapy services.

Influencing Factors that May Impact ADL/IADL Interventions and Outcomes

In the previous section, we discussed the term "barriers." What exactly are barriers? **Barriers** are obstacles that impede the completion of a task (Merriam-Webster, 2012). They negatively influence a client's functional performance and inform and guide how OT practitioners develop an intervention plan. How do OT practitioners identify factors that may negatively impact ADL/IADL treatment, interventions, and outcomes? This is an important question because as OT practitioners, it is our job to reduce these factors to improve the client's function. A skilled OT practitioner is able to look at all aspects of what it takes for their clients to complete functional tasks and from this information identify the specific components that are causing performance limitations. This varies from client to client and is the role of the OT practitioner to utilize all resources to create a series of interventions that will enhance performance. Occupational therapy practitioners need to be well aware of the co-occurring social, emotional, physical, and/or medical factors that create barriers to functional performance as well as those that support functional performance. The successful OT practitioner must consider all of these factors when developing a client-centered intervention plan. It goes without saying that interventions should be based on addressing the limiting factors and client's strengths in order to strive for successful attainment of desired client-centered goals. Do not despair. It takes time and experience to develop a repertoire of ideas and to establish appropriate interventions to achieve the desired outcomes. You will get there!

Performance Skills and ADL/IADL

When considering the bigger picture of ADL/IADLs, it is important to remember that it takes more than one skill to successfully complete each task. These actions are called performance skills (AOTA, 2014). These skills guide actual ADL/IADL tasks. As described in the *Occupational Therapy Practice Framework III*, Table 23.3 outlines the most applicable performance skills associated with various ADL/IADL tasks. For specific definitions of each task, please refer to Table 23.4, *Occupational Therapy Practice Framework III* (2014).

Goal Development for ADL/IADL Intervention

When referring to client-centered goal writing, it means that you are establishing goals that not only take into account what you feel the client needs, based on assessment results as well as an understanding of the client's postdischarge environment, but also that you are establishing goals that take into account what the client wants to achieve from the occupational therapy intervention process. Why is writing client-centered goals so important? It is important for two primary reasons. First, establishing goals that are client centered play a significant role in justifying a skilled intervention plan that targets your client's needs and helps assure reimbursement for the skilled services that you have provided. The second reason and in many respects the most important reason is that your clients will be far more likely to follow your recommended course of intervention if they have participated in its development and they are working toward goals that have importance and meaning to them.

An OT writes short-term and long-term goals as well as establishes an intervention plan that sets the path toward reaching the client's goals. The OTA, in **collaboration** with the OT, may adjust and revise the intervention plan after it has been established in order to meet the client's short-term objectives and/or long-term goals. In the event that there is a change in status and goals and objectives are no longer appropriate, it is the responsibility of the OTA to discuss this with the OT so that the intervention plan can be revised as necessary to stay on track (From the Field 23.2).

Selecting Activities for ADL/IADL Intervention

It takes a lot of work to get to this point in the intervention process. But now that you are here, it is important to recognize that selecting meaningful and purposeful activities for an intervention plan is the most essential component to consider when working with a client to improve functional outcomes. Intervention planning builds on everything that has been previously discussed in this chapter.

When establishing an intervention plan for ADL/IADL, it is critical to take into account the client's goals, age,

TABLE 23.4 ADL/IADL Domain and Performance Skills

ADL Domain	Performance Skills Needed to Complete the Task
Swallowing/eating	• Motor and praxis skills • Sensory–perceptual skills • Cognitive skills
Feeding	• Motor and praxis skills • Sensory–perceptual skills • Cognitive skills
Personal hygiene and grooming	• Motor and praxis skills • Sensory–perceptual skills • Cognitive skills
Bathing/showering	• Motor and praxis skills • Sensory–perceptual skills • Emotional regulation skills • Cognitive skills
Dressing	• Motor and praxis skills • Sensory–perceptual skills • Cognitive skills
Toileting/toileting hygiene	• Motor and praxis skills • Sensory–perceptual skills • Cognitive skills
Personal device care	• Motor and praxis skills • Sensory–perceptual skills • Cognitive skills
Sexual activity	• Motor and praxis skills • Sensory–perceptual skills • Cognitive skills
Functional mobility	• Motor and praxis skills • Sensory–perceptual skills • Cognitive skills
IADL	Performance skills
Meal preparation and cleanup shopping	• Motor and praxis skills • Sensory–perceptual skills • Cognitive skills • Communication and social skills
Care of others (including selecting and supervising caregivers)	• Motor and praxis skills • Sensory–perceptual skills • Emotional regulation skills • Cognitive skills • Communication and social skills
Child rearing	• Motor and praxis skills • Sensory–perceptual skills • Emotional regulation skills • Cognitive skills • Communication and social skills
Care of pets	• Motor and praxis skills • Sensory–perceptual skills • Emotional regulation skills • Cognitive skills • Communication and social skills
Communication management	• Motor and praxis skills • Sensory–perceptual skills • Emotional regulation skills • Cognitive skills • Communication and social skills
Safety and emergency management community mobility Driving	• Motor and praxis skills • Sensory–perceptual skills • Emotional regulation skills • Cognitive skills • Communication and social skills
Financial/Economic Management	• Motor and praxis skills • Emotional regulation skills • Cognitive skills • Communication and social skills
Health management and maintenance	• Motor and praxis skills • Sensory–perceptual skills • Emotional regulation skills • Cognitive skills • Communication and social skills
Religious and spiritual activities and expression	• Motor and praxis skills • Sensory–perceptual skills • Emotional regulation skills • Cognitive skills • Communication and social skills

American Occupational Therapy Association. Occupational therapy practice framework: domain and process (3rd ed.). *Am J Occup Ther* 2014;68(Suppl. 1):S1–S48. http://dx.doi.org/10.5014/ajot.2014.682006

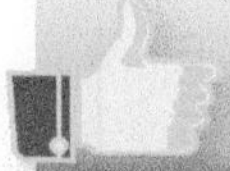

FROM THE FIELD 23.2

Measurable and Objective Goals

Measurable and objective goal writing involves knowing the following:

1. The client
2. The functional skills that the client is working toward
3. The measurement of success and/or skill level that is anticipated
4. Necessary DME or assistive devices that will help the client to achieve his/her goal(s)
5. Time frame within which to achieve the goals

Some examples of measurable goals are provided in Table 23.4. They each include the criteria as indicated above. Remember that regardless of what the setting practice you will be working in or the clients you treat, this method will help you with writing effective client-centered goals.

available support structures and services, medical status, and prior level of function. There should never be a cookie-cutter approach to intervention, that is, every client has different needs and must be provided a personally meaningful course of intervention (please also refer to Chapter 18, *Ensuring Purposeful and Meaningful Interventions*). Selecting personally meaningful **task-oriented activities** that directly enable clients to improve function cannot be stressed enough.

Plans must focus on interventions that lead to function and measurable outcomes. Consider using this checklist to guide you through developing an intervention plan (From the Field 23.3).

1. What is the functional problem area that you have identified?
2. What are the barriers or limitations that are interfering with your client's ability to be independent in with a particular skill or task?
3. Based on these barriers, what theoretical approach to intervention do you need to use to address this area of dysfunction?
4. Based on this theoretical model, what client-centered meaningful intervention activities are you going to select that will address the barriers negatively impacting client function?

A sample template for developing an effective, client-centered intervention plan for a client who has recently had a total hip replacementis found in Table 23.5.

By now, you are seeing that **intervention planning** and goals work together. You must know your client's goals in order to establish an appropriate intervention plan,

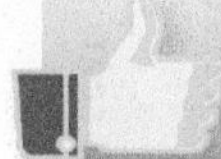

FROM THE FIELD 23.3

Front and Center

When developing your intervention plan, always keep your client's goals front and center in your mind.

and you cannot develop an appropriate intervention plan without establishing and knowing your client's goals!

Durable Medical Equipment and Assistive Devices

Durable medical equipment and assistive devices may be beneficial for clients to improve and enhance ADL/IADL skill CS1-13 (please also refer to Chapter 21, *Adaptive Equipment*, and Chapter 22, *Assistive Technology*). The equipment and devices that you may teach clients to use and/or recommend they obtain include, but are not limited to, the the information found in (Table 23.6 and Figures 23.1–23.25.

These items are just a small sampling of the commercially durable medical equipment and assistive devices that can make the difference between a client's dependence and independence. Please also refer to Chapter 21, *Adaptive Equipment*, and Chapter 22, *Assistive Technology*, for additional information. Various online companies sell DME and assistive devices as do some local medical pharmacies and bog box stores. A list of several online companies can be found at the conclusion of this chapter. Please note, the authors and publisher have no financial stake in these companies nor do they endorse any of them. The list is provided for informational purposes only.

Some insurance companies may cover the cost of the DME or assistive devices, while others may not. This varies from state to state and with individual insurance policies. Insurance companies may also request that the OT practitioner provide a letter of medical necessity to justify the need for the DME or assistive devices. Again, this varies by state and insurance companies. It is of the utmost importance for OT practitioners to be familiar with what is and is not cost covered when discussing DME and assistive devices needs with clients. Sometimes, purchasing these items is a financial hardship for the client/family. For this reason, it is equally as important to become familiar with local agencies that might provide equipment on a loaner basis. Being comfortable with all of the pieces to the puzzle of teaching, recommending, and obtaining DME and assistive devices to improve function helps the OT practitioner gain the trust of their clients and assure them that their best interest is at heart.

TABLE 23.5 A Guide to Intervention Planning

Functional Problem Area	Barriers or Limitations	Theory/Frame of Reference	Intervention Activities	Long-Term Goal
Requires assist with lower body bathing and dressing	• Total hip precautions • Decreased endurance • Decreased standing balance	• Biomechanical • Rehabilitative • Occupational adaptation • Canadian Model of Occupational Performance • Person–Environment–Occupation Performance Model • Model of Human Occupation	• Educate and train with long-handled adaptive equipment • Practice patient's sit to stand while maintaining total hip precautions • Practice **donning** and **doffing** pants and undergarments while maintaining weightbearing precautions	The client will be independent 100% of the time with lower body self-care activities with the use of long-handled adaptive equipment (LHAE) within 2 weeks.
Moderate assistance with toilet transfers	• Partial weightbearing status • Total hip precautions • Increased pain • Decreased weight shifting	• Biomechanical • Rehabilitative • Occupational Adaptation Canadian Model of Occupational Performance • Person–Environment–Occupation Performance Model • Model of Human Occupation	• Educate on weight bearing and hip precautions • Educate and practice using DME including raised toilet seat, Versaframe bars, grab bars, toileting aides • Address pain management strategies • Weight shifting activities in the parallel bars or with walker while participating in a meaningful therapeutic activity	The client will complete toilet transfers at modified independent level 100% of the time with standard walker (SW) and use of raised toilet seat (RTS) within 2 weeks.
Decreased independence with toileting	• Decreased standing tolerance • Total hip precautions • Inability to reach peri areas	• Biomechanical • Rehabilitative • Occupational Adaptation • Canadian Model of Occupational Performance • Person–Environment–Occupation Performance Model • Model of Human Occupation	• Functional activities completed in standing, increasing time as able • Educate on hip precautions • Trunk activities to increase trunk flexion and rotation to gain reaching status and if unsuccessful, discuss toileting aides and compensatory strategies	The client will be independent with toileting at a standing level with SW within 2 weeks. The client will be independent with toileting 100% of the time from a seated position on the RTS within 2 weeks.
Requires assistance with meal preparation	• Decreased activity tolerance • Decreased standing balance • Decreased safety with standard walker • Total hip precautions	• Biomechanical • Rehabilitative • Occupational Adaptation • Canadian Model of Occupational Performance • Person–Environment–Occupation Performance Model • Model of Human Occupation • Motor control and motor learning	• Functional activities to promote activity tolerance • Balance activities in standing • Written instructions for safety, place in the room and on the walker • Educate on hip precautions	The client will prepare a simple meal 50% of the time with supervision using an SW within 2 weeks. The client will demonstrate good static standing balance 75% of the time within 2 weeks for meal preparation.

From Cole M, Tufano R. *Applied Theories in Occupational Therapy: A Practical Approach*. Thorofare, NJ: SLACK, Inc.; 2008.; Sladyk et al. (2010).

TABLE 23.6 Durable Medical Equipment and Assistive Devices

Activity	Equipment/Assistive Devices	
Feeding (Figures 23.1–23.3)	• Scoop bowl/plate • Built-up utensils • Various cups • Double handle cup • One flow valve cups	• Weighted utensils • Universal cuffs • Flexible feeding arms (gooseneck) • Electric feeding devices

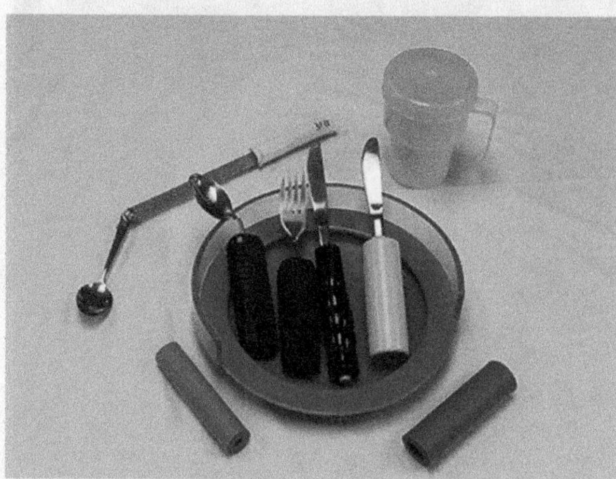

Figure 23.1 Built-up utensils, weighted utensils, plate guard. (Photos provided by Sheri Purdy and Kevin Piendak. Equipment property of New England Rehabilitation Hospital Woburn, MA. Used by permission.)

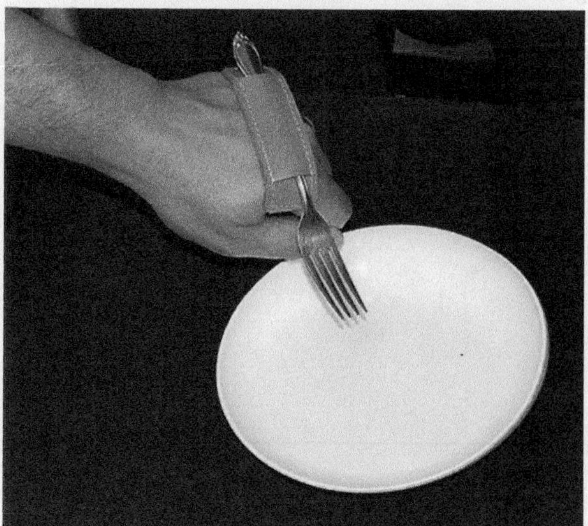

Figure 23.2 Nonskid scoop plate, universal cuff. (Photos provided by Sheri Purdy and Kevin Piendak. Equipment property of New England Rehabilitation Hospital Woburn, MA. Used by permission.)

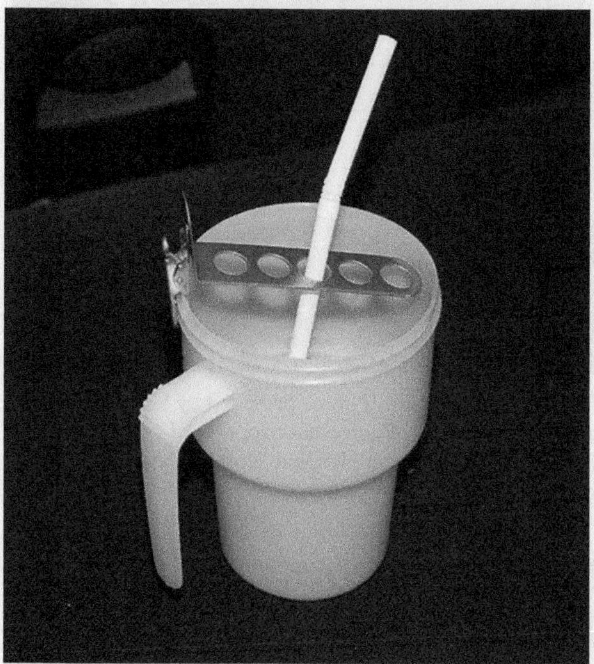

Figure 23.3 Straw holder. (Photos provided by Sheri Purdy and Kevin Piendak. Equipment property of New England Rehabilitation Hospital Woburn, MA. Used by permission.)

(*continues on page 294*)

TABLE 23.6 Durable Medical Equipment and Assistive Devices (continued)

Activity	Equipment/Assistive Devices
Grooming/hygiene (Figures 23.4–23.6)	• Built-up handle items • Suction toothbrush • Tube squeezer • Bath mitt • Foot care kit • Magnifying glass

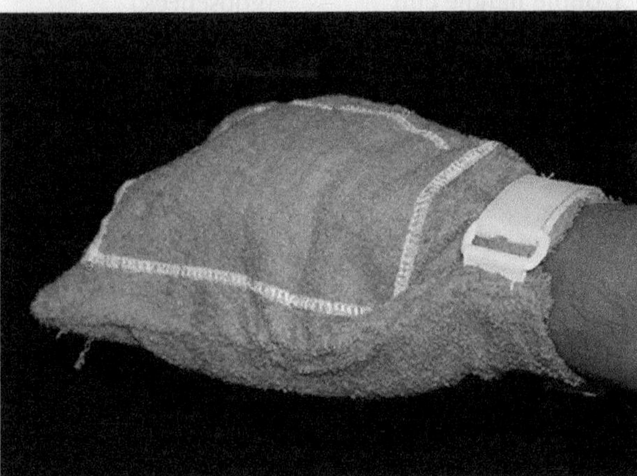

Figure 23.4 Bath mitt. (Photos provided by Sheri Purdy and Kevin Piendak. Equipment property of New England Rehabilitation Hospital Woburn, MA. Used by permission.)

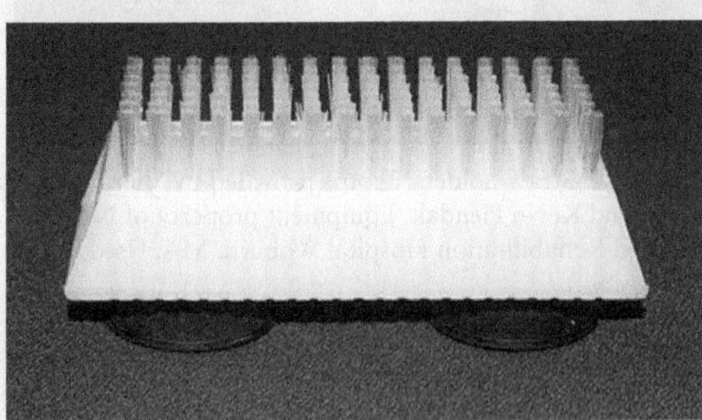

Figure 23.5 One-handed scrub brush. (Photos provided by Sheri Purdy and Kevin Piendak. Equipment property of New England Rehabilitation Hospital Woburn, MA. Used by permission.)

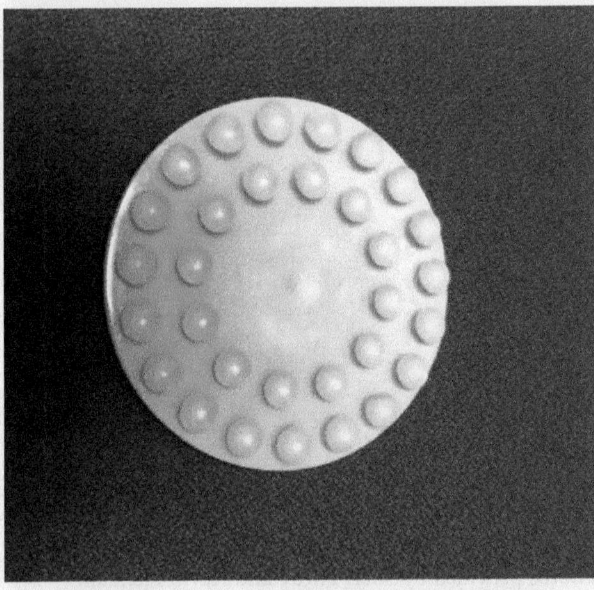

Figure 23.6 Suction soap holder. (Photos provided by Sheri Purdy and Kevin Piendak. Equipment property of New England Rehabilitation Hospital Woburn, MA. Used by permission.)

TABLE 23.6 Durable Medical Equipment and Assistive Devices (continued)

Activity	Equipment/Assistive Devices	
Bathing/dressing (Figures 23.7–23.9)	• Reacher • Sock aide • Dressing stick • Long-handled bath brush • Button hook • Zipper pull • Long-handled shoe horn	• Leg lifters • Elastic shoe laces • Lace locks • Easy fasteners • Tub seats • Tub benches • Shower hose

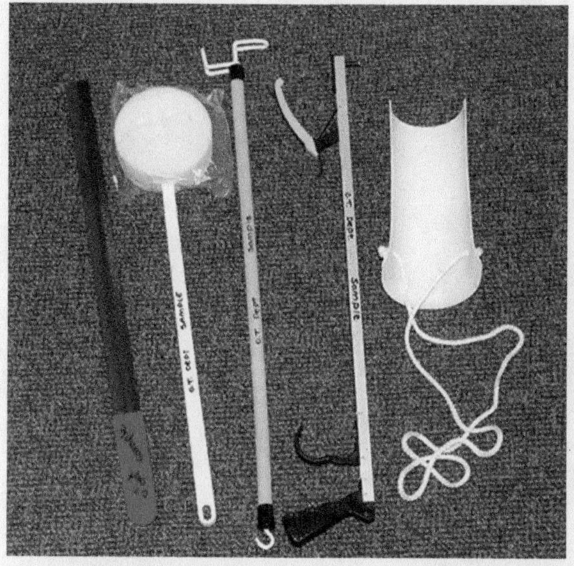

Figure 23.7 Long-handled shoe horn, long-handled scrub brush, dressing stick, reacher, sock aide. (Photos provided by Sheri Purdy and Kevin Piendak. Equipment property of New England Rehabilitation Hospital Woburn, MA. Used by permission.)

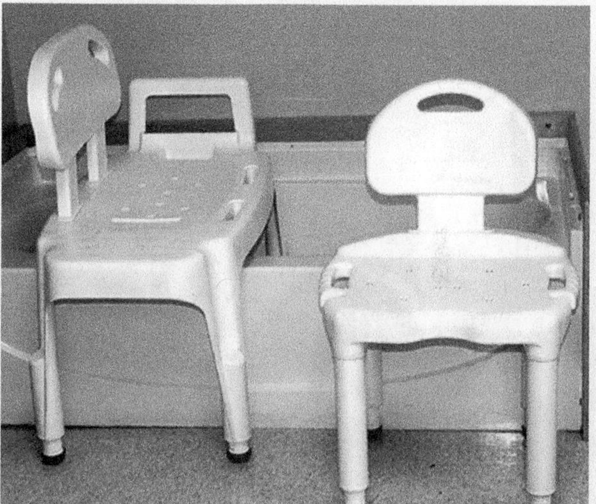

Figure 23.9 Tub seat with back transfer bench. (Photos provided by Sheri Purdy and Kevin Piendak. Equipment property of New England Rehabilitation Hospital Woburn, MA. Used by permission.)

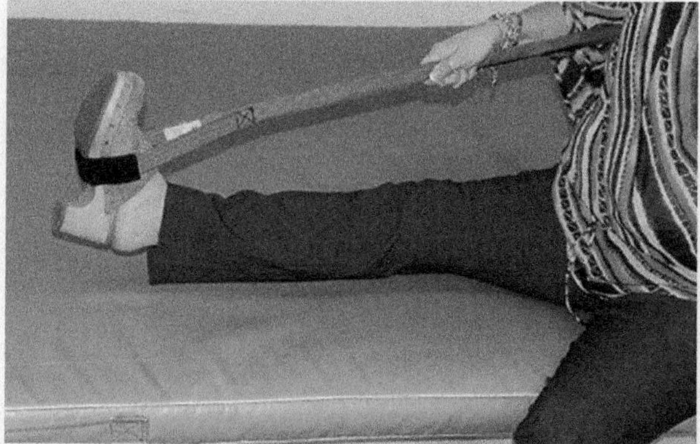

Figure 23.8 Leg lifter. (Photos provided by Sheri Purdy and Kevin Piendak. Equipment property of New England Rehabilitation Hospital Woburn, MA. Used by permission.)

(*continues on page 296*)

TABLE 23.6 Durable Medical Equipment and Assistive Devices (continued)

Activity	Equipment/Assistive Devices	
Toileting (Figures 23.10–23.13)	• Toilet tongs • Self-catheterization mirror • Pant holders • Urinals/bedpan	• Bidet spa • Raised toilet seats • Versaframe bars • Commodes

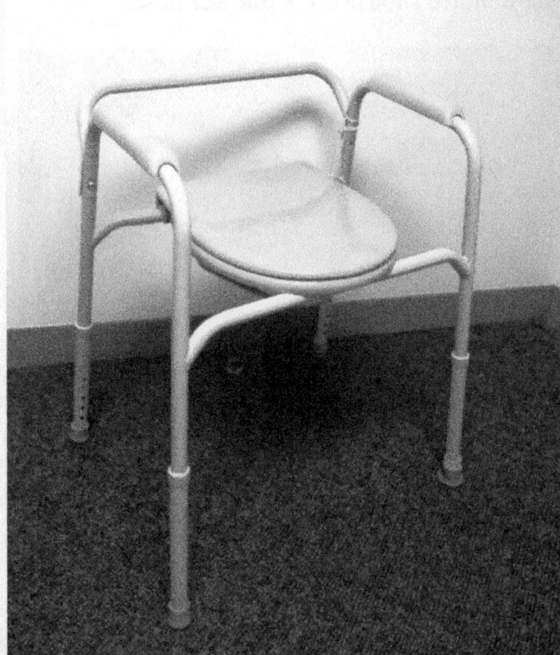

Figure 23.10 Commode. (Photos provided by Sheri Purdy and Kevin Piendak. Equipment property of New England Rehabilitation Hospital Woburn, MA. Used by permission.)

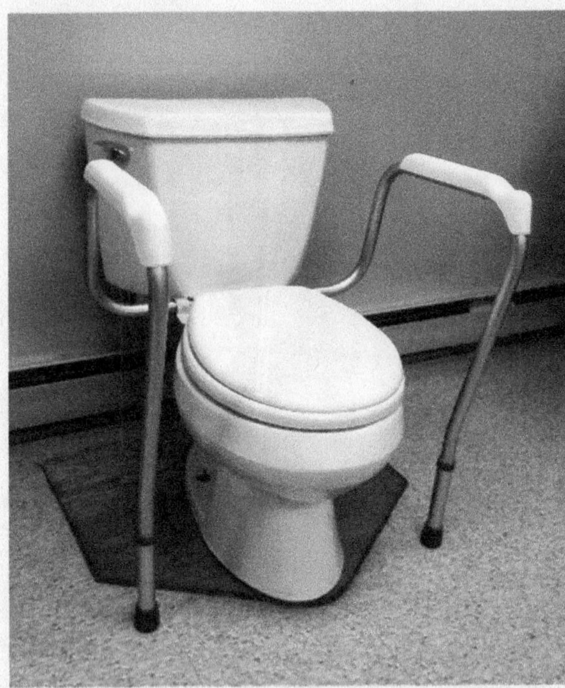

Figure 23.12 Versaframe bars. (Photos provided by Sheri Purdy and Kevin Piendak. Equipment property of New England Rehabilitation Hospital Woburn, MA. Used by permission.)

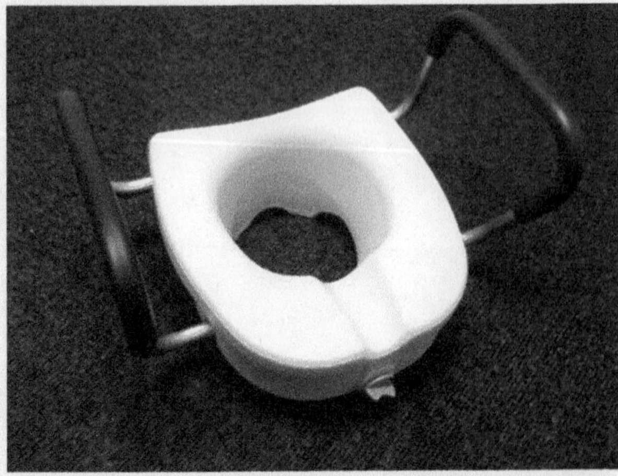

Figure 23.11 Raised toilet seat with arms. (Photos provided by Sheri Purdy and Kevin Piendak. Equipment property of New England Rehabilitation Hospital Woburn, MA. Used by permission.)

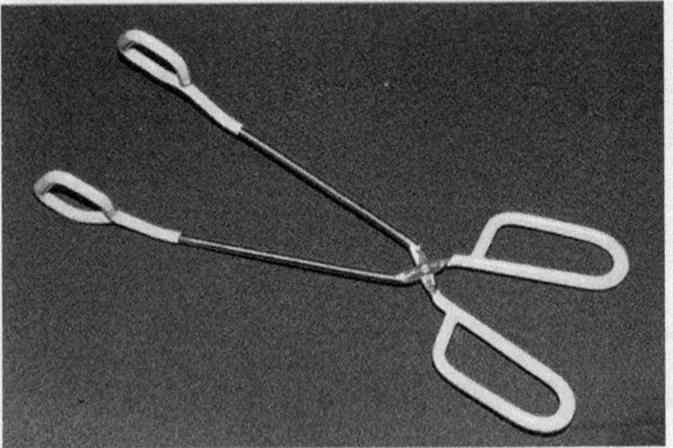

Figure 23.13 Toilet tongs. (Photos provided by Sheri Purdy and Kevin Piendak. Equipment property of New England Rehabilitation Hospital Woburn, MA. Used by permission.)

TABLE 23.6 **Durable Medical Equipment and Assistive Devices** (continued)

Activity	Equipment/Assistive Devices
Functional and community mobility (Figures 23.14–23.19)	• Cane • Crutches • Walker • Hemiwalker • Platform walker • Wheelchair • Rollators • Walker baskets and accessories • Adaptive vehicles • Transfer board • Hoyer lifts • Chair lifts

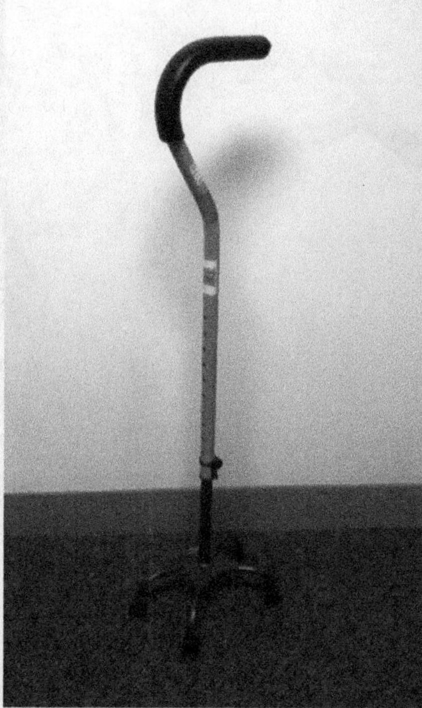

Figure 23.14 Small base quad cane. (Photos provided by Sheri Purdy and Kevin Piendak. Equipment property of New England Rehabilitation Hospital Woburn, MA. Used by permission.)

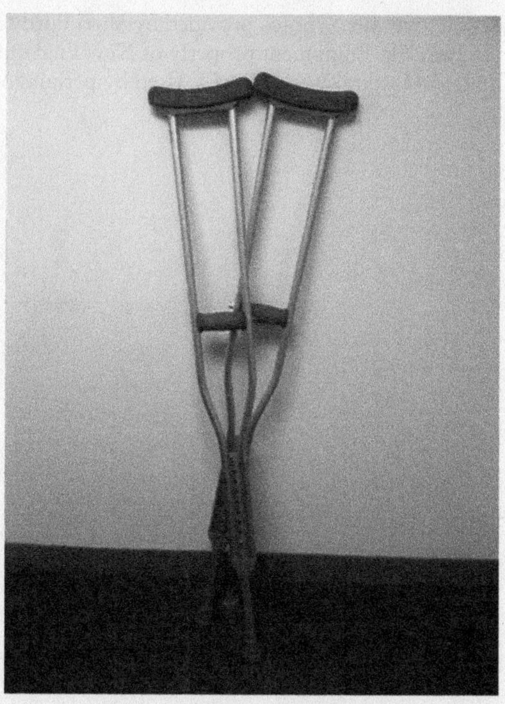

Figure 23.15 Crutches. (Photos provided by Sheri Purdy and Kevin Piendak. Equipment property of New England Rehabilitation Hospital Woburn, MA. Used by permission.)

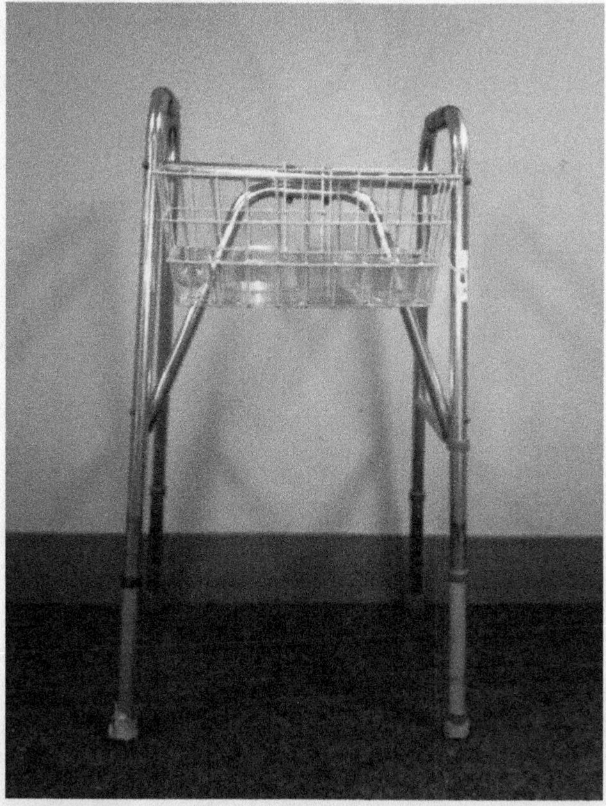

Figure 23.16 Walker with walker basket. (Photos provided by Sheri Purdy and Kevin Piendak. Equipment property of New England Rehabilitation Hospital Woburn, MA. Used by permission.)

(*continues on page 298*)

TABLE 23.6 Durable Medical Equipment and Assistive Devices (continued)

Activity	Equipment/Assistive Devices

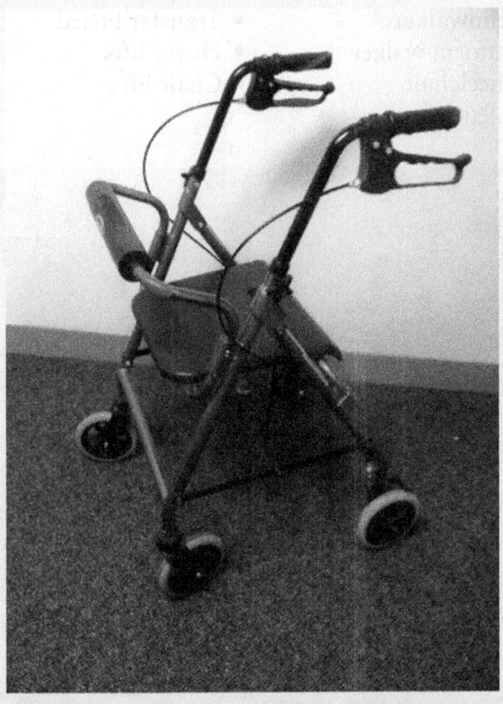

Figure 23.17 Rollator. (Photos provided by Sheri Purdy and Kevin Piendak. Equipment property of New England Rehabilitation Hospital Woburn, MA. Used by permission.)

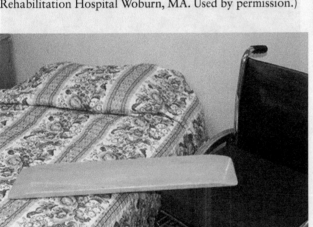

Figure 23.18 Slideboard. (Photos provided by Sheri Purdy and Kevin Piendak. Equipment property of New England Rehabilitation Hospital Woburn, MA. Used by permission.)

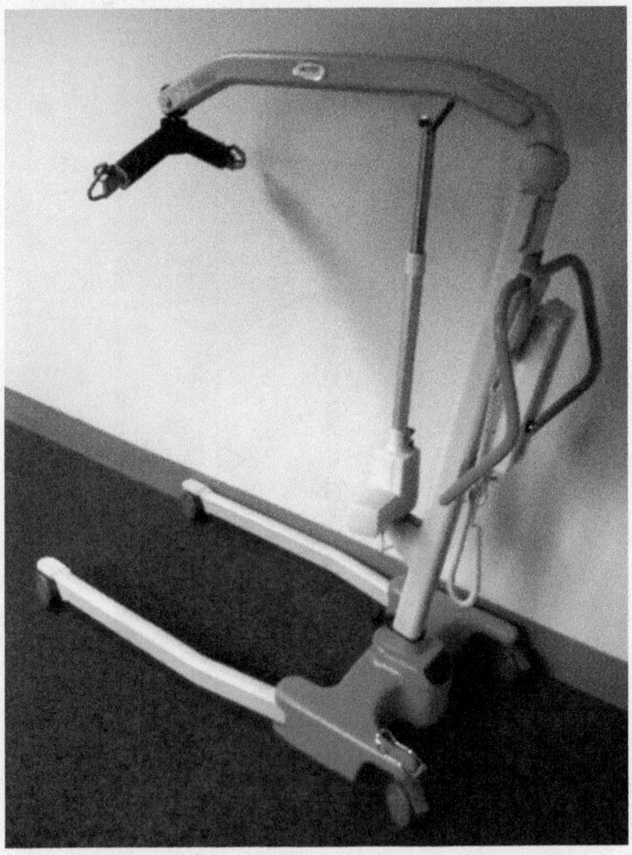

Figure 23.19 Hoyer lift. (Photos provided by Sheri Purdy and Kevin Piendak. Equipment property of New England Rehabilitation Hospital Woburn, MA. Used by permission.)

TABLE 23.6 **Durable Medical Equipment and Assistive Devices (continued)**

Activity	Equipment/Assistive Devices
Meal prep/shopping (Figures 23.20 and 23.21) 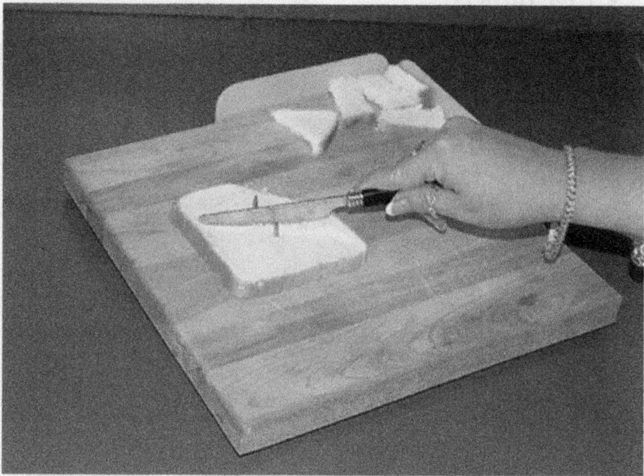 Figure 23.20 One-handed cutting board. (Photos provided by Sheri Purdy and Kevin Piendak. Equipment property of New England Rehabilitation Hospital Woburn, MA. Used by permission.)	• Stove key • Power grip • Contour turner • One-handed jar opener • Nonskid bowl • One handed cutting board • Magnifying glass • Mobility devices 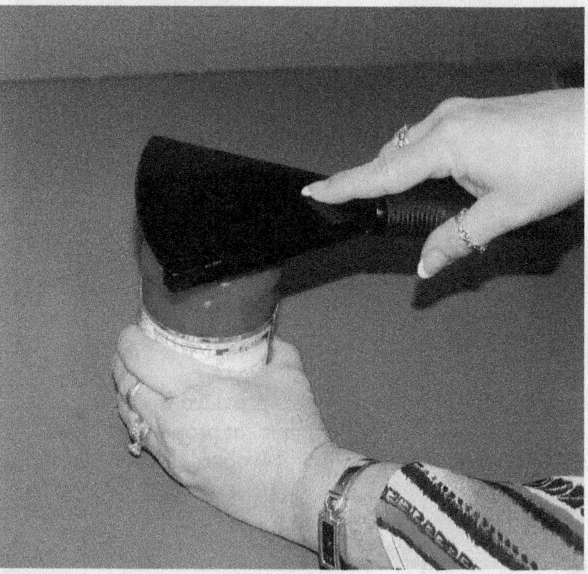 Figure 23.21 One-handed jar opener. (Photos provided by Sheri Purdy and Kevin Piendak. Equipment property of New England Rehabilitation Hospital Woburn, MA. Used by permission.)
Care of others	Situationally dependent
Care of pets (Figure 23.22) Figure 23.22 Raised food and water bowls for pets. (Photos provided by Sheri Purdy and Kevin Piendak. Equipment property of New England Rehabilitation Hospital Woburn, MA. Used by permission.)	• Raised food and water bowls • Long-handled scooper • Automatic litter replacement • Disposable litter pans

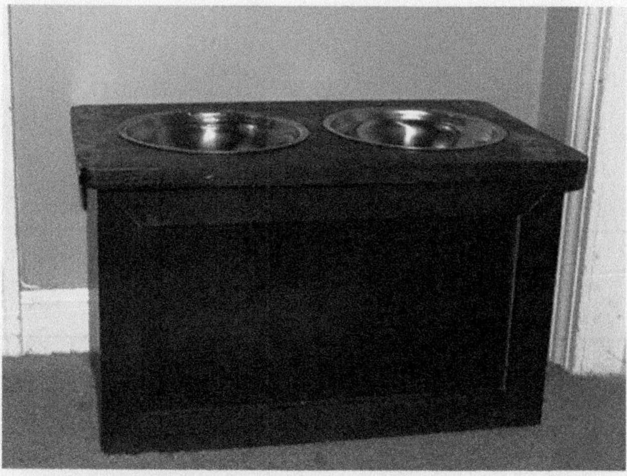

(*continues on page 300*)

TABLE 23.6 Durable Medical Equipment and Assistive Devices (continued)

Activity	Equipment/Assistive Devices
Communication management (Figures 23.23–23.25) 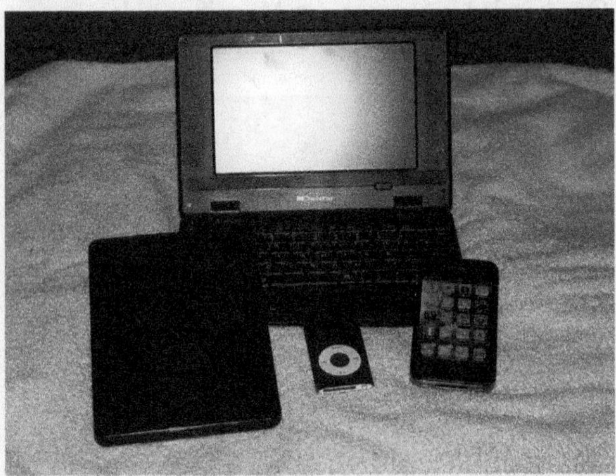 Figure 23.23 Technology. (Photos provided by Sheri Purdy and Kevin Piendak. Equipment property of New England Rehabilitation Hospital Woburn, MA. Used by permission.) 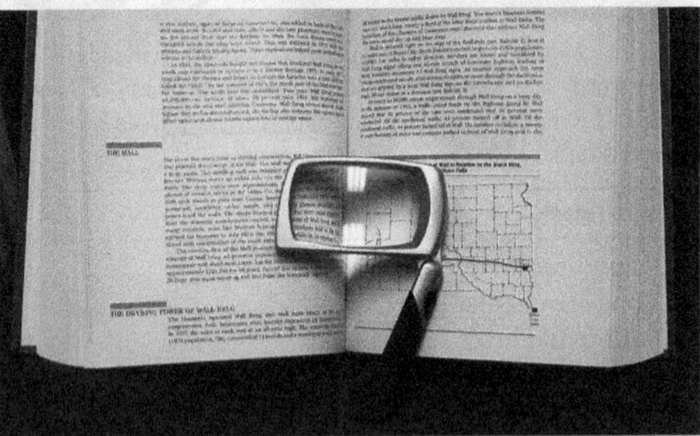 Figure 23.24 Magnifying glass. (Photos provided by Sheri Purdy and Kevin Piendak. Equipment property of New England Rehabilitation Hospital Woburn, MA. Used by permission.)	• Sip and puff devices • Head pointers/head mouse • Voice-activated devices • Book holders • Page turners • Magnifiers • Altered writing utensils • Larger print/screens • Altered styluses • Mouth stick 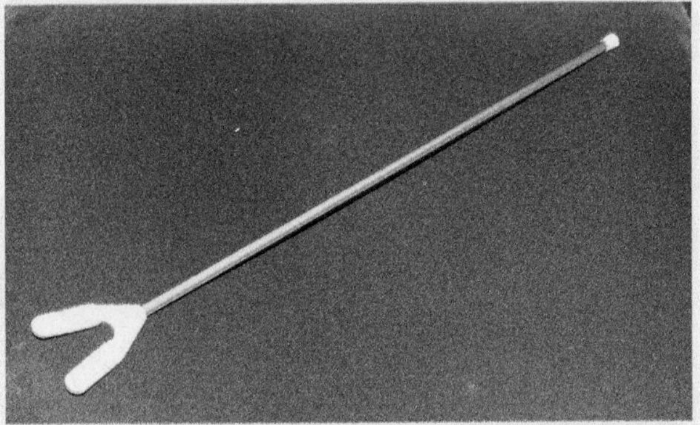 Figure 23.25 Mouth stick. (Photos provided by Sheri Purdy and Kevin Piendak. Equipment property of New England Rehabilitation Hospital Woburn, MA. Used by permission.)
Safety and emergency management	• Life line or similar emergency response alert system • Ramps • Lifts
Financial and economic management	• Large print checkbook, registers, or ledgers • Adapted writing utensils • Duplicate forms for checks • Computerized system • Ask for assistance
Religious observance	• Raised seating • Chair risers • Assess based on specific religious customs

Summary

ADLs and IADLs are the building blocks to enhancing a client's quality of life. It is what we do every day from the minute we wake up until we go to sleep. The ability to care for oneself and take part in a daily routine to the greatest extent possible enhances self-worth and identity, which in turn validates and embraces our client's individual uniqueness. This is why OT practitioners must accurately assess clients, combine this information with understanding who they are as individuals, and formulate this into goals and objectives and a intervention plan that maximizes skill level. If we are able to do this successfully, then not only are we improving a client's functional performance with a specific task but helping to provide the client the skills he or she needs to improve the job of living.

Review Questions

1. Identify three specific activities that are within the AOTA domain of activities of daily living.
   a. ____________
   b. ____________
   c. ____________

2. Identify three specific activities that fall with the AOTA domain of instrumental activities of daily living.
   a. ____________
   b. ____________
   c. ____________

3. True or false: A barrier is an obstacle that impedes completion of a task.

4. True or false: An OTA can complete the initial evaluation.

5. True or false: A standardized assessment is not valid or reliable.

6. Check off three ADL assessments that can be utilized by OT practitioners.
   _____ A-one
   _____ Amps
   _____ Assessment of Occupational Function
   _____ Functional Independence Measure
   _____ Milwaukee Evaluation of Daily Living Skills
   _____ Performance Assessment of Self-Care Skills

7. Performance skills that influence ADL/IADLs are:
   a. Motor and praxis skills
   b. Sensory–perceptual skills
   c. Emotional regulation skills
   d. Cognitive skills
   e. Communication and social skills
   f. All of the above

8. True or false: Measurable and objective goal writing involves knowing the following:
   The client
   The functional skills that the client is working toward
   The measurement of success and/or skill level that is anticipated
   Necessary DME or assistive devices that will help the client to achieve his/her goal(s)
   Time frame within to achieve the goals

9. True or false: The definition of the term "client centered" is an orientation that honors the desires and priorities of clients in designing and implementing interventions.

10. True or false: Performance skills are the abilities clients demonstrate in the actions they have the potential to perform.

Practice Activities

If your college/university's clinical lab is stocked with the following DME or assistive devices, take turns being a client and an OTA and do the following:

1. Feeding/eating
   Practice a feeding activity, such as drinking water or eating a salad with any piece of adaptive equipment (e.g., scoop plate, adaptive utensils, adaptive cups, universal cuff).

2. Dressing
   Practice donning and doffing pants with a reacher.
   Practice donning and doffing socks with a sock aide.
   Practice buttoning a shirt with a button hook.

3. Meal preparation
   Practice cutting a piece of bread/food using a one-handed cutting board and a rocker knife (with and without a universal cuff).
   Open a jar using a grip opener or a one-handed jar opener.

4. Functional communication
   Turn the page of a book using a page turner and book stand (may also use a magnifier if available).
   Use a stylus to turn a page in a book or open an application on an electronic device like a smartphone or tablet.

5. Mobility activities
   Practice walking with a walker to get from a bed/chair to a toilet.
   Practice propelling a wheelchair in order to complete self-care tasks at a sink.
   Practice transfers with a slide board or Hoyer lift from bed to chair.

After doing each of these activities, write a one-page summary of your experiences as both a client and as a practicing OTA.

Online Resources for Durable Medical Equipment and Assistive Devices

Accelerated Care Plus: www.ACPcares.com
Active Forever: www.activeforever.com
AliMed: www.alimed.com
Patterson Medical: www.pattersonmedical.com
Pmsi: www.pmsionline.com

References

American Occupational Therapy Association. Standards of practice for occupational therapy. *Am J Occup Ther* 2005;59:663–665.

American Occupational Therapy Association. *Occupational Therapy Practice Guidelines*. Bethesda, MD: Author; 2009:175–176.

American Occupational Therapy Association. Occupational therapy practice framework: domain and process (3rd ed.). *Am J Occup Ther* 2014;68(Suppl. 1):S1–S48. http://dx.doi.org/10.5014/ajot.2014.682006

Burns AP. Appendix B: assessment tool grid. In: Sladyk K, Jacobs K, MacRae N, eds. *Occupational Therapy Essentials for Clinical Competence*. Thorofare, NJ: SLACK, Inc.; 2010:542–544.

Christiansen CH, Hammecker CL. Self care. In: Bonder BR, Wagner MB, eds. *Functional Performance in Older Adults*. Philadelphia: F.A. Davis; 2001:155–178.

Cole M, Tufano R. *Applied Theories in Occupational Therapy: A Practical Approach*. Thorofare, NJ: SLACK, Inc.; 2008.

Rogers JC, Holm MB. Assessment of self-care. In: Bonder BR, Wagner MB, eds. *Functional Performance in Older Adults*. Philadelphia: F.A. Davis; 1994:181–202.

Sladyk K, Jacobs K, MacRae N, eds. *Occupational Therapy Essentials for Clinical Competence*. Thorofare, NJ: SLACK, Inc.

Uniform Data System for Medical Rehabilitation. *The Functional Independence Measure (FIM) The IRF-PAI Training Manual*. Buffalo, NY: Author; 2012:III28–III30.

US Department of Health and Human Services. National coverage determination (NCD) for durable medical equipment reference list (280.1); 2005. Retrieved from http://www.cms.gov/medicare-coverage-database/details/ncd-details.aspx?NCDId=190&ncdver=2&NCAId=3&ver=5&NcaName=Air-Fluidized+Beds+for+Pressure+Ulcers&bc=ACAAAAAAIAAA& http://www.anthem.com/medicalpolicies/guidelines/gl_pw_a053621.htm

Webster-Merriam online. *Diagnosis*; 2012. Retrieved from http://www.merriam-webster.com/dictionary/diagnosis

CHAPTER 24

Orthotics and Orthotic Fabrication

Lt. Col. (Ret) Sandra Harrison-Weaver, MHE, OTR/L, CHT and
Lt. Col. Matthew St. Laurent, MS, OTR/L, CHT

Key Terms

Dynamic orthosis—An orthosis with moving parts, typically used to apply constant tension or force to a body part or mobilize a joint in a controlled manner.

Orthosis—A rigid or semirigid device applied externally to a body part for support or immobilization.

Pressure area—A place on the skin that becomes red or irritated because a part of an orthosis is too tight or rough.

Static orthosis—An orthosis that typically is composed of one nonmoving part, typically used to immobilize and/or stabilize joints.

Static progressive orthosis—An orthosis that can be incrementally changed for slow progressive tissue and joint adjustments that usually have movable parts, such as turnbuckles or hinges.

Thermoplastic—A polymer that becomes soft or moldable above a certain temperature and solid when cooled.

Learning Objectives

After studying this chapter, readers should be able to:

- State five purposes for orthotic fabrication.
- Describe the differences between static and dynamic orthoses.
- Fabricate and fit a static orthosis, incorporating appropriate design principles.
- Educate a client on proper wear, care, and precautions of an orthotic device.

Introduction

While the history of splinting can be traced back for thousands of years, recently, and in accordance with best professional practice, what they are now referred to as has changed. Occupational therapy practitioners are recognized as leaders in fabricating custommade splints as part of a therapeutic program. A "splint" is an "orthopedic device for immobilization, restraint, or support of any part of the body" (Mosby, 2002, p. 1618). The term "splint" is often used interchangeably with the term orthosis, which as you may have surmised by now, is the preferred professional term. An **orthosis** (or orthotic device) is defined by the *Durable Medical Equipment, Prosthetics, Orthotics, and Supplies (DMEPOS) Quality Standards* as a "rigid or semirigid device used for the purpose of supporting a weak or deformed body member or restricting or eliminating motion in a diseased or injured part of the body" (2012, p. 3). Recently, federal legislative efforts have attempted to regulate and restrict payment for custom fabricated splints/orthoses to only qualified practitioners. Therefore, to more efficiently align with the terminology used by the Centers for Medicare and Medicaid Services (Coverdale, 2012) and to increase the likelihood of reimbursement for fabrication services, the term "orthosis" or "orthotic device" is preferred by OT and PT national associations. In effort to align with current trends in health care policy, from this point forward, the terms orthosis/orthotic fabrication will be used in place of splint/splinting in this chapter.

Frame of Reference

Occupational therapy practice is never complete without a theoretical explanation describing why we do what we do. Orthotic fabrication is no exception. Use of an orthotic device is a type of modality or intervention that supports or prepares the individual for engagement in occupation. Therefore, orthotic fabrication and client use of orthoses may encompass a variety of theoretical approaches as its foundation. For example, in the case of an individual who has had a stroke, a sensorimotor approach is considered when the orthosis is used to inhibit abnormal muscle tone. Whereas a rehabilitation approach may be used when applying a tenodesis orthosis used to recreate grasp and release for a client with a spinal cord injury (Coppard & Lohman, 2007). A theoretical basis or frame of reference is helpful in guiding the OT practitioner to select both the type of orthotic device to provide and the intended purpose and/or outcome of the orthotic device.

In the context of the *Occupational Therapy Practice Framework III*, an orthosis is a preparatory intervention method within the client factor domain to optimize ability and performance during occupational engagement. The use of an orthosis and its effects on pain reduction, support to the extremity, and improved function may enhance physiological ability and motivation to perform. Meaningful efforts to complete a task lead to habituation and valued outcomes for optimal performance and return to quality living (AOTA, 2014).

Purposes of Orthotic Devices

There are a multitude of reasons that an individual may require an orthosis. They include injury, disease processes, birth defects, or aging processes. The ultimate goal of an orthotic device is to allow an individual to engage in meaningful/purposeful activities such as work, leisure, self-care, and sleep safely, competently, and as independently as possible (Fig. 24.1).

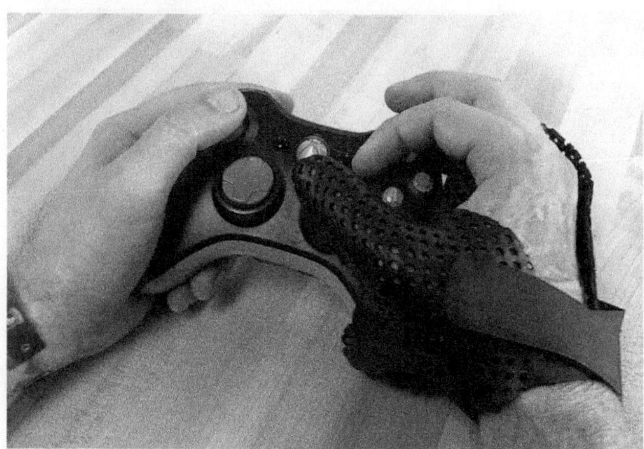

Figure 24.1 Adaptive stylus for an upper extremity amputee. (Courtesy of Erik Johnson.)

Use of sound clinical reasoning and an applicable frame of reference will help an OT practitioner determine and prioritize orthotic needs and goals. Some individuals may need a very complex orthotic device, and some may need more than one orthosis to achieve the intended goal. It is imperative that every OT practitioner tasked to fabricate any type of orthotic device thoroughly understand anatomy, biomechanical principles, and the stages of wound healing in order to properly and effectively apply an orthosis that the physician has recommended. Therefore, an OTA, working under the supervision of an OT, must demonstrate competency before fabricating orthotics for clients. A primary purpose for orthotic use is immobilization of a joint or body part, including bones, tendons, ligaments, nerves, blood vessels, fascia, and/or skin. In most cases, stabilization or immobilization is essential in order to:

- Promote healing of an injured body part and/or tissue (such as a fracture).
- Prevent further damage of the involved structures (such as a tear or rupture).
- Provide rest to inflamed tissues (such as tendinitis or rheumatoid arthritis).
- Prevent deformity (such as contractures from burns or spasticity).
- Support lax ligaments (such as after joint hyperextensions or dislocations).

Another primary purpose for orthotic use is to promote movement of a joint, body part, and/or tissue in a specific fashion. Examples include the following:

- Substitute for lost motor function (such as in radial nerve palsy or spinal cord injury).
- Correct deformities (such as elongating or stretching scar tissue from burns or joint contractures).
- Provide controlled motion (such as with flexor and extensor tendon rehabilitation in which the orthosis facilitates specific motion to promote healing while limiting any motion that may damage the tendon).
- Aid in fracture alignment (primarily providing traction in a specific direction).

Both mobilization and immobilization orthoses can be used to reduce pain or discomfort.

Creative orthotic designs are also useful for adapting equipment or environments to improve functional outcomes. An example may include application of an orthosis to an amputee's residual limb in order to use a stylus to operate a mobile phone (Fig. 24.2). While OT practitioners fabricate and/or apply orthoses primarily to the upper extremities, it should be understood that orthotic devices can be applied to lower extremities and other parts of the body as well (Coppard & Lohman, 2007).

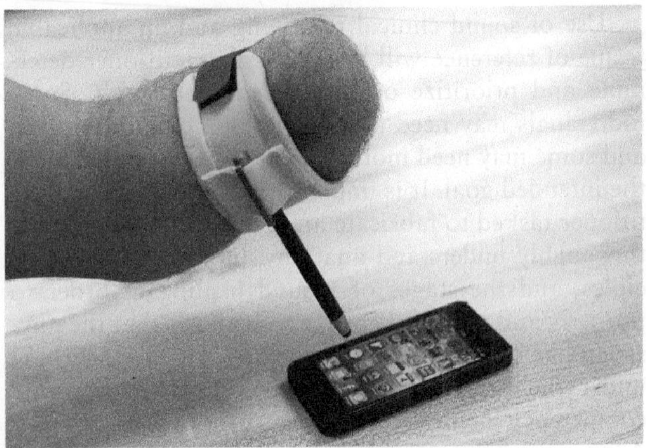

Figure 24.2 Adaptive smart phone and gaming orthosis. (Courtesy of Erik Johnson.)

Types of Orthoses

In general, there are three types of orthoses. A **static orthosis** is most often used to immobilize tissues, joints, or injured body parts. It is usually comprised of a single kind of material and has no moving parts (Fig. 24.3A,B). A **dynamic orthosis** is used to mobilize a joint or body part in a controlled manner and has some type of moveable component. It may also be used to apply constant tension or force to a body part for tissue elongation. Dynamic orthoses are primarily custom made using tension bands such as rubber bands or springs, wires, and/or hinges (Fig. 24.5A,B). However, more and more dynamic orthoses are now commercially available and can be purchased from a variety of medical supply vendors. A third type of orthosis is the **static progressive orthosis** (Fig. 24.4). It has static components that can be incrementally changed as progress is made. It is often used to correct existing deformities such as joint contractures to improve range of motion (Coppard & Lohman, 2007). Serial casting is a technique commonly used in a static progressive manner to decrease joint contractures. Casting or similar material is used to hold a joint in its most elongated position for a period of time, usually a few days. Then, the cast is removed, the joint is stretched further, and a new cast is applied (Fig. 24.6). This sequence is repeated until the desired range of motion or a plateau in progress has been reached.

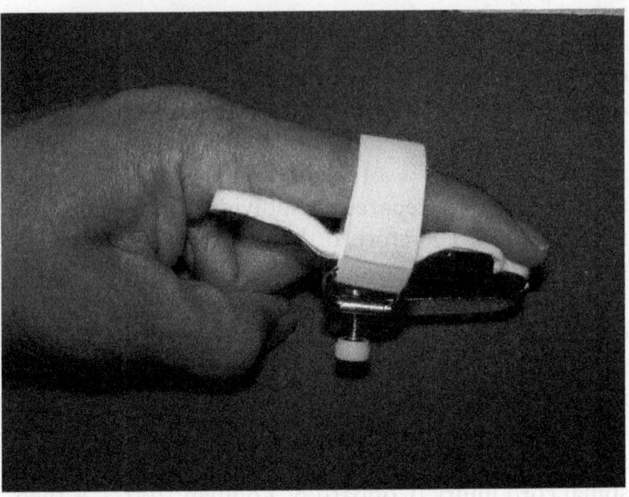

Figure 24.4 Static progressive orthosis. (Joint Jack.)

Prefabrication Concepts: Hand Function and Anatomy

Before exploring the practice of orthotic fabrication and fitting, a number of concepts need to be considered. Understanding the anatomy is a critical element of orthotic fabrication. While the OT practitioner may be called upon to fabricate and fit an orthosis for any body part, the hand and upper extremity are most common. Thus, our discussion focuses on the upper extremity. A brief description and understanding of hand creases and arches are warranted for beginner knowledge. Although understanding the anatomy beneath the skin

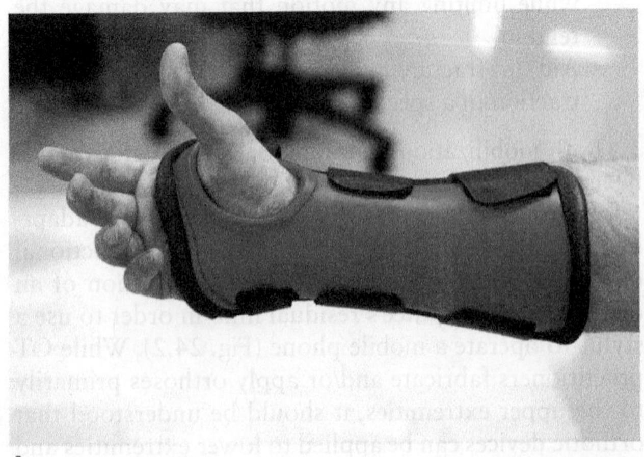

A

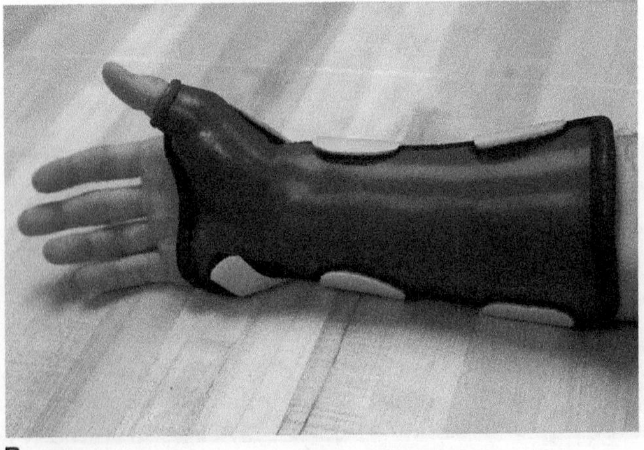

B

Figure 24.3 A: Static orthosis—wrist support. (Courtesy Erik Johnson.) B: Static orthosis—thumb spica. (Courtesy Erik Johnson.)

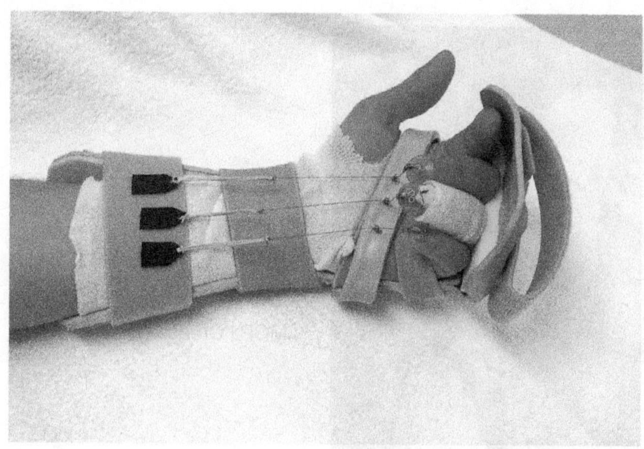

A

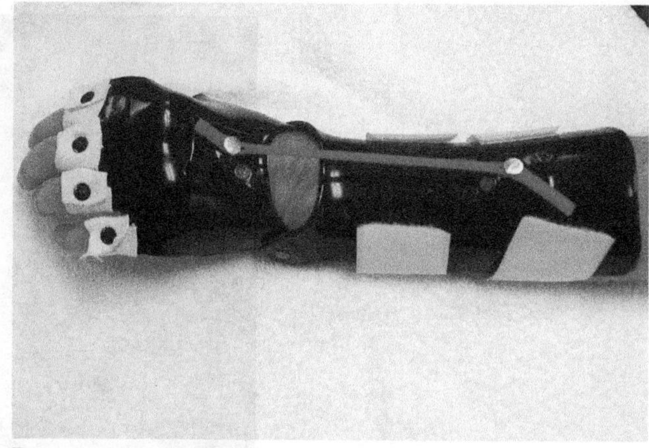

B

Figure 24.5 A: Dynamic orthosis for flexor tendon repair. (Courtesy Erik Johnson.) B: Dynamic wrist extension orthosis. (Courtesy Erik Johnson.)

is important for advanced fabrication techniques, it is beyond the scope of this chapter. You are strongly encouraged to further your knowledge base to be better prepared to fabricate orthoses.

Skin creases in the wrist, hand, and fingers represent the areas of joint mobility underneath the skin. On the palmer (or volar) aspect of the each digit, there are three main creases. One is formed by the distal interphalangeal joint (DIPJ). The second is formed by the proximal interphalangeal joint (PIPJ). And the third is formed by the metacarpophalangeal joints (MCPJs) (Fig. 24.7). On the dorsal (top/back) aspect of these joints, the skin is wrinkled when the digits are extended and stretched tight when the digits are flexed. It is critical not to block these creases/joints if the primary goal of the orthosis is to immobilize the wrist. Full active range of motion of the digits promotes hand function and allows greater independence in the performance of daily activities.

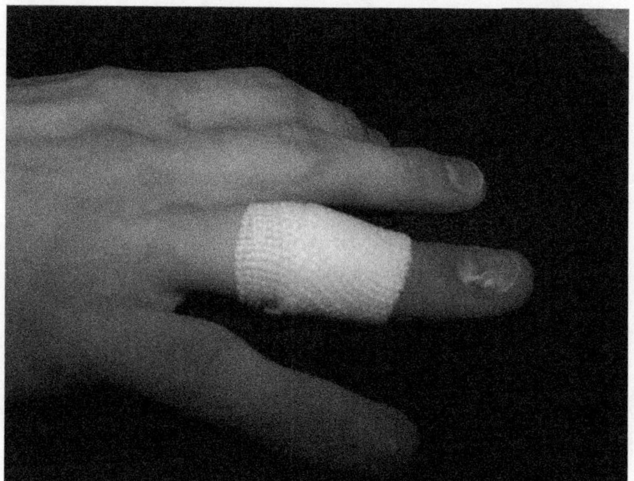

Figure 24.6 Serial cast.

The palm has four main creases to be aware of, especially when fabricating orthotic devices for the hand and wrist. The distal palmer crease is of utmost importance and indicates the space needed for the MCPJs to fully flex (Fig. 24.7). Any orthotic device fitted to the volar aspect of the hand and wrist that is intended only for wrist control should not extend beyond this crease. Otherwise, it will prevent full flexion of the MCPJs, which leads to joint stiffness. As its name implies, the proximal palmer crease is proximal to the distal palmer crease. It is anatomically less important than the distal palmer crease but contributes to the natural arches of the hand (Fig. 24.7).

The thenar crease forms the edge of the thenar muscles responsible for thumb movement and is an important landmark for orthotic fabrication (Fig. 24.7). Crossing or blocking this crease will prevent full thumb flexion and opposition and should be avoided unless specifically requested by the physician or OT. The final crease to consider is the hypothenar crease, which forms the edge of the hypothenar muscles (Fig. 24.7). It is of less anatomical importance than the thenar crease but does contribute to the natural arches of the hand.

Both the dorsal and volar aspects of the wrist have creases that indicate the articulation or movement of the wrist during flexion and extension motion. It is important not to block these creases when fabricating hand-based orthoses. However, it is expected that these creases will be blocked when applying orthoses that are intended to prevent or restrict wrist motion. Most requests for wrist support or immobilization orthoses will require that the hand be maintained in the "functional position." This means that the wrist is placed in approximately 20 degrees of extension and slight ulnar deviation with the MCPJs flexed at approximately 60 degrees. This maintains the wrist and hand in the most natural position for functional use.

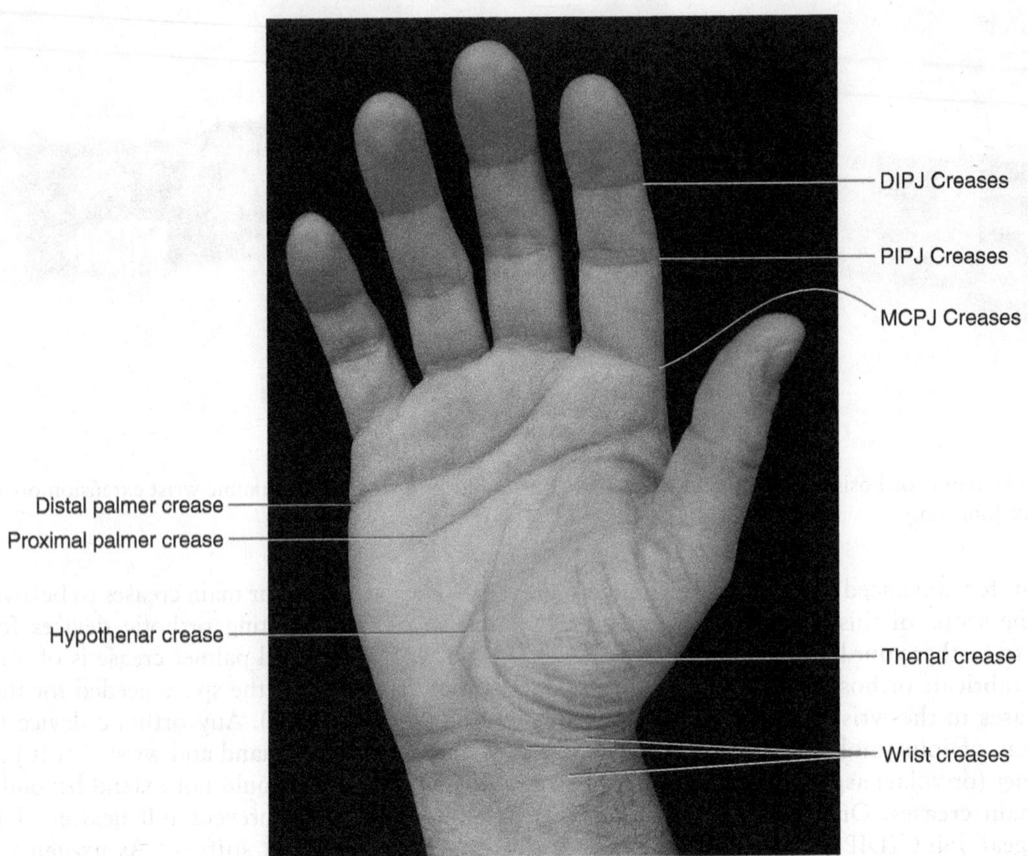

Figure 24.7 Wrist, hand, and digit creases.

Another concept to consider when applying an orthosis to the hand is the existence and orientation of the transverse and longitudinal arches of the hand. The proximal transverse arch is formed by the distal carpal row that creates a dip between the thenar and hypothenar eminences of the hand (Fig. 24.8). The distal transverse arch is formed by the metacarpal heads that shape the concavity of the palm allowing for conformity to objects placed in the hand (Fig. 24.8). The longitudinal arch extends proximally from the carpus through the palm and through the digits. Its center is formed by the 2nd and 3rd metacarpals, which are relatively stable. The more mobile 4th and 5th metacarpals rotate around this longitudinal arch forming a secure and full grasp on objects in the hand (Emerson & Shafer, 2003). Any orthosis fabricated to the hand has to accommodate and conform to these natural arches to preserve normal hand function (Fig. 24.8).

Prefabrication Concepts: Wound Healing

Since many requests for orthotic devices stem from injuries or postoperative events, a basic understanding of wound healing is necessary. There are three primary stages of healing. The first stage is the inflammatory phase, which begins immediately after the trauma and lasts for 3 to 6 days. There is usually a significant amount of edema. Healing tissue is vulnerable to further injury during stage one. A static orthosis is typically used during this stage to provide rest and protection for the involved structures.

The second stage is the proliferative or fibroblastic phase, which may begin as early as 2 to 3 days after trauma and can last up to 2 to 6 weeks. Fibroblasts, a type of cell necessary to support the healing process, begin to multiply and produce collagen. During the second stage, tissues, including skin and tendons, begin to get stronger and thus begin the scarring process. Initially, rest may be continued (via a static orthosis), or early controlled motion may be indicated (via a dynamic orthosis).

The final, third stage of wound healing is the maturation phase, which begins at approximately 3 to 4 weeks post injury and can last up to two years after initial injury. During this stage, tensile strength of tissues continues to mature and contract. This is the stage in which scar adhesions and contractures develop, thus limiting tissue excursion and joint range of motion. During this stage, dynamic or static progressive orthoses are used to reduce potential adhesions or contractions (Coppard & Lohman, 2007).

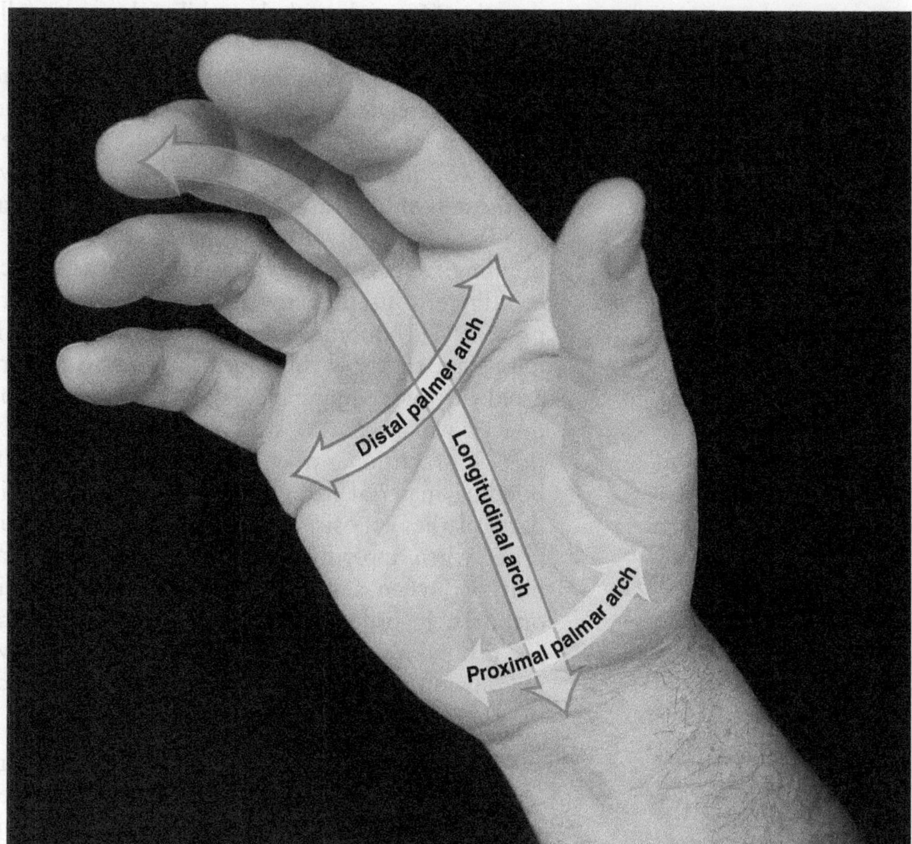

Figure 24.8 Arches of the hand.

Prefabrication Concepts: Tools for Efficient Fabrication of Orthoses

The OT practitioner must be familiar with and be able to use a variety of tools in order to fabricate a properly fitting orthosis. Typically, the client is seated in the clinic with the extremity at rest on a table or on a foam wedge. However, some clients may be too ill to sit for long periods of time or may be confined to a bed. Fabricating and fitting orthoses at the bedside are common practices in settings such as critical care units, nursing facilities, a client's home, and neonatal units (please note that OTAs do not practice in NICUs). Therefore, the OT practitioner must be prepared with a mobile tool kit. Tools include, but are not limited to, hydroculator (heating pan or skillet that allows water temperature to reach up to 180 degrees); heat gun, utility knife, scissors, tongs, or spatula (to retrieve thermoplastic materials from the heating pan); towels, hole punch, awl, pencil or pen, paper, or paper towels (for tracing a pattern); and thermoplastic materials, solvent, ace wrap, stockinette, padding materials, strapping materials, and Velcro (Fig. 24.9). Occupational therapy practitioners with advanced skills in fabricating dynamic and adaptive orthoses will require additional tools such as a hammer, pliers, anvil, crimper, rubber bands, eyelets, eyelet setter, rivets, fishing line, outriggers, turnbuckles, coil springs, bra hooks, D-rings, wire, wire bender, hinges, plaster or casting materials, and a variety of strapping materials that include Velcro hook and loop (both with and without adhesive backing), padded and nonpadded strapping, elastic strapping, and a wide variety of thermoplastic materials. The possibilities for designing orthotic devices are endless and only limited by the practitioner's creativity and experience (Coppard & Lohman, 2007).

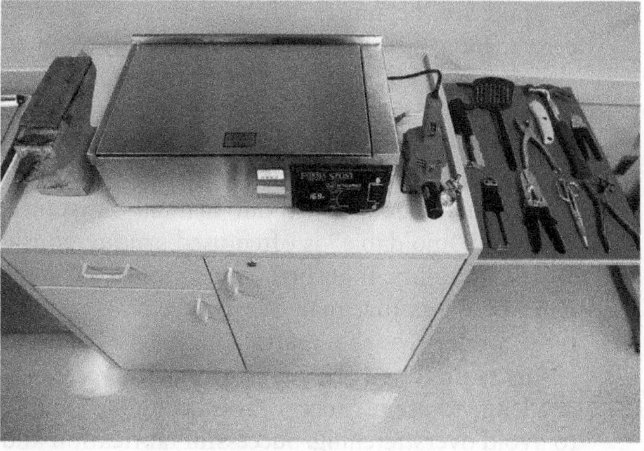

Figure 24.9 Orthotic fabrication tools. (Courtesy Erik Johnson.)

Prefabrication Concepts: Orthotic Materials and Properties

To ensure optimal effectiveness and compliance with wearing, understanding the wide variety of materials available for orthotic fabrication involves choosing one that best meets the client's comfort and needs. Occupational therapy practitioners most often work with thermoplastic materials. **Thermoplastic** is a term used to describe plastic materials that respond to heat. With advances in science and technology, there are now many low temperature thermoplastic materials available for fabrication of orthotic devices. These materials soften in water temperatures ranging from 135°F to 180°F. Thermoplastics are made from plastic or rubber-based materials. Plastic-based materials are more malleable and easier to manipulate and contour to the arches of the hand and around bony prominences. Rubber-based materials are less conforming and more rigid, hence easier to control and handle. They are more useful for larger orthoses and for areas such as forearms or elbows. Because they are easier to handle and control, rubber-based materials are not as moldable or pliable as plastic-based materials. An ace bandage or wrap may be helpful in securing the material to the extremity during the molding process (Coppard & Lohman, 2007).

Thermoplastic materials are created with different properties or characteristics that influence the ease of use. These properties are referred to as "handling characteristics." They include memory, drapability, elasticity, and bonding:

- Memory: refers to the material's ability to return to its original shape and size when reheated. Some materials have 100% memory and some have little to no memory. Most materials that have 100% memory turn clear or become translucent when heated. Memory allows an OT practitioner to reheat and reshape an orthosis many times, which is good for beginners when needing to correct errors. However, materials with memory tend to shrink when attempting to correct a small area. Thus, caution must be used not to reheat too large an area (Coppard & Lohman, 2007).
- Drapability: describes the ability to conform to the underlying structure without manual assistance. The term "moldable" is often used synonymously with drapability. If an orthosis is required for the hand or digits that may overlie prominent structures, wounds, or skin grafts, a material with drapability is preferred. This type of material can be a challenge to use because it must be handled gently to avoid overstretching. Successful fabrication and fit requires the OT practitioner to gently and constantly stoke the material while allowing gravity to assist. Materials with drapability do not usually have much memory.
- Elasticity: refers to the material's resistance to stretch and tendency to return to its original shape. The material can be handled aggressively and used when working with clients who are uncooperative or those with increased tone. Aquaplast is a thermoplastic material with this characteristic.
- Bonding: refers to the material's ability to stick or adhere to itself. Many materials are coated to prevent self-bonding, while others are not. It is important to know this ahead of time to prevent accidently overlapping pieces of the material if you do not want them to stick together. Conversely, the OT practitioner may purposefully choose self-bonding material in order to ensure that certain parts of the orthosis stick together. This situation arises when applying layers to build strength/stability or when attaching outriggers on dynamic orthoses. In order to layer thermoplastic materials, a bonding solvent may be applied to remove manufactured coatings to create a stronger bonding characteristic (Coppard & Lohman, 2007).

In addition to the characteristics above, there are many other aspects of orthotic materials to consider. They include heating time, how long it takes to become soft; working time, how long the material holds the heat and remains pliable; and self-finishing edges, edges that remain smooth when cut and shrinkage and the material's potential to shrink as it cools, which could be problematic when fabricating circumferential finger orthoses.

Orthotic materials come in a variety of thicknesses, which also influence how and when they are used. A thicker material (1/8 in.) is heavier and more rigid than a thinner material (3/32 in. or 1/16 in.). A thinner material is more useful for children or the elderly, or when fabricating a finger orthosis. Thicker materials are more useful for larger joints such as elbows, wrists, and ankles, or as the basis for dynamic orthoses (From the Field 24.1).

Orthotic materials may be perforated, meaning it has holes, to allow for increased ventilation and help decrease perspiration. It is important to understand that

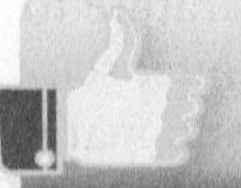

FROM THE FIELD 24.1

Choice of Colors

Thermoplastic materials now come in a wide variety of colors including white, beige, black, bright neon colors, and even camouflage patterns for military personnel.

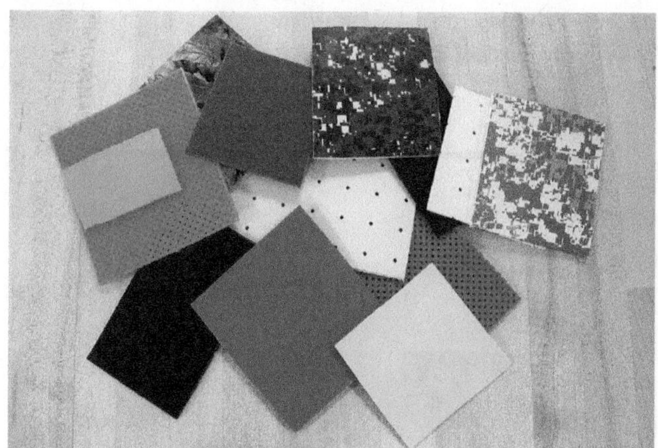

Figure 24.10 A variety of thermoplastic materials.

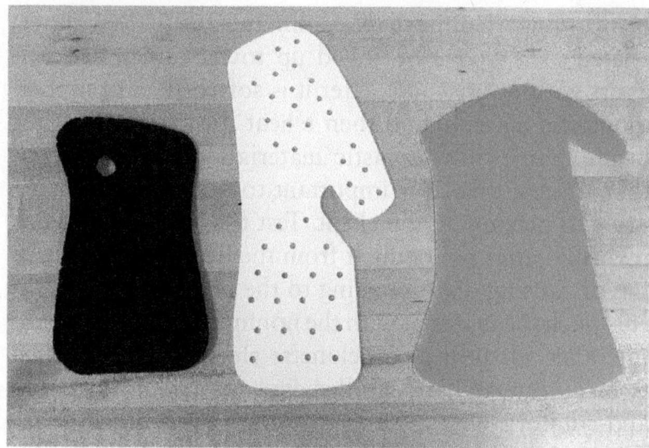

Figure 24.11 Precut thermoplastic materials.

the greater the perforation, the less rigid/sturdy a material is. You can learn more about splinting materials from manufacturer websites and catalogs (Fig. 24.10).

Fabrication of Orthotic Devices: Preparation

The OT practitioner must have a clear understanding of the reason and purpose for the orthotic prescription and should also know the client's diagnosis. The first step in preparation is to observe the client's ability to assume a position that will allow for proper fitting of the orthosis (e.g., can the client place the affected extremity on the table? Is the client bedridden?). The next step is to observe for swelling, wounds, burns, spasticity, skin grafts/flaps, or abnormalities that may require alterations during fabrication of the orthosis. Be aware that forearms are cone shaped and have circumferences that increase proximally. These factors must be considered before fabricating the orthosis (Lashgari & Yasuda, 2013).

Making a Pattern

Most practitioners begin the fabrication process by making a pattern or template (although a more advanced practitioner may choose not to use a pattern). When making a pattern, it is important to provide enough time to create a well thought-out pattern. Some clinics have premade patterns made of flexible plastic or laminated paper to use for commonly prescribed orthoses such as wrist support and resting hand orthoses. Some clinics may stock precut thermoplastic material already in the shape of a pattern, and other clinics may stock premade thermoplastic orthoses (Fig. 24.11). While precut and premade orthoses may save time, they are usually more costly than starting from scratch. Whether using a pattern, a precut material, or a premade orthoses, it should be noted that one size does not usually fit all, and some trimming and/or modification may be necessary to create a properly fitting, comfortable orthosis.

To make a pattern, trace the client's hand on a piece of paper or paper towel. If a client has significant deformities or injuries that make tracing difficult, use the limb on the contralateral side of the body to make the pattern. When drawing the pattern for the orthosis on paper, take into consideration creases, joints, bony prominences, and hand/arm length and width. Be sure to add extra length on the pattern if the orthosis will be on the dorsal surface of a joint that will be flexed, as it will require more material. A forearm-based orthosis should be 2/3 the length of the forearm and 1/2 the circumference. This is important to provide adequate support. After the pattern is cut out, resize it to the client's extremity for final shaping and preparation. Consider moistening the paper pattern before resizing it to the extremity for proper fitting (Coppard & Lohman, 2007). Once the pattern is complete, place it on a piece of thermoplastic material and trace it using a pen or grease pencil. Keep in mind that this is the point at which the OT practitioner selects the desired material with the handling characteristics most amenable to the orthosis being fabricated (e.g., drapability, memory, perforated, thickness). If the facility has a wide variety of thermoplastic colors, the OT practitioner may select one desired by the client (such as a neon color for a young child or camouflage for a service member/veteran). You will want the final product to be aesthetically pleasing to the client, as it helps increase compliance with the wearing program. At this point in the process, place the selected thermoplastic material in hot water to soften before cutting.

Fabrication of Orthotic Devices: Fitting

While the thermoplastic material is softening in hot water, preposition the client's extremity for fitting, preferably in a gravity-assisted position that is safe and as comfortable as possible. For clients with high tone or stiff joints, a heating pad or fluidotherapy may be used to warm and prepare the extremity/joints for proper positioning (Coppard & Lohman, 2007). A rubber-coated arm wedge or rolled up towel can be used to assist with positioning. After it is softened, cut the thermoplastic material and then reheat the cut material for fitting. Some thermoplastic materials retain more heat than others; thus, it is important to test its temperature prior to placing on the client. Test the material on your own skin after removing it from the heat to avoid burning or causing discomforting to the client. Have the client touch the material with the noninjured hand to assess tolerance for heat. A stockinette sleeve can be applied to an extremity, hand, and/or digit for added protection and comfort. Once a safe temperature is reached, place the thermoplastic material onto client's extremity for fitting. This is when it is important to remember the handling characteristics described earlier (e.g., drapability, elasticity). It may be helpful for a novice OT practitioner to have a second set of hands available from a colleague for assistance. Otherwise, as previously mentioned, an ace bandage can be used to help secure and shape the material to the hand, forearm, elbow, etc. It can take approximately 2 to 3 minutes for a newly heated orthosis to cool. If an orthosis needs to be cooled quickly, cold spray or cool water can be used. If a client has a respiratory condition, consider using cool water instead of cold spray to avoid exacerbating their symptoms. When the thermoplastic material has slightly cooled and hardened, carefully remove it from the client's extremity and run it under cool tap water so it can become firm.

Your thermoplastic material is now an orthosis! After cooling it, smooth and flare any rough edges to avoid areas that may cause discomfort or injury. Perforated materials can leave many rough edges at each perforation. Place the orthosis back on the client and inspect for possible **pressure areas**. A pressure area is a place on the skin that becomes red or irritated due to a part of the orthosis that is too tight or rough. This can lead to skin breakdown and/or restricted blood flow to the area. Pressure areas often occur over bony prominences such as the radial styloid, the ulnar styloid, the base of the thumb (1st CMCJ), the metacarpal heads (MCPJs), and the PIPJs. Modify any areas that appear to create pressure by either cutting away or reheating the material in the heat pan or with a heat gun and reshaping it by rolling back the edges or creating a bubble over the prominent area. Remember, some thermoplastic materials have memory and will return to their original shape if placed back in the hot water; therefore, it may be best to spot heat-specific areas using a heat gun with a nozzle. To ensure there are no rough edges, the OT practitioner should glide his/her thumb along edges of the orthosis until all edges are smooth. If full range of motion of the digits is required/allowed, such as with a wrist support orthosis, ensure the orthosis extends only to the distal palmer crease. This will allow for full flexion of the MCPJs (West-Frasier, 2005).

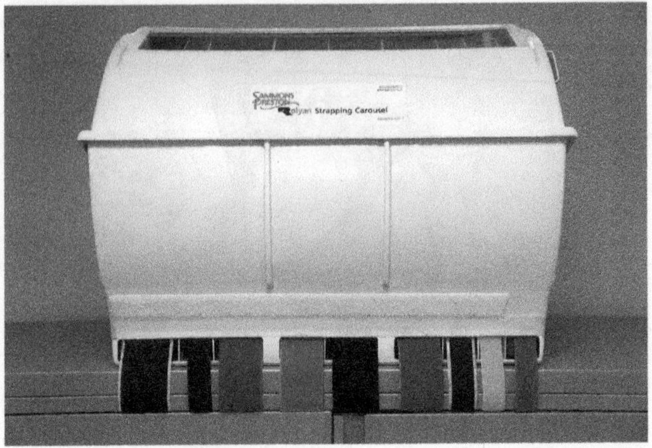

Figure 24.12 Strapping materials.

Fabrication of Orthotic Devices: Strapping

Proper strapping is important to secure the orthosis and to maintain its primary function. Strapping needs to be comfortable or compliance issues may arise. Consider using 2-inch-wide straps across the forearm and 1-inch straps across the hand and finger areas. For clients who have difficulty securing straps, consider using D-ring straps. The D-ring provides leverage, allowing for easy fastening. Strapping must secure the orthosis firmly, yet not impair circulation. When possible, straps should be placed in a diagonal fashion so as to be the least restrictive. A helpful hint is that the OT practitioner should be able to slide his/her small finger under the straps when applied to the client. To secure a finger orthoses, it is sometimes easier to use an elastic self-stick bandage wrap material. Similar to thermoplastic materials, strapping materials are now available in a wide range of colors, thicknesses, widths, and textures (Fig. 24.12).

Fabricating Orthotic Devices: Final Adjustments

Once the orthosis has been completed and fastened, make a final check for any needed adjustments. Recheck edges, potential pressure areas, straps, and overall function. Ensure that all joints that are supposed to be immobilized are immobilized and that all other joints are free to move in accordance with the referral/prescription recommendations. Ask the client for feedback regarding discomfort. If possible, have the client wear the orthosis for 15 minutes before leaving the clinic. After this trial period of wear, have the client remove the orthosis and check for redness that may indicate pressure areas. Make adjustments as needed. And finally, check to ensure that the orthosis is as aesthetically pleasing as possible, for example, no stray pen marks, no finger prints, no unfinished or rough edges, and no excess strapping. It may be necessary to line the edges of the orthosis with a soft material if rough edges cannot be smoothed. Additionally, padding may be needed in specific spots such as around bony prominences. There are a wide variety of commercially available materials to line and pad orthoses, which can be found in medical supply catalogs.

Client Instructions and Education

Educating the client and/or caregiver (e.g., family member, nursing professional, or certified nurse assistant) is perhaps the most important aspect of providing an orthotic device. The client must understand the purpose of the device and the implications if he/she does not wear it as prescribed (e.g., could it cause further injury if the client does not wear the orthosis?). The client must be educated on how and when to wear the orthosis (e.g., at night only, during activities, all the time). If the client should remove the orthosis to bathe or perform specific exercises, it should be noted as part of the wearing program as well as in chart documentation. The client and caregivers should be instructed on any specific precautions and how to monitor for pressure areas. The client needs to understand what to do if he/she has increased pain, which is to return to the clinic or call the physician. The client must be educated on how to take care of the orthosis, for example, cleaning it with mild soap and water or alcohol wipes if it becomes soiled or malodorous. And finally, before leaving the clinic, the client and/or caregiver must demonstrate the ability "don and doff" the orthosis, which means to put it on and take it off. It is suggested that the OT practitioner provides specific written instructions with all the pertinent information to the client, especially the wear schedule and clinic phone number. All aspects of client education should be documented.

Follow-Up

It is important for the OT practitioner to provide the client with instructions for follow-up. If the client is returning for intervention, then follow-up regarding the orthosis may be incorporated in that visit. However, if the sole purpose of the visit is for fabrication or issuing of the orthosis, a specific follow-up visit should be made for adjustments or modification of areas causing pressure or irritation. Follow-up orthosis appointments should include re-evaluation to assess proper fit, which may change due to changes in edema or progression in phases of certain intervention protocols, tolerance and compliance with wear, and overall functioning of the orthosis (is it still accomplishing its intended purpose?). Modifications may be needed or the OT practitioner may have to consider alternative orthotic options to improve compliance and function (West-Frasier, 2005).

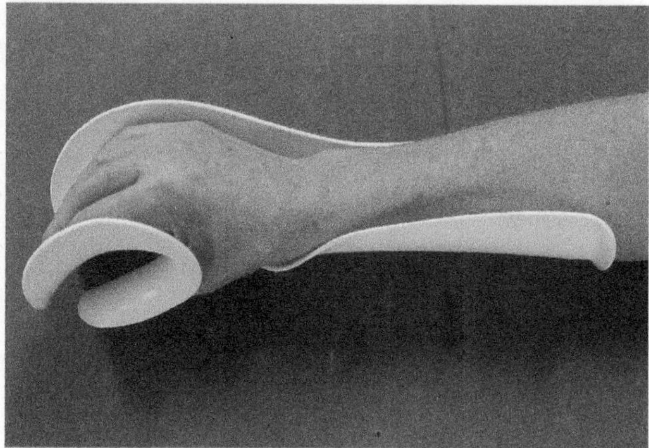

Figure 24.13 Prefabricated functional position splint.

Prefabricated Orthoses

With advanced technology and manufacturing, a wide variety of specialized prefabricated orthoses is now available to include static, dynamic, and static progressive orthoses. They come in a variety of materials such as low- and high-temperature thermoplasts, neoprene, leather, and combinations of materials. They are available from numerous vendors. Typically, prefabricated orthoses are ordered by size and may be universal or come specifically for the left or right extremity.

As discussed above, the advantages of using prefabricated orthoses include saving time and effort. There is no need to draw and cut a pattern or mold the splint. If the clinic has the orthosis in stock, it can immediately be applied to the client and assessed for proper fit. In many cases, prefabricated orthoses have a more sophisticated technology than what the OT practitioner can custom make. Additionally, many prefabricated orthoses are more aesthetically pleasing than their custom-made counterparts. This can increase the wearing compliance (Figs. 24.13–24.22).

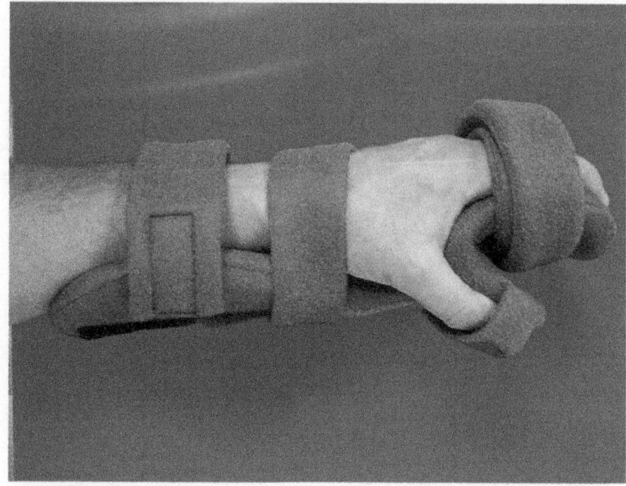

Figure 24.14 Prefabricated resting hand orthosis. (SoftPro CHAMP.)

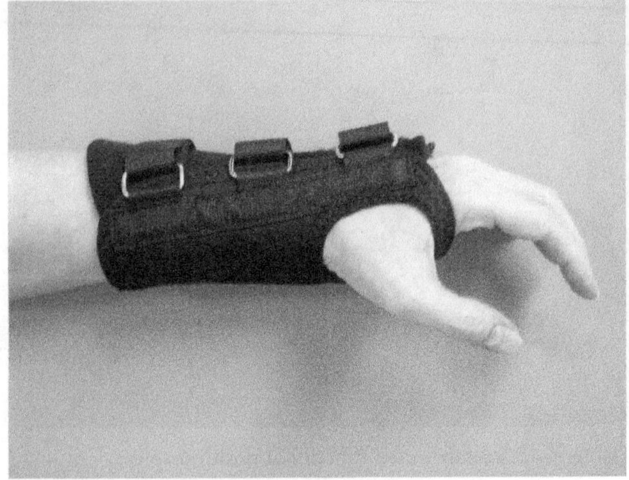

Figure 24.15 Prefabricated wrist support orthosis.

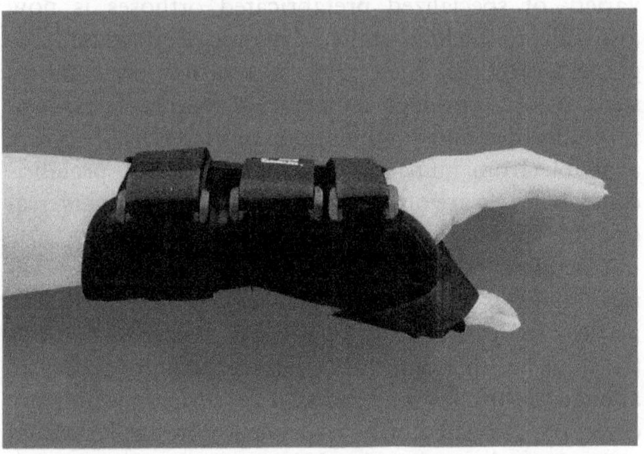

Figure 24.16 Prefabricated thumb spica. (Össur.)

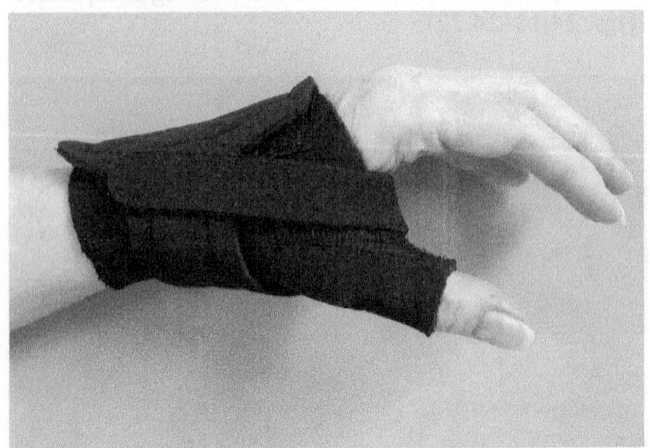

Figure 24.17 Prefabricated neoprene CMCJ restriction splint. (Comfort Cool.)

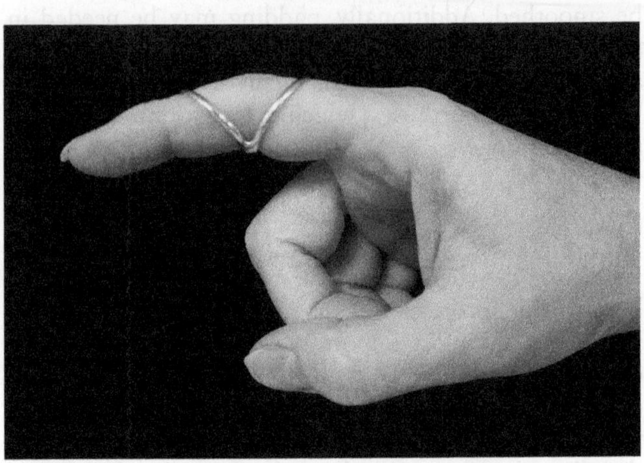

Figure 24.18 Prefabricated silver ring static V-splint.

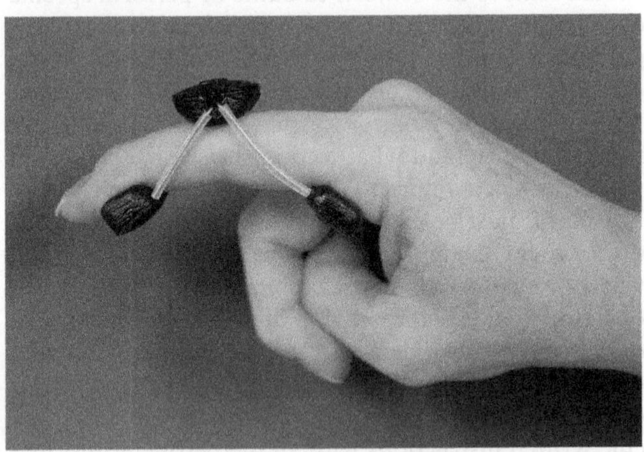

Figure 24.19 Prefabricated dynamic PIPJ extension splint.

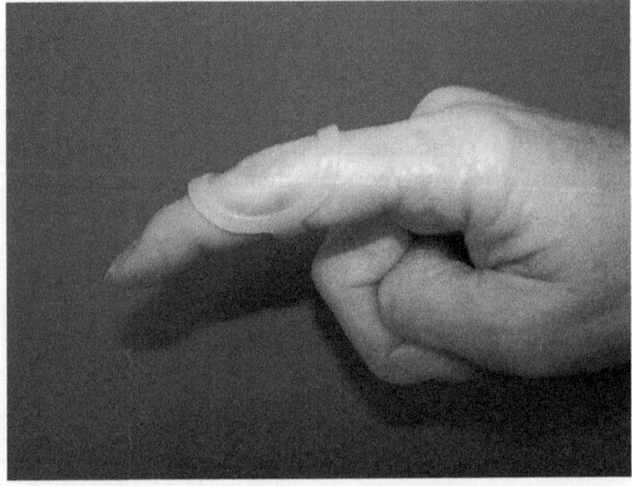

Figure 24.20 Prefabricated static splint. (Oval-8.)

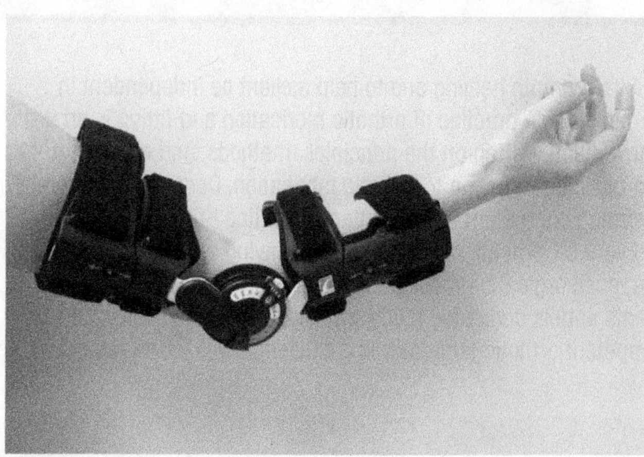

Figure 24.21 Prefabricated elbow immobilization—innovator X post-op elbow brace. (Össur.)

There are a few disadvantages to using prefabricated orthoses. Obtaining an accurate fit can be difficult if the clinic does not have a wide variety of sizes available. Some prefabricated orthoses cannot be adjusted to accommodate specific nuances of the client's extremity and/or condition, such as changes in edema, an atypical bony prominence, protruding pins, or skin grafts/wounds. It can also be costly to order enough sizes and styles of prefabricated orthoses to have just the right one for your client. Additionally, many clinics do not have enough storage space to keep an adequate supply in stock.

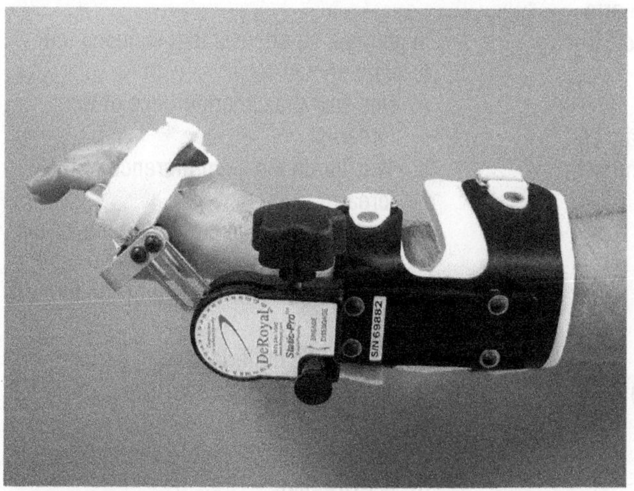

Figure 24.22 Prefabricated static progressive wrist orthosis. (DeRoyal.)

It is important to note that when issuing a prefabricated orthoses, the OT practitioner must still apply all the principles previously described. The orthosis must be assessed to ensure it achieves the prescribed outcome and function. It must allow for free range of motion of unaffected joints. It must not impair circulation or cause pressure areas. It should be aesthetically pleasing and comfortable to wear. The client must be able to don and doff the orthosis independently. Instructions should be provided for wear and care as well as follow-up and what to do if there are any issues. And all aspects of the therapeutic program need to be documented (Coppard & Lohman, 2007).

Documentation

Documentation of orthotic fabrication must be thorough to ensure third-party payment, to demonstrate efficacy of occupational therapy intervention, and to properly communicate with other health care providers. In terms of reimbursement, OT practitioners need to consult current Medicare guidelines for billing and coding regulations, which may vary from year to year. Specific elements of documentation should include the type of orthosis, purpose, anatomical location, client or caregiver education regarding the orthosis, and the wearing schedule. It should be documented whether written instructions were given to client and/or caregiver. It is also important to document that the client or caregiver demonstrates the ability to "don" and "doff" the orthosis (put in on and take it off) independently or not (Coppard & Lohman, 2007).

Summary

The ultimate goal of wearing an orthosis is to promote healing and to help a client be independent in daily activities in a safe and satisfactory manner. The practice of orthotic fabrication and fitting is an art and a science. Many books and articles have been written on the principles, methods, and efficacy of orthotic fabrication. This chapter offered a basic introduction to orthotic fabrication. Occupational therapy practitioners need to understand that becoming competent in fabricating and fitting orthotic devices takes a great deal of time and repetition. Every OT practitioner must start by having a good understanding of anatomy, biomechanics, wound healing, postsurgical protocols, and disease processes. Fabricating safe and effective orthotic devices for clients entails dedicated study, practice, confidence, and good mentoring and guidance. Becoming a competent orthotic fabricator is a challenge well worth the effort.

Review Questions

1. The length of an orthosis on the upper extremity should be:
   a. One-half the length of the forearm
   b. Three-fourths the length of the forearm
   c. Two-thirds the length of the forearm
   d. Midway between the radial styloid and the olecranon

2. When making an orthosis to maintain the wrist in the "functional" position, the wrist should be placed in:
   a. 10-degree flexion
   b. 20-degree flexion
   c. 0 degrees
   d. 20-degree extension

3. An orthosis that has moving part(s) is referred to as a:
   a. Static orthosis
   b. Dynamic orthosis
   c. Aesthetic orthosis
   d. Proper orthosis

4. To allow for full flexion of the metacarpal phalangeal joints, a volar-based orthosis should extend:
   a. To the digital creases
   b. Distal the distal palmar crease
   c. Proximal to the distal palmar crease
   d. Proximal to the proximal palmar crease

5. Thermoplastic material that goes back to its original shape when placed back into hot water is said to have:
   a. Memory
   b. Drapability
   c. Stretch
   d. Conformability

6. The purpose of an orthosis may be to:
   a. Substitute for loss of motor function
   b. Promote wound/tissue healing
   c. Immobilize an injured body part
   d. All of the above

7. In general, an orthosis that includes the forearm should be:
   a. One-half the circumference of the forearm
   b. Two-thirds the circumference of the forearm
   c. Three-fourths the circumference of the forearm
   d. The entire circumference of the forearm

8. Thermoplastic material that is perforated:
   a. Is extra heavy for better support
   b. Has metal in it
   c. Has holes in it for more ventilation
   d. Is extra thin

9. Which of the following is not a bony prominence that must be considered during the orthotic fabrication process?
   a. Heads of the metacarpal phalangeal joints
   b. Second carpometacarpal joint
   c. Ulnar styloid
   d. Radial styloid

10. When fabricating an orthosis, one must be cautious to avoid creating a pressure area that is:
    a. Caused by a part of the orthosis that is too tight
    b. Mental stress a patient feels due to having to wear an orthosis
    c. Where you place a strap to secure the orthosis
    d. A biomechanical landmark

Practice Activities

Fabricate and fit a resting hand orthosis on a fellow classmate. Have your classmate wear the orthosis for at least one hour and provide feedback on comfort, aesthetics, and function.

Fabricate and fit a wrist control orthosis on a fellow classmate. Have your classmate wear the orthosis for at least one hour and provide feedback on comfort, aesthetics, and function.

Wear a static orthosis for at least one hour during the performance of each of the following activities: self-care, vocational, and leisure. Discuss your experience, including the physical and emotional impact it had on you.

Prepare a sample wearing/care plan for a resting hand orthosis you fabricated for a 70-year-old male client who had a left CVA. He has a history of high blood pressure and type 2 diabetes.

Photograph and identify the creases on your right palm. Do the same with three classmates, as well as your instructor. Compare and contrast the similarities and differences. Share your findings with the class.

References

American Occupational Therapy Association. Occupational therapy practice framework: Domain and process (3rd. ed.). *Am J Occup Ther* 2014;68(Suppl. 1):S1–S48. http://dx.doi.org/10.5014/ajot.2014.682006

Coppard BM, Lohman H, eds. *Introduction to Splinting: A Clinical-Reasoning and Problem-Solving Approach*. 3rd ed. St. Louis, MO: Elsevier Mosby; 2007.

Coverdale JJ. An editorial note of nomenclature: orthosis versus splint. *J Hand Ther* 2012;(January–March):3–4.

Emerson S, Shafer A. Splinting and orthotics. In: Crepeau EB, Cohn ES, Boyt Schell BA, eds. *Willard & Spackman's Occupational Therapy*. 11th ed. Philadelphia: Lippincott Williams & Wilkins; 2003:676–686.

Lashgari D, Yasuda L. Orthotics. In: Pendleton HM, Schultz-Krohn W, eds. *Pedretti's Occupational Therapy: Practice Skills for Physical Dysfunction*. 7th ed. St. Louis, MO: Elsevier Mosby; 2013:755–795.

Mosby. *Mosby's Medical, Nursing & Allied Health Dictionary*. 6th ed. United States: Mosby; 2002:1618.

West-Frasier J. Basic splinting. In: Sladyk K, Ryan SE, eds. *Ryan's Occupational Therapy Assistant*. 4th ed. Thorofare, NJ: Slack Incorporated; 2005:416–427.

CHAPTER 25

Group Dynamics: Planning and Leading Effective Therapeutic Groups

Sarah G. Sieradzki, OTR/L, HTR, CDP

Key Terms

Discussion-oriented groups—Type of group that focuses on connections and communication.

Task groups—Type of group that focuses on performing various types of tasks.

Therapeutic use of self—The manner in which the occupational therapy practitioner uses his/her personality, life experiences, intuition, knowledge, and skills to develop therapeutic relationships with clients in order to encourage, inspire, communicate, and be effective in leading them to achieve meaningful therapy goals.

Learning Objectives

After studying this chapter, reader should be able to:

- Identify two major types of therapeutic groups used in occupational therapy practice as well as their main purposes.
- Compare two different group planning formats for developing effective therapeutic group occupations and select meaningful therapeutic occupations that can be used successfully in therapeutic groups.
- Systematically analyze therapeutic occupations to thoroughly understand their application to therapeutic goals and understand how to grade and adapt them.
- Explore a variety of leadership roles and responsibilities and understand how therapeutic use of self aids in leading successful intervention groups.
- Identify ways an effective group leader handles difficult participants.

Introduction

In this chapter, we explore how to plan and lead effective group intervention sessions in occupational therapy. We will identify helpful ways to select therapeutic occupations and how to adapt them for participants with differing abilities. Effective group leadership skills will also be discussed, so group participants can be provided with meaningful and accessible growth experiences.

Therapeutic Groups in Occupational Therapy

Providing intervention to clients in groups has been a part of occupational therapy since its beginnings (Schwartzberg et al., 2008, p. 235). The formats, theories, and contents of therapeutic groups have evolved throughout the profession's lengthy history and continue to evolve with the recent focus on occupational science (Schwartzberg et al., 2008, pp. 235–258). Generally speaking, therapeutic occupational therapy groups can be divided into task-oriented groups and discussion-oriented groups. **Task groups** focus on performing various types of tasks including such occupations as cooking, ADLs, arts and crafts, prevocational tasks, therapeutic exercise, and leisure exploration. **Discussion-oriented groups** focus on connections and communication and may include skill building, learning concepts, emotional expression, and group processing (Schwartzberg et al., 2008, pp. 254–255). Discussion-oriented groups may deal with personal growth topics such as communication skills, assertiveness, self-esteem, community resources, stress management, coping with grief and loss, relaxation, and life balance. Discussion groups may also concentrate on development of IADL skills such as nutrition, medication management, employment, parenting, relationships, and strategies for better sleep, money management, home care, driving safety, and caregiving CS-4,10.

Planning a Therapeutic Group Occupation Using Cole's Seven Step Format

Marilyn B. Cole literally "wrote the book" about planning and conducting groups for therapeutic purposes in occupational therapy. In her book *Group Dynamics in Occupational Therapy*, Cole provides a wealth of useful and usable information about the theories and practice of group occupational therapy intervention. Her seven step format for planning an effective therapeutic group is especially pertinent and valuable when used for discussion-type groups. Cole's seven step planning process is outlined in Table 25.1 (Figs. 25.1 and 25.2).

Planning Format and Group Leadership Evaluation for Task-Based Groups

The following is a simple and streamlined format for planning and reflecting on task-based groups (Fig. 25.3). It is derived from over 30 years of group plan-

TABLE 25.1 COLE'S Seven-Step Therapeutic Group Planning

Step One: Introduction/Warmup
• Brings the group together and prepare them for what will occur during the group session • Warmup activities or ice breakers may bring the group together. Have each group member say their first name along with a descriptive adjective that starts with the same first initial (e.g., Studious Sarah, Funny Frank, or Delightful Diana), identifies one of their best qualities or skills (e.g., Energetic Edward, Athletic Allen, Creative Cynthia, or Musical Margaret). • Another good warmup activity is to set the stage for what the group will be working on. For example, if the group is focusing on positive coping skills, each member can state their name and one thing they need to cope with in life. This may range from superficial daily irritants like waiting in line or bad drivers to more difficult stressors like panic attacks, dealing with chronic illness, or issues of grief and loss. • The concepts to be discussed as a group are introduced next. Identifying *why* the topic will be meaningful or valuable to the members helps them recognize the purpose of the therapeutic occupation. You will want to highlight the procedures the group will use, including the amount of time that will be provided for each step.
Step Two: Activity
• Create a specific plan for the therapeutic occupation that the group will engage in. The more carefully and completely the plan is executed, the easier and smoother implementation will be during the actual group. Identify which client-centered therapeutic goals will be targeted by the group activity, and ensure that the activity is age appropriate and meaningful. Think through an occupational analysis of the group activity to determine if all the clients have the necessary performance skills to successfully perform the activity. Consider how to grade the activity for clients with differing cognitive abilities in the same group and how can you adapt the activity for clients with varying physical limitations. • Plan ahead for what supplies and room arrangement will be needed. Identify how to set up the activity so group members can share supplies and equipment and have enough space to work easily. Consider any special needs that the activity requires. For example, a cookie making task requires access to a stove, water, and cooking utensils. Be responsible about the cost of materials that need to be replaced after each group, such as replacing soil and pots for a weekly horticulture group.

(*continues on page 320*)

TABLE 25.1 COLE'S Seven-Step Therapeutic Group Planning (continued)

• Reflect on how clients will be led through performing the actual activity. Will any special techniques need to be taught, and if so, will you demonstrate these techniques or use a video for instructions? Is it important that the clients remember each step independently, or will the group work together? Does each step of the activity need to be done in a particular sequence, or can they be done out of order? Think about whether or not you will show examples of completed projects. • Plan ahead for any cleanup needs and leave enough time for the group to perform cleanup duties.
Step Three: Sharing
The group will be more effective if you plan ahead about how to guide or direct individual self-expression and sharing about the task or topic involved. Create a list of questions you can use to conduct the group discussion portion of the session. If the group session uses a worksheet for individuals to take notes, each group member can share their ideas with the group at large. Please refer to Figure 25.1 for an example of a handout for group discussion.
Step Four: Processing
• In this phase, the group explores a deeper understanding of the topic or concept being addressed. You will want to help members identify and delve into whatever feelings, issues, needs, or ideas that they may have during the session's activity. Establish ground rules about confidentiality, taking turns, and what information is appropriate to reveal with the larger group. Some members will feel more comfortable about sharing than others, but most will model what you demonstrate. Ensure that members know they will be expected to communicate at a "getting to know each other" level of sharing, and not a "deep, dark secret" level of sharing. • Consider asking members how they feel about the topic, if they feel it might be helpful to them in the future, and what impact it could have on them. Deal with any communication or behavioral issues that have come up during the group to help all the members participate more fully, openly, and congenially during this processing part of the group.
Step Five: Generalizing
• After each group member has shared in the processing phase of the group, direct participants to review and explore the experience of the group discussion as a whole. Was there any consensus reached about the topic, or did members identify any new ideas or a different perspective about the topic? Did individual participants notice a change in feelings as they became aware that others have experienced similar feelings and experiences? Did group members share any helpful strategies about dealing with similar life situations in the future?
Step Six: Applying
• Once the group has reviewed their learning, help the members understand how they can actually apply what they have learned in the future. Guide members to explore how they might handle specific situations related to the topic differently in the future. Concrete examples will help members visualize using the skills and knowledge they have just discussed. Some members may find role-play examples to be useful in helping them plan how they might communicate with family or friends or better deal with a problem situation in the future. • Remind the group members to place their notes or handouts in a specific place at home so it is readily accessible if they want a reminder about the information they have learned in group (Fig. 25.2).
Step Seven: Summary
• Summarize the concepts discussed and review the general ideas shared. Reinforce the members' learning by asking each of them to summarize their own ideas, feelings, and experience to the larger group. Quickly review how members can apply their new skills and knowledge in their regular lives, both now and in the future. • Often, individuals recall their emotions in the last few moments of a group experience, so it is important to end on a positive note. Express appreciation to each member for sharing and for contributing to the others involved. This is the strength of the group experience, that members support and teach each other effectively. Thank the group, remind them about confidentiality, and end the group at the scheduled time.
Adapted from Cole M. *Group Dynamics in Occupational Therapy*. Thorofare, NJ: Slack Incorporated; 2012:3–12.

Healthy Sleep Solutions

How Health Conditions Can Affect Sleep, and How Poor Sleep Can Affect Health Conditions:

Our bodies tend to operate on a 24-hour circadian cycle. Sleep, body temperature, and alertness are all part of a daily rhythmic cycle that is regulated by our brains. Pain and other health conditions can make sleep more difficult because it can be hard to find a comfortable position for long periods, which causes increased wakefulness. Sleep deprivation can become so problematic that it can interfere with work, self-care, and relationships.

Research suggests poor sleep may either cause pain or lower pain thresholds, thus intensifying pain. Using good sleep hygiene techniques can help you establish and maintain healthier sleep/wake patterns.

Common Causes of Insomnia:

- **Change in general health conditions:** Hormonal changes (especially during menopausal years), allergies, enlarged prostate which causes men to need to urinate more frequently, GERD (gastro-esophageal reflux disorder), bruxism (teeth grinding), sleep apnea, or restless legs syndrome
- **Medical conditions that cause pain:** Osteoarthritis, fibromyalgia, diabetic neuropathies, bursitis, degenerative spinal discs, rheumatoid arthritis, back problems
- **Psychological problems:** Anxiety, depression, high stress levels or chronic stress, excessive boredom
- **Lifestyle habits:** Dieting, smoking, alcohol intake, change in work schedule or environment, eating too late in the evening, napping during the daytime
- **Personality style:** Chronic worrier, perfectionist tendencies
- **Reaction to medications, side effects of medications, or withdrawal from medications:** Some prescription drugs (ex. antidepressants, high blood pressure medication, corticosteroids) and over-the-counter medications (ex. decongestants, weight loss products, stimulants that contain caffeine, antihistamines) may interfere with sleep. Long time use of sleep medications can be habit-forming and become less effective over time.

General Sleep Hygiene Tips:

(NOTE: It may take 3-4 weeks of trying these techniques before you begin to see a noticeable improvement in your sleep amount and quality. Be persistent—these techniques are helpful!)

- **Establish a sleep schedule and stick to it.** Try to keep your bedtime and wakeup time on a consistent schedule. Avoid napping during the day.
- **Avoid or limit caffeine, alcohol, and nicotine.** Caffeine and nicotine are stimulants that can keep you awake. If you must drink coffee or other beverages with caffeine, stop at least 8 hours prior to bedtime. Alcohol can cause restless sleep and frequent awakenings.

FIGURE 25.1 An example of a handout for a discussion group addressing difficulties with sleeping. (Prepared by Sarah G. Sieradski.)

- **Don't eat or drink just before bedtime.** A light snack or meal at least two hours before bed may be okay. Avoid spicy or fatty foods if you are prone to heartburn. Limit liquid intake to eliminate the need to get up frequently during the night to urinate.
- **Exercise regularly but not within two hours of bedtime.** Regular aerobic activity can help you fall asleep faster and make your sleep more restful. However, exercising just before bedtime can interfere with sleep.
- **Make your sleep environment more conducive to sleep.** Make sure your bedroom is dark, quiet, and comfortable, and has a cool temperature. Minimize sleep interruptions by closing your bedroom door so you won't be wakened by the telephone or voices. Create a neutral background sound by using a fan to block out other disturbing noises. Set your alarm, then hide your clock or turn it face down to block intrusive light. Choose a comfortable mattress and pillow—one that is supportive, but soft enough to prevent pain. Set limits on children and pets sharing the bed with you as their movements can keep waking you up.
- **Create a relaxing bedtime routine.** Doing the same things each night prior to bedtime (especially with the lights turned down low) will signal your body that it is time to wind down. This may include listening to soothing music, reading, or practicing relaxation techniques such as meditation or guided imagery. Taking a warm bath or shower just before bedtime may feel comforting, but if the water is too hot, this may actually interfere with sleep, as the body needs to cool a degree before getting into deep sleep.
- **Go to bed when drowsy and turn out the lights.** Reserve your bedroom only for sleep or sexual activity. Don't use your bedroom for other activities such as TV watching, studying, or work. Maintain it as your sleep environment. If you don't fall asleep within 30 minutes, get up and do something else that is relaxing until you feel drowsy again. Don't agonize or worry about falling asleep—this stress will actually prevent sleep or create shallower, less restful sleep. Keep a notepad and pencil by your bed to write down any thoughts that may nag at you so you can put them to rest.
- **Keep a daily sleep log to show your doctor.** Keep track of the time you went to bed, fell asleep, woke up during the night, how you felt in the morning, and the timing of exercise, meals, and liquid intake.
- **Discuss your medications and pain issues with your doctor if they create sleep difficulties.** Check to see if medications may be contributing to your insomnia, or to increase the effectiveness of your pain reliever.
- **Use sleeping medications only as a last resort, and only for a limited time.** Check with your physician before trying a pain medication, and make sure he knows all the medicines and supplements you are taking to avoid unwanted interactions. Most sleep medications have a limited usefulness, so work with your doctor to determine the best dosage, length of time, and ways to prepare to sleep without the medication. Never mix alcohol and sleeping medications. If you get unwanted side effects from your sleep medication, be sure and consult with your physician about changing the dosage or type of medication.
- **Cool your head and neck.** Research shows that you naturally become sleepy when the temperature of your head and neck is cool. Either turn your heat down a few hours before bedtime, or use a cool washcloth on your face and neck to cool your skin.

Figure 25.1 *(continued)*

A Goal for the New Year

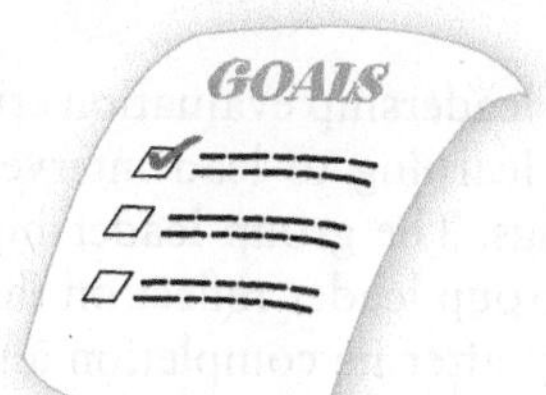

One goal I would like to accomplish in the next year is:

Benefits that would occur if I could achieve this goal include:

Physical benefits:

Emotional benefits:

Mental benefits:

Spiritual benefits:

Relationship benefits:

Other benefits:

Barriers that will make my goal more difficult include:

Ways I might solve or overcome these barriers include:

Steps I need to take to make my goal come true include:

FIGURE 25.2 An example of a worksheet designed to help group participants apply the concepts from a group discussion on goals for the New Year. (Prepared by Sarah G. Sieradski.)

GROUP TITLE ______________________

- Overall group purpose
- Group goals and objectives: the client(s) will…
- Population involved and group size
- Setting and time of group
- List of all materials needed
- List of preparation and set up tasks
- Introduce the participants
- Introduce the task including:
- Steps and instructions for the task
- Sequence of activities to perform task
- Ways to adapt the task (due to clients' physical limitations)
- Ways to grade the task (for various cognitive levels)
- Potential questions to lead the group discussion including potential follow-up questions
- Closing comments on what concepts or skills were learned and summary of the group experience
- Back up plan (in case the group plan is not working)
- Clean up tasks
- Criteria for evaluation of task and group session
- Criteria for evaluation of clients' participation

FIGURE 25.3 Group planning or protocol format. (Prepared by Sarah G. Sieradski.)

ning and leadership evaluation criteria for OTA and OT students learning to lead intervention groups in clinical settings. The group leadership checklist (Fig. 25.4) helps a group leader reflect on the successful aspects of the group after its completion and identify what might be changed in the future to make the activity more effective.

Considerations for Selecting Therapeutic Occupations for Use in Group Settings

Careful selection of tasks and topics for use in therapeutic groups is as much art as science, but will make an enormous difference in the success of the group. Luckily, with advance planning, it is relatively easy to make tasks more complex or simpler to perform. How a topic is presented is also adaptable, ranging from lecture, to group brainstorming, to completion of written worksheets. You may even want to consider using a game format, especially when it is challenging to get participants to attend. Clients in an inpatient mental health setting, for example, will more likely attend a stress management bingo activity than the usual stress management discussion. Even though the same concepts will be presented in both types of activities, they may feel the bingo activity would be more fun, enjoyable, interesting, and meaningful.

Providing handouts to reinforce concepts explored or taught in group is very helpful for participants as they try out newly learned skills and information. You might suggest a place at home where the participants can keep their handout(s) for future reference—on their refrigerator door, for example. See Figure 25.5 for a simple example of a single page two-sided handout used for a horticulture planting group with the purpose of discussing self-care issues.

Planning Meaningful and Accessible Therapeutic Groups

The following considerations, which involve several factors that are outlined in Table 25.2, are helpful in planning meaningful and accessible therapeutic group occupations.

Occupational Analysis

The purpose of using occupational analysis is to understand the therapeutic intervention possibilities and inherent characteristics of a specific occupation. It is best to actually try out the process of the occupation in order to learn the steps, sequence, and abilities needed to perform the occupation before trying to teach it to others. Once the occupation is well understood, ways to adapt or grade the occupation become possible to problem solve. Please also refer to Chapter 11, *Activity Analysis: The Jewel of Occupational Therapy*.

Group Leadership Roles and Responsibilities

An effective group leader is the ultimate multitasker as there are many roles and responsibilities involved in fulfilling the role. The number one role, of course, is management of the group process for all participants. In order to do this successfully, the leader must pay careful attention to each participant's verbalizations, body language, facial expressions, comfort level, and ability to follow the topic being discussed or perform the steps of the task. A group leader also needs to constantly monitor safety issues such as fall risk and safe use of tools and materials.

In a discussion group, the leadership role entails many responsibilities. They include teaching the desired concepts, keeping the participants on topic, validating their responses, checking for understanding, redirecting problem behaviors, and reinforcing positive ones. The leader must also model the type of interpersonal and communication skills that he or she would like the participants to use, learn, or practice. The leader may also need to adapt the format or style of the discussion "on the fly" based on the needs of an individual who is having greater difficulty following the discussion or understanding the group concepts. The leader will need to gracefully cut off some member's lengthy tangential responses and carefully elicit responses from quieter or less communicative group members. The group leader must also be prepared to handle uncomfortable situations, such as a tearful participant, an angry group member, or friction between members. A successful group leader may also serve as coach, cheerleader, advisor, confidant, teacher, confessor, and problem solver.

The leader of a task group needs to give clear concise instructions, observe each participant's ability to follow instructions, and provide any needed assistance to help each member perform the task to the best of their ability. Some members will need more assistance with organizing the task, while others will want more flexibility and freedom to experiment with the basic task to add more interest and challenge. Providing an adaptable task that gives all the group members the chance to experience the "just right" challenge is the key to keeping all participants invested. Effective task group leaders know that thoughtful planning, organizing, and preparing the task beforehand will result in a more satisfying and successful experience for all group members.

Group Leadership Reflection

	1 All the time	2 Most of the time	3 None of the time	4 Not applicable
1. All participants took part in the activity. Activity was successfully graded and adapted to meet individual members' needs.				
2. Materials were suitable and setup was well-organized.				
3. Participants were greeted and introduced by name.				
4. The purpose of the group and the task are clearly identified to clients.				
5. Directions were given clearly, briefly, and in correct order (without notes.)				
6. Group began on time. Clients were gathered for group quickly.				
7. Helped clients complete the task as independently and successfully as possible.				
8. Provided encouragement, acknowledgement, and positive reinforcement to clients. Incorporated clients' ideas for task if appropriate.				
9. Group leader demonstrated enthusiasm at all times.				
10. Leader showed no favoritism, prejudice, or judgmentalism.				
11. Leader redirected members appropriately with tact and kindness.				
12. Leader was prepared with alternate plans if task or discussion was not successful.				
13. The chosen task met clients' needs and held their interest.				
14. The leader assisted clients who needed extra help, or directed co-leader/assistant to provide assistance as needed.				
15. There was a definite ending to the task and leader thanked the clients. The purpose/meaning of group was reinforced, and clients were given opportunity to give feedback.				
16. Leaders evaluated task and noted desired changes for next time.				

Comments on client participation:	Successful and less successful aspects of task/ session:	Strengths of group leadership:

FIGURE 25.4 Group leadership reflections. (Prepared by Sarah G. Sieradski.)

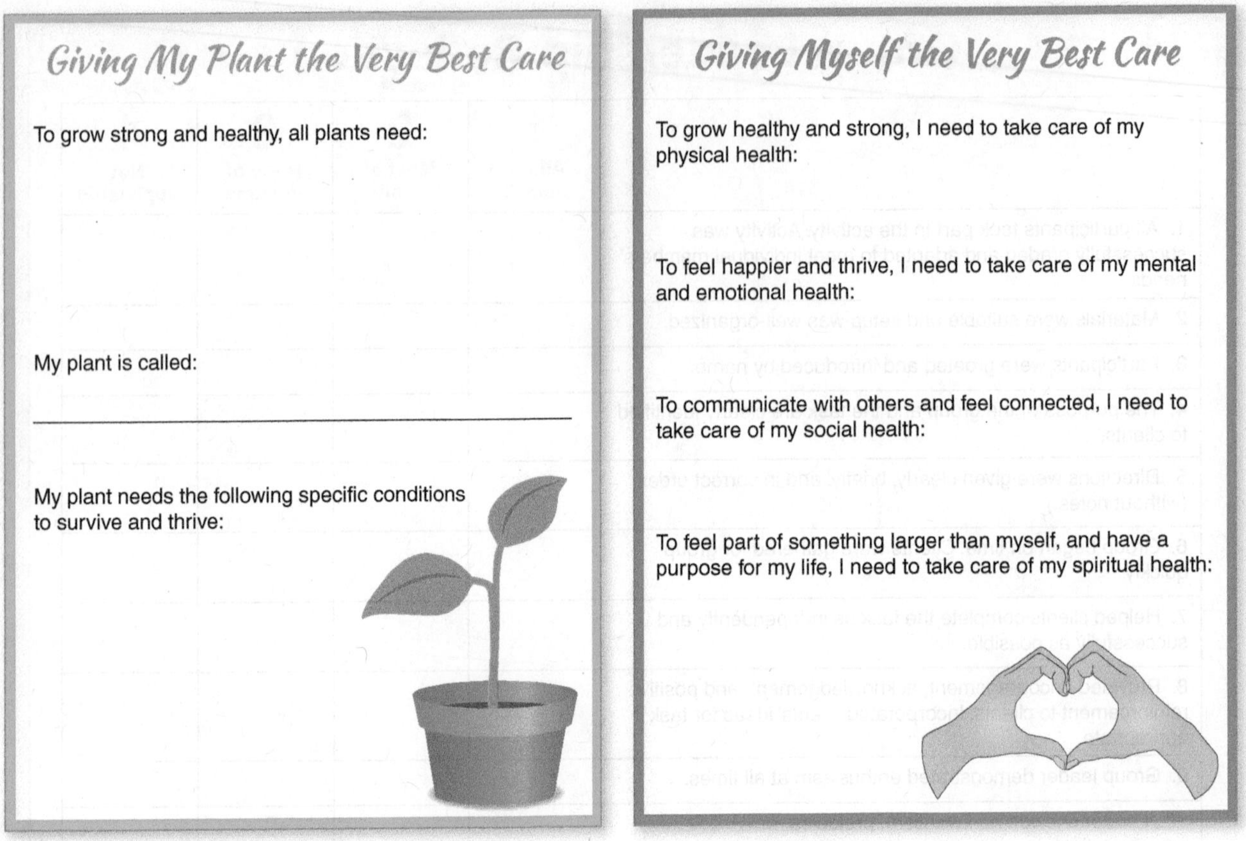

Giving My Plant the Very Best Care

To grow strong and healthy, all plants need:

My plant is called:

___

My plant needs the following specific conditions to survive and thrive:

Giving Myself the Very Best Care

To grow healthy and strong, I need to take care of my physical health:

To feel happier and thrive, I need to take care of my mental and emotional health:

To communicate with others and feel connected, I need to take care of my social health:

To feel part of something larger than myself, and have a purpose for my life, I need to take care of my spiritual health:

FIGURE 25.5 Giving my plant the very best care. (Prepared by Sarah G. Sieradski, 2004.)

In every type of therapeutic group, the leader will also have demands and responsibilities tied to his or her role as an OT practitioner (Table 25.3). The OT practitioner will need to carefully observe all interactions and behavior that members demonstrate during the task or discussion in order to clearly document each participant's level, quality, and detail of participation. The group leader (an OT or an OTA working under the supervision of the OT) performs ongoing reassessment of the member's attention span, ability to concentrate, organizational skills, ability to follow multistep directions, communication skills, understanding of the concepts presented, and other aspects related to the client's therapeutic goals. If the goals are more functional, the OT practitioner may observe coordination, range of motion, muscle strength, or endurance. The OT practitioner will want to acknowledge and reinforce any gains that each group member makes to increase or maintain their motivation.

Therapeutic Use of Self as a Group Leader

Occupational therapy practitioners who are skillful group leaders have effective ability in the area of **therapeutic use of self**. All OT practitioners bring their life experiences, knowledge, values, strengths, and desire to help others to create therapeutic relationships. For a group leader, development of a therapeutic relationship with clients may be done as part of the group rather than on a one-to-one basis. Special skills are needed to make OT practitioners into successful group leaders. These include the ability to put others at ease, sensitivity to other's feelings, a good sense of humor, patience, and the ability to redirect clients in a nonthreatening and noninsulting manner. The group leader needs to demonstrate a nonjudgmental and accepting attitude, be able to help group members establish appropriate boundaries, and help them explore their emotions, skills, and limitations in a safe and supportive environment. While all OT practitioners have a unique set of talents, experiences, strengths, and skills, those who lead successful groups often have developed a more flexible, intuitive, and insightful repertoire of professional expertise (Table 25.4).

Effective Leadership with Difficult Participants

As a group leader, you may recognize you are dealing with a difficult person when you find yourself experiencing an unpleasant and deeply negative response to his/her behavior. You may expend lots of energy either engaged in conflict with this person or desperately trying

TABLE 25.2 Planning Meaningful and Accessible Therapeutic Groups

Audience size, physical abilities, and cognitive level	• Design the occupation to provide the "just-right" challenge; not too easy, which can result in boredom, and not too hard, which can result in frustration. Selecting highly adaptable occupations will increase your ability to create successful therapeutic experiences for even a mixed audience.
Client-centered considerations	• Is it something clients have already enjoyed? • Is it something clients like and want to do? • Is it motivating? Do clients want to make it for themselves or others, for example, a family member or friend? • Will it work toward achieving therapeutic goals? • Is it something clients can do? Do they have the cognitive and physical ability to carry it out successfully? • Is it age appropriate? Gender appropriate? Role appropriate? It should not too childish for adults even if you need it to be simple, for example, not playing hip-hop music for older adults and not showing children's cartoons to adults.
Task flexibility	• Is it adaptable for individuals with varying physical limitations? • Can you grade the task for individuals with varying cognitive ability levels? • Can this level of flexibility be carried out simultaneously in a group?
Environment	• Do you have space? • Tables? • Ability to make a mess? • Special issues?
Materials needed	• Price, accessibility, and safety issues
Need for tools	• Cost, safety issues, storage needs (e.g., locked flammables cabinet?)
Need to transport materials	• Weight, size, messiness, storage
Time allotted for the task	• Set up, giving instructions, actual project time, and cleanup
Selection and seating of group members	• Random or self-selection? Sometimes, you will want to group people together who can help each other in some way. Separate potentially disruptive group members and sit them next to you. Seat individuals who will need more fards1:1 help next to staff.
Purpose or desired outcome for group	• Professional or self-development • Develop a skill or increase function • Social interaction • Explore or learn a hobby • Restore or adapt a previous occupation
Are there other therapeutic benefits?	• Relaxation? • Ability to also work on additional issues such as pain, sleep, or grief?
Add meaning and depth using metaphors	• Plan a seed starting task with a group of adults in a chemical dependency support group, and use metaphors related to the task to discuss planting the seed of change in their lives. How will they nurture the new growth of change? • What does the change (or plant) need in order to thrive and not just survive? • How will the change (or plant) deal with challenging conditions in the future?

TABLE 25.3 TASKS of an Effective Group Leader

- Carefully plan each group activity ahead of time
- Encourage each group member to contribute to the discussion or perform the task
- Keep the group on task or on topic
- Teach new concepts and provide opportunities to practice skills
- Help the less able group members perform successfully
- Be aware of any safety issues
- Adapt or grade the task/discussion to create the "just-right" level of challenge
- Validate each participant's responses
- Redirect problem behaviors
- Reinforce and celebrate therapeutic gains
- Respond to participant's needs as the group progresses
- Perform ongoing reassessment of each group member
- Observe all behavior and interaction carefully for later documentation
- Clearly document participant's progress toward therapeutic goals
- Reflect on what was learned in each group session to improve the activity for the next group session and to increase the effectiveness of the leader's therapeutic use of self

TABLE 25.4 Attributes of Therapeutic Use of Self in Occupational Therapy

- Individual values, strengths, skills
- Talents, abilities (e.g., artistic, musical, creative, technological)
- Commitment to help and serve others, advocacy, initiative
- Unconditional regard for others, nonjudgmental attitude
- Respect for others' dignity and differences, empathy
- Education, knowledge, life wisdom, clinical skills, experience
- Sensitivity, intuition, understanding, insight, holistic viewpoint
- Humor, ability to put others at ease, ability to establish rapport, make personal connections, generosity of spirit, enthusiasm
- Communication skills, interpersonal skills, emotional intelligence
- Sense of perspective, flexibility, clear boundaries
- Problem-solving ability, critical thinking skills, creative thinking skills
- Encouragement, support, ability to instill hope and motivation, validating
- Being present and mindful, attentiveness, patience
- Honesty balanced with tact and kindness in interactions
- Ethical, maintaining confidentiality, being professional, honest
- Teaching ability, excellent activity analysis ability, desire to contribute to clients and to the profession, research skills, sense of duty
- Storytelling ability, documentation skills, writing and speaking ability
- Focus on being client centered and evidence based
- Sense of spirituality, deep understanding of life's stages, connections with others, nature, and forces greater than ourselves
- Ability to work well with others, teamwork

to avoid it. You may hear yourself repeating the same directions over and over as part of a power struggle when this person refuses to listen to you.

Though the number of difficult people you will have to deal with in your career will mercifully be small, their impact on your therapeutic group activities is huge. They tend to frustrate and demoralize group leaders with their chronic habitual negative behavioral patterns. Difficult people often appear immune from our usual methods of communication, persuasion, motivation, and redirection.

Individuals who behave in a difficult manner have learned to manipulate or control others by keeping them off balance, thus making them incapable of effective action. Acceptance of untoward behavior avoids unpleasant confrontations, but it does not change an individual's behavior, it actually reinforces it. When you accept this behavior, you allow this individual to continually disrupt your groups. Other group participants may tolerate this situation at first, but they may gradually come to resent both the difficult behavior and your passive response to it.

Effective management of difficult behavior requires acting with consistent thoughtful purpose to restore the balance of power and minimize the ability of the difficult person to affect the group or activity. The intent of coping is to enable all participants, including the difficult person, to interact and work together in harmony to achieve their therapeutic goals (Adams, 2001). The following strategies are intended to help a group leader manage difficult behaviors (Table 25.5).

Identifying Why People May Demonstrate Difficult Behavior

For a group leader, understanding why an individual demonstrates difficult behavior can help you start to cope. Sometimes, difficult behavior results from the following:

- An unfulfilled need or unresolved issue
- Differing personality or communication styles

TABLE 25.5 **Goals for Coping with a Difficult Person**

Coping with a group member's difficult behavior consists of accomplishing several simple goals...

1. Try to discern the purpose or payoff of this behavior so you can select a strategy to interfere with the accomplishment or success of this purpose.
2. Enable you, the entire group, and the person disrupting the group to get on with the group activity or discussion at hand.
3. Provide this person incentives and methods to develop more positive and constructive behavior.

Adapted from Adams B. *The Everything Leadership Book*. Avon, MA: Adams Media Corporation; 2001.

- Unexpressed fear or anger
- Lack of interpersonal skills or insensitivity toward others
- Lack of interest or investment in the group activity, boredom

It is often helpful to step back and try to discern the apparent goal and implicit need behind the person's difficult behavior. This may give you a short cut to a positive solution. If you can identify what the individual is gaining from engaging in difficult behavior, the benefit or reward, you can use proactive strategies to delay or block the benefit, which may actually encourage a positive change of behavior.

Think about why the person is demonstrating a difficult behavior, why at this specific moment is this specific behavior being elicited? Often, the solution you come up with will suggest a strategy to attempt. For example, a person may become resistive at a particular moment because he/she perceives that an instruction or the entire activity is too complicated (e.g., too many steps, too complex a challenge, too demanding a rule or requirement). If so, the way to reduce the resistive behavior would be to simplify and decrease the demands on the person's abilities. This individual may need to complete one step at a time before you give another instruction. He/she may need another step-by-step demonstration or to work with another knowledgeable participant as a team.

Considerations and Guidelines for Coping with Difficult Behaviors

Once you can identify what the person has to gain, or what losses they want to prevent with their problematic behavior, you may find good strategies to help them modify or extinguish this difficult behavior. For a group leader, it is important to maintain a positive and solution-focused attitude when you find yourself dealing with a person's difficult behavior. It helps to recognize that this individual is presenting you with a chance to learn something new. If you view the situation as a learning opportunity, you can further hone your group leading and interpersonal skills. To be effective in dealing with the difficult person, you may need to change how *you* feel, think, and react when you are with this group member. You must look deep within yourself to determine *your role* in the situation. How might *your* thinking, assumptions, history, experience, or emotions contribute to the difficult situation (Brinkman & Kirschner, 2002)? Focus on the difficult individual's positive qualities—you may be able to turn them into an ally if you can keep your interactions positive. Try to keep an open mind. Remember that to others, *you* may be the difficult person (Rosen, 1998)!

Be aware that the other group members will watch closely to see how you react and respond to difficult

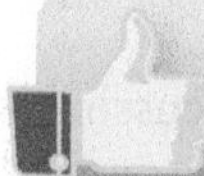

FROM THE FIELD 25.1

Benefits of Difficult Behavior

Client payoff or benefits of difficult behavior may include the following (Adams, 2001; Rosen, 1998):

- Immediate gratification
- Taking control or dominating
- Frustrating or undermining an authority figure
- Getting or deflecting attention
- Covering for feelings of insecurity or inadequacy
- Avoiding responsibility by blaming others
- Getting people to like them (acceptance)
- Feeling superior to others
- Staying in own comfort zone (avoid change or risk)
- Keeping self safe or comfortable
- Covering for fear of failure or fear of looking foolish
- Humiliating others
- Manipulating others
- Blaming others for personal shortcomings
- Taking credit for others' work or ideas
- Avoiding interaction—keeping people at a distance
- Protecting self from being hurt or rejected
- Acquiring things (values things over people)
- Concealing or continue substance abuse
- Covering for physical or cognitive symptoms they may be having

behavior. Remain calm and matter-of-fact, be fair, and always give a reason for the type of behavior that you expect as this will seem less arbitrary than "because I said so." If you can ignore some less intrusive negative behaviors, the group will usually learn to tolerate this too.

Remember that your goal is for the person to improve his/her self-control. You want to create the opportunity for the group member to demonstrate more positive constructive behavior without constantly needing cues, limits, redirection, or other forms of external control. It may be helpful to explain why the expected behavior is important for the group's activity to be successful.

Use teachable "on the spot" moments whenever possible (Vinogradov & Yalom, 1989). Stop and deal with issues of great consequence when they come up; sometimes, this is more important than the fun of a group activity. Issues to stop and process together with the group might include stigma, grief, descriptions of observed violence, coping with anger, or other critical topics. See if others in the group can relate to this issue and help the group brainstorm potential coping strategies or solutions.

Try to use nonjudgmental terms when discussing behavior. If you can, eliminate "right versus wrong," "good versus bad," and "proper versus improper" from your vocabulary or certainly when leading therapeutic groups. Instead, ask questions like "Is that working for you, or is that sometimes a problem?" or use terms such as "effective versus ineffective" or "healthy versus unhealthy." You may also say "Now *that* is the type of behavior I want to see/I like/I expect."

Recognize when a person's behavior is unintentional or is not their fault. When this is the case, you must find ways to work *with* this behavior instead of against it. Examples of clients who might exhibit difficult behavior as part of their illness or medical condition include the following:

- Individuals who have had a traumatic brain injury may demonstrate impulsivity and impaired judgment.
- Individuals who have had a stroke may demonstrate labile emotions.
- Individuals with developmental disabilities may have deeply ingrained behaviors that are often difficult to modify.
- Individuals with autism can be easily overstimulated and have difficulty screening out noise and distractions that can become upsetting.
- Individuals who have dementia may be disoriented, easily confused, repetitive, worrisome, or even easily agitated.
- Individuals with psychiatric disorders may have impaired thought processing. Delusional thinking may create paranoia or grandiosity. Disorganization may make it difficult for them to follow sequential directions or ignore distractions. You may want to limit their choices to make it easier for them to make decisions (Vinogradov & Yalom, 1989, pp. 80–82).

Sometimes, new group leaders or students worry about saying or doing the wrong thing when dealing with demanding or challenging people. Generally, if you show genuine caring, concern, and a desire to help them, even if you do not always handle situations as gracefully as you would like, people will give you the benefit of the doubt. People usually know when you are trying to be supportive; even people who are confused or ill know when they are cared about.

As you work with people, take a client-centered approach. If you know the individual's goals, hopes, and motivations, you can use these as inspiration or incentive in tough moments to remind them of their larger or long-term goals. As part of a client-centered approach, help them see the relevance of the group activity to their goals to give them a worthy reason to actively participate.

When beginning any therapeutic activity, identify the group goals up front, and tell the participants what the purpose of the activity is. This will help make the activity more meaningful and may encourage members to try harder or take it more seriously. You may want to ask the group to identify some basic rules for group behavior such as "How do we need to behave today (for children)? Or, "What do we need to do in order to accomplish this (for adults)?" Identify specific expected behaviors.

Whenever you can, validate people's feelings, even when you do not agree with them. If you reflect back the emotion they have expressed, it will help them feel as though they have been heard. Sometimes, this alone is enough to extinguish difficult behavior (Brinkman & Kirschner, 2002, pp. 35–38).

When the going gets tough, keep in mind that you may provide a life lesson to a difficult individual that will alter his/her thinking and change his/her behaviors in ways that will carry over into other life settings and circumstances (Rosen, 1998, pp. 117–118). Sometimes, you will know when this has been accomplished, but most of the time, we never know what has grown from the seeds we have planted during our therapeutic groups.

Providing Redirection to Difficult Group Participants

Make redirection time limited; make it about today's behavior. Keep discipline focused in the "here and now" moment. Tell the individual, "We can try again tomorrow." Be matter-of-fact, keep the edge out of your voice, and remember it is *not* personal. Try to be fair and treat the difficult individual as much like the rest of the group as possible (Brinkman & Kirschner, 2002, pp. 53–54).

Start any redirection as subtly and inconspicuously as possible, especially when working with adults. Try to redirect them in ways that are not obvious to the entire group. Gradually move toward more directive redirection as necessary using suggestions from the following continuum based on the work of Vinogradov and Yalom (1989). The initial steps on the continuum may help manage behaviors that are mostly irritating, while the latter steps may help you deal with more disruptive and distracting behavior. If the difficult person is doing something that is dangerous to himself/herself or others, you will need to immediately put the last few steps of the continuum into action.

A Redirection Continuum

1. *Ignore the irritating behavior if possible.*
   Often, if someone fails to gain attention with his/her distracting behavior, it may be self-extinguishing.
2. *Use proximity.*
   Walk over, stand next to, and/or sit next to the group member, as many times a person will settle down if an authority figure is nearby.
3. *Refocus attention with a gentle touch.*
   Place a hand on the individual's hand or shoulder or a hand in the center of his/her back. This is a more obvious form of proximity. (NOTE: You need to be very careful when using touch as some individuals will be agitated instead of being calmed. Individuals who have been through trauma are especially sensitive to touch, and this technique may be contraindicated.)
4. Use *"the look."*
   Sometimes, a stern glance in their direction will let the person know you are observing their behavior and are not approving!
5. *Use the person's name and ask them a question related to the activity.*
   Redirect their attention back to the task at hand. Example is as follows: "Lucie, can you guess what the next step in the project might be?"
6. *Verbally refocus their attention.*
   Ask the group member by name if he/she is able to concentrate or perform the activity.
7. *Ask for the behavior you want.*
   Use "I" statements to say what you expect rather than "you" statements that sound more like blaming. Keep a positive focus rather than using "don't," "stop," or "shouldn't." Examples are as follows: "John, I need you to listen quietly while Paul takes his turn." "Susan, I'd like you to turn around in your seat and face me so you can listen carefully while I give instructions."
8. *Enlist their help—give this member a responsibility.*
   Put your difficult individual to work—have him/her pass out materials or collect each participant's trash. When you do delegate a task, provide verbal instructions along with a demonstration of how you want the task done. Check (repeatedly) for accuracy. This step is especially valuable for restless individuals who have difficulty sitting or standing still. You may also want to give people who are restless or anxious permission to stand up and walk briefly at intervals throughout the group activity to relieve excess energy.
9. *Quietly take materials out of their hands.*
   If possible, gently remove the source of distraction without making it a verbal issue. This will cause the least upset to the group as a whole. You can even say quietly, "I'll hold this for you until you can use it according to directions."
10. *Last resort—ask other staff (or parent) to remove the difficult individual from the group* (Vinogradov & Yalom, 1989).
    Take a private moment (during or shortly after the group ends) to process the problem with the individual. Explain the reason why he/she could no longer participate *today* and that you will try again when the expected behaviors are demonstrated (Vinogradov & Yalom, 1989).

Long-Term Strategies for Difficult Participants

In the following section, we will look at general long-term strategies to help deal with disruptive group members as well as specific strategies for children and adolescents. We begin with general strategies.

1. Seek savvy advice or model other leaders' effective strategies. Find someone else who works with the difficult participant—ask for tips to better manage them. Find out what works. Even better—*watch* this colleague in action to see how he/she applies these more effective management strategies (Brinkman & Kirschner, 2002, p. 220).
2. Use reinforcements—pair the difficult person with a specific partner. Have the individual work as a team with yourself, another adult (staff or volunteer who understands and better tolerates the behavior), or even a peer who works well with the individual (Brinkman & Kirschner, 2002, p. 220).
3. Talk to the difficult individual privately ahead of time to set expectations. Use "I statements" to identify the expected behavior, not "you statements," which sound like blaming. Keep your expectations positive; tell the individual what you want him/her to do instead of what you do not want him/her to do.
4. Create a behavioral contract. Identify specific expectations and specific behaviors that are required to participate in the group. Make sure all other staff understands the expectations in order to prevent staff splitting. Have positive ways to reinforce the person's appropriate behavior such as praise and extra attention. You may also need to use natural negative consequences for inappropriate behavior.
5. Find ways to understand the purpose of the person's behavior. What need is going unfulfilled that creates this behavior? Find more positive ways to fill this

need—this may serve to extinguish the negative behavior over time (Brinkman & Kirschner, 2002, p. 22–24).

6. Use outside resources to better understand the person's behavior. Read books (the references following this chapter are a good start) or attend workshops to learn more about behavior management. This may help you look at the person's behavior in new ways and from a different perspective. When you understand it differently, you will be able to generate new ideas to problem solve it.
7. Find areas of common ground so you can align with the difficult group members rather than fighting against them. Work hard to create partnerships and allies rather than enemies and opponents.

Strategies for Dealing with Difficult Children (Adapted from Brandes & Ingold, 1997)

1. Pick your battles. Address the most important and disruptive behaviors first rather than many small nitpicky corrections. Use teachable moments wherever possible. Remember that in many instances, peers will socialize a child faster than adults.
2. Let the children establish group behavioral rules themselves. Encourage them to make the rules broad rather than very specific. Try limiting this to three rules that everyone can easily remember. Post them where the group can see it, and verbally review the rules before each group activity.
3. Have the difficult child earn the privilege of group participation. Work with the child on a 1:1 basis until he/she demonstrates the expected behaviors required for group participation. This is not a punishment; it is teaching the positive consequences of cooperative behavior.
4. Plan for a quiet area. Create a quiet spot where a child can settle himself or herself down when overstimulated. Do not call it time-out, and find a more positive term such as relaxation station. You might wish to incorporate headphones with quiet music. Use neutral warmth like a sheet, large towel, or blanket for the child to wrap up in. You may want the quiet area to face away from the rest of the group to reduce visual distractions. You can even use the quiet area for the child to work in. For outdoor activities, create a quiet spot in the garden or yard for this purpose.
5. Format the activity or behavior as a game or contest. Children respond best to fun! Which team can have their work area cleaned up first? Ready, set, go!
6. Use a behavioral modification program. Create a visual chart and specify the positive behaviors you expect or require. Have a reward that interests the child or meets an unfulfilled need. Use praise along with a positive mark or sticker on the chart—let the child place the sticker on the chart as part of his/her reward. Reinforce the positive behavior by telling other staff (or parent) about the positive behavior, or let the child convey the positive report himself/herself.

Strategies for Difficult Adolescents (Adapted from Brandes & Ingold, 1997; Goldstein & McGinnis, 1997)

1. Address behavioral issues without other adolescents present whenever possible. Remember that adolescents can be very self-conscious and desperately seek acceptance from peers. Anything that sets an adolescent apart can create a reason for others to pick on or tease them. When addressing problem behaviors, you may want to have another adult present to serve as a neutral witness.
2. Stop bullying behavior immediately. This can snowball into a much larger problem as peers take sides in a dispute. Find ways to help adolescents empathize with each other, and give experiences that reinforce natural consequences of disruptive behavior.
3. Give adolescents opportunities to try out a variety of roles within the group.
4. Adolescents are still developing their sense of identity and often do not easily move out of their usual comfort zone. Have the group rotate leadership of small teams. Give to the team leader concrete and specific duties, for example, to read a list of instructions for the rest of the team to follow. Also, rotate the membership of each team, so the adolescents mix with all of the members of the group.
5. Use fewer metaphorical therapeutic activities until the group has demonstrated more insight and ability to understand abstract thinking. Many adolescents are concrete, black-and-white thinkers and hence will benefit from step-by-step instructions and simple experiential activities. You might want to have the group brainstorm ways to apply the lessons they are learning from occupational therapy activities into other aspects of their lives as most adolescents will not easily transfer learning to other areas.
6. Involve the teens in setting standards for expected group behavior and in determining consequences. Use a small elected adolescent representative panel to assist the group leader in determining consequences for inappropriate behavior.
7. Catch them doing something right. Give praise immediately and often to reinforce positive behavior.

Summary

Many aspects of effective therapeutic group practice were discussed in this chapter. Two general methods of planning effective group occupations were shared as well as tips for selecting meaningful and accessible occupations. Occupational analysis was noted as a systematic method for identifying steps, processes, and adaptations for therapeutic tasks and topics in group practice. Ways that successful group leaders utilize therapeutic use of self to direct and encourage their clients were identified. A group leader's roles and responsibilities were discussed as well as techniques for dealing with various types of challenging group participants. Occupational therapy therapeutic groups are a cost-effective and valuable tool for providing client-centered intervention in a wide variety of practice settings. As a future OTA, you will likely have opportunities to plan and lead therapeutic groups.

Review Questions

1. Therapeutic groups are an effective way to provide intervention for:
   a. Clients in mental health occupational therapy practice.
   b. Clients in physical dysfunction occupational therapy practice.
   c. Clients in school-based occupational therapy practice.
   d. Clients in all the above areas of practice.

2. Cole's seven steps for planning successful therapeutic groups include all the following *except*:
   a. Generalizing and processing.
   b. Setting up and cleaning up.
   c. Application and summary.
   d. Introduction and activity.

3. In selecting tasks or topics for therapeutic groups, one should consider:
   a. Identifying what would be meaningful to the clients that would also help them meet their intervention goals.
   b. Finding out what materials would be least expensive to use.
   c. Picking a task that would have easy setup and cleanup.
   d. Teaching the group about a special hobby the therapist enjoys.

4. Which of the following types of individuals might need to perform tasks that are easily gradable for varying cognitive ability levels?
   a. Individuals in a cardiac rehabilitation exercise program
   b. Individuals in a school-based social skills program
   c. Individuals with schizophrenia, dementia, and Parkinson disease in an inpatient geropsychiatric program
   d. Individuals in a long-term rehabilitation post-CVA exercise program

5. Discussion-oriented therapy groups may focus on therapeutic occupations such as:
   a. Cooking.
   b. Assertiveness training.
   c. Activities of daily living.
   d. Arts and crafts.

6. Task-oriented intervention groups may focus on therapeutic occupations such as:
   a. Coping with grief and loss
   b. Communication skills
   c. Leisure exploration and community resources
   d. Activities of daily living

7. When planning a group, it is helpful to consider:
   a. The intervention goals of all the clients who will participate
   b. Having a backup plan in case the first plan is not successful
   c. Having enough staff to assist individuals who need extra assistance
   d. All of the above

8. When beginning a therapeutic group, the leader should always:
   a. Greet and introduce the participants as well as identify the group's purpose and activity
   b. Call on a favorite client more than others
   c. Quickly run through all the steps of the task at once
   d. Wait until all late-arriving participants get there

9. Effective ideas to consider when selecting therapeutic occupations include all of the following EXCEPT:
   a. Planning to have a handout available for participants to take home to reinforce the concepts that are discussed in the group
   b. Using a game format that may encourage more participation and enjoyment by clients
   c. Having the clients compete to see who can create the nicest looking project
   d. Having enough space for all the participants to work comfortably

10. Performing an occupational analysis of a therapeutic task is helpful for:
    a. Adapting and grading the task for clients with varying cognitive and physical abilities
    b. Reinforcing the proper sequence of steps as the client performs the task
    c. Redirecting the client who is using materials in an unsafe manner
    d. Being a positive role model for group participants

11. Finding the "just right" amount of challenge for a client performing a therapeutic task will prevent:
    a. Misuse of materials and tools
    b. Arguments over who gets to use the tools first
    c. Frustration if the task is perceived as too difficult by the client
    d. Acting out behavior by the client

12. The many tasks of an effective group leader include all the following EXCEPT:
    a. Performing ongoing assessment of the clients to increase the meaningfulness of documentation
    b. Reinforcing and celebrating progress gains as part of therapeutic use of self to encourage the clients
    c. Being aware of safety issues and keeping the group focused on the task or topic
    d. Making sure those clients who have difficulty must figure out solutions without the leader's assistance

13. When dealing with difficult participants, the leaders should always:
    a. Try to identify the purpose or need behind the person's problem behavior
    b. Immediately ask the difficult participant to leave the group
    c. Ignore the problem behavior until another client complains about it
    d. Express frustration directly to the difficult client

14. When redirecting a problem participant, the leader should do all the following EXCEPT:
    a. Keep the redirection in the "here and now" moment so the clients understand they can try again when they can behave more appropriately
    b. Be matter-of-fact and not take the negative behavior personally
    c. Immediately redirect the adult client in front of the entire group to show that this behavior will not be tolerated
    d. Ask for the type of positive behavior you want rather than blaming them for their negative behavior

15. Attributes of therapeutic use of self include all of the following EXCEPT:
    a. Always being consistent in your approach to clients in order to show them how something should be done correctly to ensure they successfully complete the project perfectly
    b. A therapist's individual values, strengths, skills, talents, and abilities
    c. Commitment to serve others, advocacy, initiative, and empathy
    d. Interpersonal skills, clear boundaries, flexibility, and humor

Practice Activities

Use Cole's seven step planning process to design a therapeutic discussion group for a selected population and setting of clients.

Use the group planning format to design and carry out a therapeutic task group. Use the group leadership evaluation to grade yourself and identify areas of success and things you might choose to change the next time you teach the task.

Reflect on what aspects you and your life experience may contribute to your unique therapeutic use of self when leading groups of clients.

References

Adams B. *The Everything Leadership Book.* Avon, MA: Adams Media Corporation; 2001.

Brandes BH, Ingold JB. *Get Real: A Practical Guide to Leading Adolescent Groups.* Milwaukee, WI: Families International, Inc.; 1997.

Brinkman R, Kirschner R. *Dealing With People You Can't Stand*. New York, NY: McGraw-Hill, Inc.; 2002.

Cole M. *Group Dynamics in Occupational Therapy*. Thorofare, NJ: Slack Incorporated; 2012.

Goldstein A, McGinnis E. *Skillstreaming the Adolescent: New Strategies and Perspectives for Teaching Prosocial Skills*. Champaign, IL: Research Press; 1997.

Rosen MI. *Thank You for Being Such a Pain*. New York, NY: Three Rivers Press; 1998.

Schwartzberg S, Howe M, Barnes M. *Groups: Applying the Functional Group Model*. Philadelphia, PA: F. A. Davis Company; 2008.

Vinogradov S, Yalom I. *A Concise Guide to Group Psychotherapy*. Washington, DC: American Psychiatric Press, Inc.; 1989.

CHAPTER 26

Workplace Safety

Naomi Abrams, OTD, OTR/L, CEAS

Key Terms

Administrative controls—Safety measures that are put in place through action of supervisors such as a change in job pacing or job rotation.

Engineering controls—Safety measures that make changes to tools and/or environment.

Lifting Index—Measurement of risk calculated by comparing the recommended weight limit to the actual weight being lifted.

Reach envelope—Primary, secondary, and tertiary ranges that identify how far a person is reaching and therefore what items or tasks should be completed in each range.

Recommended weight limit—A calculation of a safe weight that can be lifted in specified situations.

Root cause analysis—A systematic process of identifying method of injury as well as the context surrounding injuries.

Task analysis—A systematic method of identifying the physical, cognitive, and psychosocial demands of a given task.

Work—A task that requires physical, cognitive, and/or psychosocial effort.

Learning Objectives

After studying this chapter, readers should be able to:

- Identify how occupational therapy fits within the field of workplace safety.
- Understand how to structure an intervention to address foundation skills necessary for working safely.
- Educate clients about keeping themselves safe at work tasks.

Introduction

Throughout this book, you have been reading about pieces of a large puzzle that OTs and OTAs put together for the benefit of each of our clients or client populations. This includes our commitment to use evidence-based practices, to use meaningful interventions, and to use whatever tools we need to make a difference in a client's recovery. It is time to put some of that information together, not only to treat client injuries but also to prevent injuries from occurring. In order to do that, we need to be sure that no activity exceeds the physical, psychological, or cognitive abilities of our clients within the appropriate contexts. Much of the emphasis of injury prevention education is within the context of work-related injuries, often taking place after an injury or a series of injuries has occurred. This chapter will focus on using principles of occupational therapy and related fields to help prevent injury or prevent reinjury, specifically when related to the context of work; however, these same principles should be applied at all times in a client's daily life, whether or not they are at a job.

Where is Work?

Before we begin this chapter on workplaces and keeping them safe, we need to step back and decide what we would call a workplace. For many people, that would be an easy definition to give: a workplace is somewhere you go to do "work," which is also known as your "job" for which you get "paid." **Work**, according to the *Occupational Therapy Practice Framework III* (AOTA, 2014), is an area of occupation that includes not only activities that are completed to receive remuneration but also volunteer activities. The *Occupational Therapy Practice Framework III* (AOTA, 2014) then goes on to acknowledge that occupations can be classified differently based on their value or the perception of each individual or society.

The activity of getting dressed, according to this definition, would not be considered work, and consequently the bedroom would not be considered a workplace. However, to some people, such as a group of individuals with paraplegia, work may include these activities of daily living such as getting dressed. For the purposes of this chapter, the term "work" will be synonymous with the idea of tasks that require effort (physical, psychological, or cognitive). Each task is completed within contexts and roles. The term "work" is then able to be expanded to include all tasks. Therefore, all spaces where effort is made can be classified as workplaces.

Consider for a moment a fictitious client, Jodi. Jodi comes to an occupational therapy clinic for arm pain. She is asked a fairly common question "what do you do?" She answers "I am a lawyer." Many would consider this her "work." Alarm bells go off in the practitioner's mind: if she is a lawyer, she must work at a computer, and therefore, the risks associated with working at a computer must be addressed in order to alleviate her arm pain. However, this assumption limits the practitioner and may lead to incorrect judgments. Instead of classifying the idea of being a lawyer as her work, think of being a lawyer as a role she plays.

Even though she does not mention it in response to that specific question, she plays many different roles within her life that may influence her arm pain. She is also a mother, a daughter, a sister, a wife, an individual who cares for herself, an individual who maintains a home, an individual who participates in community activities, etc. The list of roles Jodi plays is fairly long. Each of those roles is played within many different contexts. Within each role, she does work or tasks that meet the expectations and needs of that role.

For example, refer back to the role of a lawyer. When she plays this role, she completes work tasks that accomplish the goal of meeting the needs of the clients who hired her. Some of the work tasks included in this role may be using a computer, carrying a briefcase, using a laptop, pulling books from shelves, filing, and communicating with coworkers. This work is completed within contexts or workplaces such as a court, an office, a conference room, or a client's home. Each workplace presents different opportunities for reinjury of her arm while completing the work tasks included in the role of being a lawyer.

Now look at her role as a mother. Within this role, she completes work tasks that include preparing food, assisting with baths, purchasing food or school supplies, assisting with homework, and many more. Many of these tasks are completed within the workplace of home. However, some are completed in grocery stores, shopping malls, or other environments. When developing interventions for her arm injury, we would be remiss if we did not address the risks associated with each of those tasks within each of those workplaces. As an OTA, you need to address the potential of injury in every area in which any work is completed and not allow yourself to become focused on "workplaces" only as places people go to complete paying jobs. The concepts discussed in this chapter have been focused on work tasks completed in workplaces where people play the role of worker in order to limit the number of pages required to demonstrate each concept. However, the concepts must be applied everywhere in all of the client's daily roles.

Ergonomics

An astute observer will note that this chapter is not listed as being solely about "ergonomics" even though ergonomics is often inexorably linked to workplace safety. The International Ergonomics Association (2000) defined ergonomics as "the scientific discipline concerned with the understanding of the interactions among humans and other elements of a system, and the profession that applies theoretical principles, data and methods to design in order to optimize human wellbeing and overall system" (IEA, 2000, "What is Ergonomics," para. 1). The field of ergonomics is a tool that OT practitioners use to better understand the complex interactions of person, tool, and environment CS9. The focus of this chapter will be on how OT practitioners use the knowledge gained by ergonomic research in combination with our own knowledge base to better help our clients. The concepts used in the field of ergonomics are similar to what occupational therapy has been using for years, labeled as "joint protection" or "energy conservation." Ergonomics has simply provided a scientific method and a language for studying those concepts with tools normally associated with engineering fields (such as back compression studies or force lifting measures).

Within the field of ergonomics, research is often limited by its inability to account for the transactional nature of humans within contexts (Abrams, 2011; Amick et al., 2012; Leyshon, et al., 2010). Understanding and being comfortable with addressing multiple factors such

FROM THE FIELD 26.1

OT and Ergonomics

According to industrial rehabilitation consultant Jill J. Page, occupational therapy practitioners are uniquely able to implement ergonomics consultation because the core of occupational therapy educational training is task and activity analysis (AOTA, n.d.).

as physical, psychosocial, environmental, and societal are qualities at which occupational therapy excels. In fact, addressing such factors is an integral part of our practice through the basic tenants of our profession (Abrams, 2011; AOTA, 2014) (From the Field 26.1).

Work-Related Injuries

The National Institutes for Occupational Safety and Health (NIOSH), the US federal government agency responsible for research and recommendations related to workplace safety, reports that an estimated 3.4 million emergency room visits in one year were related to workplace injuries or illnesses (NIOSH, 2007). Of those injuries, approximately 53% were categorized as sprains and strains or injuries such as lacerations and punctures. Most of the sprains and strains affected the trunk (which includes, in their definition, the shoulder as well as the back, chest, and abdomen) and lower extremity. The World Health Organization (WHO) estimates that within all industrialized countries, one-third of all health-related absences from work are related to work-related musculoskeletal disorders (WRMSD) (Luttmann et al., n.d.).

The Bureau of Labor Statistics (BLS), which collects information related to labor issues in the United States, reported that the median amount of time a worker was out of work due to an injury is eight days (Bureau of Labor Statistics, 2011). In that same report, BLS announced that the rate of WRMSDs was increasing, especially within the fields related to nursing aides.

As OT practitioners, we are well aware of the physical and psychosocial toll caring for others places on the caregiver. What can we extrapolate, based on these numbers, regarding the risks involved with other caring tasks, such as caring for children or elderly parents by laypeople? These tasks often are done without any government monitoring. Since there is no "employer," they are not seen as "work." No government-funded statistics are gathered to assess the rate of injury among mothers or fathers. It would be impossible to measure days away from work from the tasks of caring for an infant; parents cannot call in sick to that role (Griffin & Prince, 2000). Again, as OT practitioners, we must broaden our view of injury rates to include roles that are not well measured.

To make matters within the workplace even more dire, occupational injuries are not only associated with factors relating to the workplace. The workers themselves bring with them many factors that affect injury rates and the ability to avoid injuries. For example, obesity, diabetes, and heart disease are any increasing public health crisis in the US population (Ogden et al., 2012). All of these factors can influence how a person behaves at a workplace (Schulte et al., 2007). If a person in a paid workplace is obese and has diabetes that has caused peripheral neuropathy in his legs, he has an increased risk of foot injury on the job. If he also has undiagnosed sleep apnea, a condition where he stops breathing for brief periods at night due to a collapsing of the trachea, he is not getting enough rest at night to sustain optimal daily function (Thornton, 2011). This will decrease his situational awareness and therefore decrease his ability to avoid injury.

Workers also bring with them cultural and societal influences that may change how they deal with education related to injury prevention, methods of reporting injury, and ability to follow through with postinjury re-education to prevent further injury (Braveman & Page, 2012). For example, in a workplace where a majority of the workers come from backgrounds in which they were taught to work hard regardless of discomfort—because providing for the family takes priority over anything else *and* the workers are paid based on units completed—the OT practitioner has to modify all injury prevention education to fit within that belief and pay structure. The education will need to be practical and focused on allowing the worker to complete more work through increased productivity. The workers would not respond well to education focused on slowing down or reducing productivity in order to reduce injury. Seen on paper, this seems fairly obvious: if the person is paid to produce, they will not respond well to being told not to produce so as to prevent the *possibility* of later injury. However, we see it happen in clinics all the time. Occupational therapy practitioners will tell clients to stop doing tasks so that they can give their bodies time to heal. We have to be aware of what that advice does in the larger picture of that person's life.

Expanding on Jodi's story a bit, consider that she comes from a cultural environment where women are supposed to be stoic and showing weakness is considered insulting. From the perspective of injury prevention, we would need to be sure to include methods of decreasing physical stressors while completing work-, home-, and family-related tasks. Being comprehensive, our education would include injury prevention measures for the wide range of her activities, such as computer use, carrying objects, cooking, cleaning, and childcare. However, we are seeing her in our clinic because of an injury that *has already occurred*. How long did it take before she reported the injury to her doctor? Has she informed her family about her injury? Will she be willing to ask her coworkers or family for assistance? In Jodi's case, the OT practitioners may have to work with her to increase her use of culturally appropriate support mechanisms to decrease the risk of reinjuring her arm. This may not be an issue with a client who comes from a culture where all family members have the expectation of caring for one another and sharing income producing tasks equally.

Mechanisms of Injury

There are many causes of work-related injuries that are necessary to understand.

Acute Trauma

Injuries that fall under this category are traditionally related to slips, trips, falls, machine accidents, car accidents, cuts, burns, etc. On the surface, these fall outside of the realm of occupational therapy preventative action. Accidents happen and OT practitioners are there often only after the injury occurs. However, consider this: why do people slip, trip, get burned, or fall at work? Sometimes, it is as simple as grease on the ground. Sometimes, it only seems simple until examined more closely. We refer to the exercise of digging deeper into the causes of accidents as "**root cause analyses**." Occupational therapy practitioners can consult with companies and clients to educate them about environmental cognitive requirements, visual cues, increased contrast, effects of fatigue on postural reactions, or even phrasing safety material to meet the needs of different populations.

Keep your eyes and ears open for accidents that seem too simple. A client comes to you after tripping on an uneven brick walkway at work. While the fall seems simple—a brick stuck out and the person tripped—this is where you also consider things like as follows: are these people working 18-hour shifts and therefore more likely to trip because of fatigue? Is the brick walkway in an area of reduced light or shifting shadows? Is the walkway in an area with multiple other visual cues where people are unlikely to be looking down? The company's root cause analysis may end at unleveled bricks causing a trip. However, this is where occupational therapy's ability to see multiple causations is a strength not seen in other fields. It is your time to shine and let the company know that there may be more they can be doing to prevent injuries.

Consider a puncture injury caused by someone's hand going into a stamp machine. The root cause analysis could end with user error: the person did not follow safety precautions to be sure she kept clear of the moving parts. However, we can look at a much broader picture. Was she fatigued because of prolonged standing? Was she unable to distinguish the edges of the machine due to low contrast or light level? Did she have the cognitive or language skills required to understand the safety training video?

The Occupational Safety and Health Administration (OSHA), a government agency that enforces safe working conditions, provides guidelines for both keeping workplaces free of slips, trips, falls, burns, etc., as well as dictating how these injuries should be recorded. Injuries, their classification, extent, severity, and cause are recorded in an OSHA 300 Log (US Department of Labor, 2004). When working with a company on injury prevention, you may get access to that log to better understand the areas where injuries are occurring. The log is important because it influences how injuries are recorded and how root cause analyses are completed and documented. For example, strains and sprains are not documented unless "they result from a slip, trip, fall, or other similar accidents" (US Department of Labor, 2004, p. 3). In other words, there must be a discrete event that occurs in order for it to be recordable versus a repetitive strain complaint with no discernible acute injury.

Repetitive Strain

Repetitive strain injuries are often called WRMSDs although this is a bit of a misnomer since WRMSDs also can occur with acute injury. Repetitive strain WRMSDs have a multifactorial nature that makes finding root causes difficult. As a result, the study of causes often becomes controversial (Bernard, 1997). Repetitive strains are injuries that occur from repeated use of one or more body structures. The injuries that fall under this classification are related to muscles, tendons, nerves, bones, and ligaments. It is commonly understood that they occur when the workload required is greater than the capacity of the body component being used (Luttmann et al., n.d.) CS9&11. What is not often studied is how the limitations of the structures that support the area injured may also play a role in that injury. For example, a common repetitive strain disorder is lateral epicondylitis (a.k.a. tennis elbow). This injury is often associated with using the mouse for long periods. The root cause analysis often ends here: cause = using the mouse. However, we know through our understanding of the body that each structure requires a supporting structure to function (we'll talk more about this later in the chapter). Instead of blaming the lateral epicondylitis solely on the mouse, consider whether it is possible that the person's forward head posture with rounded shoulders played a role in that injury. Keep this in mind as we continue.

Risk factors for the development of WRMSDs from repetitive tasks depend on relationship of the loads being applied, the duration of the exposure, and the postural demands (Amell & Kumar, 2001; Bernard, 1997; Bongers et al., 2006) CS9. For example, if a worker is required to lift a light object three times a day, this may not be a high-risk activity. But what if we take that same light object, put it in an extremely cold environment, and have a person lift it three times per day? The risks of physical injury increase due to the environmental context. Taking the context out of the equation, if the amount a person is required to lift increases to 100 lb, even just three times per day, the risks also increase. If a person is required to lift the same 100 lb three times per day while in a twisted position, the risks increase even higher. Conversely, consider a cashier who counts thousands of bills an hour. The loads are very light, it does not take much pinch force to move bills; however, the number of times the task is completed is very high. The risk for hand injury increases, therefore, as the repetition increases.

Now, consider if that same cashier is hunched over a desk for eight hours per day while counting bills in a low-light environment. The cashier's poor posture increases the risk of hand injury because the supporting structures, the back and shoulders, are at a disadvantage even through the external loads remain low. This takes into account the idea that the weakest link is often the one that breaks and it may not be solely related to the action being performed. In order to better understand this chain, we can examine basic patterns of movement.

Basics of Movement Patterns

Movement directly impacts musculoskeletal disorders and understanding this relationship is an important component of workplace safety practice.

Stability and Mobility Intertwined

Without stability, there can be no mobility. This is a basic tenet of movement that plays a vital role in understanding WRMSDs (Chapman, 2008). However, it is often neglected when the injury seen does not relate to the body's core stabilizers such as the back and legs.

Recall that client Jodi is complaining of arm pain. The first thing that is blamed for that arm pain is usually the mouse or keyboard. After all, she complains of pain while using the mouse and keyboard and those are low load but highly repetitive tasks with her arm. Research has been unable to determine which mouse or keyboard works best to prevent arm pain or even if there is a direct link between many of the WRMSDs of the upper extremity and the keyboard and mouse (Abrams, 2011; Baker, 2009; Baker & Cidboy, 2006; Baker & Redfern, 2009; Bongers et al., 2006; Brewer, et al., 2006; Ripat, et al., 2006; Thomsen et al., 2008; Waersted et al., 2010). This is because the research fails to take into account the other factors that are influencing injury, such as the lack of stability in the structures that support the arm's mobility.

Jodi brings in pictures of herself working at her workstation. You note that, while working on her computer, Jodi is perched on the edge of her seat. Does she have good stability that allows her arm to have mobility? No. Her weakest link is her arm, and therefore, that is where the injury is seen. However, we cannot just treat her arm or we will be doing nothing to prevent the injury from recurring.

Think about stability and mobility this way: consider for a moment where you would put a ladder if you had to reach something on a very high shelf (Fig. 26.1). Would you put it on an uneven surface or on an even surface?

The smart approach would be to put the ladder on a solid base of support. What injuries would you see if the person put the ladder on an uneven base of support? Well, if he fell, the list would be very long, ranging from head injury to leg fractures. What if he did not fall but instead strained his back as a result of the lift? At no point would the injury be classified as an "uneven base of support injury to the back" although that would be a lot more accurate than classifying it as lifting injury.

The spine and core musculature are the most basic stabilizing mechanisms we have in our body, but we often ignore them when creating injury prevention programs

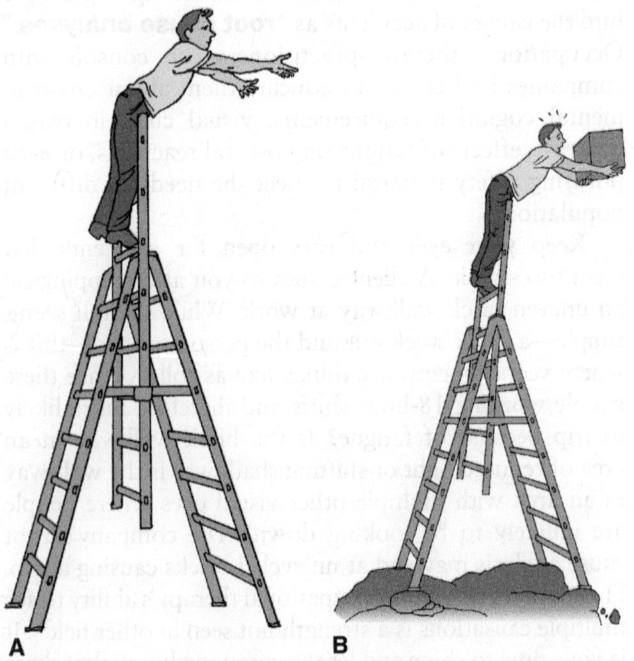

Figure 26.1 A. Reaching with a stable base of support. B. Reaching without a stable base of support. (Copyright Worksite Health & Safety Consultants, LLC, adapted with permission.)

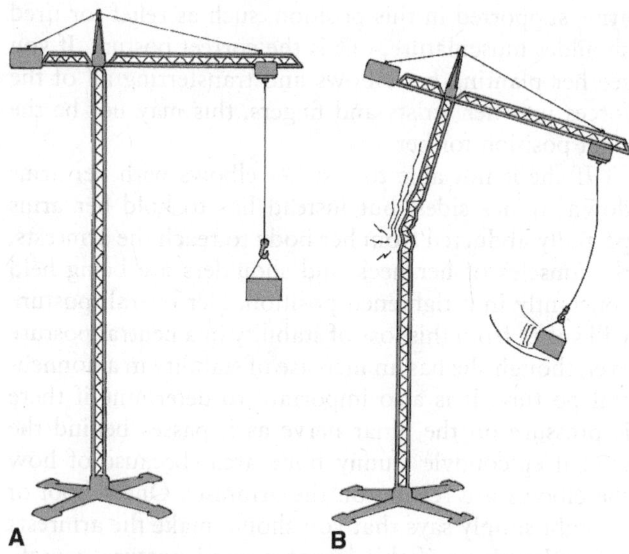

Figure 26.2 A. Stable at the core. B. Unstable at the core. (©NAOE Publishing, adapted with permission.)

unless the programs are directly related to lifting. Base of support, or having stability, is important regardless of the position being used or the task being completed. An easy way to understand this concept is to consider the spine as the core support in a large crane. So long as that crane is upright and straight, it can handle a large load (Fig. 26.2A). However, if you ever saw a crane starting to bend in the middle, you would probably run away as fast as you could (Fig. 26.2B).

When working with people to prevent injuries, we have to help them put themselves into a posture that promotes stability whenever the task requires mobility. In standing positions, this means insuring a solid, supportive, and even base of support, such as leveling floors and providing a nonslip and antifatigue mat. In sitting positions, it means providing a good seat pan (the part of the chair you sit on) and a backrest that allows for an upright supported posture.

The Reach Envelope

Base of support is only the first part of the stability to mobility relationship. The size and type of base of support also directly change the balance of the individual (Braveman & Page, 2012; Chapman, 2008). Stability, however, will be lost as the person moves into a position where the forces of the body are no longer directed toward the base of support such as leaning forward to reach something (Chapman, 2008). Ergonomic research provides us with a concept that helps delineate how far someone can safely reach. This is called the **reach envelope** (see Fig. 26.3).

With repetitive tasks or tasks requiring force, the tools or objects related to the task should be within the person's primary reach envelope. The primary reach envelope is the arc created when the person puts their

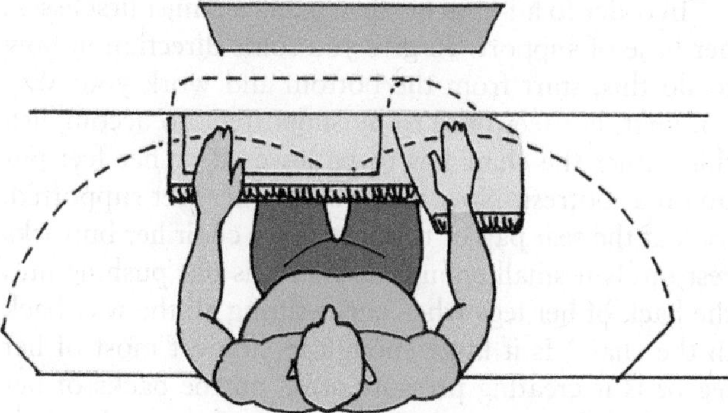

Figure 26.3 Primary reach envelope. (Adapted with permission from Abrams ND. *Why is My Office a Pain in My...?* Rockville, MD: NAOE Publishing; 2011:67. Copyright 2011 by NAOE Publishing.)

elbows up against their ribs then internally and externally rotates their shoulders (Sanders & McCormick, 1976).

As the frequency of the task decreases, the range of the envelope can increase. Objects the person uses *occasionally* can be placed in the secondary zone, which is the arc created when the person reaches forward without bending the spine and horizontally abducts and adducts their shoulders. The objects that a person *rarely* uses can be placed in the zone where he or she must climb on something while completing the reach.

Returning to Jodi in her office will help illustrate these concepts. She is sitting at her desk perched at the edge of her chair reaching forward for her keyboard and mouse. She looks something like the woman shown in Figure 26.4.

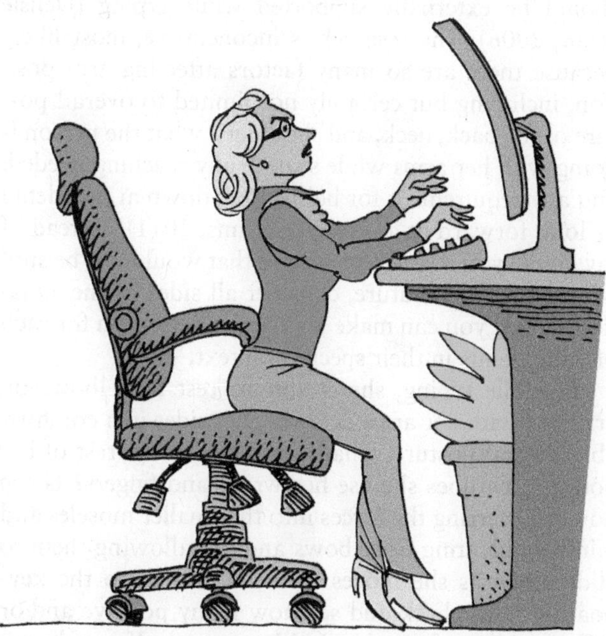

Figure 26.4 Computer user instability. (Adapted with permission from Abrams ND. *Why is My Office a Pain in My...?* Rockville, MD: NAOE Publishing; 2011:30. Copyright 2011 by NAOE Publishing.)

In order to address her arm pain, we must first assess her base of support. To give you some direction in how to do this, start from the bottom and work your way up. First, her feet need to be supported. To accomplish this, either the chair has to be lowered or her feet put up on a footrest. Now that we have her feet supported, look at the seat pan or the part of the chair her buttocks rest on. Is it small enough so that it is not pushing into the back of her legs when she is sitting all the way back in the chair? Is it large enough to support most of her leg or is it creating pressure areas on the backs of her thighs? If the answer is no to either of these, the chair has to be adjusted, modified, or adapted to better fit her leg length.

Moving up her spine, determine whether she is sitting upright but supported. When she relaxes her core musculature, does she slide down and drop her ribs into her pelvis? To support her spine, move the lumbar support to better fit her back. When she sits upright, not supported by the chair, palpate her lumbar curvature. Now, adjust the chair so that the curvature of the backrest matches the curvature of her spine in height and depth (this will take some trial and error). Have her sit back against the backrest and relax between each trial. Watch her spine and posture. She should be able to sit back against the backrest while still maintaining an upright posture.

Move the assessment out to her arms. Check her armrests, do they interfere with her arm movements or keep her from putting her elbows against her ribs (neutral posture)? There is great debate in the world of seated postures regarding whether a person's arms should be externally supported while typing (Delisle et al., 2006). The research is inconclusive, most likely because there are so many factors affecting arm position, including but certainly not limited to overall posture of the back, neck, and shoulders; what the person is doing with her arms while seated; any reaching needed; and any requirement for her to look down at fine detail or look forward at a screen (Abrams, 2011). Instead of my giving you a concrete answer that would not be supported by the literature, consider all sides of the situation so that you can make an informed decision for each of your clients in their specific context.

If, while typing, she is able to rest her elbows on armrests with her arms down by her sides in a comfortable neutral posture, what is it doing to the rest of her body? How does she use her wrists and fingers? Is she now transferring the forces into the smaller muscles and joints by planting her elbows and not allowing them to glide along as she moves from the mouse to the keyboard? Now, check and see how many positive and/or negative effects from this position you see. If you do not see any negative effects from having her arms supported in a neutral position, this may be the correct position for your client. If you see any positive effects of having her arms supported in this position, such as relief for tired shoulder musculature, this is the correct posture. If you see her planting her elbows and transferring all of the forces into her wrists and fingers, this may not be the right position for her.

If she is not able to rest her elbows with her arms down by her sides, but instead has to hold her arms partially abducted from her body to reach the armrests, the muscles of her neck and shoulders are being held constantly in a tightened position. Her overall posture will suffer from this loss of stability in a neutral posture even though she has an increase of stability in a nonneutral posture. It is also important to determine if there is pressure on the ulnar nerve as it passes behind the medial epicondyle (funny bone area) because of how the elbows are resting on the armrests. One school of thought simply says that you should make the armrests softer. However, if this is not a good posture overall, there is no real reason to simply treat a symptom and not address the root cause. This position can be useful if the chair will not adjust properly but the person really needs any support she can get. In the long term, she will tend to lean either left or right in order to incorrectly use the armrest or slump down to get more use out of the armrests.

And what if she does not have any support under her arms? Does she feel strain in her neck and shoulders? Is she able to self-correct her posture from sliding down in the chair without the armrests to boost up on? Does she need armrests to safely enter and exit the chair? Again, if you see that she has osteoarthritis in her knees and cannot safely exit the chair without the armrests, you would be causing injury to remove them even if the armrests do not promote correct postures. In general, most healthy people do not *need* support under their arms while they type if their arms can be down by their sides. The arms just do not weigh that much when the person is upright and in neutral posture.

There is also a school of thought that postulates that her entire forearm should be supported on a padded support projecting from the desk. This support is supposed to wrap around her chest similar to a wheelchair tray, which has a belly arch cutout so that it fits snuggly to the body. There is no research to support this posture (Delisle et al., 2006; Leyshon et al., 2010). However, you will encounter it so it is a good idea to break it down into its important questions: how is this posture affecting her overall posture? How is she sitting in order to allow the desk to wrap around her? What are the psychosocial issues that may arise due to this close-fitting desk? What is she moving the most when typing or using the mouse? Is it a large joint or small joint?

Only now that she has a good base of support can we address the tools she is using, namely, the computer. While it is out of the scope of this chapter to discuss the different types of keyboards and mice on the market, it is important to address the location of these devices. Remember the reach envelope. If she regularly has to reach outside of her primary reach envelope in order to reach the keyboard and mouse, she will be destabilizing herself. Her body weight is pulling her forward and down; gravity always wins. By moving the keyboard and mouse close to her, we place her weight back against the backrest and reduce the likelihood that she will slump forward.

Since it is brought up frequently, it is necessary to discuss wrist rests. The primary purposes of wrist rests are to reduce the likelihood of pressure areas against a sharp desk edge and/or to provide support for the arms. Scan back a few paragraphs and consider why Jodi may have pressure on her wrists while typing or using the mouse. Either the desk is too high and her wrists have to be protected from the desk edge or she is reaching out and has to support the weight of her arms. Again, there is no good research out there about wrist rests being definitively good or bad (Abrams, 2011; Bernard, 1997). Considering the multiple variables involved, this is not surprising. Instead of relying on rules to make the decision for your client, use the concepts above to reduce the likelihood of injuries occurring because of the use or nonuse of a wrist rest.

Do not forget that the monitor is also a tool used to complete the tasks included in being a lawyer and can directly affect posture and visual strain (Amick et al., 2012). The visual distance to read the screen can be considered her visual envelope. Jodi wears progressive lenses and has to move her head out of a neutral position to see the screen. She tends to jut her chin forward and look down her nose in an attempt to look at the monitor through her reading lenses. First, we must adjust the height of the monitor so that she can look through the middle part of her lenses, that is, the area set for middle distances. Next, we have to set the screen at an appropriate distance from her eyes so that she can see it easily without craning her neck.

Put all together, the changes listed above will make her look like the woman shown in Figure 26.5.

Here, she has a good base of support that is promoting an upright and supportive spinal alignment. Her work tools are set to reduce strain and assist her in maintaining proper posture.

There are many different variations of setups that occur within an office environment. For example, the offices may have keyboard trays; the staff may need two or more monitors; or the staff may need to reference a lot of paper while working on the computer. It is beyond the scope of this chapter to go through office arrangements in great detail. However, the basic principles described above can and should be expanded to include any arrangement and can be expanded even further to apply to any situation, such as someone with hemiplegia learning how to fold clothes or a jeweler working with diamonds.

Another important fact to remember is that there is no rule saying a person has to work sitting down. Sitting down causes higher back compressive forces than does standing, which itself causes higher back compressive forces than walking or standing with one foot propped up on a short step (Garg & Hegmann, 2006). Encourage your clients to problem solve how they can add movement into a sedentary job. Please note that the OTA does not complete an ergonomic assessment, but may, depending on demonstrated competency, assist with parts of it.

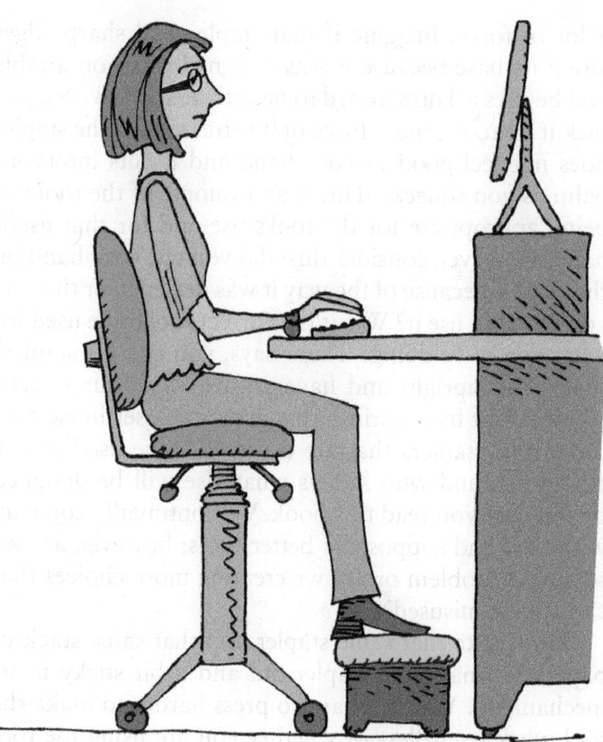

Figure 26.5 Computer user with stability. (Adapted with permission from Abrams ND. *Why is My Office a Pain in My…?* Rockville, MD: NAOE Publishing; 2011:62. Copyright 2011 by NAOE Publishing.)

Object Manipulation

Another basic movement pattern is completed when we handle and manipulate objects such as tools. When considering injury prevention, we must consider the person's ability to grip and manipulate the objects required for task completion (Woodson et al., 1992). With tool use, we must consider the size and shape of the handle, the amount of force required to activate the tool, and the tool's recoil or vibration (Sanders & McCormick, 1976; Woodson et al., 1992).

If forceful action is required to hold the tool or activate the tool, the person must be able to grip the object firmly, and the handle of the tool must be without protrusions, which may cause pressure areas on the hand (Sanders & McCormick, 1976). Consider a stapler, something we have all used. Have you ever tried to squeeze a stapler through a large stack of pages? It takes a lot of force. Imagine if that stapler had sharp edges along its base because it was designed to sit on a table and be pressed downward to be activated. However, you pick it up to get more force or a better angle. The stapler does not feel good in your hand and it cuts into your palm as you squeeze. This is an example of the tool not being appropriate for the tool's use and for that user's hand. However, consider this: did you cut your hand on the stapler because of the way it was designed or the way you chose to use it? Was it the correct tool to be used for what you were doing? These days, you can get staplers that stand upright and have grooves for your fingers, staplers that have springs that assist the user in ejecting the staple, staplers that are designed to be used with a closed fist, and who knows what else will be designed by the time you read this book. We continually come up with new and supposedly better tools; however, are we solving a problem or are we creating more choices that can still be misused?

Now, take that same stapler and that same stack of paper, but make the stapler old and a bit sticky in its mechanisms. You will have to press harder to make the tool work regardless of whether you are using the tool correctly. The lack of general tool maintenance is often the root cause of injury; more force is applied than necessary to activate the tool. There is a truism in the cooking world: a dull knife is more dangerous than a sharp one. This is because the forces being applied, the amount of times the forces have to be applied, and the angle at which the forces are applied change based on the maintenance of the tool. Sometimes, injury prevention comes down to appropriate maintenance or selection of tools that do not wear out quickly and require constant fixing.

Gloves also can affect the amount of force applied to a tool, and it is not always good to have them. Consider why gloves should be used: gloves increase friction between a handle and hand without increasing forces on the muscles and joints (Chapman, 2008; Sanders & McCormick, 1976). Gloves protect hands from sharp objects, vibration, hot or cold objects, dirty objects, or even chemically dangerous objects. However, gloves also decrease the amount of tactile input the body receives when it is using a tool. Users tend to increase the amount of force used when wearing gloves. Gloves interfere with the transfer of forces from the hand to the object (Sanders & McCormick, 1976). Also, if tactile reinforcement is needed to complete the task, gloves may hinder task completion (Sanders & McCormick, 1976). In other words, if you need to feel what is in your hand, you are more likely to put increased force into the grip or take more time with the task if you are wearing gloves.

The size of the grip should be small enough so that a person can grip the handle comfortably. Touch your fingers to your thumb, like the sign language letter "o." This is your comfortable grip size. Handles that are close to this size, but not larger than this size, will be large enough for you to grip with force (Chapman, 2008). Handles should also be shaped so that they do not slide in the user's hands or have areas where the user may pinch themselves on the tool itself (Woodson et al., 1992).

Tool vibration is also a concern if the tool is going to be used for extended periods. Hand tool vibration should be minimized whenever possible (Bernard, 1997; Sanders & McCormick, 1976). The measurement and adaptation of tool vibration is outside the scope of standard occupational therapy practice and requires continued study of physics to be fully explained; therefore, it will not be explored in great detail here. However, it is important to note that hand–arm vibration (HAV) exposure can contribute to Raynaud syndrome and nerve injury (Sanders & McCormick, 1976; Woodson et al., 1992).

On-Site Task Analysis

Your client is a group of assembly line workers who manufacture cars. While the OT will be responsible for the evaluation, OTAs are often involved in implementing the solutions, so a basic understanding of the evaluation process is recommended. You are asked to teach the workers body mechanics. You go with an OT to complete an analysis of the job components. One of the jobs you are asked to look at involves using a pneumatic ratchet to attach a side panel to a console. The workers have been complaining of neck, shoulder, and elbow pains. To analyze the work, first complete a systematic review of what the task requires or do a **task analysis**.

This task requires the worker to

1. Pick up one bolt from a bin on the left side of the table.
2. Slide the bolt through two holes, joining two pieces together. The holes are parallel to the ground so that the bolt is perpendicular to the ground.
3. Use the ratchet to fasten the two pieces together.

Then, analyze the tools themselves: the ratchet weighs 3 lb and is attached to a pneumatic hose hung from the ceiling. The ratchet itself is not hung from the ceiling. The ratchet has a handle set at 90 degrees from the bit.

Then, analyze the other items involved: the two pieces the worker is attaching to one another sit on a 30 in. high table and they weigh less than 5 lb each. The two pieces are not difficult to put together. The workers do not use gloves.

Then, analyze the timing: the worker completes this activity for seven hours total in a day. The workers are paid by the piece.

You, as the OTA, and the OT watch a few people complete the task. You video tape it so that you can continue your analysis later. You both talk to the workers and ask their opinions, what they have tried, and where they see the solutions or problem areas.

Complete your analysis of risk areas; always start with the basics and do not let the pains narrow your focus. Start with stability questions: do the workers have a solid base of support at the floor? Do they have the ability to work upright? Are they seated? If so, are the seats supportive or unstable? In this case, you see that the workers stand for the task and lean forward to work over the two pieces on the table, an inherently unstable position.

Then, move on to the task itself: how do they position themselves when using the ratchet? Is it habit or are the tools or task items forcing these postures? How much force is being used? Is there noise, vibration, tool kickback, or other effects when the tool is being activated, used, or stopped? In this case, when using the ratchet, the workers raise their elbow that holds the ratchet up toward the ceiling, bend their neck away from their arm, and lean their trunk forward and toward the holes. This allows the ratchet bit to be pointed down and allows the worker to see the bolt head while working.

Next, come up with solutions to limit risk. Consider the variety of solutions available: the job itself could be altered or adapted (what is often termed **engineering controls**); the workers could be taught biomechanics, stretching, or strengthening; the managers could implement task rotation to limit exposure (often termed **administrative controls**); or some combination of all of these could be used. The areas of concern and some methods of correcting the problems include the following:

Concerns

1. The workers are working in unstable postures: bent over while holding their arms up.
2. The tool used and the pieces being assembled are forward of the worker.
3. The tool is set at 90 degrees from the handle, which puts the force downward (which in and of itself may not be bad) and the arm upward.
4. The bolt and holes require precision work, making the workers tend to lean forward to accurately see the holes.

Possible Solutions

1. Option: Engineering control—change the pistol grip ratchet to one that has the bit and handle in line with each other so that a gross grasp with a neutral forearm can be used while still ratcheting downward. The worker can then work with his arm down by his side in a more upright posture.
2. Option: Engineering control—rotate the two pieces so that they are perpendicular to the floor and the holes are in front of the worker. The worker's arm can then go down by his side in a more upright posture.
3. Option: Engineering control—rotate the two pieces so that they are at a 45-degree angle from the floor so that the worker can lower his arm slightly into a more upright posture.
4. Option: Administrative control—change the pay structure so that job rotation is possible without pay loss.
5. Option: Training—teach the workers stretches to decrease the uneven strain on the dominant arm.

This is not an exhaustive list and there are other options to consider. In general, we like to implement engineering controls whenever possible because, in essence, it forces the users to change their methods (Garg & Hegmann, 2006). However, be careful when you change one or more tools or processes. You must remember that each change has an effect down the process chain. Also, each option has an associated cost that will influence which, if any, are implemented. There are also cultural issues such as union representation that will need to be addressed before any of these changes could take place. Notice, however, that while these changes move the worker's arm down to the side, none of the changes will be effective unless the worker is able to improve the base of support provided by the trunk through a more upright posture.

Material Handling

When working, people are often required to move objects from one location to another. The objects can be pushed or pulled, carried, or lifted. The next section deals with material handling activities.

Pushing and Pulling

Workers push and pull dollies, carts, baskets, shelves, heavy machinery, wheelchairs, gurneys, objects hanging from the ceiling, etc. While it is out of the scope of this chapter to detail the exact physics of these actions, much of injury prevention methodology uses basic body mechanics and joint protection strategies. When looking at pushing and pulling, we take into consideration the amount of force and direction of force necessary to start the movement, continue the movement, and stop the movement (Chapman, 2008). If working with something that rolls along the ground, we must also consider the forces required to overcome friction between the object and the floor necessary to get the object moving, keep it going, and then overcome inertia to stop it (Chapman, 2008). If working with something hanging from the ceiling, the forces applied must overcome friction between the rollers and the track to get the sling moving and continuing along its path. Then, inertia must be overcome to safely stop the object and keep it from swinging (if necessary).

Pushing with your body against an object, such as when you turn around and use your back to move a bookcase or heavy cart, is the best way of distributing forces. However, when exerting force on a cart, for example,

> Pulling is easier than pushing from a biomechanical viewpoint, mainly due to the difference in behavior of the arm musculature in the two activities. Contraction of the leg and trunk muscles produces forces at the shoulder joints that must be transmitted to the cart by the arms…during pushing, the elbow and wrist joints need to be kept at fixed angles by moments generated by muscles on one side of each joint…When pulling, the joints of the upper limb are automatically straightened, and both flexors and extensors can reduce stress in elbow ligaments. (Chapman, pp. 162–163)

What happens, however, when the forces cannot be applied by the large muscles of the torso and legs and must be completed by the arms, for example, when someone is working on their back under a car? What about when the floor itself does not provide adequate friction for the user to get traction to apply forces to the object being pushed or pulled? It is at the very start of the movement or when the load must be turned that the greatest amount of force is needed and this is the time when mistakes and injuries can occur (Chapman, 2008).

Also, you must take into account how each person is designed and where they have strengths and weaknesses before deciding whether to teach a push or a pull. If the person tends to arch their back when pulling an object, they are often trying to compensate for weaknesses. If they tend to rotate when pushing, they are again attempting to compensate for one-sided weakness. Both of these actions can cause injury. Therefore, no concrete rule can be applied to pushing or pulling.

Lifting and Lowering

"Lift with your knees and not with your back." This is a mantra repeated over and over again in therapy clinics and worksites around the world. However, there is much about this "rule" that isn't quite true.

The goal of keeping your back straight or more correctly, keeping your back in good postural alignment, and bending at the hips and knees to lower yourself into a squat before picking up an object is to distribute the load away from the spine (Kingma et al., 2010). However, we rarely find this technique used out in the field due to poor workplace design or object design (Garg & Hegmann, 2006). There is also conflicting data regarding the validity of this lift pattern to reduce pressures on the spine (Garg & Hegmann, 2006). If the object does not fit between the person's legs, this lift technique may in fact increase pressures on the spine (Garg & Hegmann, 2006; Kingma et al., 2010). Before we get into rules about lifting, let's use one of the most commonly applied lifting measures to better understand what goes into determining a safe lift.

The NIOSH Lifting Equation, originally designed in 1981 and revised in 1991 to reflect additional research findings, was designed to help identify risks and ergonomic solutions for manual two-handed lifting of objects (Waters et al., 1993; 1994). It is a useful tool for breaking down the biomechanical components of a lift and determining which factor may be influencing risk levels. In general, NIOSH recommends keeping lifting below 51 lb (Waters et al., 1993; 1994). The equation uses 51 lb as the maximum and then reduces the amount allowed for the lift by multiplying 51 by a fraction or "multiplier" that reflects the danger of the lift. That is, the size of the multiplier depends on how dangerous each component of the lift is for the body. This will make more sense with the example below.

By inserting the particulars of a certain lift into the equation, we get two results. First, the equation tells us what the **recommended weight limit** (RWL) is for an object at the lift's origin and destination. In other words, we know that we want to keep the compressive forces on the spine low and if we lift too much the wrong way, the compressive forces exceed recommended levels. The RWL is the object weight that would not create unsafe compressive forces while taking into consideration how you lifted the object. Second, it provides a rating for level of risk called a **Lifting Index** by comparing the amount actually being lifted with how much the equation says should be the maximum. A high Lifting Index, or score greater than three, is considered high risk and changes need to be made quickly. A Lifting Index score of one means the lift is safe with regard to back compression forces (Waters et al., 1994).

We will not get into all of the tool's intricacies and mathematics here—that would take an entire chapter of its own; however, it is important to note where the equation should *not* be used. It does not, for example, address one-handed lifts or lifts completed with a tool such as a shovel. It also does not take into account unstable footing or slippery areas that may affect risk levels (Waters et al., 1993; 1994). If you look closely, you will notice too that the calculations do not take into account whether you squatted to lift. This equation is looking at back compressive forces, not muscular strains.

We can apply this information by applying a simplified example of a postal worker delivering a package and go through the equation. It is important to note that the equation only reflects the risks at the start and the end of a lift, not what happens in between. In this example, we have a postal worker, Theo, who takes a package from the back of his truck and carries it up five stairs, into an elevator, through a door with a knob that he has to turn and push to open. Then, he delivers the package onto a receptionist's counter. The equation could be run with the origin being Theo's truck and the destination being the receptionist's counter. However, if run that way, the equation does not take into account everything that happens in between, so it will not be very useful to us. Instead, break the task down into its small components. First, Theo must get the package from the back of his truck and lift it to his waist height. We will stop there and only compute this one section.

We first take some measurements:

1. The package weighs 40 lb.
2. There are many packages in the truck, and the one Theo needs is located toward the middle. He reaches 28 in. forward to get it (his tertiary reach zone). The package is on the floor of the truck and his hands grab it 30 in. above the ground on which he is standing.
3. There are no handles and the box is a little slippery.
4. When he reaches for the box, he is a bit distracted. He noticed a man walking a dog nearby and he is keeping one eye on the dog and one eye on the package. His body is twisted to a 30-degree angle.
5. He grabs the box and lifts it so that he is standing upright. The box is now 40 in. from the ground (ground level to his hands) and 13 in. away from him (center of his mass to center between his hands).
6. There are still no handles and the box is still a little slippery.
7. He is holding the box evenly in both hands so the load is directly in front of his body and he is not twisting.
8. The overall duration of the lift is short—he has ample time to recover from this lift before going on to his next lift.
9. He does not do this lift frequently; mostly, he delivers small parcels of mail. He completes this type of lift once every hour or so for an 8-hour day.

To use this information in the equation, we convert our raw scores into a language the equation can understand, called "multipliers." This simply requires us to compare our measurements with charts provided by NIOSH. Table 26.1 shows what happens when we convert the data.

As you can see from Table 26.1, the converted score or "multiplier" is a fraction; a smaller fraction means the risks are higher. In other words, we want to get a multiplier of 1. To get the RWL for origin and destination, we multiply all of factors that may make the lift unsafe by the maximum 51 lb. The same equation is run using the destination multipliers to get the destination's RWL.

Origin RWL = 51 × horizontal modifier × vertical multiplier × distance travelled multiplier × asymmetry multiplier × frequency multiplier × coupling multiplier

The calculated RWL at origin, when Theo is getting the box from the truck, is zero pounds. The Lifting Index

TABLE 26.1 NIOSH Lifting Equation Example Data Points

	Raw Measurements	Converted Scores
Hand location at origin		
Horizontal	28 in.	0
Vertical	30 in.	1
Hand location at destination		
Horizontal	13 in.	0.77
Vertical	40 in.	0.93
Vertical distance traveled	10 in.	1
Asymmetrical angle		
Origin	30 degrees	0.9
Destination	0 degrees	1
Frequency rate (lifts/min)	<0.2 (the lowest the equation can handle)	0.95
Object coupling (how well can he hold the box)	Fair	1

is literally off the scale—it cannot be calculated and the assumption is that the risk is extraordinarily high. In other words, according to the information put into the equation, NIOSH would not recommend doing this lift at all. Think about the reach envelope for a moment. We know that the further away from the body the object is, the harder the body has to work to manipulate that object. The horizontal distance Theo is reaching to get the box from the truck is well beyond what he can reach with a stable base of support. He has to bend over to get the box at the start. That is not safe and the NIOSH equation shows us just how bad it is. According to the equation, you should not even lift a sheet of paper in that position, let alone a 40-pound box.

The RWL at destination, when he is standing with the box in his hands, is 34.7 lb. The Lifting Index at destination is 1.15. This tells us the lift has some risk, but not so much that the lift has to be changed immediately.

Look at each multiplier in Table 26.1 and decide how this lift may be corrected. By changing the raw scores into multipliers, the NIOSH equation tells us how dangerous each component of the lift is and, therefore, where we should start modifying. First, the distance Theo is reaching to pick up the box is way off the chart; the modifier of 0 immediately tells us that the lift should not be done at that distance. Let's say he instead makes sure that the box is further toward the back of the truck so that he only has to reach 20 in. to grab it. We check the chart to convert inches into a modifier of 0.5 (again, this is all on a chart that you can look up, but assume for now that that task has been done for you). When we rerun the calculation, the RWL at origin becomes 21.8 lb and has a Lifting Index score of 1.8. With this modification, the lift is now rated at a moderate-risk level where there is some concern, but not enough that it has to be changed immediately. A pretty dramatic change occurs just because Theo moved the box closer to the back of the truck before he picks it up. You could then follow the trail of scores to help eliminate risks by addressing the next worse modifier and so on.

You also will notice that this equation cannot consider what happens when two people complete a team lift, such as a two-person lift commonly used in nursing care. A two-person lift can be even more dangerous unless each party is sure he or she can lift the task and both are able to communicate effectively to keep each other out of danger (Chapman, 2008). The problem with team lifting occurs when the load becomes suddenly unevenly distributed or the people completing the lift are no longer lifting synchronously (Marras et al., 1999b). The rapid change in load can cause soft tissue injuries. We will talk more about client handling a little later.

Research on how lifting is taught in comparison to how lifting is completed is disheartening. There are limited data to show that you can teach "correct" lifting using a prescribed method, teaching one specific lifting strategy to be used always. People will complete lifts in methods that feel best (Garg & Hegmann, 2006; van Poppel et al., 1998). It is best to teach problem solving and body awareness, incorporating simple rules such as keep it close, stay smooth, do not twist, and do not throw. Lifting techniques, however, should not be seen as the primary method of decreasing injuries.

Carrying

The rules for carrying objects are the same as for lifting; keeping the object close to the body with a good grip is best. Carrying is when we transport an object without changing the height of the object. That is, carrying can be completed without lifting or lowering. For example, when you pick up a box from one table and move it to another, there is no height change of the box. People will often carry more than they can lift. However, when the load is too great, the person tends to extend his back, which compresses the posterior facets (Chapman, 2008). Think about how parents carry their children. Rarely, do you see them standing upright (Anders & Morse, 2005).

Carrying on the shoulder or asymmetrical carrying creates a lateral bend that compresses the lateral portions of the spinous processes. Also, on one side, the muscles are being strained, and on the other, the muscles have reduced tension that over time can cause muscular contractures (Chapman, 2008). Therefore, keeping the load close and as symmetrical as possible should be the goal.

We refer to Theo the postal worker again and change the object he is lifting from a box to a child. In his spare time, Theo helps out his mother who runs a day care center. Mary, his mom, looks after three children ages 2 to 4 for 4 to 6 hours per day. Each child weighs between 20 and 40 lb and has to be lifted from the ground, in and out of booster seats, on and off of the swings, etc., regularly throughout the day. She is carrying a child most of the time because of one thing or another. One of the girls, Alice, loves to jump from the couch into Mary's arms because she wants to fly when she grows up. Without even running the calculations, can you imagine what the NIOSH equation would say about this job? Would Mary's work be better or worse for her spine than Theo's postal job? The object weight has not gotten any heavier. The frequency multiplier would, however, be worse; she has to lift more often than Theo. The coupling modifier would also be worse since children do not have any solid handles. The vertical distances traveled would be worse since she is picking up from the floor and moving her hands to shoulder height. (Think about Mary grasping a child who is lying on the floor from under the child's arms and bringing the child to her chest, her hands under the child's armpits, and ending up with the child at her own shoulder height.) The horizontal distances could be worse or better depending on the child, the lift, and the cleanliness of the child (dirty diapers do not inspire squeezing the child close).

Client Lifting

This moves us into the very difficult situation many of you will face shortly, lifting and moving clients. As mentioned earlier in the chapter, the highest rate of injury in the United States is within the nursing professions (Barnes, 2007; Keller, 2009; Marras et al., 1999a; Nelson et al., 2006). Based on what you have learned so far, is that a surprise? The average male adult weighs in the vicinity of 180 lb. With the population of the United States growing even heavier, that average is likely to be increased very soon. Then, add in the factors that humans do not have handles, the body's weight is not evenly distributed, parts of the body may need to be protected while being moved (such as fracture sites), the object being lifted will sometimes fight you, and you are working 12-hour shifts on your feet, and it is actually surprising that we do not see more injuries. However, it is estimated that the caring professions have a higher injury rate than what is recorded. Within the physical therapy professionals, we estimate that over 90% will have a WRMSD although most believe that their training would keep them safe (Cromie et al., 2000; 2002). We do not have data for occupational therapy practitioners.

The belief that training will keep someone safe when handling clients is false—the calculations you already did should have convinced you of this (Waters, 2007). There is another factor that many people fail to acknowledge: when the therapy or nursing practitioner is at risk for injury, the client is at risk for injury. Dropping a client because your back just gave out is not the most sought after adventure within the hospital world. Much of the funding, and therefore motivation, for client lift devices comes from the safe client handling movements focused on reducing falls in facilities (Barnes, 2007; Collins et al., 2004; 2006). The use of a two-person lift technique, as mentioned above, does not keep people safe. The compressive forces and sheer forces on the spine often exceed maximum allowable limits.

What about helping a client to walk safely when they are doing most of the work? The therapy practitioner is just holding on to keep the client from falling, right? Look at it this way: when the client starts to fall, the therapist is responsible for most, if not all, of the client's weight. The client still weighs an average of 180 lb. However, now, the weight is not only being lifting vertically but also moving at a high rate of speed in a horizontal direction. The lift is actually a combination of lifting and pulling or pushing, depending on the direction of the fall. So, not only is the therapy practitioner attempting to keep the client from hitting the floor violently, but also she is attempting to keep her own balance. Remember the stability to mobility principle. If the therapy practitioner is unstable, it is unlikely that she will be able to create stability to manage an external force. It is highly unlikely that the therapy practitioner will have time to make sure that she has established perfect stability while attempting to control an unstable load that is talking or screaming in pain.

The good news is that there are a number of devices that are becoming more accepted within the hospital and nursing home environments to help protect the client and the caregiver (Barnes, 2007). These include transfer devices that can be used on clients who are completely dependent and transfer devices that allow clients to take some of the load or the entire load. There are also ambulation devices that can be used to provide guarding for clients who are unstable or provide assistance for clients who cannot support their own body weight.

Injury Prevention in Clinic Practices

Injuries happen at clinical settings. Learning how to prevent them will go a long way in improving the quality of care that staff can provide, not to mention being proactive in taking good care of themselves.

Risk Identification

Later in the book (*Unit Six*), you will read about the variety of places occupational therapy is practiced. For right now, take what we covered and apply it to clinical work. When we first started, we were discussing Jodi, a client who came to you because of arm pain. We talked about identifying roles that she plays and areas of risk associated with each role. How can you teach injury prevention when you cannot go to each workplace to assess risk?

First, you could work off of a client's self-report of what they do at work. A word of caution here: most people cannot accurately identify how they work, how much they lift, and how often they lift or separate what is required versus what is habit (Grandy & Westwood, 2006; Naylor & Amazeen, 2004). When using the client's descriptions, use your knowledge of the client's personality to decide whether you think the person is accurate or over- or underestimating.

Somewhat more accurate, although possibly completely inaccurate, is to go next to the company's job description. The job description within the company files may or may not be accurate or detailed. Within the current litigious environment, many companies are realizing that they need detailed and validated job descriptions. However, many do not prepare them until there is a problem. The job descriptions may be as simple as "this is a sedentary job" or as detailed as a step-by-step description of each work task. If you get a detailed job description, it is important to ask who wrote it and how they got that information. Sometimes, it is a supervisor's job to write the description, which means measurements may or may not have been taken.

Lastly, it is somewhat useful, if you are not clear on what tasks are required for a certain job description, to use the generic job descriptions available on the Occupational Information Network or O*NET (see the resources section for URL) developed by a private company in conjunction with the U.S. Department of Labor. This database has replaced the *Dictionary of Occupational Titles* book, which used to be the go to place for generic job requirements. It should be stressed that these are generic descriptions for broad job titles; however, it gives you a place to start.

Activity Simulation

One of the best ways to teach adults and children how to change movement patterns or psychosocial responses is to simulate activity or role-play (Abrams, 2010; Jarus & Ratzon, 2005). This forces the client to actually feel what movements or reactions are expected. Often, the materials needed to simulate a task are not available in the clinic or the environment cannot be accurately recreated; however, use your imagination and ask your clients to use their imaginations CS9. By asking your clients to use their imaginations, you are not only figuring out how to format the most meaningful intervention, you are also reinforcing memory through problem solving and mental practice (McDaniel et al., 2008).

When simulating tasks, you have the opportunity to force your client to address issues that make activities safe or unsafe. However, you also run the risk of oversimplification. For example, if you were working on lifting strategies with Mary, the day care owner, which would be better to simulate a child's body: using a box or using a sack filled with bags of rice? If you use a box, the weight would be evenly distributed and easy to hold. If you used a sack filled with bags of rice, the weight would not be evenly distributed and could shift midlift. The sack filled with bags of rice gives you a better simulation. Then again, it would be even better if you could use a life-sized weighted doll. Do the best you can with what you have, but do not forget that the items you choose to work with directly affect your client's experience with different risk factors.

There will be a number of activities you will not be able to simulate that require some out-of-the-box thinking. For example, what if your client is a firefighter? Many of the risks associated with firefighting involve extreme temperatures and fatigue, both physical and psychological. Firefighters have to handle very heavy loads while wearing very heavy safety gear all while working under extreme stress. If you were going to help your client problem solve safety regarding lifting victims, you have to take those external factors into consideration. However, it is not usually recommended that you set the clinic on fire. To simulate this extreme stress, you could, however, have the client first run up and down the stairs in full safety gear a few times to fatigue the muscles. Use headphones with sirens, screams, or sound of fire while practicing lifting a dummy or a volunteer to help simulate the external stressors. Just remember that you are still responsible for keeping the client safe!

That brings us to a very important point: during all of this, you have to keep the worker safe even while practicing unsafe maneuvers so that the client can self-identify issues. It can be difficult and you must control as many variables as possible when you know there is a high risk of injury. Again, using the example of the firefighter, think about how you could grade the activities to first allow the client to fail safely. Failing and feeling how his/her body is moving when that happens is very important. People do not have accurate self-awareness when it comes to body postures or body movements and that is why dancers rehearse in front of a mirror and record performances. With the firefighter, you may start with a bag of rice weighing only 5 lb, no external stressors, and no safety gear (although any limitation in mobility caused by the gear should be acknowledged and factored into the session). Allow the firefighter to practice safe lifting as if he or she were lifting a 180-pound person. Then, upgrade one or two factors and practice again. Each upgrade forces the client to problem solve what became harder and what he or she needs to be aware of when placed in different situations. Remember, as mentioned above, people will not follow prescribed patterns of movement when placed in real situations just because you told them it was safer. They have to work out for themselves the easiest and still safest movement pattern for each situation they come across.

Summary

Teaching safety in the workplace or in any situation requires that you listen as much as you teach. No matter what you know, you will never know as much about someone else's work as they do. However, you know the rules that keep them safe. It becomes a collaborative effort to problem solve how the workers can do the work while still applying as many of the safety rules as possible.

The knowledge of patterns of movement and awareness of context allows you to step back and see all areas where there may be risk. When you are treating an injury, the tendency is to just see the injury and the mechanism of injury, and the intervention become focused on fixing the symptoms. However, if you do not do a full root cause analysis for every injury, you will be missing parts of the picture. Where the client lays blame for the injury is not necessarily correct.

Early in my career, I was treating a 32-year-old man, Andy, with persistent forearm pain. His posture was good, and he was active and well-muscled. He worked at a computer for long periods and his arms hurt at the end of the day. Andy came to the clinic with the goal of learning how to set up his workstation correctly because he blamed all of his pain on his computer. He was an active participant in therapy the first week and his pain was brought under control. However, on Mondays, he would return to the clinic and say that his pain returned quickly over the weekend even though he wasn't doing anything "special." We kept working for weeks on getting his pain under control to the point where it would last more than 1 week. Needless to say, it took a few weeks before he disclosed that, for him, rock climbing every weekend was nothing "special." One weekend of not rock climbing was all it took to show that the computer was not his only problem. Shame on me for not asking more probing questions. We could have gotten his pain under control much faster if I had paid attention to all of his work tasks, not just the one he got paid for.

Review Questions

1. Ergonomics is:
   a. A set of rules to keep workers safe
   b. A science that studies the interaction between humans and the systems they interact with
   c. A type of chair
   d. A language created by engineers to explain how people use tools

2. A root cause analysis is:
   a. A method to analyze trees
   b. A system for identifying hazards
   c. A system for analyzing how injuries occurred and what factors may be involved in preventing further injury
   d. A method of recording data for OSHA

3. Risk factors for repetitive strain injuries include:
   a. Amount of the load and how long the load is carried
   b. Amount of the load, how it is carried, and how long it is carried
   c. Amount of the load, how it compares to the maximum capacity of the person carrying it, the duration of exposure, postural demands, and environmental stressors
   d. How a load is carried, how long it is handled, and exposure to the elements.

4. When analyzing movement patterns, what is important to consider?
   a. The postural stressors
   b. The amount of stability the person has relative the amount of mobility needed
   c. The person's range of motion and strength capabilities
   d. All of the above

5. A person's primary reach envelope is:
   a. The range of motion achieved when the elbows are kept against the ribs and the shoulders internally and externally rotated
   b. The range of motion achieved when a person reaches forward
   c. The place where objects frequently used should be placed
   d. A and C
   e. B and C

6. True or false: A squat lift will keep a person safe regardless of object size or weight.
   a. True
   b. False

7. When evaluating seated posture, it is important to consider:
   a. Where the feet are
   b. How well supported the feet are
   c. Whether the knees are bent or straight
   d. If the armrests support the arms

8. When lifting a client, you should consider:
   a. The weight of the client.
   b. How much assistance the person can give.
   c. How many people you can gather to complete the lift.
   d. You shouldn't be lifting clients.

9. An engineering control is:
   a. A button that doesn't need a lot of force to activate
   b. An alteration made to the job, environment, or tool to reduce risks
   c. A change made to a job that requires the help of an engineer
   d. Adapting a tool to make it more ergonomic

10. The best way to teach an adult a new pattern of movement is:
   a. Teach them in a classroom using slides.
   b. Teach them in a classroom using slides and make them answer questions about risky situations.
   c. Create safe environments for them to practice different situations they may encounter on worksites and ask them to problem solve safe movement patterns.
   d. A video of people doing the job correctly and incorrectly

Practice Activities

Consider everything you do in 1 day. List all of the roles that you play, the associated environments, and a sample of tasks completed for each role. List at least one safety concern for each task. Brainstorm with your classmates about ways to limit risk in each situation.

You are treating Alex, a 20-year-old website designer, for neck pain. He takes a picture of his workstation and brings it into the clinic (see Fig. 26.6 below, and yes, this was based on a real client). Use the picture to decide how you could address his neck pain.

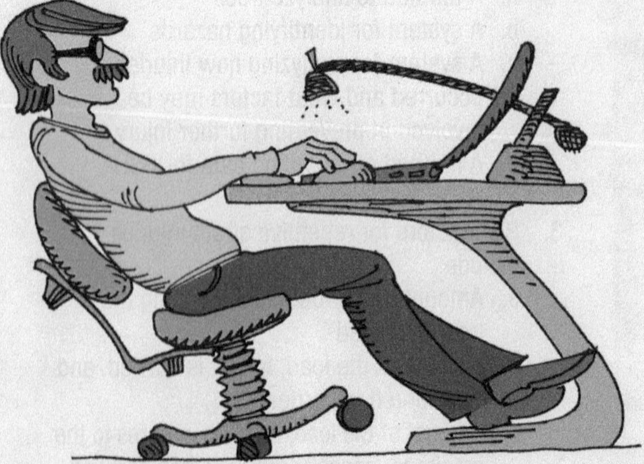

Figure 26.6 Slouched at the computer. Illustration published with permission of Work Site Health & Safety Consultants, LLC and NAOE Publishing.

You are asked by the local grocery store to work with a clerk, Janie. Janie has been complaining of forearm pain. You and the OT go out to complete a workplace review.

a. Go to your local grocery store and watch a clerk ring up and bag groceries. Note all areas of potential risk for each task (grasping items on the belt, scanning each item, manually typing in prices, bagging the items, putting the bags in the cart, etc.).
b. Create a tentative intervention plan to address the risks you found.
c. Would you modify your intervention plan based on the following and if so, how? Janie has been telling all the other clerks that they are going to have pain too if the management does not do something. That "something" is rather vague, but she is persistent and has started threatening to bring in her union representative.

Web Links and Resources

Center for Disease Control: http:\\www.cdc.gov
National Institute of Occupational Safety and Health: http:\\www.cdc.gov/niosh
Occupational Safety and Health Administration: http:\\www.osha.gov
International Ergonomics Association: http:\\www.iea.org
Human Factors and Engineering Society: http:\\www.hfes.org
O*Net: http:\\www.occupationalinfo.org

References

Abrams N. Motivation, communication, and change: ergonomic program success. *Work Ind Spec Interest Sect Q* 2010;24(2):1–4.

Abrams N. *Occupation-Based Office Ergonomics*. Rockville, MD: NAOE Publishing; 2011.

Amell T, Kumar S. Work-related musculoskeletal disorders: design as a prevention strategy. A review. *J Occup Rehabil* 2001;11(4):255–265.

American Occupational Therapy Association. Occupational therapy practice framework: Domain and process (3rd. ed.). *Am J Occup Ther* 2014;68(Suppl. 1):S1–S48. http://dx.doi.org/10.5014/ajot.2014.682006

American Occupational Therapy Association. *Ergonomics and occupational therapy: improving workplace productivity*. n.d. Retrieved from http://www.aota.org/en/AboutOccupationalTherapy/Professionals/WI/Articles/Improving-Productivity.aspx

Amick BC III, et al. A field intervention examining the impact of an office ergonomics training and highly adjustable chair on visual symptoms in a public sector organization. *Appl Ergon* 2012;43:625–631.

Anders MJ, Morse T. The ergonomics of caring for children: an exploratory study. *Am J Occup Ther* 2005;59:285–295.

Baker NA. Alternative keyboards. *Work Ind Spec Interest Sect Q* 2009;23(3):1–4.

Baker NA, Cidboy EL. The effect of three alternative keyboard designs on forearm pronation, wrist extension, and ulnar deviation: a meta-analysis. *Am J Occup Ther* 2006;60(1):40–79.

Baker NA, Redfern M. Potentially problematic postures during work site keyboard use. *Am J Occup Ther* 2009;63(4):386–397.

Barnes AF. Erasing the word 'lift' from nurses' vocabulary when handling patients. *Br J Nurs* 2007;16(18):1144–1147.

Bernard BP, ed. *Musculoskeletal Disorders and Workplace Factors: A Critical Review of Epidemiologic Evidence for Work-Related Musculoskeletal Disorders of the Neck, Upper Extremity, and Low Back*. Washington, D.C.: U.S. Department of Health and Human Services National Institute for Occupational Safety and Health; 1997.

Bongers PM, et al. Epidemiology of work related neck and upper limb problems: psychosocial and personal risk factors (Part I) and effective interventions from a bio behavioural perspective (Part II). *J Occup Rehabil* 2006;16:279–302.

Braveman B, Page JJ, eds. *Work: Promoting Participation and Productivity through Occupational Therapy*. Philadelphia, PA: F.A. Davis Company; 2012.

Brewer S, et al. Workplace interventions to prevent musculoskeletal and visual symptoms and disorders among computer users: a systematic review. *J Occup Rehabil* 2006;16:325–358.

Bureau of Labor Statistics. News release: nonfatal occupational injuries and illnesses requiring days away from work, 2010. 2011. Retrieved from http://www.bls.gov/news.release/pdf/osh2.Pdf

Chapman AE. *Biomechanical Analysis of Fundamental Human Movements*. Champaign, IL: Human Kinetics; 2008.

Collins JW, et al. An evaluation of a best practices musculoskeletal injury prevention program in nursing homes. *Inj Prev* 2004;10(4): 206–211.

Collins JW, et al. *Safe Lifting and Nursing Home Residents*. Cincinnati, OH: NIOSH-Publications Dissemination; 2006.

Cromie JE, et al. Work-related musculoskeletal disorders in physical therapists: prevalence, severity, risks, and responses. *Phys Ther* 2000;80:336–351.

Cromie JE, et al. Work-related musculoskeletal disorders and the culture of physical therapy. *Phys Ther* 2002;82:459–472.

Delisle A, et al. Comparison of three computer office workstations offering forearm support: impact on upper limb posture and muscle activation. *Ergonomics* 2006;49(2):139–160.

Garg A, Hegmann K. *Applied Ergonomics: Low Back*. Milwaukee, WI: University of Wisconsin Milwaukee; 2006.

Grandy MS, Westwood DA. Opposite perceptual and sensorimotor Responses to a size-weight illusion. *J Neurophysiol* 2006;95:3887–3892.

Griffin SD, Prince VJ. Living with lifting: mother's perceptions of lifting and back strain in childcare. *Occup Ther Int* 2000;7(1):1–20.

International Ergonomics Association. Definition of ergonomics. 2000. Retrieved from http://www.iea.cc/01_what/What%20is%20Ergonomics.html

Jarus T, Ratzon NZ. The implementation of motor learning principles in designing prevention programs at work. *Work* 2005;24:171–182.

Keller S. Effects of extended work shifts and shift work on patient safety, productivity, and employee health. *Am Assoc Occup Health Nurses J* 2009;57(12):497–502.

Kingma I, et al. How to lift a box that is too large to fit between the knees. *Ergonomics* 2010;53(10):1228–1238.

Leyshon R, et al. Ergonomic interventions for office workers with musculoskeletal disorders: a systematic review. *Work* 2010;35:335–348.

Luttmann A, et al. *Protecting Workers' Health Series No. 5: Preventing Musculoskeletal Disorders in the Workplace*. Switzerland: World Health Organization; n.d. Retrieved from http://www.who.int/occupational_health/publications/muscdisorders/en/index.html

Marras WS, et al. A comprehensive analysis of low-back disorder risk and spinal loading during the transferring and repositioning of patients using different techniques. *Ergonomics* 1999a;42(7):904–926.

Marras WS, et al. Spine loading and trunk kinematics during team lifting. *Ergonomics* 1999b;42(10):1258–1273.

McDaniel MA, et al. Implementation intentions facilitate prospective memory under high attention demands. *Mem Cognit* 2008;36(4):716–724.

Naylor YK, Amazeen EL. The size-weight illusion in team lifting. *Hum Factors* 2004;46:349–356.

Nelson A, et al. Development and evaluation of a multifaceted ergonomics program to prevent injuries associated with patient handling tasks. *Int J Nurs Stud* 2006;43:717–733.

NIOSH. Nonfatal occupational injuries and illnesses—United States 2004. *MMWR* 2007. Retrieved from http://www.cdc.gov/mmwr/preview/mmwrhtml/mm5616a3.htm

Ogden CL, et al. *Prevalence of Obesity in the United States, 2009–1010. NCHS Data Brief, No 82*. Hyattsville, MD: National Center for Health Statistics; 2012.

Ripat J, et al. The effect of alternate style keyboards on severity of symptoms and functional status of individuals with work related upper extremity disorders. *J Occup Rehabil* 2006;16:707–718.

Sanders MS, McCormick EJ. *Human Factors in Engineering and Design*. 7th ed. New York, NY: McGraw-Hill, Inc.; 1976.

Schulte PA, et al. Work, obesity, and occupational safety and health. *Am J Public Health* 2007;97(3):428–436.

Thomsen JF, et al. Carpal tunnel syndrome and the use of computer mouse and keyboard: a systematic review. *BMC Musculoskelet Disord* 2008;9. Retrieved from http://www.biomedcentral.com/1471-2474/9/134

Thornton A. Sleep apnea: what employers should know. *Am Sleep Apnea Assoc* 2011. Retrieved from http://www.sleepapnea.org/asaa-blog/sleep-apnea-what-every-employer-should-know.html

US Department of Labor. OSHA forms for recording work-related injuries and illnesses. 2004. Retrieved from http://www.osha.gov/recordkeeping/new-osha300form1-1-04.pdf

van Poppel MN, et al. Lumbar supports and education for the prevention of low back pain in industry. *JAMA* 1998;279(22):1789–1794.

Waersted M, et al. Computer work and musculoskeletal disorders of the neck and upper extremity: a systematic review. *BMC Musculoskelet Disord* 2010;11(79):1471–2474.

Waters R. When is it safe to manually lift a patient? *Am J Nurs* 2007;107(8):53–59.

Waters TR, et al. Revised NIOSH equation for the design and evaluation of manual lifting tasks. *Ergonomics* 1993;36(7):749–776.

Waters TR, et al. *Applications Manual for the Revised NIOSH Lifting Equation*. Cincinnati, OH: US Department of Health and Human Services; 1994. Retrieved from http://www.cdc.gov/niosh/docs/94-110/pdfs/94-110.pdf

Woodson WE, et al. *Human Factors Design Handbook*. 2nd ed. New York, NY: McGraw-Hill, Inc.; 1992.

UNIT

V

Common Conditions

[Evidence-based medicine] is about integrating individual clinical expertise and the best external evidence.

—David L. Sackett,
William M. C. Rosenberg,
J. A. Muir Gray,
R. Brian Haynes, and
W. Scott Richardson

CHAPTER

27 Developmental Disabilities

Wanda J. Mahoney, PhD, OTR/L

Key Terms

Activity analysis—Breaking down a task into what is required to do the task in a typical way; determining activity demands of a task.

Activity synthesis—Changing the activity demands of a task to match the skills and ability of the client.

Adaptive behavior—Age-appropriate performance of self-care, social, and other daily living skills.

Assistive technology—Adaptive devices that can range from simple to complex equipment that allows a person with a disability to engage in an activity.

Contractures—Decreased range of motion in a joint due to shortened muscles.

Developmental delay—Condition where a child (up to 9 years old) does not meet expected developmental milestones; usually requires at least 20% delay or one or more standard deviations below the mean on a standardized test of development; each state in the United States has its own definition of what constitutes developmental delay in order to qualify for services under IDEA.

Developmental disability—Conditions that exist prior to age 22, are expected to remain throughout life, and affect cognitive development, physical development, or both (AAIDD, 2012).

Developmental milestones—Expectations about what a person should be able to do at a specified age (often associated with children).

Habilitation—Services designed to help individuals establish skills that they have not previously developed.

Hyperactivity—Higher level of activity (motor or verbal) than expected based on age and developmental level.

Impulsivity—Acting prior to considering consequence of actions to a greater extent than expected for age and developmental level.

Inattention—Lower level of attention to task or shorter attention span than would be expected for age and developmental level.

Intellectual disability—Condition that started prior to age 18 with significantly lower than normal IQ scores (below 70) and considerable issues meeting performance standards expected for their age and culture in two or more areas of occupation, learning, or social participation (Schalock et al., 2010).

Muscle tone—The amount of tension in a skeletal muscle at rest.

Praxis—Motor planning cognitive aspect of movement.

Proprioception—Sensation within joints and muscles providing information about position of body in space.

Self-determination—Process of making things happen in one's own life; higher levels involve knowing one's needs and advocating to get those needs met.

Tactile—Sensation within skin about touch and pressure input.

Vestibular—Sensation within the inner ear providing information about linear and circular movement of the head through space.

Learning Objectives

After studying this chapter, readers should be able to:

- Define developmental disability, identify types of developmental disabilities, and recognize the impact of developmental disabilities across the life span.
- Describe occupational therapy interventions with individuals with developmental disabilities.
- Compare different strategies to improve the participation of individuals with developmental disabilities.

Introduction

Occupational therapy practitioners often provide services to individuals with developmental disability. According to the AOTA *Occupational Therapy Compensation and Workforce Study* (AOTA, 2010), over 25% of OT practitioners work in schools or early intervention, and most of the individuals who receive services in these settings are those with developmental disabilities. In addition, over 25% of OTAs identified children and youth aged 0 to 21 as the primary age group that they worked with (AOTA, 2010), and most children who receive occupational therapy services have developmental disabilities or delays. Although developmental disabilities are commonly associated with children, the disabilities continue across the life span. Adults with developmental disabilities may have occupational needs that would benefit from occupational therapy services although these services are often less readily available. In addition, older adults with developmental disabilities face unique challenges associated with changes related to aging combined with their developmental disability.

Defining Developmental Disability

Developmental disabilities are conditions that exist prior to age 22 (18 in some definitions), are expected to remain throughout life, and affect cognitive development, physical development, or both (AAIDD, 2012). **Developmental disability** is a broad term that includes a wide variety of conditions including intellectual disability, autism spectrum disorders (ASDs), movement disorders, and learning disabilities. Approximately 1 in 6 children in the United States between the ages of 3 and 17 have a developmental disability, and the prevalence of most developmental disabilities has increased in the last ten years (Boyle et al., 2011).

Developmental disabilities are generally due to a combination of genetic and environmental conditions. There are a variety of factors that increase the risk of a child developing a developmental disability. These risk factors include genetic abnormalities, premature birth, low birth weight, infections, poor nutrition, low socioeconomic status, or exposure to toxins such as drugs or lead. Not all children exposed to these risks will have developmental disabilities or delays. The severity of a developmental disability and its impact on occupational performance can vary greatly.

There are some conditions covered briefly in this chapter that do not fit the definition of developmental disability because they may not last throughout the life span. These include developmental delay, juvenile rheumatoid arthritis, and emotional disturbances. These conditions occur in children, so OT practitioners working with children with developmental disabilities may work with people with these disabilities. Some background information on these conditions as well as developmental disabilities is necessary in order to be successful in settings such as early intervention, schools, and pediatric outpatient clinics (From the Field 27.1).

Occupational Therapy with People with Developmental Disabilities

There are no cures for developmental disabilities although there are a variety of treatments available to assist people with developmental disabilities to lead full and healthy lives. These treatments may include medical intervention such as medication or surgery, educational services, and therapy services. Children with developmental disabilities often receive occupational therapy to address feeding, self-care, play, education participation, and other needs. The occupational needs of an individual with a developmental disability will vary greatly based on the individual's age, condition, and situation. Occupational therapy practitioners can work with

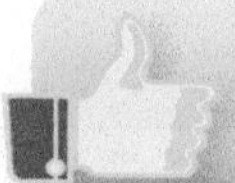

FROM THE FIELD 27.1

A Note about Language

The words we use are important and reflect how we think about something. When we say *people with* disabilities, we are acknowledging that they are *people* first, not a disability. Some language (including "handicapped" and "retarded") is considered derogatory or offensive, and OT practitioners should not use such language whether discussing people, objects, or anything else. When discussing parking spaces or restroom stalls, we can say that they are *accessible* meaning that they allow access for people with disabilities. With developmental disabilities, we use the term *typical* development rather than "normal." A person's development may be atypical or different, but the person is not "abnormal" as implied when we use the word "normal" to discuss typical development. People with disabilities may use other terms to refer to themselves, and we should respect individual preferences in those instances.

individuals throughout the life span. Once an individual with a developmental disability is an adolescent or adult, occupational therapy often focuses on instrumental activities of daily living such as home management and transportation (community mobility), education participation, and preparation for employment.

Occupational Therapy Assessments

Occupational therapy assistants can administer assessments and contribute information from observations for an evaluation once they demonstrate service competency (AOTA, 2009). Examples of assessments used with individuals with developmental disabilities are included in Table 27.1. The specific assessments used will likely depend on the practitioner's facility. The table does not include developmental assessments used with young children because there are so many different types of these assessments. In addition to standardized assessments, observation during typical activities and information that the individual and his or her caregivers provide are also essential to record and share with the supervising occupational therapist.

Purpose of Occupational Therapy with People with Developmental Disabilities

The purpose of occupational therapy is improving participation in life. Occupational therapy does not concentrate on making the symptoms of a condition better; we focus on people's participation and engagement in occupation to ensure that they can do the things they want and need to do regardless of any condition or disability (From the Field 27.2). Expectations about what children need to do often revolve around **developmental milestones** (see Chapter 8: *Human Development: Framing Who We Are*). For example, when an OT practitioner asks preschool teachers or parents what they think the child needs to do, they may state that the child needs to "walk and talk." It is our responsibility to ask more questions to get at what specific occupations are involved. In addition to acknowledging the caregiver's desire for the child to walk, we need to ask about the activities that the child may not be doing because he or she is not walking such as playing outside with classmates, getting a snack from the kitchen, or participating in other age-appropriate activities. We can offer suggestions about how to adapt these other activities so that the child is engaged in meaningful occupations regardless of his or her ability to walk.

Background on Development

All children, including those with developmental disabilities, are constantly developing. People continue to develop as adults, but the changes are generally less dramatic than during childhood, and there is more variability in the expectations regarding adult development. For individuals with developmental disabilities, development may be slower than what is typical and some developmental tasks may be different. For example, a child with spina bifida or other movement disability may need to develop skills using forearm crutches, a manual wheelchair, or a power wheelchair. These are developmental skills that improve with time and practice, but they are not the same skills that people without disabilities develop.

Individuals with developmental disabilities may need additional time, structure, or opportunities in order to develop skills. Occupational therapy practitioners train parents, teachers, and others in the client's life to provide frequent opportunities that the individual with a developmental disability can take advantage of to foster development.

Occupational Therapy Intervention with People with Developmental Disabilities

When working with individuals with developmental disabilities, OT practitioners should consider a strengths-based approach. This is not a specific occupational therapy approach; rather, it is a strategy where the professional seeks to build on what the individual does well and the positive factors influencing performance (Petrechik et al., 2011). This is in contrast to a deficit or problem-based approach that is common in medical fields. Rather than

TABLE 27.1 Examples of Assessment Tools for People with Developmental Disabilities

Participation assessments for children with developmental disabilities

- *School Function Assessment (SFA)* (Coster, Deeney, Haltiwanger & Haley, 1998)
  - School team members rate child's level of participation and amount of assistance necessary for school tasks for grades K-6.
- *Child Occupational Therapy Self-Assessment (COSA)* (Keller, Kafkes, Basu, Federico & Kielhofner, 2005)
  - Clients ages 6 to 17 provide information about how well they do activities and how important the activities are to them.
- *Children's Assessment of Participation and Enjoyment (CAPE)* (King, Law, King, Hurley, Rosenbaum, Hanna, Kertoy & Young, 2004)
  - Clients ages 6 to 21 provide information with caregiver assistance about the activities they engage in and their preferred activities.
- *Perceived Efficacy and Goal Setting System (PEGS)* (Missuna, Pollock & Law, 2004)
  - Children ages 5 to 10 report how well they think they perform activities presented on picture cards: includes parent/teacher questionnaire.

Examples of motor assessments for children with developmental disabilities

- *Peabody Developmental Motor Scales (PDMS-2 or Peabody)* (Folio & Fewell, 2000)
  - Fine motor and gross motor skills for children birth to 5 years old
- *Bruininks-Oseretsky Test of Motor Proficiency (BOT-2)* (Bruininks & Bruininks, 2005)
  - Fine motor and gross motor skills for individuals ages 4 to 21

Examples of visual motor assessments for individuals with developmental disabilities

- *Beery-Buktenica Developmental Test of Visual-Motor Integration (Beery or VMI)* (Beery et al., 2010)
  - *Visual perception, motor coordination, and visual motor skills for individuals age 2 and older (through older adulthood)*
- *Developmental Test of Visual Perception (DTVP-2)* (Hammill et al., 1993)
  - Visual perception and visual motor skills for individuals ages 4 to 9

Handwriting assessment examples

- *Evaluation Tool of Children's Handwriting (ETCH)* (manuscript/print and cursive versions available) (Amundsen, 1995)
  - Manuscript/print or cursive legibility and speed for grades 1–6
- *Test of Handwriting Skills (THS-R)* (Milone, 2007)
  - *Manuscript/print or cursive legibility and speed for ages 5–18*

Examples of assessments for adults with developmental disabilities

- *Performance Assessment of Self-Care Skills (PASS)* (Holm & Rogers, 2008)
  - Provides information about task breakdown and assistance to perform ADLs and IADLs
- *Supports Intensity Scale (SIS)* (Thompson et al., 2004)
  - In-depth assessment designed to provide an overall picture of the support and assistance an individual with an intellectual disability requires (multiple team members provide information)
- *Volitional Questionnaire (VQ)* (de las Heras et al., 2007) (Pediatric version also available)
  - Observational assessment to determine the motivation to engage for people with severe disabilities
- *Allen Cognitive Level Screen (ACLS-5)* (Allen et al., 2007)
  - Provides information about how an individual learns new tasks

looking at what is "wrong" with the person and the situation, a strengths-based approach seeks to build on what is going well. This is especially relevant for individuals with more significant disabilities where there may be a larger gap between what the person with the disability can do and what a typically developing individual can do.

A deficit-based approach places the cause of any issues on the individual, and the individual must change in order to address the issue. This is a fairly negative view of the individual and can be disheartening for the individuals with disabilities and their family. I was in a meeting discussing potential goals with a mother of an adolescent with severe autism and intellectual disability. When we started the conversation using a strengths-based approach by talking about what the youth did well and how we could build on those skills in the next year, the mother visibly relaxed and smiled. It was clear that she anticipated another meeting discussing what was "wrong" with her son. It also helped the professionals

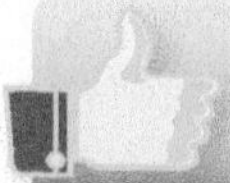

FROM THE FIELD 27.2

Something to Keep in Mind

"What I would like others, especially future OT practitioners, to know about individuals with developmental disabilities is that they are people with the same desires and needs as you and me, they can learn, and that they are not broken. When I work with OTA students, the hardest thing for them to learn is our role as OT practitioners is not about 'fixing' the individual. Our role is to support them in being the most independent person they can be by utilizing the abilities that they have or that they can learn with our intervention" (Quote from Kelli Meents, COTA/L in Illinois).

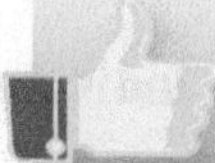

FROM THE FIELD 27.3

Debbie Gruber, COTA in New York, shared the following about her job in a private school for students with developmental disabilities. When she started, she had never worked with people with developmental disabilities.

> I worked hard to develop rapport with my students, and, with all due modesty, feel that this is one of my strengths. What I lacked in therapeutic experience, I made up for with humor and respect. What is the biggest lesson I've learned from working with my students? Doubtlessly, it is being aware of all they CAN accomplish and all they WANT to achieve, if they are just given the right training and opportunities. Many of our high school-aged students have some community work experiences through school, and occupational therapy has been involved in teaching work skills, appropriate behavior, good hygiene, grooming, and other life skills.

to see the youth's potential in spite of his significant cognitive and behavioral issues (From the Field 27.3).

Frames of Reference

Occupational therapy practitioners use multiple frames of reference when working with individuals with developmental disabilities. Common frames of reference used with this population include developmental, acquisitional, behavioral, and sensory processing or sensory integration. It is common for an OT practitioner to use two or more frames of reference when working with clients. Regardless of the frame of reference used, the overarching goal is always to enable participation in meaningful activities.

Developmental and Acquisitional Frames of Reference

Figure 27.1 illustrates the different ways of approaching a child's developmental issues with a developmental frame of reference versus an acquisitional frame of reference. In this example, a 5-year-old child has a developmental disability. The child's motor skills and cognitive skills are significantly delayed. For motor development, the child crawls on her forearms but does not yet creep on hands and knees or stand independently. She holds objects in her hands, lets the objects go, and is starting to use her fingers. Cognitively, the child finds toys hidden under a blanket and names simple pictures and objects.

Using a developmental frame of reference with this example, the OT practitioner would work on the child obtaining the next developing milestone starting from the child's current abilities. This may involve teaching the child to pick up small objects such as cereal, stack two blocks, hold a spoon for feeding, creep on hands and knees, and follow a variety of directions. The practitioner uses developmental theories such as Piaget's theory of cognitive development, Erickson's theory of psychosocial development, Vygotsky's theory of social development, or other sources of developmental milestones in order to determine the next skill that the child can develop. The developmental frame of reference assumes that development is sequential and that each skill builds on previous skills and requires a strong understanding of developmental sequence to know which skills to work on next.

An acquisitional frame of reference uses a different approach. Rather than starting with the skills that the child currently has, this frame of reference starts with the tasks that the child should be doing at her age. This frame of reference relies heavily on **activity analysis** and adapting activities to match current skills and ability (**activity synthesis**). With the child in this example, the acquisitional frame of reference would involve analyzing the activities that a typical 5-year-old participates in and ensuring that this child can participate in those same activities. Rather than focusing on getting the child to creep on hands and knees, the OT practitioner may help the kindergarten teacher set up the environment so that the child can independently access classroom items by crawling and rolling on the floor. The child may use a power wheelchair to promote independent mobility so that she can move around the school like her classmates. When the other children are learning to write, this child also needs a way

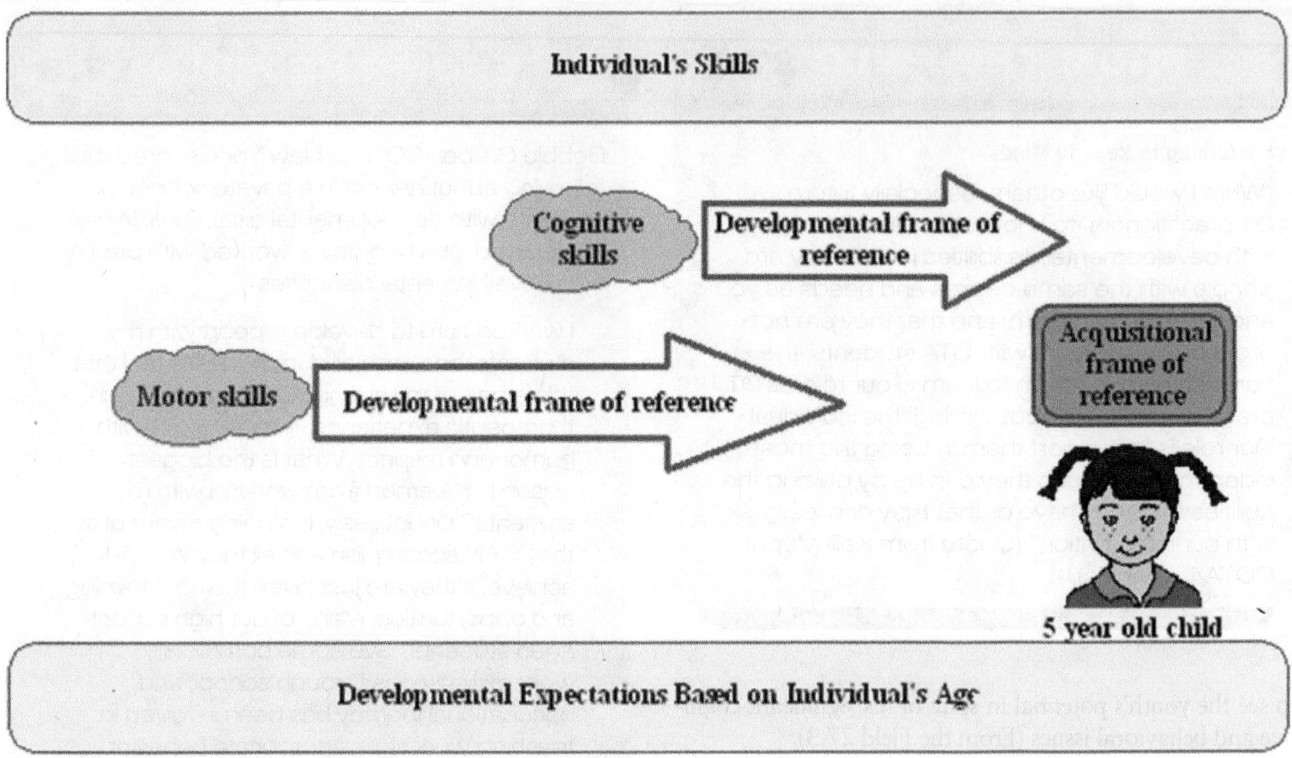

Figure 27.1 Comparing the developmental and acquisitional frames of reference.

to do this. This may involve providing a pencil like the other students, but it could also involve a name stamper or computer so the child is involved in the same developmental tasks that his/her classmates are doing such as signing in at the beginning of the day with a name stamper or "writing" letters with a keyboard. The acquisitional frame of reference often involves adaptations to the environment and the use of **assistive technology** in order to foster participation in age-appropriate activities. Parents and others may need encouragement to allow these types of accommodations, and OT practitioners can emphasize that providing a young child with a wheelchair, communication device, or computer does not mean we are "giving up" on the idea that the child will walk, talk, or write his name. There is research evidence that using augmentative communication increased verbal language in children with autism (Ganz & Simpson, 2004), and 2-year-old children using power mobility improved social and cognitive skills and did not lose motor skills (Jones, 2004).

Behavioral Frame of Reference

The behavioral frame of reference is commonly used with people with developmental disabilities to decrease problem behavior and increase desired behavior. A behavior can be any observable phenomenon, and the behavioral frame of reference involves a variety of strategies to change behavior. The most common behavioral strategies that OT practitioners use include positive reinforcement, modeling, shaping, forward chaining, and backward chaining, and using several strategies in combination is customary.

Positive reinforcement involves providing praise or small rewards when the person demonstrates a desired behavior. This can include a variety of things such as saying "good job," clapping, giving a short break with a favorite toy, or providing the opportunity to do a favorite activity. Some rewards are larger than others, and the level of the reward should match the behavior. Occupational therapy practitioners need to use caution about using food as a reward.

Modeling consists of demonstrating how to do a task and then having the individual complete the task. Modeling is often most successful when it starts with the practitioner talking the steps of the task out loud while performing them, as it provides multimodal cues to support different learning styles.

A practitioner uses *shaping* by praising close approximations of the desired behavior. For example, if working with a child on self-feeding, a practitioner may praise the child for trying to scoop the food even if it is unsuccessful.

Chaining is used with tasks that have several discrete steps such as handwashing. In *forward chaining*, the client does the first step independently, and the practitioner does the remaining steps with the client. Once the first step is mastered, the client starts to do the first and second steps independently. This process continues until the client can do the entire task. *Backward chaining* uses the same idea, but the steps are addressed in a different order. With backward chaining, the OT practitioner starts doing the task with the client, and the client does the last step independently. Once the client is successful with the last step, the client does the second-to-last and the last step. This sequence continues backward until the client is doing the entire task. Backward chaining is often useful because there is an immediate reward when the client is successful: the task is complete.

As an example of using behavioral strategies in combination, an OT practitioner may use modeling by first washing his/her hands and talking out the steps before assisting the person with the disability to do it. When the client is washing hands, the OT practitioner may use pictures to demonstrate each step and assist the client to perform each step until the client reaches the step he or she is working on. The OT practitioner may use shaping to teach that step, and then the client would complete the last step independently (backward chaining). When the task is complete, the OT practitioner would provide positive reinforcement by praising the client to increase the desired handwashing behavior in the future.

When using the behavioral frame of reference to decrease problem behavior, a practitioner needs to consider what purpose the behavior is serving. Behaviors do not "disappear;" they are replaced with other behaviors. These new behaviors need to serve the same purpose to the same or greater extent for the problem behavior to decrease.

Sensory Frames of Reference

There are two major sensory frames of reference that occupational therapy practitioners use: sensory integration primarily informed by research by Jean Ayres and sensory processing based on Winnie Dunn's work. It is beyond the scope of this chapter to cover the differences between these two sensory frames of reference. Sensory frames of reference are used when one of the underlying causes of an occupational performance issue is how the individual processes and responds to sensory information from the body and/or the environment. In addition to the basic five senses of vision, hearing, smell/olfactory, taste, and touch, sensory frames of reference expand touch sensation and consider additional sensory systems. While the sensory frames of reference address all sensory pathways, they focus on three primary sensations: **tactile** (touch and pressure), **proprioception** (position of body in space), and **vestibular** (sensing movement of head). The sensory frames of reference involve adapting the environment to compensate for the individual's different way of processing sensory information, teaching a variety of strategies to deal with controlling responses to sensations, and using equipment such as swings, scooters, and therapy balls in specific ways to promote changes in how an individual processes sensory information. For additional information about sensory systems and occupational therapy's role in addressing these issues, please refer to Chapter 28, *Sensory Processing*, in this textbook (From the Field 27.4).

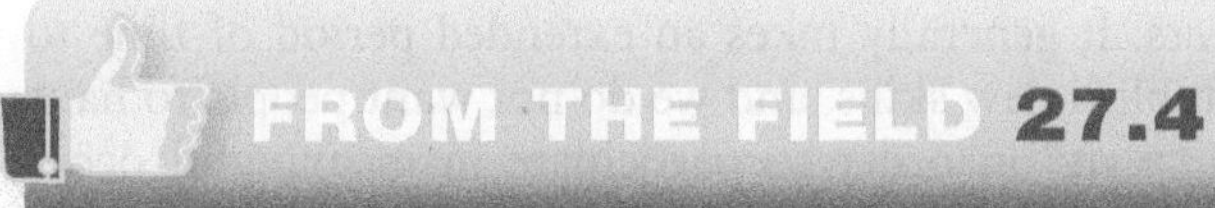

Sensory Space

Sarah Perry, COTA/L in Illinois, shared the following experience about using a sensory frame of reference in a compensatory manner to adapt the environment for adults with intellectual and developmental disabilities in a sheltered workshop setting.

> I was involved in creating a sensory room space in the sheltered workshop. This building was a large barn with fluorescent lighting, echoing noise levels, and inconsistent temperatures. The sensory room provided a calm, quieter space for individuals to use independently. The sensory room was blocked off with canvas curtains. The internal walls were painted green, known for its natural calming effects. Lavender scenting was added in addition to a beanbag, lava lamp, CD player with easy listening music, and books to complete the environment. Several individuals found the sensory room beneficial when they became sensory overloaded during their day at work.

Difficulties with processing and appropriately responding to sensory experiences are common among people with developmental disabilities. Research studies have shown inconsistent results on the effectiveness of interventions using sensory frames of reference, and intervention is most often effective when it occurs over an extended period of time and addresses multiple sensory pathways (American Academy of Pediatrics, 2012). It has worked well for some individuals, but because of the lack of strong evidence, it is essential that any practitioner using this approach in intervention closely monitor the effectiveness of the intervention with each individual and make changes as necessary.

Frames of Reference Summary

An OT practitioner often uses several frames of reference to address the occupational performance issues that a person with a developmental disability experiences. Even when we are working to establish specific skills, we must ensure that individuals with disabilities have access to meaningful occupations with their current abilities throughout development, especially if their abilities are significantly below their typically developing peers. It generally takes an extended period of time to establish new skills, and we do not want people to have to "wait" in order to participate in meaningful occupations. The individual's developmental level should not prevent participation or access to age-appropriate activities, and OT practitioners can work with the client, family, and other professionals to ensure access to meaningful participation.

Developmental Delay

Developmental disability is different from **developmental delay** although they are often grouped together. Children with developmental delays may later be diagnosed with a specific developmental disability, but it is also possible that children will "grow out of" a developmental delay especially if they receive early intervention services. Children up to nine years old may be diagnosed with developmental delay when they do not meet developmental milestones by an expected age (Individuals with Disability Education Act [IDEA], 2004). This is usually determined through standardized assessment comparing the child's development to typically developing same-age peers in five major areas: motor development, cognition, communication, social/emotional, or **adaptive behavior** (IDEA, 2004). Although OT practitioners do not often use the term "adaptive behavior" or adaptive development, it is common in developmental disability and child development literature. Adaptive behavior focuses on age-appropriate occupational performance primarily in activities of daily living and instrumental activities of daily living, a crucial aspect of the occupational therapy domain.

The Individuals with Disabilities Education Act (IDEA, 2004) allows each state to set its own definition of developmental delay. These definitions vary greatly in terms of the age of the child and the severity of the delay necessary to meet the criteria (Ringwalt, 2012). While some states use the diagnosis of developmental delay for children up to nine years old, other states only allow the developmental delay label for children up to age 3 or 5 (NICHCY, 2012). The states also determine how delayed the child must be compared to peers the same age in order to qualify for services with a developmental delay, and there is a wide range of what is considered developmental delay between different states (Ringwalt, 2012). This variety in defining the condition makes it difficult to obtain accurate data about how common developmental delay is.

Occupational Therapy with Children with Developmental Delay

Because individuals diagnosed with developmental delay are always children and there is a potential for the delay to diminish with intervention, OT practitioners

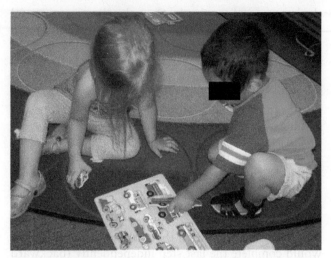

Figure 27.2 Addressing fine motor skills through play with toys and peers.

typically use a **habilitation** approach to improve performance skills that are delayed. The developmental frame of reference is most commonly used with children with developmental delay. Depending on the nature of the delay, the behavioral or sensory frames of reference may also be appropriate. The focus of occupational therapy intervention is still to improve occupational performance. If the child has delayed fine motor skills, it is not sufficient to only address fine motor skills. The fine motor skills need to be linked to play (see Fig. 27.2), feeding, or other occupations to ensure that the intervention is meaningful. It is a problem if the child's fine motor skills improve but the child's occupational performance does not change.

Developmental Disability Conditions

Many health conditions fit under the broad category of developmental disability. These include intellectual disability, ASDs, movement disorders, and learning disabilities, among others. Basic knowledge about specific disabilities helps OT practitioners know what to expect in terms of a person's client factors and performance skills. In addition, using knowledge about the disability, OT practitioners consider potential risks associated with the condition and the precautions they need to take. The following sections provide this type of information for the most common developmental disabilities encountered in occupational therapy practice.

Previous sections of this chapter covered information about occupational therapy with individuals with developmental disabilities. Some examples and additional strategies related to specific conditions are included with the categories below (From the Field 27.3).

Intellectual Disability

Intellectual disability, formerly known as mental retardation, is a disability affecting cognitive functioning and is diagnosed based on intelligence quotient (IQ) testing and adaptive behavior or occupational performance. Individuals may be diagnosed with intellectual disability when they have a disability that started prior to age 18, which includes significantly lower than normal IQ scores (below 70) and considerable issues meeting performance standards expected for their age and culture in two or more areas of occupation, learning, or social participation (Schalock et al., 2010). By definition, individuals with intellectual disabilities have impaired cognitive skills and issues with occupational performance.

The report prevalence rates for intellectual disabilities vary greatly between less than 1% up to 3% depending on the age group and method for measuring prevalence (Boyle et al., 2011; President's Committee for People with Intellectual Disabilities, 2012). Intellectual disability may be caused by a genetic condition such as Down syndrome or environmental factors such as lack of oxygen, injury, or exposure to toxins, but in many cases, no one knows what caused the disability (Centers for Disease Control and Prevention [CDC], 2010).

Genetic Conditions

There are a variety of genetic conditions that may result in intellectual disability. The most common are Down syndrome, which occurs in approximately 1 in 737 births in the United States (Parker, et al., 2010) and fragile X syndrome occurring in approximately 1 in 5000 births (Coffee et al., 2009). Individuals with fragile X syndrome may also have other developmental disabilities; the most commonly occurring are autism and attention deficit hyperactivity disorder (ADHD) (Bailey et al., 2008). An individual with Down syndrome often has distinctive facial features; low **muscle tone**, loose ligaments, and approximately 40% of individuals with Down syndrome have congenital heart defects that may require surgery during the first year of life (National Association for Down Syndrome, 2003). Some individuals with Down syndrome have atlantoaxial instability where the ligaments between the C1 and C2 vertebra allow for the bones to move too much and increase the potential for damage to the spinal cord (Alvarez & Kao, 2011). Individuals with atlantoaxial instability can participate in typical activities, but they should avoid rough sports that may cause damage to the neck. Adults with Down syndrome are at increased risk for early-onset Alzheimer dementia. The loss of skills associated with dementia can be especially challenging for individuals who may already require support to engage in occupations.

Occupational Therapy Intervention with People with Intellectual Disabilities

The occupational therapy interventions for developmental disabilities in the previous sections are appropriate for individuals with intellectual disability. In addition, occupational therapy practitioners need to foster **self-determination** in individuals with intellectual disabilities, because adolescents and adults with higher self-determination have better outcomes for independent living, employment, and other important life areas (Wehmeyer & Palmer, 2003). Occupational therapy practitioners simplify tasks, adapt the environment, and assist the individual with intellectual disability to establish skills in order to improve participation in occupations. When interacting with a person with intellectual disability, talk directly to the person; do not "baby" the individual or "talk down" to him or her. Everyone working with the individual with an intellectual disability needs to respect the person's life experience and age regardless of the person's developmental or cognitive level.

Autism Spectrum Disorders

ASDs, previously called pervasive developmental disorders, involve impaired social interaction skills and repetitive behaviors and/or interests (APA, 2013). Many individuals with ASD, also called autism, also have impaired language skills (expressive and receptive). The prevalence of ASDs has increased in recent years, and estimates vary from 1 in 68 to 1 in 150 children in the United States (Baio, 2014).

Individuals with autism learn differently than most people. Most people learn by watching others do tasks; individuals with intellectual disability or other developmental disabilities may require more time or a different way to do a task, but they generally learn in a typical fashion. The brains of individuals with autism are different; the part of the brain that is activated when typical individuals see someone do a task is not activated when a person with autism sees someone do a task (Oberman et al., 2005). Additionally, individuals with autism learn more through using proprioception sensation (feeling own body do a task) rather than visual information (watching someone else) (Haswell et al., 2009). For these reasons, individuals with autism often cannot learn through observation and need explicit instruction and possibly physical assistance to learn new tasks.

Occupational Therapy Intervention with Individuals with ASD

There are specific strategies that OT practitioners as well as other professionals use when working with individuals with autism to address how they learn.

Case-Smith and Arbesman (2008) reviewed evidence on the effectiveness of sensory-based, relationship-based, visual supports and structured teaching, specific social skill training, and intensive behavioral interventions. All of these strategies had some level of effectiveness with children with autism. The issue with specific social skill training was that the individuals often did not generalize the skills learned to new settings or situations. Strategies using applied behavior analysis often did not affect daily living skills, so OT practitioners working with individuals receiving intensive behavioral services can address these needs in other ways.

Because many people with ASD have problems with communication, they may use augmentative or alternative communication such as computerized communication devices or pictures (such as Picture Exchange Communication System, PECS, or Proloquo2Go). Occupational therapy practitioners need to be familiar with the strategies that are successful for the individual to communicate. Because people with ASD have difficulty with receptive communication and processing auditory information, it may be necessary to limit verbal directions, supplement verbal directions with visual information, or allow extra time for an individual with ASD to process auditory information. It may be necessary to count to five or even ten before repeating a cue in order to allow enough time for the individual to understand the request. Before giving a direction or providing a cue, it is necessary to get the person's attention first. Consider the two ways to present the direction to sit down:

1. Shawn (pause), sit down, please.
2. Please sit down, Shawn.

In the first example, by stating the person's name first and pausing to ensure you have his attention, it is more likely that the person will process the direction. Whether or not he follows the direction is impacted by multiple factors. With the second example, the person may not realize you are talking to him until after you have already given the direction, so you will likely have to repeat it. If the person has difficulty processing auditory information, you need to keep the directions as simple as possible, so you may leave off extra words that are usually included to be polite, such as "please" in the example.

Individuals with ASD benefit from clear structure and visual information. Written schedules and other visual supports can be very helpful for individuals with ASD, and they may require them throughout life. These supports vary based on the needs of the individual. They can consist of photographs, drawings, or written lists that range from a list of routine activities (similar to a to-do list) to a detailed sequence based on activity analysis. Written or picture cues can be paired with physical or other assistance (such as pointing to the next task to be completed), and they can be useful ways to teach new tasks using a variety of frames of reference. Occupational therapy practitioners can train others to use the picture cues with the individual with ASD and gradually fade the assistance until the person with ASD can use the pictures without assistance.

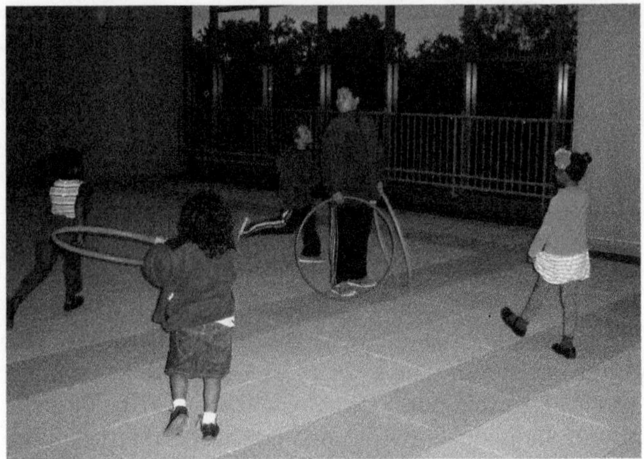

Figure 27.3 Group intervention with children with and without developmental disabilities to foster social skills development.

Individuals with autism have difficulty with social participation that can be addressed using a strengths-based approach. Highly specific interests are common among individuals with autism. Rather than casting this interest as an "obsession," an OT practitioner can use the individual's interest to enable performance. Social group interventions can involve children of different ages and abilities who enjoy similar activities in order to foster interaction skills (see Fig. 27.3). As an example, an OT practitioner can help children to start a group for people interested in trains. This group can bring people with common interests together as a way to address social participation needs rather than specific social skills training that focuses on the person's deficits and may not generalize to other settings.

Movement Disorders

Movement disorders are a category of developmental disabilities often caused by issues in the neurological or musculoskeletal systems. The major movement disorders covered in this chapter are cerebral palsy, spina bifida, muscular dystrophy, juvenile rheumatoid arthritis, and developmental coordination disorder (DCD).

Cerebral Palsy

The most common movement-related developmental disability is cerebral palsy affecting approximately 1 in 303 people in the United States (CDC, 2012a). Cerebral palsy is caused by an injury to the motor area of the brain and can occur prior to birth, during birth, or after birth. All individuals with cerebral palsy have movement difficulties, but over half of the children with cerebral palsy can walk independently (Kirby et al., 2011). Approximately 60% of the individuals with cerebral palsy have additional developmental disabilities such as intellectual disability, visual impairment, or seizure disorder (epilepsy) (Kirby et al., 2011). Seizure disorders CS1 occur in 0.67% of all children ages 3 to 17 (Boyle et al., 2011). Individuals working with people with seizure disorders need to be familiar with first aid for seizures.

There are four major types of cerebral palsy based on the type of movement and muscle tone that the person exhibits: spastic cerebral palsy, athetoid cerebral palsy, ataxic cerebral palsy, and mixed cerebral palsy. Spastic cerebral palsy is the most common type, and approximately 80% of individuals with cerebral palsy have this type CS1 (CDC, 2012b). Spasticity is increased muscle tone, the amount of tension in the muscle at rest. Athetoid cerebral palsy involves changing muscle tone (high and low) that makes movements difficult to control. Ataxic cerebral palsy is when the person has difficulty with smooth movements and balance, and the person may shake when reaching for items or have difficulty walking. Mixed cerebral palsy is a combination of different types of cerebral palsy.

Cerebral palsy may also be categorized according to the parts of the body that are affected. Quadriplegia affects both arms and legs, and hemiplegia affects one side of the body (e.g., right arm and right leg). Diplegia is a specific type of quadriplegia where the person's legs are much more significantly affected than the arms and the individual may have full use of his/her arms and hands.

Occupational Therapy Intervention with Individuals with Cerebral Palsy

There is research evidence that children with cerebral palsy participate in fewer activities than peers without disabilities (Imms, 2008) and individuals with more severe cerebral palsy have lower performance in self-care and socialization occupations (Phipps & Roberts, 2012). Therefore, OT practitioners need to address the participation needs of individuals with cerebral palsy. Training individuals to use assistive technology is a common way to do this. There are a variety of devices that can be switch adapted so that a person can participate in activities by pushing a single switch. Switch-adapted toys CS1 enable children with fine motor impairments to play with manipulative toys. Connecting a device such as a Powerlink and switch to electric kitchen devices such as an electric can opener, mixer, or blender (anything that plugs in and has an on/off switch) enables participation in cooking activities with another person (see Fig. 27.4). There are a wide variety of ADLs, IADLs, and other occupations that can be adapted with assistive technology so that people with motor impairments can participate.

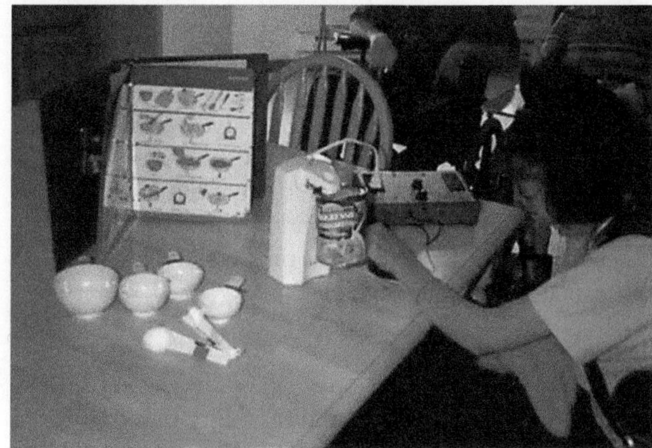

Figure 27.4 Using assistive technology devices to engage in meal preparation.

Range of motion exercises and splinting are common interventions for individuals with spastic cerebral palsy because their tight muscles can make it difficult for them to move, and **contractures** can develop over time. Positioning is an important concern for individuals with cerebral palsy (see Fig. 27.5). If they are not in a functional position, they will have increased difficulty moving and engaging in occupation. Parents often dress infants in a supine position, but this is one of the most difficult positions for a person with high or low tone to purposefully move in. Individuals with high tone may be most successful dressing while in a sidelying position, although they will have to move from side to side to dress. Individuals with low tone often perform better in

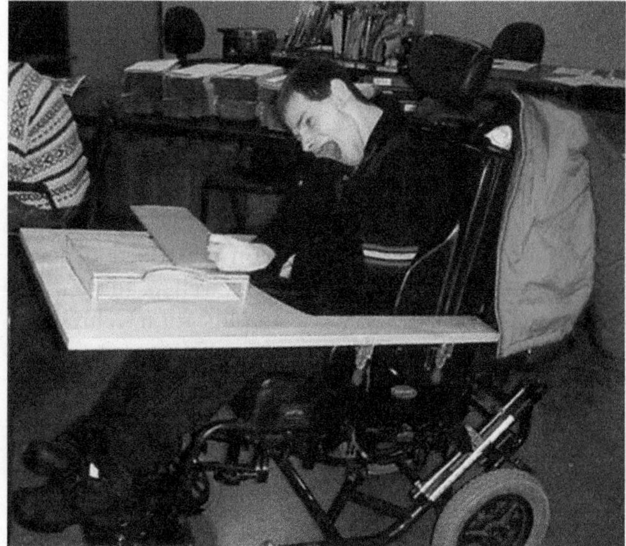

Figure 27.5 Eric uses limited range of motion in his arm and assistive technology including a customized tray and positioning equipment to stamp the date on documents that the staff members use.

a supported position such as sitting in a chair with arms or, for young children, in a caregiver's lap. Even if the individuals require assistance to engage in a task, such as dressing, they need to be actively involved in the task. For example, they can move to assist as much as possible and/or choose clothes or the order to put on the clothes (such as shirt or pants first), and as the individuals get older, they should direct the person providing the assistance as much as possible.

Spina Bifida

Spina bifida is a developmental disability that can occur as a result of atypical neural tube development during the embryonic stage of prenatal development. There has been a decrease in neural tube disorders in the United States since 1998 when the federal government required food industries to fortify cereals with folic acid, a vitamin that when taken by pregnant women decreases the likelihood of the child having a neural tube disorder (Honein et al., 2001). The prevalence of spina bifida following mandatory folic acid food fortification is now approximately 3.5 per 10,000 births (Parker et al., 2010).

Individuals with more significant forms of spina bifida often have difficulties with bladder management that require catheterization. Children with spina bifida need to learn to self-catheterize, an occupation that requires specific skills. Occupational therapy practitioners address the occupational needs of individuals with spina bifida by helping the individuals compensate for their motor impairments.

Muscular Dystrophy

There are many different types of muscular dystrophy in which the muscles get progressively weaker over time. Duchenne muscular dystrophy is the most common type, occurs in 2.9 per 10,000 males (CDC, 2009), and often leads to death by young adulthood. Because this is a progressive condition, any recommendations for equipment need to consider the decline in skills that the client will likely exhibit. Occupational therapy intervention focuses on continued participation in valued occupations through assistive technology as well as adaptation, energy conservation, and work simplification techniques. Individuals may experience frustration, fear, or other feelings related to the decline in skills, and OT practitioners can help provide an outlet for these feelings. Other forms of muscular dystrophy are usually less severe and do not result in premature death (CDC, 2009).

Juvenile Rheumatoid Arthritis

Only 40% to 45% of individuals with juvenile rheumatoid arthritis still have symptoms of the condition after 10 years (CDC, 2011), so there is inconsistency about whether or not this condition would actually be considered a developmental disability. There are a wide range of estimates for the prevalence of juvenile rheumatoid arthritis and other rheumatic conditions in children (CDC, 2011). Individuals with juvenile rheumatoid arthritis experience significant pain in their joints that can impact occupational performance. This pain can be constant and severe as noted in the following clinical example from Christopher Alterio, Dr. OT, OTR, an occupational therapist from New York.

> I was kind of shocked when I saw little tears welling up in Lacey's eyes. I didn't understand. I was moving her fingers so slowly and so gently. I was watching her closely to make sure I would have noticed the slightest change in her respiration or any other sign that would have indicated any discomfort. And then I made one of the most uninformed statements that I ever made in my therapy career that still rings in my ears all these years later:"Oh Lacey, I am so sorry. I thought I told you to let me know if I did anything to hurt your fingers when we were doing therapy."And then a little nine year old child gave me the lesson about JRA and pain that I will never forget. She said back to me through too many tears, "It's really OK. But my fingers always hurt. What am I going to say?" (Alterio, 2012).

Occupational Therapy Intervention with Individuals with Juvenile Rheumatoid Arthritis

Occupational therapy for individuals with juvenile rheumatoid arthritis is similar to strategies used with adults with rheumatic conditions. This includes teaching compensatory strategies such as energy conservation and work simplification, exercises to maintain range of motion and strength, and teaching a variety of methods for pain management. The primary differences when working with children are considering their unique developmental needs in terms of play and school participation, advocating for their needs with the adults in their lives such as parents and teachers, and helping the children to advocate for themselves.

Developmental Coordination Disorder

DCD is significantly impaired motor skills and coordination that affect occupational performance (APA, 2013). While it is a movement disorder, individuals with DCD have difficulties with motor planning (**praxis**), which is the cognitive aspect of movement, so this condition is also known as dyspraxia. Handwriting, dressing, and other tasks that require higher levels of fine motor coordination and motor planning are often difficult for individuals with this condition. Individuals with DCD often also have other developmental disabilities such as

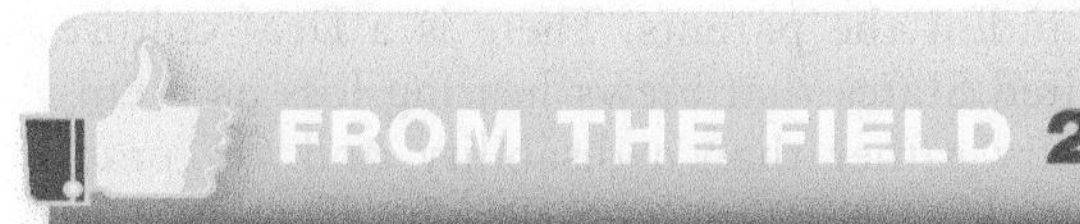

A typical day in the life of an elementary school occupational therapy assistant consists of working with all the children… (so) that the students feel that they are having fun but also working towards an educational goal. One student may be practicing handwriting skills by forming letters in shaving cream while another student is engaged in a beanbag-toss game with a partner to work on eye–hand coordination and turn-taking skills.

There is nothing more fulfilling than when the students achieve milestones, whether it (is) taking their first step or writing their name for the first time and knowing that together, you and the student have achieved something that is very meaningful to them.

Quote from Kara Kightlinger, COTA in Colorado (Kightlinger, 2004).

attention deficit hyperactivity disorder, learning disabilities, or language impairments.

Occupational Therapy Intervention with Individuals with DCD

There are three major categories for evidence-based intervention strategies with children with DCD: motor, sensory, and cognitive. Working with the child to improve motor performance, sensory strategies to address how the child processes information to the body, and cognitive strategies, such as having children talk out their problem-solving strategies to deal with a motor task, can be effective for skill development (Banks et al., 2008; Hillier, 2007). There is limited evidence about occupational therapy intervention for adults with DCD (From the Field 27.5).

Attention Deficit Disorders

The major categories of symptoms associated with ADHD are **inattention**, **hyperactivity**, and **impulsivity** (American Psychiatric Association [APA], 2013). Approximately 6.69% of children ages 3 to 17 are diagnosed with ADHD (Boyle et al., 2011). Sensory-processing issues and variability in behavior are common among individuals with ADHD (Young, 2007). Like all developmental disabilities, ADHD continues throughout the life span; however, the symptoms often decrease during adolescence and adulthood.

Although the underlying causes are different, individuals with DCD or ADHD often experience similar occupational performance difficulties. As children, they often have difficulty with academic tasks. They may have problems with self-care or IADL tasks such as tying shoes, not washing all body parts, difficulty or errors with clothes fasteners, messy eating, or difficulty keeping work spaces organized (Poulsen, 2011). These difficulties are especially evident when they are learning new tasks.

Occupational Therapy Intervention with Individuals with ADHD

There is beginning evidence supporting using cognitive frames of reference such as cognitive behaviorism and the dynamic interactional approach with children with ADHD. Hahn-Markowitz et al. (2011) found improved behavior and problem solving for children with ADHD following occupational therapy intervention focused on child-directed goal setting, parent involvement, and teaching specific cognitive strategies and building awareness of abilities and strategies. Young (2007) described using cognitive behavioral strategies to improve occupational performance for children with ADHD.

There are several recent studies supporting the effectiveness of social skills training with children with ADHD. Wilkes et al. (2011) found that play-based occupational therapy groups with typically developing peer mentors, specific modeling techniques, and parent training were effective at improving social play for children with ADHD. Gol and Jarus (2005) demonstrated improved cognitive skills and coordination skills following occupation-based social skills training for children with ADHD.

Learning Disabilities

Individuals are diagnosed with specific learning disorders, also called learning disabilities, when their reading (dyslexia), writing (dysgraphia), or math (dyscalculia) skills are much lower than what would be expected based on their intelligence, age, and previous education (APA, 2013). Although learning disabilities continue into adulthood, prevalence rates are usually based on children. Approximately 7.66% of children ages 3 to 17 are diagnosed with a specific learning disability (Boyle et al., 2011). Individuals with learning disabilities may also exhibit difficulties processing sensory information.

For children with learning disabilities, academic performance is a major occupational concern. In addition, the individuals often have difficulty with social interaction and building social relationships, and these difficulties can continue into adulthood (Poulsen, 2011).

Occupational Therapy Intervention with People with Learning Disabilities

Individuals with learning disabilities often require assistive technology to support their participation at school or work. This may include using a computer or word processor, specific computer programs that read text or assist with organizing writing, or calculators or graph paper for math. For children and adolescents, necessary assistive technology should be included in their individualized education programs (IEP). Adults with learning disabilities, including students in college, need to request reasonable accommodations that may include assistive technology from their employer or college. Occupational therapy practitioners can help to determine appropriate technology and train individuals in its setup and use.

Interventions based on sensory frames of reference can be helpful for individuals with learning disabilities and/or ADHD to improve school participation and teach students self-regulation techniques. The earliest research on the effectiveness of sensory integration intervention was with children with learning disabilities, and interventions based on sensory frames of reference continue to be commonly used in occupational therapy with this population.

Hearing Impairment and Visual Impairment

When hearing and visual impairments occur during childhood, they are often categorized as developmental disabilities because they are physical disabilities that last throughout life and can impact occupational performance. Prevalence rates for hearing impairments vary greatly, but researchers estimate that 0.45% of children ages 3 to 17 have moderate to profound hearing loss (Boyle et al., 2011). Occupational therapy practitioners are most likely to work with individuals with hearing loss when they have additional developmental disabilities such as cerebral palsy or intellectual disability. Over 50% of hearing loss is due to genetic factors (Morton & Nance, 2006). Occupational therapy practitioners working with children with hearing loss need to consider that the parents may also have hearing loss, and providing sign language interpreters would be an appropriate accommodation to make for the child and/or the parents. There is a Deaf culture in the United States that views hearing loss as a cultural identity rather than a disability, and OT practitioners working with individuals who identify with this culture need to demonstrate appropriate cultural sensitivity.

Vision loss that starts in childhood and cannot be corrected with glasses is a developmental disability. This includes individuals with low vision and blindness. Approximately 0.13% of children between 3c and 17 years old have blindness (Boyle et al., 2011), but prevalence rates for low vision are less available. Vision loss can co-occur with many other developmental disabilities including cerebral palsy and intellectual disability. For information about occupational therapy intervention with individuals with low vision, please refer to Chapter 31, *Vision*, in this textbook.

Disruptive Behavior and Emotional Disorders

Disruptive behavior disorders and emotional disturbance are mental health conditions that occur in childhood and may or may not continue throughout the life span. Therefore, they may not meet the definition for developmental disability. However, since children with these conditions can receive services in schools and other settings providing intervention with individuals with developmental disabilities, some information about these conditions is included here.

Emotional disturbance may encompass many different diagnoses including oppositional defiant disorder, conduct disorder, and other mental health issues that occur in children and adolescents such as depression or anxiety (Barnes et al., 2011). There are medical definitions for distinct disorders. IDEA (2004) includes a definition for emotional disturbance, which includes a decreased ability to learn not explained by another condition, impaired social relationships, and inappropriate behavior or mood.

Clear limit setting is essential when working with people with disruptive behavior disorders or emotional disturbances. Additional information about interventions for individuals with mental health issues is included in Chapter 29, *Psychological Conditions*, and Chapter 34, *Mental Health*, in this textbook.

Summary

Occupational therapy practitioners working with people with developmental disabilities need to address the quality of a person's life. Occupational therapy practitioners do not decide what makes a good quality of life for their clients. Only the individual and his or her family can determine what makes a good quality of life for them. Addressing participation in age-appropriate activities, ensuring that activities are personally meaningful and fulfilling, acknowledging individuality, promoting self-determination, and encouraging social inclusion are major areas for OT practitioners working with individuals with developmental disabilities.

This chapter focused on the most common developmental disabilities seen in occupational therapy practice. There are a variety of other less common developmental disabilities. Prior to working with an individual, it is essential to briefly review the conditions that the person has in order to prepare for specific precautions that may need to be taken. Being knowledgeable about the conditions helps the practitioner to ensure that intervention activities are safe and to predict appropriate intervention activities prior to seeing the individual.

Review Questions

1. What is the MOST important information an OTA needs to know in order to develop intervention activities using a developmental frame of reference?
   a. Expectations for what the person needs to do based on chronological age
   b. Current performance skills and the next developmental milestones
   c. How often specific behaviors occur and what is likely causing them
   d. How the individual responds to a variety of sensory experiences

2. What is the MOST important information an OTA needs to know in order to develop intervention activities using an acquisitional frame of reference?
   a. Expectations for what the person needs to do based on chronological age
   b. Current performance skills and the next developmental milestones
   c. How often specific behaviors occur and what is likely causing them
   d. How the individual responds to a variety of sensory experiences

3. What is the PRIMARY purpose of occupational therapy intervention with an individual with a developmental disability?
   a. Improve fine motor skills.
   b. Prevent contractures.
   c. Enhance participation.
   d. Encourage development.

4. Which is an example of positive reinforcement with the behavioral frame of reference?
   a. Give a child a toy to get her to stop crying.
   b. Show a child a picture of a task he needs to do.
   c. Take away television privileges when a child refuses to do his chores.
   d. Clap when a child washes her hands after going to the bathroom.

5. What would be the MOST correct way to describe a large restroom stall with grab bars and a wheelchair sign on the door?
   a. Handicapped restroom
   b. Disabled restroom
   c. Accessible restroom
   d. Occupational therapy restroom

6. Which condition most commonly co-occurs with cerebral palsy?
   a. Autism
   b. Learning disability
   c. Seizure disorder
   d. Osteoarthritis

7. What is the primary advantage of using visual supports with individuals with autism spectrum disorders? Visual supports can be as follows:
   a. Compensate for auditory processing and language impairments.
   b. Encourage relationship building between children and parents.
   c. Allow individuals with autism to learn in a typical way.
   d. Be used with anyone who can read at a 2nd grade level or higher.

8. Which condition in children may not be considered a developmental disability?
   a. Autism
   b. Muscular dystrophy
   c. Attention deficit hyperactivity disorder
   d. Juvenile rheumatoid arthritis

9. What is the PRIMARY difference between developmental delay and developmental disability?
   a. Developmental disability lasts throughout life span and developmental delay may not.
   b. There are universal definitions of developmental delay but not developmental disability.
   c. Developmental delay is a category with multiple diagnoses and developmental disability is one diagnosis.
   d. Developmental disabilities only affect children and developmental delay can also affect adults.

10. What is an example of a cognitive intervention used in occupational therapy that can be helpful for individuals with DCD, ADHD, or LD?
   a. Using different seating cushions to improve attention
   b. Teaching how to use computer software for schoolwork
   c. Social groups with peers with similar interests
   d. Talking out possible solutions to a problem prior to acting

Practice Activities

Think of an activity that you do on a regular basis. How could you adapt this activity for a person with a moderate intellectual disability to participate? How could you adapt this activity for a person with spastic quadriplegic cerebral palsy who has limited use of his/her hands? What are three specific strategies you could use to teach the activity to a person with autism?

Watch a documentary movie featuring people with developmental disabilities. Especially if you are a visual learner, it can be helpful to see how a person with a disability engages in occupation. Recommended movies include *Autism: The Musical*, a documentary about a group of children with autism and a wide range of functioning levels in a theater group, and *Monica and David*, a documentary about the early married life of two adults with Down syndrome.

For more information on person-first language, review http://www.disabilityisnatural.com/explore/people-first-language for examples, rationales, and handouts.

References

Allen CK, et al. *Allen Cognitive Level Screen*. 5th ed. Camarillo, CA: ACLS and LACLS Committee; 2007.

Alterio C. Lessons about pediatric pain and JRA [weblog entry]. 2012. Retrieved from http://abctherapeutics.blogspot.com/

Alvarez N, Kao A. Atlantoaxial instability in Down syndrome [website article]. 2011. Retrieved from http://emedicine.medscape.com/article/1180354-overview#a1

American Academy of Pediatrics. Sensory integration therapies for children with developmental and behavioral disorders. *Pediatrics* 2012;129:1186–1189. doi: 10.1542/peds.2012-0876

American Association on Intellectual and Developmental Disabilities [AAIDD]. FAQ on intellectual disability [website article]. 2012. Retrieved from http://aaidd.org/intellectual-disability/definition/faqs-on-intellectual-disability

American Occupational Therapy Association [AOTA]. Guidelines for supervision, roles, and responsibilities during the delivery of occupational therapy services. *Am J Occup Ther* 2009;63:797–803.

American Occupational Therapy Association [AOTA]. *Occupational Therapy Compensation and Workforce Study*. Bethesda, MD: Author; 2010.

American Psychiatric Association [APA]. *Diagnostic and Statistical Manual of Mental Disorders*. 5th ed. Arlington, VA: Author; 2013.

Amundsen SJ. *Evaluation Tool of Children's Handwriting*. Homer, AK: O.T. KIDS; 1995.

Bailey DB Jr, et al. Co-occurring conditions associated with *FMR1* gene variations: findings from a national parent survey. *Am J Med Genet* 2008;146A:2060–2069. doi: 10.1002/ajmg.a.32439

Baio J. Prevalence of autism spectrum disorder among children aged 8 years—autism and developmental disabilities monitoring network, 11 Sites, United States, 2010. *Surveill Summ* 2014;63(SS02):1–21. Retrieved from http://www.cdc.gov/mmwr/preview/mmwrhtml/ss6302a1.htm?s_cid=ss6302a1_w

Banks R, et al. Mastering handwriting: how children with developmental coordination disorder succeed with CO-OP. *OTRJ* 2008;28:100–109.

Barnes K, et al. Occupational therapy for children with severe emotional disturbance in alternative educational settings. In: Bazyk S, ed. *Mental Health Promotion, Prevention, and Intervention with Children and Youth*. pp. 207–229. Bethesda, MD: AOTA; 2011.

Beery KE, et al. *Beery-Buktenica Developmental Test of Visual Motor Integration*. 6th ed. San Antonio, TX: Pearson Assessments; 2010.

Boyle CA, et al. Trends in the prevalence of developmental disabilities in U.S. children, 1997–2008. *Pediatrics* 2011;127:1034–1042. doi: 10.1542/peds.2010-2989

Bruininks RH, Bruininks BD. *Bruininks-Oseretsky Test of Motor Proficiency*. 2nd ed. San Antonio, TX: Pearson Assessments; 2005.

Case-Smith J, Arbesman M. Evidence-based review of interventions for autism used in or of relevance to occupational therapy. *Am J Occup Ther* 2008;62:416–429.

Centers for Disease Control and Prevention [CDC]. Prevalence of Duchenne/Becker muscular dystrophy among males aged 5–24 years-four states, 2007. *MMWR* 2009;58:1119–1122.

Centers for Disease Control and Prevention [CDC]. Intellectual disability fact sheet [website article]. 2010. Retrieved from http://www.cdc.gov/ncbddd/actearly/pdf/parents_pdfs/IntellectualDisability.pdf

Centers for Disease Control and Prevention [CDC]. Childhood arthritis [website article]. 2011. Retrieved from http://www.cdc.gov/arthritis/basics/childhood.htm

Centers for Disease Control and Prevention [CDC]. Summary of 2009 national CDC EHDI data [website article]. 2012a. Retrieved from http://www.cdc.gov/ncbddd/hearingloss/2009-Data/2009_EHDI_HSFS_Summary_508_OK.pdf

Centers for Disease Control and Prevention [CDC]. Facts about cerebral palsy [website article]. 2012b. Retrieved from http://www.cdc.gov/ncbddd/cp/facts.html

Coffee B, et al. Incidence of Fragile X syndrome by newborn screening for methylated *FMR1* DNA. *Am J Hum Genet* 2009;85:503–514. doi: 10.1016/j.ajhg.2009.09.007

Coster WJ, et al. *School Function Assessment*. San Antonio, TX: Psychological Corporation/ Therapy Skill Builders; 1998.

de las Heras CG, et al. *A User's Manual for the Volitional Questionnaire (Version 4.1)*. Chicago, IL: Model of Human Occupation Clearinghouse; 2007.

Folio MR, Fewell RR. *Peabody Developmental Motor Scales*. 2nd ed. Austin, TX: Pro-ed; 2000.

Ganz JB, Simpson RL. Effects on communicative requesting and speech development of the picture exchange communication system in children with characteristics of autism. *J Autism Dev Disord* 2004;34:395–409.

Gol D, Jarus T. Effect of a social skills training group on everyday activities of children with attention-deficit-hyperactivity disorder. *Dev Med Child Neurol* 2005;47:539–545.

Hahn-Markowitz J, et al. Effectiveness of cognitive-functional (Cog-Fun) intervention with children with attention deficit hyperactivity disorder: a pilot study. *Am J Occup Ther* 2011;65:384–392. doi: 10.5014/ajot.2011.000901

Hammill DD, et al. *Developmental Test of Visual Perception*. 2nd ed. San Antonio, TX: Pearson Assessments; 1993.

Haswell CC, et al. Representation of internal models of action in the autistic brain. *Nat Neurosci* 2009;12:970–972. doi: 10.1038/nn.2356

Hillier S. Intervention for children with developmental coordination disorder: a systematic review. *Internet J Allied Health Sci Pract* 2007;5(3). Retrieved from http://ijahsp.nova.edu/articles/vol5num3/hillier.pdf

Holm MB, Rogers JC. Performance assessment of self-care skills. In: Hemphill-Pearson B, ed. *Assessments in Occupational Therapy Mental Health*. 2nd ed., pp. 101–110. Thorofare, NJ: Slack; 2008.

Honein MA, et al. Impact of folic acid fortification of the U.S. food supply on the occurrence of neural tube defects. *J Am Med Assoc* 2001;285:2981–2986.

Imms C. Children with cerebral palsy participate: a review of the literature. *Disabil Rehabil* 2008;30:1867–1884. doi: 10.1080/09638280701673542

Individuals with Disability Education Act [IDEA]. 20 U.S.C. § 300. 2004.

Jones M. *Effects of Power Mobility on the Development of Young Children with Severe Motor Impairments*. (Unpublished doctoral dissertation). Oklahoma City, OK: University of Oklahoma; 2004.

Keller J, et al. *The Child Self-Assessment (COSA) (Version 2.1)*. Chicago, IL: University of Illinois, College of Applied Sciences, Department of Occupational Therapy, Motto Clearing House; 2005.

Kightlinger K. Finding rewards in the classroom. In: *Life on the Job as an Occupational Therapy Assistant: Recent Graduates Talk About their Work*. Bethesda, MD: AOTA; 2004. Retrieved from http://www.aota.org/Educate/EdRes/StuRecruit/Working/38378.aspx?FT=.pdf

King G, et al. *Children's Assessment of Participation and Enjoyment*. San Antonio, TX: Harcourt Assessment, Inc.; 2004.

Kirby RS, et al. Prevalence and functioning of children with cerebral palsy in four areas of the United States in 2006: a report from the autism and developmental disabilities monitoring network. *Res Dev Disabil* 2011;32:462–469.

Milone M. *Test of Handwriting Skills*. (Revised ed.) Novato, CA: Academic Therapy Publications; 2007.

Missuna C, et al. *Perceived Efficacy and Goal Setting System (PEGS)*. San Antonio, TX: Psychological Corporation; 2004.

Morton CC, Nance WE. Newborn hearing screening: a silent revolution. *N Engl J Med* 2006;354:2151–2164.

National Association for Down Syndrome. Facts about Down syndrome [website article]. 2003. Retrieved from http://www.nads.org/pages_new/facts.html

National Dissemination Center for Children with Disabilities [NICHCY]. Developmental delay [website article]. 2012. Retrieved from http://nichcy.org/wp-content/uploads/docs/fs9.pdf

Oberman LM, et al. EEG evidence for mirror neuron dysfunction in autism spectrum disorders. *Cogn Brain Res* 2005;24:190–198.

Parker SE, et al. Updated national birth prevalence estimates for selected birth defects in the United States, 2004–2006. *Birth Defects Res A Clin Mol Teratol* 2010;88:1008–1016. doi: 10.1002/bdra.20735

Petrenchik TM, et al. Children and youth with disabilities: Enhancing mental health through positive experiences of doing and belonging. In: Bazyk S, ed. *Mental Health Promotion, Prevention, and Intervention with Children and Youth*. pp. 189–205. Bethesda, MD: AOTA; 2011.

Phipps S, Roberts P. Predicting the effects of cerebral palsy severity on self-care, mobility, and social function. *Am J Occup Ther* 2012;66:422–429. doi: 10.5014/ajot.2012.003921

Poulsen AA. Children with attention deficit hyperactivity disorder, developmental coordination disorder, and learning disabilities. In: Bazyk S, ed. *Mental Health Promotion, Prevention, and Intervention with Children and Youth*. pp. 231–265. Bethesda, MD: AOTA; 2011.

President's Committee for People with Intellectual Disabilities. Welcome [website article]. 2012. Retrieved from http://www.acl.gov/Programs/AIDD/Programs/PCPID/index.aspx

Ringwalt S. *Summary table of states' and territories' definitions of/criteria for IDEA Part C eligibility*. 2012. Retrieved from http://www.nectac.org/~pdfs/topics/earlyid/partc_elig_table.pdf

Schalock RL, et al. *Intellectual disability: Definition, Classification, and Systems of Supports*. 11th ed. Washington, D.C.: American Association on Intellectual and Developmental Disabilities; 2010.

Thompson JR, et al. *Supports Intensity Scale*. Washington, D.C.: AAIDD; 2004.

Wehmeyer ML, Palmer SB. Adult outcomes for students with cognitive disabilities three years after high school: the impact of self-determination. *Educ Train Dev Disabil* 2003;38:131–144.

Wilkes S, et al. A play-based intervention for children with ADHD: a pilot study. *Aust Occup Ther J* 2011;58:231–240. doi: 10.1111/j.1440-1630.2011.00928.x

Young RL. The role of the occupational therapist in attention deficit hyperactivity disorder: a case study. *Int J Ther Rehabil* 2007;14:454–459.

CHAPTER

28 Sensory Processing

Diane L. Maxson, MHA, MA, OTR/L

Key Terms

Accommodation—Changes that individuals make in interaction style, task demand, or environmental conditions to function in a specific environment or under specific conditions.

Adaptive response—An appropriate action in which an individual responds successfully to an environmental demand.

Arousal level—An individual's overall level of alertness and responsiveness to environmental stimuli.

Compensation—Changes that individuals make in interaction style, approach, and task execution in response to loss or absence of needed abilities.

Interoception—Awareness of sensation that originates inside the body, particularly the viscera.

Kinesthesia—The ability to sense the direction and extent of joint movement.

Overresponsivity—Exhibition of a more intense, more rapid, and/or longer lasting response to sensory input than is typical.

Praxis—The process of conceiving of, organizing, and carrying out intentional, goal-directed actions.

Proprioception—The ability to sense the position and location of a joint or body part.

Sensory diet—An individualized program of regularly scheduled and as-needed activities that facilitate an individual's ability to self-regulate arousal level and achieve a functional state of homeostasis.

Sensory discrimination—The ability to sense similarities and differences between sensations.

Sensory integration—The organization of sensation for use.

Sensory modulation—Sensory responses that match the nature and intensity of the sensory input.

Sensory processing—Reception and interpretation of sensory input for use.

Sensory processing disorder—Difficulty receiving, processing, and appropriately responding to sensory information from the environment and our body.

Sensory seeking—A persistent craving for sensory input that is difficult to satiate, often in ways that are socially unacceptable.

Sensory underresponsivity—Exhibition of less of a response to sensory input than the situation requires, longer response time to react to input, and/or the requirement of more intense or longer sensory input to generate a response.

Vestibular input—Information from the vestibular system about one's position in and movement through space.

Learning Objectives

After studying this chapter, readers should be able to:

- Explain the link between sensory input and learning.
- Identify the different types and subtypes of sensory processing disorders.
- Explain the different intervention approaches for sensory processing disorder.

Introduction

Everything that we know about ourselves and the world we live in can be linked to the information we receive through our senses of hearing, touch, smell, taste, movement, proprioception, and interoception. Sensory input is processed by our peripheral, central, and autonomic nervous systems and then relayed back to the body to be used in a functional manner. All of this sensory input forms the foundation for our ability to understand and interact with our world in increasingly complex ways as we mature and develop from infancy into adulthood. If the quality or quantity of this input is not a match for the requirements of the higher-level skills, there is a risk that these higher-level skills will not develop appropriately or sufficiently.

The idea that developmental and learning disabilities could be related to atypical sensory processing abilities was initially exclusive to pediatric occupational therapy practice. Over time, we have realized that sensory processing disorder (SPD) can be identified in individuals of all ages. Therefore, understanding normal and abnormal sensory processing abilities is as essential for an OTA working in a skilled nursing facility as it is for an OTA working in a school system.

Sensory Processing

Occupational therapy practitioners use the term **sensory processing** to refer to an individual's ability to detect and interpret information received from the body's sensory systems. This sensory input serves as the foundation for human development and influences motor, cognitive, social–emotional, communication, and adaptive skill development. Everyone reacts in unique ways to different types of sensory input along a continuum of sensitivity. In doing so, we develop our own patterns and strategies in response to various sensory input and events, such as an unexpected tap on the shoulder; do you slowly turn around or physically jerk and let out a little yelp? Or, at the smell of your seatmate's cologne on the subway, do you lean in to get a better whiff or tense for the headache that you know is coming? When these response patterns are consistent with the demands of everyday life and allow us to function optimally, there are no concerns CS2.

In her book *Living Sensationally: Understanding Your Senses,* occupational therapist Winnie Dunn explains the importance of sensations in everyday life and a structure for identifying our own sensory patterns. She identified four typical response profiles: bystander, seeker, sensor, and avoider (Dunn, 2008). The characteristics of each profile are summarized in Table 28.1.

Remember, these behaviors describe the range of typical or "normal" responses. Understanding our own unique response profile can help us to perform more effectively in all areas of our lives. Occasionally though, an individual's response to sensory input is at the extreme end of the continuum and their response strategies actually limit their occupational performance. In other words, life is very challenging.

Sensory processing difficulties, often referred to as **sensory processing disorder** or SPD, are often first identified during childhood as parents and caregivers begin to expand the child's involvement in activities outside of their home and family scope. Parents may find that atypical responses to common environmental events that were easily accommodated within the family network and environment may now be preventing a child from engaging with the larger world beyond the home. That is, a sensory-sensitive child who has grown up wearing only soft, stretchy clothing may refuse to put on the tights and leotards needed to attend dance lessons with his/her friends. As awareness of the lifelong functional impact of SPD is increasingly acknowledged by the medical and educational community, OTs have emerged as leaders in identifying the warning signs of SPD in very young infants, children, and teenagers and, more recently, with adults. Many OT practitioners are now applying a growing awareness of the impact of lifelong sensory coping and **accommodation** and implementing sensory-based intervention strategies with their older adult clients. The difficulties resulting from SPD can and do significantly and persistently affect function and occupational performance throughout life.

Cause and Prevalence of Sensory Processing Disorder

Little is known and still less has been proven about the cause(s) of SPD, and research is in its early stages. Some of the existing studies have shown that up to14% of

TABLE 28.1 What Is Your Sensory Profile?

Sensory Pattern	Description
Bystander	• Need extra sensory input to notice what is happening around them • Are easy going and can focus in the midst of chaos • Not bothered by drafts, messy desks, or stiff clothing • Often get lost or miss landmarks when following directions
Seeker	• Love sensation, actively work to get more • Love new things, new routines • Love to have all of their favorite things near them • Dislike routine and predictability
Sensor	• Notice everything that is happening and have definite ideas about how best to respond • Are the first to notice when you change your hair color, perfume, or cell phone • Spend a lot of time getting ready to do things • Have trouble working in noisy environments
Avoider	• Love order and routine • Need time to be alone • Have orderly homes and rarely rearrange the furniture • Prefer an intimate dinner with two or three friends over an impromptu cocktail party

Adapted from Dunn W. *Living Sensationally: Understanding Your Senses*. Philadelphia, PA: Jessica Kingsley Publishers; 2008.

school-age children demonstrate atypical responses to sensory stimulation (Ahn et al., 2004; Reynolds & Lane, 2008). Emerging research also suggests that there is a strong hereditary pattern of SPD within families, particularly between parents and children, and with identical twins (Heuler et al., 2011). A higher rate of SPD has been found with children who have experienced prenatal stress such as very low birth weight (<1,500 g), intrauterine drug or alcohol exposure, and twin or higher-order multiple births (May-Benson et al., 2009). Birth complications are also a risk factor. One study reported that 42.1% of children with SPD who were sampled had experienced birth trauma, including prolonged labor, fetal distress, forceps/vacuum assistance, or jaundice (May-Benson et al., 2009). The typical rate of birth complications in the United States is less than 10% (Miller, 2006). Environmental factors are also associated with a higher incidence of SPD. Children who have been raised in institutional environments such as orphanages that provide little environmental stimulation and personal contact have been found to demonstrate symptoms of sensory **overresponsivity** that ultimately evolved into **sensory seeking**, which are abnormal responses to sensory input (Lin et al., 2002). It has been determined that children who experience severe sexual and/or physical abuse often become extremely defensive to touch and loud sounds (Lin et al., 2002). There are also medical and psychological conditions associated with symptoms of sensory processing difficulties, including autism spectrum disorders (Cheung & Siu, 2009), anxiety disorders, attention deficit hyperactivity disorder (Hender, 2001), fragile X syndrome (Baranek et al., 2002), and developmental coordination disorders (White et al., 2007) CS2.

Occupational Therapy Services for Sensory Processing Issues

Sensory input surrounds us and is ever present, ceaseless, and constant. As you now know, everyone experiences sensations, yet we all interpret them differently. Each of us filters and interprets sensations through our own unique nervous systems. This variability accounts for things such as your love of spicy, highly seasoned food and my preference for mild, subtle flavors. Our olfactory and gustatory sensory tolerance levels are different but do not limit our health or lifestyle in any way. If my olfactory and gustatory sensitivity was such that I only wanted to eat plain pasta, one brand of peanut butter, and baked chicken nuggets, it would be an indication that my sensory sensitivity levels were limiting my health and occupational performance.

Occupational therapy practitioners become involved with individuals with SPD when it impedes their ability to function in some critical way. These specific functions differ in terms of one's occupational performance depending on client's age, yet there are qualities associated with SPD that are consistently reported as areas of concern. They may include the following:

- Dressing: ability/inability to tolerate textures, tags, seams, and decorations; preference for loose/tight

clothing; inability to secure clothing fasteners that are small or out of sight; and desire to wear minimal clothing or several layers regardless of season
- Sleep: extreme difficulty adjusting to seasonal light/time changes, difficulty falling/staying asleep, and need for very tight/very light bedding
- Eating/nutrition: extremely limited diet, reliance on processed foods, and sensitivity to cooking smells
- Movement: frequent falls/bruises; shuffling gait; difficulty standing/walking in dark; seek crashing/jumping/stomping experiences in excess; fearful of elevators/escalators; fearful of tipping head forward/back; clumsy; and constantly moving
- Hearing: hears and is bothered by sounds that others do not hear; panic at common environmental sounds such as a toilet, blender, and vacuum; and tantrums/overwhelmed in noisy environments
- Grooming: resistant to nail care; resistant to hair care; limited awareness of clothing misalignment; dislike wearing watches or jewelry; and panics at dentist

Across the life span, there are indicators of possible SPD. Table 28.2 presents an overview of indicators that can, in their extreme, impede function and participation (Table 28.2).

TABLE 28.2 Possible Indications of Sensory Processing Difficulties

Life Stage	Difficulty with Modulation	Motor Difficulty	Discrimination Difficulty
Infant	• Does not like to be held or cuddled • May be demanding, hard to calm • Needs help to fall asleep, stay asleep	• Low muscle tone • Crawls with belly on floor, does not get up on all 4's • Feels unexpectedly heavy when lifted	• Needs to be wakened for feedings • Very messy eater • Does not appear to hear, even though hearing is fine
Child	• Covers ears in response to common household noises • Does not like to play on grass, sand • Strong clothing preferences based on "feel" rather than fashion	• Loses balance easily • Low energy level, tires quickly in standing • Messy coloring and handwriting	• Having toileting accidents past age 5 (esp. BM) • Clothing often messy, twisted, rumpled • Has difficulty locating source of noises/sounds
Adolescence	• React with physical and/or verbal aggression when bumped from behind • Thrill seeker: loves going fast, jumping, crashing, banging; loves intense sports • Constantly chews on pencils, pens, clothing	• Never learned to ride a bike • Frequently drops or knocks things over • Has difficulty with fine motor tasks such as tying, using a ruler, placing cards in envelope	• Talks too loudly or too softly • Has difficulty judging distances with driving or parking a car • Cannot sleep if room is not completely dark or unless a light is on
Adult	• Wears very loose, soft clothing • Very picky eater • Has difficulty adjusting to changes in plans and routines	• Prefers slip-on shoes • Has difficulty learning new skills and routines • Avoids leisure activities involving movement	• May barely lift feet off ground when walking • Uncomfortable in visually complex spaces • Talks too softly or too loudly for setting
Elder	• Extremely particular about grooming products and routines • Eat less when eating in public • Pull away from social touch	• Intensely resistant to introduction of adapted devices or techniques • Very slow to resume daily routines following illness/injury • Tends to be sedentary when alone	• Has difficulty noticing noxious odors: spoiled food, full litter box • Loss of interest in eating • Has difficulty identifying objects in pockets by touch

Processing Sensory Information

Occupational therapy practitioners recognize that there are more than just the five basic senses (vision, hearing, touch, taste, and smell) and acknowledge the importance of the body-based senses of **proprioception, kinesthesia, vestibular input**, and **interoception** on function and performance. The sensory systems can be organized into three groups: systems that process information from the environment, from the musculoskeletal system, and from the viscera, which are based on the source of the input. As noted in Table 28.3, all of our senses provide vital information about our world and our relationship to it and form the foundation for development, learning, and function.

Sensory Systems that Process Information from the Environment

These systems include the visual, auditory, gustatory, olfactory, and tactile systems. Each will be discussed.

The Visual System

When the retina of the eye is stimulated by light, it sends information to the visual processing centers in the brain via the ocular nerve and brainstem. This information is also sent to other structures within the brain that are simultaneously processing information from the muscles that move the eyes and neck, the vestibular system about body movement, and the cortical system for shape recognition. A well-functioning visual system smoothly

TABLE 28.3 Sensory Systems

System	What It Is	It Provides Us with Information about
Visual	The visual system processes information obtained through our eyes. It is made up of two subsystems, the central and peripheral systems.	• Objects in front of us (central, discrimination) • Objects to the side of us (peripheral, movement) • Light • Movement • Spatial relationships
Auditory	The auditory system is housed within the inner ear and processes sound conducted through the air and the physical structures (bones) of the head and ears.	• Voices • Sounds • Movement • Space
Tactile	Receptors housed within our skin form the basis for our sense of touch. It is made up of two systems, the discriminative and the protective.	• Light touch • Deep pressure • Pain • Object affordances (contour, shape, texture, resilience)
Vestibular	The vestibular system is housed within the inner ear and is comprised of three fluid-filled semicircular canals, the utricle, and the saccule.	• Position in space • Orientation in relation to gravity • Movement through space • Balance • Speed
Proprioception/ kinesthesia	Receptors within our joints (tendons, ligaments, articular surfaces) provide information about joint position and movement.	• Body and joint position • Joint movement
Gustatory/olfactory	The senses of taste and smell are housed within our oral cavity and nasopharynx.	• Tastes • Smells
Interoception	Interoception refers to our awareness of sensation that originates inside the body, particularly the viscera.	• Hunger • Thirst • Bowel and bladder status • Body temperature • Breathing rate

adjusts to varying levels of light, keeps the center of the visual field focused on a target, shifts visual focus smoothly in all planes and directions, orients to changes in the peripheral field, and provides clear and complete images for the brain to process (please also refer to Chapter 31, *Vision*).

The Auditory System

Sound waves are funneled by the outer ear to structures in the inner ear. These waves are translated into nerve impulses that are then sent to auditory centers in the brainstem and the brain. Some of the auditory input is sent to other parts of the brainstem and cerebellum for coordination with input from the proprioceptive and the vestibular systems. Integration and cross-communication of auditory information with visual, tactile, and vestibular input allow us to make meaning out of what we hear and help us recognize speech, judge the distance and location of sounds, and discriminate between familiar and unfamiliar noises.

The Gustatory and Olfactory Systems

The gustatory system regulates our sense of taste and provides information about the physical and chemical properties of things that touch our mouth and tongue. Most of this information is processed by taste buds located on the surface of the tongue. The size and density of these sense organs varies from person to person. With age, our sensitivity to taste diminishes. Babies and young children are more sensitive to the flavors and temperatures of food than their parents are and may reject or dislike highly seasoned foods or extreme flavors. As we age, our taste buds become less sensitive, and because of this, we often prefer more highly seasoned foods or foods with stronger flavors.

Olfactory receptors are located within the nasal cavities and control our sense of smell. The gustatory and olfactory systems are located in close proximity, as the oral cavity and the nasopharynx are connected at the back of the throat. Disruptions in either system will impact the function of the other; our sense of taste is dependent upon a fully functioning olfactory system. Individuals who have no sense of smell will also have a severely impaired sense of taste. The olfactory system is the only sensory system that is processed within the limbic system of the brain. The limbic system is responsible for emotional regulation. Smells can create or trigger emotional memories that can influence our choices and preferences just as strongly as pictures or sounds (From the Field 28.1).

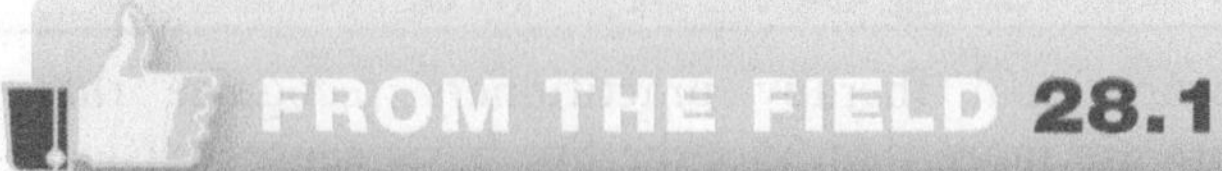

Smell and Memory

When you pass by a bakery and can smell the aromas of freshly baked bread, what comes to mind? Are they positive thoughts? Have you walked by someone wearing a fragrance that elicits some type of memory? What is it?

The Tactile System

The tactile system is the largest and one of our most important sensory systems. Divided into two functional subsystems, protective and discriminative, it plays an essential role in our ability to function both physically and emotionally. Tactile receptors within the layers of the skin let us know where we have been touched, the general size and shape of an object, its temperature, surface properties (e.g., smooth/rough, wet/dry, sticky/smooth), its threat level (e.g., pain, pressure), and whether it is familiar or unfamiliar (Fig. 28.1). Our protective system quickly determines whether this stimulus will hurt or harm us. This protective system is closely linked to muscle fibers that elicit rapid, reflexive movements away from the stimulus if needed. Think about accidentally touching a hot stove burner; your reflexive action is to quickly remove your hand from the burner. If the sensory input does not lead to a protective response because it is not interpreted as a threat, our **discriminative system** provides information about the nature of the input to support function and learning.

Systems that Process Information from our Musculoskeletal System

Our musculoskeletal system houses the receptors that provide vital information about our movement and position in space relative to gravity (the vestibular system)

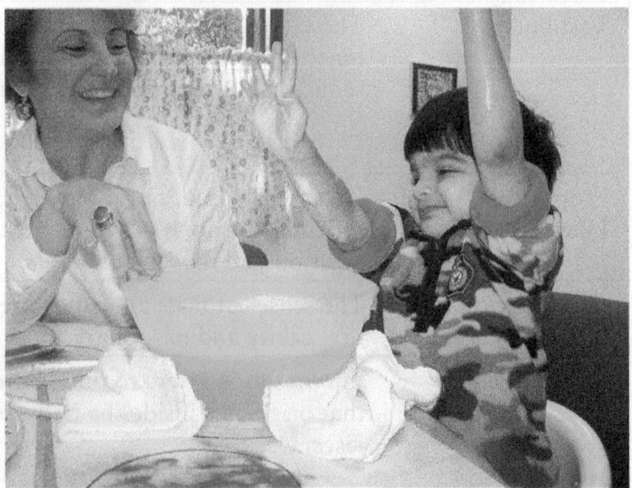

Figure 28.1 A toddler learns to enjoy the tactile sensation of things that are wet.

and about the position and movement of our limbs and joints (the kinesthetic/proprioceptive system).

The Vestibular System

Protectively nestled within the inner ear, the vestibular system is quite small. It is comprised of three fluid-filled semicircular canals, the utricle, and the saccule. The vestibular system registers movement of the body and gravitational pull. Our vestibular system helps us to know how our head is oriented in space and whether we are moving or standing still, and if we are moving, it tells us how fast. The vestibular system is intricately connected to the visual system as well as the auditory system. It supports control and refinement of our movements in and around our world, our ability to time our movements appropriately, and our ability to put sequences of movements together. Our vestibular system, working with all of our other senses, keeps us upright while skiing down a hill and helps us to slow to a stop at the bottom next to our awaiting friends.

The Proprioceptive and Kinesthetic Systems

Our proprioceptive sense tells us what position our limbs and joints are in without needing to look. Proprioception is fundamental to overall awareness of our body position in space and provides essential information and feedback for all movement. Kinesthesia refers to the sensation of the movement of our limbs and joints, including how fast, how far, and how forcefully we move. These systems are neurologically linked. The receptors for these systems are the same and are located in the muscles, ligaments, and tendons. Our proprioceptive abilities allow us to assume the same position every time we get ready to hit a golf ball and let us know that our feet are positioned under the chair we are sitting on without having to look. Our kinesthetic sense supports our ability to execute a perfect golf swing time after time and helps us walk confidently up stairs while carrying items that obscure the view of our feet. The interplay between our proprioceptive and kinesthetic senses allows us to control the speed and force of our movements.

Sensory Systems that Process Information from our Viscera

There are sensory systems that process information from the internal organs in our abdomen and thoracic cavity.

The Interoceptive System

Interoception refers to the awareness and understanding of sensations originating inside the body, especially within the viscera. These sensations include our awareness of hunger and thirst, breathing, pulse, heartbeat, and awareness of the need to urinate and move our bowels. Our internal organs include the stomach, liver, and heart and are located within the thorax and abdomen. They are innervated by the autonomic nervous system and not the central nervous system. Because of this, interoception sensations are often poorly localized and difficult to quantify and measure. Our ability to recognize and interpret them is a learned process, unlike the way the other sensory systems work in a subcortical, subconscious way. Infants are born with only a general awareness of comfort and discomfort. Over time, they learn to identify more specific internal feelings of hunger, thirst, satiety, the need to urinate and defecate, and the elevated pulse and respiratory rates associated with fear and anxiety that are associated with interoception.

Sensory Integration

The sensory information we receive from the environment and within our bodies provides the foundation for all we know about ourselves and our world. This information provides a reference point for our physical, cognitive, and emotional development and function. While each sense can be thought of and described separately, which we have already done, they are all neurologically interconnected (Fig. 28.2). Our sensory systems share and coordinate input and responses to support our ability to explain our environment and function optimally. Accordingly, if the information received from our sensory systems is inaccurate or absent, it can compromise future learning and function.

Sensory Foundations for Development and Learning

As we grow and mature from infancy through childhood, we synthesize information from all of our senses as we learn to move, first automatically in direct response to gravity, touch, or stretch on our muscles and later purposefully, as we begin to actively explore our bodies and environment. We refer to this as sensory motor learning. We use visual, tactile, and proprioceptive input when beginning to reach toward objects. Visual, vestibular, and proprioceptive input activates reflexive motor patterns that help us learn to roll over, sit, and begin to crawl. The combination of sensory input and motor movements also allows us to pull up to standing, move confidently through space, plan new motor movements, develop an awareness of our own body, and refine our automatic balance and protective reactions.

As we become more confident and skilled at controlling our bodies, we begin to be increasingly focused and interested in the larger world around us. We do

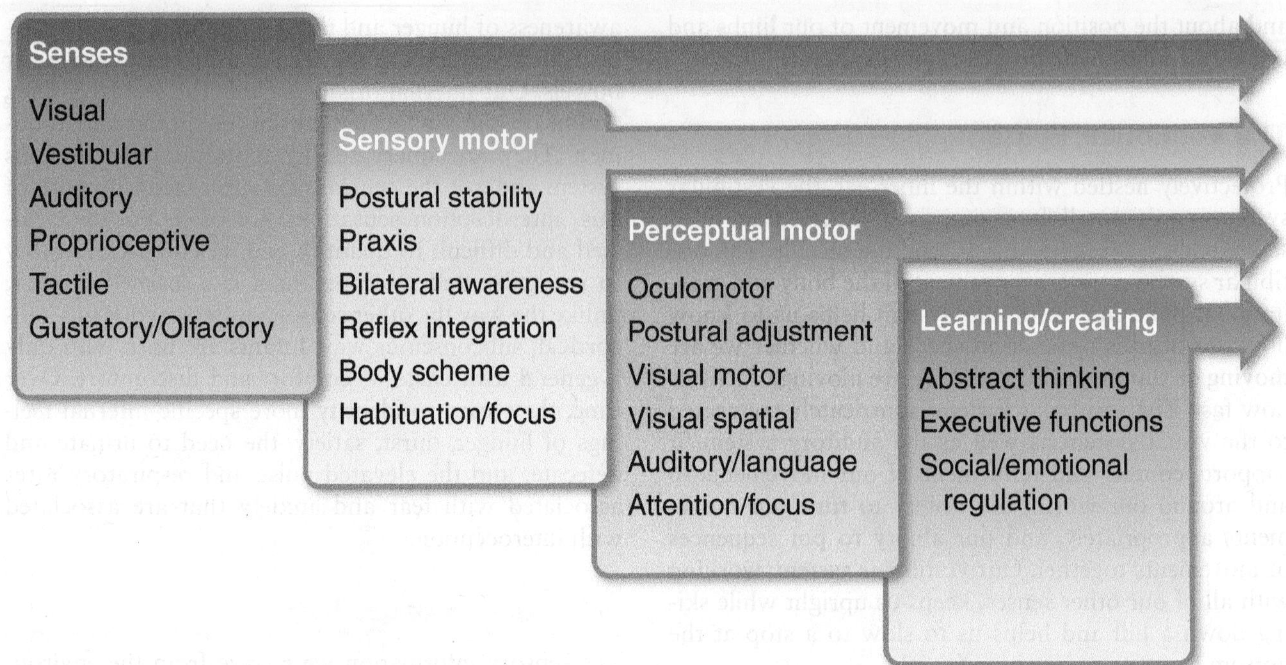

Figure 28.2 The interconnectedness of the sensory systems.

this through a process of developing perceptual motor and **adaptive responses**. Moving about through a sensory-rich environment requires us to learn to focus our attention and screen out distractions, react purposefully rather than impulsively, visually scan our environment in order to understand what we are seeing, understand and localize sounds and voices, and begin to understand spatial relationships in our immediate and larger world. During this period in early development, children are constantly refining their ability to interpret information from our senses and environment and to adapt and change their responses as needed to master developmental milestones. The highest level of learning is called **integrative** or **associative learning.** It integrates the foundational skills of sensory motor learning and perceptual motor adaptive responses. The purpose is to support the refinement of higher-order thinking skills needed for academic learning, development of executive function skills that enable us to reason and make good decisions, social/emotional growth, and behavioral regulation skills.

Sensory Integration Theory: Roots and Application

As we have already discussed, sensory input is critical for learning and development. Anything that interferes with optimal sensory processing will significantly impact function and performance. A. Jean Ayres, an occupational therapist and neuroscientist, developed **sensory integration** theory to explain what she recognized as the relationship between sensory processing difficulties and difficulties with motor and academic learning (Bundy et al., 2002). Ayres' groundbreaking work has provided the foundation for ongoing research and refinement of our understanding of neurological concepts to better understand and drive the expansion and refinement of evaluation and intervention methods for those with SPD. Ayres's foundational model of sensory integration theory (1979) contributed to development of two predominant contemporary models of sensory integration that OT practitioners use to interpret and explain SPD.

In late 2000, a group of five experts in the field of sensory integration culminated 2 years of collaboration with the publication of a position statement aimed at creating a consensus on terminology for sensory integration theory and intervention (May-Benson, 2000). Their work broadened the field and proposed establishment of clear distinctions between terminology used for discussing theory, intervention, and diagnostic labels. The theory was referred to as "sensory integration theory" based on Ayres' work, intervention was "OT using principles of sensory integration," and the diagnostic label was determined to be "dysfunction of sensory integration (DSI)" (Lane et al., 2000, p. 2). Further refinements to this nomenclature were made in 2004 when the term SPD replaced the confusing diagnostic label DSI, and a classification system of types and subtypes of SPD was introduced (Anazalone et al., 2004). This new classification system was recently refined and now clearly identifies three major sensory integrative disorder patterns and five subtypes related to the three patterns (Anazalone et al., 2007). Each is discussed below.

Sensory Modulation Disorder

Sensory modulation is the ability to receive sensory input and then to generate a response of appropriate degree, intensity, and quality for the situation. There are three subtypes of sensory modulation disorder (SMD). **Sensory overresponsivity** is characterized by extreme reactivity to external and internal stimuli in one or more sensory systems, inability to habituate to repeated stimuli, and a tendency to become quickly overloaded (Fig. 28.3). (Miller, 2006). Overresponsivity may occur in just one sensory system or in multiple systems at the same time. Many individuals with sensory overresponsivity have great difficulty with change and transitions and may be seen as controlling and rigid. When someone has sensory overresponsivity, sensory input is often experienced as painful, triggering fight-or-flight reactions. A person who is overresponsive to touch may lash out verbally or physically when bumped accidentally in a crowd or when standing in line.

Individuals with **sensory underresponsivity** process sensory input from internal systems and the external environment slowly. Those with sensory underresponsivity require increased frequency and intensity of sensory input to produce a response. These individuals often need to be reminded to eat and drink during the day as they are very slow to recognize feelings of hunger and thirst. When they do become aware, they are suddenly "dying of thirst" or ravenous.

Individuals with **sensory craving** actively crave sensation yet often become increasingly disorganized the more sensory input that they receive. An example of this is a child at the playground who ricochets from the swings to the climbing structure to the slide, moving faster and more intensely while other children struggle to avoid his erratic trail. His parents carry his tearful, sweaty form to the car over his protests that he wants to swing "just one more time!"

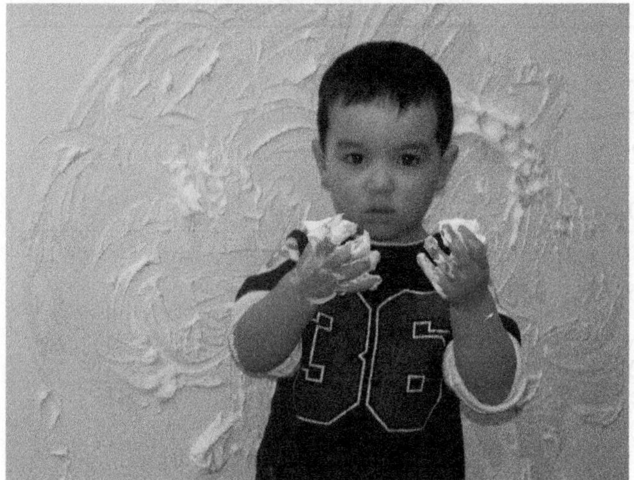

Figure 28.3 "My hands! My hands!" moans Paul, who hates messy play.

Sensory-Based Motor Disorder

Sensory-based motor disorder refers to how an individual processes sensory information to control posture and movement. There are two subtypes associated with sensory-based motor disorder. Individuals with postural disorder have difficulty processing proprioceptive and vestibular input in order to automatically manage the position and movements of the trunk and extremities. They often fail to notice that they have moved to the edge of their seat until they are on the floor. Individuals with postural disorder often have low muscle tone and poor overall strength and endurance and are generally slow to respond to physical cues. They may have difficulty judging how tightly to grip things, and objects frequently fall from their hands while they are still adjusting their grip.

Dyspraxia

Dyspraxia is a motor planning problem that affects an individual's ability to conceive of, plan, and execute new movement sequences in response to input from the environment. An example of this is what happens when we realize that we are cold and need to close the window. If we have good **praxis** skills, things go smoothly. We realize the need to cross the room to get to the window (ideation), scan the path from where we are to the window to plan the best route (feed forward), plan the complex series of muscle contractions needed to stand up, walk across the room while avoiding the sleeping dog in front of us (motor planning), close the window (motor planning), realize that we did not hear the window thump closed (feedback), push down again on the window, and walk back to our seat, still avoiding the sleeping dog. A young girl with dyspraxia may get up to walk across the room and bump into the dog because she did not lift her feet up high enough to step over it once realizing it was in front of her, may have to try a few times to reach high enough to reach the top of the window, and may slam the window closed with too much force. Walking back across the room, she may bump into the dog again because of poor use of feedback.

Sensory Discrimination

Sensory discrimination disorder refers to an individual's ability to notice and understand differences between similar internal and external sensations and apply meaning to them. Our sensory discrimination skills allow us to know whether we are moving up or down in an elevator, whether an object is too hot to drink, or whether it is Jeff or Jen that is on the phone.

Thresholds/Levels of Reactivity and Response Patterns and Self-Regulation Strategies

Thresholds, or levels of reactivity, refer to how quickly an individual's need for or ability to process a particular sensation is achieved. Individuals with high sensory thresholds need a lot of sensory input to respond or feel comfortable. Individuals with low sensory thresholds are aware of sensory stimuli more easily and earlier than those with normal sensory thresholds.

Response patterns and self-regulation strategies refer to how individuals respond to sensory input. Passive response patterns occur when there is no active effort made to change the environment or stimuli. Active response patterns occur when there is purposeful or involuntary response to change the environment or stimuli. Based on Dunn's model (2008), it is possible to characterize an individual's typical response to an activity or experience as representing a level of sensitivity or responsivity and a response pattern or strategy. High thresholds with passive response strategies reflect *low registration,* while high thresholds with active response strategies reflect *sensory seeking*. Low thresholds with passive response strategies reflect *sensory sensitivity,* and low thresholds with active response strategies are *sensory avoiding*.

Identification and Evaluation

Several standardized evaluation instruments have been developed to assess sensory processing abilities in children and adults. Like other assessments that OTs may administer, these are above and beyond assessment of neuromotor status, activities of daily living, and gross and fine motor coordination. The following is a list of standardized evaluation tools commonly used by OTs to assess sensory processing:

- *Sensory Integration and Praxis Test* (Ayers, 1989)
- *Sensory Profile: Infant/Toddler, Caregiver Questionnaire, Adolescent/Adult, or School version* (Dunn, 1999)
- *Sensory Processing Measure: Preschool or Childhood versions* (Parham & Ecker, 2007)
- *DeGangi-Berk Test of Sensory Integration* (DeGangi & Berk, 1983)

Like other assessment tools, your supervising OT will administer sensory processing assessments, but you may be called upon to participate in some capacity.

Intervention

Treating SPD requires that an OT practitioner thoroughly understand and integrate information from many sources. It has evolved into a specialized area of practice within the field of occupational therapy, and it is critical that OT practitioners take active steps to stay abreast of new developments in the evolution of theory, practice, and research.

Instruction in classical sensory integration intervention techniques or other complementary or specialized techniques is beyond the scope of this chapter. Resources for more specialized learning experiences related to the techniques and programs are cataloged in Table 28.4. What is presented here is a framework for incorporating appropriate sensory-based intervention strategies into a relevant, individualized problem-oriented intervention plan for each client (Fig. 28.4).

TABLE 28.4 Sensory-Based Intervention Techniques and Strategies

Technique	Brief Description	Where to Find More Information
Sensory integrative therapy	Classical sensory integrative therapy is provided within a sensory-rich environment, involves a balance between structure and freedom, follows the inner drive of the child, and supports the development of increasingly more complex adaptive responses (Bundy et al., 2002).	http:\\www.wpspublish.com
Therapressure Protocol	A technique developed by Patricia Wilbarger, M.Ed., OTR, FAOTA to treat sensory overresponsivity	Avanti Educational Programs, Denver, CO
Sound-based programs	Several auditory/sound-based therapy programs designed around specialized or filtered musical selections, for example • The Listening Program • Therapeutic Listening • Integrated Listening System • SAMONAS Sound Therapy	 • http:\\www.advanacedbrain.com • http:\\www.VitalLinks.net • http:\\www.integratedlistening.com • http:\\www.samonas.com

TABLE 28.4 Sensory-Based Intervention Techniques and Strategies (continued)

Technique	Brief Description	Where to Find More Information
Sensory diet	Sensory-based activities and experiences are provided at regular intervals throughout the day to meet an individual's sensory needs. May also include adaptations to the environment (Bundy et al., 2002).	http:\\www.ateachabout.com http:\\www.stickkids.com http:\\www.alertprogram.com http:\\www.pdppro.com
Astronaut Training	A intervention protocol for vestibular habilitation developed by Mary J. Kawar, MS, OTR, and Sheila Frick, OTR/L	http:\\www.VitalLinks.net
Interactive Metronome	A computer-based intervention program designed to improve sequencing and timing skills	http:\\www.interactivemetronome.com
Sensory stories	Short, customized stories written within a defined structure that instruct a child in the use of sensory strategies in everyday situations	http:\\www.sensorystories.com
Brain Gym	A set of 26 movements designed to use movement to support learning	http:\\www.braingym.org

Planning Intervention

As you are now keenly aware of, SPDs disrupt many important areas of life, often simultaneously. When planning intervention, an OT practitioner may be overwhelmed by the number and complexity of the presenting problems, so let's use a fictional client to illustrate.

Consider 4-year-old Jeff. Because of ongoing issues that Jeff's peers do not seem to have, Jeff's parents brought him to the private outpatient clinic where you work for an evaluation of his sensory processing abilities, which your supervising OT is responsible for doing. His mother needs to return to her full-time job as a teacher now that Jeff's younger sister is 2 years old; however, she cannot obtain day care for Jeff because he is still not potty trained. Jeff will only wear one particular tee shirt and one pair of sweatpants without tantruming and categorically refuses to wear socks. His grandparents would love to provide day care; however, Jeff screams upon entering their home and runs away from them yelling "no kisses!" The OT evaluation that is completed by your supervising OT indicates that Jeff has delayed gross motor, fine motor, and self-care skills. He also demonstrates severe sensory overresponsivity and has significant difficulties with emotional and behavioral regulation. So, where do you start with developing a intervention plan for Jeff?

One option is to take a three-pronged approach to help Jeff and his family. This approach involves the following:

1. Functional accommodations: Identify the most critical problem impacting the client and/or their family and develop **compensation** or accommodative strategies for immediate situational improvement.
2. Lifestyle accommodations: Assist client and/or family to prioritize the remaining functional issues or problems and develop plans/strategies to minimize the effects of problems on functional performance in the short term.

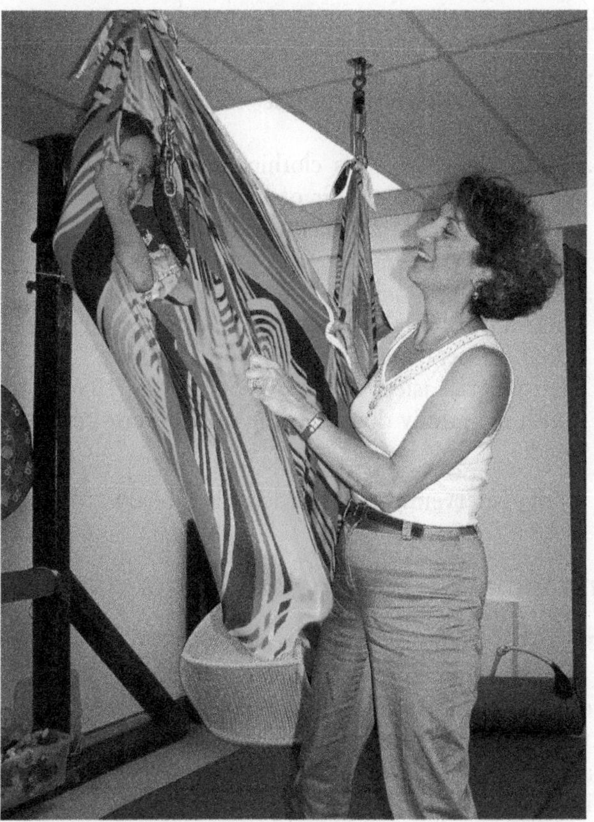

Figure 28.4 Jeff receives lots of regulating sensory input while climbing inside smooth Lycra that does not aggravate his sensitive tactile system.

3. Direct intervention: Provide occupational therapy intervention services supported by a home program to address underlying sensory processing weaknesses and enhance occupational performance. Home-based strategies may include a **sensory diet**, which is a customized selection of sensory experiences and activities that can be integrated into a client's daily routine to provide needed sensory input and promote optimal **arousal**. Intervention tools and strategies may include a variety of sensory-based techniques, some of which can be found in Table 28.4. Many of these techniques and protocols lack rigorous scientific backing, but are not necessarily ineffective. It is the responsibility of each OTA working under the supervision of an OT to monitor and assess the effectiveness of any intervention technique and make therapeutic program changes as appropriate.

Using this stepwise three-pronged approach, we can begin to assist Jeff and his family to meet their identified goals. Jeff's parents identified toilet training as their primary concern. It directly impacts the family's finances by limiting access to childcare for Jeff so that his mother can return to work. Other concerns, in descending order of importance, are as follows: his limited clothing tolerance, physical clumsiness, rejection of physical affection, tendency to tantrum when leaving or entering places, and his need to have both of the family's large dogs in his bed in order to fall asleep.

Working with Jeff and his parents, the following short-term intervention goals for Jeff are established:

1. Jeff will have fewer than three toileting accidents requiring a change of clothes for 5 out of 7 consecutive days.
2. Jeff will increase his clothing tolerance by adding one shirt and one pair of knit pants to his weekly wardrobe, wearing them without protest 80% of opportunities.
3. Jeff will approach his grandfather and offer to give him a "big hug" 5 to 10 minutes after arriving at their house, three out of five opportunities.
4. Jeff will fall asleep in his own bed within 10 minutes, with the family dogs sleeping on the floor beside his bed.

Jeff's intervention plan is described below.

Immediate Functional Accommodations

Goal 1: Toileting

It was determined that Jeff tended to urinate and have bowel movements on a regular schedule and was noted to retreat to a quiet spot when he needed to go. The bathroom in Jeff's house was drafty and located off the kitchen, far from Jeff's playroom. The toilet was older and rocked a bit and sprayed water when flushed. The cold bathroom, unstable toilet, spraying water, combined with a loud flushing noise was too much for Jeff's over-responsive sensory system. When this was pointed out to Jeff's family, they immediately installed a supplemental heater in front of the toilet. Other simple changes included fixing the toilet; the rocking, the spraying water, and reducing the noise level. During the next week, Jeff wore little clothing in the house and spent five minutes each hour sitting on a potty seat in the hallway outside of the bathroom. Jeff tried several styles of underpants before finding a style that felt right (tight, cotton knit, boxer briefs with a covered elastic waist band). Gradually, the potty seat was moved into the bathroom; at that time, Jeff agreed to transition to the regular toilet as long as it was flushed after he left the room. Jeff's day care provider agreed to allow Jeff to use the potty seat in her bathroom until he was ready to use the regular toilet.

Lifestyle Accommodations

Goal 2: Clothing

Jeff had only two items of clothing that he would willingly wear so they needed to be washed nightly. Jeff's mother purchased several shirts and pairs of sweatpants that were identical to those he wore and washed them several times before presenting them to Jeff. The new items were placed on top of Jeff's dresser where he could see them for several days before being asked to wear them. During that time, Jeff's mother varied the placement of his preferred shirt and pants within the stack so that Jeff had to see and touch the new items every day. By the end of the week, Jeff was spontaneously selecting the top item in the stack, whether old or new. As Jeff was much less resistant to getting dressed later in the day than he was first thing in the morning, he put on clean underwear and clothes before going to bed each night. When he woke in the morning, he was already dressed so that one daily stress was eliminated.

Goal 3: Family Relationships and Physical Affection

Jeff's sensory hyperresponsivity caused him to be exquisitely sensitive to sounds, smells, textures, and movement; all components of social interactions. While the ride to his grandparent's house was short, Jeff often felt queasy when he got there. Both of his grandparents met the family at the door of their compact bungalow to greet everyone and help bring in all the bundles, which parents of small children travel with. Jeff's grandmother was a great cook and usually had something special on the stove or in the oven. His grandfather worked irregular hours as a substitute bus driver and usually postponed shaving until just before he left for work.

When Jeff yelled, "no kisses!" as soon as the front door opened, his grandparents were confused and crushed. Jeff really loved his grandparents, but the immediate tidal wave of sensations, cooking smells/bustling bodies in a small space/everyone talking at once/scratchy faces immediately, overloaded his fragile system, and he instinctively moved away, physically and emotionally. Once the concept of a tidal wave of sensations was explained to Jeff's parents and grandparents, they were able to implement a few simple changes to reduce Jeff's stress level. Jeff's grandmother tried to do her cooking the day before the family arrived and have only Jeff's favorite sugar cookies in the oven when they arrived. His grandparents greeted the family outside where there was more space, and Jeff was assisted out of his car seat by his father after the rest of the family had gone inside. Jeff carried his own backpack, which had been weighted down with bottles of water. When they reached the house, the rest of the family was settled in, and Jeff was able to accept a firm side to side hug from each of his grandparents.

Goal 4: No Dogs in the Bed

As an infant, Jeff could usually be found wedged into a corner of his crib in the morning, and he continues to seek out small confined spaces to relax in. He needs close physical boundaries when resting to supplement the less intense vestibular and proprioceptive input received while he slept, and the family dogs provided that input at home. Jeff's parents reported that he often had difficulty sleeping away from home and had noticed that the aging dogs were having increased difficulty getting onto the bed. After moving Jeff's bed against the wall in a corner of his room, a few small changes created a "nest in a bed" that Jeff snuggled right into (From the Field 28.2).

The family dogs were given similar beds, placed on the floor next to his bed.

Direct Intervention

During weekly individual intervention sessions, Jeff's OT used a variety of intervention techniques to improve his ability to process vestibular input (movement), decrease his sensory sensitivity, and support his ability to manage the stress of transitioning between activities and settings. His OT created a picture-based schedule for each intervention session so that Jeff would know what he would be doing and what would come next and created a similar system for home and school. Each intervention session began and ended with the same activities, designed to support his sensory modulation abilities. Home program suggestions were modeled first in therapy, and his OT reviewed Jeff's progress each week with his family.

> **FROM THE FIELD 28.2**
>
> **Making a Nest**
>
> Some people feel exposed and disoriented when sleeping in a large bed. A "nest" can be created using one or two long "body pillows" and a stretchy fitted bottom sheet. Place the pillows in an oval on the mattress, preferably near the wall, stretch the sheet over the top, and make the bed as usual. You have now made a cozy nest to snuggle into that will gradually mold to the shape of the person sleeping in it.

Expected Intervention Outcomes

Occupational therapy intervention is not expected to "cure" SPD. Evidence-based research in support of the proposition that sensory-based intervention techniques produce measurable improvements in a client's ability to process sensory input is, at present, inconclusive. There is, however, strong evidence that sensory integrative–based occupational therapy intervention does result in measurable and lasting improvement in functional performance and independence when it is provided for a sufficient amount of time and includes the application of multiple forms of sensory input tailored to meet the needs of the client (Case-Smith & Bryan, 1999; Fazlioglu & Baran, 2008; Linderman & Stewart, 1999; Watling et al., 2011).

As previously discussed, occupational therapy goals, objectives, and intervention plans for individuals with SPD should focus on improving functional performance. In addition to achievement of individual intervention objectives and resolution of the issues that initiated occupational therapy services, improvements in the following areas of occupational performance are often observed:

- Ability to self-regulate
- Motor control
- Family and relationship stress
- Self-confidence and self-esteem
- Occupational engagement and social participation (Fig. 28.5)

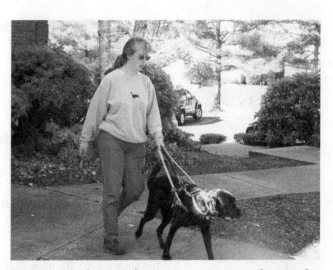

Figure 28.5 Kathy's visual overresponsivity causes her visual system to shut down in bright light; therefore, she wears tinted lenses at all times and travels with her service dog.

Summary

Sensory integration theory and SPD have traditionally been linked almost exclusively to children; however, research and clinical experience have broadened our understanding of this disorder as a neurologically based condition that persists throughout life. We now know that atypical responses to sensory input can be identified in individuals of any age and life stage. We also know that atypical responses to sensory input are often present in individuals with mental health diagnoses, many medical conditions, and some genetic syndromes. No matter the practice setting, a basic understanding of sensory integration theory and identification and SPD will assist all OTAs to gain additional insight into the children, adolescents, adults, and elders that they work with. Gaining the specialized skills to work with those with SPD is well worth the effort.

Review Questions

1. You are a sensory seeker. Which of the following activities do you avoid?
   a. Flower arranging
   b. Bungee jumping
   c. Yoga
   d. Walking barefoot

2. Which of the following senses helps you to know where your feet are in the dark?
   a. Vision
   b. Interoception
   c. Proprioception
   d. Touch

3. Which sense do we have to be taught to interpret?
   a. Gustatory
   b. Interoception
   c. Vision
   d. Auditory

4. Which diagnosis is not associated with sensory processing difficulties?
   a. Cerebral palsy
   b. Fragile X syndrome
   c. ADHD
   d. Schizophrenia

5. If you have difficulty with tactile discrimination, which task will you find most difficult to do?
   a. Thread your belt through all of your belt loops.
   b. Find a quarter in a pocket full of change.
   c. Tie your shoes tightly.
   d. All of the above.

6. The older we get, the more likely we are to:
   a. Lose our balance in the dark
   b. Be bothered less and less by itchy clothes
   c. Find food to be less flavorful
   d. Enjoy new things

7. Our vestibular sense processes:
   a. Motion
   b. Gravity
   c. Speed
   d. All of the above
   e. None of the above

8. Which is not a type of sensory modulation disorder?
   a. Sensory craving
   b. Sensory integration
   c. Sensory overresponsivity
   d. Sensory underresponsivity

9. Which is NOT an expected outcome SPD intervention?
   a. Improved attention
   b. Increased independence with ADLs
   c. Reduced irritability
   d. Improved coordination

10. Which is the current correct term used to refer to the condition characterized by atypical responses to sensory input?
    a. Sensory integration disorder
    b. Sensory processing dysfunction
    c. Disorder of sensory integration
    d. Sensory processing disorder

11. Which is NOT an appropriate goal for an individual with SPD?
    a. Will transition from home to car without tantrums
    b. Will improve ability to process vestibular input by 25%
    c. While seated in a chair will bend over to tie shoelaces without dizziness or loss of balance
    d. Will not gag when a new food is placed on dinner plate

Practice Activities

You work in a skilled nursing facility. Nursing has noticed that your newest client is unresponsive and only picks at her food and has lost 2 lb since admission 3 days ago. Think of five to seven questions to ask this woman's daughter that will give you a better understanding of her sensory-based mealtime preferences.

You work in an elementary school. A first grade teacher has noticed that even though "live wire" Jason gets lots of exercise during recess, he still has trouble sitting quietly for story time after recess. Think of two or three simple things that she can do to help Jason settle down more quickly.

Think about the people in your family. Do any of them seem to react differently to noise, movement, smells, color, texture, or taste than you do? Do any of these differences affect how they live their lives? How?

References

Ahn R, et al. Prevalence of parents' perceptions of sensory processing disorders among kindergarten children. *Am J Occup Ther* 2004;58(3):287–302.

Anazalone M, et al. Defining sensory processing disorder and its subtypes: position statement on terminology related to sensory integration dysfunction. *S I Focus* 2004:6–8.

Anazalone M, et al. Concept evolution in sensory integration: a proposed nosology for diagnosis. *Am J Occup Ther* 2007;61(2):135–140.

Ayers A. *Sensory Integration and Praxis Tests: Manual*. Los Angeles, CA: Western Psychological Services; 1989.

Ayres AJ. *Sensory Integration and the Child*. Los Angeles, CA: Western Psychological Services; 1979.

Baranek G, et al. Sensory processing correlates of occupational performance in children with fragile X syndrome. *Am J Occup Ther* 2002;56(5):538–546.

Bundy A, et al. *Sensory Integration Theory and Practice*. 2nd ed. Philadelphia, PA: F. A. Davis Company; 2002.

Case-Smith J, Bryan T. The effects of occupational therapy with sensory integration emphasis on preschool age children with autism. *Am J Occup Ther* 1999;53:489–497.

Cheung P, Siu A. A comparison of patterns of sensory processing in children with and without developmental disabilities. *Res Dev Disabil* 2009;30(6):1468–1480.

DeGangi G, Berk R. *Degangi-Berk Test of Sensory Integration*. Los Angeles, CA: Western Psychological Services; 1983.

Dunn W. *The Sensory Profile User's Manual*. San Antonio, TX: The Psychological Corporation; 1999.

Dunn W. The sensations of everyday life: empirical, theoretical, and pragmatic considerations. *Am J Occup Ther* 2001;55:608–620.

Dunn W. *Living Sensationally: Understanding Your Senses*. Philadelphia, PA: Jessica Kingsley Publishers; 2008.

Fazlioglu Y, Baran G. A sensory integration therapy program on sensory problems for children with autism. *Percept Mot Skills* 2008;106:415–422.

Hender K. *Effectiveness of Sensory Integration Therapy for Attention Deficit Hyperactivity Disorder (ADHD)*. Victoria, Australia: Centre for Clinical Effectiveness, Monash Medical Centre; 2001.

Heuler M, et al. Sensory overresponsivity: prenatal risk factors and temperamental contributions. *J Dev Behav Pediatr* 2011;32(7):533–541.

Lane S, et al. Toward a consensus in terminology in sensory integration theory and practice: part 2: sensory integration patterns of function and dysfunction. *Sens Integration Spec Interest Sect Q* 2000;23(1):1–3.

Lin S, et al. The relationship between the length of institutionalization and sensory integration in children adopted from Easter Europe. *Am J Occup Ther* 2002;59(2):139–147.

Linderman T, Stewart K. Sensory integrative based occupational therapy and functional outcomes in young children with pervasive developmental disorders: a single subject study. *Am J Occup Ther* 1999;53:207–213.

May-Benson T, et al. Creating a consensus on terminology in sensory integration: comments and reflections. *Sens Integration Spec Interest Sect Q* 2000:1–3.

May-Benson T, et al. Incidence of pre-, peri-, and post-natal birth and developmental problems of children with sensory processing disorder and children with autism spectrum disorder. *Front Integr Neurosci* 2009;3(13):1–12.

Miller LJ. *Sensational Kids: Hope and Help for Children with Sensory Processing Disorder (SPD)*. New York, NY: The Penguin Group; 2006.

Parham L, Ecker C. *Sensory Processing Measure (SPM) Manual*. Los Angeles, CA: Western Psychological Services; 2007.

Reynolds S, Lane S. Diagnostic validity of sensory over-responsivity: a review of literature and case reports. *J Autism Dev Disord* 2008;38(3):516–529.

Watling R, et al. *Occupational Therapy Practice Guidelines for Children and Adolescents with Sensory Processing and Sensory Integration Challenges*. Bethesda, MD: AOTA Press; 2011.

White F, et al. An examination of the relationships between motor and process skills and scores on the Sensory Profile. *Am J Occup Ther* 2007;61(2):154–160.

CHAPTER 29

Psychiatric Conditions

Scott A. Trudeau, PhD, OTR/L

Key Terms

Delusions—Cognitive distortions that lead the client to believe in facts that are not real and can take on a variety of characteristics such as grandiose, religious, paranoid, or persecutory depending upon the content of the beliefs not likely to improve with reality testing and orientation.

Depressive episode—Defined by some configuration of the following depressive symptoms: feeling unhappy, sad, or blue; insomnia; anxiety; hopelessness; despair; irritability; feeling worthless; poor concentration and slowed mentation; preoccupation with death, dying, or suicide; feeling tired and fatigued; decreased libido (sex drive), changes in appetite; and unexplained physical symptoms (e.g., pain).

Differential diagnosis—A process of first eliminating all possible explanations for a client's symptom configuration before settling on a psychiatric diagnosis.

Disposition planning—The plan for continuing health care of a patient following discharge from a given health care facility.

Duration—Refers to an amount of time.

Hallucinations—Sensory experiences that are not linked to an actual stimulus and may be experienced along any sensory pathway auditory, visual, tactile, olfactory, or gustatory.

Intensity—The strength or severity of (with regard to this textbook) the presenting symptom(s).

Manic episode—A period of predominant mood elevation, expansiveness, or irritation. These episodes are paired together with some combination of hyperarousal and diminished sleep, heightened self-esteem or grandiosity, talkativeness, flight of ideas, distractibility and poor concentration, hyperactivity, sexual promiscuity and possible unsafe sex practices, and impulsivity and recklessness.

Negative symptoms—Withdrawal of a trait that would normally be present such as when a range of affective states is replaced with flat affect.

Panic attack—A discrete period in which there is the sudden onset of intense fear or terror.

Positive symptoms—When describing behaviors associated with a psychotic disorder, "positive symptoms" are the addition of a symptom(s) such as hallucinations or delusions.

Psychotic symptoms—Signs or behaviors that a client is experiencing disruption of thought processes such that the individual may not maintain a complete connection with reality.

Serious mental illness—Classes of illness that are most intense and persistent in their presentation, resulting in often chronic impairment of functional performance.

Therapeutic milieu—The structure within a mental health unit that ensures patient safety, fosters agency, and enhances cohesion of the community.

Learning Objectives

After studying this chapter, readers should be able to:

- Describe the current contextual factors influencing the care of persons with serious mental illness.
- Delineate diagnostic considerations of frequently encountered clinical presentations.
- Articulate general theoretical considerations underpinning occupational therapy intervention strategies.
- Provide a rationale for occupational therapy provision in mental health settings.

Introduction

Mental health care delivery has evolved and changed significantly in the past few decades. These changes have directly impacted the practice of occupational therapy in mental health settings. We begin this chapter with an exploration of contextual factors that influence the provision of care to individuals with serious mental illness. Medical–legal and reimbursement considerations weigh prominent in this discussion. We then look at the structure of the treatment setting and the important role that occupational therapy practitioners play in the interdisciplinary team approach to treatment. We conclude with an overview of common diagnostic presentations that are experienced by clients seeking mental health treatment.

Contextual Factors

Mental illness is currently identified by the World Health Organization (WHO, 2011) as a leading cause of disability worldwide and is predicted to remain so well into the future. The American Occupational Therapy Association (AOTA, 2006) echoes this priority in the *Centennial Vision*, identifying mental health as an essential area for future practice. Future occupational therapy practice will need to emphasize mental health treatment and prevention services for children, youth, adults, and older adults while continuing to address the needs of individuals with severe and persistent mental illness. In spite of the renewed emphasis on mental health needs and the practice of occupational therapy, the recent AOTA *Workforce and Compensation Survey of the Profession* (AOTA, 2010b) reports that only 3% of practitioners identify their primary practice setting as mental health. It is a huge hurdle for our profession to attract competent providers to this practice area in order to continue to meet the needs of the population and maintain occupational therapy's professional role in mental health care. Please refer to Chapter 36, *Mental Health Practice Settings*, for further information about specific venues in which occupational therapy practitioners work with clients with mental health conditions.

The health care delivery system for people with **serious mental illness** is changing. The core of the mental health system in the United States is grounded in what is known as the diagnostic classification system. Since the 1950s, the American Psychiatric Association (APA) has published the *Diagnostic Statistical Manual of Mental Disorders (DSM)*, which has been used to standardize the criteria sets used to define psychiatric conditions. Currently in the fifth edition, the *DSM-5* (APA, 2013) describes the key symptoms that are characteristic of each diagnosis. Please note that the commonly known acronym, *DSM*, will be used to describe this book throughout the chapter. The *DSM* allows for a process of **differential diagnosis**, first eliminating all possible explanations for the symptom configuration before settling on a psychiatric diagnosis(From the Field 29.1).

Occupational therapy practitioners do not make diagnoses, but understanding the diagnostic categories in the *DSM* is important for client-centered mental health practice. Our observations of client behaviors will be an important contribution to the interdisciplinary diagnostic process. It is critical to appreciate that differential diagnosis is not an exact science; we cannot take an MRI of someone's psyche and apply a diagnosis. As such, the *DSM* is at times vulnerable to influence from political and social pressures. In fact, the current revision of the *DSM* has already been met with much debate and drawn criticisms for the changes that were implemented, including the way autism spectrum disorders are classified. Another example of this is in the history of classifying homosexuality as a disorder from the first edition of the *DSM* until it was removed in 1987. As social acceptance of gay and lesbian individuals

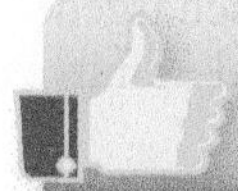

FROM THE FIELD 29.1

Differential Diagnosis

One common example of the differential diagnostic process involves an older adult being admitted through the emergency room (ER) of an acute general hospital because of an acute change in mental status. The individual might be highly confused and agitated. There may be evidence of acute psychosis with visual hallucinations and paranoia. This presentation may be explainable in someone with chronic serious mental illness, but this elder does not reveal that history. The medical workup ensues, and it is later determined that this state of delirium was caused by a urinary tract infection (UTI) and consequent dehydration. Without careful history taking and comprehensive medical workup, this could easily have been diagnosed incorrectly as a psychiatric disorder.

increased, social and political pressure were applied to declassify this sexual orientation as being pathological. One of the reasons for social and political lobbying for classification of mental disorders has to do with reimbursement structures. As the basis for classification of mental disorders, the *DSM* also serves as a source of codes used for billing for treatment. For example, there was a significant lobbying effort to get Alzheimer disease included in the *DSM* so that there would be enhanced reimbursement for treatment of this diagnosis.

The *DSM* outlines the classification system that is used in most clinical settings serving clients with mental illness (APA, 2013). The foundation of this system rests in a nonaxial documentation system of disorders with separate notation systems for psychosocial and contextual factors and for disability (APA, 2013). The diagnostic disorder categories are as follows:

- Neurodevelopmental disorders (e.g., intellectual disability, autism spectrum disorder, and attention deficit disorder)
- Schizophrenia spectrum and other psychotic disorders
- Bipolar and related disorders
- Depressive disorders
- Anxiety disorders
- Obsessive–compulsive and related disorders
- Trauma- and stressor-related disorders
- Dissociative disorders
- Somatic symptom and related disorders
- Feeding and eating disorders
- Elimination disorders
- Sleep–wake disorders
- Sexual dysfunctions
- Gender dysphoria
- Disruptive, impulse–control, and conduct disorders
- Substance-related and addictive disorders
- Neurocognitive disorders
- Personality disorders
- Paraphilic disorders
- Other mental disorders
- Medication-induced movement disorders and other adverse effects of medication
- Other conditions that may be a focus of clinical attention

It is useful to understand the previous *DSM-IV* framework of a multiaxial system, although this system is not a part of the *DSM-5*. Some practitioners may continue to organize their thoughts regarding treatment based on the five-axis system of the *DSM-IV*. The multiaxial system of the *DSM-IV* includes five areas for diagnostic consideration. These are as follows:

Axis I: Primary psychiatric condition—major mental disorder
Examples include anxiety disorders, mood disorders, dissociative disorders, substance-related disorders, attention deficit hyperactivity disorder, schizophrenia, sexual and gender identity issues, and eating disorders.

Axis II: Personality disorders and mental retardation
Examples include paranoid personality disorders, antisocial personality disorder, narcissistic personality disorder, borderline personality disorder, and dependent personality disorder.

Axis III: Contributory general medical conditions
Examples include infectious and parasitic diseases, endocrine, nutritional, metabolic, immune diseases, brain injuries, diseases of the nervous system and sense organs, and congenital abnormalities.

Axis IV: Psychosocial and environmental stressors
Examples include problems with a primary support group, problems related to social environment, educational problems, occupational problems, and housing or other economic problems.

Axis V: Global Assessment of Function (GAF) Score (APA, 2000)

The purpose of a multiaxial system of mental health diagnoses is to provide a consistent format for noting an overview of a client's clinical condition; however, the *DSM-5* (APA, 2013) captures this information in a different format to address an individual's mental health diagnosis. The *DSM-5* (APA, 2013), a nonaxial system, includes information from Axes I to III as a part of the general medical condition. Important psychosocial and contextual factors (Axis IV) and disability (Axis V) are noted separately from the diagnoses.

This nonaxial system was adopted to highlight the separation between diagnosis and functional status as it is reflected by the World Health Organization (WHO) and the International Classification of Diseases (ICD) (APA, 2013).

Diagnostic-Related Groups

As managed care has become universal across our health care system, psychiatric services are now subject to payment constraints. When diagnostic-related groups (DRGs) were first defined for managed care purposes, mental health was exempt. Insurance companies were reluctant to apply DRGs to mental health diagnoses. Instead, they had indemnity insurance plans where there would be relatively complete reimbursement for services. Eventually, behavioral health management companies proposed that they could develop a workable model of DRGs for psychiatric conditions and now often subcontract to manage mental health benefits for larger insurance providers. Typically, this model includes a preauthorization requirement, thus raising the bar in terms of who can access mental health care. One must be sicker in order to access care, and yet care delivery for this sicker population has to be more expedient. An insurance company typically authorizes a set number of days for mental health treatment based on the admission evaluation. This number of days can later be extended through a process of concurrent review. The insurance company closely monitors progress and client status as the treatment proceeds.

There are psychogeriatric and medical psychiatric wards where clients can be admitted to address the complexity of conditions with which they may present. To that end, insurance constraints have resulted in significantly decreased inpatient hospital admission rates and decreased lengths of stay. As the health care system has become increasingly length-of-stay oriented, providing access to and the quality of mental health care remain important priorities to respond to. One of the consequences of making access to mental health services difficult is increased criminal activity. People who are mentally unwell are left in crisis to the point where they may engage in behaviors that lead to arrests and incarceration. This creates a burden on prisons, which now house many mental health treatment programs.

Committing Clients

There are three types of psychiatric admission statuses:

1. Involuntary—legally committed to stay in the institution against one's will.
2. Conditional voluntary—an individual has agreed to a voluntary admission. If this person no longer wishes to stay in the institution, 72 hours' notice to the treatment team must be provided. The team then considers whether the individual can be discharged or whether he/she needs to be committed and admitted on an involuntary basis.
3. Voluntary—an individual may leave any time. This is very unusual, as people unwell enough to access mental health care are unlikely to be voluntary admits.

In order to be committed to a psychiatric institution against his/her will, a person must be an imminent danger to himself/herself or someone else (Fowler, 2012). This threat needs to be real and immediate. In order for a threat to be imminent, both means and motivation must be present. When considering the potential threat to others, practitioners must be aware of Tarasoff's law: the right to confidentiality ends when the public peril begins (Costa & Altekruse, 1994; Ewing, 2005; Sonne, 2012; Tarasoff, 1976). Despite restrictions related to confidentiality, when a third party is at risk, the professional working with the client presenting with serious mental health issues has a legal obligation to notify the party at risk as well as the police. Police are trained to assess potential mental health crises and have the right to transport individuals for a psychiatric assessment. At this stage, an assessment is done by a psychiatrist, who determines whether commitment is necessary. While OT practitioners may be involved in beginning the commitment process based on direct contact with a client, OTs are not solely responsible to make the determination whether that client is to be committed.

Milieu Therapy Approach

As has been discussed, the function of inpatient mental health units is evolving. Increasingly, people with acute and severe mental illness are admitted to inpatient units for short periods of intense treatment and are then quickly discharged to community-based care. This has resulted in a disparaging saying that mental health care is "sicker and quicker." Currently, reduced average lengths of inpatient stay for clients challenges the historical conceptualizations of the therapeutic milieu.

Milieu is a French word meaning ambience or atmosphere. In the *therapeutic* setting, it describes a concept where everything that happens within the clinical setting has the need and potential to become part of the client's therapy (Mahoney et al., 2009; Walker, 1994). Thus, the milieu must be structured with the right mix of people (staff and clients), inanimate objects (the physical setting), and opportunities for meaningful activity engagement (what OT practitioners consider as occupation). Regardless of any psychiatric diagnosis, all clients in mental health treatment settings are there for one primary reason: they are out of control. As we consider the needs of the population served, the primary demand placed on the **therapeutic milieu** is structure. Most therapeutic milieus are organized around a tightly structured schedule of treatment groups as outlined in Figure 29.1.

Sample Therapeutic Milieu Schedule

	Sunday	Monday	Tuesday	Wednesday	Thursday	Friday	Saturday
8-9 am	Community Meeting – all attend, please be properly dressed (no pajamas)						
9-10 am	Work discussion	Parenting group	Older adults	Meal planning group	Work discussion	Managing leisure	Leisure exploration
10-11 am	Plant group	Medication group	Nutrition group	Plant group	Healthy life styles	Medication group	Community outing
11-12 am	Meeting with MDs and/or primary therapist						
12-1 pm	Lunch and Free Time						
1-3 pm	Occupational Therapy Task Group						
3-4 pm	Intro to cognitive behavioral therapy	Substance abuse group	Options group	Intro to cognitive behavioral therapy	Substance abuse group	Cognitive behavioral therapy triggers	Recreation group
4-6 pm	Dinner/personal time						
6-7 pm	Music group	Life skills	Recovery group	Life skills	Community meal prepartion	Life skills	Movie group
7-8 pm	Stress management group						
8-9 pm	Community Meeting – all attend, please be properly dressed (no pajamas)						

Figure 29.1 Sample therapeutic milieu schedule.

Occupational therapy practitioners often make a direct contribution to defining and providing the structure within the milieu, seeking to promote a healthy and balanced diet of occupational opportunity. It is important to appreciate that adult clients do not always welcome this level of structure. The care staff often walks a delicate balancing act of supporting the structure of the milieu without being demeaning or infantilizing to the clients.

Thibeault et al. (2010) described this tension in a qualitative study that explored client perspectives of the milieu with people admitted to an acute psychiatric unit. The study revealed a profound tension between structure and therapeutic need: describing client experiences as rule bound, controlling, and sometimes oppressive while also noting client experiences of healing and health within that same milieu. Despite seemingly opposite interpretations, the authors suggested that the inpatient psychiatric milieu remains an important but often neglected component of psychiatric treatment.

A critical concept to understand in mental health practice is the role of OT practitioners within the therapeutic milieu. Similar to the tension experienced by the inpatients described above, OT practitioners often experience tension between being a unique discipline within the milieu and functioning as a generic milieu therapist. It could be argued that OT practitioners must advocate for and fill both roles. Occupational therapy has a unique contribution to make to the therapeutic milieu. Finding the balance between being well integrated and accepted as an integral member of the interdisciplinary milieu treatment team is a challenge that OT practitioners working in mental health practice face.

The Therapeutic Team

Ideally, OT practitioners function in mental health care as members of an interdisciplinary team in which team members work closely together toward shared goals. Depending upon the nature of the care setting, the configuration of the team may differ slightly based on the acuity of the clients. Typically, the more acute the setting, the higher the concentration of practitioners with advanced degrees. The following role descriptions provide an overview of potential team members and their unique contributions to the typical provision of care in a variety of mental health settings:

1. Psychiatrist: Has completed full medical training and a residency specializing in psychiatry. The psychiatrist is likely to lead the interdisciplinary team in client care, is responsible for admitting and discharging clients from inpatient hospital care, prescribes and monitors medication use, and may perform 1:1 or group psychotherapy.
2. Registered nurse (RN): Coordinates the day-to-day care of clients, carries out MD orders for medication and other treatments, administers medications, evaluates clients and the effects of treatment interventions, and may perform 1:1 or group psychotherapy.

In some settings, advanced practice registered nurses (APRN) or nurse practitioners (NP) provide care that blends the role of the psychiatrist and the RN.

3. Licensed practical nurse (LPN): may administer medications and treatments as prescribed but relies on the RN for in-depth evaluation of client status and responses to treatments.
4. Nurse's aide (may also be called milieu counselor): This paraprofessional role may carry out basic care activities and collect vital signs, lead both formal and informal groups within the milieu, and provide 1:1 support to clients.
5. Social worker: Assesses the social networks of clients that either support or hinder optimal mental health. This often involves direct assessment of family dynamics and community resource linkages, which are critical for **disposition planning**.
6. Occupational therapy practitioner: The OT and OTA partnership is typically directly involved in establishing the structure of the milieu program. Occupational therapy practitioners lead groups and use the daily structure of activities to both assess the clients' functional status and practice the skills necessary to progress to the next level of care. This perspective is essential to the team and to working with social workers for effective disposition planning.

Caring for clients is a high priority, but as an OT practitioner, one's own self-care is equally as important. In mental health, care can be especially challenging to a practitioner's personal and emotional well-being. The personal burden is lessened when it is shared across multiple team members (Rossen et al., 2008).

Mental Health and the Law

Medical records are legal documents that can be subpoenaed into the court system (please refer to Chapter 14, *Documentation*). This means that anything written in a client's medical record can be subpoenaed. This potentially creates a conflict between the professional Code of Ethics (AOTA, 2015) principle of nonmaleficence in which OT practitioners refrain from intentionally inflicting harm on a client and documentation requirements. Clients often have complicated social and family circumstances that might also include legal entanglements. For example, if a client was involved in custodial proceedings and you had documented negative comments about his/her parenting skills, these comments could be held against him/her if the medical record were called into court. Given the nature of mental health practice, there is increased likelihood of medical records being called in as evidence in court proceedings associated with care. Occupational therapy practitioners would do well to be very thorough and thoughtful with documentation to protect both clients and the practitioners themselves (refer to Chapter 14 *Documentation*).

An Overview of Clinical Presentations

As you may recall, psychiatric disorders are determined through a process of differential diagnosis based on the criteria defined in the most current edition of the *DSM*. Despite the fact that OT practitioners do not diagnose, it is important to review a copy of the most updated version of the *DSM* and become familiar with its content. In your work with clients with mental health conditions, this enables you to be as knowledgeable as possible about the symptoms associated with the conditions. Two considerations that permeate most diagnostic criteria sets in the *DSM* are intensity and duration. **Intensity** is considered by the determination of the strength or severity of the presenting symptom(s). **Duration** refers to the amount of time that the symptoms persist. For instance, while it may be considered normal (not pathological) to grieve over the major loss of a spouse in the weeks after her/his death, it may be considered illness if the same symptoms remain intense and persist over several months. Thus, diagnoses represent a composite of not just the symptoms, but the quality and the length of time the symptoms present and the severity of those symptoms.

Psychotic Disorders

It is important for OT practitioners to have a working vocabulary that allows for accurate reporting of and description of symptoms, no matter the practice area. The most intense symptoms that people with serious mental illness present are called **psychotic symptoms**. Psychotic refers to the disruption of thought processes such that an individual may not maintain a complete connection with reality. Clients who are considered thought disordered typically present with symptoms of hallucinations and/or delusions. **Hallucinations** are sensory experiences that are not linked to an actual stimulus. Thus, an individual may experience hallucinations along any sensory pathway (auditory, visual, tactile, olfactory, or gustatory). **Delusions** are cognitive distortions in which the client believes facts that are not real. Depending upon the content of the beliefs, delusions can take on a variety of characteristics (e.g., grandiose, religious, paranoid, persecutory). It is important to note that these symptoms are involuntary and are unlikely to respond to reality testing and orientation.

All of the diagnostic descriptions we will discuss for the remainder of this chapter are based on what can be found in the *DSM-5*. The first set of disorders or diagnoses has psychosis as the hallmark symptom. There are several types of psychotic disorders. When most people think of someone with serious mental illness, they probably picture someone diagnosed with a psychotic disorder. Symptoms of psychotic disorders are often categorized as either positive or negative. **Positive symptoms** refer to the addition of a symptom(s) such as hallucinations or delusions. **Negative symptoms** are manifested by the withdrawal of a trait that would normally be present, such as when a range of affective states or emotions is replaced with flat affect. Positive symptoms tend to respond better to pharmacological interventions than negative symptoms. Negative symptoms tend to limit an individual's ability to function and get along day to day and, in some ways, may be more disabling than positive symptoms. Generally speaking, most psychotic disorders tend to be chronic forms of mental illness that limit social and occupational function across the life span.

Schizophrenia is the most common psychotic disorder. Symptoms of schizophrenia last for at least six months (duration) and include at least one month in an active phase (intensity). During an active phase, an individual experiences two or more of the following:

- Delusions
- Hallucinations
- Disorganized speech
- Grossly disorganized or catatonic behavior
- Negative symptoms

Each of these symptoms is described in terms of severity, and symptoms can be present in varying degrees for an individual (e.g., schizophrenia with moderate hallucinations and mild paranoia). Both occupational and social functions are significantly impaired with all types of schizophrenia.

Within the classification of psychotic disorders, there are a number of diagnoses that are not as common as schizophrenia. *Schizophreniform disorder* has a similar symptomatic presentation to schizophrenia; however, its duration only lasts from 1 to 6 months and chronic functional decline is not as pronounced. In *schizoaffective disorder*, the active-phase psychotic symptoms are similar to schizophrenia and include significant changes in mood and are preceded or are followed by at least 2 weeks of psychotic symptoms with mood changes. *Delusional disorder* is characterized by at least 1 month of delusions without other active-phase symptoms of schizophrenia, whereas *brief psychotic disorder* is a disorder that lasts more than 1 day and remits by 1 month.

All causes of symptoms must be considered for each class, since some disorders may be attributable to either medical conditions or chemically induced. In *psychotic disorder due to another medical condition*, the psychotic symptoms are determined to be the direct physiological consequence of a general medical condition. For instance, a patient with lung cancer with

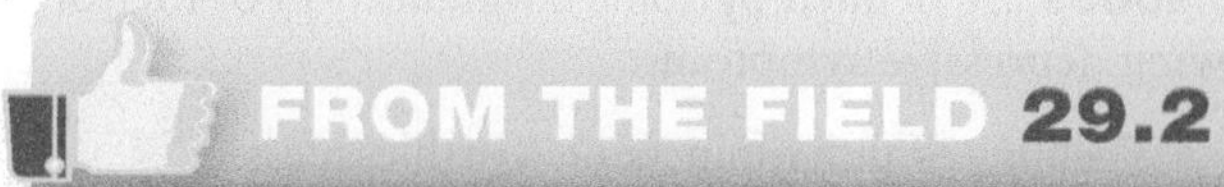

FROM THE FIELD 29.2

Complexity of Schizophrenia

The process of differential diagnosis is complicated for most psychiatric disorders but is perhaps the most complex in confirming a diagnosis of schizophrenia. This is at least in part due to the variability of symptom presentation from one individual to the next. Additionally though, it is of great consequence to the individual to receive the diagnosis of a chronic serious mental illness like schizophrenia. The interdisciplinary team must take this responsibility very seriously. I recall vividly a case when I was a recent graduate and a new OTR practicing in an acute psychiatric inpatient unit. A 19-year-old man was admitted to our unit for decompensating around fall semester midterm exam period of his sophomore year in college at a local university. The team worked diligently over the course of three or four hospital admissions to ensure that his symptoms were not accounted for by substance use/abuse, medical conditions, depressive disorder with psychotic features, or bipolar disorder with psychotic features. Finally, he received the diagnosis of schizophrenia.

metastases to the brain may experience prominent and severe psychotic symptoms due to his/her medical diagnosis. In *substance-/medication-induced psychotic disorder*, the psychotic symptoms are determined to be the direct consequence of intoxication by a drug of abuse, medication, or toxin exposure. Given that differential diagnosis is not an exact science, each diagnostic set in the *DSM* includes the categories of "unspecified" and "other specified" to capture any related disorder that does not fully satisfy the diagnostic criteria of a specific disorder. *Unspecified schizophrenia* is included for classifying psychotic presentations that do not fully fit the operational definitions of other specific psychotic disorders (From the Field 29.2)

Depressive Disorders

Like psychotic disorders, mood disorder diagnoses are based on the duration and intensity of a given presentation. It is a natural part of the human condition to experience a bad mood once in a while, but not all bad moods are diagnosable. The hallmark symptoms of interest in this category are the presence of either depressive or manic episodes. While there are always individual differences in how a client presents, **depressive**

episodes are defined by some configuration of the following depressive symptoms:

- Feelings of unhappiness or worthlessness
- Insomnia
- Anxiety
- Hopelessness
- Despair
- Irritability
- Poor concentration and slowed mentation
- Preoccupation with death, dying, or suicide
- Feelings of fatigue, decreased libido (sex drive)
- Changes in appetite
- Unexplained physical symptoms such as pain

It should be noted that it is possible for someone to also experience psychotic symptoms as part of the presentation of mood disorder, but the affective state is the hallmark symptom of the presentation.

Diagnoses falling into the depressive disorders category are marked by depressive episodes of varying intensities and durations. *Major depressive disorder* includes at least 2 weeks of depressed mood or loss of interest accompanied by at least four additional symptoms of depression from the above list. *Persistent depressive disorder* is less intense or severe than major depression but with a much longer duration of at least 2 years of depressed mood for more days than not. *Unspecified depressive disorder* is included for coding disorders with depressive features that do not meet criteria for major depressive disorder or persistent depressive disorder. Added to the *DSM-5* is *premenstrual dysphoric disorder*, which is a diagnosis that is given when a female experiences extreme mood fluctuations, irritability, dysphoria, and anxiety symptoms during the premenstrual phase of the menstrual cycle. Additionally, *disruptive mood dysregulation disorder* is a diagnosis given to children under the age of 12 who present with persistent, intense irritability.

Bipolar and Related Disorders

The *bipolar disorders* involve the presence (or history) of manic episodes, usually accompanied by the presence (or history) of depressive episodes. While a depressive episode features a sad mood, a **manic episode** consists of a period of predominant mood elevation, expansiveness, or irritation. Manic episodes are paired with some combination of the following:

- Hyperarousal and diminished sleep
- Heightened self-esteem or grandiosity
- Talkativeness
- Flight of ideas
- Distractibility and poor concentration
- Hyperactivity
- Sexual promiscuity and possible unsafe sex practices
- Impulsivity and recklessness

Similarly, there may also be psychotic features associated with a manic episode.

Bipolar I disorder is characterized by one or more manic episodes, usually accompanied by major depressive episodes. *Bipolar II disorder* is characterized by one or more major depressive episodes accompanied by at least one manic episode. *Cyclothymic disorder* is described as at least 2 years (1 year in children and adolescents) of numerous periods of hypomanic (less than full manic intensity) symptoms that do not meet criteria for a manic episode and numerous periods of less intense depressive symptoms that do not meet criteria for a major depressive episode. *Unspecified bipolar disorder* is included for coding disorders with bipolar features that do not meet criteria for any of the specific bipolar disorders defined in this section. There are also classifications for *bipolar disorder due to another medical condition*, *substance-/medication-induced bipolar and related disorder*, and *unspecified bipolar disorder*.

Anxiety Disorders

We have all felt nervous before starting an important exam or when giving a big presentation, so the profile of anxiety disorders is populated with symptoms that you may be familiar with. There are often emotional and physiological manifestations of anxiety; feelings of fear or dread may be coupled with racing heartbeat and sweating. As with all disorders previously discussed, it is the magnitude and intensity of the symptoms that determine if it is pathological. Two features associated with various forms of anxiety disorder are **panic attacks** and *agoraphobia*. Panic attacks are discrete episodes in which there is the sudden onset of intense apprehension, fearfulness, or terror, often associated with feelings of impending doom. During a panic attack, physical symptoms such as hyperventilation, chest pain, heart palpitations, difficulty catching one's breath, or gasping sensations can also be present. Agoraphobia is anxiety about and/or avoidance of circumstances from which quick departure might be difficult (or embarrassing) or that lack needed supports should panic symptoms be experienced. Most anxiety disorders have the potential to lead to avoidant behavior of circumstances that elicit a fear response.

Panic disorder features persistent anxiety and recurrent panic attacks marked by sweating, shaking, palpitations, dizziness, chest pain, and/or nausea. *Agoraphobia* is diagnosed when an individual fears two or more of the following situations:

- Using public transportation
- Being in enclosed spaces
- Being in open spaces
- Standing in line/being in a crowd or being outside of the home alone

These fears lead to active avoidance of these situations. *Specific phobia* is characterized by clinically significant anxiety prompted by the presence of a specific feared object or circumstance. For example, a client may have a specific phobia of bridges and may take an extremely long route to get somewhere in order to avoid having to go over a bridge. Another anxiety disorder is *social phobia* (social anxiety disorder), which produces major anxiety in situations demanding social performance or presentation such as meeting new people or giving a speech in front of others.

Generalized anxiety disorder is diagnosed when a client presents with persistent and excessive anxiety and worry for at least 6 months duration. *Anxiety disorder due to another medical condition*, *substance-/medication-induced anxiety disorder*, and *unspecified anxiety disorder* capture the remaining anxiety presentations that are not accounted for by other disorders in this category.

Obsessive–Compulsive Disorder and Related Disorders

Obsessive–compulsive disorder (OCD) and related disorders involve features of both obsessions (ruminative thoughts causing distress) and/or compulsions (ritualistic behavior patterns used to bind anxiety). In *OCD*, individuals may have obsessions, compulsions, or both. Although these can occur in any area of life, common behaviors include repetitive handwashing and counting (e.g., opening and closing the door five times before leaving a room). *Body dysmorphic disorder* is characterized by obsessive thoughts about a perceived flaw in physical appearance that is unnoticeable or slightly noticeable to others. Other disorders that are related to OCD are *trichotillomania* (hair-pulling disorder) and *hoarding disorder*, which is characterized by an individual's persistent difficulty with discarding items despite their lack of utility (e.g., saving daily newspapers/magazines for many years).

Trauma- and Stressor-Related Disorders

Trauma- and stressor-related disorders include *posttraumatic stress disorder (PTSD)*, *reactive attachment disorder, disinhibited social engagement disorder, adjustment disorders,* and *acute stress disorder*. PTSD features flashbacks of a major traumatic event and avoidance of triggers linked to the trauma. *Acute stress disorder* presents similarly to PTSD but is experienced immediately following the traumatic event. A child or adolescent with *reactive attachment disorder* has a pattern of emotional disturbance, and when distressed, he/she does not seek comfort or accept comfort from adult caregivers, oftentimes due to years of experiencing extreme neglect or repeated changes in caregivers (e.g., foster care system). *Adjustment disorders* are characterized by the development of emotional/behavioral symptoms in response to a clear stressor. Actual or threatened trauma can lead to a *cute stress disorders* marked by recurrent memories, flashbacks, and dissociative states that occur within a month of the event and resolve within that month.

Feeding/Eating Disorders

These disorders feature severe disturbances in eating behavior. *Anorexia nervosa* represents a profound refusal to maintain a normal body weight. *Bulimia nervosa* features episodic binging and purging of food; incorporating behaviors such as self-induced vomiting, misuse of laxatives, diuretics, or other medications; fasting; or excessive exercise to compensate for the high-caloric intake. A key element of both disorders is a distorted perception of body image (shape and weight). *Binge-eating disorder* is diagnosed when there are both recurrent episodes of excessive eating in a discrete period of time and a sense of lack of control over the eating. Occupational therapy practitioners may also encounter individuals with *pica*, who persistently eat nonnutritive, nonfood substances such as paper or chalk. An *unspecified feeding or eating disorder* category allows for coding disorders that do not meet criteria for a specific eating disorder.

Substance-Related and Addictive Disorders

The term "substance" can refer to any drug of abuse, a medication, or a toxin. The substances considered are organized into 11 classes:

1. Alcohol
2. Amphetamine
3. Caffeine
4. Cannabis
5. Cocaine
6. Hallucinogens
7. Inhalants
8. Nicotine
9. Opioids
10. Phencyclidine (PCP)
11. Sedatives, hypnotics, or anxiolytics

Many prescribed and over-the-counter medications may become abused substances. Toxic substances that may cause *substance-related disorders* include, but are not limited to

- Heavy metals
- Poisons
- Pesticides containing nicotine

- Nerve gases
- Ethylene glycol (antifreeze)
- Carbon monoxide
- Carbon dioxide

Common symptoms in response to toxic substance exposure include not only organic changes to the brain that interfere with cognition but also anxiety, hallucinations, delusions, or seizures may present.

The substance-related disorders are divided into two groups: the substance use disorders and the substance-induced disorders (*substance intoxication, substance withdrawal, substance-induced delirium, substance-induced persisting dementia, substance-induced persisting amnestic disorder, substance-induced psychotic disorder, substance-induced mood disorder, substance-induced anxiety disorder, substance-induced sexual dysfunction,* and *substance-induced sleep disorder*). The criteria sets for substance dependence, abuse, intoxication, and withdrawal are applicable across all 11 classes of substances. Additionally, excessive gambling behavior may fall into this category as an addictive disorder.

Personality Disorders

Personalities are like opinions; everyone has one even if you do not like it! Personality disorders define a persistent set of traits that endure over time, are pervasive and inflexible, presenting by early adulthood, and lead to distress or impairment. For the sake of convenience, personality disorders will be described in three clusters (A, B, and C) based on their similar characteristics. This clustering system is useful for organizing the material but does not have scientific relevance. As such, it should be recognized that individuals can present with traits across clusters.

Cluster A includes the disorders that result in odd or eccentric self-presentation. A *paranoid personality disorder* causes individuals to present with a persistent pattern of mistrust and suspiciousness interpreting other's motives as ill disposed. *Schizoid personality disorder* involves a pattern of withdrawal and isolation from social relationships with limited affective range. *Schizotypal personality disorder* includes a severe unease in close relationships; cognitive or perceptual distortions, yet not as severe as delusions and hallucinations; and eccentric behavior. Picture an individual wearing a helmet covered in tin foil to protect him/her from harmful radiation; this action may be interpreted as an eccentric behavior.

Individuals with diagnoses in Cluster B have marked difficulty establishing stable relationships and are often described as dramatic or erratic. *Antisocial personality disorder* results in profound disregard for, and violation of, the rights of others. This may result in criminal behavior for which the individual is noted to lack any empathy or remorse for the victim. People with antisocial personality disorder used to be referred to as sociopaths. Clients with *borderline personality disorder* experience pronounced instability with interpersonal relationships, impaired self-image, difficulty modulating feelings, and marked impulsivity. This symptom cluster may result in self-mutilating behavior such as cutting. *Histrionic personality disorder* describes a presentation of over-the-top emotions and drama resulting in attention-seeking behavior. *Narcissistic personality disorder* describes individuals who are driven by a need for admiration, are self-absorbed to the point where they unrealistically inflate their self-importance to grandiose levels, and possess little or no empathy for others.

Cluster C represents disorders that can be described as being rooted in the realm of anxiety and fear. *Avoidant personality disorder* individuals limit social participation due to inhibitions, feelings of inadequacy, and extreme sensitivity to criticisms from others. *Dependent personality disorder* represents a pattern of clinging to others and submitting to the desires of others for fear of offending. *Obsessive–compulsive personality disorder* symptoms are less intense than full OCD, but the individual is seriously preoccupied with order and tidiness.

Unspecified personality disorder can be considered as two conditions: (1) the individual's personality pattern meets the general criteria for a personality disorder with traits present from a variety of personality disorders, even though the criteria for any specific disorder are not met, or (2) the individual's personality pattern meets the general criteria for a personality disorder, but the individual is considered to have a personality disorder that is not included in the classification (e.g., *passive–aggressive personality disorder*).

Summary

This chapter provided an overview of occupational therapy in mental health settings. In this chapter, we explored contextual factors that influence the provision of care for individuals with serious mental illness. Medical legal and reimbursement considerations weigh prominent in this discussion. Treatment settings and the role that occupational therapy practitioners play in the interdisciplinary team were discussed along with an overview of common diagnostic presentations by clients seeking mental health treatment. While only a small portion of OT practitioners practice in mental health, the role of occupational therapy in the process of working with clients with mental health disorders is vitally important now and looking into the future.

Review Questions

1. According to the AOTA *Workforce Survey* (2010), approximately what percentage of occupational therapy practitioners report working in a mental health setting?
   a. 15%
   b. 3%
   c. 22%
   d. 50%

2. Psychotic symptoms involve:
   a. Thought disorders
   b. Hallucinations
   c. Delusions
   d. All of the above

3. Anorexia nervosa is a disorder that includes:
   a. Binging and purging
   b. Distorted self-image
   c. Obesity
   d. Malnutrition

4. Psychotic symptoms that respond best to medication are:
   a. Negative symptoms
   b. Mood disruptions
   c. Positive symptoms
   d. None of the above

5. Depressive episodes can include:
   a. Sad mood and disruption of sleep, appetite, and libido
   b. Elated mood and poor appetite
   c. Suicidal ideation
   d. a and c only

6. The criteria for diagnosing mental disorders can be found in:
   a. *The Atlas of Psychiatry*
   b. *Diagnosing Subjective Mentation*
   c. *Diagnostic Statistical Manual of Mental Disorders*
   d. The *PDM*

7. Diagnostic-related groups are useful for:
   a. Insurance and managed care reimbursement
   b. Comprehensive research programs
   c. Determining the right diagnosis
   d. Eradicating stigma

8. Personality disorders are:
   a. Persistent patterns of behavior that interfere with function
   b. No different across clusters
   c. Present in everyone we work with
   d. All of the above

9. When assessing risk in clients with serious mental illness, the practitioner must consider:
   a. Level of imminent danger to self or others
   b. Tarasoff's law and duty to warn
   c. History of violence
   d. All of the above

10. Manic episodes involve:
    a. Elevated mood
    b. Hyperarousal and diminished sleep
    c. Irritability
    d. None of the above
    e. All of the above

Practice Activities

Practice Activity 1

Read the following case study and complete the tasks at the end.

Maricelle weighed 71 lb when she was evaluated for intake into the inpatient eating disorders program. At 20 years old and 5 ft 6 in. tall, her frame appeared emaciated. She was, at times, so weak that her gait and standing tolerance were limited. Her weight loss began about 4 years ago when she started dieting to lose a few pounds. With a favorable response from others, Maricelle continued to diet and increase her exercise regime, reaching an all-time low of 59 lb. Her menses ceased about 3.5 years ago. She had a medical admission at her low weight and was treated for peptic ulcers. Within a month of discharge from that hospitalization, Maricelle was admitted to an inpatient psychiatric ward. After 8 weeks in this program, she increased her weight to 78 lb. With outpatient support and treatment, she continued to do well and was approaching 100 lb when she enrolled in college. With the increasing social and academic demands, she began dieting again, losing more than 20 lb in the 6 weeks prior to this admission.

Maricelle's eating habits are ritualized, with meticulous cutting of food and moving it around her plate. She actively avoids, resists, and refuses foods that she considers to be high in fat or carbohydrate content. She is experiencing moderate hair loss. She is excessively anxious and preoccupied with her figure. She expresses concern that as she gains weight, her "womanhood" is evident to others.

Tasks:

Identify at least three intervention strategies that an OT practitioner might employ to address Maricelle's issues.

Identify two interventions that would be inappropriate to do with Maricelle.

Practice Activity 2

Select one diagnosis from a category of the *DSM-5* and prepare a short case study that defines the diagnosis and lists its major symptoms and how an OTA working in the therapeutic milieu might work with a client with the diagnosis that you have selected, both individually and in a group. Be sure to prepare a narrative discussion about your client. Share your case study with your classmates for discussion and feedback.

Practice Activity 3

Read the following case study and respond to the task at the end.

Carlos was admitted to our locked inpatient psychiatric unit through the ER after a threatening altercation with his mom in which he threatened to kill her with a kitchen knife. Carlos was brought to the ER via the local police. Carlos has had five psychiatric admissions in the last 10 years, and he has a diagnosis of schizophrenia, paranoid type. He is admitted on a conditional voluntary. On intake, Carlos presents with limited English but readily conveys basic needs. It is unclear due to the language barrier and presence of psychotic thinking, if he has been compliant with medications, so he is given two doses of Haldol 10 mg, via intramuscular injection in the ER. Each of his previous psychiatric admissions was precipitated by similar aggressive behavior at home. His mother reports that during this incident, they were arguing over his taking medications.

Task:

Generate a list of concerns and possible strategies that you could employ to address some of the occupational deficits anticipated in this case.

References

American Occupational Therapy Association. *AOTA's Centennial Vision*. 2006. Retrieved 30 January 2013, from http://www.aota.org/News/Centennial/Background/36516.aspx?FT=.pdf

American Occupational Therapy Association. Occupational therapy code of ethics and ethics standards. *Am J Occup Ther* 2010a;64:S17–S26.

American Occupational Therapy Association. Surveying the profession: 2010 AOTA Workforce Survey points to rising demand for and commitment to occupational therapy. *OT Pract* 2010b;8–11.

American Psychiatric Association. *Diagnostic and Statistical Manual of Mental Disorders*. 5th ed. (text rev). American Psychiatric Association; 2000.

American Psychiatric Association. *Diagnostic and Statistical Manual of Mental Disorders*. 5th ed. American Psychiatric Association; 2013. doi: 10.1176/appi.books.9780890423349

Costa L, Altekruse M. Duty-to-warn guidelines for mental health counselors. *J Counsel Dev* 1994;72:346–350.

Ewing CP. Tarasoff reconsidered. *Monit Psychol* 2005;36(7):112. Retrieved from http://www.apa.org/monitor/julaug05/jn.aspx.

Fowler JC. Suicide risk assessment in clinical practice: pragmatic guidelines for imperfect assessments. *Psychotherapy* 2012;49(1):81–90.

Mahoney JS, et al. The therapeutic milieu reconceptualized for the 21st century. *Arch Psychiatr Nurs* 2009;23(6):423–429. doi: 10.1016/j.apnu.2009.003.002

Rossen EK, et al. Interdisciplinary collaboration: the need to revisit. *Issues Mental Health Nurs* 2008;29:387–396. doi: 10.1080/01612840801904449

Sonne JL. Duty to protect: reporting client threat of harm to another. In: *PsycEssentials: A Pocket Resource for Mental Health Practitioners*. pp. 151–161. Washington, D.C.: American Psychological Association; 2012.

Tarasoff v. Regents of University of California, 551 P.2d 334. 1976.

The Commonwealth of Massachusetts. *Massachusetts Law: Chapter 123*. 2012. Retrieved 12 October 2012, from http://www.malegislature.gov/Laws/GeneralLaws/PartI/TitleXVII/Chapter123

Thibeault CA, et al. Understanding the milieu experiences of patients on an acute inpatient psychiatric unit. *Arch Psychiatr Nurs* 2010;(4):216–226. Retrieved from http://www.sciencedirect.com

Walker M. Principles of a therapeutic milieu: an overview. *Perspect Psychiatr Care* 1994;30(30):5–8.

World Health Organization. *Mental Health Atlas 2011*. 2011. Retrieved 12 October 2012 from http://www.who.int/mental_health/publications/mental_health_atlas_2011/en/index.html

CHAPTER

30 Physical Conditions

Kevin Kunkel, PhD, MSPT, MLD-CDT

Key Terms

Akinesia—No movement.
Amputation—Cutting off of (e.g., a limb).
Anterior—Front.
Balance—Maintaining upright standing position during stationary and movement activities.
Bradykinesia—Slow movement.
Bursa—Protect muscles and tendons from irritation.
Cervical—Relating to the neck.
Clot—A coagulated mass of blood.
Collagen—Protein constituent of connective tissue.
Concavities—Hollowed inward.
Convexities—Bulging outward.
Disability—"An umbrella term for impairments, activity limitations, and participation restrictions" (WHO, 2012).
Fascia—Dense tissue surrounding bones.
Fibrous—Resembling fibers.
Frontal plane—Divides the body into front and back segments.
Hemopoiesis—Formation of blood or blood cells.
Horizontal plane—Divides the body in upper and lower segments.
Hypercoagulability—Tendency for blood to form blood clots.
Inflammation—Localized tissue reaction to irritation.
Intervertebral discs—Material located between vertebrae of the spine.
Ischemia—Tissue death.
Kyphosis—Spine bows posterior (backward).
Ligaments—Dense non-elastic tissue that provide bone-to-bone (joint) support.
Lordosis—Spine bows anterior (forward).
Lumbar—Relating to area between lowest ribs and the pelvis.
Metabolic—Biochemical processes required for normal functioning.
Myelin—Insulation surrounding nerve cells that speeds up conduction.
Neoplasm—New or abnormal growth.
Neuropathy—Abnormal condition of the nerve.
Paralysis—Loss of the ability to move.
Paraplegia—Paralysis of two extremities (legs).
Posture—A position of the body or of the body parts in standing or sitting.
Posterior—Back.
Quadriplegia—Paralysis of all four extremities (arms and legs).

Revascularization—Surgical procedure to correct coronary artery stenosis.
Rigidity—Quality of being stiff or inflexible.
Sacral—Relating to a triangular bone at distal end of spine.
Sagittal plane—Divides the body into left and right segments.
Scoliosis—Abnormal curving of the spine.
Synovial—Pertaining to a membrane located in joints.
Synovium—Soft tissue located inside a joint capsule that produces synovial fluid to lubricate the joint.
Tachykinesia—Fast movement.
Tendon—Tissue that attaches muscles to bones.
Thoracic—Relating to the chest.
Tone—Muscle tension.
Transient ischemic attack (TIA)—Mini stroke.
Transverse Plane—Divides the body into top and bottom halves.
Trauma—An injury to living tissue.

Learning Objectives

After studying this chapter, readers should be able to:

- Describe the basic normal anatomy needed for movement.
- Describe abnormal (pathologic) conditions that limit physical function.
- Discuss common physical conditions that occupational therapy practitioners may encounter in their clinical work.
- Understand the role of the occupational therapy assistant in working with clients with physical disabilities.

Introduction

The World Health Organization (WHO) designed the International Classification of Function (ICF) to measure health and **disability** at an individual and population level (Assembly, 2005). According to the WHO, disability is "an umbrella term for impairments, activity limitations, and participation restrictions" (WHO, 2012). The ICF model discusses three components relative to disability: body functions and structure, activity, and participation. The ICF is a framework and classification method used for physical medicine and rehabilitation. To best integrate the ICF into occupational therapy practice, knowledge of the physical structure of the human body is imperative to understand its function.

The human body is a combination of multiple systems that ideally coordinate and work in synchrony to produce movement. The major systems include musculoskeletal, neuromuscular, cardiovascular, and pulmonary. All are important for an occupational therapy assistant to understand on their own and with regard to how they interconnect with each other. Normally, the combined efficacy of the systems allows for human dynamic function. However, each system can develop pathology that individually or in combination may hinder function.

Occupational therapy assistants and occupational therapists must be able to understand normal body system structure and function and subsequently recognize and treat the abnormal/atypical when it affects function. Additionally, as medicine embraces prevention, the OT practitioner's unique role in delivering evidence-based treatment to clients with physical conditions will continue to evolve. This chapter provides an overview of body systems and several physical conditions commonly associated with each. We will also briefly highlight how the OTA will be involved in the planning and treatment of clients with physical conditions.

The Spine

The spinal column consists of four segments, the **cervical**, **thoracic**, **lumbar**, and **sacral**. Each segment contains bony structures called vertebrae. With the exception of the first and second vertebrae of the cervical region, the vertebrae are similar to each other. Every vertebra is composed of a body, an arch, a spinous process, two pedicles, and two processes. The first two cervical vertebrae lack a vertebral body and are called the atlas (recall your Greek mythology in which Atlas held up the world). The second, the axis, contains a prominent bony protuberance called the odontoid process that arises into the first vertebra, allowing it to rotate. The cervical region contains seven vertebrae. The thoracic region contains 12 vertebrae. The lumbar region contains five vertebrae. The sacral region contains five vertebrae, which are independent of each other during childhood but fuse to form one bone in adulthood. The coccygeal region contains three to five vertebrae.

Intervertebral discs are located between each vertebra except in the sacrum. They are like a cushion or shock absorber between vertebrae to absorb forces created with movement. These "discs" are formed by two parts: an annulus fibrosis, which is a ring-like structure that surrounds a nucleus pulposus, which is a gel-like structure.

The spinal column is formed by the 32 to 35 vertebrae in the four regions of the spine. The spinal column performs three important roles. It is the support for the frame of the body. It protects the spinal cord with a central canal formed by the body of each vertebra and its bilateral arch, and it allows for movement. The spine starts at the base of the skull and continues until the coccyx or tailbone. Each vertebrae is connected to the one above and/or below by a series of ligaments. Ligaments maintain the structural integrity of the spinal column and assist to limit its movement.

Atypical Spinal Conditions

The design of the spine allows it to move in three planes. Planes are two-dimensional surfaces that divide the body into sections. The **frontal plane** divides the front and rear halves of the body. The **sagittal plane** divides the left and right sides of the body. The **transverse plane** divides the body into top and bottom halves. Excessive curvature may occur in the sagittal plane with increased kyphosis or lordosis. Conversely, a decrease in either of the curves may produce a flattening of the spine.

A deformity of the spine that occurs in the frontal plane is called **scoliosis**. The (normally) straight spine becomes curved with **concavities** and **convexities** occurring in the sagittal plane. The scoliotic curve can be congenital or acquired with age or over time. Best practice rehabilitation of any part of the body requires understanding of whole body posture and alignment. For example, attempting to treat a client with a shoulder injury without observing posture and spinal mobility may limit the success of the outcome. No part of the body works in isolation; they depend on others to optimally function.

It Is All about Posture

We constantly assume various static and fluid **postures** in our daily lives. Postural alignment can be defined relative to multiple planes of movement. **Balance** refers to maintaining an upright position (Fig. 30.1). Posture and balance are integral to accomplish movement-oriented tasks in our daily activities (Wallmann, 2009) (From the Field 30.1).

The spine presents in an upright posture with three curves in the sagittal plane. The first curve is from an ascending position in the lumbar region, **lordosis**, in which the spine bows **anterior** (forward). The second curve is in the thoracic region, **kyphosis**, in which the spine bows **posterior** (backward). The final curve is a repeated lordosis of the cervical region. The primary method of determining postural alignment is from a **sagittal plane**. Posture is analyzed by using a plumb line secured from above which a weight is attached. An individual stands in a predetermined position with the feet placed symmetric to the plumb line. A visual inspection of the ascending symmetry is observed and asymmetry is noted. The significance of postural analysis relates to static and dynamic functional mobility. Normal body alignment with symmetry in all planes of movement allows for movement patterns with minimal to no restrictions.

Atypical Posture

A perfect cylinder responds to the force of gravity by equally transferring all of the force through it so that the structure maintains its integrity. However, if the cylinder has a slight bend in it, the force of gravity will create a minor lateral force. Instead of 100% of the force moving through a perfect cylinder, the slightly bent cylinder may have a 95% force moving through it, but now a 5% force is in the direction of the bend. Since all structures have

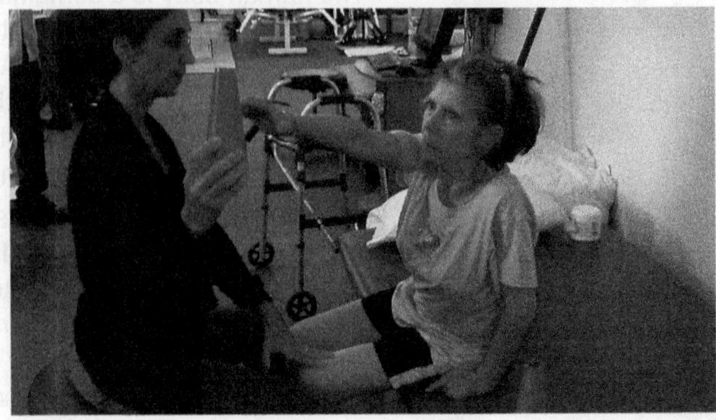

Figure 30.1 Addressing balance and stability issues following a CVA.

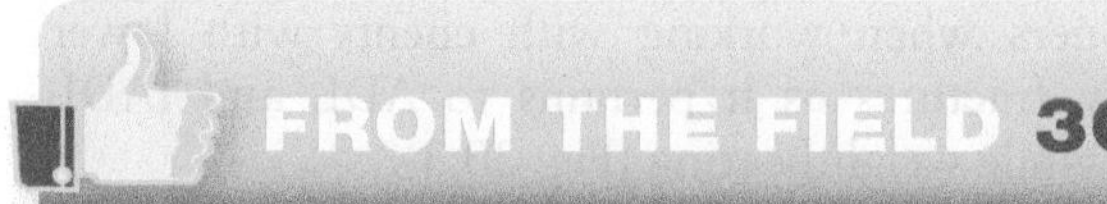

FROM THE FIELD 30.1

A Quick Way to Better Posture

Stand within a door frame and place your forearms on the doorjamb with the elbows at the same height as the shoulders. Put one foot forward and the other backward about one foot distance from each other. While holding in your stomach, bend the front leg and keep the back leg straight and move forward through the door frame until you feel a stretch across your chest muscles (pectorals), calf, and front hip area of the back leg. Hold the stretch for one minute, and then repeat, switching your legs. Repeat this every morning for better posture!

some form of malleability or ability to change based on stressors to them, a bent cylinder will continue to bend based on the stress. With regard to humans, long-term asymmetry produces abnormal forces on the body, which result in long-term adaptation of the bony, cartilaginous, ligamentous, muscle, and neurological structures.

Think about the Leaning Tower of Pisa. Its tilt makes it one of the most famous structures in the world. The tilt occurred due to the foundation settling on a base of unstable soil. As soon as the Tower was built, it began to lean due to the uneven support beneath it. Its final construction was delayed, and when it resumed years later, the wall height was increased on the tilt side to compensate and adjust for the lean. In the end, the Tower was completed, tilt and all. Alteration in the building structure was sufficient in the short term (years), but the long-term effects of the asymmetry resulted in increasing tilt.

How does this relate to the body? Consider the forces that were placed on the Tower when it was modified to correct the lean. The forces led to sideways pressure that resulted in changes to the structure. The first was continued lean, but the second was internal structural load stress and failure of the support system. Our body and spinal structure are no different in adaptation to uneven or asymmetric forces.

Forces coming through the sagittal plane of the body to the three spinal curves increase the curvatures. To optimally maintain alignment, our body fights these forces through action and coordination of multiple muscle groups. The frontal plane that divides the body side to side would ideally present without any lateral forces if the body were perfectly symmetric. However, physical development may be/have been inhibited by asymmetric growth of the lengths of the bones of the lower extremities, which misaligns the frontal plane. When asymmetry occurs, our base, like the Leaning Tower of Pisa, is uneven. While short-term effects of this asymmetry may not produce pathology, long-term effects of the moments of force on all or some of the joints may lead to compensation resulting in or contributing to physical conditions.

An example of structural asymmetry is changes in the spine. The forces of gravity and moments of force over time can accentuate spinal curves. If a structural asymmetry is present, side-to-side forces are added to the mix of moments and produce unnatural curves. The body will always attempt to maintain level eye position; however, with a longer leg on one side, the spine distorts to connect a nonlevel pelvis to a level head. When working with clients in any practice setting, it is important to recognize the structural effects of adaptation/compensation to asymmetries in the body. Long-term changes to the structure can affect movement patterns, contribute to or result in pathology, and impact occupational engagement and performance (Fig. 30.2).

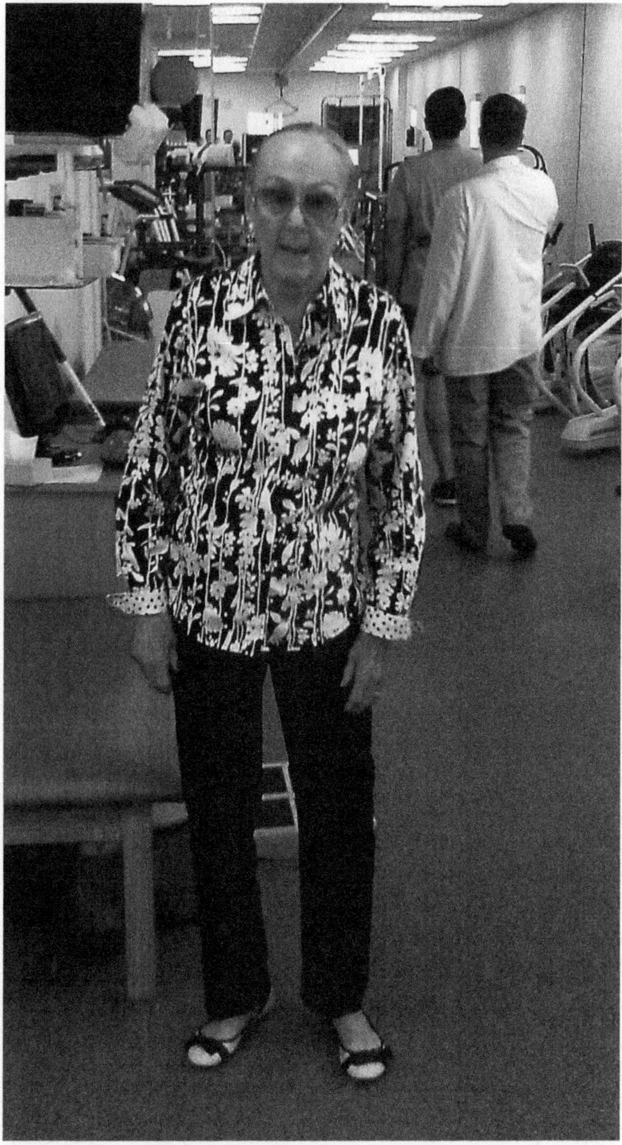

Figure 30.2 Postural asymmetry.

The Skeletal System

The adult human skeleton is comprised of 213 bones. All bones have a basic building block called mineralized **collagen** fibril. The bones provide the internal stability of the body so that it may maintain an upright posture against the force of gravity. Bone must be stiff and able to resist deformation but also flexible to absorb energy by changing shape (Seeman & Delmas, 2006). If too brittle, the energy imposed during loading (work) will result in structural failure. If bone is too flexible and bends beyond its maximal strain, it will also break (Seeman & Delmas, 2006). Bone constantly replenishes itself through a process of modeling and remodeling. During modeling, new bone is formed without reabsorption of the old bone. Remodeling occurs when reabsorption of the existing bone is followed by formation of new bone (Seeman & Delmas, 2006). As we move through our daily lives, bone is strengthened through the adaptation to physiological stresses in all planes of motion. However, excessive stress in any plane can result in structural failure.

Atypical Skeletal Conditions

There are numerous atypical skeletal conditions that you may treat in your work as an OTA. Several common conditions are discussed here.

Long Bone Fractures

The long bones in the body are located proximal to the center line and include arm and leg bones. A simple closed fracture happens when the bone continues to be in its normal anatomical alignment, but a line of damage to the bone occurs and disrupts its continuity. There is minimal damage to the surrounding tissue. The fracture is also closed since it does not penetrate the skin. When a fracture is combined with a lesion of an organ, artery, nerve bundle, or joint, it is termed a complicated fracture. A compression fracture is a collapse of a vertebra due to weakening of the bone or **trauma**, which is an injury to living tissue. A greenstick fracture is an incomplete fracture involving one side of the bone. An oblique fracture occurs at an angle to the long bone axis. A comminuted fracture occurs when a bone is broken into several pieces. An impacted fracture occurs when one fragment of the bone is wedged into another fragment. A spiral fracture runs around the axis of the bone. A pathologic fracture occurs as the result of disease that has weakened the bone. A stress fracture occurs as a result of overuse, such as in high impact sports like running and basketball.

Understanding the nature of the fracture, the healing phases, the surgical repair required to treat the fracture, and/or the safety precautions is necessary to direct the intensity and focus of the occupational therapy process. This information is especially important for OT practitioners when working with clients with lower extremity fractures as it pertains to ADL and IADL training while weightbearing (Fig. 30.3).

Congenital Malformations

Congenital bone malformations associated with genetic disorders include dwarfism and Marfan syndrome (Vanhoenacker et al., 2001). Many deformations of the bone are the result of metabolic diseases. **Metabolic** refers to the biochemical processes that the body requires for normal functioning. Metabolic diseases affecting the bone include osteoporosis, Paget disease, and hyperparathyroidism. Osteoporosis, a thinning of the bone density of the long bones and vertebrae, most commonly occurs in elderly women. Fractures may occur as a result of the density loss. Paget disease is a softening of the bone believed to occur as a result of a viral infection. It most commonly affects the skull, humeri, spine, femur, and tibia. Hyperparathyroidism is usually caused by an adenoma, a benign tumor of the parathyroid glands, or may be the result of renal failure. With hyperparathyroidism, calcium within the bone leaches out and is excreted by the urine, thus reducing bone density, which may then lead to pathologic fractures. Significant structural changes typically occur in those with metabolic disorders. The OTA will work closely with clients with bone malformations on adaptive equipment recommendations, energy conservation, and strengthening programs in order to maximize functional performance.

Neoplasms

Neoplasms are new or abnormal tissue growths in the body; a characteristic of cancer (American Heritage Science Dictionary, 2002). The three most common bone and joint cancers are osteosarcoma, Ewing sarcoma, and chondrosarcoma. Osteosarcoma is a type of bone tissue cancer that is diagnosed most frequently in teens and young adults. Ewing sarcoma is often located in the shaft of the long bone and pelvic bones and occurs most frequently in children and adolescents. Chondrosarcoma is a cancer of the cartilage cells within the bone. The risk of pathologic fractures is significant with neoplasms of the bone (Surgery, 2008).

Cancer that has spread (metastasized) is often expressed as pain in an extremity, joint, or region of the body. Since this may happen years after the initial treatment for the cancer, the pain may be diagnosed by a physician as a local musculoskeletal disorder. As an OT practitioner, it is important to be attuned to this and be aware that if treatment for the painful condition does not resolve or improve over a several weeks, a referral back to the ordering physician is indicated.

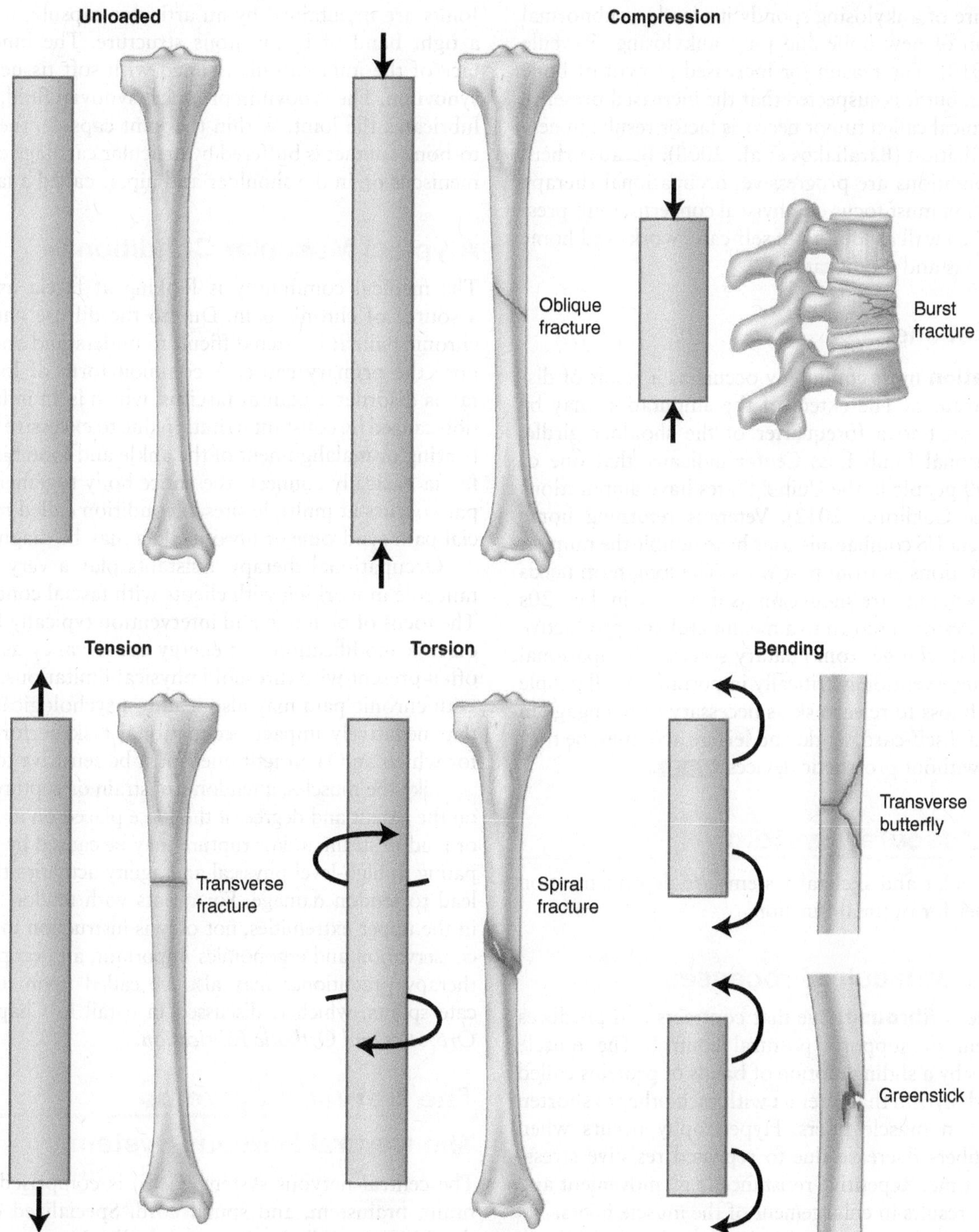

Figure 30.3 Types of fractures and the forces that cause them. (From Court-Brown C, et al. *Rockwood and Green's Fractures in Adults*. 8th ed. Philadelphia: Lippincott Williams & Wilkins; 2014.)

Rheumatic Diseases

Rheumatoid arthritis (RA) is an autoimmune disease in which the **synovial** lining of the joints becomes persistently inflamed and autoantibodies attack the tissue. It most commonly affects women and the elderly. Uncontrolled RA may lead to joint damage, disability, and decreased quality of life (Scott et al., 2010).

Acute gouty arthritis is a condition in which excessive stores of uric acid in the joint spaces result in severe pain. The pain is debilitating and requires immediate medical intervention (Naomi, 2004). Ankylosing spondylitis is characterized by **inflammation** of the spine and sacroiliac joints that causes pain and stiffness or fixing, which is a process called ankylosing. The progressive nature of ankylosing spondylitis leads to abnormal formation of new bone and joint ankylosing (Reveille et al., 2010). The reason for increased growth of bone is unclear, but it is suspected that the increased presence of a chemical called tumor necrosis factor results in new bone formation (Baraliakos et al., 2008). Because rheumatic conditions are progressive, occupational therapy intervention must focus on physical concerns, joint preservation, as well as long-term self-care, work, and home adaptations and modifications.

Amputations

Amputation most commonly occurs as a result of disease or trauma. The extent of the amputation may be a single digit to a forequarter of the shoulder girdle. The National Limb Loss Center indicates that one of every 200 people in the United States have amputations (Amputee Coalition, 2012). Veterans returning home from recent US combat missions have double the number of amputations as from past wars. The long-term needs of these veterans are significant as many are in their 20s and will desire to return to a meaningful and productive life upon discharge from military service. Occupational therapy intervention is critically important for all people with limb loss to relearn skills necessary to re-engage in meaningful self-care, work, and leisure activities, be they with or without prosthetic devices CS-5.

The Muscular System

The muscular and skeletal systems are dependent upon each other for optimal function.

Typical Muscular Processes

A muscle is **fibrous** tissue that contracts and produces movement or supports postural control. The muscle contracts by a sliding motion of bands of proteins called actin and myosin that interact with each other to shorten or lengthen muscle fibers. Hypertrophy occurs when muscle fibers decrease due to repeated resistive stressors over time. Repetitive resistance (e.g., movement and exercise) results in enlargement of the muscle fibers.

Muscles connect to each other by a layer of fibrous tissue called **fascia** that surrounds the muscle or groups of muscles. Muscles must connect to a bone in order to produce movement when it contracts. Muscle attaches to bone via a dense fibrous tissue called **tendons**. Tendons are elastic but less so than a muscle. **Bursas** protect muscles and tendons from irritation that occurs from rubbing over a bone during movement. Bursas are fluid-filled sacs that provide near frictionless movement of the tissues and bone relative to each other. **Ligaments** are dense non-elastic tissue that provide bone-to-bone (joint) support and help maintain the skeletal structure. Joints are maintained by an articular capsule, which is a tight band of ligamentous structure. The inner surface of the joint capsule is lined with soft tissue called **synovium**. The synovium produces synovial fluid, which lubricates the joint. Within the joint capsule, the bone-to-bone contact is buffered by articular cartilage called a meniscus or, in the shoulder and hip, is called a labrum.

Atypical Muscular Conditions

The medical community is looking at fascia as being a source of chronic pain. Due to the diffuse nature of chronic pain, it is often difficult to understand and diagnose the primary cause. A common form of localized fascia disorder is plantar fasciitis, which is an inflammation caused by constant irritation due to excessive weight bearing or malalignment of the ankle and foot. Since the fascia basically connects the entire body together, when pain occurs at multiple sites, a condition called myofascial pain syndrome or fibromyalgia may be diagnosed.

Occupational therapy assistants play a very important role in working with clients with fascial conditions. The focus of planning and intervention typically focuses on task modification and energy conservancy as clients often present with threshold physical limitations. Living with chronic pain may also lead to psychological issues that negatively impact occupational task performance, for which an OT practitioner must be sensitive to.

Like the muscles, a tendon can strain or rupture based on the extent and degree of the force placed on it. Muscle or tendon strain and/or rupture may be caused by participating in high-level physical and agility activities that can lead to tendon damage. For clients with tendon injuries in the upper extremities, not only is instruction in energy conservation and ergonomics important, an occupational therapy practitioner may also be called upon to fabricate splints, which is discussed in detail in Chapter 24, *Orthotics and Orthotic Fabrication.*

The Nervous Systems

The Central Nervous System

The central nervous system (CNS) is comprised of the brain, brainstem, and spinal cord. Specialized cells in the CNS are called neurons and glia. Nerve cells that carry messages away from the brain are called axons and those that deliver messages to the brain are called dendrites. The CNS initiates and delivers information to the peripheral nervous system. The brain is divided into two hemispheres by the corpus callosum. The two hemispheres of the brain are referred to as the cerebral cortex or cerebrum. The left hemisphere controls the contralateral (or opposite) right side of the body, and the right hemisphere controls the left side of the body. There is ipsilateral (same-sided) control of some elements of the nervous system, but it is minimal. The left hemisphere controls language, computation, and logical reasoning, while the right hemisphere controls spatial reasoning, facial recognition, and music. The hemispheres contain lobes. The frontal lobe is located in the anterior aspect of the hemisphere. The parietal and temporal lobes are positioned posterior with the parietal located above or superior to the temporal. The occipital lobe is located posterior to the parietal and temporal lobes.

The frontal lobes are responsible for executive functions such as higher-level thinking and reasoning. The left frontal lobe contains the Broca area, which coordinates motor activity necessary for expressive or spoken language. The left temporal lobe contains the Wernicke area, which is responsible for receptive or the understanding of language. The left parietal lobe is associated with sensation and perception. The occipital lobe is involved with vision and visual perception. The cerebellum is located in the most posterior portion of the brain and is involved with coordination and regulation of muscle activity, as well as some cognitive functions.

The brainstem is the trunk of the brain and contains the midbrain, pons, and medulla oblongata. The brainstem houses the nerve pathways from the cerebral cortex to the pons. The brainstem also contains the third and fourth cranial nerves and controls eye movement. The pons is the relay station between the cerebellum and the cerebrum. It also aids the medulla oblongata in controlling breathing. The medulla oblongata is the lowest portion of the brainstem and becomes the top of the spinal cord. It controls heart and lung function, including respiration and blood pressure.

The spinal cord is a thick bundle of nerve tissue. It is a major part of the nervous system as it conducts sensory and motor nerve impulses to and from the brain. The human spinal cord is roughly cylindrical in shape, begins at the end of the medulla oblongata, and exits the cranium via a structure called the foramen magnum into the vertebral canal (Goshgarian, 2003). The spinal cord usually terminates at L1 and L2; however, the most inferior aspect of the cord, the conus medullaris, may be found as high as T12 or as low as L2 (Goshgarian, 2003).

Atypical Central Nervous System Conditions

Stroke

Each year, approximately 200,000 to 500,000 people in the United States are diagnosed by a physician as having experienced a **transient ischemic attack** (TIA), commonly called a mini stroke (WHO, 1988). According to the World Health Organization, a TIA is defined as "rapidly developed clinical signs of focal or global disturbance of cerebral function, lasting less than 24 hours, with no apparent nonvascular cause" (WHO, 1988). Approximately 11% of those who have been diagnosed with TIA will have a cerebral vascular accident (CVA or stroke) within 90 days following the TIA, with the greatest risk noted within the first weeks (Furie et al., 2011; Johnston & Fayad, 2003; Lloyd-Jones et al., 2010). Strokes occur as a result of disruption of blood flow to an area of the brain due to a blockage. The blockage or **clot** may occur in large or small arteries, which develop arteriosclerotic plagues that eventually close off the vessel. An embolism is a free-floating mass. This mass can be lodged in a vessel and disrupt blood flow. Surgical procedures, **hypercoagulability**, or sickle cell disease may also cause an embolism (Furie et al., 2011). While lack of blood flow that leads to tissue death defines an **ischemic** stroke, a hemorrhagic stroke occurs when the blood vessel is damaged and bleeds into the areas of the brain (O'Brien et al., 2011). Whether ischemic or hemorrhagic, the location of the insult to the brain determines the extent and level of impairment of function. Damage to the right side of the brain can cause loss of function to the left side of the body and vice versa. The resultant loss is called hemiplegia or half paralysis CS-12.

The patient shown in Figures 30.4 and 30.5 has hemiplegia.

A stroke may be one of the most devastating conditions that a person experiences. Working as part of a team with other health care professionals, family, and the client, OT practitioners are integral in the rehabilitation and recovery process. Occupational therapy practitioners work with clients who have had a CVA to identify goals and based on that to reengage in occupations that are meaningful and purposeful to them.

Multiple Sclerosis

Multiple sclerosis is a disease that occurs when lesions develop in the CNS that leads to loss of nerve impulse conduction. **Myelin** is a fatty sheath that surrounds axons in the CNS and peripheral nervous system and helps to speed up nerve impulse conduction. In MS, the myelin is destroyed, which results in slow (or no) nerve conduction. The myelin is eventually replaced by scar tissue called plaques. For many individuals with MS, the course of the disease is progressive (Thompson et al., 1997). The

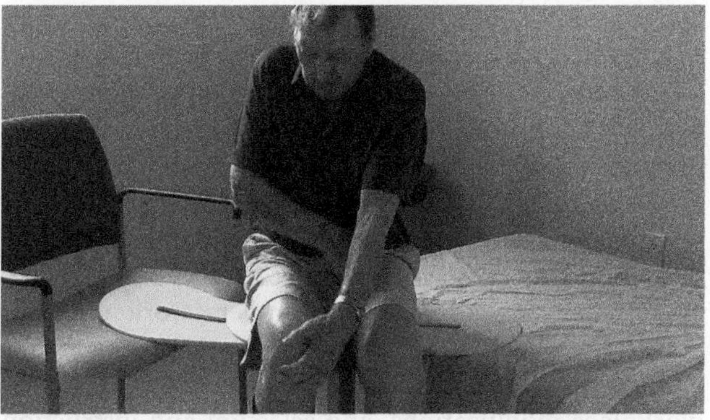

Figure 30.4 An individual with hemiplegia practices transfers using s sliding board.

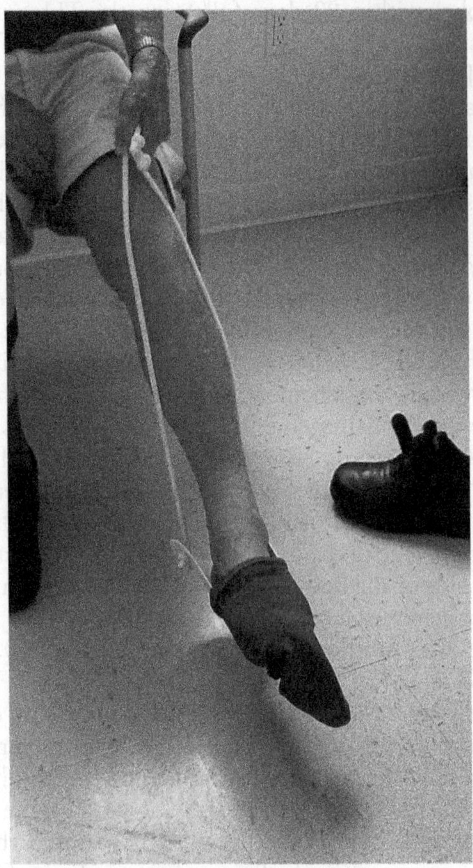

Figure 30.5 An individual with hemiplegia is learning to don socks using a stocking aid.

long-term effect of damage to the brain and spinal cord results in spasticity. Spasticity is decreased inhibition of the brain's ability to reduce reflexive actions. Individuals with spasticity demonstrate very high muscle tone. With spasticity, individuals with MS (or other condition that may involve spasticity, such as cerebral palsy or CVA) develop progressive limitations due to the high abnormal **tone** that limits movement and functional ability.

Amyotrophic Lateral Sclerosis

Amyotrophic lateral sclerosis (ALS) is a terminal disease of unknown origin. It is a neurodegenerative disorder that leads to progressive paralysis of the muscular system. Paralysis occurs due to degeneration of motor neurons in the primary motor cortex in the frontal lobe, the brainstem, and the spinal cord. Individuals with ALS may notice involuntary twitching or cramps for several months or years prior to onset of weakness and ultimately may be diagnosed with ALS (Wijesekera & Leigh, 2009).

Occupational therapy practitioners work with clients with MS or ALS on reducing spasticity, strengthening, range of motion, energy conservation, home and workplace modifications, and selection and instruction in the use of adaptive and assistive devices that address issues of independence.

Parkinson Disease

Parkinson disease, in its typical presentation, is normally an age-related progressive neurological disorder characterized by four primary motor symptoms. These features can be grouped under the acronym TRAP: tremor at rest, **rigidity** (quality of being stiff or inflexible), **akinesia** (no movement) or **bradykinesia** (slow movement), and postural instability. In addition, secondary motor symptoms of freezing, micrographia (small handwriting), mask-like expression, and unwanted accelerations like increased walking speed are common (Jankovic, 2008).

Parkinson disease is caused by a loss of cells in a structure called the substantia nigra, which is located in the midbrain and is part of the basal ganglia. The basal ganglia are similar to the processor of a computer that gathers information from many areas and then creates organized output. The substantia nigra is instrumental in basal ganglia functioning, as it is the source of a neurotransmitter called dopamine. Neurotransmitters are chemicals that transmit signals from a neuron across a synapse (small space) to a target cell. Dopamine is a chemical messenger that plays a vital role in emotional regulation and movement. Lack of dopamine results in a decrease in voluntary movement in individuals with Parkinson disease.

Because Parkinson disease is a progressive neurological condition with multiple symptoms that affect movement, the role of the OT practitioner is to work with the client to achieve optimal physical function, mobility, and independence in all areas of work, leisure, and self-care.

Spinal Cord Pathology

Spinal cord pathology includes spinal vascular disease, degenerative disease, and demyelinative spinal cord disease; infections within the spinal canal; neoplasms within the spinal canal; and traumatic injury (Kim, 2003). Traumatic injury is the most common form of spinal cord pathology. The incidence of spinal cord injury in the United States is approximately 40 per million (National Spinal Cord Injury Statistical Center, 2012).

The extent of the lesion and where the lesion occurs in the spine determine functional involvement. Injuries to one of the eight cervical vertebrae result in **quadriplegia** (all four extremities involved). **Paraplegia** (two extremities involved—legs) occurs with lesions to the thoracic, lumbar, or sacral regions (National Spinal Cord Injury Statistical Center, 2012). An injury to the spine that damages all of the spinal cord at the point of injury is termed a complete lesion, whereas partial damage is termed an incomplete lesion.

Occupational therapy practitioners work closely with clients who have experienced a spinal cord injury. Rehabilitation is team based and extensive, and like all other occupational therapy, intervention focuses on the entire person: the physical as well as psychological

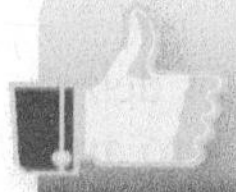

FROM THE FIELD 30.2

Recent statistics show that 42.1% of traumatic spinal cord injuries are the result of motor vehicle accidents, followed by falls and acts of violence (primarily gunshot wounds) and recreational sporting activities (National Spinal Cord Injury Statistical Center, 2012).

implications associated with, in this case, spinal cord injury. Depending on the level of the injury, clients will need to learn how to best use and protect the active motion that is available to them. Occupational therapy intervention will include strength training, adaptive equipment and assistive technology recommendations and training, home modifications, workplace adaptations, energy conservation techniques, splinting, and wheeled mobility recommendations and instruction to help clients actively engage in self-identified meaningful occupations (From the Field 30.2).

Poliomyelitis

Poliomyelitis (polio) is a viral disease that affects the CNS and may lead to partial or full paralysis (Modlin, 2009). Once contracted, there is no cure for polio. The only treatment is to alleviate the symptoms. Prior to introduction of the polio vaccine in 1955, the infection rate of polio in the United States reached a peak of 20,000 cases per annum. By the 1970s, the infection rate had been reduced to nearly zero (Garfinkel & Sarewitz, 2003). Thanks in large part to the efforts of the Gates Foundation, polio has nearly been eradicated worldwide. Today, the major concern with polio is post-polio syndrome, which is pain and progressive weakness that occurs in approximately 25% to 40% of all cases of those who, in their youth, contracted the disease. Postpolio syndrome typically manifests 30 to 40 years after the initial onset (Garfinkel & Sarewitz, 2003).

Individuals with postpolio syndrome experience bouts of significant fatigue. Occupational therapy practitioners provide clients with energy conservation techniques and ergonomic training to reduce the effects of fatigue. As well, they may be called upon to create a balanced exercise program that incorporates postural control while avoiding fatigue.

The Peripheral Nervous System

The peripheral nervous system (PNS) is located outside the central nervous system, in the periphery of the body. The PNS includes cranial nerves (except the optical) and sympathetic and parasympathetic nerves. The PNS receives information from and delivers information back to the CNS. This feed-forward and feedback loop of information permits the body's multiple systems to communicate, to coordinate, and, when functioning optimally, to seamlessly operate.

The cranial nerves consist of 12 paired nerves originating in the brain. They are as follows:

Olfactory (I)—controls smell
Optic (II)—controls vision
Oculomotor (III)—controls eyelid and eyeball movement
Trochlear (IV)—turns the eye downward and moves it laterally
Trigeminal (V)—controls chewing, touch, and pain to the face and mouth
Abducens (VI)—controls the movement the lateral rectus muscle of the eye
Facial (VII)—controls the majority of facial expression and controls taste and secretion of tears and saliva
Vestibulocochlear (auditory) (VIII)—controls hearing and equilibrium sensation
Glossopharyngeal (IX)—controls taste and also senses carotid blood pressure
Vagus (X)—controls heart rate slowing, senses the aortic blood pressure, stimulates the organs that digest food, and is involved with taste
Accessory (XI)—controls the motor activity of the trapezius and sternocleidomastoid muscles and controls the swallowing mechanism
Hypoglossal (XII)—controls the movements of the tongue

The spinal nerves arise from the spinal cord. There are 31 pairs of spinal nerves: 8 cervical, 12 thoracic, 5 lumbar, 5 sacral, and 1 coccygeal (Goshgarian, 2003). Every spinal nerve is paired so as to supply each side of the body. The spinal nerve contains both sensory nerves and motor nerves. The sensory nerves transmit information gained from the sensors located in the skin, muscles, ligaments, tendons, and joints to the brain. The motor nerves transmit information from the sensorimotor cortex of the brain through the brainstem to the muscles.

Atypical Peripheral Nervous System Conditions

Guillain-Barre Syndrome

Guillain-Barre syndrome (GBS) is a peripheral **neuropathy** with acute onset and rapid weakness of the muscular system. It is often called ascending paralysis. With GBS, the respiratory muscles may be paralyzed, and if not treated immediately with tracheal intubation (a tube inserted into windpipe to assist breathing), death may ensue. The peak level of weakness occurs within 4 weeks after onset, but most individuals reach it within two to three weeks (Doorn et al., 2010). In severe cases, total **paralysis** can occur such that the individual is unable to voluntarily move any muscle group, even the eyelids. The onset of GBS is usually preceded by infection and is considered an autoimmune disease. The treatment for GBS is intravenous immunoglobulin (IVIG); however, 25% of individuals with GBS require artificial ventilation, and 20% are unable to walk without assistance for 6 months following onset of the syndrome (Doorn et al., 2010).

During the acute phase of GBS, OT practitioners will be involved with range of motion and joint mobility. Once the peak weakness has passed and the client in no longer on a ventilator, OT practitioners will work with these clients on energy conservation techniques, strengthening as indicated, and self-care skills.

Compression

In order for a nerve to function, it must be free of any form of pressure or compression that slows conduction of impulses both outward toward the periphery as well as inward toward the spinal cord and brain. Pressure may lead to specific symptoms based on the location of the nerve root that is being compressed. Areas that are prone to compression occur at sites within the spinal column and in the periphery. Impingement of the nerve root in the spinal column may occur in several ways. Ordinary age-related changes to the intervertebral disc lead to disc degeneration. The disc may bulge, which means that the walls of the disc have weakened and pressure has forced the disc to extend into the nerve. The disc can also herniate so that the soft inner material leaks out of the disc and presses on the nerve root. The disc material can also break off and become free floating in the spinal canal and impinge the nerve root.

Spinal Stenosis

Spinal stenosis describes a narrowing of the spinal canal leading to spinal cord compression. One of the most common forms of compression is foraminal spinal stenosis, which can result in compression of the spinal cord itself. With foraminal stenosis, the opening through which the peripheral nerve root must leave the spinal column shrinks.

Thoracic Outlet Syndrome

Once a peripheral nerve leaves the spinal column, it can be compressed by restricted tissue or bony compression. Examples include thoracic outlet syndrome, sciatica, and carpal tunnel syndrome (CTS). Occupational therapy practitioners working in rehabilitation and hand clinics often treat clients with CTS. With CTS, the median nerve is compressed as it passes through the carpal tunnel at the wrist.

The tunnel is normally narrow so that any swelling or decrease in size can result in pressure on the median nerve. Symptoms include numbness and tingling to the thumb side of the hand to the middle of the ring finger. Causes of CTS are linked to repetitive use activities such as driving, painting, typing, sewing, factory assembly work, or using tools. With compression issues, the OT practitioner works with clients to reduce swelling, may fabricate splints, provide energy conservation, and to modify work or home environments to reduce the risk factors associated with causes of the compression.

The Cardiovascular System

The cardiovascular system serves as the source of delivery of gases, hormones, blood cells, and nutrients to and from our musculoskeletal system, internal organs, and nervous system. As blood leaves the heart, it is transmitted through arteries. The arteries are thick impervious tubes, which must sustain high blood pressures. As blood arrives at the tissues in the body, it moves through capillaries that allow transfer of gases (oxygen, carbon dioxide) and nutrients. Once the oxygen has left the blood stream and carbon dioxide enters it, veins return the deoxygenated blood to the heart. The heart performs these tasks by means of a pump that involuntarily contracts.

The muscle tissue in the cardiovascular system is striated or grooved/ridged to allow for mass contractions of segments of the heart, called chambers. The chambers are directed to contract through a series of electrical impulses that coordinate the heart's rhythm. The deoxygenated blood enters the right side of the heart into the atrium from the superior and inferior vena cava. The blood passes into the right ventricle through the tricuspid valve. From the right ventricle, the blood is pumped to the lungs through the pulmonary valve into the pulmonary artery. The oxygenated blood returns to the heart via the pulmonary vein into the left atrium. From the left atrium, the blood moves into the left ventricle passing through the mitral valve.

Finally, the blood is ejected from the heart through the aortic valve. The heart muscle receives oxygen by the coronary arteries, which originate immediately after the aorta leaves the left ventricle. Diastolic action of the left ventricle fills the coronary arteries, thus providing the heart muscle with oxygenated blood. The cardiovascular system is closed and maintains a blood volume of approximately 5 quarts for a 155-pound human. Contraction of the left ventricle produces a force of blood to the periphery. Blood pressure is the pushing against the walls of the vessels. Normal blood pressure in adults ranges from 90 to 120 mm Hg systolic when the left ventricle contracts to 60 to 80 diastolic when left ventricle relaxes.

When the blood volume reaches the capillaries, a small portion of the fluid leaks out into the interstitial space between tissues due to the forces of pressure (osmotic pressure) and by the process of fluid attraction to protein (oncotic pressure). The excessive fluid must be returned to the circulatory system to maintain homeostasis. The lymphatic system serves this purpose.

The lymphatic system is comprised of vessels similar to the cardiovascular system; however, it is an open system without a central pump. The lymphatic system begins in the periphery with initial lymphatics that terminate in flaps. The flaps of the lymphatics open and close via attachments called anchor filaments that surround the connective tissue. When excessive fluid accumulates in the interstitial spaces, the tissue swells and opens the flaps of the initial lymphatics. The interstitial fluid is drawn into the lymphatic vessel and now becomes lymph.

Once in the lymphatic vessels the fluid flows by body movement, a pulsating action of the nearby vascular system, and via an intrinsic pumping mechanism of the lymphangions. Since the lymphatic fluid contains protein, bacteria, viruses, cellular debris, and interstitial fluid, it needs to be consolidated before it is returned back into the circulatory system. The lymph nodes serve the purpose of removing unwanted components of the lymph. The lymph nodes house immune and white blood cells and act as filters by trapping particles. Eventually, as the lymphatic system moves and filters the lymph fluid, it deposits the lymph back into the circulatory system at the right and left subclavian veins. This process allows for a maintained balance within our blood circulatory system (Figs. 30.6–30.8). Today, many OT practitioners are seeking advanced training to become certified in lymphedema treatment. Lymphedema is an abnormal accumulation of lymphatic fluid beneath the skin that leads to edema (swelling).

Atypical Cardiovascular Conditions

The cardiopulmonary system provides the musculoskeletal system with required oxygen and removal of waste products. Endurance exercise increases the efficiency of the body, thus requiring less oxygen to produce more activity. This is called conditioning and improves as the body continues to be challenged. Lack of exercise may produce the opposite effect. Deconditioning due to lack of physical activity and exercise is one of the most common preventable causes of morbidity and mortality (Thyfault & Booth, 2011).

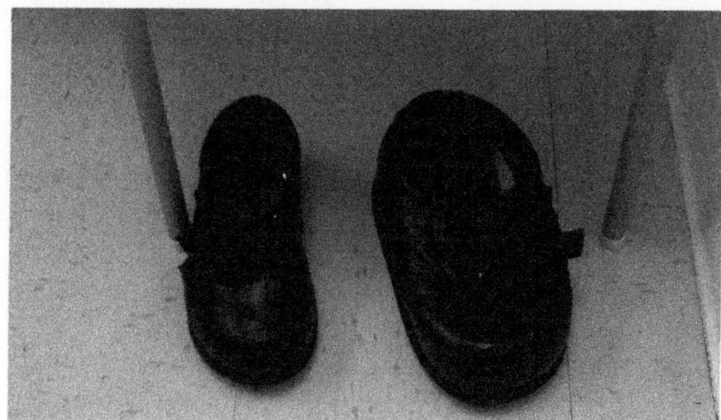

Figure 30.7 Shoes may need to be specially crafted to meet the needs of people with lower extremity lymphedema.

Myocardial Infarction

The effect of insufficient oxygenation of the cardiac muscle may lead to a myocardial infarction (MI) or heart attack. The myocardium is supplied by the coronary arteries. In the event of a blockage of blood flow, the supply is diminished and causes ischemia. Blockage is caused by a

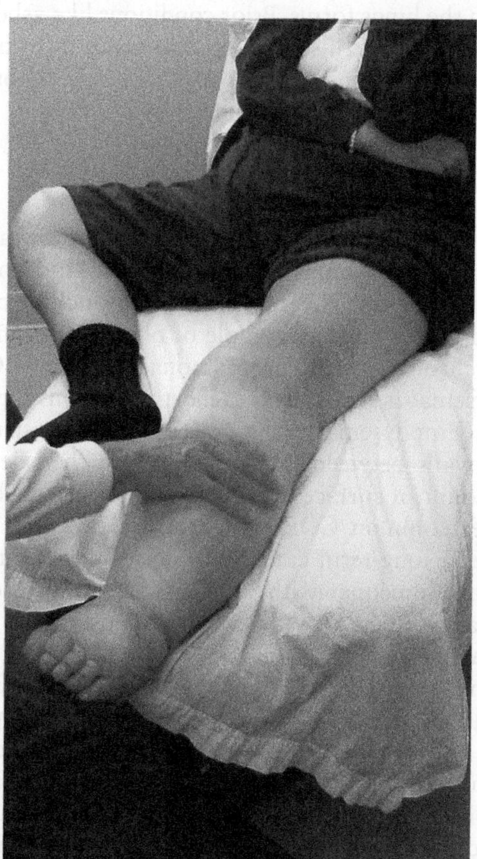

Figure 30.6 Client with lymphedema following knee surgery.

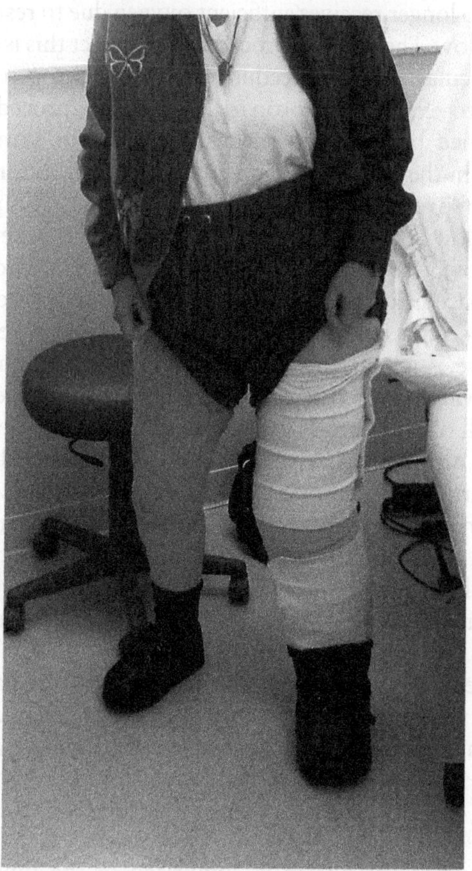

Figure 30.8 Compression wrapping is one component of lymphedema treatment.

buildup of fatty materials that form plaques on the walls of the coronary arteries. Depending on which arteries are blocked determines the extent of the damage that occurs to the myocardium. Prior to an MI, a person may experience angina, which is chest pain as a result of a lack of oxygen to the heart muscle. Coronary heart disease (CHD), also known as coronary artery disease (CAD), is a narrowing of the blood vessels in the heart and may, if untreated (or even if treated), lead to an MI.

The mechanical action of the heart is guided by electrical activity. The heart is controlled by small pacemaker cells that depolarize spontaneously to produce an electrical impulse. The impulse travels via electrical conducting cells that carry the current rapidly and efficiently through the heart. Eventually, myocardial cells, which comprise most of the heart, contract synchronously as one unit. First, the atria contract and then are followed by the ventricle thus making the sound "lubb-dubb" when listening with a stethoscope.

Any heart valve can fail. They can fail if they do not open sufficiently because of stenosis or they fail to close tightly because of insufficiency. By failing to close sufficiently, regurgitation occurs and returns blood to the prior chamber. The heart must work harder to deliver sufficient blood to the body. The heart muscle can hypertrophy due to overwork and in time decrease efficiency of the cardiac pump.

Coronary artery stenosis can be so extensive that the heart no longer receives sufficient oxygen due to restricted blood flow. The surgical procedure to correct this is called a **revascularization** procedure and requires open heart access to expose the coronary vessels. The procedure is performed by harvesting a healthy artery or vein, usually from the leg, which is then attached to the coronary artery above and below the blocked segment. This procedure allows the blood flow to "bypass" the blocked area and provide successful oxygenation to the myocardium.

A pacemaker and/or defibrillator may be inserted into the upper chest if the conducting system of the heart becomes defective. A wire is positioned from the device through the vessel walls back to the heart. The end wire is inserted into the wall of the heart. Pacemakers are specifically designed to treat arrhythmias, which are rate or rhythm problems of the heart. A heart beating too slowly is termed bradycardia and conversely too fast is **tachycardia**. If it is determined that an arrhythmia may cause life-threatening situations, a defibrillator may be inserted. It delivers a high-energy pulse to normalize the heart's electrical activity. Devices are available to perform both functions.

The OTA role in working with clients with cardiac conditions will be developing realistic exercise programs, teaching relaxation techniques, as well as energy conservation.

The Pulmonary System

The pulmonary system is comprised of the lungs and muscles of breathing including the diaphragm and the intercostal and accessory muscles. The function of the lungs is to act as an exchange system: to draw air in to the blood stream and remove carbon dioxide from the blood stream. The lungs are divided into lobes that house the smallest component of the gas exchange called the alveoli. Millions of small alveoli are present in the lungs to create significant surface area by which to allow exchange of gases.

Atypical Pulmonary Processes

There are several atypical pulmonary processes that your clients may present with. They may significantly impact function and participation and are discussed below.

Restrictive Lung Disease

Lung expansion requires that structures surrounding it are able to move. Restrictive lung disease occurs when expansion of the lungs is limited by extrapulmonary structures that result in decreased lung volume. The main symptoms of restrictive lung disease are shortness of breath and coughing. Asbestosis is caused by the long-term exposure to asbestos. Decades ago, when asbestos was installed or removed, there was no indication of the extent of damage it could incur. Today, strict procedures must be followed when removal is performed. Another restrictive lung disease condition occurs when individuals are treated for cancer and a fibrosis (hardening) of the tissue in the lungs forms. Prior conditions like asbestosis and cancer are intrinsic factors that result in restrictive lung disease. Extrinsic factors may include GBS or even structural conditions like kyphosis or obesity.

Obstructive Lung Disease

Obstructive lung disease is characterized by airway obstruction. The lungs may be inflamed and collapse and block airflow. The major symptoms include coughing and wheezing. An example of obstructive lung disease is chronic obstructive pulmonary disease (COPD). Emphysema is one of the most common types of COPD. Emphysema is characterized by a destruction of the walls between the alveoli, which then decrease the amount of surface area available for gas exchange. Another common COPD is chronic bronchitis, which involves a long-term cough with excessive mucus production. Someone with obstructive lung disorders may have difficulty with exhaling and require many hospitalizations.

Lung disease may limit occupational performance regardless of the condition. Occupational therapy practitioners will work with clients with pulmonary conditions to enhance postural awareness and chest wall expansion or respiratory muscle activation. Developing strengthening and conditioning program as well as education on energy conservation are also areas that OT practitioners address when working with this population.

Summary

This chapter provided a broad overview of general physical conditions that an OTA may encounter in their practice. The discussion was by no means all inclusive, but it touched on the general aspects of each category by describing typical and atypical physiology and conditions. It is important to understand that loss of physical function leads to loss of identity. Being able to move enables us to go about our daily routines. The overarching role of the OTA in working with clients with a broad spectrum of physical conditions is to address strength, range of motion, mobility, energy conservation, home and workplace modifications, assistive technology, and adaptive equipment needs and to always be cognizant that loss of physical function often, if not always, impacts a client's sense of self-identify. The role of the OTA in working with clients with physical disabilities is very important in helping them lead full and enriching lives, despite any limitations that they may have.

I would like to thank Richard Rinehart, BSHCA, PTA, for taking the photographs included in this chapter.

Review Questions

1. The major body system describing the respiratory organ is:
   a. Musculoskeletal
   b. Neuromuscular
   c. Cardiovascular
   d. Pulmonary

2. The postural plane that divides the body in left and right segments is:
   a. Sagittal
   b. Frontal
   c. Transverse
   d. Horizontal

3. The portion of the spinal column that refers the area between the lower ribs and the pelvis is:
   a. Sacral
   b. Cervical
   c. Lumbar
   d. Thoracic

4. A curvature of the spine in the frontal plane only is called:
   a. Kyphosis
   b. Concavity
   c. Scoliosis
   d. Convexity

5. Congenital refers to occurring at:
   a. Birth
   b. Puberty
   c. Adolescence
   d. Adulthood

6. The form of arthritis that affects the synovium of the joint is:
   a. Acute gouty
   b. Ankylosing spondylitis
   c. Rheumatoid
   d. Osteoarthritis

7. The structure that connects the bone to another bone is:
   a. Muscle
   b. Tendon
   c. Ligament
   d. Cartilage

8. All of these components comprise the central nervous system EXCEPT:
   a. Brain hemispheres
   b. Cerebellum
   c. Brachial plexus
   d. Spinal cord

9. The system responsible for "rest and digest" is:
   a. Sympathetic
   b. Enteric
   c. Parasympathetic
   d. Central

10. An ischemic stroke is defined as:
    a. Lasting less than 24 hours
    b. Occurring as a result of a blockage
    c. The result of an emboli
    d. Vessel rupture in the brain

11. Parkinsonism presents with many symptoms including akinesia, which means?
    a. Small handwriting
    b. Lack of movement
    c. Mask-like presentation
    d. Unwanted accelerations

12. The disease that can result in acute total paralysis of the body is:
    a. Postpolio
    b. Guillain-Barre
    c. Amyotrophic lateral sclerosis
    d. Neurogenic claudication

Practice Activities

Assess the posture of another person by attaching a string with a weight from the ceiling. Position the person with the feet equally distant on both sides of the string and have them stand erect.

a. What do you observe when looking at the body relative to the string?
b. Are there curvatures in the spine?
c. Does one side of the body have a different joint position than the other?
d. Document all the changes you see between the two sides of the body.

When you are out in public, observe the uniqueness of every person and consider that many may have one or some of the conditions that are listed in the chapter. From your observations, consider how your future role as an OTA may impact their lives (in a positive way).

Select one major system discussed in the chapter and an atypical condition associated with it, for example, spinal stenosis. Locate several online resources that a client could go to learn more about the condition. Prepare a small but interesting brochure that outlines the condition itself and resources to learn more about it that you could share with this client.

References

Assembly WH. *Resolution R114: Disability Including Prevention, Management and Rehabilitation*. Geneva, Switzerland: World Health Organization; 2005.

Baraliakos X, et al. (2008). The relationship between inflammation and new bone formation in patients with ankylosing spondylitis. *Arthritis Res Ther* 2008;10(5):104.

Doorn P, et al. IVIG treatment and prognosis in Guillain–Barré syndrome. *J Clin Immunol* 2010;30(1):74–78. doi:10.1007/s10875-010-9407-4

Furie KL, et al. Guidelines for the prevention of stroke in patients with stroke or transient ischemic attack: a guideline for healthcare professionals from the American heart association/American stroke association [Practice Guideline]. *Stroke* 2011;42(1):227–276. doi:10.1161/STR.0b013e3181f7d043

Garfinkel M, Sarewitz D. Parallel path: poliovirus research in the vaccine era. *Sci Eng Ethics* 2003;9(3):319–338. doi:10.1007/s11948-003-0028-7

Goshgarian H. *Spinal Cord Medicine*. New York: Demos Medical Publishing; 2003.

Jankovic J. Parkinson's disease: clinical features and diagnosis. *J Neurol Neurosurg Psychiatry* 2008;79:368–376.

Johnston SC, Fayad PB. Prevalence and knowledge of transient ischemic attack among US adults. *Neurology* 2003;60(9):1429–1434.

Kim R. *Spinal Cord Medicine*. New York: Demos Medical Publishing; 2003.

Lloyd-Jones D, et al. Executive summary: heart disease and stroke statistics—2010 update: a report from the American Heart Association. *Circulation* 2010;121(7):948–954. doi:10.1161/CIRCULATIONAHA.109.192666

Modlin J. *Principles and Practice of Infectious Disease*. Philadelphia: Elsevier Churchill Livingstone; 2009.

Naomi S. Management of acute and chronic gouty arthritis: present state-of-the-art. *Drugs* 2004;64(21):2399–2416.

National Spinal Cord Injury Statistical Center, B., Alabama. Spinal Cord Injury Facts & Figures

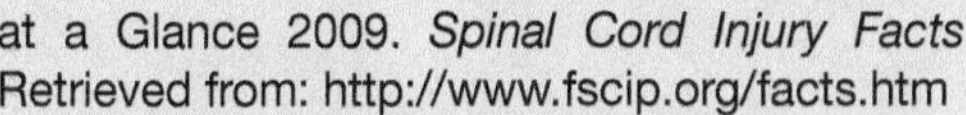

at a Glance 2009. *Spinal Cord Injury Facts*. Retrieved from: http://www.fscip.org/facts.htm

Neoplasm (n.d.). The American Heritage Science Dictionary. Retrieved from http://dictionary.reference.com/browse/neoplasm

O'Brien EC, et al. Stroke mortality, clinical presentation and day of arrival: the Atherosclerosis Risk in Communities (ARIC) study. *Stroke Res Treat* 2011;2011:383012. doi:10.4061/2011/383012

Reveille JD, et al. Genome-wide association study of ankylosing spondylitis identifies non-MHC susceptibility loci. *Nat Genet* 2010; 42(2).

Scott DL, Wolfe F, Huizinga TWJ. Rheumatoid arthritis. *Lancet* 2010;376(9746):1094–1108. doi:10.1016/s0140-6736(10)60826-4

Seeman E, Delmas PD. Bone quality—the material and structural basis of bone strength and fragility. *N Engl J Med* 2006;354(21):2250–2261. doi:10.1056/NEJMra053077

Surgery AAoO. *The Burden of Musculoskeletal Diseases in the United States* (Vol. 1). Rosemont, IL: American Academy of Orthopaedic; 2008.

Thompson AJ, et al. Primary progressive multiple sclerosis [Review]. *Brain* 1997;120(Pt 6):1085–1096.

Thyfault JP, Booth FW. Lack of regular physical exercise or too much inactivity. *Curr Opin Clin Nutr Metab Care* 2011;14(4): 374–378.

Vanhoenacker FM, et al. Congenital skeletal abnormalities: an introduction to the radiological semiology. *Eur J Radiol* 2001;40(3):168–183. doi:10.1016/s0720-048x(01)00398-9

Wallmann HW. Physical matters: the basics of balance and falls. *Home Health Care Manage Pract* 2009. doi:10.1177/1084822309337189

Wijesekera L, Leigh PN. Amyotrophic lateral sclerosis. *Orphanet J Rare Dis* 2009;4(1):3.

World Health Organization. The World Health Organization MONICA Project (monitoring trends and determinants in cardiovascular disease): a major international collaboration. WHO MONICA Project Principal Investigators. *J Clin Epidemiol* 1988;41(2):9.

World Health Organization. *Disability and Health Fact Sheet*. 2012. Retrieved from http://www.who.int/mediacentre/factsheets/fs352/en/index.html

National Limb Loss Information Center. Retrieved from http://www.amputee-coalition.org/limb-loss-resource-center/. http://www.fscip.org/facts.htm

CHAPTER 31

Vision

Jennifer Kaldenberg, MSA, OTR/L, SCLV, FAOTA

Key Terms

Astigmatism—An irregular shape of the eye that causes light to focus improperly on the retina.

Diplopia—Double vision, which can be caused by deficits in an individual's binocular visual status or neurological insult.

Functional vision—Refers to an individual's ability to use vision for functional activities.

Myopia—Nearsightedness, a refractive state where light is focused in front of the retina.

Nystagmus—A rapid, rhythmic, involuntary motion of the eye usually caused by congenital visual impairment or neurological insult.

Ophthalmologist—A medical doctor who specializes in the care of the eye and diagnosis and management of eye disease.

Optometrist—A doctor of optometry who is trained in the diagnosis and management of eye disease and refractive error.

Presbyopia—Loss of accommodation of the eye, typically begins around age 40.

Vision therapy—Exercises or treatment with lenses to enhance visual development, typically used for binocular visual deficits in children.

Visual acuity—Level of visual clarity or how well one can see.

Visual field—The area or perimeter of one's vision or how much one can see.

Visual function—Function of the ocular system, usually described as visual acuity, visual field, and contrast sensitivity measurements.

Learning Objectives

After reviewing this chapter, readers should be able to:

- Define visual impairment and describe its impact on occupational performance.
- Describe common visual conditions throughout the life span.
- Identify the personal and environmental factors that support or inhibit occupational performance.

Introduction

No matter what area of practice (pediatrics, geriatrics, home health, or mental health) OT practitioners themselves in, at some point, they will encounter individuals with vision loss. Vision is a complex sensory system that provides information about our world and provides support

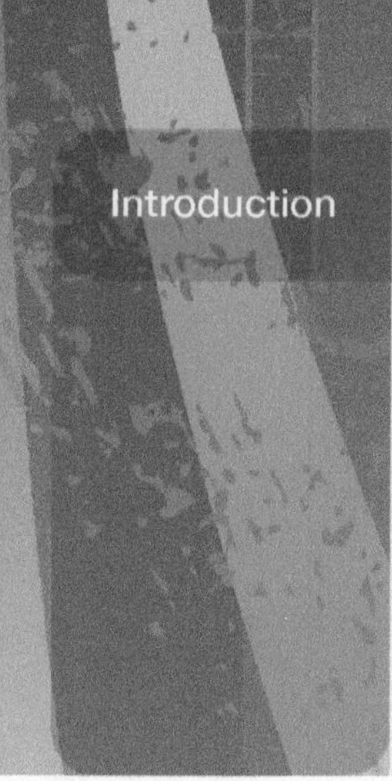

Introduction

for essential functions, such as balance, posture, and communication (Crews & Campbell, 2004; Hatzitaki et al., 2002; Soto-Faraco et al., 2004). Vision impairment can significantly impact an individual's ability to participate in meaningful occupations. For a child, this may mean difficulty meeting developmental milestones and difficulty learning and playing with peers, while for adults, it may interfere with work and engagement in leisure pursuits or impair social participation. In this chapter, we discuss the impact of vision loss on occupational performance and common visual conditions across the life span and identify the interaction of personal and environmental factors that either support or inhibit occupational performance for individual's with visual impairment.

Vision

An OT practitioner must take into account the ocular health of the client including the condition and the visual function; however, the **optometrist** or **ophthalmologist** is responsible for the medical management of the health condition and assessment of the visual function. An OT practitioner is concerned with the **functional vision** or how the visual condition and **visual function** impacts occupational performance (Colenbrander, 2003).

Person

Person or intrinsic factors comprise an individual's abilities and skills: neurobehavioral, physiological, cognitive, physiological, emotional, and spiritual. When working with an individual with a visual impairment, it is important to consider all these factors and how they contribute to participation in desired activities. Of course, one key personal factor for those with vision loss is what an individual can actually see. Therefore, understanding the anatomy of the eye and the visual system, visual development, and common visual conditions is the first step in providing best practice to those living with vision loss.

Anatomy of the Eye and Visual System

Before we can understand how the visual system impacts occupational performance, it is necessary to first understand normal anatomy and function of the visual system and normal visual development (Fig. 31.1). The eye functions much like a camera. Light enters the eye and is focused onto the retina by the cornea and lens. The iris, or colored portion of the eye, contains muscles responsible for managing the amount of light that enters the eye. In bright light, the muscles of the iris constrict the pupil, and in dim illumination, the pupil dilates allowing more light to enter the eye. The light must then pass through the vitreous, a gel-like substance that fills much of the interior of the eye in order to form the image on the retina. The retina is comprised of two types of receptor cells, rods and cones. The rods are responsible for night vision and the cones for color and detail vision. The central portion of the retina, the macula, has increased numbers of cone cells and is responsible for central detailed vision, and the fovea, the central portion of the macula, is the area of the retina with the most acute vision, 20/20 or better. Once light is focused onto the retina, the energy is converted into electrical impulses that are brought back to the brain via the optic nerve where the image is interpreted. Table 31.1 provides a description of the structures and functions of the eye.

Visual Development

Our visual system can be divided into two pathways, peripheral and central. The peripheral system provides us with information about our environment and supports mobility, while the central system is responsible for our detailed information about our environment, including color vision (Atkinson & Braddick, 2003; Warren, 1994). When we are born, our visual system is immature, and the only system that is fully developed is our peripheral visual system. When the infant is held, he/she is able to fixate and track their mother's face from a distance of approximately 18 in. However, by 6 months of age, the central system begins to develop, resulting in improved visual acuity, visual field, and oculomotor skills. It is essential for a developing child to integrate these systems in order to complete everyday activities throughout life (Atkinson & Braddick, 2003; Warren, 1994). Refer to Table 31.2 for visual developmental milestones.

As we age, normative changes within our visual system may influence our participation in life. Although these changes may not lead to a diagnosis of visual impairment, they may impair an individual's occupational performance, such as being able to read a menu in a restaurant with low lighting (refer to Table 31.3). In addition, physiological factors such as an individual's

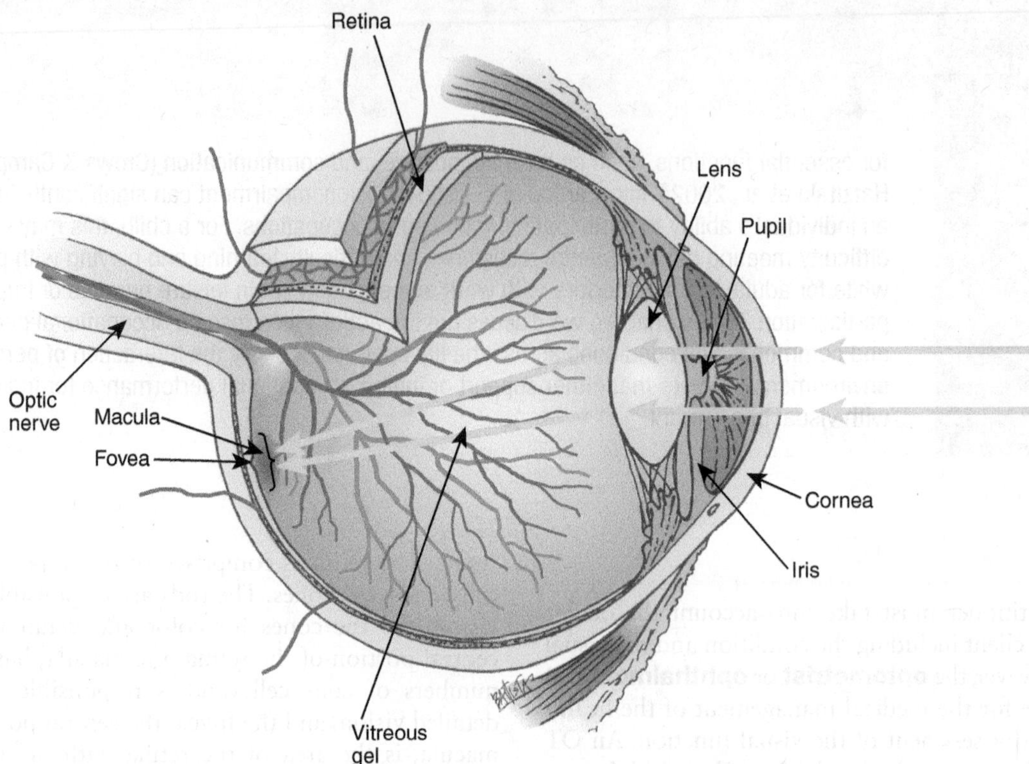

Figure 31.1 Diagram of the eye and visual system. (Image adapted from Weber JR, Kelley JH. *Health Assessment in Nursing*. 5th ed. Philadelphia, PA: Lippincott Williams & Wilkins; 2013.)

premorbid health or prior activity level can impact intervention strategies to support occupational performance. This includes people with a past medical history (PMH) of hypertension, diabetes, and chronic obstructive pulmonary disease. The OT practitioner must consider the functional implications of the individual's PMH in addition to the complications of any visual impairment in order to develop an effective plan of care.

TABLE 31.1 Structures and Function of the Eye

Structure	Function
Cornea	A transparent avascular layer of the eye responsible for focusing light.
Sclera	The white portion of the eye that serves as protection and an insertion point for extraocular muscles.
Iris	The muscular colored portion of the eye.
Pupil	A hole in the iris that works to regulate the amount of light that enters the eye.
Lens	A clear structure located behind the iris that is responsible for focusing light on the retina.
Vitreous humor	The clear gel that fills the inside of the eye. Light must be able to pass through the vitreous to fall on the retina.
Retina	The back portion of the eye responsible for receiving light and transmitting the neural signal to the optic nerve and into the brain.
Macula	A small area in the retina where photoreceptors are more densely packed. Responsible for central vision.
Fovea	A small depression in the center of the macula responsible for central vision.
Optic nerve	Carries visual information from the retina to the brain.

TABLE 31.2 Visual Development

Structure	Function
Visual pathways	• Developed by 24 weeks gestation but continues to develop until about 6 months.
Retina	• Continues to develop until 1 year old. • Visual function (visual acuity and contrast sensitivity) continues to develop until about school age.
Cortical function and binocular vision	• Continues to develop until about 3 months.
Optic nerve	• Fully myelinated at about 7 months.
Oculomotor control	• Fixation improves over first 3 months of life but does not mature until teen years. • Pursuits and saccades begin at 2–3 months but continue to improve through childhood. • Accommodation is mature by around 3 months.
Visual acuity	• 1 month: 20/400[a] • 3 months: 20/200[a] • 1 year: 20/60[a] • 2 years: 20/30[a] • Maturity at about 18 and then begins to decline after that.
Visual fields	• Full visual fields by 6–7 months.

[a]Estimations (Todd V, Tsurumi K. A second look: visual perceptual disorders in children. *Conference conducted in Woodbridge, NJ*, 1993; Glass P. Development of visual function in preterm infants: implications for early intervention. *Infants Young Child* 1993;6(1):11–20; Atkinson J, Braddick O. Neurobiological models of normal and abnormal visual development, 2003. Retrieved from http://www.psychol.ucl.ac.uk/vdu/pdf/neuro_development.pdf).

Warren (1994) discusses a hierarchy of visual skills that build on one another (Fig. 31.2). The foundational skills of visual acuity, visual field, and oculomotor control are often impacted in ocular disease. In addition, when foundational skills are impaired, higher-level skills, such as visual attention, visual scanning, pattern recognition, visual memory, and visuocognition, are also influenced. An individual's visual and visual perceptual disorder(s) can significantly impact his/her ability to perform occupations of choice.

Visual impairment is typically categorized by those foundational skills of **visual acuity** and **visual field**.

TABLE 31.3 Normative Aging Changes

Structure	Changes with Aging
Lens	Thickens, becomes yellow and more rigid. Loss of accommodative ability (presbyopia). Problems with glare, changes in perception of colors. Development of cataracts. Decrease in contrast sensitivity
Pupil	Pupil becomes smaller and less light can reach the retina, necessitating increased illumination.
Tear glands	Fewer tears are produced, leading to drier eyes and irritation.
Peripheral retina	Difficulty with night vision and light/dark adaptation due to problems with photoreceptors
Cornea	Increased light scatter leads to increased glare.

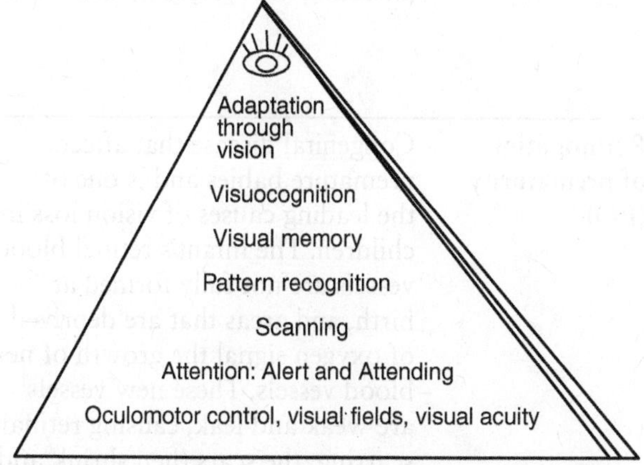

Figure 31.2 Hierarchy of visual perceptual skill development. (Reprinted with permission from Mary Warren. Warren M. A hierarchical model for evaluation and treatment of visual perceptual dysfunction in adult acquired brain injury. Part 1. *Am J Occup Ther* 1993;47:42–54.)

Visual acuity is a measure of how well one sees or the clarity of their vision. It is typically measured for both distance and near tasks. You are probably familiar with the term 20/20, which represents the distance at which an individual is able to identify a specific sized object, that is, distance/size of object. Visual field is a measure of how much one sees. This is typically measured for central and peripheral vision. A normal visual field is 60 degrees upward, 60 degrees inward, 70 to 75 degrees downward, and 100 to 110 degrees outward (Nougier et al., 1998; Zoltan, 2007). Refer to Table 31.4 for a list of common visual disorders.

TABLE 31.4 Visual Disorders

Visual Disorder	Description	Functional Implication	Medical Intervention
Amblyopia	The eye and brain are unable to work together to form a single image, due to one of three causes: an eye turn (strabismus), unequal refractive error (anisometropia), or a physical blockage of the eye (form deprivation or occlusion). One eye is suppressed, resulting in a permanent decrease in vision not correctable by lenses or surgery.	Loss or reduction of depth perception, spatial acuity, contrast sensitivity, and/or motion sensitivity.	Medical interventions are most effective before age 5; the eye disorder is corrected, and the patient is forced to use the nondominant eye. Perceptual learning and **vision therapy** can be used as long-term treatments.
Cortical visual impairment	A vision problem that affects the visual pathway and visual cortex of the brain where the brain misinterprets visual information. It can be caused at birth due to a hypoxic–ischemic event, when the baby is deprived of oxygen, or a disease or injury after birth.	Temporary or permanent mild to severe vision loss may occur. Patients may also experience motor **nystagmus**, short attention span, difficulty maintaining fixation, compulsive light gazing, variable visual acuity, and/or reduced depth perception. Patients may see best with peripheral vision.	Vision treatments are typically not given until the patient is medically stable and in an educational environment. Vision stimulation can be used but must also be used outside of therapy sessions to be effective. Often, vision loss is associated with other neurological defects.
Ocular albinism	The eye's retinal pigment epithelium lacks pigment; can be ocular or oculocutaneous (affecting the eyes, hair, and skin).	Patients can experience reduced visual acuity, high **astigmatism**, nystagmus, strabismus, and/or light sensitivity.	No current treatment exists for the condition itself, but symptoms can be treated. Lenses, vision therapy for strabismus, and low vision interventions.
Retinopathy of prematurity (ROP)	Congenital disease that affects premature babies and is one of the leading causes of vision loss in children. The infant's retinal blood vessels are not fully formed at birth, and areas that are deprived of oxygen signal the growth of new blood vessels. These new vessels are weak and leak, causing retinal scarring; the scars then shrink and can cause retinal detachment. Can also increase risks of developing **myopia**, strabismus, glaucoma, and cataracts.	Substantial or total loss of vision. Can impact all areas of visual function.	ROP is currently treated with peripheral destruction of the avascular retina using a laser to stop the growth of new blood vessels in the periphery and thus reduce leaks, scar tissue formation, and retinal detachments

TABLE 31.4 Visual Disorders (continued)

Visual Disorder	Description	Functional Implication	Medical Intervention
Retinitis pigmentosa	Group of ocular conditions in which the loss of photoreceptor cells leads to decreased vision and blindness. It is a genetic disorder in which the rods are affected first and then the cones.	Night blindness followed by peripheral vision loss and eventually total vision loss.	No current medical treatment, but many areas are being researched
Age-related macular degeneration (AMD)	Resulting from a breakdown or atrophy of photoreceptors in the macula, AMD involves the irreversible and progressive loss of central vision. There are two forms, dry, or nonexudative, and wet, or exudative, with wet AMD being the more severe form due to the formation of new, weakened blood vessels in the macula that can leak and cause damage and vision loss.	Loss of central vision, typically does not impact peripheral visual field.	Treatments include laser surgery or injections for wet AMD and nutritional and behavior changes to reduce the risks of AMD and vision loss.
Glaucoma	Glaucoma is a group of diseases that affect the optic nerve to cause peripheral vision loss. Damage occurs due to a buildup of fluid that presses on the optic nerve, caused by the closure of the eye's anterior angle or decreased drainage through the anterior chamber.	Progressive loss of peripheral field.	Treatments differ depending on whether the angle is open or closed; if closed, immediate action is required to prevent blindness. If the angle is open, medication and/or surgery can be used to treat primary open angle glaucoma.
Cataracts	Cataracts affect the clarity of the eye's crystalline lens by causing light entering the eye to scatter and produce glare and discomfort.	Cataracts can cause decreased visual acuity, **diplopia**, decreased contrast sensitivity, and difficulty driving at night.	Treatment for cataracts is surgery to remove the crystalline lens and replace it with an intraocular lens implant.
Diabetic retinopathy	Diabetic retinopathy involves the occlusion of retinal blood vessels, causing oxygen deprivation in parts of the retina and consequent growth of new, weakened vessels. These new vessels can leak blood or fluid resulting in scotomas, blurred vision, and even blindness. Diabetic retinopathy occurs in 40%–45% of diabetic patients and has two forms, proliferative, the more severe form, and nonproliferative.	Diabetes may impact all aspects of visual function.	Treatments include laser treatments, surgery, and vitrectomy.
Hemianopia	Hemianopia is the loss of vision in half of the visual field. It is associated with strokes and traumatic brain injuries and is a type of significant visual field loss.	Loss of visual field. Area of visual loss is dependent upon the area of the brain that is involved.	No medical interventions exist for the condition itself, but the symptoms can be treated with lenses, visual scanning and visual skills training.

TABLE 31.5 Visual Perception

Visual Perceptual	Description	Examples of Functional Implication
Visual scanning	The ability to move visual attention from one object to another.	• Miss objects on one side when ambulating • Skip lines when reading
Visual attention	The ability to focus on an object and its details.	• Lose attention to task • Unable to gather important information from the environment for safety
Pattern recognition	The ability to identify an object based on its features or details.	• Inability to match items • Difficulty completing puzzles or reading and writing activities
Visual memory	The ability to store visual information.	• Inability to remember phone numbers from the phonebook • Unable to recall walking directions (mental map)
Visuocognition	The ability to use visual information for learning or problem solving. Includes form constancy, visual closure, figure ground, position in space, and depth perception.	• Difficulty with matching (form constancy) • Difficulty with puzzles or tasks presented in incomplete form (visual closure) • Identifying object from its background (figure ground) • Poor sense of personal space (position in space) • Walking up or down stairs (depth perception)

Additionally, individuals may also have deficits in higher-level visual skills. Deficits of visual perception and visual cognition can impact all areas of occupation. For example, deficits in visual scanning may impact one's ability to identify and avoid hazards within the physical environment or be able to read efficiently. Table 31.5 provides examples of how impairment in visual perception may impact occupational performance.

Interventions

When determining appropriate interventions for a client with visual impairment, the OT practitioner must consider personal and environmental factors, as well as the (client's) desired occupation in order to meet the client's goals. Please refer to Table 31.6 for further information about intervention strategies.

TABLE 31.6 Considerations for Interventions

Person	Environment	Occupation
Use of remaining vision • Eccentric viewing (requires advanced training) • Scanning training (teach systematic scanning of the environment or task) **Visual substitution** • Sensory substitution • Organizational/cognitive strategies **Psychosocial and emotional factors**	**Social** • Self-advocacy • Peer support groups (e.g., problem-solving self-management) **Physical** • Contrast • Lighting • Low vision devices and/or assistive technology **Economic** • Resources availability and access • Role of advocacy	**Task** • ADL • IADL • Rest and sleep • Education • Work • Play • Leisure • Social participation

Personal Factors

It is important that OT practitioners determine the most appropriate intervention strategies, keeping in mind safety as a foremost factor. Is it in the client's best interest to use their residual vision or would it be safer to use visual substitution? If the client is able to use their remaining vision, then potential strategies could include eccentric viewing and scanning training.

Eccentric viewing is a viewing technique used with individuals with central visual field impairment, such as macular degeneration. The client is trained to use a healthier portion of the retina for central viewing. To simulate this, place your fist at the bridge of your nose and look across the room. If you move your head up, down, left, or right, you can find an area to look around the scotomas (blind or blurred area). Some clients with central visual field loss can learn to use eccentric viewing for distance and near viewing tasks, such as watching TV or reading. However, eccentric viewing can be a difficult skill to learn especially if an individual is not motivated or has cognitive impairment. Teaching eccentric viewing requires advanced training.

Individuals with central and peripheral field impairments may benefit from scanning training, and teaching clients systematic scanning techniques is another important visual skill to be learned. Teaching a client to systematically scan their environment or the task may improve safety and independence and decrease frustration. Scanning is a simple technique of using head and/or eye movements to locate objects or hazards in the environment or locate the text on a page. For example, a client with peripheral field impairment from glaucoma wants to be independent in getting around in his/her home. The OT practitioner begins by instructing the client to scan to the farthest left corner of the room using eye and/or head movements. Once the corner has been found, the client begins to scan to the right, until the end of the wall. He then moves his gaze slightly down and begins to scan back to the left. This left-to-right scanning continues until the room has been scanned and all hazards have been identified. By creating a mental map of the environment, the client is able to understand where the potential hazards are before moving through his environment. If the client is unable to rely on his/her vision to complete desired occupations, then visual substitution strategies can be used. Use of tactile, auditory, and organizational/cognitive strategies may be used to adapt the task or environment. Tactile strategies may be used to mark items for identification. Rubber bands, safety pins, puff paint, and commercially available marking tools can be used to improve identification of items within the home and community. For example, a bump dot can be used to mark 350 degrees on the oven so that a client can feel for the marking instead of having to put their face close to the burner and risk an injury. It is important to remember that many conditions including diabetes may impact sensation. Assessment of sensation is important before using the strategies discussed below. See Figure 31.3 for examples of tactile marking strategies.

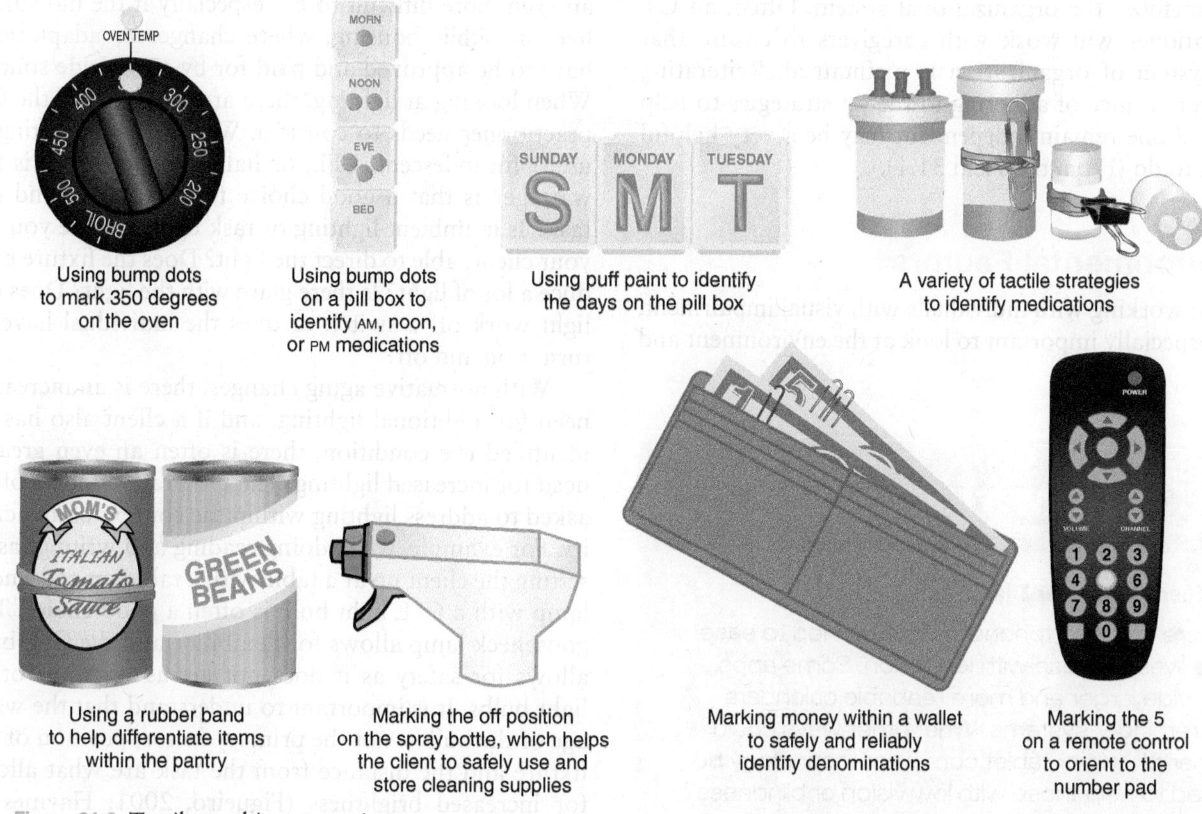

Using bump dots to mark 350 degrees on the oven

Using bump dots on a pill box to identify AM, noon, or PM medications

Using puff paint to identify the days on the pill box

A variety of tactile strategies to identify medications

Using a rubber band to help differentiate items within the pantry

Marking the off position on the spray bottle, which helps the client to safely use and store cleaning supplies

Marking money within a wallet to safely and reliably identify denominations

Marking the 5 on a remote control to orient to the number pad

Figure 31.3 Tactile marking strategies.

Another type of sensory substitution is auditory strategies. There are a number of commercially available items on the market that can be used to facilitate participation in desired activities. They include talking glucometers, scales, calculators, clocks, thermostats, and even some ATM machines. Most of these products are out-of-pocket expenses for clients that must be considered when planning interventions. Additionally, there are talking services that are free to individuals with visual impairment such as books on tape, which are available through the Library of Congress and/or reading services such as the Talking Information Center. It is important to keep in mind that the majority of visual impairment occurs as one ages and hearing impairment is also very prevalent in older adults. Trialing of several different types of voices may be helpful when addressing dual sensory impairment to make sure a client is getting the most out of a talking service.

As people are losing their vision, they often rely on and compensate with cognition and organization to complete daily activities. For example, if someone leaves his/her keys in a reliable place, they can be counted on to be there when heading out the door. Likewise, if someone enjoys baking and organizes the pantry in a very systematic way, there is no need to read labels to know where things are placed. These strategies rely on the individual and those around him/her to maintain the organizational strategy, as well as cognition to remember the organizational system. Often, an OT practitioner will work with caregivers to ensure that the system of organization is maintained. Reiterating the importance of adhering to the set strategies to help a loved one remain independent may be a very helpful thing to do (From the Field 31.1).

Environmental Factors

When working with individuals with visual impairment, it is especially important to look at the environment and how social, physical, and economic factors support or inhibit engagement in occupations. Although the OT completes a comprehensive assessment of the environment, there are a few factors that you as an OTA will need to know when working with people with vision loss.

When looking at social factors, determine whether the client is able to self-advocate or ask for help if needed. Teaching a client to self-advocate is an important skill. For example, if a client is in an unfamiliar environment and trying to cross a busy intersection, it is important that he/she is able to ask for help and instruct the volunteer in appropriate sighted guide (a technique to guide someone safely through the environment). Similarly, instructing a client to be able to help himself/herself and others by participating in active problem solving can be helpful in finding strategies to meet goals. There are many peer support groups as well as support groups led by practitioners that can address active problem solving and can be great social and functional resources for individuals with visual loss.

The physical environment may significantly impact people's ability to participate in desired occupations. Depending on where one lives, an individual may or may not have control over making accommodations to meet these needs. When looking at the physical environment, it is important to pay special attention to lighting and contrast. Lighting is not a simple issue and is often an even more difficult to fix, especially if the individual lives in public housing, where changes or adaptations have to be approved and paid for by an outside source. When looking at lighting, there are many things the OT practitioner needs to consider. What type of lighting is used? Incandescent, CFL, or halogen? And what is the wattage? Is that a good choice for the fixture and the task? Is it ambient lighting or task lighting? Are you (or your client) able to direct the light? Does the fixture produce a lot of light? Is there glare with the light? Does the light work off a switch or does the individual have to turn it on and off?

With normative aging changes, there is an increased need for additional lighting, and if a client also has an identified eye condition, there is often an even greater need for increased lighting. The OT practitioner is often asked to address lighting within the context of an activity. For example, when doing reading and writing tasks, setting the client up at a table with a tabletop gooseneck lamp with a CFL light bulb is often a good choice. The gooseneck lamp allows for flexibility, and the CFL bulb allows for safety as it does not get as warm as other light bulbs. It is important to understand that the wattage of the bulb is not the primary factor; position of the fixture and the distance from the task are what allows for increased brightness (Figueiro, 2001; Haymes & Lee, 2006).

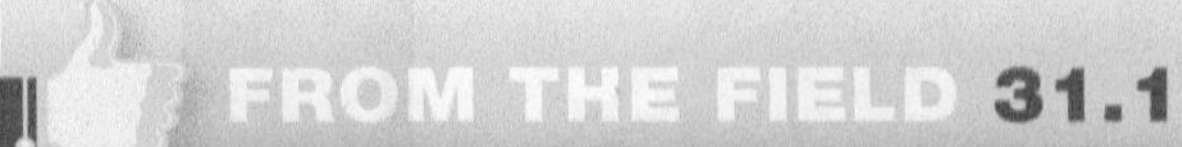

Is There an App for That?

There are smartphone apps designed to ease the lives of those with low vision. Some apps provide larger and more readable calendars or reminder systems. What other ways could smartphone or tablet computer technology be used to help those with low vision or blindness?

With increased lighting, there is often an increase in glare, which may be uncomfortable or even disabling to an individual with a visual impairment. A client may complain of issues related to glare or you may notice that he/she is squinting. It is important to make sure that all light bulbs are covered by a shade or housing, windows have shades or blinds, and highly reflective surfaces such as TVs or computers are positioned away from windows. Other interventions for glare may include wearing wide-brimmed hats, filters, or sunglasses; using nonwax polish on floors, or even placing a table cloth on a shiny table.

The majority of individuals with visual impairment will use some type of low vision device and/or assistive technology to remain engaged in occupations of choice. An optometrist or ophthalmologist prescribes low vision devices (LVD), while the OT practitioner is often called upon to train the client in the use of the LVD. As technology advances and as individuals become more accustomed to using technology in their daily lives, we will see changes in what types of devices are being used by individuals with vision loss. Table 31.7 illustrates various types of LVDs and assistive technology and their pros and cons.

When using LVD and assistive technology, it is important to be aware of the client's strengths and weaknesses and explore ways to adapt the task or the device in order for the client to be successful in its use. For example, an OT practitioner is working with Mrs. Clay, a client with macular degeneration and degenerative joint disease. Mrs. Clay would like to be able to read her magazines. Due to the significance of her visual loss, a pair of glasses was not an option. The optometrist prescribed a hand and stand magnifier for reading tasks. Because she would like to read for a prolonged period of time, the hand magnifier was not optimal for reading her magazines. It would have been difficult for her to maintain the position in order to maintain the focal distance. When exploring the options for use of the stand magnifier, the OT practitioner found that in her current setup, Mrs. Clay was unable to maintain a good posture because she had to lean forward to look through the magnifier. It was determined that by adding a pillow and a clipboard, she was able to

TABLE 31.7 Low Vision Devices and Assistive Technology

Device	Description	Pros	Cons
Spectacle or microscope	High plus lens mounted in a spectacle frame (binocular up to +14 D and in monocular up to 20× magnification)	• More acceptable/familiar • Acceptable in lower powers • Can be used for reading and writing tasks • Hands free in lower powers • Portable • Wide variety of powers	• In higher powers, requires reduced working distance • Must be maintained at the focal distance
Stand magnifier	A convex lens mounded in a housing that maintains the correct focal distance (powers of 2–15×)	• Fixed focal distance • Most times has own light source • Can drag along to read • Wide variety of powers	• In high powers, very small field of view • Difficult to carry due to size • Does not work well on nonflat surfaces • May need a reading prescription
Hand magnifier	A convex lens that is mounted in a frame that is held and the focal distance must be maintained by the individual (powers of 2–15×)	• More acceptable/familiar • Portable • Illuminated and nonilluminated • Wide variety of powers	• Must maintain focal distance • Requires a steady hand • In higher powers, very small field of view

(continues on page 430)

TABLE 31.7 Low Vision Devices and Assistive Technology (continued)

Device	Description	Pros	Cons
Telescope	A lens system that is used for viewing objects typically in the distance but can be modified to view at near ranges In its reverse position and at low power (0.5–2×), a telescope can be used for orientation. By making everything appear smaller, it provides greater awareness of visual field.	• Binocular or monocular • Can be hands free if mounted in glasses • Can be used for distance and near tasks • In reverse and in low powers can be used for visual field awareness and orientation	• Limited field of view • Requires coordination to focus • Cannot be used when walking around • Costly
CCTV	Closed circuit television or electronic magnification enlarges an object using a camera. Magnifies objects up to nearly 100 times Comes in portable and tabletop versions	• Wide field of view • Larger ranges of magnification possible • Can control lighting and contrast • Can be used for reading and writing tasks	• Portability • COST
Screen magnification software/text to/from speech software	Computer software that can magnify the text, read aloud the text, or recognize your own speech to complete a variety of computer tasks	• Wide field of view • Can be used on current computers • Wide range of magnification options • Text to speech options • Can be used for a variety of IADL tasks	• Portability • Learning may be difficult if unfamiliar with technology. • As items are magnified, the individual must scan across the screen. • COST
Text to speech	Reading machines or document readers, document is scanned and then read aloud.	• No vision is required for use. • Can be used for a variety of purposes at home, work, community	• Portability • Learning may be difficult if unfamiliar with technology. • COST

maintain a good body position and continue to view the text through the magnifier. It is important to assess and maintain good ergonomics when using LVDs and assistive technology.

As previously mentioned, one of the greatest barriers to many of these environmental interventions is resource availability and access. As the majority of these interventions are out of pocket expenses, many individuals will go without the needed adaptive devices due to an inability to pay. This is why advocacy and finding resources become a big part of working with individuals with visual impairment. Check with your local social service agencies to see what is available for clients with low vision in your community.

Occupational Factors

When addressing the occupational goals of your client, it is important to assess the personal and environmental factors and determine those that will support or inhibit occupational performance. In this section, we look at examples of interventions specific to the client's occupational goals and factors that may support or inhibit performance.

Sue is a 76-year-old woman with bilateral cataract who would like to be independent in putting on her makeup. An OT and OTA worked together and evaluated the environment in which Sue completed her occupation and determined potential strategies that could facilitate participation. Because Sue has cataracts in both eyes, which creates general blur and often difficulty with glare, the OT practitioners looked at the setup at her bathroom vanity. They noticed that the shade to the light fixture had been removed, and there was considerable glare on the vanity. The OT practitioners also noticed that there was clutter throughout and Sue had difficulty locating her items within the bathroom and did not use any adaptive devices or strategies. After discussing potential strategies (magnified, lighted mirror, organizing tray, improved lighting fixture, self-advocating for assistance), the OT practitioners and Sue decided to replace the shade to the light fixture; purchase a magnified, lighted mirror; and organize the bathroom. The lighted mirror was placed on the vanity and Sue sat to apply her makeup. She also used the organizational strategies that were taught to her to remain organized in the bathroom. With simple adaptations, Sue was able to return to managing her own makeup application.

Bob is a 45-year-old man with retinitis pigmentosa who would like to be independent in finding items in the grocery store aisles. Retinitis pigmentosa affects peripheral visual field and impairs Bob's ability to safely navigate within the environment, locate aisle markers, and locate items on the shelves. After discussing potential strategies, the OT practitioner and Bob decide to work on scanning training, training with use of a reverse telescope, which was prescribed by the optometrist, and referral to an orientation and mobility specialist, for further training in safe community mobility and long travel. Bob was trained in a systematic scanning technique to use in all unfamiliar environments to identify hazards and landmarks within the space. In addition, Bob utilized a reverse telescope for assisting in his orientation. He used the same systematic scanning technique with the reverse telescope while standing still. After training in the use of scanning techniques and with the telescope, Bob was able to use those skills in the grocery store to find items on the shelf. However, Bob does have days when his vision fluctuates. On those days, Bob is able to self-advocate and ask for help at customer service to have personal assistance for shopping.

Lilly is an 8-year-old child with albinism who would like to play with her peers on the playground. Because Lilly has albinism, the outdoor glare has prevented her from playing comfortably outdoors, and she has been staying in the shade. The OT practitioner has been working with Lilly and her friends to explore opportunities to include Lilly in activities on the playground that are safe and comfortable. The OT practitioner has also contacted the family to see if Lilly has sunglasses that she could use during school to help with the outdoor glare problems.

Tom is a 63-year-old lawyer with macular degeneration who would like to remain employed by his practice. He has self-modified his activities at work but would like to be able to read the results of the trials that the younger members of the firm have engaged in. Tom has been using computer technology for years and would like to explore computer software options. Tom was shown a variety of software options, all with pros and cons, and he decided to purchase ZoomText, a screen magnification software with reading option. With training in the use of the adaptive technology, Tom was able to read transcripts independently. On days when Tom in fatigued, he is able to use the reading option and have the text read to him instead of reading himself.

Margaret is a 93-year-old woman who previously socialized with her friends and played bridge at her senior center several times a week. About a month ago, Margaret had a significant change in her vision as a result of macular degeneration and glaucoma. She is fearful of leaving her apartment and is embarrassed that she can no longer recognize people's faces. It is important for the OT practitioner who is working with Margaret to understand the risk of depression in individuals with vision loss, be able to screen for it, and make appropriate referrals as necessary. Coping with vision loss and the progressive nature of many acquired visual impairments is often very difficult to deal with. For Margaret, understanding she is not alone and that there are many things that can be done to improve her ability to complete tasks that are important to her can assist in her adjustment process. The OT practitioner discusses and practices potential strategies of modifying the task or environment, such as using large print playing cards for playing bridge or eccentric viewing for seeing faces.

Summary

An OT practitioner may find himself/herself working with an individual with visual impairment in any practice setting and throughout the life span. It is for this reason that all OT practitioners need to develop the skills in order to address the client with visual impairment and his/her occupational needs. Consideration of the client's person and environmental factors and understanding how these factors support or inhibit engagement in occupations are essential for occupational therapy practice. This chapter provided a review of the anatomy of the eye and the visual system, visual development, and common visual conditions as well as intervention strategies to support a client's engagement in desired occupations. Through the use of intervention strategies addressing the person, environment, and occupation, the OTA can assist a client to meet his/her desired goals.

Note

The author and publisher have no financial stake in the products or companies discussed in this chapter, nor do they endorse any of them.

Review Questions

True or False

1. Visual impairment can impact an individual at any time throughout the life span.
   a. True
   b. False

2. The OT practitioner is primarily interested in visual function NOT functional vision.
   a. True
   b. False

3. At birth, the visual system is fully developed.
   a. True
   b. False

4. Vision loss in a normative part of aging.
   a. True
   b. False

5. If we all live long enough, we will all develop cataracts.
   a. True
   b. False

6. Depression is common in adults with vision loss.
   a. True
   b. False

7. The primary complaint for an individual with retinitis pigmentosa is difficulty reading.
   a. True
   b. False

8. Mary is an 80-year-old woman with macular degeneration, what would you expect for Mary to have difficulty with:
   a. Getting around in her home
   b. Seeing colors
   c. Reading the newspaper
   d. Visiting with friends

9. Tristan is a 5-year-old boy with difficulties with visual scanning, the best activity to facilitate environmental scanning would be:
   a. A puzzle
   b. Writing activities
   c. I Spy Game
   d. Tying shoes

10. Bob is a 73-year-old man with diabetes and a history a proliferative diabetic retinopathy and peripheral neuropathy. Bob's goal is to be independent in medication management. What strategy would NOT be recommended for Bob?
    a. Auditory strategies
    b. Magnification strategies
    c. Tactile strategies
    d. Organizational strategies

Practice Activities

Adapt a play activity for a child with visual impairment. How do your interventions strategies change with the different diagnoses?

Adapt a cooking activity for an adult with visual impairment. How do your interventions strategies change with the different diagnoses? If the client also has one of the following conditions (diabetes, multiple sclerosis, stroke), how does that impact your interventions?

Develop a resource guide of national and local organizations that provide services for individuals with visual impairment.

References

Atkinson J, Braddick O. Neurobiological models of normal and abnormal visual development. 2003. Retrieved from http://www.psychol.ucl.ac.uk/vdu/pdf/neuro_development.pdf

Colenbrander A. Aspects of vision loss: visual functions and functional vision. 2003. Retrieved from http://www.ski.org/Colenbrander/Images/Aspects_of_Vision_Loss.pdf

Crews JE, Campbell VA. Vision impairment and hearing loss among community-dwelling older Americans: implications for health and functioning. *Am J Public Health* 2004;94(5):823–829.

Figueiro MG. Lighting the way: a key to independence; 2001. Retrieved from http://www.lrc.rpi.edu/programs/lightHealth/AARP/index.asp

Glass P. Development of visual function in preterm infants: implications for early intervention. *Infants Young Child* 1993;6(1):11–20.

Hatzitaki V, et al. Perceptual-motor contributions to static and dynamic balance control in children. *J Mot Behav* 2002;34(2):161–170.

Haymes SA, Lee J. Effects of task lighting on visual function in age-related macular degeneration. *Ophthalmic Physiol Opt* 2006;26: 169–179.

Nougier V, Bard C, Teasdale N. Contribution of central and peripheral vision to the regulation of stance: developmental aspects. *J Exp Child Psychol* 1998;68(3):202–215.

Soto-Faraco S, Ronald A, Spence C. Tactile selective attention and body posture: assessing the multisensory contributions of vision and proprioception. *Percept Psychophys* 2004;66 (7):1077–1094.

Todd V, Tsurumi K. A second look: visual perceptual disorders in children. *Conference conducted in Woodbridge, NJ*. 1993.

Warren M. A hierarchical model for evaluation and treatment of visual perceptual dysfunction in adult acquired brain injury. Part 1. *Am J Occup Ther* 1993;47:42–54.

Warren M. Evaluation and treatment of visual perceptual dysfunction. *Presentation conducted in Boston*. Rocky Mount, NC: Advanced Rehabilitation Institutes; 1994.

Zoltan B. *Vision, Perception, and Cognition*. 4th ed. Thorofare, NJ: SLACK, Inc.; 2007.

CHAPTER 32

Cognitive Disabilities

Michael J. Urban, MS, OTR/L, CEAS, MBA, CWCE

Key Terms

Agnosia—Difficulty interpreting visual, auditory, and/or sensory stimuli even though the sensory system is intact.

Apraxia—The inability to formulate the plan needed to carry out movements or tasks that are needed to participate in daily living.

Attention—Being able to focus on one specific stimulus to the exclusion of others. (Greenberg et al., 2002).

Cognition—The mental process of knowing; that which comes to be known; and processes and systems through perception, awareness, attention, memory, intuition, and knowledge (Farlex, 2009).

Cognitive impairment (CI)—The inability to remember, to formulate ideas, and/or to organize and recall information that impacts the person's safety and overall ability to complete everyday tasks (Australian Government, 2011).

Executive functions—The brain's ability to execute and regulate complex cognitive functions such as motor planning, organizing information, time management, safety awareness, and regulate behaviors (Kielhofner, 2009).

Neuron—Specialized kind of cell located in the central nervous system.

Subcortical—Unconscious—not within voluntary control.

Learning Objectives

After studying this chapter, readers should be able to:

- Define cognition, cognitive impairments, and executive functions.
- Identify the three components of cognition related to function.
- Understand basic theoretical models guiding occupational therapy cognitive rehabilitation.

Introduction

Cognition is defined as "the mental process of knowing; that which comes to be known; processes and systems through perception, awareness, attention, memory, intuition, and knowledge" (Farlex, 2009). The *Occupational Therapy Practice Framework III* (AOTA, 2014) lists cognition under the classification of client factors as grouped into mental functions. The classifications and components listed within the *Occupational Therapy Practice Framework III* (AOTA, 2014) are an excellent resource for documentation and to help to identify components of daily functioning for practice.

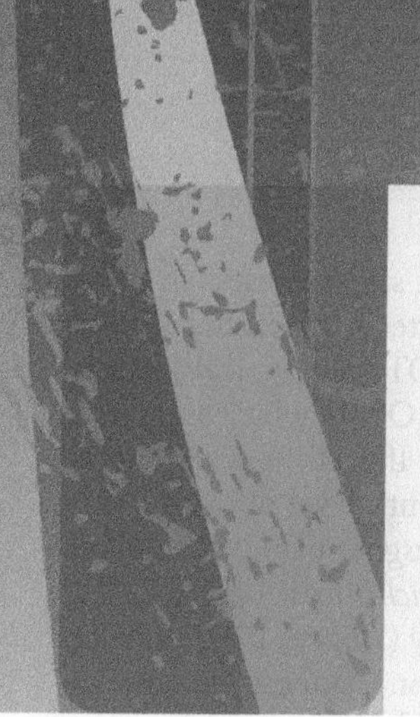

Cognition plays a vital role in our ability to carry out everyday occupations. **Cognitive impairment (CI)** is the inability to remember, to formulate ideas, and/or to organize and recall information to an extent that it impacts a person's safety and overall ability to complete everyday tasks (Australian Government, 2011). As an OTA, your awareness of the main components of cognitive functional performance will help guide clients through therapeutic interventions and functional tasks. Doing this entails, at a minimum, a basic knowledge of brain function and theories that drive occupational therapy's skilled interventions (please also refer to Chapter 7, *Occupational Therapy Theories and How They Guide Practice*). A strong foundation of the core components of cognition will guide you in treating individuals who may be demonstrating some level of CI, such as those with acquired brain injury, stroke, or dementia.

Neuroanatomy of Cognition

Understanding cognition first and foremost entails understanding brain structure and how it is structured with regard to thought processes (Fig. 32.1). The brain is comprised of billions of **neurons**, specialized cells found in the central nervous system, which form central areas responsible for different bodily functions, thoughts, and emotions. The cerebrum (also referred to as the cerebral cortex and will be referred to as such interchangeably within the chapter) is responsible for higher mental functions associated with consciousness, learning, speech, thought, and memory. The cerebral cortex is the largest structure in the brain and is divided in to two hemispheres by the corpus callosum. Each hemisphere of the cerebral cortex controls the opposite side of the body. The cerebrum contains four right- and left-sided lobes, each of which contains specialized structures that govern physical performance and cognitive functioning (Parsons & Osherson, 2001). The limbic system, an essential structure of the cerebral cortex, is located just under the cerebrum on either side of the thalamus. Figure 32.1 provides an illustration of the left cerebral cortex. To help you learn the brain structure

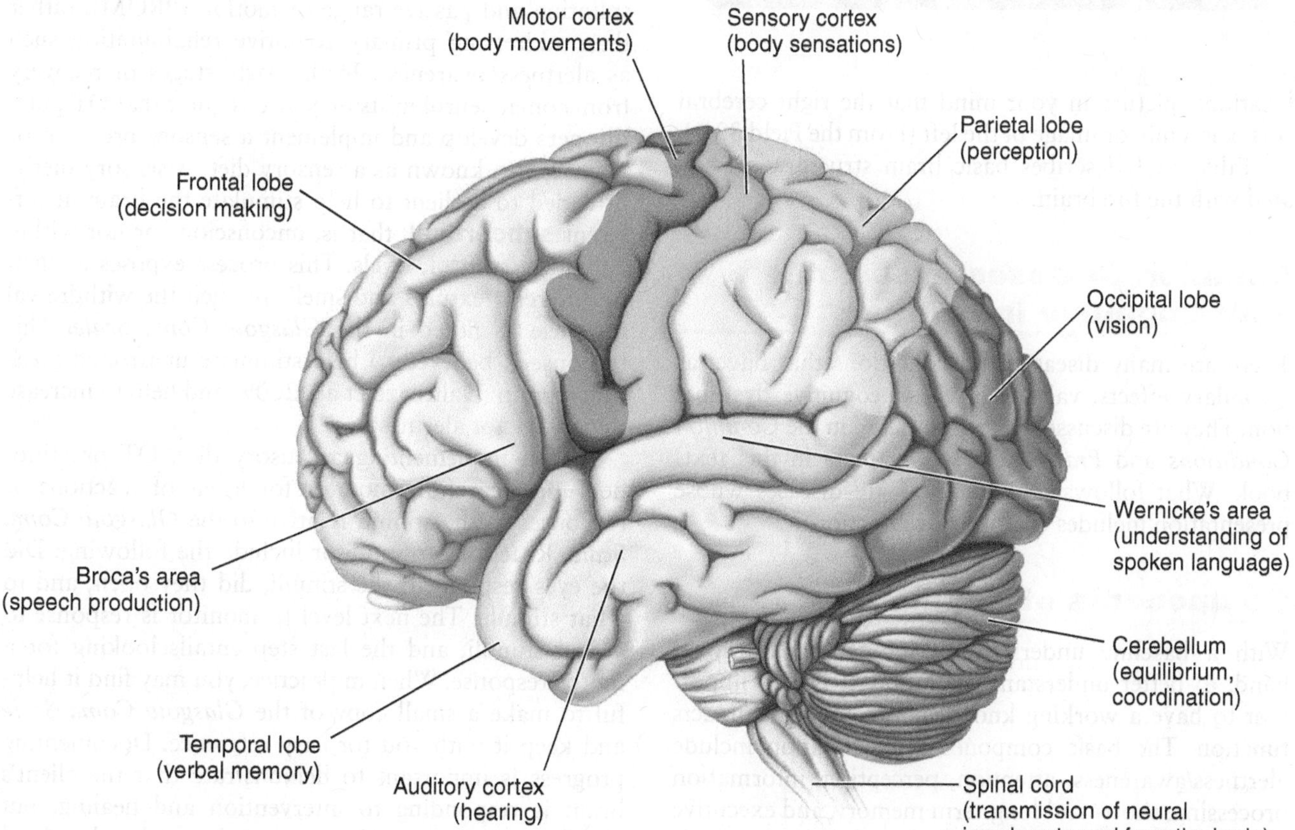

Figure 32.1 Lateral view of the left cerebral cortex.

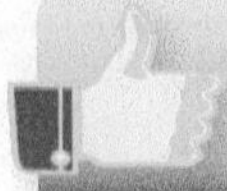

FROM THE FIELD 32.1

Contralateral Neglect

The term contralateral control describes how the left side of the brain controls the right side of the body and vice versa. Left-sided neglect is the most common form of contralateral dysfunction and is seen following a stroke (CVA) or other brain insult (Greenberg et al., 2002). With contralateral neglect, the client is not aware of body parts and environmental objects on the involved side. This leads to dysfunction with engaging in daily tasks and risk of injury to the involved side. A classic example of this occurs with people who are post-CVA. When the affected arm dangles off a side of a wheelchair/chair, the individual may be unaware of the upper extremity's location. Left-sided neglect requires individuals to be cued to look at the position of the limb because they lack perception that the arm is theirs. Contralateral neglect also impedes bilateral integration or the ability to cross the body's midline to engage in tasks. Impaired bilateral integration significantly impedes daily living skills.

locations, picture in your mind that the right cerebral cortex is a mirror image of the left (From the Field 32.1).

Table 32.1 describes basic brain structures associated with the forebrain.

Common Diseases Associated with Cognitive Impairment

There are many diseases and conditions that have, as secondary effects, varying levels of cognitive dysfunction. They are discussed in greater detail in the *Common Conditions* and *Practice Setting* chapters in this textbook. What follows in Table 32.2 are diseases whose presentation includes cognitive dysfunction.

Components of Cognition

With a baseline understanding of neuroanatomy in hand,.to better understand cognition, it is also important to have a working knowledge of how CI impacts function. The basic components of cognition include alertness/awareness, attention, perception, information processing, short- and long-term memory, and executive functions. Collectively, they all play a vital role in our everyday daily occupations.

Alertness/Awareness

Alertness or awareness is the first step to assess in terms of cognitive functioning. No matter the practice setting, in every initial evaluation, the OT will typically document: alert and orientated ×3 (A&O ×3), which stands for A&O to person, place, and date. If a client is not A&O ×3, it is documented as to the client's level of orientation, as A&O ×2 or A&O ×1. The *Glasgow Coma Scale* (Hill, 2000; Rowlett 2001) and the *Rancho Los Amigos Levels of Cognitive Functioning (Revised)* (Hagen, 1998; Rancho Los Amigos National Rehabilitation Center, 2006) are two examples of scales frequently used in acute care settings or a neurological rehabilitation units to determine level of alertness following brain injuries such as CVA, acquired brain injury, or brain tumor. The *Glasgow Coma Scale* is important to administer when documenting a client's progress in the acute stages of coma. The *Glasgow Coma Scale* helps to monitor and demonstrate a client's response to therapy interventions and progress. Alertness is an essential part of cognition because if a person is not alert, then he/she is not aware of or unable to respond to stimuli.

Individuals who are in comas can sometimes process information, but may have no voluntary control over their actions (Daltrozzo et al., 2009). At this stage of the recovery process, the OTA may be called in to work with a client primarily to address vital issues such as prevention of joint contractures through the use of splinting and passive range of motion (PROM), rather than addressing primary cognitive rehabilitation such as alertness/awareness. In the early stages of recovery from coma, neurologists may also request that OT practitioners develop and implement a sensory program or what is also known as a sensory diet. A sensory diet is provided to a client to help stimulate the brain at different **subcortical**, that is, unconscious or not within voluntary control, levels. This process exposes a client to different textures and smells to elicit the withdrawal response as noted in the *Glasgow Coma Scale*. This response is believed to help stimulate unaffected areas of the brain (Daltrozzo et al., 2009) and help to increase the process of alertness.

When implementing a sensory diet, OT practitioners must carefully monitor for levels of reactions or responses to the stimuli relative to the *Glasgow Coma Scale*. Reactions to monitor include the following: Did the eyes respond to the stimuli, did they open, and to what stimuli? The next level to monitor is response to verbal stimuli, and the last step entails looking for a motor response. When in practice, you may find it helpful to make a small copy of the *Glasgow Coma Scale* and keep it with you for easy reference. Documenting progress is important to demonstrate that the client's brain is responding to intervention and healing, but also for insurance reimbursement. Once a baseline level of consciousness is established and the client is alert,

TABLE 32.1 Brain structures associated with the forebrain

Structure	Location	Function	Dysfunction	Occupational Therapy Intervention
Frontal lobes	Most anterior portion of the cerebrum	Speech production and **executive functions**; the ability to execute and regulate complex cognitive functions such as motor planning, time management, safety awareness, and regulate behaviors and emotions. Executive functions play a vital role daily functioning and influence decision making and planning.	Poor safety awareness, disinhibition/initiation difficulties, motor planning difficulties, and **apraxia**; an inability to formulate the plan needed to carry out movements or tasks that are needed to participate in daily living.	• Environmental adaptations such as unplugging the stove. • Pictorial cues to sequence steps for a basic ADL task such as brushing teeth. • Caregiver education. • Recommend auditory/visual alert systems for medication reminders or other to-do routine care functions. • Teach skills in concise, familiar, and clear simple one- or two-step directions to complete a process. • Break down tasks into smaller components.
Temporal lobes	Located just above the ears	Perception and recognition of auditory stimuli, memory, and speech. The left temporal lobe is more closely associated with memory, recall of auditory and visual stimuli, and verbal processing. The right temporal lobe is associated with nonverbal processing and recognition of visual stimuli.	Memory impairment, **aphasia**, the inability to speak, inability to recognize written words and faces, and visual perceptual issues.	• Create client memory books. • Use current technology to compensate for memory deficits. • Close collaboration with speech therapists to develop a consistent communication system to reduce client frustration.
Parietal lobes	Located posterior to the frontal lobe and superior/medial to the temporal lobes	Assists in orientation, recognition, and perception of sensory stimuli. Holds the motor homunculus, which is an area of the brain responsible for limb movement for each respective side of the body.	Difficulty with interpreting visual, auditory, and or sensory stimuli known as **agnosia**. Dysfunction results in the misperception of objects and/or left right laterality confusion. May present as a functional physical inability to complete a task, but also cognitively (e.g., a client is presented with a toothbrush and uses it to comb his/her hair or does not know what to do with the toothbrush). Laterality issues impact knowing where objects are located within a person's visual field.	• Remediation and compensatory training such as visual scanning techniques to locate objects, placing photos of the client using objects as they are intended to do in an easily visible place to help regain mastery in everyday occupations. • Motor relearning and compensation.

(continues on page 438)

TABLE 32.1 Brain structures associated with the forebrain (continued)

Occipital lobes	Most posterior and inferior region of the cerebrum	Receive and process visual information.	Complete or partial loss of vision, visual field cuts, misperception of visual stimuli, and/or color discrimination.	• Falls prevention training and education. • Develop safe systems to carry out ADLs. • Use of contrast and good lighting to improve visual input client such as deficits secondary to macular degeneration
Corpus callosum	Separates the brain into right and left hemispheres. The fibrous structure runs in an anteroposterior direction	Interhemispheric communication.	Impedes cognitive functions, such as executive functioning, auditory comprehension, and visual processing. Dysfunction results in safety concerns and physical impairments.	• Global ADL and IADL training and compensatory techniques as noted with frontal lobes.
Limbic system	Located just inferior to the cerebrum alongside the thalamus	Regulates emotions and motivation.	Poor emotional control, lack of motivation.	• Anger management techniques. • Stress management and education. • Organizational planning for daily routines
Thalamus	Located in the center of the brain just inferior to the cerebrum	Guides motor control and is the relay system for the limbic system—receives auditory, somatosensory, and visual signals and relays them to cerebral cortex.	Pain hypersensitivity Neuropathic pain	• Sensory desensitization. Electrical stimulation for pain management. • Compensatory techniques and remediation with global ADLs and IADLs secondary to varying pain levels.
Hypothalamus	Located inferior to the thalamus and superior to the brain stem	Regulates body temperature (homeostasis), hormone balance, and bodily function drives (hunger, thirst, and sex drive).	Impaired vision, dizziness, sleep, weight problems, and temperature control.	• Education on ADL/IADL adaptations to regulate body temperature. • Development of sleep routine and stress management to limit impact of stress upon daily occupations. • Visual compensatory retraining. • Balance retraining and compensatory techniques with daily living tasks.
Reticular formation	Located within in the brain stem	Controls body function states such as sleep, alertness, and attention.	Poor sleep cycles, inability to filter out environmental distractions, altered levels of alertness.	• Compensatory techniques, adaptations, and remediation to improve attention to tasks. • Sleep pattern retraining, adaptations, and education on effect of lack of sleep upon daily functioning. • Sensory stimulation and purposeful activity.

Sources: Greenberg et al. (2002); Gutman (2008); Just et al. (2007); Kielhofner (2009); Morgane et al. (2005); Sammler, 2102; Witgert et al. (2010).

TABLE 32.2 Commonly Seen Diagnoses/Conditions That May Impact Cognition

Acquired brain injury/traumatic brain injury
Alzheimer disease and other dementias
Attention deficit hyperactivity disorder (ADHD)
Illicit drug use
Malnutrition
Metabolic disorders
Multiple sclerosis (late stages)
Polypharmacy
Stroke/cerebral vascular accident (CVA)
Down syndrome
Parkinson's (late stages)
Anxiety
Alcohol abuse
Hypoxia (low oxygen)
Depression (moderate to severe)
Dehydration
Psychiatric conditions
Brain tumor

helping a client regain function may begin with intervention initially focusing on attention.

Attention

Attention is defined as the ability to sustain focus on a particular stimulus while excluding of other stimuli (Greenberg et al., 2002). There are five areas of attention: focused attention, sustained attention, selective attention, alternating attention, and divided attention (Gehring et al., 2011). Impairment in any one of these areas may impede a client's ability to carry out his/her daily occupations.

Focused attention (Gehring et al., 2011) is the ability to focus on one stimulus while ignoring others. Typically, focused attention applies to short stimuli, such as a ringing telephone. If the stimulus is longer in duration, then focused attention transitions into sustained attention.

Sustained attention is the ability to maintain focus in order to complete a task (Gehring et al., 2011). Examples include studying your notes for a test or washing a fragile glass by hand. Sustained attention allows us to learn and acquire new skills. When a client has a dysfunction with sustained attention, learning or relearning new skills can be significantly impacted because a longer duration attention is needed to do a multistep process. Becoming skilled in task and activity analysis and understanding how to break down an everyday tasks such as donning a shirt into its smaller components are critical, as is providing extra time and patience to allow a client to complete a task (please also refer to Chapter 11, *Activity Analysis: The Jewel of the Occupational Therapy Profession*). This is critical to help decrease client frustration and ensure positive outcomes to OT interventions.

As an OTA, knowing your client's limits to maintain sustained attention on a task is important. For example, if you have a client who can only attend to a task for 2 minutes, then you will need to modify your planned intervention to help increase his/her ability to attend to the task for a longer duration of time. If the task requires 15 minutes to complete and he/she can presently attend for two minutes, you must grade the task to gradually increase his/her attention from 2 minutes up to the 15 minutes necessary to complete the task. This process will strengthen a client's skills and self-confidence by grading the activities from simple to increasingly complex to allow for successful completion. Using the just-right challenge approach, in which the tasks are not too easy or not too difficult, but still engage the client, should incrementally require him/her to increase sustained attention by short durations (i.e., 1 minute), to ensure successful outcomes.

Selective attention is the ability to filter out opposing stimuli (Gehring et al., 2011). An example of this is studying while at a busy coffee shop or while listening to music. A client with dysfunction related to selective attention will have a difficult time attending to directions or a task in a busy clinic setting. Cognitive rehabilitation needs to begin in a controlled environment, free of external distractions. The goal would be to slowly increase the level of distractions to provide appropriate cognitive challenge. The grading of the process to slowly reintroduce the client to multiple simultaneous stimuli will help support selective attention and decrease frustration.

Alternating attention is the ability to shift attention between two different stimuli while completing a task (Gehring et al., 2011). A good example of this occurs when in the classroom. You must be able to effortlessly shift attention between the auditory stimuli of the lecturer or visual stimuli of a chart or PowerPoint presentation and note taking. Imagine how poorly you might perform in school if every time you switched your attention from the lecturer to your notes, you lost your place (in your notes). The distraction ensuing from being unable to locate your position in your notes morphs into being unable to refocus on the lecturer, thus missing critical information. Many people have alternating attention issues, which may negatively impact not only academic performance but also daily living skills. As an OTA, helping a client regain these skills requires teaching compensatory techniques to learn location skills and/or doing exercises to slowly regain a mastery of these skills. For instance, one compensatory technique is to record information to listen to at a later time as frequently as needed. Additionally, an example of an exercise to help strengthen alternating attention is the *Stroop* effect (Fig. 32.2). For this exercise, a client reads the words as they appear and then repeats the exercise by saying the colors the words are written in while ignoring the words. Try it; this is not as easy as it sounds.

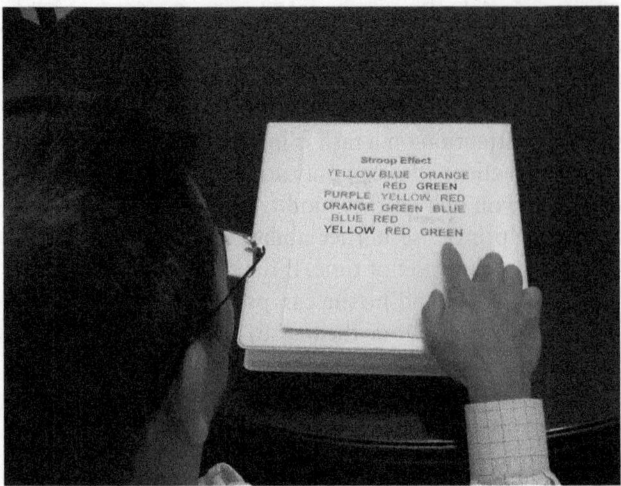

Figure 32.2 A client is working on the Stroop effect. (Photo Credit, Amy Wagenfeld.)

The *Stroop* effect requires the brain to process information the first time by blocking out the color the word is written in while the second time the brain must ignore the word and process the color name. This effect can also be addressed by presenting words such as big and small in different sizes as illustrated in Figure 32.3.

When implementing this activity, you can time and track the number of errors to monitor improvement, but the true purpose of the *Stroop* effect is to serve as a precursor to build basic skills necessary to be translated into functional activity requiring alternating attention. Once mastery of the basic *Stroop* effect is achieved, the task can be further graded up to challenge the client's ability to focus and alternate between two different types of stimuli while simultaneously counting the number of words or colors presented. These are higher-level skills necessary to be successful with tasks that require divided attention or multitasking.

Divided attention is the ability to simultaneously attend to two stimuli or, in other words, to multitask (Gehring et al., 2011). An example of divided attention is to attend to a recipe while cooking and at the same time engaging in a conversation with someone about an entirely different topic. In today's world, we are constantly bombarded with stimulation; hence, multitasking has become a basic necessity. We like to think we are all masters of this skill, but if you were to closely observe someone being a poor multitasker, it would likely make you think of *your* shortcomings with multitasking. For instance, this person you are observing could make a serious mistake in balancing the check book if also busy trying to listen to a conversation in the room at the same time. As OT practitioners, we use divided attention in our work with clients: we give clients a routine task such as completing a set of repetitive tasks to do while simultaneously asking them to report on pain levels. This sequence of events requires clients to keep track of the number of repetitions they are completing while maintaining focus on their technique while answering your question. A client who has difficulty with divided attention will either lose count and/or technique with the task in order to stop to process the question that was posed and to formulate a response.

BIG small big SMALL BIG Small
SMALL BIG small Big big SMALL
Big SMALL big SMALL small BIG
Small SMALL BIG Big SMALL big

Figure 32.3 Stroop effect example size/words.

Having a sound understanding of your client's ability to attend to a task is essential to properly plan and implement intervention, including educating clients and their families. Understanding how different states of attention impact performance is the basic building block to develop sound intervention plans. As well, understanding that attention is also impacted by changes in medication, lack of sleep, pain, depression, and/or other medical conditions gives you further insight into how to best set up your intervention program. Dysfunction in any area of attention has the potential to limit a client's ability to safely complete IADLs and ADLs and, in turn, impact his/her ability to either return home after hospitalization or to remain at home.

Perception

Perception is noted to be the "*discrimination of sensations (e.g., auditory, tactile, visual, olfactory, gustatory, vestibular-proprioception)*" (AOTA, 2014, p. 822). Perception guides our ability to assess and develop a spatial awareness of our environment. Incoming multisensory cues impact perception. We must properly interpret the different stimuli to help guide our cognitive functions. That is, what we perceive helps us understand our world. When there is misperception, information has been improperly interpreted and stored in short- and long-term memory. This leads to poor outcomes with regard to retrieval of information and overall daily function.

When the body misinterprets or misperceives the sense of light touch as being painful, engaging in daily tasks is greatly impacted. Imagine if every time you petted a little cute puppy, it felt like you were rubbing your hand across a pile of broken glass. Despite watching other people playing with and touching the puppy, because of your misperception, would you most likely stop petting the puppy? The brain's perception of what is soft has somehow been altered through injury or illness. As an OTA, helping your client to relearn this sensory processing is vital to allow them to be able to carry

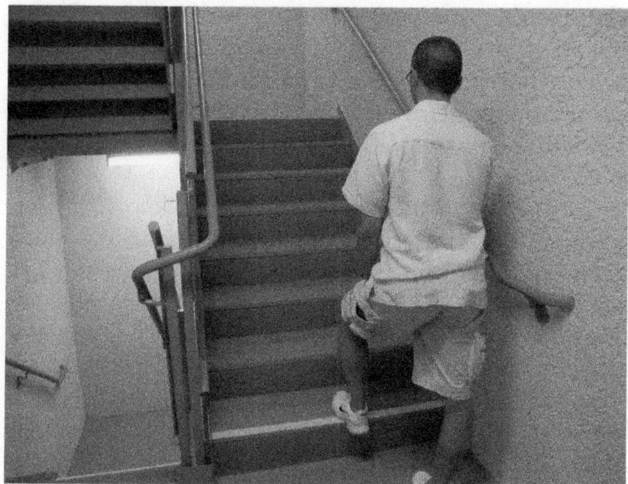

Figure 32.4 A color contrasting strip helps identify the edge of the step. (Photo Credit, Amy Wagenfeld.)

out his/her daily tasks (please also refer to Chapter 28, *Sensory Processing*).

Visual perception impairments may lead to increased risk of falling because of a misperception that something was closer to them than it really was. While this often occurs in people with visual impairments, those with various psychiatric disorders and dementia may often experience similar misperceptions. This commonly occurs in individuals with dementia with Lewy bodies. Clients with this form of dementia have well-formed visual hallucinations and depth perception issues (Greenberg et al., 2002). These two factors contribute to behavioral issues and place the client at a greater risk for falls.

Depth perception dysfunction is a major contributor to falls and is not exclusive to those with dementia. People with depth perception dysfunction need a variety of compensatory techniques to help make up for the dysfunction. An example of a compensatory technique for those with depth perception issues includes boldly color contrasting stair risers to identify the edges of steps or other transitions (Fig. 32.4).

The misperception typically ensuing from poor contrast sensitivity, which is the inability to distinguish an item of similar color against another item of same color, may lead a person to think that a carpeted stair case is just a straight walk way. In this case, a compensatory technique of adding a contrasting color to the edge of each step increases the individual's ability to safely negotiate the stairs to, for instance, access a second floor bathroom or bring laundry to an upstairs bedroom.

Information Processing

The brain is the information processing powerhouse (Kielhofner, 2009). As previously discussed, the different regions of the brain receive, interpret, and process a constant stream of information in order for the body to function and interact with the environment. To properly process information, the nerve endings in the peripheral nervous system located throughout the body must connect with the spinal column to send stimuli to and from the brain. A newborn is an inefficient information processor. As the baby learns new motor, sensory, and/or social skills, the body takes in information from the environment and continually sends it via the sensory pathways of the peripheral nervous system to the spinal column and up to the brain for interpretation and then sends it back to the body in order to appropriately respond. This process happens throughout every moment of our lives. With practice and experience, sensory motor feedback loops and pathways become increasingly refined. Pathways that are laid down in childhood directly impact future function as an adult. When the effect of disease or disability impacts this seamless process, OT practitioners work with clients to remediate the process. Sometimes though, the old pathways are completely lost, as is the case of the brain damage incurred following a stroke. In this situation, the task of the OT practitioner is to work with a client to learn to use associated areas that were not affected by the stroke to compensate for the loss of function. Let's think about this.

Picture a field full of tall grass, grass so tall that you cannot see over it. Now, picture that you need to cross through this field in order to get to the food you must eat every day. The first time you walk through the field, it takes you 2 hours to make it through, due to having to detour around streams, swampy fields, muck, and so on. At the next attempt to get your food, you try a different path so as to avoid the swampy fields, stream, and other hazards encountered on the previous attempt. Going forward, each time you walk through the field, you slightly alter your previous pathway to avoid hazards and save time and to be more efficient. Before you know it, you are crossing that same field in 10 minutes to get your food. This process illustrates how throughout life, the brain develops efficient sensory and motor pathways to make a task easier.

Now, imagine that one day you are walking along that path and a huge tree crashes down and, because of the hazardous terrain, blocks your path for what seems like a mile in either direction. This tree is the equivalent to a CVA a client you may treat has had. In order to get your daily food, you must learn a new pathway through the field to avoid the new hazard. This time, though, would the amount of time it takes to find that new path be as long as 2 hours? It could be, but there is stored memory of the other hazards, which in turn helps you, with some trial and error, to find an alternative path in less than 2 hours.

This alternative path is a successful rehabilitation process. Finding this alternative path is the client's ability to rely on old areas of the brain that remain intact and can, with help from the therapy team, be accessed in order to relearn an old route or pathway around the hazard. This notion is referred to neuroplasticity of the brain, which is the brain's innate ability to heal itself after insult to regain function through use of associated areas in the brain. Occupational therapy intervention may help facilitate this process so a client can master new skills and relearn old ones. This process could be fast or very slow, depending on many environmental and contextual factors and other comorbidities. No two clients are ever the same. Therapeutic intervention must reflect this.

With regard to information processing, sometimes, other brain regions compensate for damage to the actual brain structure impacted by stroke, acquired brain injury, and/or certain medical diseases. Neuroplasticity does not factor into recovery for those with diseases such as dementia and psychiatric conditions. In these cases, learning a new skill can be difficult. Therapy focuses on teaching compensatory techniques that are very simple and concrete. Alternatively or in addition to, educating and training caregivers on how to properly supervise and promote the client's optimal and safe level of functioning will be an important therapeutic goal.

Memory

Memory is the "process of storing and retrieving information" (Shaffer & Kipp, 2009, p. 315). There are three general types of memory, short-term, working, and long-term memory. We will look at all three types of memory.

Short-Term Memory

Short-term memory is the ability to temporarily store information within seconds after learning it (Kielhofner, 2009). Working memory is the ability to hold this information for immediate recall and processing. Information moves from working to long-term memory (and not from short-term to long-term memory). You may come across information in which working memory and short-term memory is used interchangeably, but they are not the same. Working memory allows for the manipulation of information through the temporary storage, organization and processing of information. Short-term memory is the stepping stone to facilitate working memory and long-term memory.

Short-term memory is limited in its capacity to learn and recall to an average of seven items (plus or minus two). When activating short-term memory to process information to go to working memory, we often use a process called chunking (of information) to allow us to remember a range of five to nine pieces of information. Chunking information per an individual's capacity can lead to carryover of learning from working into long-term memory (Gabakes & Birney, 2011; Kielhofner, 2009). Putting this into context, when you are studying, trying to learn between five to nine facts at a time in rapid succession should lead to moving this information from short-term to working and on to long-term memory. Can you remember what it is you memorized 1 week later? Challenge yourself to do this.

Because we work with many clients, knowing each one's specific short-term memory capacity is an important consideration for intervention planning as each client is different and has different intervention needs. Many disease processes can impair short-term memory. Dementia, acquired brain injury, brain tumors, stroke, certain metabolic conditions, and even dehydration or low oxygen levels can impact cognitive processes, including memory. Although certainly not the only factor to consider, a client's diagnosis will shed some light on to what might be expected in terms of cognitive (memory) status. If short-term memory is impaired, breaking tasks down to simple steps, and not expecting a client to follow multiple steps without redirection is a given. For example, when dressing, you may begin your session by asking the client to sit at the edge of the bed as a precursor to remove his/her nightclothes and then be cued through the multiple steps of getting dressed (please also refer to Chapter 11, *Activity Analysis: The Jewel of the Occupational Therapy Profession*). Clients with short-term memory deficits may need rescuing after the first couple of words in your initial directions. Breaking the task into its simple chunked components may also aid the client to be successful and motivated to continue to relearn skills.

Long-Term Memory

Long-term memory reflects information that can be recalled after short period of time and also after days, weeks, months, or even many years. Long-term memory is broken down into explicit and implicit memory (Fu & Anderson, 2008). Explicit memory is the storage of conscious memories and information. This is broken down into episodic memory, which is memory for specific events in time, and semantic memory, which is memory for facts such as learning the meanings of key terms in this textbook. Implicit memory is memory associated with body parts, such as learning to ride a bike and write your name (Fu & Anderson, 2008; Kielhofner, 2009). This information is understood to be encoded and stored in the different structures of the brain such as the basal ganglia, associated cortex areas, and even the frontal cortex (Fu & Anderson, 2008).

Executive Functions

Executive functions are in many ways an essential part of our everyday occupations (Kielhofner, 2009). Recall that executive functions are governed by the frontal lobes. **Executive function** is a broad term used to describe the processes of planning, working memory, attention, problem solving, verbal reasoning, inhibition, mental flexibility, multitasking, and initiation and monitoring of actions. Executive functioning allows us to plan a simple task such as getting dressed and how to process stimuli to assure that the environment we are working in is safe. Executive functions are what allow us to behave within expected social norms and to problem solve. These functions allow us to plan our tasks and complete them safely and with good insight.

Clients with executive function deficits present very differently depending how early or late in the deficit process they are. In the early stages, a client can be independent with most tasks but may start to have problems with anything that alters his/her daily routine. With minimal guidance, these clients can work with an OT practitioner to navigate potential hazards. If the deficit progresses such as with dementia <CS-13>, that person will ultimately lose executive functioning, that is, the ability to complete even the simplest tasks because of inability to plan, problem solve, and/or even identify hazards in his/her environment.

A good example of self-imposed impaired executive functioning happens when people go out to a party or a bar with friends and drink <CS-7>. After having one or two drinks, an individual's overall reaction time and judgment diminishes. If they continue to drink and become intoxicated, judgment becomes significantly negatively impacted, which impairs their ability to motor plan in order to negotiate and interact safely within the environment. People who are intoxicated may slur their words and have trouble initiating a task or monitoring what they say or do.

Individuals with all types of dementia may elicit similar characteristics, but for them, the cause is beyond their control. People with concussions, acquired brain injuries, and/or strokes may also demonstrate impaired executive functioning. As an OTA, you will help these clients relearn or compensate in order to safely function within their environment. This includes providing sequential visual cues that will remind them what tasks they need to complete, to, for instance, initiate and complete the task of washing and dressing. In extreme cases when cognitive damage is irreversible, and for safety reasons, unplugging the stove, removing the car battery, and locking cellar doors are all good recommendations to make to family members caring for those with irreversible cognitive damage.

Commonly Used Cognitive Screening Tools and Assessments

There are a number of standardized cognitive assessment tools that OTs may use when evaluating and reevaluating clients. Results of these assessments, along with other information generated from the overall evaluation, observation, and client/family interview, help shape the intervention plan. Table 32.3 illustrates several cognitive assessments that a supervising OT may use to guide and develop the client's intervention program.

TABLE 32.3 Cognitive Assessments Used by OTs to Guide and Develop a Treatment Program

Commonly Used Cognitive Screen/Test	Further Information
Mini-Mental Status Exam (MMSE)	www.minimental.com/ www.nlm.nih.gov/medlineplus/ency/article/003326.htm
Saint Louis University Mental Status (SLUMS) Examination	http://medschool.slu.edu/agingsuccessfully/pdfsurveys/slumsexam_05.pdf
Montreal Cognitive Assessment (MoCA)	http://www.mocatest.org/
Lowenstein Occupational Therapy Assessment (Lotca)	http://www.lotca.com/
Canadian Occupational Performance Measure (COPM)	http://www.caot.ca/copm/questions.html
Allen's Cognitive Level Screen/Allen Battery	http://www.allencognitivelevelscreen.org
Cognitive Assessment of Minnesota (CAM)	http://metaot.com/node/972
Clock Draw Test	http://www.aging.ufl.edu/files/pdf/tools/clockanalysis.pdf
Kohlman Evaluation of Living Skills (KELS)	http://myaota.aota.org/shop_aota/prodview.aspx?TYPE=D&PID=300&SKU=1972

Veterans and Active Duty Military Clients: Thoughts from the Clinic

When working in different practice areas with various people with myriad conditions, you may find that some clients who on the surface do not appear to have any deficits may, in fact, be struggling to carry out their everyday occupations. An example are veterans, who upon returning home from combat start to experience memory issues, isolation, anger management issues, and/or even withdrawal from social situations. In the United States, we became aware of this trend with veterans returning home from the Vietnam War and again with the return of veterans from the conflicts in Iraq and Afghanistan who fought in Operation Iraqi Freedom and Operation Enduring Freedom (OIF/OEF). Due to the extreme stressors and dangerous situations, these veterans experienced on a daily basis, and especially at the height of the conflict, some returned home with difficulty readjusting to civilian life. For instance, during their tours of duty, these veterans may have found that what appeared to be an abandoned car on the side of the road was actually a fully functioning car that was booby-trapped and intended to kill his/her fellow soldiers. Based on that experience and upon returning home, seeing an abandoned car on the side of the road may trigger memories of the veteran's past experiences. It may spiral into a domino effect, negatively impacting his/her overall cognitive and physical functioning: eliciting anger, fear, and physiological overarousal such as sweating and elevated heart rate.

These veterans may be diagnosed (or undiagnosed) with post-traumatic stress syndrome (PTSD). As an OT practitioner, your work may take you into veterans hospitals or military outpatient clinics. You may also encounter other clients with PTSD whose trauma is not related to military service but is the result of an accident, family situation, or other traumatic event. Knowing that many veterans (or civilians) have undiagnosed PTSD, making certain that they are receiving the appropriate supports is critically important.

In your role as an OTA, you will also use your skills to identify and address client factors and performance skills that may be impacted by PTSD, such as attention, memory, anxiety and stress management, and organizational skills, which all impact global ADL and IADLs. This may include teaching skills to manage anger or stress that is limiting memory, which in turn will increase daily functioning. With regard to veterans, many are working, attending school, and living in your community, but do not know how to seek help and often go untreated. At the end of the day, your ability to link a veteran in crisis to his/her local veteran's hospital for much needed care may be all the intervention you may have to provide, but it may be the most important thing ever for that veteran.

When you see a veteran on the street, always remember to thank him/her for all they do and have done. The following are good resources for information to help veterans receive the proper care they need and deserve to address cognitive, social–emotional, and physical needs.

Veterans and Military Resources

Veteran Crisis Help Line (for those who are still serving and those who have served):
http://www.realwarriors.net/livechat

Department of Veteran Affairs main Web site (for those out of service):
http://www.va.gov/

Department of Defense Healthcare main Web site (for those still serving):
http://www.health.mil/default.aspx

After Deployment a Wellness Center for those who are to be and are returning from service
http://afterdeployment.org/

Theoretical Models Related to Cognition

To this point, we have discussed brain structure and functioning related to cognition and the basic core components of cognition in relation to our everyday daily occupations. Cognitive rehabilitation requires a strong understanding of these concepts as well as knowing how theoretical models related to cognitive rehabilitation drive the occupational therapy intervention process. These theories provide a solid foundation to help develop an evidence-based practice. We will briefly discuss the following theories: cognitive disabilities, dynamic interaction approach, and cognitive rehabilitation theory. These are just a sample of many theories and models to be used interchangeably to help guide occupational therapy intervention in order to achieve optimal outcomes.

Cognitive Disability Model

The cognitive disability model was developed by Allen, Levy, and Burns and focused on clients with severe psychiatric illness and dementia (Kielhofner, 2009). This theory is based upon Piaget's concept of cognition and reformulated to embrace concepts from cognitive neuroscience. The cognitive disability model views cognition in a hierarchical formation related to overall functioning and limitations due to neurological injury or disease. The goal of assessment is to identify and monitor the level of cognition based upon a classification of six levels related to cognitive functioning. Intervention focuses on the client's present capabilities to adapt the environment and to provide the "just-right challenge."

Dynamic Interactional Approach

The dynamic interactional approach is a dynamic systems theory developed by Toglia (Kielhofner, 2009). This theory views cognition as a product of the dynamic interaction between the person, activity, and environment by examining the client's abilities and limitations. An intervention approach based on this theory consists of changing the person's strategies and self-awareness along with modifying external factors. By alternating the environment and other external variables, the client enhances his/her ability to process, monitor, and use information to carry out tasks.

Cognitive Rehabilitation

The cognitive rehabilitation theory was developed by Averbach and Kazt for clients with CIs due to traumatic brain injuries or stroke (Kielhofner, 2009). This theory incorporates the notion of neuroplasticity, which enables a client to create alternative cognitive strategies and improve his/her ability to assess and be aware of his/her abilities so as to not enter into situations beyond his/her capabilities. Based on this theory, during a therapy assessment, an OT practitioner could look at the client's self-awareness, executive functions, functional performance, and preferred learning patterns. Occupational therapy interventions should enhance the client's capacity to process and generalize information to functional areas of daily living.

TABLE 32.4 Examples of Occupational Therapy Cognitive Approaches

Theory	Creator(s)
Cognitive Rehabilitation	Averbach and Katz
Neurofunctional Approach	Giles
Cognitive Orientation to Daily Occupational Performance	Polatajko and Mandich
Dynamic Cognitive Intervention	Hadas-Lidor and Weiss
Cognitive Disabilities	Allen, Levy, and Burns
Dynamic Interactional Approach	Toglia
Higher-Level Cognition	Katz and Hartman-Maeir
Quadraphonic Approach	Abreu

As part of your continual lifelong professional development, it will be helpful to research as many different types of cognitive theories to help enhance your skills. The list of theories and models found in Table 32.4 provides such a starting point.

Summary

No matter the practice setting, understanding a client's cognitive status is very important. This knowledge is vital to develop a client-centered relationship. Cognition is not static and may shift because of medications, psychosocial issues, or changes in health, so staying on top of monitoring a client's cognition is crucial. Being aware of whether your client demonstrates signs of a deficit in short-term or long-term memory or in executive functions helps you plan interventions that will lead to positive outcomes.

Because cognition impacts all aspects of daily functioning, ongoing professional development in the area of cognition is critical for your professional career. An OT practitioner who has a strong understanding of how cognition impacts daily functional performance will be better able to recognize clients with mild impairments more efficiently. Remember, this chapter is only a brief introduction into what will be a lifelong professional learning process. Use this chapter as means to lay the foundation to build upon for the rest of your professional career.

Review Questions

The following are areas of attention:

1. Focused attention (true/false)

2. Sustained attention (true/false)

3. Choosing attention (true/false)

4. Divided attention (true/false)

5. The mental process of knowing is called:
   a. Knowledge
   b. Cognition
   c. Attention
   d. Memory

6. The inability to remember, to formulate ideas, and/or to organize and recall information that impacts safety and overall ability to complete everyday tasks is called:
   a. Short-term memory
   b. Long-term memory
   c. Cognitive impairment
   d. Attention

7. The ability to focus on a particular sensory stimulus while ignoring other stimuli is called:
   a. Memory
   b. Alertness
   c. Awareness
   d. Attention

True or False:

The following are components of executive functions:

8. Safety awareness (true/false)

9. Regulate behaviors (true/false)

10. Motor planning (true/false)

Practice Activities

Develop three functional intervention activities for a client with impaired short-term memory.

Identify three compensatory techniques that someone with an acquired brain injury can use to adhere to a schedule and budget.

Research two types of dementia and prepare a list of functional impairments typically related to each type of dementia.

Choose a theory from Table 32.4 and develop an intervention plan for the following individual with a cognitive impairment:

- *Demographics*: Male, 30 years old, married with two children ages 3 and 6, working as a production line factory manager, enjoys hunting and fishing.
- *Problem list*: Impaired attention span of 5 minutes or less, impaired short-term memory, able to recall two items after 1 minute, irritable in crowded places, overwhelmed by loud prolonged noises after 10 minutes, forgets to take medication, forgets appointments, and impulse buying due to inability to follow a schedule or budget.

References

American Occupational Therapy Association. Occupational therapy practice framework: domain & process (3rd edition). *Am J Occup Ther* 2014, 68(Suppl. 1):SI–S48.

Australian Government. *Cognitive Impairment*; 2011. Retrieved from JobAccess: An Australian Government Initiative: http://jobaccess.gov.au/Advice/Disability/Pages/Cognitive_Impairment.aspx

Chris Hagen PC-S. *The Rancho Levels of Cognitive Functioning*. 3rd ed. 1998. Retrieved June 30, 2012, from rancho.org: http://www.rancho.org/research/cognitive_levels.pdf

Daltrozzo PJ, et al. Cortical information processing in coma. *Cogn Behav Neurol* 2009; 22(1):53–62.

Farlex. *Cognition*; 2009. Retrieved from Thefreedictionary: http://www.thefreedictionary.com/Cognitive+processing

Fu W-T, Anderson JR. Solving the credit assignment problem: explicit and implicit learning of action sequences with probabilistic outcomes. *Psychol Res* 2008;72:321–330.

Gabakes L, Birney DP. Are the limits in processing and storage capacity common? Exploring the additive and interactive effects of processing and storage load in working memory. *J Cogn Psychol* 2011;23(3):322–341.

Gehring K, et al. A description of a cognitive rehabilitation programme evaluated in brain tumor patients with mild to moderate cognitive deficits. *Clin Rehabil* 2011;25(8):675–692.

Greenberg DA, Aminoff MJ, Simon RP. *Clinical Neurology*. 5th ed. New York City: Lange Medical Books/McGraw-Hill: Medical Publishing Division; 2002.

Gutman SA. *Quick Reference Neuroscience 2nd edition for Rehabilitation Professionals. The Essential Neurological Principles Underlying Rehabilitation Practice*. Thorofare, NJ: Slack Incorporated; 2008.

Hagen C. Rancho Levels of Cognitive Functioning, 3rd ed. Downey, CA: Rancho Los Amigos.

Hill RR. *How Many? A Dictionary of Units of Measure*; 2000. Retrieved June 30, 2012, from http://www.unc.edu/~rowlett/units/scales/glasgow.htm

Just MA, et al. Functional and anatomical cortical under connectivity in autism: evidence from an fMRI study of an executive function task and corpus callosum morphometry. *Cereb Cortex* 2007;17(4):951–961.

Kielhofner DO. Cognitive model. In: Kielhofner DO, ed. *Conceptual Foundations of Occupational Therapy Practice*. Philadelphia: F.A. Davis Company; 2009:84–107.

Morgane PJ, Galler JR, Mokler DJ. A review of systems and networks of the limbic forebrain/limbic midbrain. *Prog Neurobiol* 2005;75(January):143–160.

Parsons LM, Osherson D. New evidence for distinct right and left brain systems for deductive verses probabilistic reasoning. *Cereb Cortex*, 2001;11(October):954–965.

Rancho Los Amigos National Rehabilitation Center. *Patient Information: Family Guide to The Rancho Levels of Cognitive Functioning*; 2006. Retrieved from Rancho Los Amigos National Rehabilitation Center: http://www.rancho.org/research/bi_cognition.pdf

Sammler D, et al. Prosody meets syntax: the role of the corpus callosum. *Brain* 2010;133:2643–2655. Retrieved August 17, 2012

Shaffer D, Kipp K. *Developmental Psychology: Childhood and Adolescence*. 8th ed. Clifton Park, NY: Cengage Learning; 2009.

Witgert M, et al. Frontal-lobe mediated behavioral dysfunction in amyotrophic lateral sclerosis. *Eur J Neurol* 2010;17:103–110.

UNIT

VI

Practice Settings: Traditional and Emerging

The promise of occupational therapy lies in our ability to continuously combine the mandates put forth in the early tenets of our discipline with our constantly changing practice environments.

—ANN P. GRADY

CHAPTER 33

Rehabilitation, Disability, and Participation and the Discharge Planning Process

Dawndra Meers Sechrist, OTR, PhD

Key Terms

Acute hospital—A hospital that provides inpatient medical care and other related services for surgery, acute medical conditions, or a short-term illness.

Assisted living facility—"A long-term care option that combines housing, support services, and health care, as needed. Assisted living is designed for individuals who require assistance with everyday activities such as meals, medication management or assistance with bathing, dressing, and transportation" (Assisted Living Federation of America, n.d.).

Comprehensive outpatient rehabilitation facilities (CORF)—"A facility that is primarily engaged in providing outpatient rehabilitation for the treatment of Medicare beneficiaries who are injured, disabled, or recovering from illness" (U.S. Department of Health and Human Services, Centers for Medicare and Medicaid, 2010, p. 1).

Disability—"An umbrella term for impairments, activity limitations, and participation restrictions" (WHO, 2012).

Home health care—Home health care services are provided by home health agencies to clients who are homebound and need skilled care.

Inpatient rehabilitation facility (IRF)—A freestanding facility or a rehabilitation unit in an acute care hospital that provides intensive rehabilitation services to patients after an injury, illness, or surgery.

Long-term acute care hospital (LTCH)—Hospital-based inpatient care (certified as an acute care hospital) for those who require a longer than the usual hospital stay (usually more than 25 days) because of the severity of illness or the chronic nature of the disease process.

Medicare—A federal program that pays for certain health expenses for people 65 years of age or older; people under age 65 with certain disabilities; and people of all ages with end-stage renal disease (Centers for Medicare and Medicaid Services [CMS], 2014).

Nursing facility (NF)—A nursing home or nursing facility is a residence facility that provides room and meals and helps with activities of daily living and recreation. Generally, nursing home residents require 24-hour care for an indefinite period of time and have impairments that keep them from living on their own.

Participation—An outcome that "naturally occurs when clients are actively involved in carrying out occupations or daily life activities they find purposeful and meaningful in desired contexts" (AJOT, 2008, p. 660).

Rehabilitation—"A set of measures that assist individuals who experience, or are likely to experience, disability to achieve and maintain optimal functioning in interaction with their environments" (WHO, 2011, p. 96).

Skilled nursing facility (SNF)—Skilled nursing facilities or skilled nursing units (SNUs) are "primarily engaged in providing skilled nursing care and related services for residents who require medical or nursing care; or rehabilitation services for rehabilitation of injured, disabled, or sick persons" (U.S. Department of Health and Human Services, Centers for Medicare and Medicaid, 2007, p. 45).

Learning Objectives

After studying this chapter, readers should be able to:

- Differentiate between Medicare reimbursements for different rehabilitation settings.
- Define the differences between an acute hospital care and a long-term acute care hospital.
- Explain the differences between a skilled nursing facility and a nursing home.
- Compare and contrast rehabilitation facilities so occupational therapy practitioners can make appropriate discharge recommendations for the next level of client care.

Introduction

Occupational therapy practitioners have the opportunity to work with clients to be successful in achieving health and participation in life in a wide variety of settings as part of the rehabilitation process. The World Health Organization (WHO) defines the **rehabilitation** of people with disabilities as "a set of measures that assist individuals who experience, or are likely to experience, disability to achieve and maintain optimal functioning in interaction with their environments" (WHO, 2011, p. 96). Rehabilitation addresses improvements with individual functioning and includes possible changes to the individual's environment. The *International Classification of Functioning, Disability and Health* (*ICF*) defines **disability** as "an umbrella term for impairments, activity limitations, and participation restrictions" (WHO, 2012). In 2010, approximately 56.7 million people living in the United States had some type of disability and 38.3 million people (12.6%) had a severe disability (U.S. Department of Commerce, 2012). *The Practice Framework III* explains **participation** as an outcome that "naturally occurs when clients are actively involved in carrying out occupations or daily life activities they find purposeful and meaningful in desired contexts" (AOTA, 2014, p. S4).

This chapter will focus on the different practice areas that deal specifically with traditional rehabilitation settings. Occupational therapy practitioners must be familiar with these settings to understand the context of therapy for the specific setting and to make appropriate discharge recommendations for the next level of care. We begin this chapter by looking at discharge planning in order to set the stage for providing interventions that will lead to appropriate client-centered recommendations for the next level of care.

Discharge Planning and the Role of the Occupational Therapy Practitioner

Occupational therapy practitioners play an important role in providing input in discharge planning for clients in all types of rehabilitation settings. Discharge planning is the "process by which the patient is assisted to develop a plan of care for ongoing maintenance and improvement of health care (even after he or she may be discharged from the acute care hospital)" (Felong, 2008, p. 1). The OT practitioner will make discharge recommendations based on the client's current status and feedback from other health care team members treating the client. According to *Guidelines for Supervision, Roles, and Responsibilities During the Delivery of Occupational Therapy Services,* the occupational therapist (OT) is "responsible for selecting, measuring, and interpreting outcomes that are related to the client's ability to engage in occupations" (AOTA, 2009, p. 801). The OT monitors client's response to intervention and modifies and grades the treatment and discharge plans as needed. The OT collaborates with the occupational therapy assistant (OTA) to provide valuable information related to the client's current status, and discharge planning is addressed throughout the intervention process. The OTA may "implement outcome measurements and provide needed client discharge resources" (AOTA, 2009, p. 801).

Smith-Gabai (2011) identifies the following elements as primary issues affecting discharge planning:

a. Client's function and level of disability
b. Client's and family's desires and needs
c. Client's life context, including caregiver support and ability to help care for the client
d. Health care regulations and institutional procedures
e. Resource availability and accessibility
f. Durable medical equipment needs and adaptive devices

An additional factor to consider is that most facilities and Medicare (primary payer in rehabilitation settings) require a qualifying stay in the hospital before being discharged to another facility. A qualifying hospital stay is an inpatient hospital stay of three consecutive days (U.S. Department of Health and Human Services, Centers for Medicare and Medicaid, 2007).

Case Example of Discharge Planning

A 72-year-old retired teacher who is widowed and has two adult children living locally has been admitted to the hospital with a left cerebral vascular accident (CVA). She has resultant right-sided weakness and aphasia. She has been in the acute hospital for 4 days. Prior to her hospitalization, she lived alone and was independent with all activities of daily living (ADLs), including driving and volunteering at the local hospital gift shop. During the initial evaluation in an acute care hospital, the OT has a difficult time understanding the client and realizes the patient is inaccurate with "yes" and "no" responses. The client requires maximal assist with all basic ADLs and demonstrates decreased endurance with the 20-minute evaluation. The daughter is gone to the cafeteria, but nursing reports she should be back in the room shortly.

The admitting physician has asked the OT to recommend a discharge destination as part of the evaluation. The OT needs additional information from the family before making a final recommendation, but is considering several discharge destinations to continue rehabilitation services. These possible discharge destinations include the following:

a. Long-term acute care
b. Skilled nursing facility
c. Inpatient rehabilitation facility
d. Assisted living facility
e. Home with home health and full-time supervision
f. A family member's home

As we progress through the chapter, consider the possible discharge settings for this client. Later in the chapter, we will get more information from the client's daughter and will discuss the optimal setting for this client.

Medicare

Fortunately, occupational therapy services are reimbursed today in many settings, and it is important for OT practitioners to be aware of how occupational therapy services are reimbursed. Reimbursement is a method of payment, usually by a third-party payer, for a service rendered. Fees are typically based on a formula or a fee schedule. The Centers for Medicare and Medicaid Services (CMS) is the largest health care payer in the United States, and in 2010, there were 47.5 million people enrolled in Medicare (U.S. Department of Commerce, 2012). **Medicare** is a federal program that pays for certain health expenses for (a) people 65 years of age or older, (b) people under age 65 with certain disabilities, (c) and people of all ages with end-stage renal disease (U.S. Department of Health and Human Services, Centers for Medicare and Medicaid, 2012c).

Medicare is not an automatic benefit. Individuals meeting the requirements must apply for the program and pay premiums, deductibles, and coinsurance payments. Medicare is a payer for all of the rehabilitation settings listed in this chapter and reimburses for "skilled" occupational therapy services. CMS defines skilled care as "health care given when you need skilled nursing or rehabilitation staff to manage, observe, and evaluate care" (U.S. Department of Health and Human Services, 2007, p. 4).

It is important for OT practitioners to have a basic understanding of Medicare reimbursement. The original Medicare plan has Part A and Part B, and recipients are responsible for paying a deductible and coinsurance (typically 20%). Medicare Part A insurance pays for care that involves an inpatient stay in a hospital, inpatient rehabilitation, skilled nursing facilities, some home health care, and hospice. Medicare Part B covers certain physician services, outpatient services, durable medical equipment, and preventative services. Medicare Part D is the prescription drug coverage and is an optional program for beneficiaries (From the Field 33.1).

Medicare uses a prospective payment system (PPS) to motivate providers to deliver patient care effectively, efficiently, and without overutilization of services. The PPS is a predetermined flat rate, and Medicare PPS is a

FROM THE FIELD 33.1

Checking for Updates

It is important for OT practitioners to stay abreast of current Medicare regulations and guidelines and Conditions of Participation (CoPs). One way to do so is through regular reviews of the governmental Web site, Medicare Costs at a Glance.

http://www.medicare.gov/your-medicare-costs/costs-at-a-glance/costs-at-glance.html

prepayment that is based on an assessment classification of each patient and covers a defined period. Throughout the chapter, specific Medicare rules will be discussed with regard to each rehabilitation setting.

Acute Hospital Care and Long-Term Acute Care Hospital

Hospitals are designed to meet the health care needs of the surrounding population and can include teaching hospitals, specialty hospitals, private hospitals, public hospitals, Veteran's Administration hospitals, and community hospitals (CS7, 12). The **acute hospital** provides inpatient medical care and other related services for surgery, acute medical conditions, or a short-term illness. Patients are admitted from emergency room, direct admission, or transfer from another facility. The average length of stay for an acute hospital stay in the United States is less than 5 days (Organization for Economic Cooperation and Development [OECD], 2011). Hospitals are licensed by individual states and may participate in regulatory accreditations such as the Joint Commission (formerly known as the Joint Commission on Accreditation of Healthcare Organizations and prior to that, the Joint Commission on Accreditation of Hospitals). Occupational therapy services can be direct or consultative and typically include equipment recommendations and discharge recommendations for continued services at the next level of care. Specialized training is required for OT practitioners working in the critical care unit (CCU) or intensive care unit (ICU) in the hospital.

Medicare pays the hospital for occupational therapy services as part of a bundled rate that includes all services performed during the hospital stay. Medicare has designed a per-case per diem rate based on diagnostic categories called diagnosis-related groups (DRGs) and includes over 500 diagnostic categories. The rate includes room and board, nursing services, medication and supplies, diagnostic services, and other services, including occupational therapy. If a patient is able to leave the hospital earlier than usual, the hospital may make money, but if the patient stays longer than anticipated, the hospital may lose money. In 2010, 4,800 hospitals were paid under the Medicare Prospective PPS and payments for roughly 10 million Medicare inpatient admissions were around $153 billion (Medicare Payment Advisory Commission [MedPAC], 2012a). Patients are admitted to the acute care hospital from a variety of places, and there are several discharge options from acute care (Fig. 33.1).

A **long-term acute care hospital** (**LTCH** or LTACH) is hospital-based inpatient care and certified as an acute care hospital. Patients often transfer to LTCHs from CCUs or ICUs in traditional hospitals. LTCH is for those who require a longer than the usual hospital stay (usually more than 25 days) because of the severity of illness or the chronic nature of the disease process. Services provided in LTCHs usually include comprehensive rehabilitation, respiratory therapy, and pain management (U.S. Department of Health and Human Services, 2012a). Medicare is the predominant payer for most LTCHs, accounting for about two-thirds of LTCH discharges. In 2010, Medicare spent $5.2 billion on care provided in roughly 412 LTCHs nationwide (MedPAC, 2012a).

Skilled Nursing Facility (SNF) and Nursing Facility (NF)

Skilled nursing facilities (SNFs) or skilled nursing units (SNUs) are also referred to as subacute rehabilitation or transitional care. CMS defines SNFs as a distinct institution certified to provide SNF services and are "primarily engaged in providing skilled nursing care and related services for residents who require medical or nursing care; or rehabilitation services for rehabilitation of injured, disabled, or sick persons" (U.S. Department of

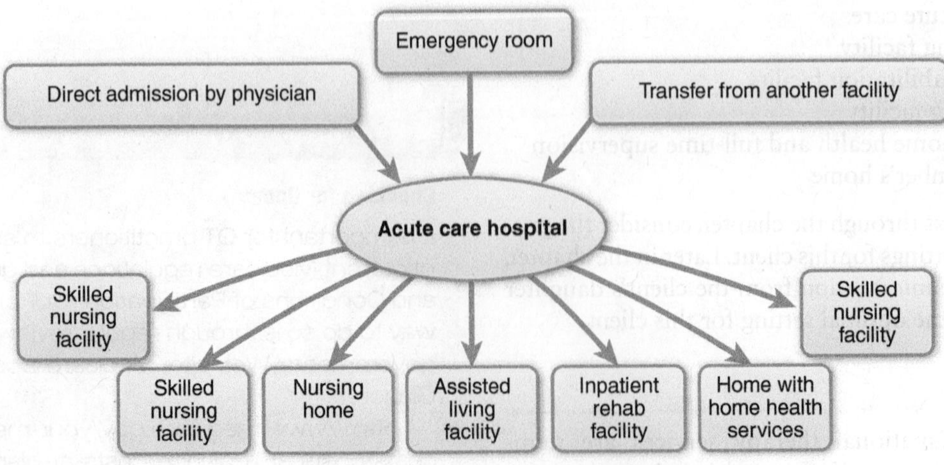

Figure 33.1 Admission to acute care and discharge from acute care.

Health and Human Services, Centers for Medicare and Medicaid, 2007, p. 45). An SNF can be part of a nursing home or hospital, but must have specifically designated rooms or beds to provide SNF services. Medicare Part A covers up to 100 days in an SNF and generally reimburses for occupational therapy for a short-term stay. Medicare pays for the first 20 days, but there is a daily coinsurance fee for days 21 to 100. In 2009, the average Medicare length of stay in an SNF was 20 days (The Alliance for Quality Nursing Home Care, 2011).

Of all Medicare beneficiaries who require ongoing postacute care after discharge from a hospital, 50% go directly to a skilled nursing facility for care and services, and just over one-third returns to their prior living situation (American Health Care Association, 2011). In 2010, more than 15,000 SNFs furnished covered care to almost 1.7 million beneficiaries, and in 2011, Medicare spent almost $32 billion on SNF care (MedPAC, 2012a). Jette et al. (2005) found that higher intensity occupational therapy during rehabilitation in an SNF is associated with shorter length of stay and functional improvements in ADLs for a variety of diagnoses.

The minimum data set (MDS) is used to assess clinical and functional status elements to help determine payment for SNF residents. Based on results from the MDS, resource utilization groups (RUGs) are determined using mutually exclusive categories that reflect different levels of resources needed for residents. A specified number of therapy minutes per week are established for each RUG based on MDS score and rehabilitation team (occupational, physical, and speech therapists) estimates.

A nursing home or **nursing facility** (NF) is a residence facility that provides a room and meals and helps with activities of daily living and recreation. Generally, nursing home residents require 24-hour care for an indefinite period of time and have impairments that keep them from living on their own. The distinction between an SNF and a nursing facility is based primarily on whether skilled medical care, nursing care, or rehabilitation is required. Custodial care (nonskilled care) is care that helps with ADLs and is common in nursing facilities. Medicare does not cover custodial care.

For nursing home care to be covered under Medicare services, (a) the care must be considered medically necessary, for a limited period of time, (b) provided by a Medicare SNF, and (c) and occur within a short time (generally 30 days) after a qualifying inpatient stay of at least three days (U.S. Department of Health and Human Services, Centers for Medicare and Medicaid, 2007). Patients are admitted to the SNF after a qualifying acute care hospital stay, and there are several discharge options from SNF (Fig. 33.2). For Medicare beneficiaries in a noncovered stay in the Medicare-certified part of the NF (not a designated SNF stay), Medicare Part B therapy services (physical therapy, occupational therapy, and speech–language pathology) must be billed by the facility. No other therapy service may be billed by another setting, such as an outpatient hospital setting (U.S. Department of Health and Human Services, Centers for Medicare and Medicaid, 2012b). SNFs and NFs are subject to federal regulations and also strict state regulations. State surveyors will inspect facilities for compliance with licensing (state regulations) and certification (federal Medicare regulations).

Assisted Living Facility

An **Assisted living facility** is "a long-term care option that combines housing, support services, and health care, as needed. Assisted living is designed for individuals who require assistance with everyday activities such as meals, medication management or assistance with bathing, dressing, and transportation" (Assisted Living Federation of America, n.d.). Occupational therapy practitioners are trained experts in working with clients who have difficulties with ADLs and can provide services to clients who are experiencing a decline in their level of safety or independence. The average assistive living resident is an 87-year-old widow who requires assistance with two or more ADLs and stays in assisted living for 28 months (Assisted Living Federation of America, n.d.). Medicare does not cover the cost of the assisted

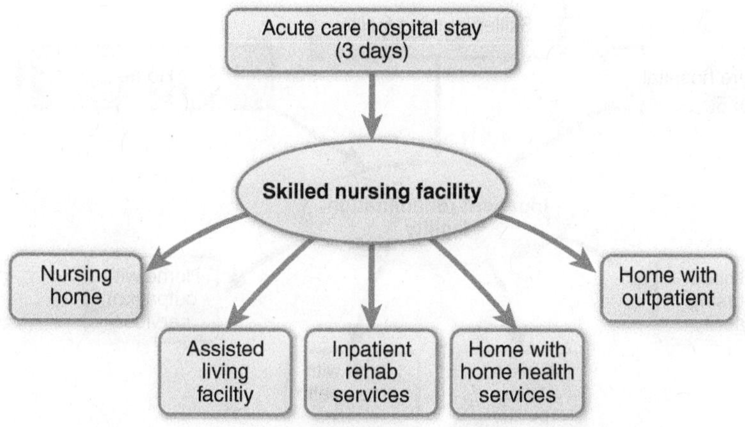
Acute care hospital stay
(3 days)
Skilled nursing facility
Nursing home
Home with outpatient
Assisted living faciltiy
Inpatient rehab services
Home with home health services

Figure 33.2 Admission to skilled nursing facility and discharge from skilled nursing facility.

living facility. Occupational therapy in an assisted living facility is typically provided by home health services, or residents are taken to an outpatient facility.

Inpatient Rehabilitation Facility

Inpatient rehabilitation facility (IRF) can be a free-standing facility or a rehabilitation unit in an acute care hospital that provides intensive rehabilitation services to clients after an injury, illness, or surgery CS7, 12. Approximately 80% of IRFs are hospital-based facilities (MedPAC, 2012b). IRFs are supervised by rehabilitation physicians and staffed by professionals including occupational and physical therapy (PT) practitioners and speech–language pathologists (SLP). Clients must be able to tolerate and benefit from intensive rehabilitation therapy, which consists of at least 3 hours of therapy a day (from at least two therapy disciplines, one of which must be physical or occupational therapy) for at least 5 days a week (MedPAC, 2012b). The average length of stay in an IRF is approximately 12 to 13 days (Jackson et al., 2013).

Beginning in January 2002, IRFs were required to follow a PPS. The IRF patient assessment instrument (IRF-PAI) is based on the functional independence measure (FIM) and determines assignment of patient in an IRF to assigned into a category called case mix groups (CMGs). The CMG is based on 92 intensive rehabilitation categories (MedPAC, 2012b). The 60% rule is used to define inpatient rehabilitation facilities reimbursement. The rule requires that at least 60% of cases an IRF have one or more of the following 13 qualifying conditions: (a) stroke; (b) spinal cord injury; (c) congenital deformity; (d) amputation; (e) major multiple trauma; (f) hip fracture; (g) brain injury; (h) neurological disorders (e.g., multiple sclerosis, Parkinson disease); (i) burns; (j) three arthritis conditions for which appropriate, aggressive, and sustained outpatient therapy has failed; and (k) hip or knee replacement when bilateral, when body mass index is greater than 50, or when age 85 or older (Medicare Payment Advisory Commission, MedPAC, 2012b, p. 3). The IRF-PAI helps in tracking compliance with the 60% rule. In 2010, almost 360,000 Medicare fee for service (FFS) received cared in IRFs, and Medicare FFS expenditures were $6.32 billion (MedPAC, 2012b). Patients are admitted to IRFs from a variety of places, and there are several discharge options from IRF (Fig. 33.3). The goal is to discharge the patient to least restrictive environment and preferably to the level of care prior to the disability.

Home Health Care

Home health care services are provided by home health agencies (HHA) to clients who are homebound and need skilled care. A client is considered homebound if "(a) leaving your home isn't recommended because of your condition; (b) your condition keeps you from leaving home without help, and (c) leaving home takes a considerable and taxing effort" (Medicare.gov, n.d.) CS8. There are several requirements to qualify for the Medicare home health benefit. A Medicare beneficiary needs to be

a. Confined to the home under the care of a physician;
b. Receiving services under a plan of care established, certified, and periodically reviewed by a physician;
c. In need of skilled nursing care (other than solely venipuncture) on an intermittent basis;
d. On physical therapy;
e. On speech–language pathology;
f. On continued need for occupational therapy;
g. Medicare certified (U.S. Department of Health and Human Services, Centers for Medicare and Medicaid, 2010).

For occupational therapy to be involved, a nurse, physical therapist, or speech–language pathologist must open the case. After the case is open, occupational therapy can be a stand-alone skilled service.

A PPS has been used in the home health setting by CMS since October of 2000. Clients are assigned to one of 153 home health resource groups (HHRGs), and assignments are made based on the data collected in the Outcomes

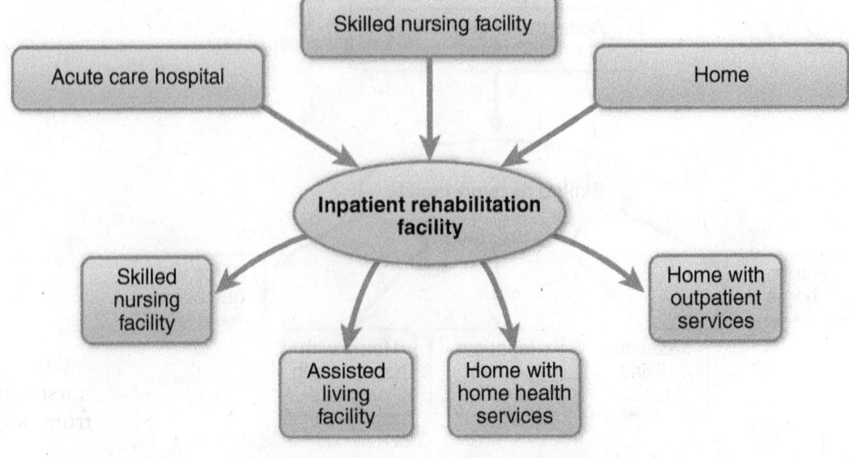

Figure 33.3 Admission to inpatient rehabilitation facility and discharge from inpatient rehabilitation facility.

and Assessment Information Set (OASIS) (MedPac, 2012c). The OASIS includes a broad array of functional measures, including instrumental activities of daily living (IADLs). The OASIS is required for each 60-day episode of care and is completed by a nurse or therapist. In 2011, about 3.4 million Medicare beneficiaries received home health services from almost 11,900 home health agencies, and Medicare spent about $19.4 billion on home health services in 2010 (MedPAC, 2012a).

Outpatient Rehabilitation

Outpatient rehabilitation (therapy) is provided in many different settings:

a. Therapists in private practice (who may work in a physician's office, but bill independently)
b. Nursing homes
c. Hospital outpatient departments
d. Physicians' offices
e. Comprehensive outpatient rehabilitation facilities (CORF) CS9-11

Services furnished in physical therapists' private practices and in nursing homes account for about two-thirds of Medicare Part B therapy payments (MedPAC, 2012d). Outpatient therapy services include PT, OT, and SLP services. Payment for services may come from private insurance, Medicaid, or Medicare. In 2011, Medicare spending on outpatient services was about 5.7 billion dollars, and occupational therapy services make up about 19% of beneficiary therapy (MedPAC, 2012d). Medicare pays for outpatient therapy according to the physician fee schedule, and there are annual spending limits ("therapy caps") on Medicare payments for outpatient therapy services. In 2012, Medicare set the cap at $1,800 for physical therapy and speech–language pathology services and $1,800 for occupational therapy services (MedPAC, 2012d). However, the Medicare Tax Relief and Job Creation Act of 2012 extended an exceptions process through December 31, 2012 (MedPAC, 2012d).

A **comprehensive outpatient rehabilitation facilities (CORF)** is a "facility that is primarily engaged in providing outpatient rehabilitation for the treatment of Medicare beneficiaries who are injured, disabled, or recovering from illness" (U.S. Department of Health and Human Services, Centers for Medicare and Medicaid, 2011, p. 1). Minimum services required by regulation are CORF physician services, physical therapy services, and social and/or psychological services. CORF skilled rehabilitation services can include the skills of OT practitioners, speech–language pathologists, and/or respiratory therapists (who are eligible to provide services under the CORF benefit), in addition to the required physical therapy services. The CORF physician (or referring physician for physical therapy, occupational therapy, and/or speech–language pathologists) must review the plan of care once every 90 days (U.S. Department of Health and Human Services, Centers for Medicare and Medicaid, 2011). CORF services are paid under Medicare Part B using the Medicare Physician Fee Schedule.

Case Example: Conclusion

Discharge planning in a variety of rehabilitation settings is an important role as an OT practitioner. It is complex and requires an interdisciplinary approach to determine the best setting for the next level of care. When the client's daughter returns to the hospital room, the OT finds out that the patient has Medicare and a complementary policy that pays the deductible on Medicare. The daughter reports she works full-time, is a single mom with four children, and does not have extra vacation or sick leave to care for her mother. Her brother lives in the same city, but is in the military and is currently deployed out of the country for nine months. The OT explains the different options for discharge planning:

a. Long-term acute care
b. Skilled nursing facility
c. Inpatient rehabilitation facility
d. Assisted living facility
e. Home with home health and full-time supervision
f. A family member's home

The client would not be able to tolerate three hours of therapy in an inpatient rehabilitation facility, and she is not sick enough to go to a long-term acute hospital. Going home or to a family member's home is not possible because family cannot provide 24-hour care. An assisted living facility would not be a viable option at this point because the client would need to be more independent with ADLs to qualify for this level of care. Given the above information, the best option would be for the client to continue rehabilitation services in a skilled nursing facility.

Summary

A coordinated discharge plan with client and family involvement will make the transition to a new level of care smoother for everyone involved in the process. The most important person in the discharge planning process is the client, but the client and family rely heavily on the OT practitioner's knowledge of different rehabilitation settings. In addition, Medicare rules for coverage and reimbursement change frequently, which require OT practitioners to be proactive in staying updated on the latest changes. Occupational therapy practitioners will continue to have an important role in making discharge recommendations to facilitate participation in occupational engagement for adults and older adults in rehabilitation settings.

Review Questions

1. What is the required length of stay in acute care hospital before being admitted into a skilled nursing facility?
   a. 12 hours
   b. 24 hours
   c. 2 days
   d. 3 days
2. What tool is used to collect admission data in the home health setting?
   a. Diagnosis-related groups (DRG)
   b. Minimum data set (MDS)
   c. Outcome and Assessment Information Set (OASIS)
   d. The patient assessment instrument (PAI)
3. Which of the following service is not one of the required minimum services for a CORF?
   a. Occupational therapy
   b. Physical therapy
   c. Physician services
   d. Social services
4. LTCH is for those who require a longer-than-usual hospital stay. The length of stay is typically longer than how many days?
   a. 5 days
   b. 10 days
   c. 15 days
   d. 25 days
5. Which of the following is the type of Medicare insurance that pays for care that involves an inpatient stay in a hospital?
   a. Medicare Part A
   b. Medicare Part B
   c. Medicare Part C
   d. Medicare Part D
6. In an SNF, the resource utilization groups (RUGs) are determined based on information from which of the following admission tools?
   a. Diagnosis-related groups (DRG)
   b. Minimum data set (MDS)
   c. Outcomes and Assessment Information Set (OASIS)
   d. The patient assessment instrument (PAI)
7. Which of the following is the type of Medicare insurance that pays for physician services, outpatient services, durable medical equipment, and preventative services?
   a. Medicare Part A
   b. Medicare Part B
   c. Medicare Part C
   d. Medicare Part D
8. A patient had bilateral knee replacements and is being discharged from an acute hospital. The patient currently receives therapy twice a day and requires minimal assist with all ADLs, but was independent prior to this hospitalization. The patient lives alone, does not have any family to assist at discharge, and will not be released to drive for 6 weeks. What discharge disposition would the OT practitioner recommend for this patient?
   a. Home with outpatient therapy
   b. Inpatient rehabilitation
   c. Long-term acute care hospital
   d. Nursing home

9. A patient had a traumatic brain injury two weeks ago and is being discharged from the intensive care unit in an acute hospital. The patient currently requires the use of a ventilator and is able to tolerate 10 minutes of therapy a day. What discharge disposition would the OT practitioner recommend for this patient?
   a. Home with home health services
   b. Inpatient rehabilitation
   c. Long-term acute care hospital
   d. Skilled nursing facility

10. A patient had a hip replacement six days ago and is being discharged from an acute hospital. The patient is independent or modified independent with all basic ADLs and requires minimum to maximum assist with IADLs. The patient has a supportive wife who will be able to provide 24-hour care. What discharge disposition would the OT practitioner recommend for this patient?
    a. Assisted living facility
    b. Inpatient rehabilitation
    c. Home with home health services
    d. Home with outpatient services

Practice Activities

Go to the American Occupational Therapy Association Web site http://www.aota.org and type "Medicare" in the search section. Look up the most current *Physician Fee Schedule*. How do the most recent rulings impact occupational therapy?

Develop a flow sheet of possible discharge settings for a client who has a total hip replacement. What would be factors in determining discharge dispositions?

Go to the World Health Organization (WHO) Web site http://www.who.int and identify disparities in worldwide rehabilitation versus rehabilitation services in the United States.

Read over the five "Types of OT Interventions" in the *Occupational Therapy Practice Framework III* (AOTA, 2014, pp. S29–S31). Pick two rehabilitation settings and describe how the "Types of OT Interventions" would be similar or different in each setting.

Helpful Websites

American Occupational Therapy Association: www.aota.org
Centers for Medicare and Medicaid Services: www.cms.gov
Medicare Payment Advisory Commission: www.medpac.gov
The Official U.S. Government Site for Medicare: www.medicare.gov
World Health Organization: www.who.int/en/

References

American Health Care Association. *2011 Annual Quality Report: A Comprehensive Report on the Quality of Care in America's Nursing and Rehabilitation Facilities*. 2011. Retrieved from http://www.ahcancal.org/quality_improvement/Documents/2011QualityReport.pdf

American Occupational Therapy Association. Guidelines for supervision, roles, and responsibilities during the delivery of occupational therapy services. *Am J Occup Ther* 2009;63(6):797–803.

American Occupational Therapy Association. Occupational therapy practice framework: domain and process (3rd ed.). *Am J Occup Ther* 2014;68(Suppl 1):S1–S48. http://dx.doi.org/10.5014/ajot.2014.682006

Assisted Living Federation of America. *What is Assisted Living?* n.d. Retrieved from http://www.alfa.org/alfa/Assisted_Living_Information.asp

Felong B. *Guide to Discharge Planning*; 2008. Retrieved from http://www.unm.edu/~dpayment/dow/N424D/pages/GuideToDischargePlanning.pdf

Jackson JP, Whisner S, Wang EW. A predictor model for discharge destination for inpatient rehabilitation patients. *Am J Phys Med Rehabil* 2013;92(4):343–350.

Jette DU, Warren RL, Wirtalla C. The relation between therapy intensity and outcomes of rehabilitation in skilled nursing facilities. *Arch Phys Med Rehabil* 2005;(86):373–379.

Medicare Payment Advisory Commission (MedPAC). *Report to the Congress: Medicare Payment Policy*; 2012a. Retrieved from http://www.medpac.gov/documents/Mar12_EntireReport.pdf

Medicare Payment Advisory Commission (MedPAC). *Inpatient Rehabilitation Facilities Payment System*. 2012b. Retrieved from http://www.medpac.gov/documents/MedPAC_Payment_Basics_12_IRF.pdf

Medicare Payment Advisory Commission (MedPAC). *Home Health Care Services Payment Systems*. 2012c. Retrieved from http://www.medpac.gov/documents/MedPAC_Payment_Basics_12_HHA.pdf

Medicare Payment Advisory Commission (MedPAC). *Outpatient Therapy Services Payment System*. 2012d. Retrieved from http://www.medpac.gov/documents/MedPAC_Payment_Basics_12_OPT.pdf

Medicare.gov. *Glossary*. n.d. Retrieved from http://www.medicare.gov/glossary/h.html

Organization for Economic Cooperation and Development (OECD). Average length of stay. *Health at a Glance 2011: OECD Indicators*. 2011. Retrieved from http://dx.doi.org/10.1787/health_glance-2011-33-en

Smith-Gabai H. *Occupational Therapy in Acute Care*. Maryland, MD: AOTA Press; 2011.

The Alliance for Quality Nursing Home Care. *Care Context: Nursing Facilities Cost-Effectively Treat an Increasingly Complex Patient Population, Benefiting Seniors and Taxpayers*. 2011, September. Retrieved from http://www.aqnhc.org/pdfs/care-context-2011-09.pdf

U.S. Department of Commerce United States Census Bureau. *The 2012 Statistical Abstract: Health & Nutrition: Medicare, Medicaid*; 2012. Retrieved from http://www.census.gov/compendia/statab/cats/health_nutrition/medicare_medicaid.html

U.S. Department of Health and Human Services, Centers for Medicare and Medicaid. *Medicare Coverage of Skilled Nursing Facility Care* (CMS Publication No. 10153). 2007. Retrieved from http://www.medicare.gov/Pubs/pdf/10153.pdf

U.S. Department of Health and Human Services, Centers for Medicare and Medicaid. *Medicare and Home Health* (CMS Product No. 10969). 2010. Retrieved from http://www.medicare.gov/Pubs/pdf/10969.pdf

U.S. Department of Health and Human Services, Centers for Medicare and Medicaid. *Comprehensive Outpatient Rehabilitation Facility* (ICN 904085). 2011. Retrieved from http://www.cms.gov/Outreach-and-Education/Medicare-Learning-Network-MLN/MLNProducts/downloads/Comprehensive_Outpatient_Rehabilitation_Facility_Fact_Sheet_ICN904085.pdf

U.S. Department of Health and Human Services, Centers for Medicare and Medicaid. *What are Long-Term Care Hospitals?* (CMS Publication No. 11347). 2012a. Retrieved from http://www.medicare.gov/Pubs/pdf/11347.pdf

U.S. Department of Health and Human Services, Centers for Medicare and Medicaid. *Your Medicare Benefits* (CMS Publication No. 10116). 2012b. Retrieved from http://www.medicare.gov/Pubs/pdf/10116.pdf

U.S. Department of Health and Human Services, Centers for Medicare and Medicaid. *Medicare and You* (CMS Product No. 10050); 2012c. Retrieved from http://www.medicare.gov/Pubs/pdf/10116.pdf

World Health Organization. *World Report on Disability*. 2011. Retrieved from http://www.who.int/disabilities/world_report/2011/chapter4.pdf

World Health Organization. *Disability and Health Fact Sheet*. 2012. Retrieved from http://www.who.int/mediacentre/factsheets/fs352/en/index.html

CHAPTER

34 Mental Health Practice Settings

Ann Chapleau, DHS, OTR/L

Key Terms

Client-centered practice—A collaborative intervention approach based on the principle of empowering the client as an active partner in the intervention process rather than a passive recipient.

***Diagnostic and Statistical Manual of Mental Disorders* (DSM-5)**—A diagnostic manual published by the American Psychiatric Association to standardize psychiatric diagnostic categories.

Forensic mental health—The field of mental health practice provided within the legal system. Occupational therapy practitioners working in forensic mental health provide services to individuals accused or convicted of crimes, assisting them in developing life skills for coping with mental illness and/or transitioning back into the community following a period of incarceration.

Medical model—The traditional approach to assessment and treatment, focused on remediation of pathology. In a medical model approach, the physician or other health care provider is generally regarded as the expert, while the client, usually referred to as a "patient," is a recipient of services.

Milieu—The therapeutic environment, including the group setting that provides opportunities for development of social skills and peer support.

Psychoeducation—A form of verbal therapy that involves providing the client with information about their condition and/or tools for managing related life challenges.

Psychotropic medication—Medications that are used to treat mental and emotional disorders and behavior.

Recovery model—An approach to treatment of mental illness or substance dependence that focuses on supporting the individual in his/her journey of recovery. Key concepts include client empowerment, a collaborative partnership between the therapist and client, and a goal of facilitating social participation and client-driven goal attainment.

Severe mental illness (SMI)—Diagnosed disorders with serious and persistent symptoms such as psychotic, mood, anxiety, and autism spectrum disorders. Symptoms of SMI can be life threatening if not treated and can significantly impact occupational performance.

Learning Objectives

After studying this chapter, readers should be able to:

- Understand the history of mental health treatment and funding in the United States and its impact on the mental health occupational therapy practitioner.
- Define the role of the occupational therapy practitioner in various mental health practice settings.
- Describe the occupational therapy *process* within mental health practice settings, particularly intervention.

Introduction

The profession of occupational therapy in the United States is deeply rooted in mental health practice. During World War I, the profession was formally established in response to the need to provide care to returning soldiers who often suffered from physical and mental disorders. Early occupational therapists, called reconstruction aides, learned the value of using occupations, such as crafts, games, and gardening, to help soldiers rehabilitate and return home (American Occupational Therapy Association [AOTA], 2012). After the war, a majority of all occupational therapists continued to work in large, long-term institutions for people with chronic illness such as **severe mental illness (SMI)**, epilepsy, and syphilis. These institutions were often referred to as insane asylums. As **psychotropic medications** had not yet been developed, there was no effective treatment available. Patients were often housed for the remainder of their lives. A lack of public funding for these large-scale operations required psychiatric hospitals to be self-sustaining. Usually located on large parcels of land, many of these institutions functioned as working farms, producing their own food. Patients were expected to work daily jobs, often tending to crops, managing dairies, making meals, and doing laundry. For those whose symptoms were too severe, the common practice was isolation; locking patients in separate rooms, or cells; and sometimes placing them in restraints for indefinite periods of time.

After World War II, many OTs switched employment from the state psychiatric institutions to new and expanding medical and rehabilitation programs. This resulted in a shortage of OTs working in psychiatry. By the mid-1950s, census at large-scale state hospitals was at an all-time high, with a total US population of over 500,000 (U.S. National Library of Medicine, 2012). In response to this OT shortage, the AOTA created the occupational therapy assistant category of practitioner. In 1958, the AOTA implemented a three-month academic program in psychiatry (Hussey et al., 2007).

During this time, the movement to provide more localized mental health services had been growing, and in 1963, President John F. Kennedy called for Congress to pass legislation to support mental health services. The resulting legislation, the Community Mental Health Centers Construction Act, supported funding for the construction of facilities that would provide local, community-based care. A second federal law, enacted in 1965, designated funding for staffing, research, training, and the development of treatment, including **psychotropic medications**, electroconvulsive therapy (ECT), psychosurgery such as lobotomy, and psychoanalytic therapy (National Institute of Mental Health, 2012).

The Community Mental Health Centers Construction Act was enacted to ensure that adults with mental illness received care in the least restrictive environment, with a coordinated community reintegration. Intended to provide more coordinated care through local mental health services, but enacted before a community mental health system was solidly in place, this policy eventually resulted in a massive deinstitutionalization of the state hospitals throughout the country, without the needed community support system to absorb the population (The Kaiser Commission on Medicaid and the Uninsured, 2007). As a result, large numbers of mentally ill people became homeless. Another casualty of this flawed policy was the loss of occupational therapy positions, as the profession failed to successfully advocate for inclusion on the community mental health treatment team. Mental health funding cuts enacted in the 1980s and 1990s further reduced reimbursement for acute care inpatient and community-based services, resulting in additional loss of occupational therapy positions. Currently, only 3% of OTs and 2.4% of OTAs identify mental health as their primary work setting (AOTA, 2010a, 2010b, 2010c).

Despite this reduction, OT practitioners continue to work in both institutional and community-based mental health settings, providing services to adults, older adults, children, and adolescents. Opportunities in traditional and emerging community-based practice settings

include hospital-based treatment, outpatient programs, case management, homeless shelters, clubhouse programs, prisons and community correctional facilities, after-school programs, and supported employment and education programs. The passage of the Affordable Care Act of 2010, which has the potential to provide mental health insurance coverage for up to 10 million additional people (Brown, 2010), may provide yet another opportunity to expand the mental health OT workforce. Roles of the mental health OT practitioner include clinician, manager, administrator, consumer advocate, and consultant. For the purposes of this chapter, the role of the clinician will be the primary focus.

The Client

Depending on the role of the OT practitioner, the client may be an individual, a group, an organization, or a community. Throughout this chapter, "client" will refer to an individual. Although the roots of mental health practice are imbedded in a **medical model** approach to care, in which the client is a recipient of diagnosis-driven treatment focused on pathology, current practice supports a **client-centered** approach. Client-centered practice emphasizes a collaborative relationship between the client and the OT practitioner. The client is an active participant in the treatment process, working with the OT practitioner to prioritize goals and guide treatment choices (Law, 1998). Client-centered practice is consistent with the **recovery model**, a growing movement that supports the individual's personal journey toward well-being, occupational engagement and community inclusion (Stoffel, 2012).

Throughout this chapter, clients refer to those individuals who have been diagnosed with a mental illness according to the ***Diagnostic and Statistical Manual of Mental Disorders*** **(DSM-5).** The *DSM-5* provides a classification system (American Psychiatric Association [APA], 2013) to identify type and severity of symptoms using universal terminology (Table 34.1). Dual or multiple diagnoses are not uncommon. For example, an individual with major depressive disorder may have a co-occurring diagnosis of substance dependence.

The Occupational Therapy Process

In some settings, the OT practitioner may be hired to function as a generalist, perhaps as a case manager or an activity therapist. In these cases, the OT practitioner does not provide skilled occupational therapy services. For practitioners who are hired to provide occupational therapy services, the process may be comprehensive or specialized. For example, an OT practitioner may be hired as a consultant to provide evaluation and treatment recommendations only, while an OT practitioner hired as a member of a multidisciplinary treatment team may see the client from admission and evaluation through the intervention phase to discharge.

Evaluation

In most settings, the occupational therapy process begins with a referral, usually by the psychiatrist or physician who heads the treatment team. In order to provide skilled interventions, the OT must first complete an evaluation of the client. This ensures that intervention is individualized, safe, and relevant to the client. The OT, often working with the OTA, will evaluate the client, using various standardized and/or nonstandardized tools as well as clinical observation and interview. As people with SMI are more likely to have cognitive and behavioral limitations, evaluations often need to be modified or limited in use.

TABLE 34.1 The DSM-5 Classification of Disorders
Neurodevelopmental disorders
Schizophrenia spectrum and other psychotic disorders
Bipolar and related disorders
Depressive disorders
Anxiety disorders
Obsessive–compulsive and related disorders
Trauma- and stressor-related disorders
Dissociative disorders
Somatic symptom and related disorders
Feeding and eating disorders
Elimination disorders
Sleep–wake disorders
Sexual dysfunctions
Gender dysphoria
Disruptive, impulse–control, and conduct disorders
Substance-related and addictive disorders
Neurocognitive disorders
Personality disorders
Medication-induced movement disorders and other adverse effects of medication
Other mental disorders

Many facilities develop their own program-specific evaluation reports, which are often based primarily on clinical observations, interview, and chart review. Assessments of IADL skills, however, are best performed through task observation rather than client report, to ensure accuracy (Brown et al., 1996). The occupational therapy evaluation should reflect the client's physical, cultural, and social environment or contexts, as well as the client's level of motivation, habits, routines, and desired roles. Table 34.2 lists examples of mental health assessment tools.

Treatment Planning

Following the evaluation process, a treatment plan is developed for each client. In settings in which a client-centered approach is used, the client participates in the development of his/her plan of care, often attending the treatment planning conferences along with other members of the team. In child and adolescent programs, parents or other caregivers may be included as well. In settings in which the client is acutely symptomatic or demonstrates severe cognitive impairment, the client may not be included in the treatment planning process. The occupational therapy treatment plan usually contains both long-term and short-term goals and identifies interventions that will be used to best meet these goals. This written plan becomes a "road map" to follow throughout the course of treatment. It is important that the OT communicates with the OTA to ensure that all interventions are targeted toward the client's treatment goals.

Intervention

The OT practitioner uses meaningful occupations and activities to improve mental health functioning and social participation. The process involves task analysis and modification as well as environmental modifications to promote opportunities for task mastery.

TABLE **34.2** **OT Mental Health-Related Assessment Tools**

Type	Examples
ADL/IADL	*Performance Assessment of Self-Care Skills (PASS)* *Comprehensive Occupational Therapy Evaluation (COTE)* *Kohlman Evaluation of Living Skills (KELS)* *Kitchen Safety Assessment*
Role performance	*Canadian Occupational Performance Measure (COPM)* *Role Checklist* *Occupational Self-Assessment version 2.2 (OSA)* *Assessment of Occupational Functioning (AOF)* *Self-Description Questionnaire (SDQ III) (young adults)* *Occupational Circumstances Assessment Interview and Rating Scale (OCAIRS)* *Occupational Performance History (OPHI-II)* *Model of Human Occupation Screening Tool (MOHOST)* *Social Interaction Scale (SIS)* *Evaluation of Social Interaction (ESI)* *School Function Assessment (SFA)* *Knox Preschool Play Scale*
Vocational	*Worker Role Interview (WRI)* *Work Environment Impact Scale (WEIS)*
Cognition	*Allen Cognitive Level Screen (ACLS-5)* *Routine Task Inventory (RTI)* *Cognitive Performance Test (CPT)*
Sensory processing	*Sensory Profile (versions: adult/adolescent, infant/toddler, school companion)* *Sensory Defensiveness Checklist (Sensory Connection Program)*
Self-concept	*Piers-Harris 3 (pediatric)* *The Body Image Scale (pediatric)* *Stress Management Questionnaire (SMQ)*

People with SMI typically struggle with multiple impairments in ADL and/or IADL performance, due to symptoms of their illness, co-occurring medical conditions, difficulty retaining employment, and limited education (Baron & Salzer, 2002; Colton & Manderscheid, 2006; Kessler et al., 2008). Prioritizing interventions is a collaborative process between the OT practitioner and the client. In addition, the treatment setting often determines which goals are selected. For example, in acute care settings, in which the client is unable to safely care for self, intervention may focus on basic ADL, increasing opportunities for social participation, and **psychoeducation** in the form of cognitive–behavioral strategies such as training in coping skills/relaxation and emotion awareness and regulation CS7. Gross and fine motor activities may also be incorporated to counteract side effects of psychotropic medications, which can include drowsiness, tremors, or restlessness. In community-based settings, intervention may include IADL interventions such as home maintenance, parenting, supported education, and employment programs (Arbesman & Logsdon, 2011). There is also growing work in the area of providing structured interventions, such as food preparation, money management, and reading, writing, and computer use, for cognitive remediation for people with schizophrenia (Katz & Keren, 2011).

Depending on the setting, interventions can be provided individually or in a group. Group is the primary mode of intervention in most mental health settings in which increasing social participation and developing social skills are common goals. The OT practitioner must be proficient in leading groups and understanding group dynamics, to ensure that the needs of all participants are met (please also refer to Chapter 25, *Group Dynamics: Planning and Leading Effective Therapeutic Groups*). The OT practitioner should be skilled in active listening and comfortable providing feedback; setting limits on disruptive, intrusive, or unsafe behavior; and providing positive reinforcement and support for client effort and improvement in goal areas. A conceptual practice model, the Intentional Relationship, defines various modes of therapeutic interaction to meet the individualized needs of clients (Taylor, 2008). Research supports the value of utilizing these modes based on therapeutic use of self in developing rapport and increasing treatment compliance and participation (Taylor, 2008) (From the Field 34.1).

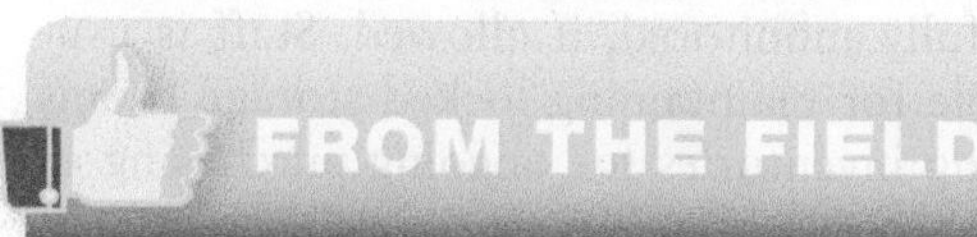

Mental Illness

According to the World Health Organization, mental illness is a growing cause of disability worldwide. It predicts that in the future, depression will be a top cause of disability.

Discharge

Throughout the treatment process, the client's response to interventions is continually evaluated and documented. Once the client has accomplished his/her treatment goals, demonstrating an ability to return to a less restrictive or community living arrangement, discharge occurs.

Occupational therapy practitioners may play an important role in the discharge process. For short-term settings, it is imperative that planning for discharge begins upon admission. Occupational therapy practitioners may provide caregiver training for significant others and professional caregivers, such as case managers and group home staff, to promote a successful transition to a new environment. This training may include a home safety evaluation and/or an assessment or reassessment of functional skills including ADL, IADL, cognition, balance and mobility, and/or work skills. In addition, the OT practitioner may provide referrals to community programs and resources to assist the client in working toward goals in health promotion, employment, education, recreation, and social participation.

In any setting, even with a target discharge date, it is not uncommon for the client to be discharged suddenly, without prior notice. Reasons for unanticipated discharge can include the client signing himself/herself out of treatment against medical advice, the client "eloping" from a secured facility program, or a change in the discharge plan. The OT practitioner must be prepared for these changes, able to adapt the plan for group and individual interventions each day, as clients unexpectedly come into and leave the program.

Practice Settings

There are numerous practice settings in which an OTA may work with clients with mental health diagnoses. Several are discussed below.

State Hospitals

Despite a 95% reduction in US state psychiatric hospitals over the past 50 years, more than 200 remain in operation today (Fisher et al., 2009), providing services to individuals who are unable to receive and/or benefit from short-term or less intensive outpatient treatment. These individuals often have severe psychiatric symptoms that do not respond to psychotropic medications or other treatment, which place them and/or others at risk of harm. The general goal of treatment within a state hospital setting is to reduce the client's psychiatric symptoms enough to allow the client to return to his/her community in a less restrictive treatment environment or to house the individual who is committed for legal purposes until such a time as they are considered competent to stand trial or are released from further legal detainment. Some individuals are involuntarily committed through the criminal court system as they have been found either incompetent to stand trial or not guilty by reason of insanity.

State hospitals provide services to adults, older adults, adolescents, and children. Some state hospitals limit services to only certain age groups, and those that offer multiple age-specific programs provide separate units or buildings. Length of stay can vary greatly, but this practice setting represents the lengthiest treatment period, ranging from days to months and, in some cases, even years. Funding for state hospitals is generally provided through both state and federal funds, such as Medicaid and Medicare.

The Treatment Team

The OT practitioner is a member of a comprehensive, interdisciplinary treatment team, which varies from facility to facility. The core team usually consists of the client, a psychiatrist, nurse, and social worker. Additional disciplines may include psychology and any number of activity therapies such as music, art, recreation, or dance/movement therapists. The psychiatrist usually heads the multidisciplinary treatment team but is most focused on prescribing, monitoring, and adjusting dosages of medications and other treatments such as electroconvulsive therapy (ECT). Nursing staff work closely with the psychiatry staff, administering medications, providing medication education, and monitoring for medical issues. They may supervise support staff who work directly throughout the day with clients, assisting with meals, self-care tasks, and general **milieu** activity. Often, the psychologist will provide testing services, while social workers, activity therapists, and aides provide the bulk of the daily programming, which is primarily group intervention. In some state hospitals, OT practitioners are employed as activity therapists, providing generalized services such as leisure and social interaction groups and one-to-one intervention.

Implementing the Treatment Plan

The goal of occupational therapy treatment in a state hospital setting is to help clients improve the quality of their lives, through improving their occupational performance skills in self-care, productive roles, leisure, and communication/socialization. Interventions include psychoeducation and opportunities to practice these skills for daily living. Many of the interventions are provided in a group setting CS7. There is a growing movement to provide sensory-based treatment in state hospitals as well. Recent research supports that people who have access to sensory materials, including a sensory room, and are taught how to use sensory and motor activities to self-regulate their emotional state require fewer physical restraints and chemical (medication) restraints (Champagne & Stromberg, 2004) (Fig. 34.1).

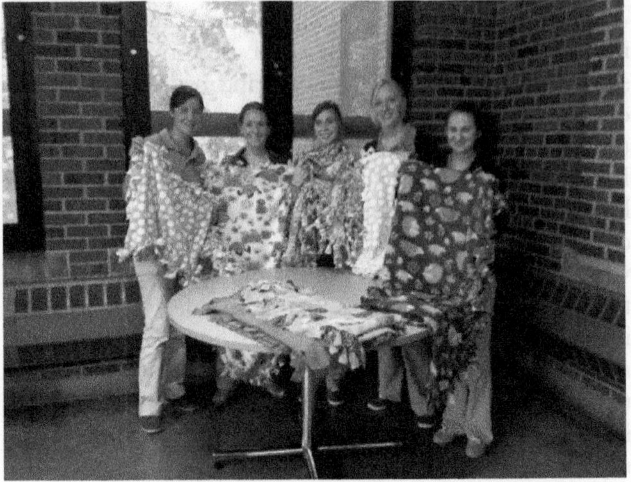

Figure 34.1 Fieldwork students at Western Michigan University display the sensory blankets made by female clients at the Kalamazoo Psychiatric Hospital. Blankets were precut and fringed so that clients could double knot around the perimeter of the fabric for a successful project completion. Clients were encouraged to bring their blankets with them to future sensory groups.

For individuals committed through the criminal court system, there may be groups for clients to learn the legal terms and processes that apply to their case. Often, the OT practitioner may address self-care/ADL issues through group education as well as individual treatment. State hospitals that retain their original floor plans are often quite spacious, with multiple rooms available for various activities. There is typically a dayroom available, which may have a television, various chairs and sofas, and tables. The dining room may also serve as a space for working on tabletop activities. Some facilities have a kitchen and even separate rooms designated for crafts, woodworking, and relaxation. Many are also equipped with a gymnasium. Clients who are not an immediate safety risk may have ground privileges for walks or other outings (Fig. 34.2). As safety is always a concern, all group materials that could be hazardous, such as scissors, paints and stains, and tools must be carefully monitored, if allowed. Staff is usually responsible for maintaining locked storage rooms and monitoring inventories for ongoing purchasing of supplies.

Documentation in the state hospital system varies from facility to facility but, in general, is completed for each treatment session. Because of the longer length of stay for many of the clients, there may also be lengthier, more comprehensive progress summaries completed at intervals such as weekly or monthly.

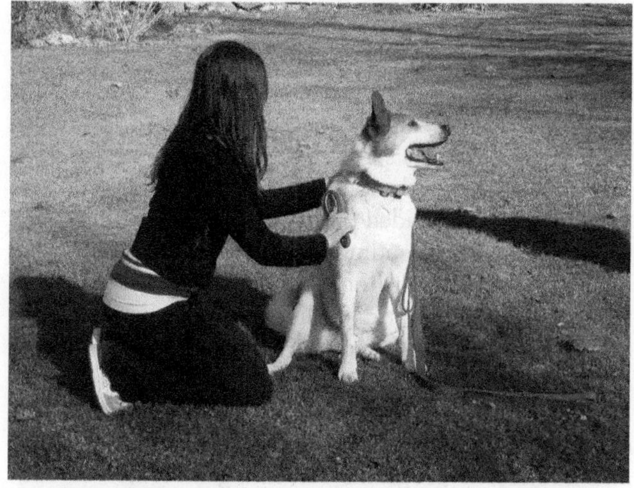

Figure 34.2 "In a highly restrictive treatment setting, clients have little control over their environment or opportunities to learn how to nurture and be nurtured. Animal assisted therapy provides opportunities for clients to practice these developmental tasks while building self-esteem." (Brenda Marshall, MA, OTR/L.)

Hospital-Based Settings

Acute care, hospital-based programs are designed to provide rapid admission and crisis intervention for those individuals experiencing acute mental health symptoms that pose a danger to themselves or others. Examples include an individual with major depressive disorder who is suicidal; a person diagnosed with schizophrenia, actively psychotic, and unable to care for himself/herself; or a child with conduct disorder who is acting out aggressively toward siblings and peers and is unable to be safely managed at home. The inpatient psychiatric setting may be located on a unit within a general medical hospital or may be a freestanding facility. The inpatient setting is highly restrictive, regardless of whether or not the individual has voluntarily admitted himself/herself or are involuntarily committed through the court system. Most often, the doors to the units are kept locked, and the clients are not allowed to have access to items that could be considered potentially harmful, such as glass objects and belts and even pencils, paperclips, and staples. Visitation hours are also limited.

The length of stay in hospital settings has decreased significantly in the past 30 years, due in great part to limited reimbursement for services. Inpatient hospital programs are primarily funded by Medicare and Medicaid and may receive additional funds through other state subsidies and private insurance. The current, average length of stay is 7.5 days (Centers for Disease Control and Prevention, 2012). For those with substance use disorders such as substance dependence, length of stay is shorter, averaging 4.8 day, but often limited to a 23-hour detoxification with no rehabilitative treatment (The Piper Report, 2011). The result is a challenging situation in which the mental health care providers are working in a crisis situation with clients experiencing severe symptoms, but with very limited time to establish rapport, complete the evaluation process, and work with clients to reduce symptoms and provide education in lifestyle changes for postdischarge CS7. Because of this quick-paced treatment process, it is imperative that members of the multidisciplinary treatment team work together on common goals and strategies for intervention.

The Treatment Team

The core treatment team usually consists of a psychiatrist, nurse, and social worker. In some settings, an OT practitioner is also a member of the team. Psychologists may be on the team either as direct care providers or to provide psychological testing and recommendations. Dieticians may also be consulted, if the client has dietary or eating disorder issues. There may be additional activity therapy representatives from music, recreation, art, or dance/movement. Occupational therapy practitioners may be employed as activity therapy staff, providing milieu programming and documenting progress, but they do not provide or bill for occupational therapy services. They may or may not participate in the treatment planning process, depending on the policies of the facility. The comprehensive treatment plan becomes the focus of intervention for all of the team members, and treatment notes are written after each session to reflect progress toward these goals. Because the length of stay in an inpatient setting is brief, even the initial evaluation process is focused on discharge, with recommendations for follow-up care and support.

Implementing the Treatment Plan

In the inpatient hospital setting, daily programming revolves around a group schedule. Some programs offer a daily community meeting, in which clients can voice concerns, comments, or questions related to their program. Community meetings may be co-facilitated by representatives from all of the treatment team disciplines. Social workers usually provide a daily verbal group that may focus on group process or planning for discharge. Nursing staff may provide a medication education or other health topic group. Occupational therapy practitioners and/or activity therapists such as recreational, music, art, and movement/dance therapists provide programming that includes exercise or other movement groups, arts and crafts, games, cooking groups, music, animal-assisted therapy, psychoeducation, or focus groups. Focus groups may involve an educational component, such as learning assertive communication styles, followed by role-play opportunities, or reviewing worksheets about coping skills, then practicing relaxation techniques. In addition to group intervention, occupational therapy practitioners work individually with clients as needed, toward achievement of treatment plan goals. All treatment sessions are documented using facility-specific forms to describe the intervention provided, the client response, progress toward treatment plan goals, and plans for future treatment.

Programs that are housed on a unit within a general hospital often have limited activity space. There is usually a dayroom, which may have a television, seating, and tables. There may be a kitchenette and dining area within the dayroom or in a separate room. A separate group or conference room may be available, sometimes shared with social work staff, for psychoeducation groups. There may or may not be a designated space for exercise. Some facilities may have accessible grounds or an enclosed courtyard to enable outdoor activities and exercise, but due to the brief length of stay and third-party reimbursement requirements, opportunities for community outings are limited. When space is limited, OT practitioners must be creative in scheduling and modifying the environment to be conducive for each chosen activity (Fig. 34.3).

Partial Hospitalization Programs

Some hospitals offer a step-down program from 24-hour hospitalization to partial hospitalization (PHP). The PHP program, often referred to as day treatment, can be an option for those with mental illness and/or a substance abuse disorder who still require intensive services but are no longer considered to be a safety risk outside the hospital. Although PHP programs may vary, they typically meet Monday through Friday. The Centers for Medicare and Medicaid Services (Centers for Medicare and Medicaid Services, Department of Health and Human Services, 2010) require a minimum of 20 hours per week of therapy services and identify occupational therapy as a covered service. Partial hospitalization services are often provided on the same hospital unit, with the patient/client attending the same daily programming, but returning to their homes at night. Other PHPs continue to provide multidisciplinary assessments, groups, and individual therapy in the hospital facility but in a separate location. Programs are typically specialized by age or specific disorder treated. Examples include an older adult program for treatment of dementia, adult and adolescent programs for eating disorders or substance abuse, and child and/or adolescent programs that may include an on-site school. Funding for adult PHPs is primarily through managed care plans, Medicare, and Medicaid.

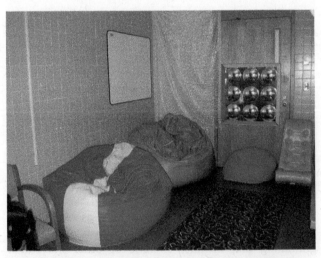

Figure 34.3 Occupational therapy practitioners use creativity to develop a sensory space. This area was created as a "drop-in" room for clients, to be used with OT staff supervision. Soft seating and lighting, a rocker chair, and weighted stuffed animals can be used safely by clients on an inpatient unit. (Photo by Karen Moore, OTR/L, Founder of the Sensory Connection Program.)

Intensive Outpatient Programs

Intensive outpatient programs (IOPs) are also used as a step-down from acute care, hospital-based treatment. Like PHPs, IOPs provide structured programming Monday through Friday but provide fewer hours of service, usually about 3 hours per day (Association for Ambulatory Behavioral Health, 2007). IOPs may be specialized for mental health or chemical dependency or various age groups, and hours of operation may include evenings for those who work during the day or attend school.

Involvement of family, residential care providers, and even employers can be an important part of the client's recovery process. In group and 1:1 intervention, the OT practitioner may help clients learn practical strategies for daily living that they can immediately implement in their home, work, school, social, and community environments.

Psychosocial Clubhouse

The psychosocial clubhouse model is a community-based, recovery-oriented program to provide mental health consumers with a supportive environment to improve opportunities for employment and social participation. The clubhouse model grew out of an early movement in the 1940s, with formerly hospitalized patients forming a support network to help one another adjust to community life. In 1948, they purchased a home, which they called Fountain House, to provide housing for recently discharged patients and rooms for recreation, study, and work. Since that first house, the clubhouse model has become an international organization, with over 330 certified clubhouses in 30 countries and 36 states (International Center for Clubhouse Development [ICCD], 2012a).

Membership is voluntary and open ended for any adult with a diagnosis of mental illness. Membership is not restricted based on ability to function or type of diagnosis. The clubhouse model is based on the principle that members and staff work in an equal partnership, responsible for all aspects of operation. The clubhouse program is not a clinical program; there are no therapy groups or other clinical interventions. Certified clubhouses operate at least 5 days a week and focus on a work-ordered day, which includes various work units, an external employment program, social/recreational activities, and opportunities for education, including assistance in preparing for the GED or other adult education courses. In-house work units may include clerical or computer work and snack bar and/or lunch preparation. There are usually separate rooms for the various work units, such as a computer lab, an education room, a kitchen or kitchenette, and a dayroom or dining room for multipurpose use. The work-ordered day also includes administrative functions such as orienting new members, participating in the hiring and training of staff, public relations, research, and program evaluation (ICCD, 2012b).

The Multidisciplinary Team

Each clubhouse program includes an administrative position of manager, who is required to hold a professional degree in a health or human services field, and various staff who work to assist members in the work units. There are no requirements listed in the accreditation standards for professional staff; however, additional staff positions may include social workers, case managers, vocational rehabilitation counselors, nurses, and OT practitioners. One ICCD requirement is that there is only enough staff to assist the members in completing the work of the clubhouse (ICCD, 2012b).

Role of Occupational Therapy

Occupational therapy practitioners are ideally suited to assist the members in carrying out the goals of the clubhouse program. Empowering members to engage in meaningful occupations of work and recreation while facilitating opportunities for social participation is consistent with the *Occupational Therapy Practice Framework III* (AOTA, 2014). In the clubhouse model, there is not a traditional OT process of referral, evaluation, treatment planning, intervention, and discharge. Instead, OT practitioners work as generalists, alongside other staff, in assisting the members in engaging in work and social roles at the clubhouse or in the local community. Staff do not bill for individualized, skilled intervention services. The OTA can work without the supervision of an OT in providing this direct support to members. The primary funding sources for clubhouse programs are Medicaid and Medicare. In addition, a sliding scale fee may be available for those members who do not receive state or federal entitlements.

Case Management Services Through Community Mental Health Programs

People with SMI who are living in the community while receiving mental health and housing services typically receive case management services as their primary intervention (Ziguras et al., 2002). Case management is a specialized practice that can include practitioners from a variety of backgrounds (Fisher, 1996). Case managers work individually with clients to coordinate care by linking them to community resources, advocating for services, and providing support as needed. The goal of case management is to ensure that the client has access to needed community services and resources to enable the client to meet his/her goals. Most case management programs provide a centralized office where staff meet with clients, participate in treatment planning conferences, and complete and submit documentation. Often, this centralized facility functions as a drop-in center for clients.

There are various models of case management. Mueser et al. (1998) identified six models: broker, strength-based, clinical, rehabilitation, intensive, and assertive community treatment (ACT). The broker model focuses on assessing needs and linking the client to service providers. The strengths-based model focuses on building client strengths by facilitating community supports to promote community integration. The relationship between the client and the case manager is primary and essential. The clinical model utilizes the case manager as a clinician, providing assessment, treatment planning, and direct intervention in life skills training. In addition, the case manager links the client with community resources and supports. The rehabilitation model is unique in its focus on assessment and remediation of skills for community living. Intensive case management provides more individualized and flexible services, with lower case loads than traditional case management.

The ACT model, like the intensive case management model, provides more intensive, flexible services, with smaller caseloads, but also includes the use of a multidisciplinary team to provide case management services as needed, 24 hours a day, 7 days a week.

The ACT model has been widely used and researched throughout the two decades. Findings support that this model is effective in reducing hospitalizations and improving housing stability among those with SMI who are most at risk for rehospitalization or homelessness due to the severity and complexity of their symptoms (Mueser et al., 1998; Tsemberis & Stefancis, 2007; Tsemberis, Gulcur & Nakae, 2004; Zigarus & Stuart, 2000).

The ACT program provides case management services as well as other needed services directly to the individual, using the expertise of the treatment team. This is in contrast to other case management models that refer clients to outside agencies and programs for needed services. When a client is admitted to the ACT program, they participate in a comprehensive evaluation process to determine needs and strengths. Assessment and treatment planning guidelines, as well as documentation requirements, vary from state to state. Funding is primarily provided through Medicaid. Not all states offer ACT programs, relying instead on other case management models through the community mental health continuum of care approach.

The Treatment Team

Ideally, an ACT team consists of 10 to 12 staff who share responsibility for an overall case load of approximately 100 consumers (SAMHSA, 2012). The ACT team typically includes an ACT leader, psychiatrist, psychiatric nurse, employment specialist, substance abuse specialist, mental health consumer/peer specialist, program assistant, and additional mental health professionals such as social workers, OT practitioners, rehabilitation counselors, or psychologists (SAMHSA, 2012). While all team members share in providing the interventions, each member can provide interventions related to their scope of practice. For example, the nurse may travel to the client's home to administer injection medications and to provide education on medication effects and side effects.

Role of Occupational Therapy

The OT practitioner's role may include assessing ADL/IADL skills and safety of community living arrangements and proposing strategies for self-care activities including hygiene, home and money management, and social integration (Meyers, 2001). For cost-saving purposes, an ACT program may utilize a part-time OT consultant to provide professional supervision to an OTA who may carry out specialized treatment interventions. In the absence of an OT on the team, the OTA should check with his/her state regulatory agency to determine if they meet the educational qualifications to carry out generalized case management services.

Homeless Shelters

Most people with SMI are at continual risk of homelessness, due to a variety of factors, including poverty, lacking of affordable housing, unemployment, and lack of access to mental health and addiction services (Morell-Bellai et al., 2000: Wilson, 2003). In fact, approximately 26% of all people in shelter facilities have SMI, and 34% have chronic substance abuse issues (SAMHSA, 2011).

There are numerous and interwoven barriers to ending homelessness, including a disjointed health care system (Burt et al., 2007; United Sates Department of Housing and Urban Development, 2010). People with SMI are often in poor physical health and lack transportation, phone, or proper identifying documents, which makes it difficult to navigate the complex system of obtaining assistance from various agencies that are often geographically separated throughout communities (Folsom et al., 2005).

Homeless shelters provide safe, temporary housing to those in need, with the length of stay varying greatly. Typical shelters may provide one night to 30 days, while homeless centers, with more comprehensive services offered, may extend the length of stay to 1 year or longer for those progressing through a treatment program that may include adult education, parenting, life skills training, and employment training and placement.

The homeless population may include

- Adults with mental illness
- Families with children
- Women seeking shelter from domestic violence
- Youth

The Treatment Team

Homeless shelter staff can vary widely, depending on the type of shelter and services provided. Intake coordinators may be responsible for the initial screening process to determine eligibility for services and general admission. Much of the daily operation of the shelter may be conducted by administrative staff, volunteers, and senior residents who function as supervisors, ensuring that all residents are following facility rules and fulfilling expectations for shared work or assigned chores.

Specialized program staff can include case managers, social workers, medical personnel, OT practitioners, and certified alcohol and drug abuse counselors. Programs that provide on-site job training may employ or contract with employment counselors. Legal advocates may also work with residents who need assistance in resolving criminal charges, custody issues, or, in cases of domestic abuse, initiating protective orders.

Role of Occupational Therapy

Due to the wide range of populations served in homeless shelters and centers, assessment and treatment interventions for the OT practitioner will vary. Occupational therapists may conduct a comprehensive evaluation and plan of care that will enable successful participation in appropriate shelter programs as well as provide recommendations and/or referrals related to housing, employment, education, and sober leisure/social participation. The role of the OT consultant in conducting cognitive and home safety assessments, leading activity-based groups, and providing treatment recommendations to case managers has also been found to be useful (Chapleau et al., 2012). Occupational therapy practitioners may also provide direct intervention in life skills training (Helfrich et al., 2006), employment skills training (Munoz et al., 2006a, 2006b), parenting skills, and time management (Schultz-Krohn et al., 2006). Families with children often receive on-site day care for children. This creates additional opportunities for OT practitioners to provide early intervention services to infants and toddlers who are at risk for developmental delays and mental illness.

Working in a homeless shelter can present challenges for space, supplies, and other resources. Funding for OT services may be provided through government or local foundation grants. Housing and Urban Development (HUD) is a major funding source for housing-related programs. State funding for community-based services, particularly those that serve individuals with SMI and/or substance abuse disorders who are at risk of homelessness may be available through the Projects for Assistance in Transition from Homelessness (PATH) program.

Correctional Systems

The goal of the US justice system is to protect society from dangerous criminals. In addition, there is a secondary goal of rehabilitation, to ensure that those who are eventually released can reintegrate into society as productive citizens. There are various levels of correctional supervision, including probation, parole, jail, or prison. In 2011, nearly 5 million adult offenders were supervised on probation or parole, while approximately 2.2 million were incarcerated in prisons or jails (Bureau of Justice Statistics, 2012). These numbers, while high, represent a decline of 98,900 offenders in the US correctional population and mark the third consecutive year of declining numbers. Juvenile incarcerations, however, have been on the rise. In 2006, 92,854 juvenile offenders were housed in residential facilities (Office of Juvenile Justice and Delinquency Prevention, 2012).

Of great concern is the startling numbers of individuals with SMI who are incarcerated. In the United States, people diagnosed with SMI are three times more likely to be in jail or prison than in a psychiatric hospital. Moreover, at least 16% of all inmates in prisons and jails have SMI (National Alliance to End Homelessness, n.d.). Unfortunately, there are minimal mental health services available within the correctional system, and many individuals lack proper medications and medication monitoring, counseling, and life skills training. The rise in the number of people with SMI who are incarcerated is related to the continued shortage of available mental health beds and other community-based treatment options. This disturbing practice of placing those with SMI in the correctional system, as well as the nursing home system, is known as transinstitutionalization, as described in the following case.

Case: Transinstitutionalization

Jesse is a young adult with untreated schizophrenia. He is experiencing his first "psychotic break." He has delusions that he is the Messiah. He believes he needs to "save" others by preaching to the public. He proceeds to shout his message in front of a private business, disrupting the customer traffic. When he will not leave after a request by the owner, the police are called. He resists the officers who attempt to physically remove him. He is charged with unlawful trespassing, resisting arrest, and assaulting a police officer. In his community, there is no mental health court available and no mental health beds for treatment. His case is processed through the criminal court and he is sentenced to incarceration. He may or may not receive mental health services, he is at risk of being victimized while incarcerated, and his criminal record will make it difficult for him to achieve future employment.

Think about and discuss the potential outcomes for Jesse if the following occurred:

1. He was sent to prison.
2. He was sent via involuntary admission to an inpatient psychiatric setting.
3. He was assigned to a community clinic.

The Treatment Team

Staffing in the correctional system can vary greatly, depending on the type of facility and level of security. Personnel, in addition to guards and correctional officers who provide oversight and monitoring of the prison milieu, can include mental health nurses, physicians, psychiatrists, social workers and other social services staff, certified alcohol and drug abuse counselors (CADAC), and legal counselors.

In the jail setting, offenders are typically awaiting sentencing or transfer to another facility. The length of stay is shorter than in the prison setting. Screening for mental illness is required. There may be separate areas and staff offices for various mental health, medical, and drug and alcohol programs, as well as designated activity and exercise spaces. In addition, some jails provide separate mental health beds. In the prison system, basic mental health services typically consist of initial screening and medication administration and monitoring. Unlike the jail setting, prisons are less likely to provide separate beds for those with mental illness. Some jails and prisons provide general rehabilitation services such as counseling to address issues of substance abuse, anger management, adult education, and job training.

Community reentry centers provide transitional support services to offenders who are preparing for their release. Although a supervised residential program, offenders are able to obtain passes to leave the facility for work or housing or job searching purposes. Personnel work with offenders to help them develop a support network of community resources.

Role of Occupational Therapy

Occupational therapy practitioners may play an important role in addressing the rehabilitative needs of both adults and juvenile offenders. With 67% of released prisoners rearrested within three years (Gibbons & Katzenbach, 2006), the need is great for a comprehensive approach to community reintegration. One strategy using animals is discussed in From the Field 34.2. OT services in **forensic mental health** may include evaluation and treatment of ADL and IADL skills, functional cognition, and evaluation of physical and social environments, for both ability to navigate prison life and future community reintegration.

The OT practitioner working in forensic mental health must be culturally competent in working with diverse populations, as offenders are typically racial and ethnic minorities, with a history of poverty, substance abuse, and often a learning disability. They are likely to have come from and will return to a high-crime community, with limited resources and opportunities for employment. Female offenders are likely to be single parents and have been exposed to violence, particularly domestic abuse. They are disproportionately diagnosed with mental illness, especially PTSD and substance abuse disorders, and their convictions are more likely to be related to drug offenses (Goff et al., 2007).

FROM THE FIELD 34.2

Animal-Assisted Programs

Over the past 25 years, numerous studies have been conducted in correctional facilities using animal-assisted training programs. Results support the value of these programs in positively impacting adult and youth offenders' social behavior, self-esteem, morale, and recidivism rates. Examples include the following:

- Puppies Behind Bars: http://www.puppiesbehindbars.com/
- Project POOCH: Oregon Youth Facility: http://www.pooch.org/
- Pound Puppies: http://www.vadoc.state.va.us/resources/events/aca-poundpuppies.pdf
- Project Second Chance: http://www.societyandanimalsforum.org/sa/sa9.2/harbolt.shtml

After-School Programs for Youth

During the past 15 years, after-school programs (ASPs), sometimes referred to as out-of-school programs, have continued to grow in response to the need to actively engage and support learning and development for youth, from kindergarten through high school. In the United States, approximately 6.5 million youth, from kindergarten through 12th grade, participate in ASPs (Little et al., 2008). The goals of ASPs are to improve academic, social, and leisure skills through engagement in meaningful activities (Fig. 34.4). Most programs include adult-directed social and recreational activities as well as an academic component such as tutoring or assistance with homework (Durlak & Weissberg, 2007).

There is substantial evidence that children who are unsupervised after school are at a greater risk of developing academic and behavioral problems and that children engaged in ASPs have better academic and social/emotional outcomes and prevention outcomes such as less alcohol and drug use; decreased incidences of juvenile delinquency, violence, and crime; and avoidance of sexual activity (Little et al., 2008).

Specialized ASPs for youth with mental health or behavioral problems are designed to promote opportunities for social participation in a safe and structured environment. There is less outcomes research on these programs but a growing number of examples of programs geared to youth with autism spectrum disorder and mental illness and those at high risk due to poverty.

After-school programs can be conducted in school settings or other community facilities such as YMCA; YWCA; Boys and Girls Clubs; faith-based organizations such as local religious facilities, including

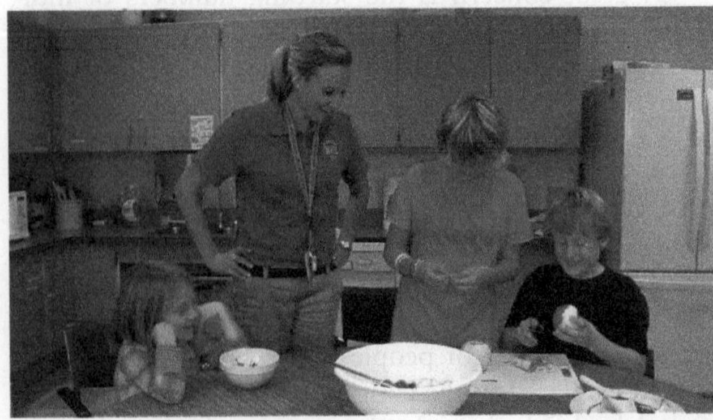

Figure 34.4 At the Skills for Living Clinic at Western Michigan University, an after-school program for children and adolescents diagnosed with mental illness, OT faculty and students provide structured group activities to develop social skills, sensory modulation, and daily living skills.

churches, mosques, and synagogues; and homeless shelters. Funding is often through community and state-funded grants and private donations, as well as federal funding. Reimbursement for clinical services for youth with mental illness may be provided through community mental health funds.

The Treatment Team

After-school program staffing varies based on goals of the program, the population served, and funding. Programs that focus on general activities, tutoring, and/or homework assistance may utilize recreation therapists and paraprofessionals. For programs that serve high-risk youth or those with mental illness, staffing may also include professionals such as social workers, psychologists, educators, and OT practitioners. Difficulties providing quality staffing for programs that serve at-risk youth have been documented (Frazier et al., 2007).

Role of Occupational Therapy

The OT practitioner may address occupational performance issues related to academic performance as well as social, emotional, and physical needs. The role of the OT practitioner may vary, depending on the focus of the ASP. In a program specifically designed for improving academic success, the OT practitioner may develop learning strategies and assist the child in time management techniques for organizing and completing homework. In more generalized programs, the OT practitioner may provide social activities, games, education, and role-play interventions to improve social participation and age-appropriate social skills and to promote emotion awareness and expression. For children with sensory processing impairments related to specific diagnoses such as autism, treatment may focus on provision of sensory experiences to improve self-regulation. Developing a positive, trusting, and collaborative relationship with the child, parents, teachers, and other care providers is also essential to the treatment process.

Veterans Administration Settings

The Veterans Administration (VA) system serves US military veterans who are experiencing mental illness and/or substance abuse issues. The VA has a network of treatment facilities throughout the United States, consisting of regional medical centers, which provide both inpatient and outpatient services, and community-based outpatient clinics. Common mental health problems for veterans include depression, substance abuse, and post-traumatic stress disorder (PTSD). Treatment settings include the following (Sullivan et al., 2011):

- Inpatient hospital
- IOP
- Outpatient services within a psychosocial rehabilitation and recovery center (PRRC)
- Outpatient services that can include telemedicine
- Residential treatment programs particularly focused on issues related to obtaining housing, employment, and education. The VA offers residential programs for treatment of substance abuse disorders as well. These programs are typically 30 to 90 days.

For veterans with mental health issues, treatment includes psychosocial rehabilitation services, peer support, and work therapies such as transitional work experience, supported employment, and incentive therapy, which provide opportunities for work at VA Medical Centers (Sullivan et al., 2011). Psychosocial rehabilitation services may include psychoeducation, health promotion programs, and family education. Examples of specialized services include treatment programs for veterans who are returning from a recent deployment, those with SMI, and women who have been sexually abused while in military service.

The Treatment Team

The team consists of the principal care provider, who is typically a physician, nurse, or counselor who is responsible for mental health care coordination, psychiatrist, social worker, counselor, and supported employment professionals. Many VA facilities have chaplains available as well, for spiritual or religious counseling.

Role of Occupational Therapy

The OT practitioner works with the multidisciplinary treatment team to evaluate, develop, and implement a plan of care and to assist the veteran in preparing for discharge by making appropriate referrals through the VA network or other community resources. Occupational therapy practitioners are able to assist veterans with PTSD, depression, anxiety, and other mental illness by utilizing cognitive–behavioral interventions such as teaching relaxation and other coping strategies. Interventions may be provided individually or in a group setting. The OT practitioner may also provide services in the work therapies programs, assessing vocational skills and providing interventions to enable opportunities for supported or competitive employment.

Summary

Mental health services in the United States have evolved greatly over the past 50 years, in response to advances in science, changing public policies, and funding. While the number of OT practitioners in traditional mental health settings has declined significantly, there are many opportunities to bring functional, occupation-based focus to a variety of practice settings. Moreover, with an estimated 25% of all adult Americans experiencing mental illness in any given year (National Institute of Mental Health, 2009), OT practitioners need the skills to address psychosocial dysfunction in nonmental health settings as well. Understanding the various treatment programs and roles of the OT practitioner in mental health practice is an important part of developing competency as a holistic practitioner.

Review Questions

1. An example of client-centered practice is:
   a. The client is a recipient of treatment provided by a mental health expert.
   b. Treatment is based on the diagnosis of the client.
   c. The client and the therapist collaborate to prioritize treatment goals.
   d. None of the above.
2. People with SMI typically struggle with multiple impairments in ADL and/or IADL performance, due to symptoms of their illness, co-occurring medical conditions, difficulty retaining employment, and limited education *(true/false).*
3. Clients who are taught how to use sensory and motor activities to self-regulate their emotional state require fewer physical and chemical restraints *(true/false).*
4. What is the current average length of stay in the inpatient hospital setting?
5. What is the primary difference between the PHP and IOP settings?
6. The clubhouse program is clinically based with daily therapy groups or other clinical interventions provided as needed *(true/false).*
7. List the six types of case management models:
8. Approximately 30% of those who are chronically homeless are mentally ill *(true/false).*
9. Research supports the positive benefits of ASPs, including better academic and social/emotional outcomes. Identify three prevention outcomes that have also been reported in the literature.
10. List four examples of group activities that could be used in various mental health settings.

Practice Activities

Visit a local homeless shelter. Determine what treatment programs are offered, and write a proposal for an occupational therapy program to meet the occupational performance needs of a target group of residents.

Look in the local want ads to find community mental health jobs that do not specify occupational therapy. Compare the job description to the occupational therapy scope of practice and write a rationale for hiring an OT practitioner for the position.

Activity-based interventions in mental health settings include crafts, cooking, art, games, sports, and music. Choose an activity to learn. Complete an activity analysis of the task, determining what psychosocial, physical, and cognitive skills are needed.

References

American Occupational Therapy Association. Occupational therapy practice framework: domain and process (3rd ed.). *Am J Occup Ther* 2014;68(Suppl. 1):S1–S48. http://dx.doi.org/10.5014/ajot.2014.682006

American Occupational Therapy Association. *AOTA: A Historical Perspective*. 2012, November 24. Retrieved from http://www.aota.org/About/39983.aspx

American Occupational Therapy Association. Specialized knowledge and skills in mental health promotion, prevention, and intervention in occupational therapy practice. *Am J Occup Ther* 2010a;64:S30–S43.

American Occupational Therapy Association. Occupational therapy services in the promotion of psychological and social aspects of mental health. *Am J Occup Ther* 2010b;58:669–672.

American Occupational Therapy Association. *Occupational Therapy Compensation and Workforce Study*. Bethesda, MD: Author; 2010c.

American Psychiatric Association. *Diagnostic and Statistical Manual of Mental Disorders*. 5th ed. Washington, DC: Author; 2013.

Arbesman M, Logsdon DW. Occupational therapy interventions for employment and education for adults with serious mental illness: a systematic review. *Am J Occup Ther* 2011;65:238–246. doi:10.5014/ajot.2011.001289

Association for Ambulatory Behavioral Health. *Fast Facts about Partial Hospitalization*. 2007. Retrieved from http://aabh.org/

Baron RC, Salzer MS. Accounting for unemployment among people with mental illness. *Behav Sci Law* 2002;20:585–599.

Brown C, et al. Influence of instrumental activities of daily living assessment method on judgments of independence. *Am J Occup Ther* 1996;50:202–206.

Brown EJ. Grabbing the brass ring: how OT is making its way back into mental health. *Advance for Occupational Therpay Practioners* 2010;28(12):8.

Burt MR, Pearson C, Montgomery AE. Comunity-wide strategies for preventing homelessness: recent evidence. *J Prim Prev* 2007;28;21–228.

Bureau of Justice Statistics. Probation and parole in the United States, 2011. 2012. Retrieved from www.bjs.gov/content/pub/pdf/ppus11.pdf

Centers for Disease Control and Prevention. *FastStats: Mental Health*. 2012. Retrieved from http://www.cdc.gov/nchs/fastats/mental.htm

Centers for Medicare and Medicaid Services, Department of Health and Human Services. Part 410.43—Partial hospitalization services: conditions and exclusions. 2010. Retrieved from http://cfr.vlex.com/vid/410-partial-hospitalization-exclsuions-19805614

Champagne T, Stromberg N. Sensory approaches in inpatient settings. *J Psychosoc Nurs Ment Health Serv* 2004;42:35–44.

Chapleau A, et al. The effectiveness of a consultation model in community mental health. *Occup Ther Ment Health* 2012;28:379–395.

Colton CW, Manderscheid RW. Congruencies in increased mortality rate, years of potential life lost, and causes of death among public mental health clients in eight states. *Prev Chron Dis* 2006;3:1–14. Retrieved at www.pubmedcentral.nih.gov/articlerender.fcgi?tool=pubmed&pubmedid=16539783

Durlak JA, Weissberg RP. *The Impact of After-School Programs That Promote Personal and Social Skills*. Chicago, IL: Collaborative for Academic, Social, and Emotional Learning; 2007.

Fisher T. Roles and functions of a case manager. *Am J Occup Ther* 1996;50:452–454.

Fisher WH, Geller JL, Pandiani JA. The changing role of the state psychiatric hospital. *Health Affairs* 2009;28:676–684.

Folsom DP, Hawthorne W, Lindamer L, et al. Prevalence and risk factors for homelessness and utilization of mental health services among 10,340 patients with serious mental illness in a large publics mental health system. *Am J Psych* 2005;162:370–376.

Frazier SL, Cappella E, Atkins MS. Linking mental health and after school systems for children in urban poverty: preventing problems, promoting possibilities. *Adm Policy Ment Health Ment Health Serv Res* 2007;34:389–399.

Gibbons JJ, Katzenbach NB. *Confronting Confinement: A Report of the Commission on Safety and Abuse in America's Prisons*. 2006. Retrieved from http://www.vera.org/content/confronting-confinement

Goff A, et al. Does PTSD occur in prison populations? A systematic literature review. *Criminal Behav Ment Health* 2007;17:152–162.

Helfrich CA, et al. Life skills interventions with homeless youth, domestic violence victims and adults with mental illness. *Occup Ther Health Care* 2006;20:189–207.

International Center for Clubhouse Development. *History*. 2012a. Retrieved from http://www.iccd.org/recent_research_iccd_ch_outcomes.html

International Center for Clubhouse Development. *International standards for clubhouse programs*. 2012b. Retrieved from http://www.iccde/org/quality.html

Katz N, Keren N. Effectiveness of occupational goal intervention for clients with schizophrenia. *Am J Occup Ther* 2011;65:287–296. doi:10.5014/ajot.2011.001347

Kessler RC, et al. Individual and societal effects of mental disorders on earnings in the United States: results from the National Comorbidity Survey Replication. *Am J Psychiatr* 2008;165:703–711. doi:10.1176/appi.ajp.2008.0801026

Law M. *Client-centered practice in occupational therapy*. Thorofare, NJ: Slack; 1998.

Little P, Wimer C, Weiss HB. *After school programs in the 21st century: their potential and what it takes to achieve it*. (Issues and Opportunities in Out-of-School Time Evaluation No. 10). 2008. Retrieved from http://www.hfrp.org/publications-resources/browse-our-publications/after-school-programs-in-the-21st-century-their-potential-and-what-it-takes-to-achieve-it

Meyers S. *Defining a role for occupational therapy in community mental health*. Paper presented at the 81st Annual American Occupational Therapy Association, Philadelphia, PA; 2001, April.

Mueser KT, Bond GR, Drake RE, et al. Models of community care for severe mental illness: a review of research on case management. *Schizophr Bull* 1998;24(1):37–74.

Munoz JP, Dix S, Reichenbach D. Building productive roles: occupational therapy in a homeless shelter. *Occup Ther Health Care* 2006a;20:167–187.

Munoz JP, Garcia T, Lisak J, et al. Assessing the occupational performance priorities of people who are homeless. *Occup Ther Health Care* 2006b;20:135–148.

National Alliance to End Homelessness. The criminalization of people with mental illness. (n.d.) Retrieved from http://www2.nami.org/Template.cfm?Section=Court_Watch1&Template=/TaggedPage/TaggedPageDisplay.cfm&TPLID=15

National Institute of Mental Health. *Important events in NIMH history*. 2012. Retrieved from http://www.nih.gov/about/almanac/organization/NIMH.htm

National Institute of Mental Health. *Statistics*. 2009. Retrieved from http://www.nimh.nih.gov/health/topics/statistics/index.shtml

O'Brien J, Husey S. Introduction to Occupational Therapy. ed 4. St. Louis, MO: *Elsevier*;2011.

Office of Juvenile Justice and Delinquency Prevention. *Correctional facilities*. 2012. Retrieved from www.ojjdp.gov/mpg/progTypesCorrectional.aspx

Schultz-Krohn W, Drnek S, Powell K. Occupational therapy intervention to foster goal setting skills for homeless mothers. *Occup Ther Health Care* 2006;20:149–166.

Substance Abuse and Mental Health Services Administration. *Assertive community treatment: Building your program*. DHHS Pub. No. SMA-08-4344, 2012. Retrieved from http://store.samhsa.gov/shin/content/SMA08-4345/BuildingYourProgram-ACT.pdf

Substance Abuse and Mental Health Services Administration. *Current statistics on the prevalence and characteristics of people experiencing homelessness in the United States*. 2011. Retrieved from http://homeless.samhsa.gov/ResourceFiles/hrc_factsheet.pdf

Sullivan G, Arlinghaus K, Edlund C, et al. Guide to VA mental health services for veterans and families. 2011. Retrieved from www.mentalhealth.va.gov/docs/Guide_to_VA_Mental_Health_Srvcs_FINAL12-2-10.PDF

Stoffel VC. Recovery. In: Brown C, Stoffel VC, eds. *Occupational therapy in mental health: a vision for participation*. Philadelphia: F.A. Davis; 2012:3–16.

Taylor R. *The intentional relationship: occupational therapy and use of self*. Philadelphia, PA: F.A. Davis; 2008.

The Kaiser Commission on Medicaid and the Uninsured. *Learning from history: deinstitutionalization of people with mental illness as precursor to long-term care reform*. 2007. Retrieved from http://www.kff.org/medicaid/7684.cfm

The Piper Report. *Hospitalizations for mental health and substance abuse disorders: costs, length of stay, patient mix, and payor mix*. 2011. Retrieved from http://www.piperreport.com/blog/2011/06/25/

United Sates Department of Housing and Urban Development. Strategies for improving homeless people's access to mainstream benefits and services. 2101. Retrieved from http:/www.huduser.org/portal/publications/pdf/Strategies-AccessBenefitsServices.pdf

U.S. National Library of Medicine. *Diseases of the mind: highlights of American psychiatry through early psychiatric hospitals and asylums*. 2012. Retrieved from http://www.nim.nih.gov/hmd/diseases/early.html

Wilson MC. Health practices of homeless women. Unpublished manuscript, Duquesne University, Pittsburgh, Pennsylvania. 2003.

Ziguras SJ, Stuart GW. A meta-analysis of the effectiveness of mental health case management over 20 years. Psychiatr Serv 2000:11:1410–1421.

Ziguras SJ, Stuart GW, Jackson AC. Assessing the evidence on case management. Brit Psychiatr 2002;181:17–21. doi:10.1192/

CHAPTER

35 Health and Well-Being

Carla A. Chase, EdD, OTR/L

Key Terms

Health—A level of emotional resources, social resources, and physical abilities a person has and is able to use to successfully meet their needs.

Health promotion—A plan or program that facilitates a person taking control of and improving his/her health.

Occupational imbalance—When the balance of habits, routines, and activities are negatively impacted by life-changing or stressful situations such as loss of a job, loss of a loved one, an illness, or injury.

Universal design—The design of products and environments to be usable by all people, to the greatest extent possible, without the need for specialized design.

Well-being—An emotional satisfaction with life in general

Wellness—Taking control of choices to increase satisfaction in life and improve overall health.

Learning Objectives

After studying this chapter, readers should be able to:

- Identify health and well-being concepts that are applicable to people of all ages as well as concepts unique to those at specific life stages.
- Recognize the role of occupation in health promotion.
- Describe the role of the occupational therapy assistant in promoting the health and well-being of individuals and communities.
- Design client-centered interventions that support health and wellness.

Introduction

Occupational therapy has at its core a fundamental belief that we should promote and support the health and well-being of each and every person. Through the use of a therapeutic relationship, OT practitioners strive to see a person as a whole being whose overall health and sense of well-being can be impacted by their past and present social, physical, and emotional environments. In this chapter, we will discuss the role of the OTA in health promotion for those at all ages and life stages. Connections to occupational therapy terminology and philosophical threads will be introduced to provide guidance and continuity. Although this chapter is not designed to be an in-depth research report, studies will be described that represent various types of successful health and wellness interventions. Along the way, we encourage you to "take a moment" from time to time, because your health is important, too! (From the Field 35.1).

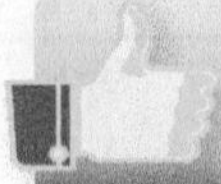

FROM THE FIELD 35.1

Five Ways to Take a Moment

Solve this word scramble:

1. *A key philosophical focus of the profession of occupational therapy is to find and maintain a good____________ (lacenba) of ____________ (realspue), productivity, and restoration in life.*
2. Close your eyes and take a slow, deep breath in through your nose and out through your mouth (with lips pursed). Do this two or three times.
3. Reach up toward the ceiling with both arms, slowly letting the stretch reach all the way down your spine.
4. Watch a short video that makes you smile. One suggestion of an uplifting video is *Crayola Doesn't Make a Color for Your Eyes,* sung by Kristin Andreassen. Perhaps then, you should get out your crayons!
5. Consider this quote by Jonathan Lockwood Huie: "The essence of life is not in the great victories and grand failures, but in the simple joys." List three simple things that bring you joy.

Definitions

Even though the word **health** is a commonly used word, a clear and consistent definition can be challenging to find. The *Occupational Therapy Practice Framework III* (AOTA, 2014) uses a version of the World Health Organization's definition that describes health in a positive way and includes consideration of what emotional and social resources as well as physical abilities a person has and is able to use to meet his/her needs. What makes this definition even more difficult to fully analyze is that it can be subjective. One person may describe himself or herself as being in good health, even if he/she has a long list of medical diagnoses, yet someone else with one minor medical condition may say he/she is in poor health. Thus, an important starting point when working in **health promotion**, or working to support a person taking control of and improving their health, is to determine the client's view of their health situation. A big part of health promotion includes injury and illness prevention strategies to promote good health and well-being and includes the client's goals.

The term **well-being** includes a quality of life or emotional satisfaction component that sets it apart from the word health. A person will likely say that he/she has a sense of well-being when satisfied with his/her life balance, if he/she feels he/she has some control of his/her life, or when he/she is content with his/her place in life. Occupational therapy, as a client-centered profession with a holistic focus, can work to facilitate an expansion or growth of this sense of well-being.

More than just being free from illness or injury, **wellness** includes making choices to be in better health, to have a better quality of life, and to actively pursue balance, according to the *Occupational Therapy Practice Framework III* (AOTA, 2014). The terms health, well-being, and wellness are often used in partnership with each other to describe a bigger picture or a broader scope of a person's feelings about his/her physical abilities, emotional satisfaction, and social resources, as he/she attempts to do what he/she needs or want to do in life.

According to the American Occupational Therapy Association (AOTA), **occupational imbalance** occurs when habits, routines, and activities are negatively impacted by life-changing or stressful situations such as loss of a job, loss of a loved one, an illness, or injury (AOTA, 2008). More focus or time and attention is spent on fewer occupational tasks, so other tasks of equal importance receive less attention. A mild form of occupational imbalance takes place every semester when instructors see new students early in the semester nicely dressed, looking as though they took the time to consider what they would wear that day. By midterm, sweatpants and baseball hats over ponytails appear to have been thrown on quickly as students go out the door leaving home for school. A more severe example of occupational imbalance is one of a single mother who is attempting to take care of a child with special needs while trying to learn new wheelchair skills following a spinal cord injury that she sustained. Occupational imbalance (in these examples, it is an increase in time spent in one or two occupations that takes time from self-care, health management, work, and so forth) may lead to impaired rest and sleep, poor eating habits, increased smoking or alcohol use, or other stress-induced behaviors, especially if prolonged. So in short, a life out of balance may cause an occupational imbalance, and prolonged imbalance can lead to health issues and an impaired sense of well-being. Helping to restore occupational balance is one possible path for the OT practitioner to start making a difference in the lives of clients we work with.

Intervention Strategies

What can OT practitioners do to support and promote the health and well-being of our clients? Since what sets occupational therapy apart from all other health care professions is the use of occupation as a goal and as a key intervention strategy, we will begin there in the exploration of the role of the OTA in promoting health and well-being. The *Occupational Therapy Practice*

Framework III (AOTA, 2014) states that the focus of occupational therapy is "promoting the health and participation of persons, groups, and populations through engagement in occupation" (p. S2). The World Health Organization agrees with this occupational therapy philosophy that participation in meaningful occupations, which they refer to as "activities," is central to improved health and well-being (WHO, 2007).

Since it is about balance in life, it is important that we, as OT practitioners, help avoid or at least minimize the negative effects of an occupational imbalance. Teaching someone who has anxiety to do a relaxation technique that takes just a few minutes each day is an example of promoting a health management and maintenance occupational task. Teaching someone with diabetes to prepare a healthful meal in the kitchen with more efficiency or with less pain is an example of promoting an instrumental activity of daily living occupation to help create health and well-being. Encouraging a youngster who has been inactive to get outside and ride a tricycle or make snow angels with friends is promoting more involvement in the joy-filled occupation of play (Figures 35.1, 35.2, and 35.3).

Even adults should play whenever possible as the health benefits of an activity like swinging on a swing are numerous and powerful as it works the vestibular system, brings back childhood memories, and is fun! Descriptions of health promotion and wellness programs at different life stages are provided here in hopes of inspiring creative ideas for addressing our goal of helping others experience a better quality of life.

In Childhood

Occupational therapy practitioners work with children in a wide variety of settings from school systems and medical settings to private practices that specialize in specific techniques such as those used in interventions for autism spectrum disorder. Community-based interventions are also very important when addressing the health and wellness needs of children and adolescents. Occupational therapy assistants are strong providers of interventions following an evaluation plan and are creative, frontline team members. This creativity is helpful when addressing the challenges facing children today.

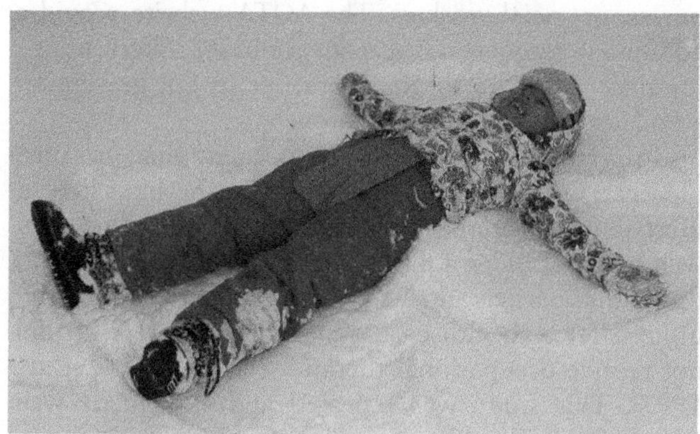

Figure 35.1 Play can take many forms. (Photo courtesy of S. McDaniel.)

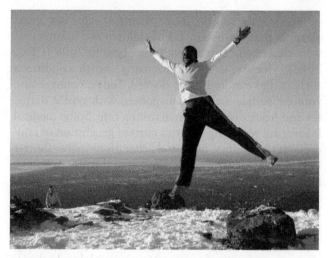

Figure 35.2 "Find ecstasy in life; the mere sense of living is joy enough."—Emily Dickinson. (Photo courtesy of P. Barnes.)

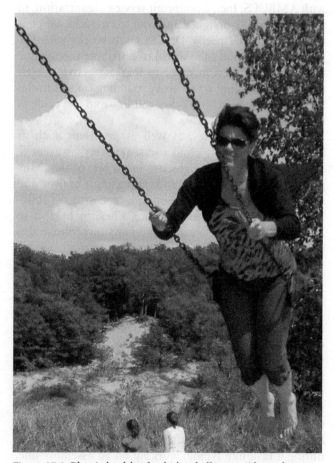

Figure 35.3 Play is healthy for kids of all ages. (Photo from the private collection of C. Chase.)

The Centers for Disease Control expresses great alarm in that more than 1/3 of children and adolescents were described as overweight or obese in 2008 (CDC, 2012). Obesity is linked to many health conditions such as diabetes and heart disease. Today, younger and younger people are being diagnosed with type 2 diabetes and heart disease at an alarming rate. Some medical leaders are reporting that this current generation of children may be the first in several generations to live shorter lives than their parents. Occupational therapy practitioners, by doing what they do best and using occupation as an intervention, can facilitate more active play and help modify habits and routines to address this health issue. For instance, Cahill and Suarez-Balcazar (2009) report that occupational therapy and occupational therapy assistant programs are partnering with local schools in an urban area to provide services that promote activity through fun and games, educational information to increase awareness for parents, and experiences with gardening to encourage eating healthier foods. One of these programs was then expanded to include other partners in the community, such as local businesses who donated play equipment and prizes.

Fred Sammons, a pioneer in the field of adaptive equipment development and sales, now works tirelessly with AMBUCS, Inc., a nonprofit service organization, to provide specially designed and adapted tricycles for children with special needs. Dr. Sammons works with OT practitioners around the world to distribute therapeutic tricycles to children in order to increase activity levels through bike riding while also expanding opportunities for them to interact with other children and feel pride in their accomplishments.

These opportunities, as well as programs such as backpack awareness, child car seat safety awareness, and antibullying campaigns, are just a few of the many possibilities for promoting and supporting a healthy and safe childhood for our little ones. By focusing on childhood occupations and encouraging a healthy balance in life, OTAs can be leaders in their community (please also refer to Chapter 40, *Emerging Practice Areas*).

In Adulthood

All life stages have their own types of stress, but those in early to midlife are often associated with multiple layers of responsibility and come at the peak time of people's work lives. Strategies to prevent injury and illness are necessary to help handle stress, to prevent cumulative trauma injuries from repetitive motions (like typing and texting), and to encourage a balance in life. Not an easy task when many times the pressures are piled on from all directions! Even small positive changes in body position during a task like typing, working on an assembly line, cooking, or in creation of and practicing healthy habits and routines may lead to positive lifelong changes. Any help for people at this stage of life almost always has a positive domino EFFECT on those for whom they are responsible. With changes in how tasks are done and practicing healthy habits, lost work days can be minimized and individuals will have more energy and mental stamina to handle what life sends their way. Helping people make these positive life changes is an important opportunity for the OT practitioner to provide guidance and to help make a difference.

Researchers studying the impact of modifications of work tasks on pain, productivity, and physical functioning for persons with osteoarthritis or rheumatoid arthritis found that those who received occupational therapy interventions had positive outcomes (Baldwin et al., 2012). Interventions provided included recommendations in modifying body positions, environmental changes, adaptive equipment use, and regular periods of stretching or gentle movement.

In Older Adulthood

Because the CDC has predicted that the cost of treating older adults who experience falls will reach 54.9 billion dollars by 2020, much research and exploration has gone into fall prevention (CDC, 2012). Occupational therapist and researcher, Elizabeth Peterson, was part of a team that started a program called *A Matter of Balance*, designed to address the needs of older adults through a series of facilitated classes. Her work has led to other successful programs across the country (Peterson, 2003). The National Council on Aging has identified this multifaceted team approach as an important and effective intervention for preventing falls for older adults (NCOA, 2012). *A Matter of Balance* includes strategies such as home modification recommendations to increase safety and user-friendly environments in and around the home, balance and strength exercises, and social support, all through a series of classes provided by local people who have received training and may include occupational and physical therapy practitioners, nurses, or social workers. The AOTA website provides additional resources and evidence-based interventions for their members to guide practice in fall prevention strategies (www.aota.org).

In a landmark study led by occupational therapist Florence Clark, researchers evaluated the impact of a lifestyle intervention program on the independence and well-being of older adults living in the community and found that participants had a slower rate of decline and utilized fewer health care dollars than those who did not receive occupational therapy services (Clark et al., 1997). This study was repeated and expanded (Well Elderly Study II) and was again found to make a significant difference in the lives of participants. Participation in the program decreased their rate of decline, allowing these community-dwelling older adults to maintain their independence longer and experience fewer medical complications than the control groups (Clark et al., 2011). The main intervention strategy included in this program is the use of facilitation rather than control of the content to be discussed. The older adult participants guide and control the topics with an underlying focus that is always on occupations and avoiding occupational imbalance. For instance, one group may express a desire to learn more about avoiding arthritis pain during daily chores while another group may want to learn to write poetry to deal with loss.

An important role for OT practitioners who work in all settings, medical and community based, is helping older adults live where they want to live and how they want to live as they face the challenges of aging. Given that most older adults want to remain in their home (AARP, 2010) and that, according to the United States Census Bureau (2012), the percentage of the population over 65 is expanding rapidly, the need for occupational therapy services for this group has the potential to increase for years to come. Many life situations can cause occupational imbalances for older adults as they face potential loss of independence. However, in no way is the picture as bleak as it may at first sound. For 78% of the younger members of this group, those who are 65 as of 2011 report that overall, they are satisfied with their lives, and those between 65 and 80 years old report having a higher sense of well-being and happiness than young adults (Urry & Gross, 2010). Where occupational therapy typically plays an important role in the lives of older adults is when they are facing an occupational imbalance from an injury, the onset or worsening of an illness, the loss of a loved one, or other major life-changing event. Through occupational therapy's whole-person approach, we can impact the lives of older adults in a positive way and promote health and well-being with education, emotional support, and creative interventions.

For All Age Groups

There are concepts related to health and well-being that are appropriate to discuss for those across the lifespan. One such concept is **universal design**. Although the overall concept has been around for well over a quarter of a century, the term universal design (UD) has been credited to the late Ronald L. Mace, who was an architect with a physical disability and his colleagues at NC State University. Universal design, comprised of seven principles, refers to the design of services, products, and environments that are usable by the widest range of people possible, regardless of age, ability, social status, or preference (The Center for Universal Design, 2008). Universal and accessible design are not interchangeable concepts. Everything universally designed is accessible, but not everything accessibly designed is universal. For instance, an accessible ramp at a building may be located in the rear and be fabricated of steel. A universally designed ramp will be located in the front of a building, ideally located next to the stairs. It will be aesthetically pleasing and may be made of the same materials as the building and/or be well integrated into the design scheme. It does not stand out and appear to be stigmatizing.

Occupational therapy practitioners, especially those working in the field of home and environmental modifications, can use this wellness-focused concept to support and promote design elements that make a home attractive, easy to use, accessible to most, and flexible in its use of space to support changing needs. Homes and objects that are created or modified using UD concepts can support occupational independence and enhance general health and well-being. It does so by eliminating barriers to function in a way that is visually pleasing and easy to use by those with a wide range of abilities.

Clinical Implications

If, as you read this chapter, you are telling yourself that these ideas for health and wellness promotion are only for those practitioners working in the community, please reconsider. Most OTAs do work in medical settings that dictate the types of goals to be addressed in order to meet the immediate rehabilitation needs of the clients and to accommodate the demands of the funders. Yet, it is still possible (and important) to consider your clients' *overall* health and well-being while helping them meet functional goals based on their medical situation. Every time you talk to a client to problem solve positions for them to sleep better at night, you are addressing their rest/sleep area of occupation and promoting their overall health and well-being. Whenever you take a moment during your session with a client who is very anxious to share a brief relaxation technique, you are supporting his/her mental health. Anytime you help someone figure out a menu to practice new techniques for cooking while using a new walker, you have an opportunity to promote healthy food choices based on his/her individual health needs.

Summary

As we explored early in this chapter, but it is important to revisit now, OTAs use occupation as a way to promote health and well-being of those we serve, regardless of age, life stage, or therapeutic setting. No matter where you work, consider your task to be more than meeting client-based functional goals. Help your clients achieve occupational balance. You have the tools to make a difference.

Review Questions

1. Which of the following does not pertain to an OT practitioner's role in health promotion?
   a. Injury and illness prevention strategies to promote good health and well-being
   b. Factoring in the client's goals
   c. Prioritizing family goals over client's
   d. Helping clients take control of their lives

2. People are said to experience well-being if they are:
   a. Satisfied with their life balance
   b. If they feel they have some control of their life
   c. When they are content with their place in life
   d. All of the above

3. Occurs when habits, routines, and activities are negatively impacted by life-changing or stressful situations such as loss of a job, loss of a loved one, an illness, or injury describes:
   a. Occupational participation
   b. Occupational imbalance
   c. Occupational justice
   d. Occupational context

4. A program that provides education and advice on how to establish a good work/life balance to minimize stress is an example of:
   a. Occupational balance
   b. Occupational performance
   c. Occupational context
   d. Occupational participation

5. Who is more likely to describe themselves as "being in good health?"
   a. Someone who has a strong sense of health and well-being and experiences occupational balance
   b. Someone who has major medical issues and is a single parent
   c. Someone with minor medical conditions and stress and anxiety
   d. Someone with minor medical conditions and occupational imbalance

6. Which of the following is the best example of an OTA incorporating health promotion education into a traditional, medically based treatment session?
   a. A client who has a shoulder fracture, adding padding to his/her sling
   b. A client who has a shoulder fracture, telling client that pain is to be expected and to ignore it
   c. A client who has a shoulder fracture, teaching client restorative breathing techniques
   d. a and c

7. What set of signs might you notice that would lead you to suspect that a person is experiencing occupational imbalance?
   a. Rapid weight loss or gain, late for appointments, nail biting, and sloppy appearance
   b. On time for appointments, tidy appearance, and nail biting
   c. Timely, well organized, calm demeanor, reports of playing cards with friends over the weekend
   d. Dirty nail beds, slightly disarrayed but peaceful, and reports gardening for several hours yesterday

8. An important aspect of the *Well Elderly Study I and II* that helped it be successful is that:
   a. The elders helped decide what they wanted to learn or to do
   b. The facilitator set the agenda prior to meeting with the participants
   c. Only OT practitioners facilitate the program
   d. Only elders who are deemed to be in good health can participate

9. When facilitating a group of older adults, as in the *Well Elderly Study I and II*, it is important to:
   a. Have a prepared list of topics for each session
   b. Follow established protocols for the class topics
   c. Allow the older adults to select the topics to be discussed or learned
   d. Make sure that you have control of the pace and take charge and unilaterally make all decisions

10. If you are have a life change or life situation that causes a major shift in the time spent on occupations that are typically important to you, it may mean that you are experiencing ____________.
    a. Health impairment
    b. Occupational imbalance
    c. Healthy sense of well-being
    d. Health and wellness

11. What might be ways to encourage a healthier lifestyle for a family whose child you are treating is obese and has been the victim of bullying?
    a. Healthy food options
    b. Noncompetitive outdoor exercise such as family walks in the woods
    c. Yoga
    d. Journaling while laying prone over a bolster
    e. All of the above

12. Homes and objects that are created or modified using _______ concepts can support occupational independence and enhance general health and well-being by eliminating barriers to function in a way that is visually pleasing and easy to use by those with a wide range of abilities.
    a. Accessible design
    b. Adaptive design
    c. Universal design
    d. Handicapped design

Practice Activities

You are working with a retired woman who has just had a hip replacement. From her overall mood and motivation, you suspect that she has some mild depression. When reviewing her evaluation prior to your session, you noticed that she had adult-onset diabetes. How could you incorporate her overall health and well-being needs into a session while addressing the goals specific to her hip surgery? Work with a partner to develop several strategies to share with your classmates.

The manager of the cafeteria in your facility has asked you and your occupational therapy team to provide safety and injury prevention training to those who work in the kitchen area. What topics might be helpful to this group of workers? Make a list of at least 10.

The nurse for the school district in your neighborhood has asked you to run a backpack safety booth during a health festival. What key concepts would you want to teach the children to help prevent back and shoulder problems? What activities would you plan to engage them in the learning process? Prepare a poster with your findings.

References

AARP. Approaching 65: a survey of boomers turning 65 years old. 2010. Retrieved from http://www.aarp.org/personal-growth/transitions/info-12-2010/approaching-65.htm

American Occupational Therapy Association. Occupational therapy services in the promotion of health and the prevention of disease and disability. *Am J Occup Ther* 2008;62:694–703.

American Occupational Therapy Association. Occupational therapy practice framework: domain and process (3rd ed.). *Am J Occup Ther* 2014;68(Suppl. 1):S1–S48. http://dx.doi.org/10.5014/ajot.2014.682006

Baldwin D, et al. Randomized prospective study of a work place ergonomic intervention for individuals with rheumatoid arthritis and osteoarthritis. *Arthritis Care Res* 2012;64(10):1527–1535.

Cahill SM, Suarez-Balcazar Y. The issue is—Promoting children's nutrition and illness in the urban context. *Am J Occup Ther* 2009;63:113–116.

Center for Disease Control. Cost of falls among older adults. 2012. Retrieved from http://www.cdc.gov/healthyyouth/obesity/facts.htm

Clark F, et al. Effectiveness of a lifestyle intervention in promoting the well-being of independently living older people: results of the Well Being 2 Randomized Controlled Health. *J Epidemiol Public Health* 2011;66(9):782–790.

Clark F, et al. Occupational therapy for independltly living older adults. A randomized controlled trial. *JAMA* 1997;278(16):1321–1326.

National Council On Aging. Center for health aging. 2012. Retrieved from http://www.ncoa.org/improve-health/center-for-healthy-aging/a-matter-of-balance.html

Peterson EW. Evidence-based practice: case example: a matter of balance. *OT Pract* 2003;8(3):12–14.

The Center for Universal Design. *About UD*. 2008. Retrieved from http://www.ncsu.edu/www/ncsu/design/sod5/cud/about_ud/about_ud.htm

United Stated Census. Population projections. 2012. Retrieved from www.census.gov/population/projections

Urry HL, Gross JJ. Emotion regulation in older age. *Curr Dir Psychol Sci* 2010;19(6):352–357.

World Health Organization. *Family of International Classifications: Definition, Scope and Purpose*. 2007. Retrieved from http://www.who.int/classifications/en/

CHAPTER 36

Children and Youth

Lisa Van Gorder, OTR/L, CEIS

Key Terms

Early intervention (EI)—Program created in 1986 to provide services for families with young children who are developmentally delayed or at risk for delays from birth until age 2.

Individualized Educational Plan (IEP)—A written document that is developed after a child has been evaluated and found eligible for services in a school environment.

Individualized Family Service Plan (IFSP)—A written document that is developed after a child has been evaluated and found eligible for services through early intervention.

Individual with Disabilities Educational Act Part B—Legislative Act that is part of the Americans with Disabilities Act (ADA) that legislates and regulates school-based services.

Individual with Disabilities Educational Act Part C—Legislative Act that is part of the Americans with Disabilities Act (ADA) that legislates and regulates early intervention services.

Mainstreaming—Placement of children with identified disabilities or delays in a regular classroom settings with peers who are typically developing.

Play—Activities performed for their simple intrinsic value with the focus on participation to create feeling of happiness.

Private practices—Private clinics in which therapy services are typically provided in an outpatient setting and typically funded by third-party payers (insurance companies) and are not legislated.

Learning Objectives

After studying this chapter, readers should be able to:

- Understand the legislative history and its importance to the current practice of occupational therapy and children.
- Appreciate the concept of play and how its forms, functions, and outcomes are related to occupational therapy and children.
- Recognize how to identify and utilize the right treatment activity to facilitate and obtain outcomes and goals.
- Understand the different venues where occupational therapy practitioners work with children, whom they work with, and the primary focus of each.

Introduction

In August of 1959, a California family welcomed twins to their current household of three boys. Added to this busy home were another son and their first daughter. Their joy slowly turned to concern as their youngest son showed physical delays in addition to a seizure disorder. As the years passed, their son would outgrow the seizures, but in its place, he would require leg braces and hours of physical therapy to assist him to walk. Eventually, he would be diagnosed with cerebral palsy, and his mother would be advised to either keep him home while his sister attended public school or place him in a setting devoid of any formal education.

I happen to know this story intimately since the son and mother in question are my uncle and paternal grandmother. Fortunately for my uncle, my grandmother was not going to allow her son to be pushed aside just because he had a "disability." My grandmother was all of 4′9″, had the tenacity of a bull dog, and never took "no" for an answer. She took her displeasure to the local school board and insisted that since she paid taxes, the school was required to give him an education. My uncle was enrolled in school that year, and though he did not receive the same supports that we have come to expect from today's educational system, he would graduate from high school the same year as my aunt.

Though this story has a positive ending, this was more of a rare occurrence than the norm in the early 1960s and 1970s. Until the passage of the Rehabilitation Act of 1973, OT practitioners traditionally provided services through medical settings like hospitals, institutions, and local health departments. With this Act, and the amendment of the Education of the Handicapped Act in October of 1986 to include **early intervention (EI)**, the role of the OT practitioner would be forever altered. As the need for services for children with identified needs grew, OT practitioners became an increasingly important part of the treatment team. Today, the role of the OT practitioner is a fluid one and is continually influenced by legislation, economics, and research trends.

We begin this chapter with a review of the history and important legislative changes that transpired to create the landscape we see today. It should be noted that the legislative changes that took place not only affected children's educational and home environments but also influenced the rise and way in which private practices and outpatient pediatric clinics are run today. This chapter discusses each of these areas of clinical practice, whom and how the treatment teams are formed, and what the roles of the OT and OTA are in pediatric practice. Furthermore, because of advances in neuroscience and research techniques, health care providers and educators are now able to better identify children's needs and how they are motivated to learn new skills. Because play is a primary occupation of childhood and it is through it that children learn about their world, play theory and how to incorporate it into treatment sessions is also discussed.

History: A Change in Outlook

To fully understand the types of educational and therapeutic interventions that are currently available to children in the United States, we must first review the history that influenced current practices. It was estimated that by the early 1970s, almost three million children were not receiving appropriate educational services (Imber & van Geel, 2004), with almost 200,000 persons labeled as having significant disabilities living in state institutions (*History: Twenty-Five Years of Process*, 2007). The concept of segregating children with disabilities centered on the belief that not only did it remove stressors placed on the child or others in the classroom, but it would also save the government undue expenses by not funding specialty services for children with disabilities (Imber & van Geel, 2004; Rothstein, 1995).

Because the belief that "separate but equal" was, for many years, a cornerstone of the US psyche, many educational programs during the late 1800s and early 1900s for children with disabilities were typically composed of very basic academic or manual job training (Trent, 1995). In addition to substandard academics, there was general consensus that children with disabilities should stay home because it was feared they would be disruptive in the classroom (Rothstein, 1995). It was not until the landmark 1954 Supreme Court ruling of *Brown v. Board of Education (Brown)* that the concept of integration and access to the educational system was mandated for all children. Though *Brown's* focus was race and ethnicity, it set the stage for **mainstreaming** and educating children with disabilities in regular classrooms settings CS-3 (Rothstein, 1995). Thus, it was not by chance that changes in how the US dealt with its treatment of children with disabilities occurred concurrently with the civil rights movement.

Six years after the passage of *Brown*, then President Kennedy established the President's Panel on Mental Retardation to study how the US dealt with individuals

TABLE **36.1** Historical Snapshot of the IDEA

Date or Period	Milestone
The early 1900s to midcentury	No established legalized service for children with disabilities, families advised that children stay at home or be placed in institutions
1954	Brown vs. Board of Education
1961	President Kennedy establishes the President's Panel on Mental Retardation
1971	Pennsylvania Association for Retarded Children (PARC) v. Pennsylvania
1972	Mills v. Board of Education
1973	Congress passes the Rehabilitation Act of 1973 (RHA)
1975	Congress passes Education of the Handicapped Act (EHA)
1986	Part H is added to the EHA establishing early intervention
1990	Congress passes Americans with Disabilities Act—EHA renamed the Individuals with Disabilities Education Act (IDEA)

with disabilities. At that time, it was typical to advise families to place individuals with disabilities into state or regional institutions. These institutions tended to be in rural areas out of sight and set apart from general public awareness (*History: Twenty-Five Years of Process, 2007*; Smith et al., 2011; Trent, 1995). With the establishment of this panel, concerns surrounding the poor treatment and substandard living conditions of individuals with disabilities were brought to the forefront of the political stage, and the movement to deinstitutionalize and find alternative supports for individuals began to take on traction (*History: Twenty-Five Years of Process, 2007*; Smith et al., 2011; Trent, 1995).

Unfortunately even with these groundbreaking events, during the early 1970s, special education was still being implemented in a haphazard and inconsistent manner. What was considered acceptable education and what was provided continued to vary by state, regional districts, and individual schools (Rothstein, 1995). Not uncommon was the practice of excluding children with disabilities from public education, placing ethnic groups disproportionately into special education programs, and a general discouragement of parent involvement (Imber & van Geel, 2004; Rothstein, 1995).

It was this environment of haphazard education that sparked a number of federal lawsuits. Two suits made their way to the U.S. Supreme Court, becoming the landmark cases that would ultimately forever change the educational system. In *Pennsylvania Association for Retarded Children (PARC) v. Pennsylvania* and *Mills v. Board of Education*, the Supreme Court determined that governmental exclusion of children with disabilities from schools was not legitimate and a violation of the Equal Protection Clause of the Fourteenth Amendment of the U.S. Constitution (Imber & van Geel, 2004; Rothstein, 1995). Additionally, the *Mills* decision addressed the concept that families and children have protected rights and final say when working with the treatment team to create a treatment plan (Rothstein, 1995).

It is hard for someone born after 1970 to comprehend how dramatically the makeup of our educational system changed. Yet, within three years of the 1972 *Mill v. Board of Education* Supreme Court ruling, two major laws would be passed, addressing the responsibility of the federal educational system with regard to children with disabilities. In 1973, the Rehabilitation Act of 1973 (known as "Section 504") and in 1975 the Education for All Handicapped Children Act (EAHCA), also known as the Education of the Handicapped Act (EHA), came into fruition (Imber & van Geel, 2004). By 1986, Part H would be added to the EHA, thereby establishing an entirely new comprehensive program for children under the age of three, which came to be known as **early intervention (EI)**. A mere fifteen years later, the EHA would be renamed the Individuals with Disabilities Education Act (IDEA) and was rolled into the sweeping reforms associated with legislation of the Americans with Disabilities Act (ADA) (*Building the Legacy*, 2004; Imber & van Geel, 2004; Rothstein, 1995) (Table 36.1).

Early Intervention

As previously noted, EI was created to provide services for families with young children, from birth to age two who are developmentally disabled or at risk for delays. Within **Part C** of **IDEA** is a clearly defined process of identifying and supporting those infants and toddlers who are found to qualify for these services (Table 36.2). The role of the OT practitioner is broad in EI. Occupational therapy for EI services addresses a child's functional needs, adaptive behavior, play,

TABLE 36.2 Comparison of IDEA Programs

	Part C Early Intervention, 0–2.11 years	Part B Special Education, 3–21 years
Environment	• Natural settings	• Home, center, or school based
Eligibility	• Child is diagnosed with a disability • Established risk for delays via diagnosis • Developmental delay via appropriate assessment tool • Child is found to be at risk for delays	• Child found as having at least 1 of 11 identified disabilities • Noted decreased in academic performance as compared to their peers via standardized evaluations and structured observation
Services provided	• 16 primary services depending on needs • Interdisciplinary and transdisciplinary teams • Individualized Family Service Plan (family centered) • Service coordination	• Special education services to support access to the educational environment and curriculum • Individualized Education Program (child centered)

sensory, motor, and postural development (IDEA Part C § 303.5 (8)). Included in the OT practitioner's role is to adapt the environment, select, design, and fabricate assistive and orthotic devices to facilitate development and promote the acquisition of functional skills while preventing or minimizing the impact of initial or future impairments (IDEA Part C § 303.13). Additionally, OT practitioners have the opportunity not only to work directly with young child on mastering their activities of daily living but also to play a major role in assisting the family with implementing and carrying out strategies to achieve these goals. A study by Schaaf and Mulrooney (1989) suggested that when including occupational therapy as part of the team within a family-centered framework, positive changes were noted in children's play and their ability to interact with the environment as a whole. Since EI sessions occur in a "natural environment," OT practitioners have the opportunity to work in environments (e.g., parks, markets, local pools, community groups) that are not typically available in outpatient clinical settings. Additionally, EI is "family centered," thus allowing the clinician the opportunity to work closely with the family in identifying and making immediate changes for their young child in their home.

Eligibility

An important aspect of EI is making consumers aware of it through state Child Find initiatives. This is a comprehensive system that identifies children who are at risk for developmental delays and would benefit from EI or preschool special education. This system includes standard referral procedures used by all involved agencies. Anyone, including the family, can make a referral for services (IDEA Part C § 303.115).

Infants and toddlers are found to be eligible for EI services based on any one of the following three categories:

1. *Established risk*: Those infants or toddlers who have a diagnosis associated with a developmental disability, such as an autism spectrum disorder (ASD) or cerebral palsy (see also Chapter 27, *Developmental Disabilities*).
2. *Developmental delays*: Infants and toddlers are to be assessed through an "appropriately" diagnostic instrument, procedure, or clinical judgment for one or more of the following developmental areas: cognitive, motor, communication, social–emotional, and adaptive. Since each state defines what they consider qualifying criteria, the determination of what is an "appropriate" instrument or procedure tends to differ. With regard to occupational therapy services, evaluations are carried out by the OT.
3. *At risk*: This refers to a child who would be at risk of experiencing a substantial developmental delay if not provided with services. States are also given the discretion to include biological or environmental factors to qualify children for EI services (e.g., infants born with a diagnosis of intrauterine growth retardation (IUGR) or small for gestational age (SGA) or substance abuse in the home) (IDEA Part C § 303.101).

Evaluation and Assessment Process

For all children referred to EI, an initial evaluation is performed by a comprehensive multidisciplinary team of service providers who are qualified to determine a child's eligibility. These service providers include developmental specialists, occupational therapists, physical therapists, speech and language pathologists, psychologists, social workers, educators, and nurses. Once the need for services has been established, those professionals who actually work with the child must ensure that the services are appropriate and continue to meet the child's identified needs. No single procedure is used as the sole criterion for determining a child's eligibility. Determination must include the following: an evaluation instrument, review of the child's history including caregiver interview, identification of the child's level of function in each of the development areas (cognitive, motor, communication, social–emotional, and adaptive), information gathering from additional sources, and review of pertinent records (IDEA Part C § 303.321).

The Individualized Family Service Plan

A major component of EI is the **Individualized Family Service Plan (IFSP)**. The IFSP is a written document that is developed after a child has been evaluated and found eligible for services CS-1. It is considered a working document that can be amended at any time to reflect the current needs and goals of the child and family. It represents a collaboration by the service providers and family members and is based on findings from the evaluation and any additional assessments that the service providers administer (IDEA Part C § 303.344).

The initial screening, evaluation, assessment, and writing of the IFSP must be completed within 45 days from the date of first referral (IDEA Part C § 303.310). The measurable IFSP outcomes are as follows:

- The outcomes the family and child are expected to achieve
- The strategies and activities for those outcomes
- Which professional(s) will be providing these services
- How often, when, and in what environment will these services be provided

An important aspect of the IFSP is that it names the service coordinator. This key individual is typically from the profession that is most immediately relevant to meet the needs of the child and family. The service coordinator is responsible for implementing all of the EI services identified on the IFSP, coordinating with other agencies and individuals, and assisting with transition planning from EI to preschool services. Service coordinators not only help educate the family on the EI process but also often help the family to learn how to be an advocate for themselves and their child (IDEA Part C § 303.12).

Early Intervention Services

All EI services are selected in collaboration with the parents and are provided at either no cost or via a payment system based on a sliding scale established by the state. Qualified EI personnel can provide up to 17 distinct services to address a child's needs as identified through the evaluation and IFSP process CS-3. These services are as follows: (1) assistive technology services; (2) audiology services; (3) family training, counseling, and home visits; (4) health services; (5) medical services; (6) nursing; (7) nutrition; (8) occupational therapy; (9) physical therapy; (10) psychological services; (11) service coordination; (12) sign language and cued language services; (13) social work; (14) special instruction; (15) speech and language therapy; (16) transportation; and (17) vision services. These services take place in the family and child's *natural environment*, that is, the setting that is natural or typical for a same-aged infant or toddler without a disability, and include the home as well as some other community settings such as day cares, playgrounds, or the local pool (IDEA Part C § 303.13).

Early Intervention Team

Two team models are typically used in EI settings. They are interdisciplinary and transdisciplinary practice models.

Interdisciplinary

Interdisciplinary models in EI settings encompass professionals from different disciplines working together with the family and child to develop and implement an intervention program. The advantage of an interdisciplinary model is that each specific team member brings their unique professional expertise to the table. This gives the team a rich depth of knowledge and a large range of ideas, thus typically making problem solving easier. That said, issues may arise with an interdisciplinary approach because this type of team must coordinate their efforts to maximize the benefits for the child and family. Pitfalls may occur if team members do not agree or if there is poor communication. Since children with significant disabilities often have multiple issues, it is easy for team members to work in isolation, focusing only on their own goals and outcomes. When this happens, the service coordinator is essential to coordinate the team to maintain and provide consistent and overlapping treatment strategies (see also Chapter 39, *Management and Education*). Furthermore, it is very easy for families to be overwhelmed by the large number of team members providing services via an interdisciplinary model.

Transdisciplinary

A transdisciplinary model in an EI setting entails having a single team member carry out the strategies that have been developed by the rest of the team. Various disciplines remain on the team acting as consultants and advising the primary service provider. The idea of a transdisciplinary model is that through consultation, the primary service provider develops a more comprehensive knowledge base and is better able to more effectively incorporate different strategies into the treatment plan. Additionally, with the ability to synthesize this information, the service provider is better able to educate and teach the family in an organized manner that avoids splintering of information. For example, a service coordinator may be able to help the family better incorporate both fine motor and language concerns during bath time. During this activity, the provider may suggest that the child and caregiver draw with bath crayons while the parent uses simple language to describe the activity. In this instance, the provider has incorporated concerns from two separate disciplines into a functional combined activity. Since all team members contribute to the assessment and development of the outcomes and planning, the team continues to benefit from their experiences. For this model to be effective, the primary service provider must be accomplished at analyzing and recognizing problems as they occur. Issues arise with transdisciplinary practice when the service provider has difficultly figuring out the next steps of activities or fails to identify important needs that are outside their scope of practice (From the Field 36.1).

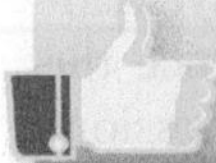

FROM THE FIELD 36.1

Through the Eyes of an Early Intervention Practitioner

Joni Kamstra, COTA/L, has been working for 29 years, nine years in a school and private practice setting and 20 years in EI. When she was a junior in high school, her class took a tour of the local hospital. She explained that when they arrived at the physical rehabilitation area, there was an OT practitioner in the room playing with a child. Joni stayed in the room while the rest of her class left, amazed that the practitioner got to "play with the child." She was hooked. When she got back to school, she spoke with her school counselor only to discover that there was a college five miles away that had an OTA program.

Rewards: Joni expresses that she enjoys the ability to see wide variety of diagnoses (cerebral palsy, preemies, sensory integration needs, developmental delay, rare genetic disorders, etc.). Additionally, she loves working with families. "When family tells you they took their child to a restaurant for first time ... you cannot but just feel wonderful."

Challenges: Though Joni is allowed to attend team meetings, the state in which she practices does not compensate OTAs for attendance. Because of this, the team attempts to hold meetings during her treatment time so she can "listen in and be part of the conversation." She expressed that this is also hard on the families since she is the one treating the child and they feel she knows the child best.

Advice: "Use your occupational therapists as much as you can, especially if you only meet with them once a month. Come ready with your questions and comments, and use those other team members to do cotreatments as much as you can. I find that speech and occupational therapy work wonderfully together since occupational therapy can get the sensory system going!" Joni also advised that the more that an OT practitioner can learn from continuing education, the better, along with taking the time to watch children who are typically developing.

Transitioning Out of Early Intervention

Just as treatment planning is a key to EI, so too is timely discharge planning. This gives the team and the family enough time to put relevant supports in place to insure that progress made is maintained. Not all children will qualify and be transitioned into a local educational agency (LEA). Some will have reached their age-appropriate developmental milestones and no longer need services. In this case, the team, and especially the service coordinator, must ensure that the family has a well-developed home program, clear understanding of the next phase(s) in the child's development, and identified community resources. Additionally, though once qualifying out of EI, families typically do not return, so the team must provide the family with clear instructions that if new concerns arise, the child can be referred for additional assessments. If the child is referred to the LEA, this process should be made 6 months (but not less than 90 days) before his/her third birthday (e.g., at 30 months of age). This helps the school system review all pertinent information, determine if further testing is warranted, and put in place those supports that the child may require (IDEA Part C § 303.209).

Schools

As previously mentioned, **Part B of IDEA** governs how services for children with disabilities will be provided. Within this law are clearly defined policies that address the environment, environmental access, education plans, due process, and funding for children from the age of three until their twenty second birthday (or those who have graduated from high school with a regular high school diploma). The purpose of the IDEA is to "ensure that all children with disability have available to them a free appropriate public education that emphasizes special education and related services designed to meet their unique needs and prepare them for further education, employment, and independent living" (IDEA Part B, subpart A § 300.1). At its core, the primary principle of the IDEA is that schools are to educate children with disabilities in the same environment as children who are not disabled (Rothstein, 1995).

With this in mind, OT practitioners have the opportunity to make a significant difference in the educational performance of children who qualify for services. Dunn (1990) found that not only did direct occupational therapy intervention help students but that collaborative consultation between the OT practitioner and teacher was effective in assisting students in achieving their goals. Case-Smith (2002) found positive results with regard to improving handwriting skills when OT practitioners collaborated with other professionals in the classroom. Thus, the overarching goal of the OT practitioner as part of a treatment team in a school setting is to improve the student's performance of tasks and activities that affect their abilities to function successfully within the school environment. This is through adaption, modification, functional skill building (e.g., seating, writing aid, fine motor activities), and collaboration CS-3.

Eligibility

Part B of IDEA spells out a comprehensive system that identifies children who may qualify for services. Whereas in Part C, the focus is on the child and the environment (e.g., those children who are considered at risk), Part B focuses on the child's ability to access their academic program. Again, state-run Child Find programs help to identify children with disabilities, children who are suspected having a disability, those who need special education even if they are advancing from grade to grade, or are highly transient (e.g., migrant children) for school services (IDEA Part B, subpart B § 300.111). Eligibility for school services is based on the child being identified as having any one of the following: mental retardation; a hearing, speech or language, or visual impairment (including deafness or blindness); serious emotional disturbances; orthopedic impairment; autism; traumatic brain injury; other health impairments; a specific learning disability; or deaf–blind (IDEA Part B, subpart B § 300.8). It should be noted that while many preschool-aged children show a developmental delay, because they are so young, they cannot be identified by one of the categories listed above. Because of this, the IDEA Improvement Act of 2004 clarified that a state may apply the term developmental delay to the age range 3 through 9, or any subset of that range, including ages 3 through 5 (IDEA subpart B § 300.619), thus making it easier for children to receive services.

Although the least restrictive environment (LRE) is one of the major principles of the IDEA, it also takes into account that for some children, such placement may not always be appropriate. Regulations are in place to define when it is appropriate to place a child with disabilities into a different setting. Hence, separate classrooms as well as separate schools are still part of the educational system's landscape.

Evaluation and Assessment Process

To initiate the evaluation process to determine if a child qualifies for services, the parent or guardian of the child or a public agency can request an initial evaluation. The school is required to "use a variety of assessment tools and strategies to gather relevant functional, developmental, and academic information" and conduct the evaluation within 60 days of receiving signed consent (IDEA subpart B § 300.304). As with EI, no single measure or assessment is to be used as the sole criterion for determining whether a child has a disability or to determine an appropriate educational program for the child. Additional requirements for the evaluation process also include reviewing existing assessments or evaluations that may be provided by school or outside sources (e.g., private practice clinicians, physicians) or classroom-based observations by teachers or other related service providers. For these observations to be considered valid in assessing the child's academic performance and behavioral issues, the child must also be observed in his/her learning environment, including the regular classroom setting. For those children who are not of school age or out of school, a team member observes the child in an age-appropriate environment.

The Individualized Educational Plan (IEP)

Creating an effective **Individualized Educational Plan (IEP)** takes into consideration the most recent evaluations, past and present education performances, and identification of the student's strengths and needs. The best IEPs are developed out of open and honest dialogue between the parent, educational team, and at times the student. The goal is to not only identify those items that are priorities but also to create functional and achievable interventions and goals. Within this framework, the team is able to consider all factors that may affect the child's progress and ability to be successful in school. An IEP has several parts that help to describe and define the concerns and needs of the child in order to succeed in the school environment. Furthermore, it gives those working with the student a good understanding of his/her current functional level and goals and how to achieve them.

The IEP is comprised of the following:

- Statement of present levels of educational performance: This statement includes academics, life skills, physical functioning, social and behavioral skills, and any other areas of concern affecting the child's ability to learn. Typically, this statement includes formal assessments or observations used to determine the child's level of function and to establish a baseline of performance.
- Statements of measurable annual goals: The IEP must contain a statement of the child's goals, which are updated at least annually. Goal statements spell out what the child will be expected to learn and do in the coming year. Additionally, the IEP must also contain measurable short-term objectives that will be used to determine the child's progress toward reaching these annual goals.
- Explanation of progress measurement: The IEP must contain an explanation of how the progress toward goals and objectives will be measured and how that information will be reported to parents.
- Description of special education services: The IEP must include a description of the student's special education program, specially designed instructions, and related services the child will receive to help him/her progress toward meeting those educational goals. The amount of time allocated to receive services and in which setting they occur must also be described.
- Statement of participation in the regular education program: The IEP must specify the amount of time a child will participate in regular education programs and explain the rationale for that decision.
- Statement describing testing adaptations and modifications: If required, the IEP must explain why testing adaptation and modification are to be used and why they are necessary. Additionally, if the child will be participating in alternative assessment situations, the rationale for that decision must be included in the IEP.
- Statement of length and duration of services: The IEP must include a projected beginning and ending date of services, the frequency of the services, where they will be delivered, and how long they will be provided.
- Statement of transition: Beginning no later than age 16, the IEP must include measurable goals for the student's anticipated postsecondary program and a description of the services needed for the child to reach those goals (IDEA Part B, subpart D, §300.320).

School Services

The school-based educational team is made up of those professionals that assist a child with a disability to access and benefit from special education (Table 36.2). The role of occupational therapy is to improve, develop, or restore function and improve the child's ability to perform task for independence in the school environment (IDEA Part B, §300.34) (From the Field 36.2).

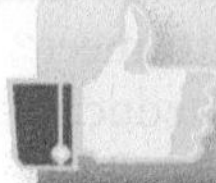

FROM THE FIELD 36.2

Through the Eyes of a School Practitioner

Leah Nyberg, COTA/L, has been practicing since 2008. She currently works at a private not-for-profit school in Southborough, MA, with children diagnosed with ASD. What led her to working with children were her previous experiences of being a nanny and working as a direct service provider at a residential school for young boys. After working closely with the OT, she came to realize that not only was she interested in occupational therapy, but a good portion of what she was doing with the children at the residence seemed to align with the occupational therapist's goals.

Rewards: The great thing about this job is that "[I] get to spend a lot of time with each child. I can swim with the same child three weeks in a row, and each session is different. I also like to see [the] functional changes and explain why things are being done. Because we are considered the motor people at our school we can explain to [the staff] what is going on and why what we are doing can help. Also seeing it carried over to the class room setting is rewarding."

Challenges: Some of the challenging aspects of the job are that "it's kind of nonstop. I enjoy it, but I feel it is a little rushed [at times], and I can't get done as much as I would like. We also have a lot of other disciplines who teach self-help skills. I feel [these skills] are very much a part of occupational therapy, and not being the primary person involved in them is hard."

Advice: If anyone is interested in working in pediatrics, they should do "observations and interactions on volunteer basis to be more familiar with the population." Finding a mentor who has worked with pediatrics is helpful. Additionally, in working with children in general, Leah advised you should be "... able to be flexible and be able to respond to changing situations (since) things with kids just change so quickly. Being able to know what to say to redirect them and keep them on track is important. Know what to do. Be able to respond. Know what adaptation to make and how to grade whatever activity it is that you are focusing on with a student."

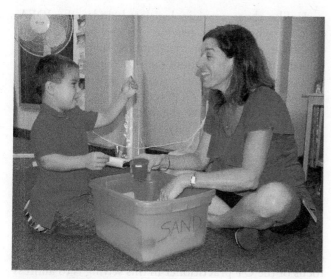

Figure 36.1 Sharing success in activity.

Therefore, the focus of the school-based occupational therapy is typically to address functional and educational skills (e.g., handwriting, manipulating and organizing materials, participating in educational instruction) that effect access and performance within this environment CS-3. A child who may have a specific diagnosis will not be automatically be eligible for occupational therapy services if they perform at the same age-appropriate level as their peers (Fig. 36.1). For example, a child who has hemiparesis from a birth incident on his/her nondominant side but is still able to perform at age level will not automatically be provided therapy because of the diagnosis. If this disability does not interfere with the ability to learn, the child is ineligible for occupational therapy in school, despite the fact that the nondominant hand is not fully functional (Table 36.3).

Transitioning Out of School

Like EI, it is important for the student's educational team to plan for the termination of services. To ensure termination is in the best interest of the child, termination of a program is more cumbersome than initiation. As with EI, for those children whose services are discontinued, if the family or the LEA identifies future concerns, a reassessment and possible return to services may occur. It is appropriate to discontinue services when the following happens:

- The student met established goals and objects.
- The student performs at the same expectations of his/her typical peers.
- The student is no longer making significant progress despite intervention.
- The student is gaining but a particular service is no longer relevant to those gains.

TABLE 36.3 IEP Service Providers and Related Services

- Speech and language pathology
- Audiology
- Interpreting services
- Psychological services
- Physical and occupational therapy
- Recreation, including therapeutic recreation
- Early identification and assessment of disabilities in children
- Counseling services, including rehabilitation counseling
- Orientation and mobility services
- Medical services for diagnostic or evaluation purposes
- School health and nursing services
- Social work services in schools
- Parent counseling and training

IDEA Part B subpart A, §300.34.

- The identified skills are no longer a concern within the educational setting.
- The student or family expresses a desire to discontinue services.

For those students who continue to need services, post postsecondary planning beginning no later than age 14, including course of study, is necessary. This discussion should consider living situation, career goals, and postsecondary education. By age 16, the IEP should include a vision statement and transition plan, and by age 18 or one year prior to graduation, the school recommendations for adult services should be identified.

Private Practice

Another major pediatric setting where OT practitioners work is in **private practices**. Whereas EI and school-based therapy grew out of legislation, outpatient settings emerged to answer the need for additional specialty services. Families seek private occupational therapy services for a variety of reasons. Oftentimes, they are looking to supplement the services the child is receiving from EI or at school. Sometimes, services are sought because the child did not qualify for various reasons (e.g., concerns are not relevant to the educational environment, a child does not show enough of a delay). Other times, additional private practice services are recommended because a specific specialty service is not offered (e.g., feeding therapy, sensory integration therapy). Whatever the reasons, services in the private sector have increased dramatically over the past 20 years (From the Field 36.3).

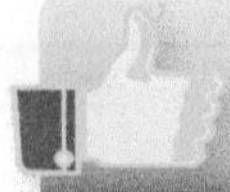

FROM THE FIELD 36.3

Through the Eyes of a Private Practice Practitioner

Vicki Sawyer, COTA/L, has been practicing since 2009 and has additional experience in school environments. Currently, she works at a private practice in Haverhill, MA, that services children with a variety of diagnoses. Vicki's path to becoming an OTA was not straightforward. While interviewing for a special education tutoring position, the interviewer suggested she would be a great OTA. A year later, she was again introduced to occupational therapy because of her mother's failing health. Her sports medicine background and working with children in the community, including incorporating functional goals into daily activities, were the inspiration for Vicki to become an OTA.

Rewards: There are "never dull moments, never mundane, or too repetitive, (and) I like to mix it up so that it is never the same thing." She expressed that she finds it "is a lot of work but it is very nice to see progress and see the kids reach their milestones." "Sometimes it is the most difficult ones that you get to see that make the best progress..." Vicki went on to say "[my] favorite things working in private practice is the ability to educate parents about skills and developmental milestones."

Challenges: Vicki expressed that working with the families is sometimes difficult. "Parents sometimes compare school to the center and I am continually working on educating them. This can be difficult because certain things are not as easy to understand when it comes to occupational therapy." Other challenges she identified is that "sometimes (I) have worked hard to make a plan, but because of kids being kids, that plan changes, so I need to quickly accommodate what needs to be done for the session to be successful instead of what was originally in my head."

Advice: "(You) need to be flexible .... And put a lot of thought into what you are going to do, look on line, use text books, and try to be creative. I am always going to conferences and special interest group meetings, it always worth the drive and I always come back with something." Lastly Vicki expressed, "you need to like kids and not just tolerate them, and you need to be personal, be playful and patient, and really committed. [You] also need to be a good communicator with the parents, school and other colleagues I would recommend that [you] job shadow, and know how to explain what occupational therapy is so to be an advocate for your profession."

Unlike those services legislated under the IDEA, children who receive private services have different qualifying criteria for determining eligibility. That is, unlike in EI and school settings, the private practice OT practitioner must simply see a need to treat a child. Additionally, OT practitioners in private practice settings do not have the same restrictions that are placed on EI or school services; thus, different criteria for eligibility are applied. Depending on the practice, clinical observation, parent report, and a decreased ability to participate in ADLs are typically the criteria used to determine need. Formal assessments are not required for private practice occupational therapy services, though it is not unusual for parts or a shortened standardized evaluation to be used to assist the OT to establish a baseline and create goals and outcomes. The focus of the OT practitioner in this setting is to address not only children's functional independence with ADLs but also their ability to regulate and participate in all environments. Thus, the child we previously mentioned who had a diagnosis of hemiparesis would typically be seen in this setting for increased strengthening, coordination, and tactile registration.

The private practice environment is usually different than those found in EI and schools. Typically, private clinics have large treatment areas designed to use suspension equipment (e.g., swings, hammocks), in addition to other structures to allow children to seek out movement activities. Additionally, it is not uncommon to incorporate the use of other treatment modalities (e.g., listening programs, vestibular and ocular motor control programs, tactile play activities) when working on identified needs (Fig. 36.2). In this setting, children still are brought to the table for fine and visual motor tabletop activities, though in this environment, the focus is more on addressing building block skills that the child may have missed.

As with all settings, private practice presents with its own challenges. One of the primary challenges faced in treating children in a private setting is the limited ability to collaborate and communicate with other members on the child's team. In these instances, it is often the private practitioner who takes the initiative to seek out and discuss the child's goals and current strategies with the other professionals.

Another issue that can impact private treatment is third-party reimbursement for services. Furthermore, depending on the payer's policy, some have exclusions for any services that can or are seen as best to be addressed in a school setting. Additionally, occupational therapy is considered a short-term therapy based on an adult outpatient medical model. Because of this, most health maintenance organizations (HMOs) policies are limited either by time (e.g., all treatments are to occur within 60 days of initiation per diagnosis per lifetime) or by allowed visits (e.g., treatments are to occur within

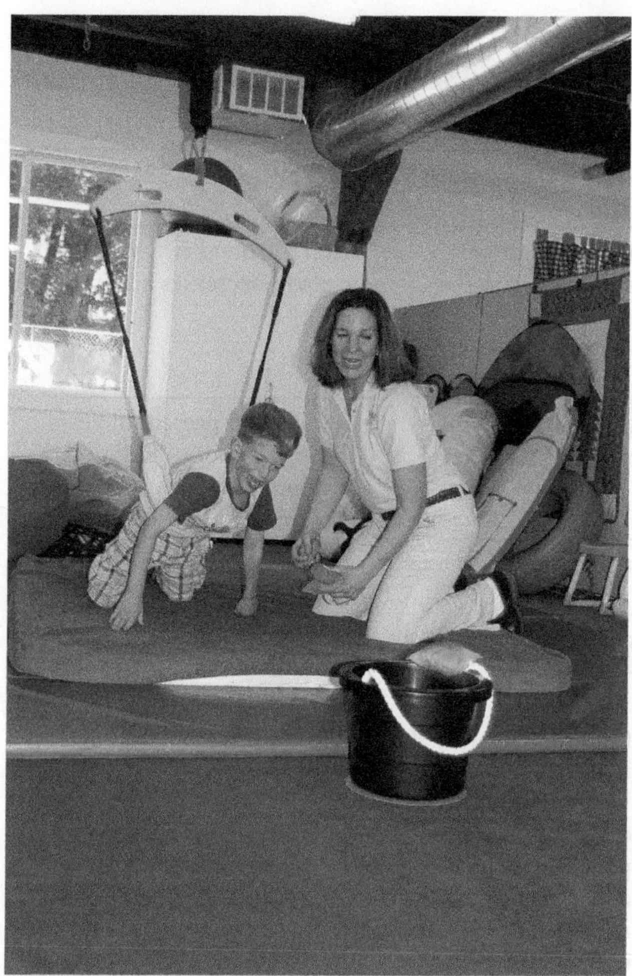

Figure 36.2 OT and child are working together on postural stability, eye–hand coordination, timing, sequencing, and ocular control.

an 8- to 12-week period and are therefore typically used weekly). Because of the time limitations in this practice setting, the OT practitioner must work effectively with the family to establish a well-defined home program (Fig. 36.3).

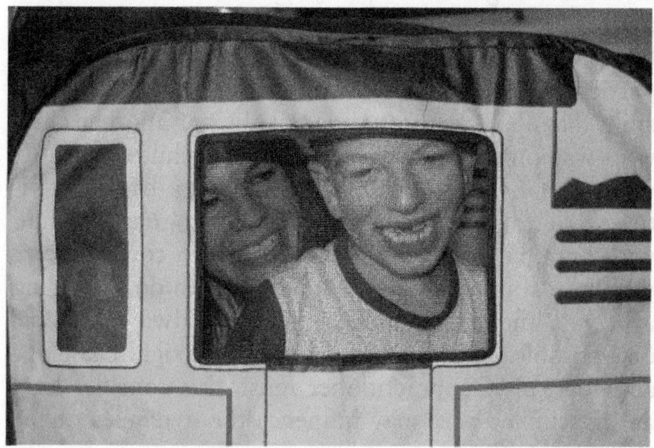

Figure 36.3 Enjoying pretend play.

Play: How Children Learn

Understanding what an OT practitioner's duties are in a pediatric setting is part of, but not the whole, a story about how to work with children. Simply put, one cannot work effectively with children without comprehending the primary occupation of childhood: **play**. This concept is so vital that whenever pediatric treatment is discussed, play is typically identified as one of the cornerstones for learning new skills. Couch et al. (1997) surveyed OT practitioners on how the role of play was used in their work with preschoolers. They found that play was very important and used as a treatment modality or reinforcer by 91% of the respondents. Additionally, of the 222 respondents, "205 (92%) answered that they used play as a modality to elicit motor, sensory, or psychosocial outcomes in their clients" (Couch et al., 1997, p. 113).

Play is often defined as exploration and experimentation for its simple intrinsic value with a focus on participation to create feeling of happiness and create opportunities to be actively involved in the world (Ayres, 2005; Garner, 1998; Mooney 2006; Singer & Revenson 1996). Play is also the process of taking known and new information and combining them to understand the world and to develop a sense of self. Most of all, a child's play is all about learning. Please see Table 36.4 and Figures 36.4 and 36.5.

Treatment: The Art of Working with Children

In 2007, the National Board for Certification in Occupational Therapy (NBCOT) and Castle Worldwide, Inc., conducted an analysis of the type of facilities in which OTAs were employed and what their responsibilities were in these locations. The goal of this study was to gain insight into what OTAs were experiencing out in the field in order to establish a baseline for the development of an appropriate credentialing examination. Of the 111 participants, 21% worked with children and youth, with 16% of the respondents reporting working in schools. Though a majority of the respondents reported working with adults, it is interesting to note that almost a fourth of the respondents were employed in pediatric settings (*Executive Summary for the Practice Analysis Study*, 2008).

When speaking with anyone who works with children, you often hear how satisfying and rewarding it feels. From my own experience, working in pediatrics has allowed me to see, firsthand, incredible progress and provided me an amazing sense of accomplishment. In saying this, pediatrics can also be one of the most challenging fields in which to work. Playing with children does not always come naturally to all adults. Typically, we tend to be rigid and linear in our adult leisure activities. Understanding that treatment is more like a dance, where being the leader is passed back and forth

TABLE 36.4 The Developmental Sequence of Play

Type of Play	Description	Age Range
Sensorimotor	Exploratory play of self and how to affect the world. This stage tends to be object centered	Infancy up until 18 months
Imaginative/pretend play	Incorporate social themes to better understand the world, relate to others, and understand societal roles. Begins with objects and transforms to take place with other children with specific play themes and complex ideas	Begins around two years of age and decreases around age of 8
Constructional play	Helps to develop fine motor and cognitive skills while manipulating objects to discover new uses for them	Develops in preschool years through middle childhood and into adolescence when it becomes more abstract
Games/group play	Shapes what are to be the important rules and how to comply with the wishes of others	Preschool through adolescence

Sources: Garner (1998); Johnson (1998); Knox (2005); Manning (1998); Piaget and Inhelder (1969).

between the OT practitioner and child, is vitally important. The role of the pediatric OT practitioner is that of a guide, teacher, and participant. Children tend to be less concerned with different goals or particular outcomes than adults. They also tend to be motivated by different aspects of an activity than adults. For example, an adult may be motivated to work on motor tasks so that they can be independent with daily living skills, whereas a child is more apt to be concerned with success, such as making a basket or grabbing a toy from a swing (Miller & Kuhaneck, 2008).

In interviewing several of the OTAs for this chapter, a recurring theme emerged. One of the most important tools in a therapeutic tool box was flexibility while simultaneously creating a supportive and therapeutic environment. When planning a treatment session, the OT practitioner needs to take in consideration not only the needs of the child but how an activity can be motivating. This is the concept of the "just-right challenge," reflecting the important balance between grading an activity to match the ability level of the child and creating an appropriate difficulty level that is motivating (Ayres, 2005).

Miller and Kuhaneck (2008) identified several core characteristics about what influenced children in choosing and participating in a particular activities. The characteristics included the activities themselves, who participated in them, what was the child's level of success, and the environment in which it was performed (Miller & Kuhaneck, 2008). Activities need to be challenging yet designed to enable children to experience success. Further, grading the parts of an activity from easy to more challenging also increases the fun factor (and motivation) for children (Miller & Kuhaneck, 2008).

In addition to the above items, it is important to consider the power of peer interaction. Vygotsky proposed that through participation in social engagement, children discuss, correct, and are exposed to novel ideas that they eventually internalize to become their own (Cross & Coster 1997, Mooney, 2006; please also refer to Chapter 8, *Human Development: Framing Who We Are*). This concept is relevant for OT practitioners who work in settings where treatment is primarily one to one. In my experience as an EI and private practice clinician, I have witnessed children at a range of developmental levels motivate one another to participate in an activity. While working in EI, I observed this most while running a feeding group. Children who were making slow progress at home with individual treatment were willing to engage with nonpreferred food items after watching another peer try them. Additionally, in the private practice setting, I have often been surprised by the children who gravitate toward each other. One particular pairing always comes to mind. A very social child diagnosed with apraxia sought out another child who was on the autism spectrum. The child with ASD was more inclined to participate in motor-based activities while taking on the task of encouraging the child with apraxia to increase her attempts to communicate with him about what she wanted them to do. Including a peer in the treatment session is not always possible or advisable. Thus, as with creating just-right challenge activities, an OT practitioner must also consider how an age-similar peer may influence the dynamics of the treatment session.

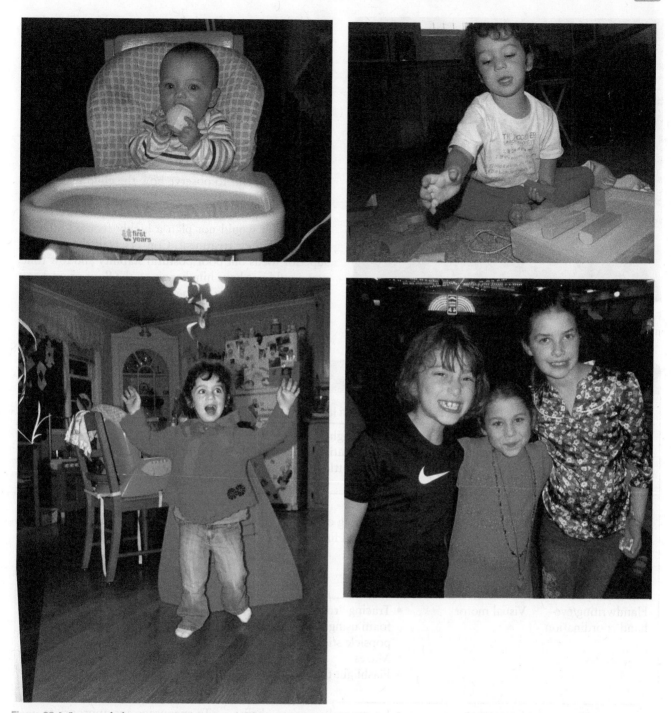

Figure 36.4 Stages of play: sensorimotor (**top left**), construction (**top right**), imaginative/pretend (**bottom left**), games/group (**bottom right**). (Photos courtesy of *Sarah Ford*.)

Another motivating aspect for children is that activities with movement are considered to be more fun than activities without (Miller & Kuhaneck, 2008). This may be difficult to incorporate into treatment depending on the environment and child's motor abilities. Creating a playful environment for children with disabling conditions is never easy (Bundy, 2002). Occupational therapy practitioners always need to be aware of how the child responds to movement and how the experience can be different for children with different diagnoses (e.g., sensory processing disorder vs. developmental disabilities with limited movement such as cerebral palsy). In several instances, I have treated children with limited motor control who have shown intense joy with movement experiences, whereas I have also had children with sensory processing issues who

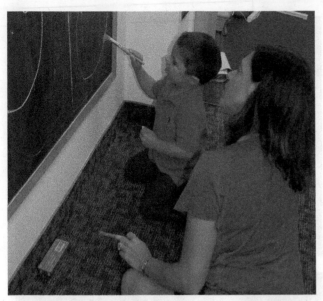

Figure 36.5 An OTA and child are working together on fine motor and visual motor activities.

avoided or even refused the same activities. Therefore, it is always imperative that any movement-based program be implemented under the direct supervision of an OT skilled in sensory integration since they are able to assess the child's primary regulatory state (focus, attention, and arousal) and ascertain the baseline of their discriminatory skills (motor planning, coordination, body awareness) (please also refer to Chapter 28, *Sensory Issues*).

Lastly, when choosing a treatment activity, it is always important to observe how the child is functioning on that particular day and at that particular moment. For example, if a child is unable to sit for more than a minute, you would not plan a highly focused tabletop activity for their treatment. Conversely, if the child has superior focus but poor postural stability and low tone, you would not have him/her sit on the floor or on a soft chair while working at the table. Table 36.5 lists some suggested treatment activities.

TABLE 36.5 Suggested Treatment Activities

Category	Skill Enhancement	Activity Item Ideas	Purpose
Fine motor/hand dexterity	Hand strengthening and development	• Play dough/clay • Manipulative (e.g., legos) • Spray bottles	To increase a child's ability to manipulate and use items that encourage use of the whole hand and not just the fingers
Visual identification	Visual perception	• Puzzles • Matching or sorting games • Seek and find pictures	To help a child to identify and recognize objects and shapes in their environment. Note: Remember to make sure to start by grading the activities by using only two or three items
Handwriting/eye–hand coordination	Visual motor	• Tracing "roads" in sand or foam using a finger, pencil, or popsicle stick • Mazes • Flashlight tag	The end goal is for a child to replicate a mental picture onto the written page. Activities should involve tracing, copying, or motor imitation of objects
Fine motor/ handwriting	Grasp patterns	• Using small crayons, chalk, and markers on a variety of writing surfaces • Children's chopsticks, oversized tweezers • Pencil grips	To encourage age-appropriate grasp; patterns encourage children to use their fingers to manipulate objects
Core strengthening and stability	Posture	• Scooter board • Therapy ball • Appropriate seating	The focus should be to encourage doing activities in prone and supine while performing other motor movements since trunk stability is a key aspect of being able to focus and attend

TABLE 36.5 Suggested Treatment Activities (continued)

Category	Skill Enhancement	Activity Item Ideas	Purpose
Eye–hand coordination	Timing and sequencing	• Balloons with striking objects (e.g., rackets, bats) • Clapping to rhythms • Ball games	These activities help with a child's ability to plan an action for a desired motor goal. They should be graded to allow a child enough time to process and initiate the movement (e.g., hitting a balloon with their hand, then an object, then using a ball)
Coordination of all quadrants of the body (e.g., left and right/top and bottom)	Bilateral movement	• Reaching across the body to grab or hit an object • Song and finger play movements that require crossing midline • Propelling self on swing or glider	The focus of these activities is to enable a child to coordinate movements of their upper and lower body for symmetrical and asymmetrical movements

Summary

The role of the OT and the OTA is an important one in assisting children to succeed in achieving their developmental milestones. By understanding how the ideological landscape has changed over the past 50 years, with the treatment of children with disabilities, it is easier to comprehend how OT practitioners fit into it today. As with all things, the stage in which treating pediatrics is set is ever changing. Current economic, health care legislation, and alterations to the ADA affect how and by whom children will receive services. Whatever the setting or parameters, the incorporation of and communication with caregivers and other team members are vital in a child's ability to reach his/her identified outcomes. Additionally, always remembering how children are motivated and interpret the world helps to maintain the blossoming therapeutic relationship as a partnership full of new ideas.

Review Questions

1. What are the two landmark cases related to children with disabilities that were ruled on by the Supreme Court? What were their findings?
2. What two Acts passed by congress legislated early intervention and schools?
3. What is the purpose of the IDEA?
4. What six treatment items does occupational therapy address in early intervention (EI)?
5. What are the two team models in EI, and how do they function?
6. What is the role of occupational therapy in a school-based setting?

7. What does occupational therapy typically address in the school environment?

8. List three reasons why a family would seek occupational therapy in a private practice setting?

9. What is the focus of the OT practitioner in the private practice setting?

10. Name the four types of play.

11. What are the four characteristics about play that influence children in choosing and participating in a particular activity?

12. What five principles should be followed when creating the play environment?

Practice Activities

Develop three treatment activities that a family can incorporate into their daily routines with a toddler child who is able to sit up with support, but has difficulty grasping an age-appropriate toy.

Develop three treatment activities for a child in a school setting who has trouble crossing midline and has difficult correctly holding a writing implement.

Develop three treatment activities for a child in a private practice setting who has poor postural strength and tends to slouch when sitting.

References

Ayres AJ. *Sensory Integration and the Child: 25th Anniversary Edition*. California: Western Psychological Services; 2005.

Building the Legacy. *IDEA 2004* (part B & part C). 2004. Retrieved from http://www.idea.ed.gov/

Bundy A. Play theory and sensory integration. In: Bundy AC, Lane JS, Murray AE, eds. *Sensory Integration: Theory and Practice*. 2nd ed., pp. 227–240. Pennsylvania, PA: F.A. Davis; 2002.

Case-Smith J. Effectiveness of school-based occupational therapy intervention on handwriting. *Am J Occup Ther* 2002;56(1):17–25.

Cross AL, Coster JW. Symbolic play language during sensory integration treatment. *Am J Occup Ther* 1997;51(10):808–814.

Couch JK, et al. The role of play in /pediatric occupational therapy. *Am J Occup Ther* 1997;52(8):111–117.

Dunn W. A comparison of service provision models in school based occupational therapy services. A pilot study. *Occup Ther J Res* 1990;10:300–320.

Executive Summary for the Practice Analysis Study. 2008. Retrieved from http://www.nbcot.org/pdf/Executive-Summary-for-the-Practice-Analysis-Study-COTA.pdf?phpMyAdmin=3710605fd34365e380b9ab41a5078545

Garner PB. Play development from birth to age four. In: Fromberg DP, Bergen D, eds. *Play from Birth to Twelve and Beyond Context, Perspectives, and Meanings*. pp. 137–145. NY: Psychology Press; 1998.

History Twenty-Five Years of Progress in Educating Children with Disabilities through IDEA. 2007. Retrieved from http://www2.ed.gov/policy/speced/leg/idea/history.html

Johnson EJ. Play Development from four to eight. In: Fromberg DP, Bergen D, eds. *Play*

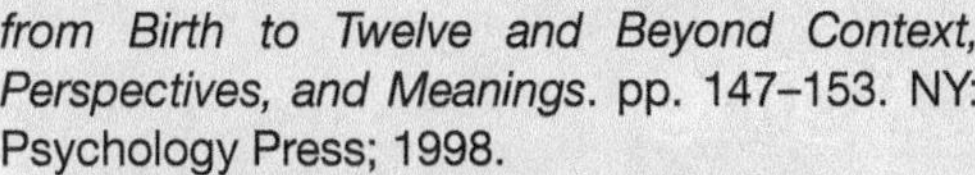

from Birth to Twelve and Beyond Context, Perspectives, and Meanings. pp. 147–153. NY: Psychology Press; 1998.

IDEA Subpart A, B, D, & E. Retrieved from http://nichcy.org/laws/idea

Knox S. Play. In: Case-Smith J, ed. *Occupational Therapy for Children*. 5th ed. pp. 571–586. Missouri: Elsevier Mosby; 2005.

Imber M, van Geel T. *Education Law*. 3rd ed. New Jersey: Lawrence Erlbaum Associates; 2004.

Manning LM. Play development from eight to twelve. In: Fromberg DP, Bergen D, eds. *Play from Birth to Twelve and Beyond: Context, Perspectives, and Meanings*. pp. 1154–1161. NY: Psychology Press; 1998.

Miller E, Kuhaneck H. Children's perceptions of play experiences and play preferences: a qualitative study. *Am J Occup Ther* 2008;62(4):407–415.

Mooney GC. *An Introduction to Dewy, Montessori, Erikson, Piaget & Vygotsky*. New Jersey: Pearson Education; 2006.

Piaget J, Inhelder B. *The Psychology of the Child*. New York: Basic Books; 1969.

Rothstein FL. *Special Education Law*. 2nd ed. New York: Longman Publishers USA; 1995.

Schaaf CR, Mulrooney LL. Occupational therapy in early intervention: a family-centered approach. *Am J Occup Ther* 1989;43(11):745–754.

Smith M, et al. *Sustaining Family Involvement in Part C Policy and Services*. pp. 39–44. Washington, D.C.: ZERO TO THREE Policy Center; 2011.

Singer GD, Revenson AT. *A Piaget Primer: How a Child Thinks* (rev ed). England: Plume; 1996.

Trent WJ. *Inventing the Feeble Mind: A history of Mental Retardation in the United States*. pp. 225–268. Berkeley & Los Angeles, CA: University of California Press; 1995.

CHAPTER 37

Productive Aging

Stacy Smallfield, DrOT, MSOT, OTR/L, FAOTA and
Sue Berger, PhD, OTR/L, BCG, FAOTA

Key Terms

Aging in place—Living in the same environment, typically one's home, as one ages.

Nontraditional or emerging areas of practice—Areas of practice that are not typically reimbursed by the traditional health care system and/or are new areas of practice for occupational therapy practitioners.

Normative aging changes—Changes that are an accepted part of aging. If you live to a certain age, you will experience these changes.

Productive aging—Used to describe the societal contributions of older adults, including paid employment, volunteer activities, caring for others, and daily activities.

Learning Objectives

After studying this chapter, readers should be able to:

- Describe the sociopolitical context in which older adults live today.
- Distinguish the normative changes associated with aging from the nonnormative disease processes or medical conditions that increase in prevalence with age.
- Describe the current areas of practice in which occupational therapy practitioners work with older adults.
- Discuss the emerging areas of practice in which occupational therapy practitioners can continue to grow and develop.

Introduction

In the health and social sciences, we commonly use the term **productive aging** to describe the societal contributions of older adults, including paid employment, volunteer activities, caring for others, and daily activities (Butler, 2002). Engagement in these meaningful activities as one ages promotes health, life satisfaction, and longevity (Rath & Harter, 2010); it also may decrease overall health care costs (Butler, 2002). It is in this positive view of the contributions that older adults have on society that we consider their influence in America and discuss the role of OT practitioners in promoting their health and well-being.

The American Occupational Therapy Association (2012) states that there will be an increasing need for occupational therapy services within the practice area of productive aging. There are several reasons for this, including the ever-growing numbers of older adults in the United States, longer life spans, and older adults' desires for person-centered care and high quality of life. Older adults represent the fastest growing segment of the population (United States Census Bureau, 2011). The first baby boomers, or those born between 1946 and 1964, have started turning age 65. In fact, beginning in 2011, they are turning age 65 at the rate of 10,000 per day. This means that while there were about 40 million older adults in

2009, this number will grow to 72 million older adults in 2030 (Triple Tree, 2011). They then will comprise almost 20% of the US population (Administration on Aging, 2011) (From the Field 37.1).

An important health goal for older adults is to improve their health, function, and quality of life (HealthyPeople.gov, 2012). Approximately 90% of those age 65 and older state they would like to stay at home as long as possible and over 80% of them state that they do not plan to move from their current home (Farber & Shinkle, 2011). Older adults' ability to remain at home and live alone depends largely upon their ability to complete everyday self-care activities independently (see Fig. 37.1). However, even without any formally diagnosed chronic or medical conditions, several factors can test the independence of older adults (Leland & Elliott, 2012). These include normal age-related changes, the built environment, changes in transportation options, and potential limitations to formal and informal caregiving resources, among others. Occupational therapy practitioners can continue to support productive aging by maximizing older adults' ability to engage in meaningful activity, by designing environments that promote full participation, and by providing resources and strategies that minimize the impact of normative age-related changes and chronic conditions on function.

In this chapter, we will explore the sociopolitical context in which older adults live today, distinguish the normative changes associated with aging from the nonnormative disease processes or medical conditions, describe the current areas of practice in which OT practitioners work with older adults, and discuss the emerging areas of practice in which OT practitioners can continue to grow and develop. We begin by discussing the sociopolitical context of aging in America.

Sociopolitical Context of Aging

In the United States, we now live in a society that sees another person reach age 65 at the rate of one every 8 seconds. By 2030, there will be twice the number of older adults living in this country as there was in the year 2000 (Triple Tree, 2011). Born just after World War II when America was flourishing, these baby boomers are hard-working, goal oriented, rebellious, and independent. Because of their large numbers, they believe their generation is changing society as they age. They saw the first man on the moon, lived through the assassinations of John F. Kennedy and Martin Luther King, Jr., and were involved in other historical events including the Cuban Missile Crisis, the Cold War, the civil rights movement, and Watergate.

With the average life expectancy in the United States now at age 78 (Administration on Aging, 2011), this generation is living longer, but they are doing so at a price, as about 80% of them manage one or more chronic health conditions (Triple Tree, 2011). At the same time, the cost of health care is soaring and the Patient Protection and Affordable Care Act of 2010, many components of which as of this writing have not been fully implemented, is bringing an added level of uncertainty to the delivery of health care today. Furthermore, due to the financial crisis of 2008 to 2012 and the gradual decline of employer-sponsored pensions, many baby boomers have not adequately saved for retirement.

FROM THE FIELD 37.1

Rewarding Work

Until you try working with an older adult population, you won't understand the rewards. I treat all of the older adults I work with as if they were my grandparents. I am their advocate. Be confident and be their advocate.

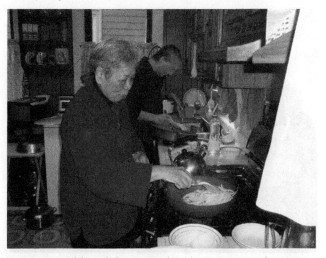

Figure 37.1 Older adults engaged in the instrumental activity of daily living of meal preparation.

In combination, it will be financially difficult to care for this generation of Americans.

There are two federally funded programs available to older adults that assist them in financing their retirement years. Social Security is the federally funded retirement benefit program, which the federal government pays to retirees on a monthly basis based upon the retiree's earnings and the age at which the retiree decides to start to receive benefits. All workers fund the program by paying a payroll tax. Medicare is the federal health insurance program created in 1965 for those 65 and older. It also is funded by a payroll tax paid by both workers and their employers. Medicare insurance is intended to cover the majority of health care costs, including hospital expenses, some home health care, and some hospice care (Part A), outpatient medical expenses (Part B), and prescription drugs (Part D). However, it is important to note that Medicare health insurance does not pay for long-term care in a skilled nursing facility (except for a short duration when followed by a hospital stay) or for assisted living expenses (Centers for Medicare and Medicaid Services, n.d.a). Because of the large number of baby boomers who will receive Social Security, the solvency of the Social Security program is in question without major reform. Likewise, the federal government regularly proposes reimbursement rate cuts to health care providers who service Medicare insurance recipients due to the rising cost of operating this federal insurance program.

As the baby boomer generation ages, their need and desire for amenities and services in their older years will continue to emerge and evolve. After their primary basic needs are met, older adults are most interested in living in a community that promotes health and wellness, integrates current technology, is equipped to allow for transitions to increased care and services without moving, and provides appealing methods of transportation (American Seniors Housing Association, 2011). Baby boomers are looking for communities where they can easily access restaurants, entertainment, culture, retail, volunteer, and productive opportunities (see Fig. 37.2). In other words, they want to be engaged with not only their community of seniors, but their community in general (American Seniors Housing Association, 2011). Seniors and their families will expect a seamless transition between phases in their lives with little difference in service delivery and customization that they have come to expect in other aspects of their lives.

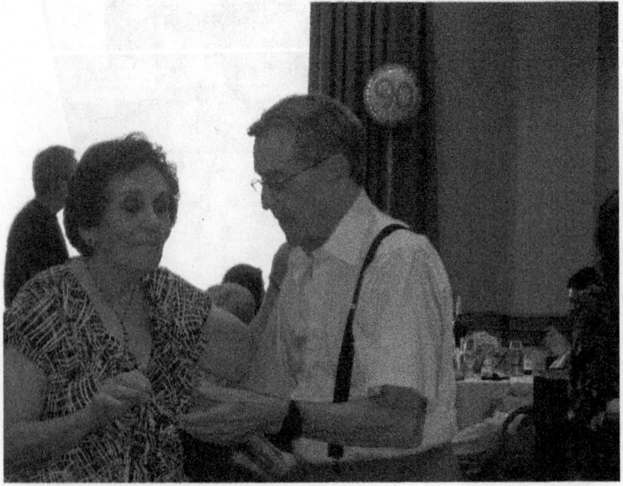

Figure 37.2 Older adults engaged in the leisure activity of dancing.

Normative Aging Changes

A colleague, now 55 years old, remembers when she was turning 40 and everyone was telling her it was a big birthday. She was thinking, *it is just a number, what is the big deal.* She was feeling good about where she was in her life and was looking forward to this milestone. To this individual, age 40 implied wisdom and confidence. And then, a week before her 40th birthday, she went down a waterslide and hurt her back. As she was in pain and going to doctors and getting tests, she realized why each birthday decade *is* a big deal and understood why people do not want to age. If pain and illness are associated with aging, it makes perfect sense why we all envy Peter Pan.

Aging, however, does not need to be associated with pain and illness. Many illnesses one associates with getting older, such as heart attack, stroke, cancer, and Parkinson disease, are not **normative aging changes**. These conditions do increase in prevalence with age, but there are many ways to decrease the risk associated with these conditions and to stay healthy into later decades of life (please also refer to Chapter 35, *Health and Well-Being*). There are certain normative changes, however, that do occur with age. Although sometimes we can slow down these changes, if we live long enough, we will all have to face them.

Cardiopulmonary Changes as One Ages

As we age, tissues throughout the body lose elasticity. When decreased elasticity occurs in the small vessels of the lung, the lung becomes less efficient at exchanging gas. Mechanical changes also occur in the cardiac muscles, which lead to the heart pumping less effectively as one gets older. These changes of the heart and lung result in reduced capacity for oxygen transport at rest and even more so in response to activity. Even low-demand activities, such as brushing teeth, can be physically demanding as one ages. With age, we also lose respiratory and abdominal muscle mass, which limits the ability to produce a forceful cough, increasing risk of aspiration and resulting in pneumonia.

Some cardiopulmonary conditions that increase in prevalence with age but are not normal age-related changes include the following:

- Coronary artery disease (CAD): This is a degeneration of the arteries that supply nutrients to the heart. CAD can lead to heart attack and other coronary conditions.

- Hypertension: Commonly referred to as high blood pressure, hypertension produces no outward symptoms. Despite the seriousness of this condition, compliance with medication is challenging because individuals often *feel fine*. Hypertension leads to an increased risk for heart disease, stroke, and other cardiovascular conditions.
- Emphysema: Air sacs of the lung are destroyed, making oxygen exchange limited, which leads to breathing difficulties.

Sensory Changes as One Ages

Many sensory changes occur with aging, including change in sensation to touch, smell, taste, pain, and temperature, as well as a decrease in vision and hearing. As one ages, there is a decrease in the number of peripheral receptors and nerve fibers, which is thought to lead to increased sensitivity to pain. Difficulty with temperature regulation occurs with aging and has functional implications. For example, older adults are more susceptible to heat stroke and frostbite as they cannot regulate their body temperature. Changes to taste and smell also occur, which influences nutritional intake. Most notably, however, are changes to the visual and auditory system, and they deserve further discussion.

Vision

It is common to see those who are in their 40s holding reading material at arm's length. Some joke that they wish they had longer arms. Because they cannot grow their arms, they purchase reading glasses and for most, this works just as well. As we age, the lens of the eye loses elasticity and therefore has less ability to change shape, which is needed to adjust to distance of item viewed. The lens stays focused for items further away, so when doing near work such as reading, glasses are needed. This difficulty in focusing on near objects begins around age 40 and is called presbyopia.

The pupil of the eye gets smaller as one ages and, similar to the lens, is less able to adapt its size. Smaller pupils mean less light getting in and so it is harder for older adults to see in low-light situations. It is also harder for older adults to adjust quickly to lighting changes. For example, it takes a longer time to adjust to a darkened room as one ages, which has implications for safe mobility.

Decreased tissue elasticity affects all parts of the body, including the eyes. You may notice the eyes of older adults appear sunken and this is due to this decreased elasticity of the tissue along with loss of subcutaneous fat. Older adults often talk about *dry eye*, and this occurs because tear production decreases with age.

Cataract is an increase in the opacity of the lens of the eye; the lens appears cloudy and yellow. This leads to decreased acuity and contrast and an increased sensitivity to glare. Cataract is a normative part of aging and if we live long enough, we will develop cataract. There are things one can do to slow the progression of cataract including wearing sunglasses and stopping smoking as ultraviolet rays and nicotine are two factors that speed up the development of cataract. In most situations, cataracts can surgically be removed and vision restored.

Some eye conditions that increase in prevalence with age but are not normal age-related changes include the following:

- Age-related macular degeneration: This condition destroys the macula, the central part of the retina that provides sharp vision. This results in the development of a scotoma (blind spot) leading to loss of central vision.
- Glaucoma: An increase in pressure in the eye leads to damage of the optic nerve and results in peripheral vision loss.
- Diabetic retinopathy: This condition, caused by an extended, unmanaged diabetes mellitus, is the result of damage to the blood vessels of the retina leading to scattered blind spots and varying vision loss.

Hearing

Being able to hear has significant implications for social participation. Engaging with grandchildren, other family, and friends can be strained when conversation is difficult. Hearing loss leads to isolation and depression (Teixeira et al., 2010). Thirty percent of those 65 to 74 have hearing loss and this increases to 47% when considering those 75 and older (National Institute on Deafness and Other Communication Disorders, 2010). Presbycusis is defined as age-related hearing loss and is the most common diagnosis of hearing loss with older people. Hair cells of the cochlea are lost or damaged as a result of presbycusis.

Other conditions of hearing loss that increase in incidence with age but are not normal age-related changes include the following:

- Sociocusis: Hearing loss due to noise exposure from years of work in loud environments.
- Ototoxicity: Hearing loss as a side effect of medication.

Musculoskeletal Changes as One Ages

Changes that occur with age to the musculoskeletal system can lead to an increased risk of falling, decreased independence, and pain. Bodies continually rebuild bone to compensate for bone reabsorption, but the balance between this bone formation and reabsorption changes as we age and this decreased balance eventually leads to a decrease in bone density. Up until age 50, bone loss

FROM THE FIELD 37.2

Meeting the Client Where She Is

I worked with a woman who was deconditioned. It was her goal to put a girdle on. Despite the fact that she could have been independent in dressing without wearing her girdle, we worked several weeks on this goal because it was important to her. She had always worn her girdle and I wasn't going to convince her otherwise.

occurs very slowly (at about 0.7% to 1% a year) but increases with age, especially in women after menopause.

Additionally, as one ages, decreased muscle mass occurs from a decrease in the number and size of the muscle fibers. This loss of muscle mass and strength is called sarcopenia. Because an older adult has a decrease in number and size of muscle fibers, the muscles are slower to react as one ages. A decrease in strength leads to difficulty in daily tasks such as opening jars and turning keys. Although sarcopenia is considered a normative aging change, decreased muscle strength is related to inactivity. No one is too old to build strength and muscle mass. Exercise and activity at any age are important, but especially for older adults, as sarcopenia leads to increased risk of falls, dependence, and pain (From the Field 37.2).

Along with changes in the bones and the muscles, joint changes occur with age. The water content of cartilage decreases, causing wear and tear on the joints during repetitive activity. Ligaments that connect bone to bone lose elasticity and joint space narrows, leading to pain and stiffness. As water content in ligaments decreases, causing less elasticity, older adults lose flexibility and range of motion. Although it is understandable that these changes might lead to inactivity and pain, it is really important that older adults remain active and use their joints and muscles as much as possible.

Some musculoskeletal conditions that increase in prevalence with age but are not normal age-related changes include the following:

- Osteoporosis: Loss of bone density is a natural progression of aging but can lead to osteoporosis, especially in weightbearing joints, if preventive measures such as engaging in weightbearing activities and assuring calcium (via food or vitamins) and vitamin D (via food or sun exposure) intake are not taken.
- Degenerative joint disease/osteoarthritis: As the cartilage between bones decreases, bones rub against each other, wearing out and causing pain and limited motion.

Neurological Changes as One Ages

As with other body systems, the central nervous system (CNS) goes through many changes during the aging process. Specifically, brain cells die, leaving a smaller number of brain cells to perform the same, important daily routines. Fewer brain cells mean slower mental processing. The nerves conduct at a slower rate, decreasing reaction and processing time. Therefore, older adults often struggle with tasks that require quick responses. However, if given time, it has been shown that they perform as well as younger adults (Eckert, 2011). A decrease in nerve cells also correlates with a decrease in ability to maintain balance, leading to an increased risk of falling.

Some neurological conditions that increase in prevalence with age but are not a normal part of aging include the following:

- Stroke: This occurs when blood flow to the brain is blocked (ischemic stroke) or when a blood vessel in the brain bursts (hemorrhagic stroke). Symptoms vary depending on location of the stroke but may include motor and sensory loss on one side of the body, communication difficulties, and perceptual and cognitive changes.
- Alzheimer disease: This disorder of the brain causes a progressive death of brain cells and results in memory loss, personality changes, impaired judgment, and confusion.
- Parkinson disease: This progressive disorder is caused by a decrease in dopamine production leading to slowed movement, rigidity, and tremors along with a myriad of other symptoms and functional challenges.

Genitourinary Changes as One Ages

The genitourinary system is not exempt from changes related to aging. Although incontinence is not a normative part of aging, the capacity and muscle tone of the bladder decrease with age and these changes can cause problems in holding urine. The urethra gets shorter and the sphincter that controls urine flow has less control, especially after menopause. These many changes in the urinary system can lead to incontinence or leakage. Bladder exercises and changes in routine, however, can prevent this. It is important to address incontinence as urinary urgency leads to rushing and potential falls.

Prostate enlargement is very common in men, especially those 70 and older. An enlarged prostate can cause an increased need to urinate and/or difficulty fully emptying the bladder. Hormonal changes in older women can lead to vaginal dryness, causing itching and discomfort.

Despite decreased levels of estrogen in women and testosterone levels in men, sexual pleasure can continue throughout the life course. Decreased hormones can lead to a need for change in sexual activity to achieve pleasure, however. Decreased estrogen levels in women can require more effort to achieve orgasm. Lubrication can help address dryness that often occurs after menopause. Older men may need more time to achieve an erection and erections may be less firm. Decreased testosterone levels can affect overall energy and strength, as well.

Some genitourinary conditions that increase in prevalence with age but are not a normal part of aging include the following:

- Urinary tract infection (UTI): Due to the normative aging changes listed above, older adults are at an increased risk of having UTIs, an infection that begins in the urinary system.
- Dehydration: This occurs when an individual does not drink enough water to replace what is lost through daily activity and though anyone can develop dehydration, older adults are at an increased risk. Initial symptoms include thirst, dry mouth, decreased urine output, headache, and light-headedness but can progress to delirium, fever, low blood pressure, and rapid breathing.

Mental Health Conditions

Widowhood, retirement, change in financial status, chronic health conditions, death of peers, and social isolation can all lead to psychosocial challenges for older adults. Also, with age, there is a decline of neurotransmitters, such as serotonin and dopamine, which may increase older adults' vulnerability to depression.

Mental health conditions associated with aging but are not a normal part of aging include the following:

- Late life depression: This is the most frequently occurring mental health condition in older adults and is the result of the many changes listed above such as loss of friends and spouse and living with multiple health conditions. Suicide rates increase in older adults as well, especially white males over the age of 85 (National Institute of Mental Health, 2007).
- Alcohol abuse: Although statistics show about 10% of older adults abuse alcohol, this number is likely higher as many older adults who abuse alcohol live alone and drink in the privacy of their home; therefore, they are less likely to be noticed or reported (Dar, 2006).
- Anxiety disorder: Although often overlooked, older adults have an increased risk of developing chronic anxiety due to the many daily stressors they are juggling.

Other Challenges that Increase in Prevalence with Age

There are numerous challenges that older adults face. Their likelihood of occurrence increased with age. Some are discussed in this chapter.

Falls

Many normative aging changes along with the conditions that increase in incidence with age can increase the risk of falls. The incidence of falls among older adults has become a public health concern as it can lead to injury and death. There is extensive literature regarding fall prevention and OT practitioners play a large and important role in this area (Leland et al., 2012; Peterson et al., 2012). It is important to understand that falls occur not due to one thing (e.g., poor vision) but due to multiple risk factors occurring simultaneously (e.g., poor vision combined with decreased strength, poor reaction time, and a cluttered environment). The more risk factors one has, the higher the risk of falling. These risk factors are divided essentially into intrinsic and extrinsic factors.

- *Intrinsic factors* include age, history of previous falls, living alone, number and type of medications, chronic health conditions, sedentary behavior, mental health status, nutritional status, cognitive status, visual impairments, and foot problems.
- *Extrinsic factors* include unsafe environments (e.g., poor lighting, slippery floors), footwear and clothing, and inappropriate ambulation device.

Polypharmacy

After understanding the normative aging changes along with the conditions that increase in prevalence with age, it should be no surprise that older adults are often taking multiple medications daily. It is common for older adults to take multiple pills several times a day. Although each pill has a purpose, the combination and interaction of pills have its own challenges. For example, data show that older adults taking five or more medications a day are at an increased risk for falls and the risk increases exponentially as the number of medications increases (Freeland et al., 2012).

Additionally, to be effective, medications need to be taken at certain times in certain ways (e.g., with or without food). Managing a medication routine can be challenging and is made even more difficult when managing age-related changes such as decreased vision, strength, and sensation. Occupational therapy practitioners, in conjunction with nursing, can play an important role in facilitating compliance with a medication routine. Providing large-print labels, helping to establish routines, and working to build up hand strength are just a few of the ways to assure that an individual can safely manage their medications.

Current Occupational Therapy Practice Settings

Table 37.1, Current Occupational Therapy Practice Settings for Working with Older Adults, provides an overview of the many possible environments in which OT practitioners may work with older adults. For each

TABLE 37.1 **Current Occupational Therapy Practice Settings for Working with Older Adults**

Acute Care: A hospital stay focused on medical needs	
Typical length of stay	One week or less
Frequency and duration of occupational therapy intervention	Variable, but typically 1×/day, 5–7×/wk for 30 min
Occupational therapy performance areas commonly addressed	The focus of occupational therapy in this setting is to evaluate the patient to make appropriate recommendations for discharge to a lower level of medical care and to provide education and training in ADLs for safety and independence.
OT/OTA role delineation	Because of the frequency of evaluations requiring written plans of care and high patient acuity, OTAs work closely with OTs in this practice setting. About 15% of OTAs work in hospital settings (American Occupational Therapy Association [AOTA], 2010).
Typical team members	Physicians; physician assistants; nurse practitioners; nurses; nurse assistants; pharmacists; dieticians; other rehabilitation professionals including physical, speech, and respiratory therapists and assistants; social workers; family members; and other caregivers
Inpatient Rehabilitation Facility (IRF): A hospital stay focused on intense skilled rehabilitation therapy	
Typical length of stay	2–6 weeks, but variable based on medical condition, functional challenges, progress toward therapy goals, and other factors
Frequency and duration of occupational therapy intervention	2 sessions per day (for a total of 1.5 h per day); 5–7 days per week. Individuals in inpatient rehabilitation must be able to tolerate a total of 3 hours of therapy per day.
Occupational therapy performance areas commonly addressed	ADLs, IADLs, sleep and rest, work[b], leisure, and social participation
OT/OTA role delineation	Both OTs and OTAs work in inpatient rehabilitation units. The OTA is primarily responsible for implementing the plan of care established by the OT following the initial evaluation. The OTA can also complete components of the evaluation as directed by the OT.
Typical team members	A physiatrist and/or other consulting physicians; physician assistants; nurse practitioners; nurses; nurse assistants; pharmacists; dieticians; other rehabilitation professionals including physical, speech, recreational, and respiratory therapists and assistants; social workers; family members; and other caregivers
Long-Term Acute Care (LTAC): An extended hospital stay due to prolonged medical needs	
Typical length of stay	A minimum of 3 weeks
Frequency and duration of occupational therapy intervention	Variable, but typically 1–2 times a day for a total of 30–60 min, 5–6 days per week
Occupational therapy performance areas commonly addressed	ADLs, IADLs, sleep and rest, leisure, social participation
OT/OTA role delineation	Because of high patient acuity and complexity, OTAs work closely with OTs in this practice setting, implementing plans of care as directed by the OT.
Typical team members	Physicians; physician assistants; nurse practitioners; nurses; nursing assistants; pharmacists; dieticians; other rehabilitation professionals including physical, speech, and respiratory therapists and assistants; social workers; family members; and other caregivers

TABLE 37.1 Current Occupational Therapy Practice Settings for Working with Older Adults (continued)

Long-Term Care (LTC)/Skilled Nursing Facility (SNF): Institutionalized, residential care due to skilled rehabilitation, nursing, and/or medical needs	
Typical length of stay	Residents can stay in skilled nursing facilities either on a short-term or long-term basis. Short-term stays can vary from approximately 10 days to 3 months, with a goal of transitioning to a lower level of care. Long-term stays can last from months up to several years and a resident's length of stay can exceed the duration of therapy.
Frequency and duration of occupational therapy intervention	Residents in SNFs may receive occupational therapy 1–2 times per day for a total of 30–60 minutes per day 3–6 days per week when a need exists. Not all residents of SNFs need skilled occupational therapy.
Occupational therapy performance areas commonly addressed	ADLs, sleep and rest, leisure, and social participation. When a resident is planning to transition to a lower level of care, such as to home or to assisted living, IADLs may be addressed. Occupational therapy practitioners may also be involved in fall prevention, low-vision rehabilitation, exercise, and other types of programming.
OT/OTA role delineation	The OTA is primarily responsible for implementing the plan of care established by the OT following the initial evaluation. The OTA can also complete components of the evaluation as directed by the OT. According to AOTA (2010), 45% of OTAs work in long-term care/SNFs.
Typical team members	Nurses; nursing assistants; dieticians; other rehabilitation professionals including physical, speech, recreational, and respiratory therapists and assistants; social workers; family members; and other caregivers. Physicians, physician assistants, nurse practitioners, and pharmacists are also vital team members; however, they are typically off-site.
Dementia Care/Memory Units: Institutionalized, residential care, in a separate, secured area, due to declining intellectual and social abilities	
Typical length of stay	Length of stay in a memory unit is similar to that of a long-term skilled nursing facility stay; it can vary from months to years. The length of stay can exceed the duration of skilled therapy services.
Frequency and duration of occupational therapy intervention	Residents in memory units may receive occupational therapy services 1–2 times per day for a total of 30–45 minutes per day 3–5 days per week when a need exists for skilled occupational therapy services. Not all residents of memory units need skilled therapy services.
Occupational therapy performance areas commonly addressed	ADLs, IADLs, sleep and rest, leisure, and social participation. Occupational therapy practitioners may also be involved in fall prevention, exercise, and other types of programming.
OT/OTA role delineation	Both OTs and OTAs work in memory units. The OTA is primarily responsible for implementing the plan of care established by the occupational therapist following the initial evaluation. The OTA can also complete components of the evaluation as directed by the OT.
Typical team members	Nurses; nursing assistants; dieticians; physical, speech, and recreational therapists and assistants; social workers; family members; and other caregivers. Physicians, physician assistants, nurse practitioners, and pharmacists are also vital team members; however, they are typically off-site.

(*continues on page 510*)

TABLE 37.1 Current Occupational Therapy Practice Settings for Working with Older Adults (continued)

Hospice: Supportive care focused on quality of life for those who are terminally ill; can be provided in the home, hospital, skilled nursing facility, or a stand-alone hospice facility	
Typical length of stay	Hospice care is provided for those with a life expectancy of 6 mo or less and continues until end of life.
Frequency and duration of occupational therapy intervention	Variable, but typically 1 session per day, 30–60 minutes per session, 1–3 sessions per week
Occupational therapy performance areas commonly addressed	Any area of occupation of importance to the individual with an emphasis on quality of life, pain control caregiver training and support, and facilitating the individual to remain in environment of choice
OT/OTA role delineation	The OTA is primarily responsible for implementing the plan of care established by the occupational therapist following the initial evaluation. The OTA can also complete components of the evaluation as directed by the OT.
Typical team members	Physicians, nurses, nursing assistants, pharmacists, dieticians, social workers, physical therapists and assistants, pastoral staff, volunteers, family members, and other caregivers
Assisted Living Facility (ALF): A residential facility that provides assistance with basic self-care and homemaking needs but does not provide skilled medical services	
Typical length of stay	Assisted living is a residential setting; length of stay can range from months to years. Skilled therapy services may or may not be needed in an assisted living setting.
Frequency and duration of occupational therapy intervention: facility	If skilled therapy is needed, it may be provided as home health care or as an outpatient service. Occupational therapy services are not typically located on site in an assisted living residence unless the assisted living is on the same campus as a skilled nursing.
Occupational therapy performance areas commonly addressed	ADLS, IADLs, sleep and rest, work, education, leisure, and social participation. Occupational therapy practitioners may also be involved in fall prevention, low-vision rehabilitation, exercise, and other types of programming.
OT/OTA role delineation	The OTA is primarily responsible for implementing the plan of care established by the OT following the initial evaluation. Occupational therapy practitioners may also serve as consultants for accessibility and universal design in assisted living settings.
Typical team members	Nurses, medication assistants, activities staff, family members, and other caregivers
Home Health Care: Nursing, rehabilitation, and other medical care provided in the home	
Typical length of stay	Older adults receiving home health care typically have skilled therapy services for 2–6 weeks.
Frequency and duration of intervention	Variable, but typically 1–3 days per week, 30–60-minute sessions
Occupational therapy performance areas commonly addressed	ADLs, IADLs, sleep and rest, work, education, leisure, social participation

TABLE 37.1 Current Occupational Therapy Practice Settings for Working with Older Adults (continued)

OT/OTA role delineation	The OTA is primarily responsible for implementing the plan of care established by the OT following the initial evaluation. The OTA can also complete components of the evaluation as directed by the OT. Less than 5% of OTAs work in this practice setting (AOTA, 2010).
Typical team members	Care coordination is often completed at a distance with physicians; physician assistants; nurse practitioners; nurses; home health aides; pharmacists; other rehabilitation professionals including physical, speech, and respiratory therapists and assistants; social workers; family members; and other caregivers.
Outpatient Therapy: Rehabilitation provided in a therapy clinic	
Typical length of therapy	Variable; 2–6 weeks
Frequency and duration of intervention	Variable, but typically 1–3 days per week, 30–60-min sessions
Occupational therapy performance areas commonly addressed	Basic and instrumental ADL, sleep and rest, leisure and social participation, work (volunteer activities)
OT/OTA role delineation	The OTA is primarily responsible for implementing the plan of care established by the OT following the initial evaluation. The OTA can also complete components of the evaluation as directed by the OT.
Typical team members	Care coordination is often completed at a distance with physicians; physician assistants; nurse practitioners; nurses; pharmacists; other rehabilitation professionals including physical, speech, and respiratory therapists and assistants; social workers; family members; and other caregivers.
Continuing Care Retirement Community (CCRC): A community in which an older adult can transition from independent living to assisted living to skilled care all on one campus depending upon their care needs	
Occupational therapy at a CCRC may be provided as home health service to an older adult who is living in an independent residence or an assisted living residence within the community or occupational therapy may be provided as outpatient therapy. As an older adult transitions to skilled care at a CCRC, occupational therapy would be provided as needed per physician orders in that setting.	

Note: ADLs, activities of daily living; ALF, assisted living facility; CCRC, continuing care retirement community; IADLs, instrumental activities of daily living; IRF, inpatient rehabilitation facility; LTAC, long-term acute care; LTC, long-term care; OT, occupational therapist; OTA, occupational therapy assistant; SNF, skilled nursing facility.

[a]While there are multiple occupational therapy performance areas that could be addressed in all of the current practice areas listed, often, third-party reimbursement of occupational therapy evaluation and intervention influences the actual performance areas addressed. For example, Medicare is a primary payer of occupational therapy services for adults over age 65, but Medicare only reimburses therapy that is deemed medically necessary (Centers for Medicare and Medicaid Services, n.d.b). Therefore, performance areas of ADLs, IADLs, and rest and sleep are most commonly addressed in skilled therapy because these areas are reimbursable by third-party payers. Work is a performance area that is typically not covered by Medicare, since Medicare is a federally funded program intended for retirees.

[b]The performance area of work, as defined by AOTA (2014), includes volunteer activity and adjustment to retirement.

practice setting, this table includes the approximate length of stay, typical frequency and duration of occupational therapy intervention, the occupational therapy performance areas commonly addressed, the role delineation between the OT and OTA, and the interdisciplinary team members involved in the care of these older adults. We emphasize the words *typical* and *approximate* and *commonly addressed*, as many of these features of practice settings vary based on insurance, state regulations, and organizational philosophy.

Emerging Areas of Practice Associated with Productive Aging

There are many other potential practice settings not included on Table 37.1. Occupational therapy practitioners call these additional environments **nontraditional** or **emerging areas of practice** (please also refer to Chapter 40, *Emerging Practice Areas*). Traditional third-party (insurance) reimbursement often does not cover nontraditional areas of practice; rather, these services are covered through grant funding, private pay, individual companies or organizations, or other innovative mechanisms.

A variety of life events occur with age, many of which include significant loss. For example, retirement leads to loss of a job, loss of proximity to a social network, and possibly loss of financial security. Widowhood means loss of a spouse; and relocation often involves loss of a home. Loss of friends and family through death and loss of a healthy and active lifestyle may also occur with age.

Occupational therapy practitioners can play a large role in enabling older adults to adjust to these many transitions and losses.

As baby boomers age, they will advocate for occupational therapy to help them work longer, age in place, and remain active and healthy for years to come. Some of the areas of practice below are well established while others are truly emerging and there are many areas not included. The opportunities for OT practitioners to practice in nontraditional areas are limited only by their ability to think outside of the box.

Home Modification

The majority of older adults want to remain home (AARP, 2011), commonly referred to as **aging in place**. In order to remain active, productive, and independent in one's home as he/she ages, modifications may be needed. For some, renovations to have a living space on the first floor, including a bathroom, may be necessary. Grab bars and other safety features might be needed in the bathroom. Additional lighting, lever door handles, and eliminating thresholds are just a few of the possible adaptations that might facilitate aging in place for some older adults (Fig. 37.3). Providing consultation to families and working in collaboration with architects are two nontraditional practice models used when addressing environmental modifications (please also refer to Chapter 21, *Adaptive Equipment*, and Chapter 22, *Assistive Technology*) (From the Field 37.3).

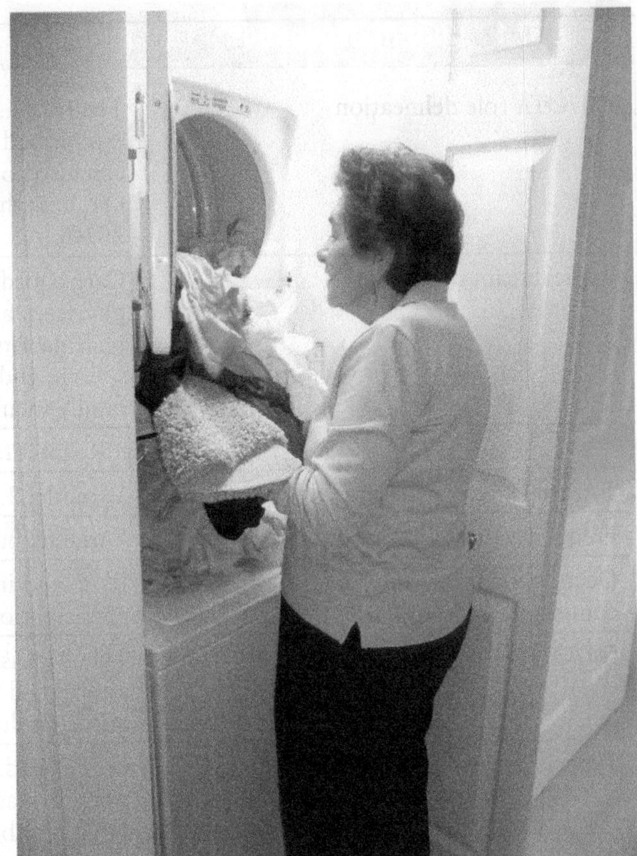

Figure 37.3 Following home modifications, this older adult performs laundry tasks in a well-lit area using principles of body mechanics.

Workplace Modification

Many older adults want and/or need to work beyond the traditional 65-year retirement age. To remain competitive in the workforce, older adults may require certain adaptations including a modified work schedule (e.g., shorter days), a modified work environment (e.g., improved lighting, supportive seating), and/or modified tasks (see Fig. 37.4). An OT practitioner is the ideal clinician to analyze the job, the environment, and the schedule and work with the client and the employer to facilitate continued employment.

Senior Centers and Adult Day Programs

Many older adults access neighborhood senior centers or attend day programs to receive nutritional meals, participate in social activities, engage in exercise, and learn new skills. Adult day programs also provide respite for caregivers. These are ideal settings for OT practitioners to provide consultation or direct services to groups of individuals focusing on prevention. For example, OT

FROM THE FIELD 37.3

Home Adaptation

There is so much more to a comprehensive home evaluation (note: this is completed by an OT) than removing throw rugs and installing grab bars. Use all your knowledge and skills when helping to enable an older adult to remain at home safely and independently. As an OT practitioner, you have knowledge about how client factors such as vision loss, decreased strength, or decreased cognition influence participation. As an OT and OTA team, consider partnering with a contractor who has the knowledge of materials (e.g., types of tiles that provide friction) to make the best recommendations for home adaptations and renovations.

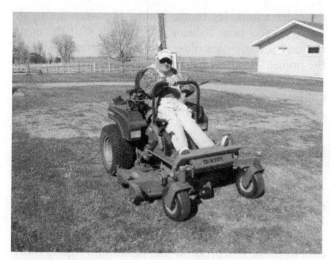

Figure 37.4 A 69-year-old farmer with a disability uses a lawn mower with an adapted foot plate and extended levers on the control panel.

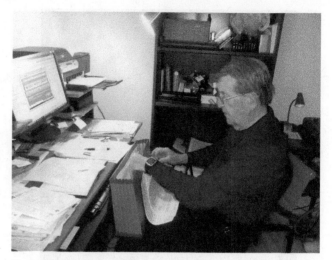

Figure 37.5 In retirement, this older adult remains independent in his financial affairs.

practitioners have the appropriate skill set to lead a fall prevention group and are skilled in developing and leading groups that facilitate social participation. Walking groups and healthy cooking groups are two other examples of relevant groups that an OT practitioner might organize at a senior center or adult day program. If one has expertise in teaching yoga or tai chi, teaching these Eastern skills adapted for older adults is popular and has been shown to improve balance and overall health (Lee & Ernst, 2012). Organizing support groups, such as a monthly low-vision group, provides education, support, and socialization for older adults living with vision loss. As many older adults who attend day programs have dementia, practitioners must be creative in adapting activities to support participation by adults with varying cognitive abilities. The role of the OT practitioner at senior centers and adult day programs is broad and varied based on the needs of the specific environment and the individuals who attend.

Retirement

Leaving a job, even a job one did not enjoy, is rarely easy. Retirement can come with a change in social connections and social status, a change in financial status, and a change in productivity. Helping individuals and groups explore previous and/or new interests and finding ways to remain productive and engaged are important to assure a positive transition to retirement (see Fig. 37.5). Occupational therapy practitioners have the skills needed to analyze the factors that might support and the barriers that might limit continued participation past retirement.

Low-Vision Rehabilitation

Although no longer "emerging," this area of practice with older adults is growing and is less traditional than a facility-based environment. Older adults with vision loss deal with unique challenges in occupational performance and benefit from an OT practitioner skilled in this specialty area. Working in conjunction with an optometrist in an outpatient setting, going into the homes of older adults, or providing talks on strategies to help continue participation at senior centers or adult day programs are all within the scope of OT practice (please also refer to Chapter 31, *Vision*).

Driving Rehabilitation and Community Mobility

Many older adults choose to continue to drive well into their retirement years. Driving rehabilitation can help maintain independence in this area of occupation. Additionally, many older adults need help deciding when to retire from driving and finding other methods of transportation that will fit their skills and lifestyle and enable them to continue to engage in their occupations of choice. Occupational therapists work in programs that provide assessments for older adults to determine if they are able to continue to drive safely. There is an important role for OT practitioners to advocate for transportation options including arm-to-arm paratransit, taxi voucher programs, and other accessible public transportation options.

Health and Wellness/Prevention

Older adults are living longer (United States Census Bureau, 2011) but as importantly, they want to remain healthy during those additional years. Evidence shows that it is never too late to begin exercising (Jette et al., 1999). Helping older adults remain active and find ways to incorporate safe exercise into their daily routine is within the scope of occupational therapy practice (see Fig. 37.6). We understand that exercise comes in all shapes and sizes just as older adults do. OT practitioners are well suited to help older adults find the best match for an exercise/activity program.

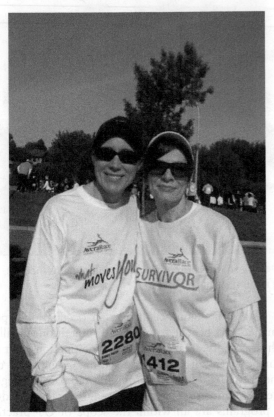

Figure 37.6 This woman who is a survivor of cancer celebrates her health by participating in her first 5-km walk/run event at age 60 with her daughter.

Along with exercise, eating a healthy diet is important to staying healthy. Many older adults struggle to continue cooking and eating habits and preferences may change. Promoting healthy nutrition through fun recipes, social eating environments, daily logs, and routines are just a few of the ways an OT practitioner may address the nutritional needs of older adults.

Sleep is an area of occupation within the *Occupational Therapy Practice Framework III* (AOTA, 2014). Frequent bathroom trips, lack of exercise during the day, medications, and chronic health conditions are just a few of the reasons older adults may struggle to get the amount of sleep their body needs. Occupational therapy practitioners are skilled in analyzing the situation to understand the underlying cause and addressing this to promote healthy sleep habits.

All of these *health and wellness* interventions are relevant to older adults in many practice settings including traditional and nontraditional settings. The environment of the practice setting will determine how addressing healthy aging might be reimbursed.

Community Design

To remain active and engaged, it is important for older adults to participate in community activities, yet often, community environments are not accessible or safe for older adults. Icy roads, limited opportunities to sit and rest, and poor lighting are just a few of the environmental challenges older adults encounter outside of the home. Occupational therapy practitioners have the skills to consult with and advocate to private businesses, public employers, and community organizations for safe and senior-friendly community environments.

Grief and Loss

As previously mentioned, older adults face many losses, not the least of which is dealing with the loss of their spouse or other aging family members and friends. These losses can lead to social isolation. As OT practitioners, we understand the value of participation in valued activities to prevent depression and isolation. Helping older adults find avenues to express their grief and ways to move forward is an important role. Although grief and loss is part of aging, depression and social isolation do not need to be.

Animal-Assisted Therapy

As with people of all ages, many older adults find the company of a pet or other domesticated animal to be comforting and, in some cases, a means of achieving physical activity. Occupational therapy practitioners who are specifically trained in animal-assisted therapy use animals as an intentional part of the intervention process in order to address therapy goals. Animals can be used in therapy to achieve improvements in physical, social, emotional, and cognitive well-being and have been used with older adults across a range of therapy settings, including long-term care, dementia units, hospice, inpatient rehabilitation, and outpatient programs, among others. For example, animals can assist in therapy to address activity tolerance by having the patient complete a pet grooming activity; they may also be integrated into a therapy session addressing bimanual upper extremity function by completing brushing, grooming, and other pet care activities that force the use of both extremities at the same time. Animal-assisted therapy is another method that OT practitioners can use to achieving positive outcomes with the clients they serve (From the Field 37.4).

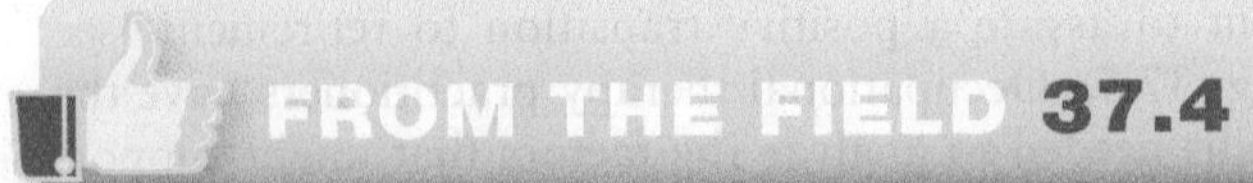

The "Most Important Thing"

It is not about a specific therapy as much as it is that I care for them. Whatever their goals are, I want that for them. My patients spend time with me because I treat them as the most important thing.

Summary

Older adults have stories, experience, and wisdom to share with OT practitioners. We must take the time to truly listen to our clients to understand their abilities, their routines, their goals, and even their dreams. By carefully listening and observing, we can facilitate their participation in their occupations of choice. As one ages, physical, social, and financial changes can influence one's ability to do those activities that are important and meaningful. Yet, older adults want to remain engaged; they want to give to others; they want to be productive. As a future OTA, you have the knowledge and skills to help them achieve these goals!

Review Questions

1. All of the following are normative age-related changes EXCEPT:
   a. Sarcopenia
   b. Decrease in elasticity in tissues throughout the body
   c. Difficulty with temperature regulation
   d. Congestive heart failure

2. Which of the following is a government-funded income program relevant for retired older adults?
   a. Social security
   b. Medicare
   c. Medicaid
   d. Older Americans Act

3. Which of the following might prevent an older adult from aging in place?
   a. Physical environment of their current home
   b. Social support
   c. Medical status
   d. All of the above

4. The role of the OT practitioner in emerging practice areas is dependent upon which of the following?
   a. Scope of practice
   b. Reimbursement
   c. Creativity of practitioner
   d. All of the above

5. Which of the following is a true statement regarding hospice?
   a. Hospice care can be provided in the home, hospital, long-term care facility, or in a stand-alone hospice facility.
   b. Hospice care is appropriate for those with a terminal illness, when a physician believes the individual has one year or less to live.
   c. The key role of the OT practitioner working with a client on hospice is to improve strength and endurance, facilitating independence.
   d. OT intervention is typically provided on a daily basis for the duration of time the client is on hospice.

6. Which of the following is a normative age-related change?
   a. Age-related macular degeneration
   b. Cataract
   c. Osteoporosis
   d. Urinary tract infection

7. Which of the following settings might be considered an emerging practice area for occupational therapy practitioners working with older adults?
   a. Skilled nursing facility
   b. Providing home care in the older adult's freestanding home
   c. Senior center
   d. Outpatient clinic

8. Although the makeup of interdisciplinary teams varies depending on the needs of the client, typically, at a rehabilitation hospital, along with the OT practitioner, the team includes all of the following EXCEPT:
   a. Physiatrist
   b. Volunteers
   c. Social worker
   d. Recreational therapists

9. Reducing falls and injury resulting from falls in older adults has become a major public health initiative. Many risk factors increase the likelihood of falling and it is important to consider these in fall prevention programs. Which of the following is NOT a major risk factor?
   a. Marital status
   b. Cognitive status
   c. Visual impairment
   d. Unsafe environments

10. There is an increasing need for OT practitioners to work in the area of productive aging for several reasons including all of the following EXCEPT:
    a. The number of older adults is growing, due to the baby boomer population.
    b. The number of opportunities for OT practitioners to work with kids is decreasing.
    c. Individuals are living longer.
    d. Older adults want to remain in their home for as long as possible.

Practice Activities

Read one book about aging, such as *Still Alice* by Lisa Genova or *Old Friends* by Tracy Kidder. After you have read the book, reflect on the following questions:

a. What might an OT have done to enable the individual to participate more fully in occupations of choice?
b. How do you think the individual would have defined "productive aging"..., that is, what was important to him/her?

Learn a hobby from an older adult. Teach it to your classmates. Identify at least three ways the activity might be adapted or modified for a variety of functional impairments such as upper extremity hemiplegia, decreased bilateral fine motor coordination, or decreased activity tolerance.

Spend several hours with an older adult that you know. First interview them, asking them about their daily routines, their interests, and the people they spend the day with. Carefully observe how they perform their activities in their home environment. Document your observations. Repeat the same activity with an older adult living in a skilled nursing facility. Compare and contrast your observations. In what ways were they similar? In what ways were they different?

Acknowledgments

We gratefully acknowledge Jacqueline Dobson, Karen Duncan, and Jeanette Justice, occupational therapy assistants who shared *From the Field* notes with us.

References

AARP. *Aging in Place: A State Survey of Livability Policies and Practices*; 2011. Retrieved from http://www.aarp.org/home-garden/livable-communities/info-11-2011/Aging-In-Place.html

Administration on Aging. *A Profile of Older Americans: 2011*; 2011. Retrieved from http://www.aoa.gov/aoaroot/aging_statistics/Profile/2011/docs/2011profile.pdf

American Occupational Therapy Association. *2010 Occupational Therapy Compensation and Workforce Study*; 2010. Bethesda, MD: AOTA Press, Inc.

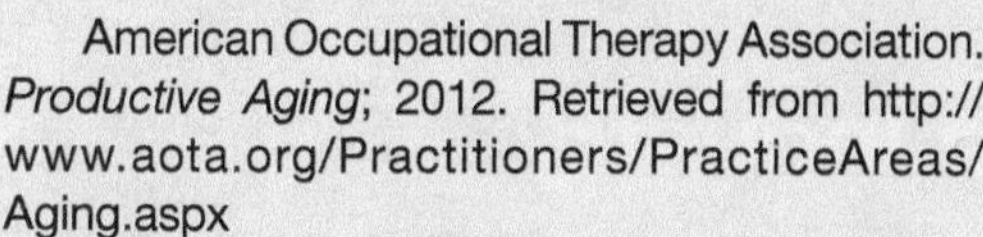

American Occupational Therapy Association. *Productive Aging*; 2012. Retrieved from http://www.aota.org/Practitioners/PracticeAreas/Aging.aspx

American Occupational Therapy Association. Occupational therapy practice framework: domain and process (3rd ed.). *Am J Occup Ther* 2014;68(Suppl. 1):S1–S48. http://dx.doi.org/10.5014/ajot.2014.682006

American Seniors Housing Association. *Senior Living for the Next Generation: A View Through the Lens of the Experienced Adult Child*. Washington, DC: Author; 2011.

Butler RN. The study of productive aging. *J Gerontol B: Psychol Sci Social Sci* 2002;57:323.

Centers for Medicare and Medicaid Services. *What's Not Covered by Part A & Part B?*; n.d.a. Retrieved from http://www.medicare.gov/what-medicare-covers/not-covered/item-and-services-not-covered-by-part-a-and-b.html

Centers for Medicare and Medicaid Services. *What does Medicare Part A Cover?*; n.d.b. Retrieved from http://www.medicare.gov/what-medicare-covers/part-a/what-part-a-covers.html

Dar K. Alcohol use disorders in elderly people: fact or fiction. *Adv Psychiatr Treat* 2006;12:173–181.

Eckert MA. Slowing down: age-related neurobiological predictors of processing speed. *Front Neurosci* 2011;5(25). doi:10.3389/fnins.2011.00025

Farber N, Shinkle D. *Aging in Place: A State Survey of Livability Policies and Practices*; 2011. Retrieved from http://assets.aarp.org/rgcenter/ppi/liv-com/aging-in-place-2011-full.pdf

Freeland KN, Thompson AN, Zhao Y, et al. Medication use and associated risk of falling in a geriatric outpatient population. *Ann Pharmacother* 2012;46(9):1188–1192.

HealthyPeople.gov. *Older Adults Objectives*; 2012. Retrieved from http://www.healthypeople.gov/2020/topicsobjectives2020/overview.aspx?topicid=31

Jette AM, Lachman M, Giorgetti MM, et al. Exercise—it's never too late: the strong-for-life program. *Am J Public Health* 1999;89(1):66–72.

Lee MS, Ernst E. Systematic reviews of t'ai chi: an overview. *Br J Sports Med* 2012;46:713–718. doi:10.1136/bjsports80622

Leland NE, Elliott S. Special issue on productive aging: evidence and opportunities for occupational therapy practitioners. *Am J Occup Ther* 2012;66:263–265.

Leland N, Elliott SJ, Johnson E. *Occupational Therapy Practice Guidelines for Productive Aging Community-Dwelling Older Adults*. Bethesda, MD: AOTA Press; 2012.

National Institute of Mental Health. Older adults: depression and suicide facts; 2007. Retrieved from http://www.nimh.nih.gov/health/publications/older-adults-depression-and-suicide-facts-fact-sheet/index.shtml

National Institute on Deafness and Other Communication Disorders. Research to improve the lives of people with communication disorders. 2010. Retrieved from http://www.nidcd.nih.gov/health/statistics/Pages/quick.aspx

Peterson EW, Finlayson M, Elliott SJ, et al. Unprecedented opportunities in fall prevention for occupational therapy practitioners. *Am J Occup Ther* 2012;66(2):127–130.

Rath T, Harter J. *Well-Being: The Five Essential Elements*. New York: Gallup Press; 2012.

Teixeira AR, Goncalves AK, Freitas CDLR, et al. Association between hearing loss and depressive symptoms in elderly. *Int Arch Otorhinolaryngol* 2010;14(4):444–449.

Triple Tree. *Innovation & the Health Care Needs of Seniors*. 2011. Retrieved from http://www.triple-tree.com/research/innovation-and-the-health-care-needs-of-seniors

United States Census Bureau. *The Older Population: 2010*. 2011. Retrieved from http://www.census.gov/prod/cen2010/briefs/c2010br-09.pdf

Additional Resources

Span P. *When the Time Comes: Families with Aging Parents Share their Struggles and Solutions*. New York: Springboard Press; 2009.

Vaillant GE. *Aging Well*. New York: Little, Brown and Company; 2002.

CHAPTER 38

Work and Industry

Michael J. Urban, MS, OTR/L, CEAS, MBA, CWCE

Key Terms

***Dictionary of Occupational Titles* (DOT)**—A two-volume set that describes the general characteristics and physical job demands in relation to lifting weight requirements and frequency ratings.

Functional capacity evaluation (FCE)—A systemized, intensive, short-term evaluation that focuses on major physical tolerance abilities related to musculoskeletal strength, endurance, speed, and flexibility.

Maladaptive behavior—The client's inability to adjust or adapt to a particular situation.

Occupational Information Network (O*NET)—Online resource for obtaining information about job requirements.

Work conditioning (WC)—An "intensive, work-related, goal orientated conditioning program designed specifically to restore systemic neuromusculoskeletal functions, motor function, range of motion, and cardiovascular/pulmonary functions" to help the client return to work (APTA, 2009).

Work hardening (WH)—A "highly structured, goal-orientated, individualized intervention program designed" to return the client back to work (APTA, 2009).

Learning Objectives

After studying this chapter, readers should be able to:

- Define the difference between work hardening, work conditioning, and FCE.
- Explain occupational therapy's role in work and industry.
- Understand key components to a successful industrial rehabilitation program.

Introduction

As occupational therapy practitioners, our diverse skill set helps clients engage in their daily occupations across the life span and allows us to work in unique environments. One area of specialization is the field of industrial rehabilitation, also commonly referred to as return-to-work programs or work and industry. As we explore this practice area, you will learn about the different components that make up industrial rehabilitation programs. You will also read about different skill sets an OT practitioner needs to be successful in this practice area.

Occupational Therapy's Role in Industrial Rehabilitation

The *Occupational Therapy Practice Framework III* defines **work** as "labor or exertion; to make, construct, manufacture, form, fashion, or shape objects; to organize, plan, or evaluate services or processes of living or governing; committed occupations that are performed with or without financial reward" (Christiansen & Townsend, 2010, p. 423 in AOTA, 2014, p. S20). As we age, the primary area of play in childhood is replaced by work in adulthood and shapes how we go about interacting with our environment. Many people define who they are in adulthood through the work they do. It is for this reason that when individuals suffer an injury requiring a significant amount of time to return to work, the greater the risk is for developing depression and other maladaptive behaviors, which may limit their success in returning to work in their previous capacity (Franche & Krause, 2002). As an OTA, your level of understanding of psychosocial and physical impairment will help you to increase clients' self-efficacy and regain confidence to perform their job after injury. When practicing in the area of work and industry, you must also understand the whole body, and not just treat the upper extremity region as may be the norm in other practice settings in which physical therapy practitioners treat the lower body and occupational therapy practitioners treat the upper body. For instance, a thorough understanding into the biomechanics of how the muscles work in the legs and how dysfunction can impact the ability to lift an item is crucial in the work and industry practice setting. It is more than an in-depth understanding of body mechanics. In the work and industry setting, you must also have a strong sense of psychological processes to provide a holistic approach in your treatments.

When working in the industrial rehabilitation practice area, you may find yourself working outside the parameters of a traditional outpatient setting. You may travel between different employers on a daily basis and provide treatments in-house versus off-site at a therapy clinic. On-site (on the job) treatment is ideal as you can apply real life intervention and help employee and employer create a safer work environment. To note, the first time you go to a client's workplace, it is incumbent upon you to learn the job-related safety requirements to keep you and the employee or client (both terms will be used interchangeably) safe. It is also strongly recommended that you request a general tour of the facility to learn what may be available on-site to use for "real-time" treatment.

Examples of industrial rehabilitation settings that you may work in include warehouses, manufacturing plants, science labs, office spaces, surgical rooms, construction sites, and military bases. A complete understanding of what tasks the employee is responsible for per their job description is essential. Today, you will likely find that

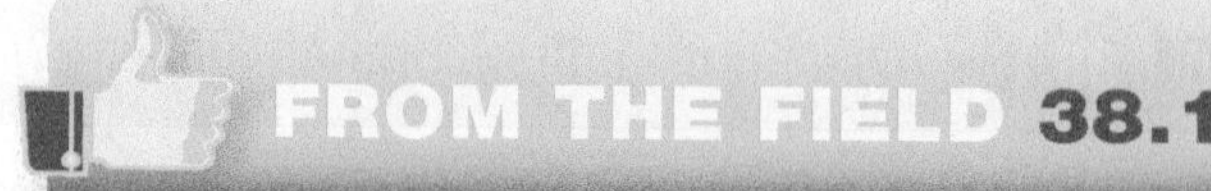

O*NET

For those with easy Internet access, the Occupational Information Network (O*NET) now replaces the *DOT*. It was developed by a private company in conjunction with the US Department of Labor. The *DOT* is discussed in this chapter because some facilities continue to use it as a reference tool.

many employees will be required to perform certain job functions outside of their job descriptions. Prior to any site visit, you or the supervising OT who conducted the evaluation should have already asked the client's supervisor or human resources representative for a complete job description. If you are unable to obtain one, ask the employee to describe his/her job functions. Even if you do obtain a description, go ahead and ask the employee to describe his/her job duties so you can understand what is expected of the client from his/her perspective. It may be quite different than the written description. Once this information is obtained, you will need to reference the job description with the ***Dictionary of Occupational Titles* (DOT)** (DOL, 1991), which is a two-volume set that describes the general characteristics and physical job demands in relation to lifting weight requirements and frequency ratings. **The Occupational Information Network (O*NET)** is an online resource that contains this same information (From the Field 38.1).

The chart in Table 38.1 was created by Leonard N. Matheson, who worked closely with the Department of Labor (DOL) to develop a classification system for rating job functions and frequency of characteristics. This chart used in conjunction with the *DOT* and O*NET work classification and employee job description provides you with valuable information as to the capacity you need to train your client to achieve in order to have a safe return to work.

Case Example for Using the *DOT*

Mr. Sparks is a 32-year-old firefighter for the city of New York who sustained a lower back injury while rescuing a victim from an apartment building fire. Mr. Sparks has had 12 weeks of traditional physical therapy and now has mild to no pain, but still lacks the overall strength and confidence to return to work. The doctor and worker's compensation case manager have referred him to your industrial rehabilitation program to further condition and strengthen his body (and mind) to return to work. A full job description was provided and the client shared additional information about his daily job functions. The

TABLE 38.1 Physical Demand Characteristics of Work

Physical Demand Level	Occasional (0%–33% of the workday)	Frequent (34%–66% of the workday)	Constant (67%–100% of the workday)	Typical Energy Required
Sedentary	10 lb	Negligible	Negligible	1.5–2.1 METS
Light	20 lb	10 lb and/or walk/stand/push/pull of arm/leg controls	Negligible and/or push/pull of arm/leg controls while seated	2.2–3.5 METS
Medium	20–50 lb	10–25 lb	10 lb	3.6–6.3 METS
Heavy	50–100 lb	25–50 lb	10–20 lb	6.4–7.5 METS
Very heavy	Over 100 lb	Over 50 lb	Over 20 lb	Over 7.5 METS

Matheson LN (1993). Reproduced with permission by L.N. Matheson, PhD. Understanding METS and MET Testing (June 17, 2010). Retrieved from: blog.matheson.com/blog/bid/24928/Understanding-METS-and-MET-Testing

supervising OT conducted the evaluation and asked you to begin a work hardening (WH) program. The focus is to be on strengthening the client's cardiovascular health and core strength with the aim to return to work in four weeks. Results of the initial occupational therapy evaluation reported his core strength to be about a 4/5 with no complaints of pain with testing, but noted the client could only lift 20 lb from the floor to waist level. What the evaluating therapist and job description did not tell you is how much a firefighter should be able to lift. This is very important information to have in order to strengthen Mr. Sparks' back to be able to handle the demands that could be expected upon the job (Table 38.1). The *DOT* description of a firefighter is as follows:

> **373.364-010 FIRE FIGHTER** (any industry)
>
> Controls and extinguishes fires, protects life and property, and maintains equipment as volunteer or employee of city, township, or industrial plant: Responds to fire alarms and other emergency calls. Selects hose nozzle, depending on type of fire, and directs stream of water or chemicals onto fire. Positions and climbs ladders to gain access to upper levels of buildings or to assist individuals from burning structures. Creates openings in buildings for ventilation or entrance, using ax, chisel, crowbar, electric saw, core cutter, and other power equipment. Protects property from water and smoke by use of waterproof salvage covers, smoke ejectors, and deodorants. Administers first aid and artificial respiration to injured persons and those overcome by fire and smoke. Communicates with superior during fire, using portable two-way radio. Inspects buildings for fire hazards and compliance with fire prevention ordinances. Performs assigned duties in maintaining apparatus, quarters, buildings, equipment, grounds, and hydrants. Participates in drills, demonstrations, and courses in hydraulics, pump operation and maintenance, and firefighting techniques. May fill fire extinguishers in institutions or industrial plants. May issue forms to building owners, listing fire regulation violations to be corrected. May drive and operate firefighting vehicles and equipment. May be assigned duty in marine division of fire department and be designated Firefighter, Marine (any industry).
>
> *GOE: 04.02.04 STRENGTH: V GED: R4 M2 L3 SVP: 6 DLU: 81* (DOL, 2012).

Looking at and understanding all the information you have, both the subjective client function and the objective information provided in the *DOT* or *O*NET* may be very overwhelming to some. But the objective information is essential for comparison to the information provided by the employer and client. The last line of the description (*GOE: 04.02.04 STRENGTH: V GED: R4 M2 L3 SVP: 6 DLU: 81*) contains many pieces of valuable information to help summarize the job characteristics. "GOE" (DOL, 2012) stands for guide for occupational exploration, which lists out a broad interest of the occupation; in the case of firefighter, 04 represents protective. The next category listed is the strength required for the job. A firefighter is listed as a "V," which refers to very heavy (see Table 38.1). This translates to being aware that you will need to train Mr. Sparks to be able to occasionally handle over 100 lb at various levels on the job.

The "GED" (DOL, 2012) refers to general education development, which are the formal and informal job education requirements expected of an individual. "SVP" stands for specific vocational preparation, which, when looking at the coding, explains the time required to learn the skills for the job performance. "DLU" represents the date of the last update to the job description

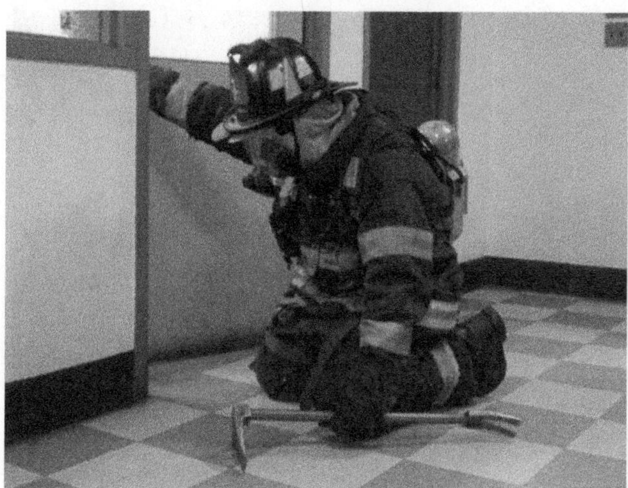

Figure 38.1 A firefighter conducting a simulated search and rescue in full turnout gear, respirator mask, oxygen tank, and Halligan tool.

in the book. Taking this information in hand, if Mr. Sparks' job title was different, such as fire chief or fire inspector, different classifications would be noted. It is very important to make sure you are accurately selecting the appropriate job classification from the *DOT* or from O*NET in order to train a client to the necessary work level (Fig. 38.1).

When the Job Title Is Not Listed

When consulting the *DOT* or *O*NET*, you may find that the job title you are looking for is not listed. So, then what do you do? You must select and use a listed title that is close to the client's job description. Then you must document what and how you decided upon the particular job's physical demand classification for which you are training your client. This discovery process is important and must be immediately conveyed to your supervising therapist and all members of the interdisciplinary team you will be working with.

Members of the Rehabilitation Team

When working in the work and industrial setting, you will be working as part of an interdisciplinary team. It is important to know who is on this team and what their roles are in this process. Some states may require certain disciplines to be involved in the treatment team. Being aware of and following your state and local laws and regulations when working in a program to avoid being out of compliance are critically important. Working with the team, you will be one of many to help a client return to work. Members of an interdisciplinary team may consist of any of the following:

1. Physicians (other than psychiatry)
2. Worker's compensation case manager
3. Employer
4. Client
5. Occupational therapist/occupational therapy assistant
6. Physical therapist/physical therapy assistant
7. Social worker/psychologist
8. Nurse
9. Psychiatrist

These are just a few team members who you may see or interact with to help a client return to work. Being clear of your role in the entire process will enable you to be an important part of the client return-to-work process.

Work Hardening

Treating a client requires a general understanding of the two main types of treatment approaches typically seen in industrial rehabilitation programs. The two programs are work hardening (WH) and work conditioning (WC) programs. **Work hardening** (APTA, 2009) is defined as a "highly structured, goal-orientated, individualized intervention program designed" to return the client to work. WH programs are interdisciplinary and use real or simulated work activities to retrain the client to return to work. Activities must be designed to address and restore the "physical, behavioral, and vocational functions of the client by addressing the safety, productivity, physical tolerances, and behavioral components of the injured worker" (APTA, 2009). Either type of program can be run at the employer's work site if space is allocated or in a private clinic setting.

WH program treatment sessions are typically provided 5 days per week for up to 8 hours a day. The client may work directly with you for a whole day or for a portion of it. WH programs incorporate a component of real or simulated work activities and positions designed to strengthen the client (APTA, 2009). Client safety must be at the forefront of the OT practitioner's mind throughout the entire WH rehabilitation process.

To be enrolled in a WH program, a client should have a targeted job or job plan for return to work. Clients must be committed to the program and view their attendance and participation in the program as if they were going to work. If the program is part of a worker's compensation claim, the client is being compensated for time missed from work (From the Field 38.2).

Work Conditioning

Work conditioning (WC) is defined as an "intensive, work-related, goal orientated conditioning program designed specifically to restore systemic

FROM THE FIELD 38.2

Clients and the Clock

From the outset and as a requirement for attendance, it is strongly suggested that you and your team members have clients "clock" in and out. When a client frequently shows up late or misses scheduled treatment sessions, sit him/her down and have a talk. You may find out that the client may be missing appointments for reasons such as having trouble paying for transportation to the clinic because a worker's compensation check was late or did not come at all.

And if a client is to be at therapy at 8 AM and continually shows up at 8:30 AM without calling to let you know that he/she is going to be late, you need to track this and directly address the client with your concerns. Ask the client if this was typical behavior when at work and if it was acceptable and tolerated. When clients miss appointments or cancel frequently, the physician and case managers need to be aware of this, for the client might be deliberately delaying treatment or having legitimate financial difficulties that impact getting to therapy.

neuromusculoskeletal functions, motor function, range of motion, and cardiovascular/pulmonary functions" to help a client return to work (APTA, 2009). WC focuses on restoring a client's physical capacity and function to work. The team intervention process does not usually include many other disciplines than those who are usually associated with WH. A typical WC treatment process generally ranges from 3 to 5 days per week for up to 4 hours per day (APTA, 2009).

WC programs typically do not have the job simulation component that comes with WH. But, as an OTA, you may want to trial clients in certain job-required positions in order to help a client feel secure about his/her ability to return to work (Fig. 38.2). WC is sometimes used as a transition from traditional therapy into WH when a client needs to focus less on manual therapy provided in traditional therapy and more on strengthening and job skill retraining. When a client cannot tolerate a full day of treatment, or even a simulated 5-day work week, a WC program is often indicated. The purpose of WC is to help increase a client's physical tolerance to transition into a WH program and ultimately progress

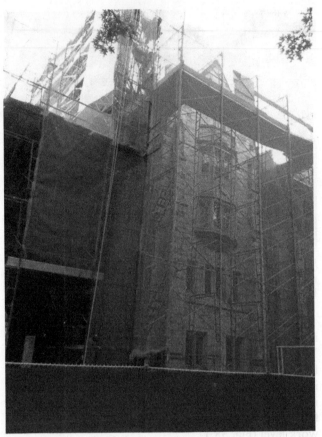

Figure 38.2 Clients may have to return to adverse climates and work environments for which they will need to feel confident to complete.

toward the end of goal of returning to work. If the client is unable to complete this transition, a functional capacity evaluation may be ordered.

Functional Capacity Evaluation

Functional capacity evaluation (FCE) are used at various points throughout the rehabilitation process. The FCE (Matheson, 2003) is a systemized, intensive, short-term evaluation focusing on major physical tolerance abilities related to musculoskeletal strength, endurance, speed, and flexibility. The FCE tracks a client through a full day of testing completed by an OT, which can range from 2 to 8 hours, depending upon a variety of client and environmental factors. These factors may include functional cumulative tolerance throughout the testing day based on the physical demands of the task like weight or positioning. Although testing will be completed by an OT and/or other discipline, as an OTA working on an interdisciplinary team, you must understand the purpose of this evaluation and be able to pull valuable information from the report. Figure 38.3 is a sample page from an FCE report, which ranges in length from 5 to 20+ pages.

Summary of Sitting, Standing, and Sustained Working Tolerances

Mr.Xxxxxxxx demonstrated sitting, standing, and sustained working tolerances which suggests that he is capable of performing 8 hours of work in the light work strength category. Mr.Xxxxxxxx is capable of ligting in the light category for 26 minutes with increased reports of discomfort and functional pain. Mr.Xxxxxxxx used good body mecharics and positioing to minimize neck and low back imitation.

Job Simulation

Mr.Xxxxxxxx completed an assortment of functional job simulation tasks to assess his tolerance levels and ability to complete the tasks. Mr.Xxxxxxxx completed stair climbing with a high-rise hose pack, uncharged hose drag, equipment carry forcible entry, confined search, adn rescue. Mr.Xxxxxxxx did not the a additional 50 pound weighted vest

Stair climbing consisted of Mr.Xxxxxxxx removing a high-rise hose pack (58 lbs) off its testing shelf of a height of 56 inches and then proceeds to descend and ascend four flights of stairs. Mr.Xxxxxxxx was instructed to descend and ascend the stairs at his own pace. He completed the task with a confidence level of 2/10 with 10 equal to total codidence to perform job function and a 9/10 paing rating.

Uncharged hose dragrequires Mr.Xxxxxxxx to drag an uncharged fire hose and multitask fog nozzle down a conidor for 94 feet with one 90 degree bend till he crosses a marked line. At this point Mr.Xxxxxxxx is was asked to drop to one knee and pull 100 feet of uncharged hose a cross the line. He completed the task with a confidence level of 3/10 with 10 equal to total confidence to perform job function and a 7/10 pain rating.

Equipment carry requires Mr.Xxxxxxxx to unload a reciprocal saw (31.5 lbs) and a simulated chain saw (31 lbs) off its resting place of 26 inches tall one at a time and place on the ground. Mr.Xxxxxxxx is then asked to pick up the equipment and carry them around two 90 degree bends and around one cone to then return the equipment on the shelf. The total carrying distance is 138 feet with 62.5 pounds. He completed the task

Figure 38.3 Example section of a functional capacity evaluation report.

In this report, a summary of a client's sitting, standing, and sustained working tolerances proceeds each section, which explains in detail how the client was evaluated and his/her overall performance on the testing. The report also notes if testing was conducted over a 1- or 2-day period and if any portion of testing was stopped due to either safety factors that would have further harmed the client due to the nature of his/her diagnosis or physical demands required by the task. A good FCE will also report on factors noted to further screen for any underlying depression, self-limiting behaviors, and lack of effort with testing. There are well-documented standards and methods that dictate how to administer the FCE based upon different methodologies the clinician was trained to do. When following a client in a WH or WC program, if it has not already been done, you may suggest an FCE be conducted early on in the program if there are doubts regarding evaluation results due to **maladaptive behaviors.**

Maladaptive behavior is a client's inability to adjust or adapt to a particular situation. This should not be interpreted that the client is being untruthful about his/her limitations and impairments. Instead, maladaptive behavior can be viewed as due to the severity and/or nature and duration of the injury, there is a misperception on the part of the client as to what he/she is able to perform. Maladaptive behavior can also be noted in terms of client reports of pain and disability. As an OT practitioner, it is critical to establish good client rapport with a client in order to gain his/her trust to help a client understand this misperception of the disability and help him/her learn what are, in fact, within reasonable limits to perform (From the Field 38.3).

Further Training and What You Need to Know

Being successful in this specialty area of practice requires a strong background in common orthopedic conditions, general anatomy and physiology, general cognitive/psychological interventions, and principles in whole body exercise training. It is also important to learn about local and state insurance and worker compensation laws and to review common job functions related to industries in your community that you may frequently be dealing with. And finally, in order to better understand the job performance demand, do not hesitate to ask a client's employer if you can go to the work site to observe someone doing the same job as your client (Fig. 38.4).

It is also important to be aware if a client has legal counsel involved in his or her work-related injury

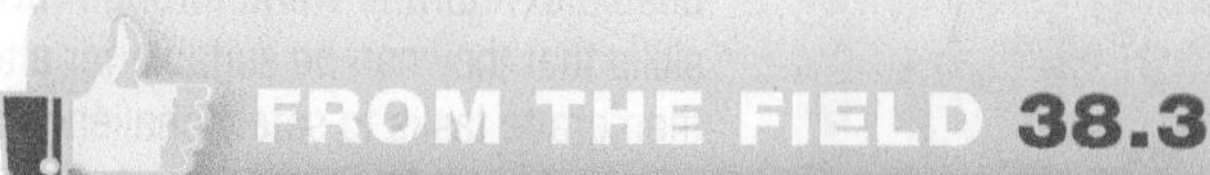

The Role of Depression in Work-related Injuries

The longer an individual is out of work, the less likely they are to return to work. Literature also supports the relationship between depression and higher rating on perceived pain and disability (Wasan et al., 2010). Knowing this is the case with work-related injuries, early identification of underlying depression and provision of meaningful opportunities to achieve skills needed for successful return to work early on in a safe manner is imperative.

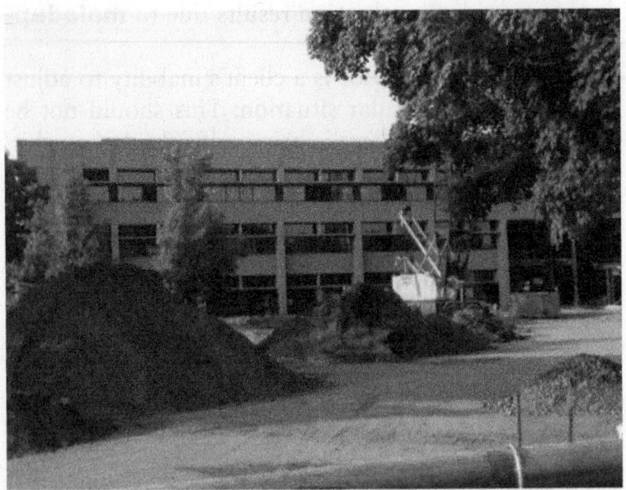

Figure 38.4 Some jobs such as construction workers, factory workers, and even firefighters and police will face workplace environments that are ever-changing.

case. This may potentially lead to interference between worker's compensation case managers, employers, and the client's ability to communicate and progress through the rehabilitative process in a timely manner. This may also mean that you may potentially be subpoenaed as witness for either side regarding things you document, so *documentation must be clear, concise, detailed, and objective*. If your notes are brief, subjective, and/or vague, when you review them to prepare for testimony, you may not be able to recall important facts. You need to be knowledgeable in all things you are administering and documenting on for every client you work with. If you are not, when being questioned in a court of law, there is high potential to appear foolish and to be open for potential legal matters and, in extreme cases and depending on your state regulatory board policies, to loss of professional licensure.

Summary

As an OTA, you have the exciting opportunity to work in a collaborative environment to help clients in the final stage of rehabilitation regain the necessary skills to return to work. Blending a strong background in psychosocial well-being and in total body workout approaches, your role in the process will help a client initially regain work tolerance stamina and strength in a WC program or progress to the more rigorous demands of a WH program. In a WH program, you will have the opportunity to educate the client in lifelong skills to use at work and to help master key job functions after sustaining an injury. You will use your knowledge of human anatomy and mental health to help retrain these individuals. For those who are unable to return to work, through review of a functional capacity evaluation, you will help them seek other skills that they can be suitable for alternative employment. Your skills as an OTA will help you choose and then grade tasks to safely challenge clients and help them overcome any maladaptive behaviors that may impact their ability to perform to their fullest potential in the programs. For further detailed information to support occupational therapy's role in industrial work program settings, please refer to the American Occupational Therapy Association (AOTA) official statement titled *Statement: Occupational Therapy Services in Facilitating Work Performance* that can be found in the AOTA's official documents.

Review Questions

1. What is the difference between work hardening and work conditioning?
2. Who can be members of a work hardening program?
3. What vital information does the *Dictionary of Occupational Titles* or O*NET tell an OT practitioner?
4. Define maladaptive behaviors.
5. What is physical job classification category for someone who has to occasionally lift between 20 and 50 lb?

True or False:

6. Occupational therapist assistants can perform an FCE.
   a. True
   b. False
7. Firefighters are classified as a heavy physical job classification.
   a. True
   b. False
8. Occupational therapy assistants should have a strong background in total body workouts when working in a work hardening/work condition program.
   a. True
   b. False
9. Work condition programs have a psychiatrist working as part of the main interdisciplinary team.
   a. True
   b. False
10. Obtaining a job description for your client's job functions is not an important piece of information to gather.
    a. True
    b. False

Practice Activities

Go to the Department of Labor's Web site and locate the *Dictionary of Occupational Titles*. http://www.oalj.dol.gov/libdot.htm

a. Look up the job description for 2 to 3 jobs that are common in your community.

b. Identify what physical job demand classification the job falls into.

c. Create a job simulation and exercise program for each of the jobs researched for a client with a lumbar disc herniation at L4–L5.

Develop/list a job simulation flow sheet of activities for a client with lower back injury. Use the Department of Labor's *Dictionary of Occupational Titles* or O*NET for job reference of any job selected.

Research depression and the effect upon human functional performance. Prepare a list of signs and symptoms of depression related to Table 1 of the *Occupational Therapy Practice Framework III* (AOTA, 2014) components to create a job simulation activity for a firefighter with a shoulder injury and medically diagnosed depression.

References

American Occupational Therapy Association. Occupational therapy practice framework: domain and process (3rd ed.). *Am J Occup Ther* 2014;68(Suppl 1):S1–S48. http://dx.doi.org/10.5014/ajot.2014.682006

APTA. *Guidelines: Occupational Health Physical Therapy: Work Conditioning and Work Hardening Programs BOD G03-01-17-58*. 2009, December 14. Retrieved from APTA.org: http://www.apta.org/uploadedFiles/APTAorg/About_Us/Policies/BOD/Practice/OccupationalHealthWorkConditioningHardening.pdf

DOL. *Dictionary of Occupational Titles Fourth Edition, Revised 1991*. 1991. Retrieved from United States Department of Labor (DOL): http://www.oalj.dol.gov/libdot.htm

Franche R-L, Krause N. Readiness for return to work following injury or illness: conceptualizing the interpersonal impact of health care, workplace, and insurance factors. *J Occup Rehab* 2002, December;12(4):233–265.

Matheson L. The functional capacity evaluation. In: Andersson G, Demeter S, Smith G, Andersson G, Demeter S, Smith G, eds. *Disability Evaluation*. 2nd ed. Chicago, IL: Mosby Yearbook; 2003:1–35. Retrieved July 14, 2012, from http://www.epicrehab.com/abstracts/ama-fce.pdf

Roy Matheson and Associates, Inc. *Matheson Philosophy on Workplace Safety and Work Injury Evaluation: Understanding METs and MET Testing*. 2010, June 17. Retrieved from roymatheson: http://blog.roymatheson.com/blog/bid/24982/Understanding-METs-and-MET-Testing

Wasan MM, et al. Differences in pain, psychological symptoms, and gender distributions among patients with left- vs right-sided chronic spinal pain. *Pain Med* 2010;11:1373–1380.

CHAPTER 39

Management and Education: Career Options for the Occupational Therapy Assistant

Tia Hughes, DrOT, MBA, OTR/L

Key Terms

Academia—The community of faculty and students within higher-level educational.

Education—The act of receiving information, knowledge, or skills through a learning process.

Leadership—The act of leading others through influence and guidance for a common purpose. Leadership requires one to create energy and motivation in such a way that others choose to follow.

Management—The act or system of governing, directing, or controlling individuals in a work environment in order to achieve objectives.

Mentoring—The interaction that takes place between individuals with the goal of elevating a less experienced individual through the sharing of skills, knowledge, and perspectives.

Supervision—The process of overseeing the work of others. This often includes the acknowledgment of responsibility for those individuals who are under one's care.

Teaching—The act of imparting knowledge or skills to others.

Learning Objectives

After studying this chapter, readers should be able to:

- Define the management and educational career roles for the occupational therapy assistant.
- Demonstrate an understanding of the skills and aptitudes required of the occupational therapy assistant in the areas of management and education.
- Determine the additional education and expertise required of the occupational therapy assistant wishing to transition to a full-time managerial or educational role.

Introduction

How many times as an OTA student have you been asked where you wish to work after graduation? Most find this simple question a challenge. There are so many options in the clinical, community, and school settings to choose that narrowing it down to a population is often the best that most students can determine while in their studies. Few feel comfortable in this stage of their career considering positions in **management** or in **academia**. Why should you consider these career options? Because the art and occupation of a manager is a component of many jobs that do not even include the title of "director." You should consider it because all practitioners should be educating others: clients, family members, other professionals, and the community. It is only natural that this gift for **teaching** transitions into the academic environment.

What Is a Manager?

Merriam-Webster defines a manager as "one that manages" and "a person who directs a team or athlete" (Merriam-Webster, 2012). For those working in occupational therapy, control is needed in a number of ways. Client scheduling, program marketing, billing, quality control, equipment and space management, and personnel **supervision** are only a few of the areas that practitioners may be responsible for. Could someone with a degree in management be a better option to control these areas? Possibly, but someone without a comprehensive understanding of therapy may not be able to connect with employees, market to stakeholders, or manage the flow of therapy services in an acceptable way (Jacobs, 2011). The ideal situation and the choice of most agencies is promotion of practitioners to managers. Practitioners who show management potential or better have management experience often find themselves in official management positions. Ask any boss, and they will tell you that their position creates different stressors than the clinic, but the satisfaction that comes with leadership is extremely fulfilling. Being able to foster an environment that runs smoothly, offers quality therapy services, creates financial sustainability, and engages team players can override those stressors that may accompany a management role. One of those stressors is management ethics.

Since many managers in occupational therapy are also practitioners, there may be dilemmas that arise because of dual responsibilities. The manager is in a sandwich of responsibility: answering to both the practitioners and the upper management. Decisions made to improve productivity will have a direct effect on the day-to-day clinical practices. Following the *Occupational Therapy Code of Ethics* (AOTA, 2015) may help practitioners focus on the ultimate target of the position: quality patient care. Managers often have to challenge themselves by asking if a company practice will meet this goal. If the manager finds that patient care can be upheld, they must then determine how to integrate change into a system of individuals who may have been comfortable working in a status quo manner. Convincing good employees that there may be another effective and efficient way to conduct business requires empathy, communication, and patience (From the Field 39.1).

Ethical dilemmas can also arise from conflicts of interest. Conflict of interest errors are common when there are financial incentives that involve diminished or compromised patient care. Market pressures on administration can translate to increased productivity pressure on practitioners. It is critical that the occupational therapy manager find the best balance between meeting the financial needs of the business, providing exceptional care for clients, and creating an enjoyable work environment for employees. In order to do this, a good manager will need to make regular adjustments depending upon financial statements, client population, and the personalities and needs of staff. These challenges may be difficult to envision while completing your academic program, but it should not be. Whether you ultimately take on a role of leadership or remain a strong supporter of your managers, an understanding of the role will benefit the entire team (From the Field 39.2).

The therapy team is often made up of individuals who work well with one another and like one another. What happens when you manage your friends? It is very common for a practitioner to take on a management role in a department in which he or she was working. A practitioner who was a coworker on Friday may be a subordinate on Monday. Although some individuals may find this to be an easy transition, others struggle with the ethical and personal challenges of managing one's friends. It is important that you, as a new manager, are able to support and discipline all employees in a fair and equitable fashion. Showing favoritism can take place in many forms: giving better shifts, promoting, allowing attendance exceptions, or following exclusion behaviors. In occupational therapy, we value having a variety of roles. It is more difficult when we experience this role conflict. Honest communication with one's friend prior to and during the transition takes maturity, patience, and compassion. These are some of the qualities of a good leader.

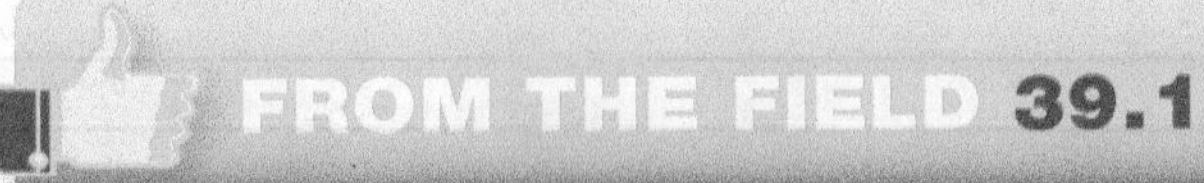

FROM THE FIELD 39.1

Acknowledge Others

Make a point to acknowledge employee strengths. Weaknesses should be addressed with plans of actions and not with criticism.

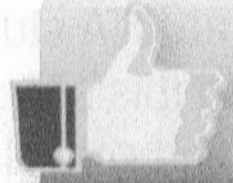

FROM THE FIELD 39.2

Loyalty

Loyalty is a tricky business. One of the challenges that come with leadership is the issue of loyalty. Are you loyal to the employer or your team? The answer should be "both." Shielding loyalties, acting secretly, or appearing two faced is a quick way to lose the respect of both administration and the therapy team.

What Is a Leader?

You could spend thousands of dollars purchasing books related to understanding leadership, leadership styles, training principles, and ways to improve one's leadership skills. **Leadership** is a concept that has been studied throughout history. If you consider your own upbringing, you can identify those individuals you were drawn to, whom you would follow, and who you wanted to be more like. These individuals may or may not have had an official management job. Here, we see one of the most important findings in the world of business management; not all managers are good leaders, and not all leaders are identified as managers. Managers hold an official job designation, whereas leaders have a combination of natural and learned leadership skills (From the Field 39.3).

What kind of leader will you be? Many theorists have identified continuum models of leadership (Schneider et al., 2009). These models span from a style of managerial control to a style of employee control (Fig. 39.1). Why would someone choose one extreme or another? Those who choose an autocratic style of leadership may do so because of their personal beliefs surrounding how management should take place. It may also be affected by the environment that the leadership occurs in. If there is a "lack of control" in the occupational therapy department with apparent issues with attendance, quality, timeliness, attitude, or policy compliance, a manager may need to use more of a heavy-handed approach. On the other hand, a manager may oversee a number of highly motivated and independent practitioners who do well with a more stand back approach to supervision. The "free-rein" style would be more suited for this environment. It is important for managers to note that leadership styles may change over time based upon staffing and situational context. You may be more authoritative at times and more laid back at others. Being able to change over time and not hold onto a rigid standard of behaviors is important. This ability to change over time is one of those characteristics often cited as a true leadership skill. Flexibility and awareness will guide you as a leader in determining which leadership style to rely upon (Fig. 39.1).

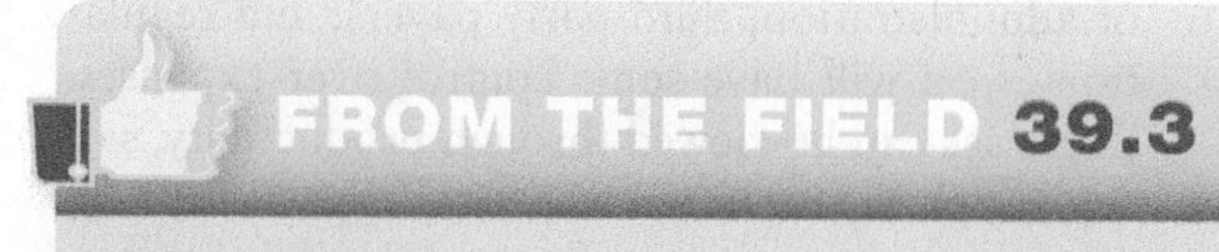

Leadership Skills

Skills necessary for leadership in occupational therapy:

- Organization
- Interpersonal communication skills
- Clinical competence
- Information literacy
- Time management
- Fairness and impartiality
- Honesty
- Budgeting and basic accounting
- Interviewing skills
- Flexibility

Management in Occupational Therapy

There are several domains in occupational therapy management. As is with most roles, individuals may be stronger in certain areas and weaker in others. Recognizing these areas of weakness and taking the steps to grow in them is part of the lifelong learning process that all practitioners are expected to follow. These domains will be addressed briefly below:

- Budgeting: as a manager, your department will have to show financial responsibility. This comes from the ideal balance between income and expense. Although client billing may be the result

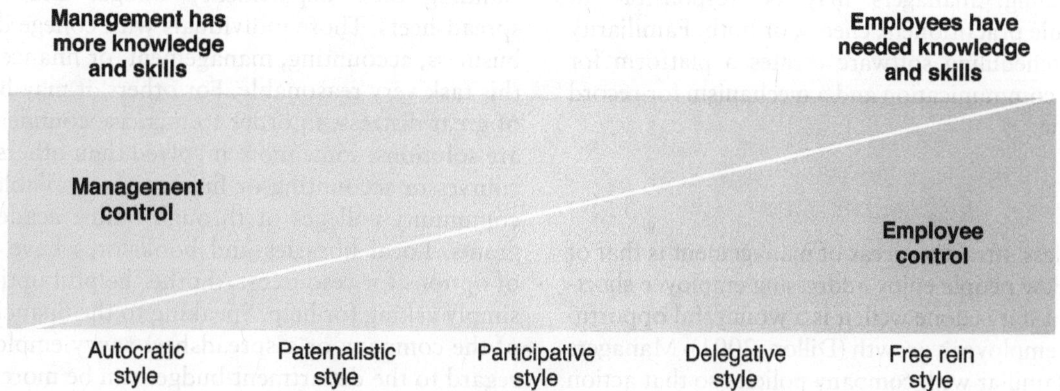

Figure 39.1 Management style continuum. (Source: U.S. Army Handbook. *Military Leadership*. 1973.)

of administration, third-party payers, and regulations, you will have some control over expenses. Expenses can be viewed through productivity, salary, supplies, and benefits.

- Staffing: managers are often responsible for hiring and firing staff. Being familiar with reading resumes, understanding legalities related to interviewing, and perfecting interview skills are crucial for hiring. If the situation arises that a staff member needs to be let go, there will need to be administrative support to ensure that disciplinary processes were followed following company policy, federal regulations according to the Equal Employment Opportunities Commission (EEOC), and possible union rules.
- Marketing: who is better at marketing a program than the individuals that know it best? Managers may be required to participate in formal and informal marketing strategies. Formal marketing includes market needs assessments, community perception studies, advertising, and follow-up satisfaction reviews. Informal marketing can take place in a number of ways. Participation in community events, visits to referral sources, speaking in the community, student intern programs, and organizing tours in your department are just a few ways to market and show off your organization.
- Supervision: managers are expected to observe the working habits of employees, oversee documentation, ensure a safe work environment, and address problems in those areas if and when they arise.
- Education: staff education may occur formally through organized training sessions or informally in individual or small group interactions. Managers are responsible to ensure that practitioners are competent and current in intervention practices. Managers should also be proactive in continuing their own education in the area of management. Courses, seminars, and readings are extremely helpful for those practitioners who do not have a degree in management.
- Scheduling: managers may be responsible to schedule practitioners, clients, or both. Familiarity with scheduling software creates a platform for easier communication and a mechanism for record keeping.

The Role of Discipline

One of the less attractive areas of management is that of discipline. Few people enjoy addressing employee shortcomings, but if it is done well, it is a wonderful opportunity for the employee's growth (Dillon, 2001). Managers need to be familiar with company policies so that action plans can address specific policies or shortcomings. The field of occupational therapy affords therapy managers with a familiar process. Much like the process of client care, goal achievement comes from identification of problems followed by a measurable action plan with which to achieve those goals. Making areas for improvement and goals that are behavioral and associated with outcomes will minimize personality differences and impartiality in the clinic.

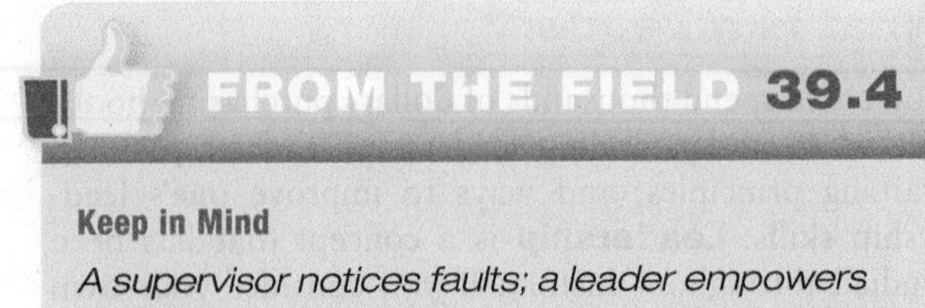

Keep in Mind

A supervisor notices faults; a leader empowers change.

How can you reduce the amount of discipline that occurs in your facility? One way is through early **mentoring**. Employees who have a designated mentor to assist in company orientation and modeling have fewer difficulties related to expectations in the work environment (Burtner et al., 2009). Direct mentoring does not need to be the responsibility of the manager. Instead, the manager should delegate reliable role models to be mentors for new employees. This offers the ideal level of attention for the new employee while acknowledging the work and expertise of the more experienced employee. When you are mentored by someone other than your manager, there is a sense of safety and privacy. This safe zone allows the new employee to make mistakes without fear of discipline or job risk (From the Field 39.4).

Preparing for the Occupation of Management

The world of personnel management is a more familiar territory to OT practitioners than the world of accounting. Managers are often responsible for understanding their department's budget and respective spreadsheets. Those individuals with college degrees in business, accounting, management, or finance will find this task very reasonable. For others, it may be a cause of great distress. In order to increase confidence, there are solutions; some more involved than others. College courses in accounting or finance are available at local community colleges or through online academic programs. Local libraries and bookstores have a wealth of options for resources. Another helpful option is just simply asking for help. Speaking to the financial officer of the company or a spreadsheet-savvy employee with regard to the department budget can be more personal and helpful.

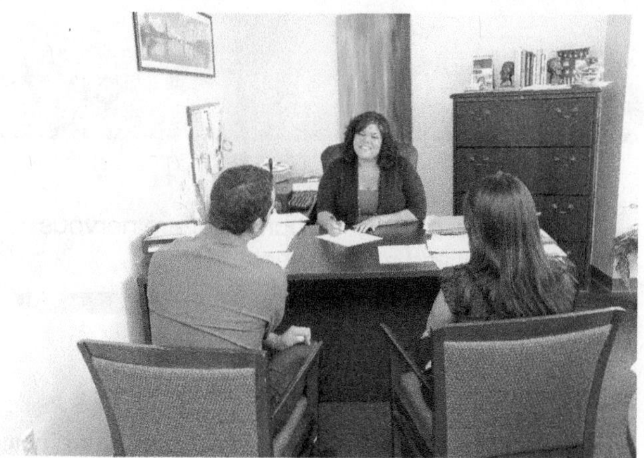

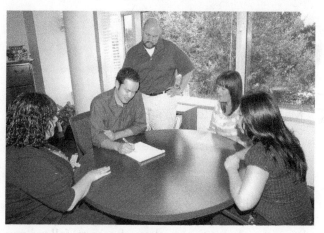

Figure 39.2 Managers who make a point of sharing company information with staff build loyalty and camaraderie.

Not all management work is budgeting and discipline (Figs. 39.2–39.4). Managers are chosen by the interpersonal skills that are noticed by others. These interpersonal skills need to be relied upon for empowerment and conflict resolution. The ability to communicate with a team to create an atmosphere of respect, interest, and enthusiasm is as critical as understanding a department budget. To enhance this ability, it is important to know your own style as well as that of others. Interacting with others in an intentional and respectful manner will lend more positive outcomes no matter the actual leadership styles of those involved. Understanding the culture and history of the organization is also a key to a good working relationship. Assessing oneself using tools such as *StrengthsFinders* can be beneficial in identifying strengths and weaknesses related to the job (From the Field 39.5).

In today's environment of outcome driven businesses, it is critical that managers in occupational

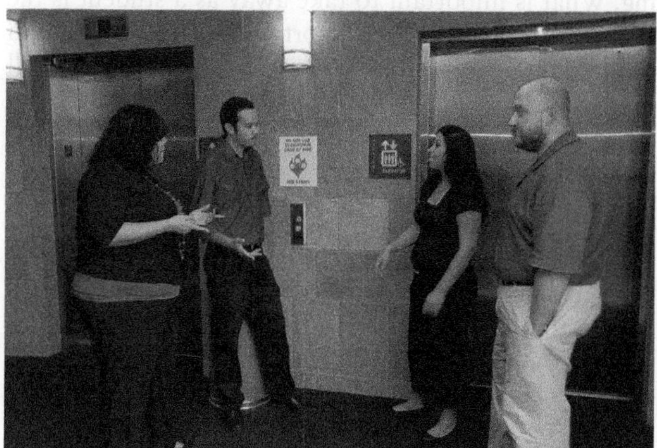

Figure 39.3 Management and leadership happen in the halls. You don't need formal meetings and scheduled retreats to make meaningful impact on your team. Be the "everyday mentor."

Figure 39.4 A team working at a table together.

therapy settings participate in organizational assessment strategies. You may be familiar with the terms "quality assurance" or "continuous quality improvement." These are processes that organizations use to assess a process, identify areas for improvement, implement strategies, and assess the outcome of those strategies. This comprehensive plan shows internal and external shareholders that the organization is indeed guided by a focus on quality. Volunteer to be on one of these committees as a member to better understand the process and participate in solution.

An area that may be a role of the occupational therapy manager is that of research support. Depending upon the setting and the mission of the setting, there may be research activities that take place within the occupational therapy department. If this is the case, the manager must understand the client safety and confidentiality policies related to research at the site. If a manager feels that participation in research may compromise the safety or benefit of the client, it is the manager's responsibility to discontinue the research (From the Field 39.6).

After graduation, OTA students will be introduced to a number of opportunities in various settings, traditional and emerging practice areas. Regardless of the setting, there are needs in each of them for individuals

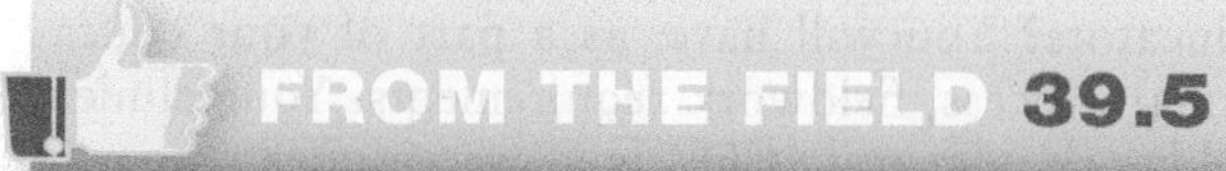

Team Inventory

Do a team inventory: have your team participate in a learning style inventory, a personality inventory, or a strength inventory. Consider the *Myers-Briggs Personality Inventory, True Colors,* or *StrengthsFinders.*

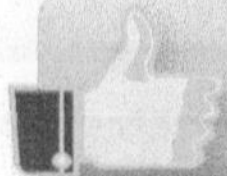

FROM THE FIELD 39.6

Open-Door Policy

Managers need to have an open-door policy that allows staff members to share their concerns and ideas when issues arise.

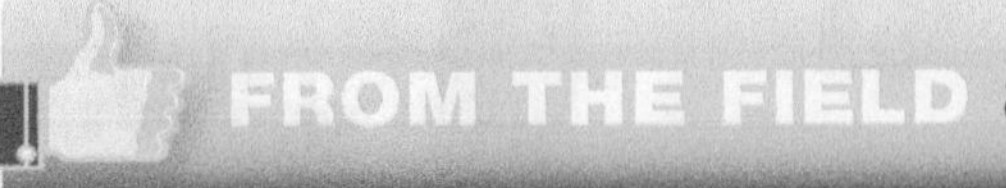

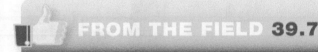

FROM THE FIELD 39.7

Ask for Help

If you want to present a course but are nervous the first time, find a copresenter.

in leadership roles. Whether you aspire to hold an official company position as a manager or you simply want to be a person others choose to follow, you will need to identify and enhance those skills that are seen by others as worthy of following (Townsend et al., 2011).

What Is an Educator?

We have all had educators from the time that we were old enough to participate in classroom activities. We have had educators in public or private schools. We may have had educators as a component of religious training. What about music teachers or dance instructors? These are all educators, and as consumers of **education**, we can all think of characteristics that make a good educator. It may seem premature to consider a role in education while you are still in school, but it is not. You should understand the ever-present need for quality educators in the field of occupational therapy and begin to prepare yourself for that opportunity when it arises.

Education in OT takes a number of forms that we will review. In the simplest of terms, all OT practitioners are educators. The teaching–learning process occurs when we teach a client how to dress following a stroke. We teach family members and caregivers when we explain a sensory diet to a parent or teacher. We teach other health care professionals when we show them how to position a client to avoid contractures. Occupational therapy is, by its very nature, a profession of teaching (Roley et al., 2008).

Where else do OT practitioners use their skills as educators? You will have, as a part of your educational process, fieldwork requirements. Your clinical fieldwork educator (CFE) is a practitioner who will be working with your academic institution to educate you within a clinical setting in order to complement the classroom experiences you have. Within the clinical environment, practitioners may be responsible for occupational therapy staff training. Other opportunities may include corporate training, professional lectures, or interdisciplinary learning modules. Then of course, there are roles within the academic environment.

Academia

Academia refers to those activities that take place within an institution of higher education. Career prospects in academia are almost as varied as the clinical environment. You can participate as a guest speaker, a lab assistant, or an advisory committee member. If you find that you want a larger role in an academic institution, you may start as an adjunct instructor (From the Field 39.7).

An adjunct instructor is an educator who is not a permanent employee of a school, but instead fills a need of the institution. Most adjunct instructors have limited academic responsibilities. They are hired to teach a course, whereas institutional faculty members will have other responsibilities such as advising, committee work, and scholarship.

Faculty may be full time or part time, and appointments may be based upon semesters or a specified number of months per year. These are all terms that would arise in the hiring negotiation phase of employment. Within some academic institutions, faculty will be classified as clinical or academic. What this usually refers to is the type of coursework being taught by the individual. It is even possible to be hired by a college or university to teach students within the clinical environment. You can see how the maze of academics can be confusing. What is important to take away as a student is the fact that there are great opportunities to participate in occupational therapy education for practitioners at all levels of experience. What does it require to be a good educator?

Expectations of an Educator

Something every student will agree with: educators need to know their topic. Fewer things are more frustrating to a student than the feeling that their educator is not competent in their area of discussion. Clinical competence and knowledge of current treatment practice are necessary prerequisites to teaching in occupational therapy. Being an evidence-based practitioner begins in the educational setting. If you are interested in teaching, it is critical that you are able to share current evidence that supports the interventions that you are teaching students to use.

FROM THE FIELD 39.8

Technology

Use technology in the classroom that enhances your topic—don't add technology just to do it.

Those OT practitioners in academia will tell you that the teamwork expectations are no different than they are in the clinical arena. Faculty members must work with other therapy educators in order to ensure a strong, cohesive curriculum. They must also work closely with the other educators on campus for projects related to general education improvement and for institutional enhancement.

What is the workday like? Duties in the educational environment are much different than those of a practitioner. The ebb and flow of workload is less consistent than found in the clinics. For most OTAs, the day in the field is made busy by the expectation of productive client intervention time. There is little "down time" during the day, but clocking out means that the OTA is done for the day. Those who teach must create their entire course prior to the course beginning. This takes a great deal of organizational skill and planning. Successful lectures are a combination of good objective development, clinical competence, awareness of student knowledge, and good public speaking skills (Sladyk, 2001). Think back to an instructor you have had that knew a great deal of information but was not gifted in delivery. You knew they had "book smarts" but struggled in sharing their knowledge in a practical and engaging way. Classes are not meant to be entertainment, but all practitioners should understand that an engaged audience will learn better than one that is disengaged (From the Field 39.8). This is how we address client education in the field of occupational therapy. We must consider the client's interest and motivators as we create a therapy plan of action. In the classroom, there are just many more individuals to consider, but the process is much the same (Figs. 39.5 and 39.6).

Figure 39.5 A teacher laughing with students.

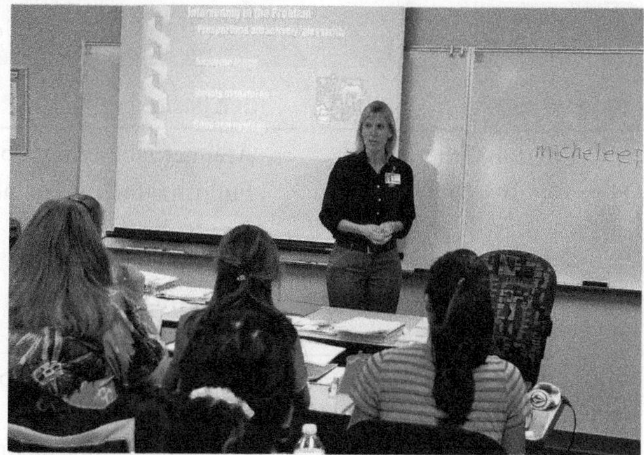

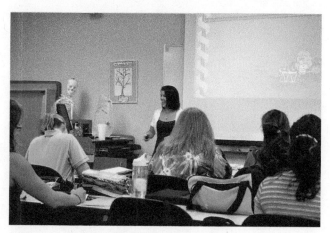

Figure 39.6 Leading a class lecture.

Other tasks of an educator include the development of assessments, choosing supplemental learning materials, tutoring, advising, and grading (Bradshaw, 2011). Many of these tasks do not take place during the workday. Few educators are able to complete grading and lecture development during the day and perform these tasks at night. This is especially true for adjunct instructors who come on campus to teach and then leave. Students must realize that the individual must perform these tasks in their personal time. By the same token, applicants to a teaching position should realize that the day will not necessarily end when they will leave the school. So, what if you did want to take this route after graduation? What would you need to do to obtain a position in an educational setting after becoming an OTA?

Path to a Career in Education

At the time of this publication, the requirements for faculty members in occupational therapy education are identified in Table 39.1.

As you can see, full-time positions require at least a bachelor's degree. For OTA graduates who wish to become teachers in the future, it is necessary to begin work toward a bachelor's degree. For those individuals who decide to return to school, it is suggested that the bachelor's degree is chosen for reasons that improve clinical skills or address leadership skills. Common degrees are in the areas of psychology, sociology, education, health sciences, public health, business, and health care administration.

Do you need to wait until you complete a bachelor's degree before you can start to work on your educator career path? The answer is a resounding "no." Even if you need to start classes toward further collegiate work, there are a number of steps that

TABLE 39.1 Qualifications for Instructors in Occupational Therapy Education

Type of Setting	Job Desired	Qualifications
Occupational therapy assistant program	Adjunct faculty member	Content expert
	Full-time faculty member	Bachelor's degree
	Academic fieldwork coordinator	Bachelor's degree
	Program director	Master's degree and 1 year of FT teaching experience
Entry-level occupational therapy program	Adjunct faculty member	Content expert—graduate work recommended
	Full-time faculty member	Doctoral degree recommended—majority of faculty must have doctoral degree; remainder may have a master's degree.
	Academic fieldwork coordinator	Minimum of master's degree—may be doctoral depending upon make up of faculty
	Program director	Doctoral degree

Source: AOTA. *Accreditation Council for Occupational Therapy Education Standards and Interpretive Guidelines.* 2012. Retrieved from http://www.aota.org/Educate/Accredit/StandardsReview/guide/42369.aspx?FT=.pdf

will improve your chances of becoming an academic instructor:

- Become a clinical fieldwork educator for level I and level II fieldwork students.
- Act as the clinical fieldwork coordinator at your facility.
- Participate in presentations at your facility.
- Offer to present a poster, workshop, or lecture at your state, regional, or national occupational therapy conference.
- Write an article for submission in your local paper, a trade magazine, or a scholarly journal.
- Contact your local occupational therapy school and ask to assist with labs or provide a guest lecture.
- Familiarize yourself with current evidence in the field of occupational therapy.

If you can accomplish some of these steps, you will be able to present a robust resume to the academic institution showing your diligence and perseverance regarding a career in education (From the Field 39.9).

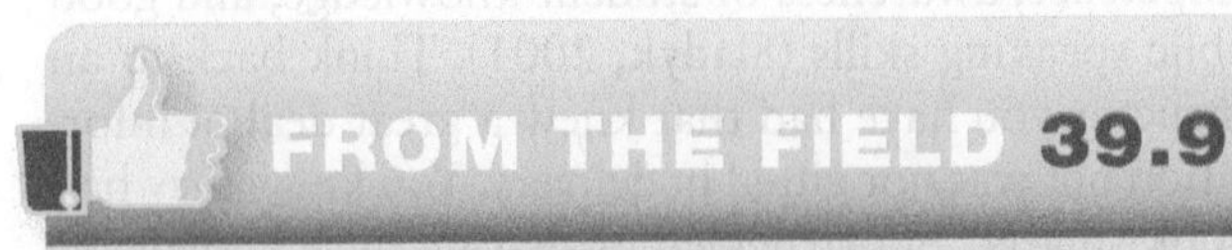

FROM THE FIELD 39.9

Sharing

Don't be afraid to share personal clinical stories with students. Your experiences combined with textbook readings help students to grasp concepts.

Summary

You may be like most OTA students and long for the day when you can begin your career in the clinical setting. You are currently learning about all of the roles and duties you will undertake as you care for your clients. Roles that may you may not have considered are those of manager and educator. The skills that you need to succeed in these roles will serve you in other areas of your life. There is a longstanding question as to whether leaders are born with or learn their skills. Most studies have found that it is indeed a combination. Use those leadership skills you have, and learn more skills that you may not currently have. Share your passions and your experiences on the many paths of education. You are joining a profession that values its entry-level education. Just as important is the value our profession places on the ability to educate our clients, caregivers, health care professionals, and the general public. Embrace the fact that you will walk into the clinic as an educator. Allow the opportunities that await you in the field of occupational therapy to inspire the manager and educator that resides inside of you.

Review Questions

1. Which of the following management style allows for the most employee control?
   a. Participative
   b. Free rein
   c. Paternalistic
   d. Delegative

2. Which of the following ethical dilemma is also a legal dilemma?
   a. Supervising a friend
   b. Having to discipline someone with disabilities
   c. Having a different personality type than a subordinate
   d. Enforcing productivity expectations based on corporate budget only

3. An effective leader:
   a. Is the individual identified as the department manager
   b. Is the individual who employees feel compelled to follow
   c. Is the individual who has a degree in management
   d. Is someone who was born with those skills

4. Which of the following is a responsibility of a manager but not necessarily a leader?
   a. Being a good role model
   b. Following departmental policies
   c. Hiring and firing staff
   d. Communicating with team members

5. Who is the most effective mentor?
   a. The newest employee
   b. Your immediate supervisor
   c. A registered occupational therapist
   d. Someone who can empathize and communicate

6. An OTA with a bachelor's degree is able to teach:
   a. As a guest lecturer
   b. As an adjunct instructor
   c. As an academic fieldwork coordinator
   d. All of the above

7. Which of the following OTA educators are required to have at least a master's degree?
   a. Guest speaker
   b. Adjunct instructor
   c. Program director
   d. Academic fieldwork coordinator

8. Which of the following is most important in an OTA educator?
   a. Professional competence
   b. Public speaking skills
   c. A master's degree in occupational therapy
   d. At least 5 years of experience

9. Which of the following tasks is required of an adjunct instructor in most settings?
   a. Student advisement
   b. Test writing
   c. Committee involvement
   d. Scholarship

10. Which of the following organizations are responsible for occupational therapy education?
    a. NBCOT
    b. AOTA
    c. ACOTE
    d. WFOT

Practice Activities

Create a training module for your classmates. As you create a 10-minute lesson, modify your plan based on the three major learning styles: auditory, visual, and tactile. Consider how you would address the same information as you teach someone who learns in one of these three ways.

Plan your educational path. Considering the degree-level expectation for educators in occupational therapy, use the Internet to locate an educational institution and degree that appeals to you and helps to meet the requirements for a faculty member.

Using the management style continuum in Figure 39.1, consider an employee who is not turning in documentation in a timely manner. Choose three different styles of management, and for each, determine the method you would use to address this disciplinary challenge.

Strengths and weaknesses. Make a list of five strengths and five weaknesses you have regarding leadership. For the weaknesses you list, develop a plan to eliminate or diminish them.

References

American Occupational Therapy Association. *Accreditation Council for Occupational Therapy Education Standards and Interpretive Guidelines*. 2012. Retrieved from http://www.aota.org/Educate/Accredit/StandardsReview/guide/42369.aspx?FT=.pdf

Bradshaw M. Effective learning: what teachers need to know. In: Bradshaw M, Lowenstein A, eds. *Teaching Strategies in Nursing and Allied Health Professions*. 5th ed., pp. 3–21. Sudbury, MA: Jones and Bartlett; 2011.

Burtner P, et al. A model of mentorship in occupational therapy: the leadership of A. Jean Ayres. *Occup Ther Health Care* 2009;3:226–243.

Dillon T. Authenticity in occupational therapy leadership: a case study of a servant leader. *Am J Occup Ther* 2001;55(4):441–448.

Jacobs K. *The Occupational Therapy Manager*. 5th ed. Bethesda, MD: AOTA Press; 2011.

Merriam-Webster. Merriam-Webster Dictionary. 2012. Retrieved from http://www.merriam-webster.com/

Roley S, et al. Occupational therapy practice framework: domain and practice, 2nd edition. *Am J Occup Ther* 2008;62(6):625–683.

Schneider B, et al. Creating a climate and culture for sustainable organizational change. In: Burke W, Lake D, Paine J, eds. *Organizational Change; A Comprehensive Reader*. San Francisco, CA: Josey-Bass; 2009.

Sladyk K. *Clinician to educator: what experts know in occupational therapy*. Thorofare, NJ: Slack Inc.; 2001.

Townsend E, et al. Introducing the leadership in enabling occupation model. *Can J Occup Ther* 2011;78(4):255–259.

U.S. Army Handbook. *Military Leadership*. 1973.

Helpful Websites

1. Accreditation Council for Occupational Therapy Education—http://www.aota.org/Educate/Accredit
2. American Occupational Therapy Association—http://www.aota.org
3. Myers-Briggs Type Inventory—http://www.myersbriggs.org/my-mbti-personality-type/mbti-basics/
4. StrengthsFinder—http://strengths.gallup.com/default.aspx
5. What color is your brain?—http://www.whatcolorisyourbrain.com/

CHAPTER

40 Emerging Practice Areas

Amy Wagenfeld, PhD, OTR/L, SCEM, CAPs

Key Terms

Emerging practice—A multifaceted concept [that] encompasses diverse professional roles, a variety of contexts for the provision of services, as well as the development of innovative business models (Holmes & Scaffa, 2009, p. 81).

Entrepreneur—A person who brings resources together that are needed to start a business (Cole, 1959).

Learning Objectives

After studying this chapter, readers should be able to:

- Understand how keeping current with occupational therapy practice may lead to identification of and implementation of emerging practice areas.
- Extrapolate how the traditional occupational therapy practice areas are uniquely suited for innovation.
- Appreciate the role of entrepreneurism on emerging practice areas.
- Begin to think about new emerging practice areas.

Introduction

As we conclude this unit on practice areas, we have, arguably, covered a great deal of ground with regard to occupational therapy starting with history, to foundations and fundamentals, and to applications, specific conditions, and, in this unit, the broad practice areas identified by the AOTA. As part of the *Centennial Vision*, the AOTA identified the six practice areas you have just read about. Within each practice area are emerging trends. Aligning with their respective traditional practice areas, these trends have been identified to help OT practitioners be poised to respond to society's occupational needs (Yamkovenko, n.d.). We will look carefully at the trends that the AOTA has identified, so please do refer back to the practice area chapters for in-depth information about each traditional practice area. In this chapter, we expand on these traditional practice areas to include unique niche and emerging practice areas that occupational therapy practitioners work within and look at how the scope and fluidity of occupational therapy supports out-of-the-box thinking that may lead to yet more emerging practice areas that are eligible for third-party reimbursement and/or introduce people to the value and importance of occupational therapy who might not otherwise be aware of our profession.

Framing Emerging Practice Areas

Emerging practice can be described as "a multifaceted concept [that] encompasses diverse professional roles, a variety of contexts for the provision of services, as well as the development of innovative business models" (Holmes & Scaffa, 2009, p. 81). An OT practitioner who is an innovator and develops an idea and takes it to market could be called an entrepreneur (Fig. 40.1).

As defined by Cole (1959), an **entrepreneur** is someone who brings resources together that are needed to start a business. The concept of entrepreneurship was first presented by economists in the 18th century and by the 20th century had become closely associated with "free enterprise and capitalism" (Kuratko & Audretsch, 2009, p. 4). Today, entrepreneurship is associated with economic growth and development (Kuratko & Audretsch, 2009). According to the U.S. Small Business Association (SBA, n.d.), qualities that are associated with entrepreneurship include the following:

- Creative
- Inquisitive
- Driven
- Goal oriented
- Independent
- Confident
- Calculated risk taker
- Committed
- Avid learner
- Self-starter
- Hard worker
- Resilient (able to grow from failure or change)
- High-energy level
- Integrity
- Problem-solving skills
- Strong management and organizational skills (http://www.sba.gov/content/entrepreneurship-you)

While an entrepreneur need not have all of the abovementioned qualities, the more he/she does have, the greater the likelihood the business endeavor will succeed. And certainly, an aspiring entrepreneur can learn and adapt some of the skills associated with an entrepreneurial spirit in order to launch a successful idea (From the Field 40.1).

There is a strong relationship between innovation, entrepreneurship, and emerging practice areas. Why? Emerging practice areas identified by the AOTA come into their own because of the OT practitioners working in traditional roles whose vision and innovative ideas enable them to see a better way forward to serve the clients they work with. For instance, what may be seen as mainstream occupational therapy practice today, such as work and industry, was not much more than 30 years ago, novel and "out of the box." As you read this chapter, begin to formulate ideas for entrepreneurial roles within current emerging practice areas, as well as new emerging practice roles that have yet to be fully explored. Think about how you may take some of the ideas that will be discussed below and turn them into your future career path. Or, how you can expand upon

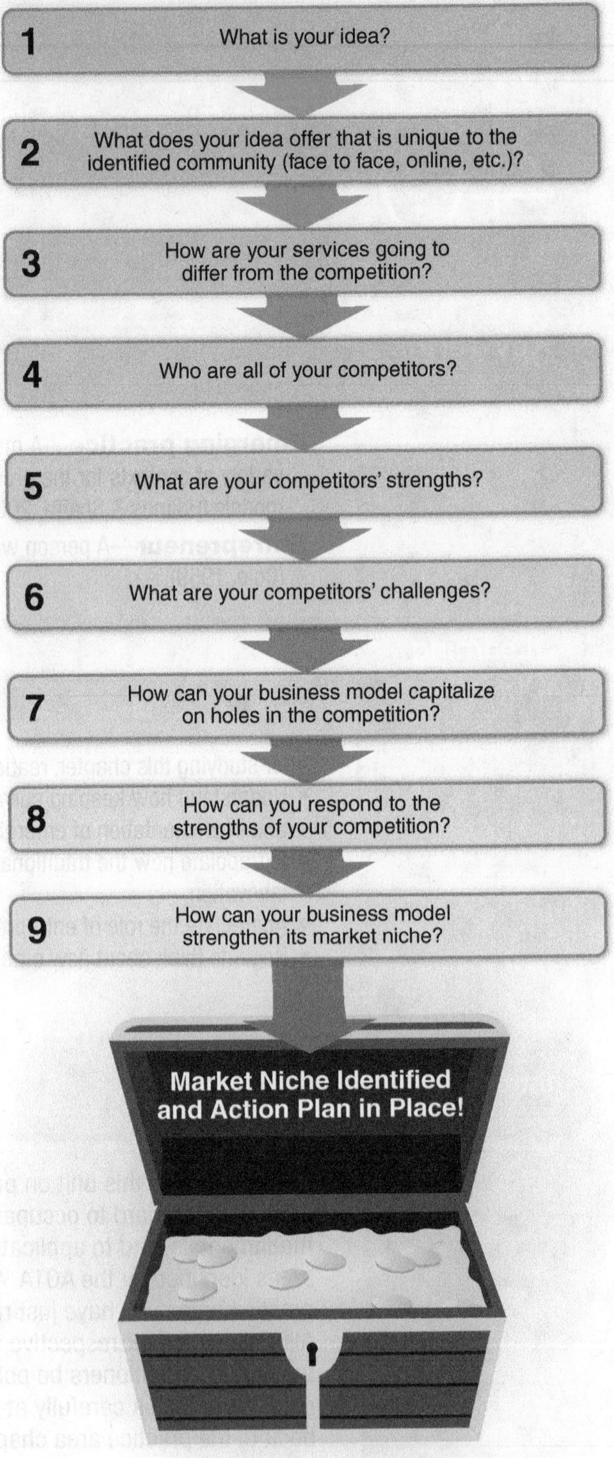

Figure 40.1 Action steps for exploring a market niche. (Adapted from Prabst-Hunt W, ed. *Occupational Therapy Administration Manual*. pp. 63–80. Clifton Park, NY: Delmar, Cengage Learning; 2001.)

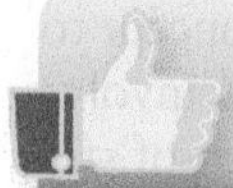

FROM THE FIELD 40.1

Score

The SBA offers a free online or in-person service to anyone interested in starting or growing a business. It is called Service Corps of Retired Executives (SCORE). SCORE is "dedicated to entrepreneur education and the formation, growth, and success of small businesses nationwide." The URL for SCORE is http://www.score.org. As well, the SBA (http://www.sba.gov) provides important information for anyone interested in information about starting and running a small business, including online resources, funding sources, and seminars.

them or use them as a springboard to develop new ideas. Then think about how you will market your ideas and ultimately implement them in your role as an OTA.

And, to keep you apprised of these emerging trends, keep in mind that the AOTA website (http://www.aota.org) contains up-to-date information about traditional practice areas for OT practitioners and the emerging trends within each. Some information is for the general public and others for members only. You are strongly encouraged to explore these sites. Emerging trends may influence the professional path you take as a future OTA.

Traditional Practice Area: Rehabilitation, Disability, and Participation—Traditional Practice Venues: Hospitals, Clinics, Nursing Facilities, Hospice, Home Health, and Day Treatment Facilities

Emerging Trends

Autism in Adults

The *Allsup Disability Study: Income at Risk* showed that for the second quarter of 2011, people with disabilities experienced an unprecedented unemployment rate more than 80% percent higher than people with no disabilities (Allsup Foundation, 2012, http://www.allsup.com). Data from the *National Longitudinal Transition Study Two,* a 10-year study of youth who received special education services, suggests that young adults with autism spectrum disorder (ASD) are less likely to work than most other disability groups (National Center for Special Education Research, 2012). Autism Speaks (2012), the United States largest autism science and advocacy organization for people with autism and their families, reported that regardless of IQ, 9 out of 10 adults with autism are unemployed, with the number of adults with ASD expected to rise to half a million over the next decade. Clearly addressing the needs of adults with autism is a high priority for society, with meeting occupational needs at the forefront.

An emerging role for OTAs might be[1]...vocational horticulture. While there is limited research focused specifically on vocational production-oriented gardening programs for people with ASD, there is a growing body of research supporting the efficacy of such vocationally oriented programs with adults with chronic mental illness and those with physical and intellectual challenges. Similar benefits may hold for individuals with ASD, providing them with much-needed opportunity to learn transferable job skills while being engaged in a meaningful and purposeful occupation.

Cancer Care and Oncology

According to the National Cancer Institute (2015), there are more than 100 types of cancer. It is a leading cause of death (8.2 million people) annually worldwide (Stewart & Wild, 2014). The estimated annual cost of cancer to the United States, excluding incalculable psychosocial costs, is $110 billion, or approximately 2% of the GNP (Cancer Prevention Coalition, UIC, n.d.). About 70% deaths from cancer occur in low- to middle-income countries. Throughout the world, for men, the most common cancer fatalities are (in order) lung, stomach, liver, colorectal, and esophagus. For women, the most common cancer fatalities are breast, lung, stomach, colorectal, and cervical. Tobacco use is the largest preventable cause of cancer in the world. More than 30% of cancers might be cured if detected early and treated adequately. This means not using tobacco, eating a healthy diet, staying physically active, and preventing infections that may lead to cancer. All cancer survivors seeking pain relief might be helped if what we now know about pain control and palliative care were applied (Ten Facts About Cancer, 2006, http://www.who.int/features/factfiles/cancer/10_en.html). Managing pain associated with cancer and cancer treatment includes addressing lymphedema, which is often a side or aftereffect of cancer treatment. Lymphedema management is an area of practice that OT practitioners are increasingly engaging in. In addition to understanding the disease process itself and addressing pain and lymphedema issues, working in oncology entails understanding how psychosocial, fatigue, and cognitive factors also strongly influence a client's functional abilities (Yamkovenko, n.d.).

An OTA might consider creating a family-centered palliative care program in a hospice or care treatment center to improve the quality of the client and family's

[1]Please note that this and all other potential emerging roles for the OTA described in this chapter (and book) are to be carried out under the supervision of an OT.

lives. As well, becoming certified in lymphedema treatment may be another option to explore.

Hand Transplants and Bionic Limbs

Technological advances and ongoing research have made the previously unthinkable a reality. Bionic limbs that are operated via volitional thought and hand transplants are now enriching the lives of those with limb loss and making the impossible, possible (Yamkovenko, n.d.). There are nearly 2 million people living with limb loss in the United States (Limb Loss Awareness, 2012; Ziegler-Graham et al., 2008). About 185,000 new amputations occur each year in the United States. The main causes of limb loss are vascular disease, which includes diabetes and peripheral artery disease (54%), trauma (45%), and cancer (2%) (Limb Loss Awareness, 2012; Ziegler-Graham et al., 2008).

For OTAs interested in this area of practice, designing adapted equipment to make the transition to using prosthetic limbs easier and more palatable to those who have lost a limb may be an option to pursue. Despite the indisputable need for OT practitioners to become involved with this emerging practice area, it requires in-depth expertise and an extensive understanding of neuroanatomy of the upper extremity. It is not a practice area well suited for new graduates of OT or OTA programs.

New Technology for Rehabilitation

Who among us is not in some way shape or form connected to technology? Some of you may be reading this on an e-reader. Some may be texting or tweeting about tomorrow's assignment. Some of you have grandparents or parents who use personal emergency response systems (PERS), "I have fallen and cannot get up" devices. Whether we deem it a blessing or a curse, technology influences all of our lives. For many of our clients, assistive technology may make the difference between independence and dependence. It is also an important and motivating therapy tool. For instance, many applications (apps) seem to have been tailor made for OT practitioners working in most every practice area (Yamkovenko, n.d.). Yet, there is real room for us to create tailor-made therapy apps and to help clients maintain an independent lifestyle.

An OTA can become a therapy application designer. Choose a specialty area and make it happen. Or, integrate smart technology into your practice and measure the outcomes. Remember, evidence is critically important to continue to move our profession forward.

Emerging Niche: Telehealth

As defined by the American Telemedicine Association, telemedicine is "the use of medical information exchanged from one site to another via electronic communications to improve patients' health status" (American Telemedicine Association, 2012, http://www.americantelemed.org). The term is a broader concept to define "remote healthcare that does not always involve clinical services. Videoconferencing, transmission of still images, e-health including patient portals, remote monitoring of vital signs, continuing medical education and nursing call centers are all considered part of telemedicine and telehealth" (American Telemedicine Association, 2012, http://www.americantelemed.org). Telemedicine is not a separate medical specialty. It is important to know that reimbursement fee structures are usually the same for on-site or remote services and that telehealth does not require different billing codes (American Telemedicine Association, 2012, http://www.americantelemed.org). The potential to increase health care access in rural and underserved areas via telehealth has very important positive implications. It expands our scope and potential to provide services to a far wider reaching population. As well, interprofessional communication can be greatly enhanced through telehealth models.

Consider alternating face-to-face therapy sessions with virtual sessions. Think about how best you could involve your clients as active participants in this process. What kind of virtual documentation could you and your supervising OTs develop to keep your clients engaged in the therapy process in between face-to-face visits?

Veteran and Wounded Warrior Care

As of May 2011, the total number of US-active duty military personnel was 1,431,403 (DOD, 2011). The U.S. Department of Veteran's Affairs (VA) reported that there are nearly 25 million veterans (US Department of Veteran's Affairs, 2012). Ongoing US VA research finds that among veterans returning from recent conflicts, post-traumatic stress disorder (PTSD) is diagnosed at ranges from 10% to 18%, which incurs a cost of 4 to 6.2 billion dollars over a two-year period for treatment (Rosenthal et al., 2011). Included within those diagnosed with PTSD are those with additional diagnoses including traumatic limb amputation and mild traumatic brain injury (Dougherty, et al. 2010; Rosenthal et al., 2011). These wounded warriors are in need of complex and ongoing care, not only for themselves but also for their families.

An OTA might work as a civilian or military OTA at VA hospitals or outpatient veteran's treatment centers (From the Field 40.2).

Mental Health—Traditional Practice Venues: Hospitals, Clinics, Rehabilitation Facilities

Emerging Trends

Depression

There is more to depression than simply feeling sad. People with depression often feel a lack of interest or

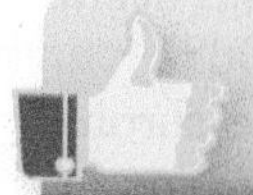

FROM THE FIELD 40.2

Gardening for Wounded Warriors

Recently, I had the honor of spending the day with a group of wounded warriors and veterans at Veterans Farm in Jacksonville, Florida. They have created an accessible farm that specializes in growing blueberries in wheelchair-height containers and a greenhouse for growing hot peppers. The wounded warriors come to the farm to learn farming skills, which they can take home and start their own farming endeavors. The founder of the farm, Adam Burke told me that they value and need OT practitioners to help them with all aspects of the process. You can find out more about the farm is available by viewing the video at http://www.growingagreenerworld.com/episode308/

joy in participation in daily activities and experience symptoms such as:

Significant weight loss or gain
Insomnia or excessive sleeping
Lack of energy
Inability to concentrate
Feelings of worthlessness or excessive guilt
Recurrent thoughts of death or suicide (APA, 2012; 2013)

Depression is the most common mental disorder, but it is treatable (APA, 2012). The most common treatments for depression are medication and psychotherapy, but exercise, a third adjunctive treatment for depression is proving to be very effective in combating depression (APA, 2004). It has been noted that aerobic exercise works quickly and equally as well as medication and talk therapy for men and women with moderate depression over the long-term. The older a person is, the greater the decrease in depressive symptoms (when engaged in an exercise program) (APA, 2012). The greater the duration of an exercise program, the more beneficial it is, and combining exercise and psychotherapy produces the greatest antidepressant effect (APA, 2004). Other studies have shown that a combination of exercise and medication produce positive results, but aerobic exercise itself also has very positive long-term effects on the reduction of depression that surpass the effects of medication alone (Babyak, et al., 2000).

An emerging role for OTAs might be working with mental health clinicians to set up and implement an inpatient exercise program for people with depression. Because we are OT practitioners, the expectation would be that the program has occupational relevance for the participant, that is, meaning and purpose and not just exercise for exercise sake. To that end, it is important to consider the context and environment in which the exercise program would be implemented as well as what the exercise itself would be.

Another role might be working in an outpatient mental health clinic as a community reintegration coordinator or case manager: planning excursions that work to reconnect clients with meaningful community resources, such as public transportation, shopping, medical appointments, and social events.

Recovery and Peer Support Model

Substance abuse (and addiction) is a chronic illness. Substance abuse and addiction are widespread and have a significant negative impact on human health as well as the national economy (Substance Abuse and Mental Health Services Administration, 2011). In 2007 and with regard to crime, health, and productivity, the economic cost of illicit drug use totaled more than $193 billion in the United States (National Drug Intelligence Center, 2011). The most common treatment for substance abuse and addiction is a combination of medication and psychotherapy (American Psychiatric Association, 2007).

Because there is a link between substance abuse and mental health issues, developing a novel way of working in a substance abuse treatment venue to implement therapeutic yoga or tai chi programs that are individualized and client centered is an option. Both of these approaches are an introspective form of exercise, which you now know has positive implications for individuals diagnosed with depression.

Sensory Approaches to Mental Health

Use of physical restraints or placing people with severe mental health challenges in seclusion is physically and psychologically damaging, not to mention dangerous. Many injuries and deaths have been linked to restraint and isolation procedures, yet they are not closely regulated in the United States (Steel, n.d.). While facilities may have policies and procedures, there are no federal guidelines for the use of restraints and isolation in mental health facilities (Steel, n.d.). An alternative to restraint and seclusion methods that is receiving a great deal of positive recognition is sensory integrative-based therapies and sensory rooms.

When a supervising OT deems an OTA competent and skilled with regard to understanding trauma and sensory integration and sensory regulation theory, an OTA may want to plan and implement interventions that are rich in sensory experiences to help clients better self-regulate.

Veterans' and Wounded Warriors' Mental Health

One of the prominent mental health concerns that veteran's face is PTSD. Symptoms associated with PTSD include intense feelings of fear and anxiety that may lead to avoidance of people, places, or situations that could cause re-experience of the trauma (American Psychological Association, 2015). People with PTSD experience self-regulation issues that limit the ability to logically set and achieve goals, to prioritize, and to deal with environmental demands (Tangney et al., 2004). Presenting symptoms of PTSD include thought intrusions, self-absorption, emotional numbing, and hyperarousal. Veterans are also at significant risk for other mental health issues including depression, substance abuse, self-regulation issues, interpersonal issues, and suicide.

An OTA may get involved with service animal training programs that link wounded warriors and veterans with service animals. There is extensive research supporting the mental and physical health benefits that can be derived from connecting people with animals.

Health and Wellness—Traditional Practice Venues: Hospitals, Clinics, Nursing Facilities, Schools, Home Health

Emerging Trends

Chronic Disease Management

According to the Centers for Disease Control and Prevention (CDC), chronic diseases are "noncommunicable illnesses that are prolonged in duration, do not resolve spontaneously, and are rarely cured completely" (CDC, 2009, http://www.cdc.gov). Heart disease, cancer, stroke, diabetes, and arthritis are a few examples of chronic disease (cdc.gov, CDC, 2009). The CDC reports that:

> Chronic diseases cause 7 in 10 deaths each year in the United States. About 133 million Americans—nearly 1 in 2 adults—live with at least one chronic illness. More than 75% of health care costs are due to chronic conditions. Approximately one-fourth of persons living with a chronic illness [also] experiences significant limitations in daily activities. The percentage of children and adolescents in the United States with a "chronic health condition has increased from 1.8% in the 1960s to more than 7% in 2004" (2009).

While older people tend to have a greater tendency to develop chronic diseases, they are increasingly affecting people of all ages and are recognized as a serious health concern in the United States (cdc.gov, CDC, 2009).

An OTA can work with clients who have chronic diseases on community access as well as energy conservation techniques and activity prioritization techniques. The purpose of this role will be to help clients to better manage their lives and optimally participate in what is most meaningful to them.

Obesity

Over the past two decades, the rate of obesity has been rapidly rising (cdc.gov, CDC, 2012a). The cost of obesity in both human and financial terms is enormous. Roughly 37.5% of all Americans are obese, and in 2008, the medical costs associated with obesity were approximately $147 billion (cdc.gov, CDC, 2012a). The CDC notes that medical costs paid by health insurance providers for people who are obese were $1,429 higher than those of normal weight (CDC, 2012c).

An OTA might run goal-oriented graded exercise programs for men and women (not a mixed group, to avoid unintended competition or discomfort) in underserved areas. In doing so, it is important to get community buy-in for the program, so that no member of the program feels marginalized or unwelcomed. Eliciting the support of community leaders is an important way to garner support for any program like this.

Prevention

"An ounce of prevention is worth a pound of cure." While this saying has been around since Benjamin Franklin coined it, it still makes good sense. Basically, this idiom translates into, if people take care of themselves now, there is a higher probability that they will not develop chronic diseases or other negative health conditions later. While it is not an absolute, it is prudent to eat well, exercise, and, otherwise take good care of yourself, to the greatest degree possible relative to one's life circumstances. Today, more than ever, we as a society and policymakers in particular are realizing the importance of prevention, from a personal as well as economic standpoint. Prevention is a concept the occupational therapy profession has long advocated and practiced.

An emerging role for an OTA might be to become a community advocate or become well versed in the prevention programs that your community has to offer and convey this information to clients you work with, no matter the practice area. Throughout life, having access to and the ability partake of prevention programs is critically important for individual, community, and societal health. Well-run prevention programs may help to curtail rising health care costs.

Children and Youth—Traditional Practice Venues: Hospitals, Schools, Private Practice, Home Settings

Emerging Trends

A Broader Scope in Schools

Generally speaking, OT practitioners maintain a strong presence working with children and youth in educational, health care, outpatient, and home-based settings. In fact, one of the more common venues for an OTA to be employed are school (educational) settings. As you may recall from Chapter 1, *Historical Perspectives of Occupational Therapy*, with the passage of several federal laws, provision of free and appropriate educational services for all children was mandated. The laws opened the door for occupational therapy services in the schools. Today, we have come a long way from working with children on handwriting skills (Yamkovenko, n.d.). The role of the OT practitioner working with children and youth has moved in new and exciting directions, especially with regard to the Response to Intervention (RTI), which is a "multilevel prevention system that maximizes student achievement and to reduce behavioral problems." With RTI, "schools use data to identify students at risk for poor learning outcomes, monitor student progress, provide evidence-based interventions and adjust the intensity and nature of those interventions depending on a student's responsiveness, and identify students with learning disabilities or other disabilities" (National Center on Response to Intervention, 2010, http://www.rtiforsuccess.com; Yamkovenko, n.d.).

An OTA might consider developing an inclusive, developmentally appropriate, client-centered, and holistic study skills group for children with identified learning disabilities.

Autism

As of 2014, the CDC suggested that 1 in 68 children (11.3 per 1,000) have been identified with an ASD (Baio, 2014). ASD is five times more common in boys (1:54) than girls (1:252) (cdc.gov, CDC, 2012b). It is the fastest growing serious developmental disability in the United States (http://www.autismspeaks.com). This rise in diagnosis represents a 23% increase since the 2009 report and 78% since the first report was published in 2007. One explanation for the rise in diagnosis is the new way in which children are diagnosed and receive services, but the extent to which these criteria explain the rise in diagnosis is not fully understood. The greatest rises in incidence of diagnosis were among Hispanic children (110%) and black children (91), which are attributed to greater awareness and better identification within these groups (CDC, 2012b, http://www.CDC.gov). This finding does not fully explain the dramatic rise in diagnosis, as across the board there is a rise in diagnosis of ASD among all groups of children. Diagnosis is more frequently being made before age 3, but still, most are not diagnosed until after age 4. There is no medical test to diagnose it, and there is at present no cure for autism (Autism Speaks, n.d.); the diagnosis is based on observable symptoms and parent and teacher report measures.

An OT practitioner could develop and run a social club for children with ASD. A group such as this would address social skills that are often lacking with this population. There might be on site and field trips into the community based on the needs and skills of the group. Autism is a complex disorder and intervention of any type must be carried out with a complete understanding of what is being done and why.

Bullying

No longer is bullying being swept under the rug as a problem that children and teens need to simply work out among themselves. As described by Young and Leventhal (2008), bullying is "an aggressive behavior in which individuals in a dominant position intend to cause mental and/or physical suffering to others, with a prevalence worldwide ranging from 9% to 54%" (p. 133). Whether a child is the recipient, or perpetrator, all are at substantially high risk of mental and physical problems. According to Klomek et al. (2011), "Victims of bullying consistently exhibit more depressive symptoms than nonvictims; they have high levels of suicidal ideation and are more likely to attempt suicide than nonvictims" (p. 3). Cyberbullying has become a serious public health concern, in part because of a recent spate of highly publicized youth suicides following episodes of cyberbullying.

Those OT practitioners employed by school districts or, for that matter, anyone who is interested may join antibullying task forces to help raise awareness of the ways in which occupational therapy's focus on positive occupational performance can help in the fight to reduce face-to-face bullying and cyberbullying.

Childhood Obesity

According to the 2007 to 2008 *National Health and Nutrition Examination Survey* (NHANES), since 1980, the prevalence of childhood obesity has nearly tripled (CDC, 2012b). Approximately 17% (or 12.5 million) of children and adolescents ages 2 to 19 years are obese (CDC, 2012d, http://www.cdc.gov). Additionally, NHANES results indicated that significant racial and ethnic disparities in obesity prevalence among US children and adolescents. In 2007 to 2008, the survey results showed that "Hispanic boys, aged 2 to 19 years, were significantly more likely to be obese than non-Hispanic white boys, and non-Hispanic black girls were significantly more likely to be obese than non-Hispanic white girls" (Ogden & Carroll, 2012).

Consider developing noncompetitive, motivating, and positively focused programs to get children to get up and move at school. OTAs can work with teachers to carve out short duration periods to take movement breaks. The OTA could lead these mini movement sessions or prepare a handbook of process-oriented movement ideas for teachers to implement.

Driving for Teens with Disabilities

A highly anticipated event for teens, whether or not they have disabilities, is learning to drive. It represents a rite of passage on the way to independence. With modifications and specialized driving instruction, many teens with disabilities can earn a full or limited driver's license. The Association for Driver Rehabilitation Specialists (ADED) website (ADED, n.d., http://www.driver-ed.org) contains fact sheets with information about driving assessments for potential drivers with physical and intellectual disabilities. Noteworthy is that the majority of the members of ADED's board of directors are OTs. Of additional interest with regard to driving for teens with disabilities is that a recent study showed that teen drivers with ASD showed better safety records than their typically developing peers (Heasley, 2012).

An OT practitioner could work with a local driving school to develop specialized training and services for teens with disabilities, as well as recommend adaptations for classrooms and training vehicles to best meet these teen's needs. As well, becoming an advocate for including driver's education as part of the transition process toward graduation might also be an important role to consider.

Transitions for Older Youths

Whether a child has disabilities or not, the transition from school to higher education or college or work is a time of great emotional transition for them as well as their parents. Arguably, for children with disabilities, the options tend to be fewer and often less desirable. Although the transition process often begins in the early high school years, when a child ages out of special education services, parents often find themselves uncertain about what comes next for their child.

An emerging role for OTAs might be working as part of the transition team as a child prepares to age out of the educational system. For most families, this is a highly charged time in their lives as, up to this point, their child has been provided with services. It is equally or not more so emotionally charged for the child himself/herself. As part of the team, an OTA may work with families to identify their child's strengths and challenges and recommend postgraduation options that will help him/her reach their highest potential. This type of practice entails keeping an ongoing pulse on community resources that would be of benefit to older children with disabilities.

Productive Aging—Traditional Practice Venues: Hospitals, Skilled Nursing Facilities, Home Health

Emerging Trends

Community Mobility and Older Drivers

How dependent are you on an automobile? How about your parents and grandparents? Does your community have an efficient and affordable public transit system? Do you live in a walkable city? With a rapidly aging population reluctant to give up the privilege of driving, despite perhaps not being well suited to remain behind the wheel, addressing driving needs and alternative modes of transportation for the aging population is very important.

Consider getting involved with the CarFit program, which is a joint venture between the American Automobile Association, the AARP, and AOTA. CarFit is "an educational program that offers older adults the opportunity to check how well their personal vehicles 'fit' them" (CarFit, 2012, http://www.car-fit.org/).

Aging in Place and Home Modifications

Currently, over 28% of the US population is aged 50+ and comprises what is known as the baby boomer generation. Most boomers (nearly 90%) indicate a strong desire to age in place in their homes and communities (AARP Oregon, 2012). Despite this desire to remain at home and independent, many are not looking into what home modifications need to be made, now, in order to be in place when the need arises for them to be used. Home and environmental modifications will go a long way to help those who need them to enjoy and continue to participate in activities that are meaningful to them, at home.

OTAs can register for the American Association of Retired Persons/National Association of Home Builders Certified Aging in Place (CAPs) course and can team with CAPs-certified contractors on specialty areas of design such as aging in place kitchens or bathrooms. Further, working with HomeFit or Rebuilding Together (Table 40.1) may be another way to get involved with the home modifications emerging practice area.

Low Vision

According to the National Eye Institute, the definition of low vision is "… even with regular glasses, contact lenses, medicine, or surgery, people find everyday tasks difficult to do" (National Eye Institute, 2012, http://www.nei.gov). Low vision typically occurs because of specific eye diseases such as glaucoma, macular degeneration, cataracts,

TABLE 40.1 Home Modification Resources: Their Missions, Your Commitment

Resource, Website	Description
The HomeFit Program http://assets.aarp.org/www.aarp.org_/articles/families/HousingOptions/200590_HomeFit_rev011108.pdf	Originally a guide developed by the AARP to help people stay safely in their homes and communities. The guide contains comprehensive advice, tips, and checklists for getting a home in top form for comfort, safety, and long-term livability. HomeFit has expanded and is now a free seminar that helps individuals assess and make modifications to their current dwelling so that they can remain in their home independently as they age. Today, OT practitioners are becoming involved by leading HomeFit workshops.
Rebuilding Together http://www.rebuildingtogether.org/whoweare/	Rebuilding Together is the nation's leading nonprofit organization providing critical home repairs, modifications, and improvements for America's low-income homeowners, rebuilding the homes of the nation's most vulnerable homeowners and families at no cost to those served. Their work extends beyond the four walls of a home to impact the health and vibrancy of entire communities.
CAPs http://www.nahb.org/category.aspx?sectionID=686	The Certified Aging-in-Place Specialist (CAPs) designation program teaches the technical, business management, and customer service skills essential to competing in the fastest growing segment of the residential remodeling industry: home modifications for the aging in place.

or chronic diseases such as diabetes. Some people are diagnosed with low vision secondary to birth defects or eye injuries. While normal changes in vision are common with age and, typically, what is lost cannot be restored, many individuals with low vision are now seeking the expertise of OT practitioners skilled in low vision practice for assistance with modifications to make their lives easier so that they can make the most of the vision they still have.

One project that might be interesting to an OTA is to work with an OT to set up a mobile low vision occupational therapy specialty clinic that services low-income senior citizens.

Alzheimer Disease and Dementia

Dementia is a group of symptoms that significantly and negatively impact a person's life and includes memory loss, loss of reasoning and judgment, and language skills (McKhann & Albert, 2002). Alzheimer is the most common cause of dementia. Upward of 5.1 million Americans have been diagnosed with Alzheimer disease, and that number is projected to double in the coming years (U.S. Health and Human Services, 2012). Researchers have found that Alzheimer disease "involves progressive brain cell failure, but why the cells fail is not clear" (Alzheimer's Association, 2012, http://www.alz.org). While Alzheimer disease or other forms of dementia are not a normal part of aging, the risk increases with age. According to the Alzheimer's Association, the risk of Alzheimer doubles every 5 years after age 65 and by the age of 85 is nearly 80% (Alzheimer's Association, 2012). Family history is also a risk factor for Alzheimer. A person whose parents, sibling, or child has Alzheimer is more likely than someone without a family history of Alzheimer disease to develop the disease (Alzheimer's Association, 2012, http://www.alz.org).

As part of your practice, you may want to start a memory support group. Plan meaningful and purposeful movement-based activities that will help clients feel engaged and focused. Meet at the same time and in the same place on a regular basis. Remind clients what happened last time and discuss what will be done at the current meeting. As much as possible, plan and implement sensory-based movement activities (From the Field 40.3).

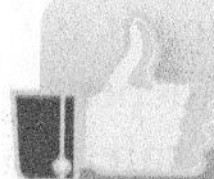

FROM THE FIELD 40.3

As part of a service learning project for an introductory OTA course, I scheduled a series of workshops for my students to plan and implement under my direct supervision at a nearby skilled nursing facility. We worked with a small group of residents with varying levels of dementia. One of our most positive sessions was making sachets with the residents. Not only did they enjoy filling their bags with fragrant herbs like lavender and lemon verbena, the smells elicited positive memories. I clearly remember one woman taking a deep inhalation and pausing to smile and sigh and say, "This so reminds me of Mother's sock drawer."

Work and Industry—Traditional Practice Venues: Hospitals, Clinics, Job Sites

Emerging Trends

Aging Workforce

Be it for personal or financial reasons, a greater number of older people are choosing to continue to work than ever before (Yamkovenko, n.d.). According to the Bureau of Labor Statistics, from 1977 to 2007, employment of workers 65 and over increased 101%, compared to a much smaller increase of 59% for total employment (16 and over). The number of employed men 65% and over rose 75%, but employment of women 65 and older increased by nearly twice as much, climbing 147%. While the number of employed people age 75 and over is relatively small (0.8% of the employed in 2007), this group had the most dramatic gain, increasing 172% between 1977 and 2007 (Bureau of Labor Statistics, 2008).

Consult with employers to help create environments that best meet the needs of the aging population, including addressing lighting, seating, auditory distractions, instruction in use of technology, and selection of optimal tools to make the job simple and safe.

New Technology at Work

With consistent advances in technology come seemingly endless opportunities to change the way we work (Yamkovenko, n.d.). Technological advances including tablet computers, smartphones, and other communication devices, as well as workspace adaptations, may lead to greater opportunities for people with differing abilities to be equal players in the workforce.

Consider becoming a technology expert. Develop the skills necessary to work with people of all ages and abilities to maximize use of technology when it is deemed to lead to the best possible outcomes: independence, increased production, and, most of all, safety. Remember, though, sometimes, despite the appeal of technology, a low-tech solution may in fact be the best option for a client.

Management and Education—Traditional Practice Venues: Colleges and Universities, All Other Practice Venues

Emerging Trends

Distance Learning

We have come a long way from the settlement house to the traditional classroom throughout the evolution of the profession. With a high demand for occupational therapy services, today's aspiring OT practitioners are receiving their education in new ways that best meet their lifestyles. While no entry-level occupational therapy or occupational therapy assistant programs are fully online, over 50% of all programs do have a distance learning component (AOTA, 2010; Yamkovenko, n.d.). For many, the flexibility that distance or hybrid programs offer is very appealing.

An emerging role for OTAs might be to teach. Current ACOTE rules state that "All OTA faculty who are full-time must hold a minimum of a baccalaureate degree awarded by an institution that is accredited by a USDE-recognized regional or national accrediting body" (AOTA, 2012). The same holds true for an OTA serving as the academic fieldwork coordinator. An OTA may teach on an adjunct or part time basis without holding a baccalaureate degree. Teaching part time or if you have an advanced degree to teach full time in a program that offers distance education is an exciting opportunity for OTAs. A word of advice, practice for several years first. Having actual field experience will make you a better instructor.

Coming Back to the Profession

By now, you are now aware that OTAs and OTs rank in the top 15 fastest growing professions (Bureau of Labor Statistics, 2012). For some who have left the profession, the allure of a secure and often flexible career has drawn them back (Yamkovenko, n.d.)

An emerging role for an OTA might be to mentor OTAs who are contemplating returning to the field or have recently returned. Once in the field, by taking on the role of mentor above and beyond your duties as an OTA, you will have much to offer those who are thinking of or recently returned to practice. As you have learned, a good mentor is worth his/her weight in gold.

Other Examples of Possible Emerging Practice Areas: Where Do They Best Fit?

Results of a qualitative study of 22 occupational therapists in Montreal, Canada, showed that a potential emerging practice for OT practitioners is working with the homeless population as case managers, outreach workers, and advocates (Grandisson et al., 2009). Because of the extensive physical and psychosocial challenges facing this marginalized population, it is difficult to pigeonhole which practice area working with the homeless falls within. Nonetheless, it is a good example of assessing societal occupational needs and taking necessary first-step action to consider working with the homeless population as an emerging practice area for OT practitioners.

Occupational therapy practitioners are also uniquely qualified to thoughtfully integrate task-oriented gardening and horticultural activities into clinical practice and measure its effectiveness with almost all clients we treat, no matter the practice area (Wagenfeld, 2012). In fact, many of the earliest occupational therapy interventions were based on gardening and farming. The Health Through HOrTiculture model (Wagenfeld, 2012) goes one step further. It propels OT practitioners beyond the realm of traditional practice to forge entrepreneurial and meaningful collaborative relationships with landscape professionals on the design of human-centered therapeutic and healing outdoor spaces (Winterbottom & Wagenfeld, 2015).

Service dog training for people with disabilities, as well as for veterans, represents yet another potential emerging practice area. Service animals can be trained to alert owners to impending seizures or other health issues, to help reduce anxiety, and to assist with daily living tasks. AOTA's OT Connections contains links to several groups of OT practitioners who are interested in or practicing within this potential emerging area.

Summary

As we conclude this unit on practice areas and this chapter on emerging practice areas and prepare to move into applying what you have learned to case studies, think about the myriad ways and places that OT practitioners work with clients. What we have explored is only a tiny sampling of the vast opportunities that await you or have yet to be explored. Think big and look to a very bright future filled with many opportunities to help clients achieve their maximum occupational performance levels, through your work in either traditional or emerging practice areas.

Review Questions

1. Which of the following emerging practice areas does AOTA not link with children and youth?
   a. Obesity
   b. Transitions
   c. Autism
   d. Restraint and isolation

2. Which of the following emerging practice areas requires an in-depth understanding of trauma and sensory regulation and integration theory?
   a. Autism
   b. Home modifications
   c. Restraint and isolation
   d. Wounded warrior and veteran care

3. The economic cost of substance abuse and addiction on an annual basis (United States) is about:
   a. 100 million dollars
   b. 200 billion dollars
   c. 200 million dollars
   d. More than 500 billion dollars

4. A student receives a series of perplexing and threatening text messages over a 7-day period from five different people in her social studies class. This may be an example of:
   a. Bullying
   b. Pranks
   c. Miscommunication
   d. Research study

5. Which of the following is not consistently associated with aging in place and home modifications?
   a. HomeFit
   b. Habitat for Humanity
   c. CAPs
   d. Rebuilding Together

6. The obesity epidemic:
   a. Impacts only minority populations
   b. Is always the fault of the person
   c. Is declining
   d. Impacts people of all ages, SES, and races

7. With regard to the emerging practice areas and the OTA:
   a. No supervision is necessary to pursue these roles.
   b. In the role of an OTA must work under the supervision of an OT.
   c. Different supervisory capacities apply to emerging practice areas as defined by the AOTA Centennial Vision.
   d. There is no distinction made between occupational therapist and OTAs in emerging practice areas.

8. Providing instruction in use of a tablet computer and the proper desk setup for a client with cerebral palsy who works in an office setting would be an example of which emerging practice area(s)?
   a. Restraint and isolation and home modifications
   b. Home modifications and mental health
   c. Home modifications and new technology for rehabilitation
   d. New technology for rehabilitation and chronic disease management

9. Six people came together to discuss the possibility of opening a restaurant that grows its own food and trains youth with mental health issues as cooks and wait service staff. Which of the following is the best example of an entrepreneurial endeavor?
   a. Line cook at a local table to harvest restaurant
   b. Grower for a local table to harvest restaurant
   c. Public relations director for a local table to harvest restaurant
   d. All of the above

10. Which of the following provides the best explanation for new and expanded roles for occupational therapy practitioners working in schools?
   a. Response to Intervention
   b. Individuals with Disability Act
   c. PL92-142
   d. Civil Rights Act

Practice Activities

Select one emerging practice area that seems to be most interesting for you. Locate additional information about this practice area on the AOTA website. Prepare a short PowerPoint presentation that provides a more in-depth discussion about the area. Discuss why this area is most appealing to you. Share your presentation with your class. Additionally, find a community resource that would benefit from knowing more about the role of occupational therapy in this area. Make an appointment to discuss this with the program director or arrange to speak at a meeting at the community organization.

Prepare a grid that outlines the emerging practice area and show how they cross traditional practice area lines and link to each other.

Come up with an emerging practice area that has yet to be proposed in the occupational therapy community. Present your concept to your class and program director. As a class, consider presenting your idea at a state conference as a roundtable discussion.

References

AARP Oregon. *Focusing on your home—Get the HomeFit guide*. 2012. Retrieved from http://www.aarp.org/home-family/livable-communities/info-06-2012/home-fit-guide-or1859.html

Allsup Foundation. *Allsup disability study: income at risk*. 2012. Retrieved from http://www.allsup.com/Portals/.../allsup-study-income-at-risk-q2-11

Alzheimer's Association. What we know today about Alzheimer's disease. 2012. Retrieved from http://www.alz.org/research/science/alzheimers_disease_causes.asp

American Occupational Therapy Association. *Academic programs annual data report: Academic year 2009–2010*. 2010. Retrieved from http://www.aota.org/Educate/EdRes/OTEdData/42026/46508.aspx?FT=.pdf

American Occupational Therapy Association. *2011 Accreditation Council for Occupational Therapy Education (ACOTE®) standards and interpretive guide (effective July 31, 2013) January 2012 Interpretive guide version*. 2012. Retrieved July 26, 2012, from http://www.aota.org/Educate/Accredit/Draft-Standards/50146.aspx?FT=.pdf

American Psychiatric Association. Exercise helps keep your psyche fit. 2004. Retrieved from http://www.apa.org/research/action/fit.aspx

American Psychiatric Association. *Let's talk facts about substance abuse and addiction*. 2007. Retrieved from http://www.healthyminds.org/Document-Library/Brochure-Library/Substance-Abuse-and-Addiction.aspx

American Psychiatric Association. *Depression*. 2012. Retrieved from http://www.apa.org/topics/depress/index.aspx

American Psychiatric Association. *Diagnostic and Statistical Manual of Mental Disorders DSM-IV-TR*. 5th ed. Washington, D.C.: American Psychiatric Publishing, Inc.; 2013.

American Psychological Association. *Post-traumatic stress disorder*. 2015. Retrieved from www.apa.org/topics/ptsd/index.aspx

American Telemedicine Association. *Telemedicine defined*. 2012. Retrieved from http://www.americantelemed.org/i4a/pages/index.cfm?pageid=3333

Association for Driver Rehabilitation Specialists. n.d. http://www.driver-ed.org

Autism Speaks. *Adult employment: New allies come on board*. 2012. Retrieved from http://www.autismspeaks.com

Autism Speaks. *Facts about autism*. n.d. Retrieved from http://www.autismspeaks.com

Babyak MA, et al. Exercise treatment for major depression: maintenance of therapeutic benefit at 10 months. *Psychosom Med* 2000;62:633–638.

Baio J. Prevalence of autism spectrum disorder among children aged 8 years—autism and developmental disabilities monitoring network, 11 sites, United States, 2010. *Surveill Summ* 2014;63(SS02):1–21. Retrieved from http://www.cdc.gov/mmwr/preview/mmwrhtml/ss6302a1.htm?s_cid=ss6302a1_w

Bureau of Labor Statistics. *Older workers*. 2008. Retrieved from http://www.bls.gov/spotlight/2008/older_workers/

Bureau of Labor Statistics. *Occupational Outlook Handbook, 2010–11 Edition*. 2012. Retrieved from http://www.bls.gov/oco/ocos166.htm

Cancer Prevention Coalition. *Facts you need to know about cancer*. n.d. Retrieved from http://www.globalhealingcenter.com/truth-about-cancer/facts-you-need-to-know-about-cancer

CarFit. *Goals and objectives*. 2012. Retrieved from http://www.car-fit.org/

Centers for Disease Control and Prevention. *The power to prevent, the call to control:at a glance 2009*. 2009. Retrieved from http://www.cdc.gov/chronicdisease/resources/publications/AAG/chronic.htm

Centers for Disease Control and Prevention. *Adult obesity facts*. 2012a. Retrieved from http://www.cdc.gov/obesity/data/adult.html

Centers for Disease Control and Prevention. 2007–2008 *National health and nutrition examination survey*. 2012b. Retrieved from http://www.cdc.gov/nchs/data/nhanes/nhanes_07_08/overviewbrochure_0708.pdf

Centers for Disease Control and Prevention. *Overweight and obesity facts*. 2012c. Retrieved from http://www.cdc.gov/obesity/data/adult.html

Centers for Disease Control and Prevention. *Obesity rates among all children in the United States*. 2012d. Retrieved from http://www.cdc.gov/obesity/data/adult.html

Cole A. *Business Enterprise in its Social Setting*. Cambridge, MA: Harvard University Press; 1959.

Department of Defense. *Military strengths*. 2011. Retrieved from https://kb.defense.gov/app/answers/detail/a_id/253/session/L3RpbWUvMTM0MzQwOTMwMy9zaWQvZm1UQ2RjMmw%3D

Dougherty PJ, et al. Multiple traumatic limb loss: a comparison of Vietnam veterans to

OIF/ OEF servicemembers. *J Rehabil Res Dev* 2010;47(4):333–348.

Grandisson M, et al. Occupational therapists' perceptions of their role with people who are homeless. *Br J Occup Ther* 2009;72(11):491–498.

Heasley S. *Should teens with autism be allowed to drive?* 2012. Retrieved from http://www.disabilityscoop.com/2012/01/10/should-teens-autism-drive/14743/

Holmes WM, Scaffa ME. An exploratory study of competencies for emerging practice in occupational therapy. *J Allied Health* 2009;38(2):81–90.

Klomek AB, et al. Bullying and suicide: detection and intervention. *Psychiatr Times* 2011;28(2):1–13. Retrieved from http://www.psychiatrictimes.com/pdf?p_p_id=PDF_CONTENT&articleId=1795797&groupId=10168

Kuratko DF, Audretsch DB. Strategic entrepreneurship: exploring different perspectives of an emerging concept. *Entrepreneurship Theory Pract* 2009:1–17. Retrieved from http://www.pogc.ir/Portals/0/maghalat/890707-8.pdf

Limb Loss Awareness. *Limb loss statistics* 2012. Retrieved from http://www.limblossawareness.org/about-limb-loss/limb-loss-statistics/index.php

McKhann G, Albert M. *Keeping Your Brain Young: The Complete Guide to Physical and Emotional Health and Longevity*. Hoboken, NJ: Wiley; 2002.

National Cancer Institute. *What is Cancer?* 2015. Retrieved from www.cancer.gov/about-cancer/what-is-cancer-cancer#typesofcancer

National Center for Special Education Research. *National Longitudinal Transition Study Two*. 2012. Retrieved from http://www.nlts2.org/

National Center on Response to Intervention. *Essential components of RTI—a closer look at response to intervention*. 2010. Retrieved from http://www.rti4success.org

National Drug Intelligence Center. *The Economic Impact of Illicit Drug Use on American Society*. Washington D.C.: United States Department of Justice; 2011.

National Eye Institute. *What you should know about low vision*. 2012. Retrieved from http://www.nei.nih.gov/health/lowvision/index.asp

Ogden C, Carroll M. *NCHS Health E-Stat. Prevalence of obesity among children and adolescents: United States, trends 1963–1965 through 2007–2008*. 2012. Retrieved from http://www.cdc.gov/nchs/data/hestat/obesity_child_07_08/obesity_child_07_08.htm

Prabst-Hunt W, ed. *Occupational Therapy Administration Manual*. pp. 63–80. Clifton Park, NY: Delmar, Cengage Learning; 2001.

Rosenthal JZ, et al. Effects of transcendental meditation in veterans of Operation Enduring Freedom and Operation Iraqi Freedom with posttraumatic stress disorder: a pilot study. *Mil Med* 2011;176(6):626–630.

Small Business Administration. *Is entrepreneurship for you?* n.d. Retrieved from http://www.sba.gov/content/entrepreneurship-you

Steel E. *Seclusion and Restraint Practice Standards: A Review and Analysis*. National Consumer Supporter Technical Assistance Center. n.d. Retrieved from http://www.ncstac.org/index.php?option=com_content&view=article&id=94%3Aseclusion-and-restraint-practice-standards-a-review-and-analysis&catid=34&Itemid=53

Stewart BS, Wild CP. *World Cancer Report 2014*. In: Stewart BS, Wild CP, eds. Chapter: Cancer Worldwide. Geneva, Switzerland: World Health Organization. International Agency of Research on Cancer; 2014:pp. 16-69.

Substance Abuse and Mental Health Services Administration. *Results from the 2010 National Survey on Drug Use and Health: Summary of National Findings*. NSDUH Series H-41, HHS Publication No. (SMA) 11–4658. Rockville, MD: Substance Abuse and Mental Health Services Administration; 2011.

Tangney JP, et al. High self-control predicts good adjustment, less pathology, better grades, and interpersonal success. *J Pers* 2004;72: 271–322.

Ten Facts About Cancer. 2006. Retrieved from http://www.who.int/features/factfiles/cancer/10_en.html

U.S. Health and Human Services. *Obama administration presents national plan to fight Alzheimer's disease*. 2012 Retrieved from http://www.hhs.gov/news/press/2012pres/05/20120515a.html

US Department of Veteran's Affairs. *National Center for Veteran's Analysis and Statistics. Veteran Population*. 2012 Retrieved from http://www.va.gov/vetdata/Veteran_Population.asp

Wagenfeld A. Health through HOrTiculture™: a natural innovation. *Home Community Health Spec Interest Sect Q* 2012;19(2):1–4.

Winterbottom D., Wagenfeld A. *Therapeutic Gardens: Design for Healing Spaces*. Portland, OR: Timber Press; 2015.

Yamkovenko S. *The emerging niche: what is next in your practice area?* n.d. Retrieved from http://www.aota.org/Practitioners/PracticeAreas/EmergingAreas.aspx

Young SK, Leventhal B. Bullying and suicide. A review. *Int J Adolesc Med Health* 2008;20(2):133–154.

Ziegler-Graham K, et al. Estimating the prevalence of limb loss in the United States: 2005 to 2050. *Arch Phys Med Rehabil* 2008;89(3): 422–429.

UNIT

VII

The Occupational Therapy Assistant in Action: Putting Theory into Practice

Authentic occupational therapy is based upon a commitment to the client's realization of his own particular meaning.

–ELIZABETH JUNE YERXA

Introduction to the Case Studies

In this unit, you are presented with 13 case studies that cover the life span. The cases are representative of what you may see when you are practicing as an OTA. What you are provided with is background information about the case study topic and a fictitious clinical narrative about a client with the issue at hand. While each chapter builds on and contains information about what you need to know to work through the case studies, you are directed to cross-reference specific chapters in this book that are particularly relevant to each case study. There are also several no-noccupational therapy specific Internet resources included in each case study to help you learn more about the case topics. Please note though, a very important first Internet resource to consult is www.aota.org.

The process of working through the case studies will involve in-depth evidence-based research searches, a good deal of diligence, and creativity. The information provided in the background section, and clinical presentation may not cover some of what you are asked to fill in to complete the case summations. And, some cases have no specific conclusions. This is to allow you to build on what information has been presented to you and create your personal case summation, based on existing evidence relevant to the case study topic.

At the end of Case Study 1, you will find a sample Case Summation and Activity Analysis.

The case summation forms are designed to correspond to parts of the Domain of the *Occupational Therapy Practice Framework III* (AOTA, 2014). It is strongly recommended that you also refer to *The Occupational Therapy Practice Framework III (AOTA, 2014)* regarding key concepts that you will be asked to respond to in the case study summations. Enjoy this unique learning experience!

Reference

American Occupational Therapy Association. Occupational therapy practice framework: domain and process (3rd ed.). *American Journal of Occupational Therapy* 2014;68(Suppl. 1):S1–S48. http://dx.doi.org/10.5014/ajot.2014.682006

CASE STUDY 1

CHAPTER

41 My Baby Has Cerebral Palsy

Amy Wagenfeld, PhD, OTR/L, SCEM, CAPs

Background Information

Cerebral palsy (CP) is one of the most common congenital disorders of childhood. About 500,000 children and adults of all ages in the United States have CP (Nemours, n.d.). The symptoms of CP vary, but all people with CP have difficulty with movement and posture (CDC, 2012). Many people with CP also have related issues such as cognitive disability, speech and language issues, hearing loss, visual issues, scoliosis, joint contractures, and seizures (CDC, 2012). It is usually caused by brain damage occurring before or during a child's birth, or during the first 3 to 5 years of a child's life (CDC, 2012). Premature babies are at greater risk for CP, as are low-birth-weight and multiple babies (CDC, 2012; Nemours, n.d.). Postnatal factors such as trauma, lead poisoning, or meningitis may also lead to CP (CDC, 2012).

There are four main types of CP:

- Spastic cerebral palsy, the most common form of CP, affects 80% people with the disorder.
- Dyskinetic cerebral palsy, which includes athetoid, choreoathetoid, and dystonic cerebral palsies
- Ataxic cerebral palsy
- Mixed cerebral palsy

There is no cure for CP, but therapy, special equipment, and, in some cases, surgery is often how the disorder is managed (CDC, 2012).

Traditional Practice Area: Children and Youth

Cross-References: Chapters 19, Spirituality; Chapter 27, Developmental Disabilities; Chapter 31, Vision; Chapter 36, Children and Youth.

CLINICAL PRESENTATION

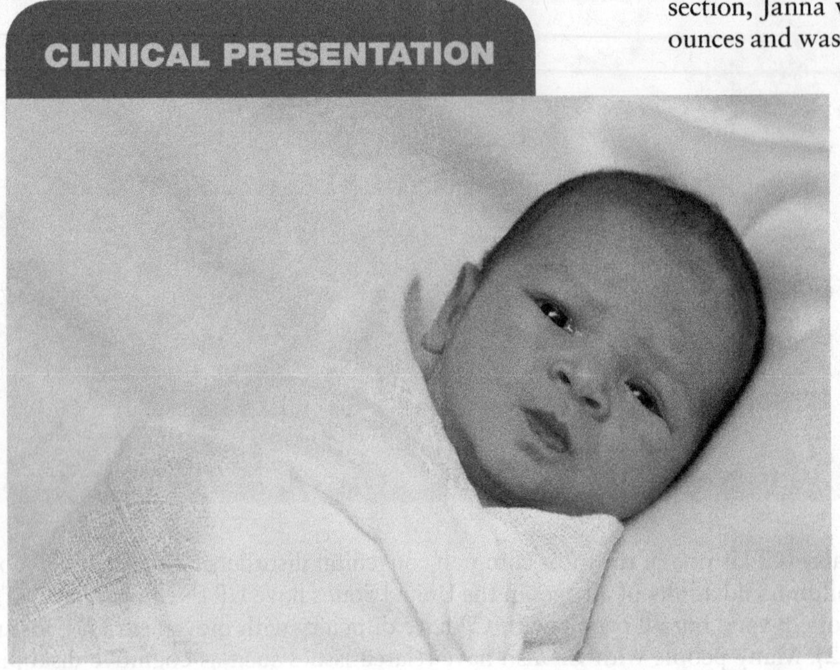

Janna was a much-anticipated baby. Her parents, Caryn and Martin, had tried for 10 years to conceive. After multiple rounds of in vitro fertilization, they got the good news that Caryn was pregnant. At the time of conception, Caryn was 41 years old and Martin was 46. Caryn is Hispanic, and Martin is White. Both of them are practicing Unitarians. Caryn has four siblings, and Martin is the eldest of three. They live 5 hours away from either family. While Caryn experienced the typical symptoms of pregnancy, including morning sickness and fatigue, all was progressing well. Because Caryn was over age 35, her pregnancy was carefully monitored. She had regular ultrasounds and prenatal testing. All signs indicated that the fetus was developing perfectly. Once Caryn started regaining her energy and the morning sickness passed, she was back to her usual busy lifestyle. Her work as a hair stylist, kept her on her feet for long hours, but she balanced this with swimming four times a week and going to prenatal yoga classes. Martin, an insurance agent, did most of the cooking and cleaning. On the weekends, they enjoyed bike riding and going to flea markets. They spent many hours talking about their baby, even wondering what the sex would be, as they opted to not know.

One morning, Caryn woke up just not feeling right. She was experiencing strong abdominal cramps at regular intervals. Caryn was 28 weeks pregnant. Alarmed, Martin called Caryn's doctor, who upon hearing Caryn's symptoms, urged them to go to the local hospital, immediately. Caryn was seen quickly in the emergency room and admitted to the labor and delivery unit. Things happened very quickly. Caryn was in active labor, and there was no stopping it. Following an emergency cesarean section, Janna was born. She weighed 1 pound and 14 ounces and was 12 in. long. Janna was unable to breathe on her own and shortly after birth had a seizure as well as other serious medical complications. Her parents were shocked and shattered.

Janna spent 20 weeks in the NICU, growing, albeit slowly. Her reflexes were sluggish. Her muscle tone was very high, and she kept her fists tightly closed. She had retinopathy of prematurity (ROP). She was diagnosed with spastic cerebral palsy 4 weeks after her birth. As soon as Janna was medically stable, she began receiving occupational and physical therapy services. As part of the discharge planning, early intervention services were arranged and an IFSP was developed with the family. Janna was to receive occupational therapy three times a week and physical therapy two times a week in her home. Caryn decided to give up her hair stylist job and remain home with the baby.

On the first home visit, the occupational therapy team (an OT and OTA) came together. After the evaluation, the OTA would be implementing a majority of the treatment sessions under the supervision of the OT. The OT evaluated Janna and noted delays with gross motor skills. She had a great deal of difficulty turning her head from side to side when placed prone and did not unfist her hands. Janna had trouble localizing the sound of a noisy rattle and was very fussy unless she was tightly swaddled in a blanket. She was having trouble latching on to a nipple on a bottle.

By the time Janna was 9 months old, her gross and fine motor skills delays were obvious. She was not yet sitting unsupported and was not purposely reaching for and grasping objects with her hands. She had begun to develop better oral motor control, so would take a bottle without incident. She was not eating pureed food, and caloric intake had to be carefully monitored, because Janna was not gaining weight at an appropriate rate. She continued to be fussy unless she was held and had not yet established a regular sleep or feeding schedule. Janna did not visually track objects, and while she had begun to smile, it seemed to be a random, rather than a social smile. She was not babbling. Caryn and Martin were physically and emotionally exhausted and worried about what life with Janna was going to be like as she grew up. Would she be able to learn like her typically developing peers? Would she ever walk, ride a bike, or paint a picture? Would she be able to feed herself? Would she talk? These were only a few of the many issues that Caryn and Martin had to face as parents of a child with CP.

On the following pages you will find a Case Summation.

Internet Resources

Centers for Disease Control and Prevention—www.cdc.gov
United Cerebral Palsy—www.ucp.org
National Institute of Neurological Disorders and Stroke (NIH)—http://www.ninds.nih.gov/disorders/cerebral_palsy/cerebral_palsy.htm

References

CDC. *Facts about cerebral palsy*; 2012. Retrieved from http://www.cdc.gov/ncbddd/cp/facts.html
Nemours. *Cerebral palsy*; n.d. Retrieved from http://kidshealth.org/parent/medical/brain/cerebral_palsy.html

A note to readers: Responses are constructed from case study information and conclusions drawn from relevant existing evidence on topics related to this case. The sample Case Summation and Activity Analysis were contributed by Karie Carbone, OTS.

Case Summation—by Amy Wagenfeld, PhD, OTR/L, SCEM, CAPs

Context, Environment, and Clinical Presentation

Personal Information: *Janna is 9 months old and the first child of Caryn and Martin. She was born at 28 weeks of gestation and weighed 1 pound 14 ounces and was 12 in. long. Mother had multiple rounds of failed in vitro fertilization; this was the first to progress to a live delivery. She was 41 years old at delivery and father was 46. Janna is diagnosed with cerebral palsy and retinopathy of prematurity. She also shows signs of sensory and oral motor concerns.*

Cultural Background: *Janna's mother is Hispanic, of Honduran heritage, and her father is White, of Germanic and Norwegian heritage. Both are proud of their respective cultural backgrounds and look forward to sharing them with Janna as she grows up. They plan to do so by visiting their respective countries of cultural origin and exposing her to foods and festivals that embrace their heritages. Since both sets of grandparents are still alive, Janna's parents want to try to do a photo voice diary of each for Janna to enjoy when she gets older.*

Physical Environment(s): *Janna lives with her parents and pet dog, Glacier, in a two story home in a small community of about 15,000 people. Janna's nursery is on the second floor on the north side of the house. The house has an attached garage with two steps up to the kitchen door. There are six steps up to the front porch. The house is in a neighborhood with sidewalks, and the town center is less than a mile away. The local elementary school is accessible via bus, and the church is 3 miles away.*

Social Context(s): *Janna's mother is now home with her and her father works full time. Mother has been trying to find a babysitter to stay with Janna so she can have some time off, but so far no one that she interviews is willing to care for her because of her complex health and behavioral issues. Janna's parents have not gone out for a date since she was born. Because Janna's grandparents live 5 hours away, they are seldom there to be with Janna. Janna's mother would like to take her to a mom and baby playgroup but is scared that they will be rejected or shunned.*

Janna does not interact consistently with adults or children.

Temporal Context(s): *Janna naps erratically and has not established a predictable sleep routine. She will only sleep in her crib and must be rocked to sleep.*

Virtual Context(s): *On occasion, Janna's grandparents will attempt "face time with" her, while Caryn holds her in her lap. Janna does not seem to be interested in this.*

Client Factors

Values: *(Parental) Janna's parents pride themselves on being hard-working, honest, compassionate, and generous to others in need.*

Beliefs: *(Parental) Janna's parents are firmly rooted in the just treatment of all people. Prior to Janna's birth, they had little contact with people with disabilities, but being who they are, intend to serve in some type of advocacy role.*

Spirituality: *(Parental) Janna's parents are active members of the local Unitarian church. They attend at least three times a month. Janna's father is on the education committee. They are also deeply connected with nature and enjoy being outside, biking, walking, or hiking.*

Body Functions: *(Janna's) Cardiovascular, musculoskeletal, sensory, respiratory complications.*

Body Structures: *Janna's heart and blood vessels are impaired, as is Janna's central and peripheral nervous system.*

Performance Skills

Sensory Perceptual Skills: *Janna is showing signs of sensory defensiveness and sensory processing issues. She enjoys being rocked but does not like the baby swing. She startles easily and appears disoriented in brightly lit environments. She cries when Glacier the family dog "kisses" her and startles when she barks.*

Motor and Praxis Skills: *Janna is demonstrating deficits with motor planning and praxis skills; developmental milestones are delayed, bilateral upper extremity skills are impaired.*

Emotional Regulation Skills: *Janna is fussy and does not self-regulate consistently. She likes to be tightly held, swaddled, and rocked. She calms when her mother (not father) sings her lullabies. She does not calm when her mother plays a CD of lullabies.*

Cognitive Skills: *Janna is having trouble with visual tracking and is not babbling.*

Communication and Social Skills: *Janna does not appear to socially smile; rather her smile is random and not directed at a specific person. She has not yet established her primary attachment figure (typically one's mother). She is not babbling.*

Performance Patterns

Habits: *Janna does not have a regular sleep–waking cycle or feeding schedule.*

Routines: *Jana has no established routines other than negative responses to Glacier's attempts at affection or barking.*

Roles: *Janna is the first born child of Caryn and Martin.*

Rituals: *None have been established, although parents have expressed interest in getting assistance to plan sleep rituals to help Janna develop a regular sleep schedule.*

Areas of Occupation

Activities of Daily Living (ADL):

1.	Self-feeding	
	Occupational Participation:	*Drinking from a bottle*
	Observed and Measured Occupational Performance:	*Can hold and drink from a bottle, but it is a reflexive action due to persistent grasp reflex.*
2.	Feeding	
	Occupational Participation:	*Eating pureed foods*
	Observed and Measured Occupational Performance:	*None, refuses food*

3.	Bathing	
	Occupational Participation:	*Bathing in infant tub with seatbelt, tub placed on countertop in kitchen to align with good body mechanics for parents.*
	Observed and Measured Occupational Performance:	*Cries when water is too cool, recoils when lotion is rubbed on her body after a bath.*
4.	Dressing	
	Occupational Participation:	*Donning one piece jumpsuits (dependent).*
	Observed and Measured Occupational Performance:	*Challenging due to high tone, takes a great deal of effort on mother's part; Janna is most comfortable when swaddled with just a diaper and tee shirt on beneath the swaddle.*

Instrumental Activities of Daily (IADL):

1.	Occupational Participation:	*N/A*
	Observed and Measured Occupational Performance:	*N/A*
2.	Occupational Participation:	*N/A*
3.	Observed and Measured Occupational Performance:	*N/A*
4.	Occupational Participation:	*N/A*
	Observed and Measured Occupational Performance:	*N/A*

Rest and Sleep:

Occupational Participation:	*Naps and night sleep*
Observed and Measured Occupational Performance:	*Needs to be rocked to sleep, prefers to be swaddled, startles awake easily, likes to be sung to, prefers room to be darkened when sleeping.*

Education:

	Janna is receiving early intervention services.
Occupational Participation:	*Receives services a total of five sessions per week from OT and PT.*
Observed and Measured Occupational Performance:	*Parents are deeply invested in Janna's therapy and consistently follow home programs that the therapists provide.*

Work:

Occupational Participation:	*N/A*
Observed and Measured Occupational Performance:	*N/A*

Play/Leisure:

1.	Play	
	Occupational Participation:	*Reach, grasp, release of toys.*
	Observed and Measured Occupational Performance:	*Not engaging in play, reflective grasp pattern is just beginning to integrate.*
2.	Occupational Participation:	*N/A*
	Observed and Measured Occupational Performance:	*N/A*
3.	Occupational Participation:	*N/A*
	Observed and Measured Occupational Performance:	*N/A*

Social Participation:

Occupational Participation:	*Interactive pre language; No Babbling*
Observed and Measured Occupational Performance:	*Babbling is not purposeful or used to engage other in conversation. Social skills are limited.*

Desired Outcomes (Client)

Janna will reach her maximum potential and always know that she is loved.

Summary of Identified Function and Strengths

Caregivers are deeply committed to meeting Janna's needs; Janna is able to hold her bottle, likes deep pressure and being sung to.

Summary of Identified Weaknesses

Limited social skills and communication; multiple physical challenges; sensory issues; feeding and weight gain concerns; visual and visual perceptual issues.

Measurable Goals and Objectives

LTG

Janna will demonstrate improved sensory processing skills by discharge from early intervention services.

STG

Janna will self-soothe using a transitional object such as a soft blanket to snuggle with and fall asleep for nap time 3 of 5 consecutive days within 2 months.

Janna will tolerate play with a textured ball while in supported sitting; grasping it, mouthing it, and rolling it purposely to therapist or parent 50% of the time within the next 12 weeks.

Janna will tolerate room temperature lotion being applied to her body by either parent after a bath without complaint 50% of the time within the next 2 months.

Janna will sit in baby swing with gentle rocking motion for 5 minutes without crying 100% of the time within 6 months.

Intervention Plan

Activities of Daily Living (ADL):

Address self-feeding as primary ADL intervention.

Increase tolerance to pureed foods.

Exploration of food with fingers.

Bring fingers to mouth.

Progress to finger foods as tolerated.

Instrumental Activities of Daily (IADL):

N/A

Rest and Sleep:

Develop set of sleep rituals for Janna's parents to implement to help Janna learn to fall asleep on her own, in her crib.

Education:

Parent education—ongoing.

Work:

N/A

Play/Leisure:

Increase tolerance and interest in toys and social interaction with caregiver during play.

Social Participation:

Improve reciprocal social interactions.

Equipment Needs

Assistive technology: Positioning devices for sitting and/or wheelchair or stroller, adapted feeding chair.

Low-tech: Bolsters for positioning, Boppy pillow for sitting on floor.

Adapted equipment: Ring seat for bathtub as sitting balance improves, "peanut" or other therapy ball, weighted blanket.

Durable medical equipment: See adapted equipment.

Home Programming

Educational information: Provided parents with AOTA fact sheets on cerebral palsy, toy selection, and early intervention.

Resources: Recommended that parents contact the local cerebral palsy foundation, feeding group run through the EI agency, infant–parent play groups run through local community education center, support groups for children with developmental disabilities facilitated by local school district, respite service organizations (so they can get out and leave Janna in the care of a qualified care provider).

Discharge Plan

Janna is currently receiving EI services 5 times per week in her home. If her mother were to return to work and put Janna in daycare, EI team will, at parent request, coordinate with parents and also treat Janna at daycare. If Janna were to continue with EI services, she will do so until age 2 years, 364 days. Upon her third birthday, she will transition to preschool services in her local school district. Transition to preschool will begin 6 months prior to Janna's third birthday with communication with the local school district special services. She will transition from having an Individualized Family Service Plan (IFSP) to an Individualized Education Program (IEP).

Documentation Note

S: Janna was happy today. She had just awakened from her nap before OTA arrived.

O: Janna was dressed in a long sleeved/legged cotton jumpsuit. Janna tolerated being positioned prone on elbows over the peanut for 3 minutes with mom in front of her while shaking a jingly rattle and talking with her. Janna attempted to track from midline to the left and back to midline x2. When positioned in supported ring sitting on mom's lap facing the OTA, did not show signs of discomfort when a textured ball was rubbed up and down upper and lower extremities with pressure equal to the weight of a nickel, with arms and legs covered in clothing. Finger plays to passively range upper and lower extremities.

A: Janna appears to be tolerating positional changes and textures with less complaint.

P: Continue to see Janna for occupational therapy services in her home three times per week. Provided mom with carry over activity; to continue to roll the textured ball up and down Janna's arms and legs (while covered with clothing) with gentle pressure (the weight of a nickel) and to watch for signs of discomfort; grimacing, wriggling, drooling, crying, faster and more shallow breathing. Note and discontinue if aversive responses are observed.

Activity Analysis Form—by Karie Carbone, OTS **Page 1**

Activity Peek-a-Boo

Area of Occupation:

- ___ Activities of Daily Living
- ___ Instrumental Activities of Daily Living
- ___ Rest and Sleep
- ___ Education
- ___ Work
- X Play
- ___ Leisure
- X Social Participation

Brief Activity Description:

A time honored game that involves reciprocal social interaction between (typically) an adult and infant. The game is a building block for the developmental concept of object permanence.

Describe how the activity is done: (Add more space and steps if necessary.)

Step 1 Infant and adult sit facing one another.

Step 2 The adult ensures he/she has the infant's attention: eye contact and ideally, still and quiet body posture.

Step 3 The adult covers his/her face with his/her hands and waits 2-3 seconds.

Step 4 The adult pulls his/her hands away from face while simultaneously exclaiming "Peek-a-Boo!" while smiling and making eye contact with infant.

Step 5 Repeat steps 2-4 until infant's attention has waned.

Step 6 Increase time adult's face is covered as infant's attention and tolerance increase.

Step 7 ___

Step 8 ___

Step 9 ___

Step 10 ___

Sequencing and Timing:

How much time will the activity take? 1 to 5 minutes

Can it be broken down and done for short periods of time? Yes How? Adult can adjust the number of times that they do step 5.

Does activity have to be done in a specific sequence? Yes Why? The adult's face needs to first be covered and then uncovered in order to properly contribute to the infant's early experience with object permanence.

Do certain parts of the activity have to be done in a specific time frame? Yes If so, which ones? Each step needs to be completed nearly immediately after one another in order to not lose interest and to help establish object permanence.

Does this activity require the client to plan parts of the activity? No If so, which parts? ___

Method of Instruction:

- Verbal: ___ Oral
- Visual: ___ Pictures ___ Written Words ___ Video X Demo ___ Diagram
- Tactile Cueing: ___
- Group Instruction: ___
- Individual Instruction: X

Activity Demands:

Objects Used	Properties	Where purchased/found	Cost
None			

Activity Analysis Form (continued)

Page 2

Qualities of the Activity:

Does the activity allow for creativity? *Yes* Which parts? *Can vary activity by placing a light cloth over adult or infant's face and carrying out the Peek-a-Boo sequence by removing the cloth from adult or child and exclaiming "Peek-a-Boo!" Infant can also be encouraged to remo ve the cloth with hand over hand assist and grading to do so independently.*

Is the activity structured or unstructured? Explain why. *Structured, because the steps need to be followed in a particular order and require the full attention of both the infant and adult.*

Does the activity have repetitive parts? *Yes* What are they? *Steps 2-4 are repeated.*

Environmental Requirements: ____ Indoors ____ Outdoors _X_ Either

Room size *Any size* Seating *Any type that allows for facing one another and is safe for the infant.*

Furniture *None required, high chair or other infant seating system may be preferred if sitting on the ground/floor is contraindicated.*

Lighting *Daylight or overhead lighting, enough to see each other clearly.*

Ventilation *Normal* Temperature *Comfortable* Floor surface *Soft for the infant*

Table surface *None required* Noise level *Low, to prevent distractions* Visual Stimuli *Few, to prevent distractions*

Safety Precautions: *Infant safety: have infant seated in an approved high chair/seat or on a carpet or rug away from hazards (choking, electrical, heat source, etc.). Infant should not be left unattended.*

Social Demands: Age level: *6-12 months* Educational level needed: *None*

____ Male
____ Female
_X_ Either

_X_ Group activity *(infant adult pair)*
____ Individual activity

Group membership needed? ____ Yes _X_ No

Activity is done: ____ Alone _X_ Group ____ Parallel activity

If with others, a minimum of how many people are needed? *2*

Required Actions/ Performance Skills:

	Performance Skills/ Required Body Actions & Functions for Activity	Performance Skills/ Client's Body Function/ Structure	Client Precautions	Adaptations/Grading
Body position and motion	*If needed, infant can be positioned for this activity at step one and will not need to move. The infant can also be repositioned as needed.*	*Janna is unable to position or reposition herself. She has gross motor delays.*	*Janna needs to be carefully supervised to reposition her if she slips into an unsafe position and is unable to move herself.*	*Grade down by having Janna sit in a Bumbo seat or a similar sitting support system in order to encourage proper body positioning.*
Trunk control	*If on floor, infant needs to be able to sit up. If in chair, needs enough trunk stability to remain upright and centered in seat.*	*Janna is currently unable to sit unsupported.*	*Janna needs support during sitting activities to prevent injury.*	*Seat supports on the anterior and lateral surfaces of seating system can help to grade down the level of trunk control needed.*
Trunk endurance	*Needs to be able to sit upright for 1 to 5 minutes.*	*Janna is currently unable to sit unsupported.*	*Janna needs support during sitting activities to prevent injury.*	*Allow for frequent breaks and position changes for a less strenuous activity. Increase intervals of sitting time to grade up the activity.*
Crossing midline	*Not required*			
Head movement	*Infant needs to be able to turn toward and/or follow adult with eyes and head.*	*Janna does not visually track objects, but is able to move her head.*	*None*	*Grade down by having the adult positioned in Janna's midline. Grade up by having the adult sit off to the side so that Janna has to turn their head to see the adult.*
Shoulder movement	*Not required*			

Activity Analysis Form (continued)

Page 3

Required Actions/ Performance Skills (continued):

	Performance Skills/ Required Body Actions & Functions for Activity	Performance Skills/ Client's Body Function/ Structure	Client Precautions	Adaptations/Grading
Elbow movement	Not required			
Wrist movement	Not required			
Hand skills	Not required			
Upper extremity strength	Not required			
Upper extremity endurance	Not required			
Upper extremity coordination	Not required			
Fine motor manipulation	Not required			
Unilateral task	Not required			
Bilateral task	Not required			
Hip movement	Not required			
Knee movement	Not required			
Ankle movement	Not required			
Lower extremity strength	Not required			
Lower extremity endurance	Not required			
Lower extremity coordination	Not required			
Muscle tone	Not required		None	None
Motor reflexes	Not required			
Motor planning	Not required			
Cardiovascular/hematological function	Not required		None	None
Immunological function	Not required		None	None
Respiratory function			None	None
Digestive function	Not required			
Excretory function	Not required			
Dermatological function	Not required			
Visual function	Client must be able to see the adult and to track the adult's actions with his/her eyes.	Janna has difficulty visually tracking objects.	None	Position the adult infant's field of vision to decrease complexity of activity. Position the adult outside child's field of vision to increase difficulty of activity.
Visual-perceptual function	Client must be able to see and interpret visual information.	Janna's visual-perceptual skills seem to be intact.	None	None
Auditory function	While not required, as hand gestures can suffice, the typical way the game is played is for the child to respond to visual and auditory (adult says "Peek-a-Boo") cues.	Janna has difficulty localizing sound.	None	By accompanying the auditory cue with the hand motion of the adult uncovering his/her face, the infant will still be able to visualize the action despite any auditory deficits. Position the adult outside child's field of vision to increase difficulty of activity.

Activity Analysis Form (continued)

Page 4

Required Actions/ Performance Skills (continued):

	Performance Skills/ Required Body Actions & Functions for Activity	Performance Skills/ Client's Body Function/ Structure	Client Precautions	Adaptations/Grading
Taste function	Not required			
Smell function	Not required			
Proprioceptive function	Not required			
Touch function	Not required			
Pain function	Not required			
Temperature function	Not required			
Emotional control/regulation	The infant needs to be able to regulate her emotions long enough to participate in this 1 to 5 minute activity.	Janna is often fussy unless she is being held.	None	The adult/parent can hold the infant in their laps facing them while playing Peek-a-Boo if necessary.
Impulse control	The infant needs to be able to control impulses long enough to participate in this 1 to 5 minute activity.	Janna's impulse control is typical of an infant (sporadic and susceptible to visual and auditory distractions).	None	Remove visual and auditory stimuli to grade down, add stimuli to grade up.
Expressive communication	An appropriate response during this activity would be for an infant to smile or laugh after step 4.	Janna is able to smile, but it seems to be random rather than social.	None	None
Receptive communication	The infant needs to be able to understand visual and verbal (volume, tone) communication.	Janna has difficulty visually tracking objects and localizing sounds.	None	None
Oral motor control	Not required			
Collaboration with others	Not required			
Judgment/safety awareness	Not required			
Executive functions	Not required			
Reading	Not required			
Calculations	Not required			
Memory				
Organization skills	Not required			
Multitasking	Not required			
Others as needed:				

Additional Client Factors:

How does the activity provide the opportunity to express the client's values? The infant client has multiple opportunities to make a social connection with the adult. If the adult is the parent, the adult client has the opportunity to learn a new method to create a meaningful connection with their child.

How does the activity interest the client? Infants are interested in activities that are new and exciting and meet their needs. Parents are interested in activities that they can share with their child and activities that contribute to their child's healthy development.

Activity Analysis Form (continued)

Page 5

Additional Client Factors (continued):

How is the client motivated to participate in this activity? *The infant is motivated to participate in this activity because of the opportunity to interact and connect with another human being.*

How does the activity have any spiritual meanings for the client? *This activity could contain spiritual meaning for the client if they feel it is allowing them to experience their connectedness with others.*

How could the activity positively contribute to the client's self-esteem? *For the infant, developing a new skill and sharing the joyful experience of Peek-a-Boo with an adult can contribute to their self-esteem. For the parent, helping their child to develop this skill and to meet a milestone promotes self-esteem and creates a shared moment with their child.*

How does the activity offer opportunity for affective expression? *At the completion of step 4, both adult and infant celebrate the discovery that the adult's face is present.*

____ Aggression ____ Sadness __X__ Happiness ____ Love ____ Others

How does the activity provide an opportunity for the client to test reality? *In step 3, to the infant, the adult's face seems to have disappeared. In step 3, to the infant, the adult's face seems to have disappeared. In step 4, reality is tested when the adult's face seems to reappear. The infant's perception of reality is challenged and the concept of object permanence begins to develop.*

Performance Patterns:

How does the performance of this activity reinforce useful habits? *This activity can help to reinforce the habit of maintaining attention with other people.*

How does the performance of this activity reinforce poor habits? *This activity does not require much purposeful movement or action from the infant, so it may indirectly reinforce a habit of neglecting to initiate actions.*

How does the performance of the activity utilize, reinforce or help create routines? *Performance of this activity could help to create or reinforce a routine of the adult and infant participating in a social interaction with one another.*

How does the activity reinforce a customary role for the client? *This activity reinforces the role of parent for the adult and the role of child for the infant. The infant plays the role of the child because she is learning from her parent. The adult plays the role of parent because they are facilitating an activity that is contributing to their child's development.*

How does the activity help establish a new role for the client? *The activity helps the infant to establish a new role as a social participant.*

How does the activity reinforce rituals performed by the client? *This activity could reinforce the rituals performed by the client because Peek-a-Boo may hold cultural or social meaning for the parent. Playing Peek-a-Boo is a classic activity that may act as a symbol representing parenthood to the adult.*

Context and Environment (describe):

Physical *The physical environment may include a large range of settings, however it must be void of hazards for infants and and free of or limited visual and auditory distractions.*

Social *The social environment typically includes one to three adults (an OT, OTA, and parent) and one infant.*

Temporal *Time of year, month or week does not have significant relevance to this activity. Time of day should be considered in light of the sleep schedule of the infant.*

Cultural *The cultural context needs to be one in which peek-a-boo is an accepted and valued activity.*

Personal *Age, gender, and socioeconomic status of the parent are highly flexible. The child should be approximately 6 to 12 months old to participate in this activity.*

Virtual *A virtual context is not applicable in this activity.*

Additional Information:

CASE STUDY 2

CHAPTER 42

A Diagnosis of Autism: The Role of Sensory Integration and Applied Behavioral Analysis in OTA Practice

Amy Wagenfeld, PhD, OTR/L, SCEM, CAPs

Background Information

Autism spectrum disorders (ASDs), also referred to as autism, are developmental disabilities that may lead to significant social, communication, and behavioral challenges (CDC, 2012). ASDs include autism, Asperger's, Rhett syndrome, and pervasive developmental disability (PDD)-not otherwise specified. The rate of diagnosis of ASD has risen to 1 in 68 children and 1 in 54 boys (Baio, 2014; CDC, 2012). Boys are four times more likely to have an ASD than are girls (Baio, 2014). Autism is the fastest growing serious developmental disability in the United States (Autism Speaks, 2012a, 2012b).

The federal costs associated with autism are about $137 billion per year. Research has found a strong genetic link to ASD within families. For instance, if one identical twin is diagnosed with an ASD, the other has a 36% to 95% of also being diagnosed. If a fraternal twin is diagnosed, the other has up to a 31% chance of being diagnosed. If a sibling has an ASD, there is a 2% to 18% chance that other children in the family will be diagnosed. Additionally, research suggests a strong relationship between the age of the father at time of conception and an increased incidence of autism in offspring (Stefansson et al., 2012). About 62% of children with an ASD are not intellectually impaired (IQ ≤ 70). The CDC (2012) reported that the typical yearly medical costs for Medicaid-enrolled children with an ASD were $10,709, which is approximately six times higher than costs for children without an ASD, which was $1,812. Medical costs are 4.1 to 6.2 times greater for children with ASD as compared to those without (Shimabukuro et al., 2008). Above and beyond medical costs, behavioral interventions such as applied behavioral analysis may cost between $40,000 and $60,000 per year (Amendah et al., 2011).

A specialized treatment method called applied behavior analysis (ABA) is often used with children with ASDs. It is important to note that there is an ongoing debate in the autism community about the efficacy of ABA and/or sensory integration treatment methods. Behavior analysis is focused on principles, such as positive reinforcement that offer an explanation for how learning occurs (Autism Speaks, 2012a, 2012b). From a behavioral perspective, if a behavior is rewarded, it is more likely to reoccur. ABA is the application of techniques and principles that lead to positive and purposeful changes in behavior and a reduction in undesired ones (Autism Speaks, 2012a, 2012b). ABA treatment is extremely intense and involves a strong commitment on the part of the families of children with an ASD.

Sensory integration or sensory processing is the means by which the nervous system receives information coming into the senses and processes in order to elicit the desired motoric and behavioral responses (SPD Foundation, 2012). For children (and adults) with sensory processing disorders, there is a disconnection between appropriate processing and motor and behavioral outcomes that limit functional skills and engagement in occupations. Please refer to Chapter 28, *Sensory Issues*, for a more detailed discussion about sensory integration.

Traditional Practice Area: Children and Youth

Emerging Practice Area: Autism

Cross References: Chapter 27, *Developmental Disabilities*, Chapter 28, *Sensory Issues*, Chapter 36, *Children and Youth*

CLINICAL PRESENTATION

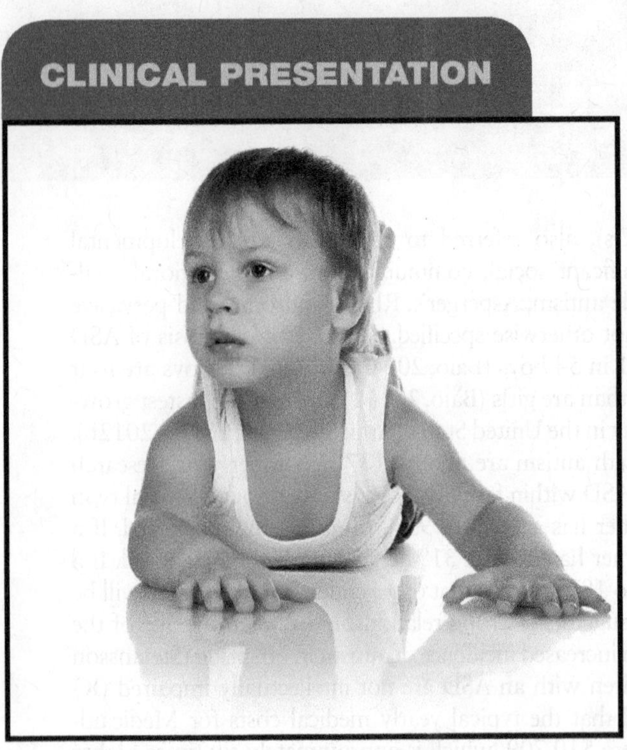

Luke is a 4-year-old white boy who lives with his family in a high rise condominium building in a central business district in a large city. Luke's mom, Lisa, is 34 years old and works part time as a radio talk show host. Luke's father, Charles, is 60 years old and employed as a research scientist. It is a first marriage for Lisa and a second for Charles. Charles has three adult children who live within a 1-hour radius from Charles and Lisa. Charles' adult children are all employed in the governmental sector. Luke has one full sister, Maura, who is 8 years old. Maura is a very high spirited young girl. She has one close friend but spends most of her time outside of school running around the family condo, often crashing into furniture, and then getting up and starting again. She cries easily and easily gets frustrated.

Luke was a full-term baby. Unlike his sister, Maura, Luke was a placid and easy going baby, who smiled frequently, was social, self-soothed with ease, ate without incident, and by 9 months had begun to say his first words. Luke took his first steps at 12 months and loved to play with toys and share them with his family. Lisa and Charles felt that Luke was an easy baby and that their family was complete. With the exception of dealing with a high spirited daughter, life was rosy. Luke was thriving.

When Luke was about 3 years old, Lisa started to notice that Luke seemed to be losing his words and was not speaking as much as he had in the past. Concerned, she took him to the pediatrician because she worried that there was something wrong with Luke's hearing. Testing showed his hearing to be normal. One weekend not long after, the family was off doing what they liked most, to play in the large park about a 10-minute walk from their condo. Luke seemed to be fixated on the hand-operated merry-go-round, watching it spin for what seemed like hours. Charles and Lisa thought it was odd, but dismissed it as just a passing thing. As the weeks and months progressed, Luke seemed to retreat into himself. He no longer sought out others for company or comfort. He was no longer saying any words and started to refuse all the foods he had previously enjoyed. He now only ate white bread, white rice, chicken, and hot dogs. He began to scream a high-pitched sound for hours on end. The only time it stopped was when Luke was asleep, which lately had been very little. He was awake for 18 of a 24-hour period, day after day. Luke recoiled from touch and responded negatively to baths.

Alarmed, Lisa and Charles brought Luke back to the pediatrician. Following an extensive interview and observations, Luke was diagnosed with autism. Completely caught off guard, Lisa and Charles set out to find out what was necessary to help Luke achieve his fullest potential. They read everything they could about autism and learned that scientific evidence now suggests that genetics (nature) contribute to autism. In doing their research, they learned that based on the IDEA, Luke was eligible for preschool services. They enrolled him immediately. He was placed in a mixed preschool classroom with typically developing and atypically developing children.

Working as a transdisciplinary team within the classroom, the teachers, OT and PT practitioners, speech and language therapist, and social worker at Luke's new school prided themselves on respecting that children have myriad learning styles and strived to understand how to nurture each child's skill acquisition styles. Through their research, Lisa and Charles learned that two common approaches to working with children with autism are sensory based and ABA. They wondered what the preschool team would do, and how they could support the team. The team developed a behavioral program that focused on positive reinforcement for desirable behaviors such as making eye contact. They strove to avoid negatively reinforcing undesirable behaviors in an effort to extinguish them. Punishment was used as little as possible.

Over the next 6 months, Luke showed minimal improvements. He had begun to use an electronic communication system on an IPad and was able to make eye contact for 3 seconds when cued to do so. While pleased that Luke was making small gains, they were anxious and unsure that ABA was the best and only therapeutic approach for Luke. They explored the evidence on sensory integration and felt it was important for Luke to receive this type of therapeutic intervention.

After much discussion with the team, it was determined that Luke was eligible for a sensory evaluation, and an OT certified to administer the *Sensory Integration and Praxis Test* was located and brought in to test Luke. Luke demonstrated significant sensory processing disorder, and accordingly, the OT developed a sensory diet that the team and parents administered at school by the OT team and at home. Luke was also approved to receive outpatient sensory integrative therapy through the family's private insurance company. The private OT worked with the school's OT practitioners to carry over some techniques in the classroom. Meanwhile, Luke was continuing to receive ABA services. Gains were noted. Luke began to eat new foods and was able to tolerate new textures with only minimal resistance. And they began to adjust to life with a child with autism—a lifetime journey had only begun for Charles and Lisa. ■

Internet Resources

Association for Behavior Analysis International—www.abainternational.org
Autism Speaks—www.autismspeaks.org
Centers for Disease Control and Prevention—www.cdc.gov
National Autism Association—www.nationalautismassociation.org
National Institutes of Health—www.nih.gov
National Institute of Neurological Disorders and Stroke—http://www.ninds.nih.gov/disorders/autism/detail_autism.htm
Sensory Integration International-Spiral Foundation—http://www.thespiralfoundation.org/
Sensory Processing Disorder Foundation—http://www.spdfoundation.net/

References

Amendah D, Grosse SD, Peacock G, et al. The economic costs of autism: a review. In: Amaral D, Geschwind D, Dawson G, eds. *Autism Spectrum Disorders*. Oxford, UK: Oxford University Press; 2011:1347–1360.

Autism Speaks. *Applied behavior analysis*; 2012a. Retrieved from http://www.autismspeaks.org/what-autism/treatment/applied-behavior-analysis-aba

Autism Speaks. *Facts about autism*; 2012b. Retrieved from http://www.autismspeaks.org/what-autism/facts-about-autism

Baio J. Prevalence of autism spectrum disorders—Autism and developmental disabilities monitoring network, 14 sites, United States. *Morb Mortal Wkly Rep* 2014;61(SS03):1–19. Retrieved from http://www.cdc.gov/mmwr/preview/mmwrhtml/ss6103a1.htm?s_cid=ss6103a1_

Centers for Disease Control and Prevention. *Autism spectrum disorders*; 2012. Retrieved from http://www.cdc.gov/ncbddd/autism/index.html

Sensory Processing Disorder Foundation. *About sensory processing disorder*; 2012. Retrieved from http://www.spdfoundation.net/about-sensory-processing-disorder.html

Shimabukuro TT, Grosse SD, Rice C. Medical expenditures for children with an autism spectrum disorder in a privately insured population. *J Autism Dev Disord* 2008;38(3):546–552.

Stefansson S, et al. Rate of de novo mutations and the importance of father's age to disease risk. *Nature* 2012;488:471–475.

CASE STUDY 3

CHAPTER 43

Fine Motor Skills Issues and Challenges with Mastering School Readiness Skills

Amy Wagenfeld, PhD, OTR/L, SCEM, CAPs

Background Information

Fine motor skills enable people to be effective tool users. Fine motor skills build onto a foundation of gross motor skills. By the time children enter school, the expectations are high that they be skilled tool users. For some, this is not possible. Children and adolescents' self-perception of fine and gross motor skills suggest a direct correlation between perceived level of ability and competence in terms of academics and scholastic endeavors (Piek et al., 2006). Further, research suggests that poor handwriting skills, which depend in part on fine motor skill, may also negatively influence self-esteem (Brossard et al., 2008). Younger children with higher perceived scholastic skills do in fact have better fine motor skills than their peers with less fine motor skill (Piek et al., 2006). Evidence strongly point to the necessity of providing individualized strategies to address the multilayered implications of fine motor skills as they influence self-perception of academic ability as well as self-esteem (Tseng & cHOW, 2000). It is important to intervene and implement strategies to enhance children's fine motor skills before they experience needless failure (McHale & Cermak, 1992).

Traditional Practice Area(s)—Children and Youth

Emerging Practice Area(s)—A Broader Scope in Schools

Cross Reference—Chapter 20, *Arts and Crafts*; Chapter 21, *Adaptive Equipment*; Chapter 25, *Group Dynamics: Planning and Leading Effective Therapeutic Groups*; Chapter 27, *Developmental Disabilities*; Chapter 31, *Vision*; Chapter 36, *Children and Youth*; Chapter 40, *Emerging Practice Areas*

CLINICAL PRESENTATION

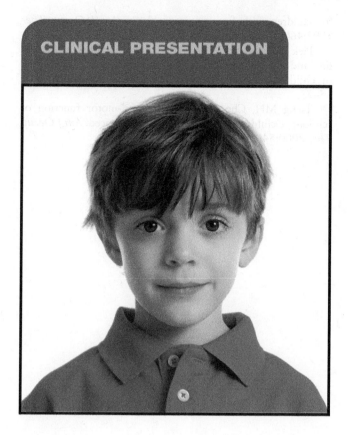

Mikey is a 6-year-old white boy who attends first grade in his suburban town's public elementary school. Normally sunny and cheerful Mikey is the oldest of three boys, who live with their mom, Ariel. In addition to Hebrew school, Mikey plays soccer, takes piano lessons, and just loves to play and rough house with his brothers and his many friends. Mikey's family has an electronic game box system, which he does not like to play, even if his friends or brothers invite him to do so. Life is very busy in Mikey's household. Ariel works full time as an accountant. The boys go to a home day care provider, who takes Mikey to and from school. His younger brothers do not yet go to school.

In kindergarten, Mikey's teacher noted that he spent most of his free play time in the building center creating fabulous castles and roads. He was eager to build with friends and to show his teacher what he created. Mikey's teacher tried to gently direct him to the painting or fine motor centers. Eager to please, Mikey would spend a few moments there and then retreat to the block center, telling her. "I can't do this so well." The teacher was quick to redirect Mikey to feel good about himself, and he seemed to shake off his negative self-commentary. When the class was engaged in learning to write, Mikey rushed to finish his and tended to be somewhat disruptive, often reaching over to tickle his friends seated nearby. Mikey had trouble setting up his snack and always asked his teacher to help him.

Recently Mikey's piano teacher told his mom that Mikey does not seem to enjoy his lessons and often tries to redirect the lesson to a conversation about a recent television show he had watched. He seems to not be able to coordinate his fingers to move along with his eyes as he reads the musical notes. Mikey would rather sing or talk about television than play piano. Mikey told his mom that he is "bad at piano."

In first grade, the stakes are higher, and Mikey is expected to be writing his letters and using scissors and other school tools with greater proficiency. He is resistant and spends a great deal of work time sharpening his pencil or wandering about the classroom. His work product is of poor quality, when he does it. Many of his friends have become obsessed with Legos, but Mikey has thus far avoided playing with them. At home, he has begun to be aggressive toward his brothers. He complains that he is dumb and stupid. He does not want to play soccer anymore. Alarmed, Mikey's mom makes an appointment with the first-grade teacher. Both agree that Mikey's self-esteem is at risk and that because of his reluctance to write and do other fine motor skills, an occupational therapy evaluation was in order.

After going through the necessary procedures to obtain an evaluation, the school-based OT evaluated Mikey. The OT determined that based on results of several motor and handwriting evaluations, discussion with Mikey's mom about his motor development history, and in combination with his plummeting self-esteem that Mikey would benefit from occupational therapy services once weekly. The district's OTA added Mikey to his caseload and, in recognizing the importance of nurture in helping Mikey improve his fine motor skills and associatively, self-esteem, also worked with the teacher and mom to develop a home program, involving things such as having Mikey write the dinner menu on the whiteboard hung on the refrigerator at home. In school, at the OTA's recommendation, the entire class began to participate in a fine motor skills school readiness program (Brook et al., 2006) three times a week. By the end of the school year, Mikey's skills had significantly improved and he no longer was self-disparaging. The sunny and cheerful Mikey had returned. ■

Internet Resources

Fingergym Fine Motor Skills School Readiness Program—http://www.fingergym.info/

Medline Plus—http://www.nlm.nih.gov/medlineplus/ency/article/002364.htm

References

Brook G, Wagenfeld AE, Thompson C. *The Fingergym™ Fine Motor School Skills Readiness Program*. Brisbane, Australia: Australian Academic Press; 2006.

Brossard Racine M, et al. Handwriting performance in children with attention deficit hyperactivity disorder (ADHD). *J Child Neurol* 2008;23(4):399–406.

McHale K, Cermak SA. Fine motor activities in elementary school: preliminary findings and provisional implications for children with fine motor problems. *Am J Occup Ther* 1992;46(10):898–903.

Piek JP, Baynam GB, Barrett NC. The relationship between fine and gross motor ability, self-perceptions and self-worth in children and adolescents. *Hum Mov Sci* 2006;25(1):65–75.

Tseng MH, Chow SMK. Perceptual-motor function of school-age children with slow handwriting speed. *Am J Occup Ther* 2000;54(1):83–88.

CASE STUDY 4

CHAPTER 44

Experiencing Poverty, Obesity, and Bullying in School

Amy Wagenfeld, PhD, OTR/L, SCEM, CAPs

Background Information

The statistics are sobering. Most Americans (51.4%) will live in poverty at some point before age 65 (McKernan et al., 2009). Today, 15.1% of people living in the United States are living in poverty (World Hunger, 2012). This is equivalent to one in seven people. More than 1 in 5 or 16.2 million children are part of households struggling to put food on the table (Coleman et al., 2011). In the United States, upward of 44% of children live in low-income working families (US Census Bureau, 2011). Minority groups, such as African Americans and Latinos, experience childhood hunger at a rate of one in three children (Coleman et al., 2011).

The 2007–2008 *National Health and Nutrition Examination Survey* (*NHANES*) indicates that childhood obesity has nearly tripled since 1980 (2012). Approximately 17% (or 12.5 million) of children and adolescents aged 2 to 19 years are obese (Centers for Disease Control and Prevention, 2012). Results of the *NHANES* indicated significant racial and ethnic disparities in obesity prevalence among U.S. children and adolescents. In 2007–2008, the survey results showed that "Hispanic boys, aged 2 to 19 years, were significantly more likely to be obese than non-Hispanic White boys, and non-Hispanic Black girls were significantly more likely to be obese than non-Hispanic White girls" (Ogden & Carroll, 2012).

Young and Leventhal (2008) indicated that bullying is "an aggressive behavior in which individuals in a dominant position intend to cause mental and/or physical suffering to others, with a prevalence worldwide ranging from 9% to 54%" (p. 133). Whether the recipient, victim, or perpetrator of bullying, all are at substantially high risk of mental and physical problems. According to Klomek et al. (2011), "Victims of bullying consistently exhibit more depressive symptoms than nonvictims; they have high levels of suicidal ideation and are more likely to attempt suicide than nonvictims" (p. 3). Cyber-bullying is a serious public health concern, in part because of a recent spate of highly publicized youth suicides following episodes of cyber-bullying.

Traditional Practice Area(s): Children and Youth and Health and Wellness

Emerging Practice Area(s): Obesity and Bullying

Cross Reference: Chapter 16, *Working Together: Clinical Reasoning and Collaboration*; Chapter 25, *Group Dynamics: Planning and Leading Effective Therapeutic Groups*; Chapter 35, *Health and Well-Being*; Chapter 36, *Children and Youth*; Chapter 40, *Emerging Practice Areas*

CLINICAL PRESENTATION

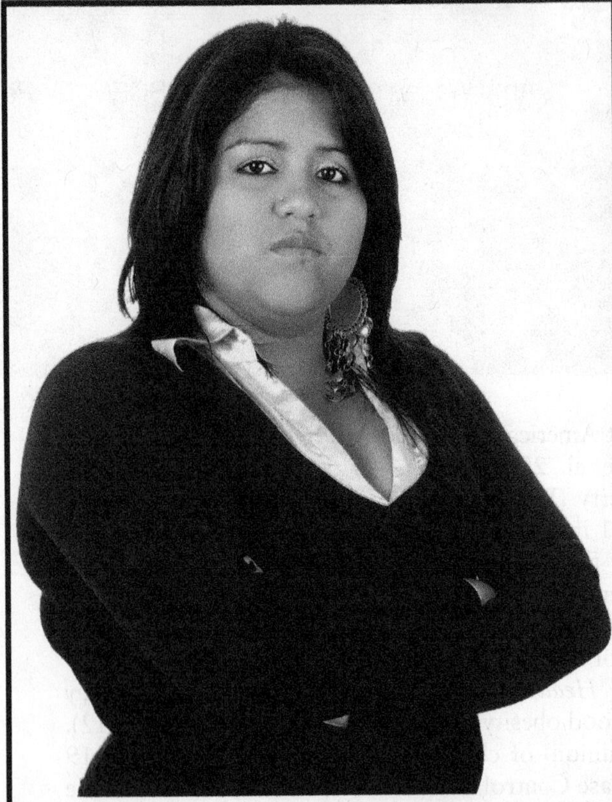

Stella is 11 years old. Her father, who is deceased, was Hispanic. Her mother is no longer in the picture. She is Muslim. Stella and three siblings live with her grandmother and uncle and his family in a two bedroom apartment in a housing project in a major metropolitan area. Stella's uncle is on disability because of an accident he had at his job as a waiter. Her aunt works full time at a minimum wage job. Her grandmother receives a social security check. Stella's siblings, who are both under age 5, receive financial support for healthy foods through the Federal Governmental Women Infants and Children Program. Money is very tight. There are no grocery stores close-by, and since the family has no car, they rely on public transportation or rides from friends. Stella receives free breakfast and lunch at school, but often, she only eats the things she likes and is familiar with, such as cookies or muffins. There is a small bodega store that sells convenience foods a block away, and now, a mobile farmers' market truck comes by weekly to sell fresh produce at a cost well below grocery store prices. Up until the vegetable truck arrived, Stella's family relied on the bodega for their food supply. This meant eating a great deal of canned meats and unhealthy snack foods, as the store does not stock fresh produce. Consequently, Stella and her siblings, while always hungry, are obese. There are high hopes that with the arrival of the vegetable truck, having low cost, healthy food options will help to reduce the obesity issue in the family. A confounding factor to the obesity is that there is no playground or park nearby Stella's apartment. The only open space is over-run with garbage and gangs. It is not safe to be outside.

School used to be Stella's haven. She dreaded school vacations because that meant she had to be home. Now that she is 11, she has started middle school. She is a top notch student, and because of her academic aptitude, was recommended to attend an elite public middle school in an affluent, mostly white suburb at no cost. She does not know anyone in her classes because her friends all go to the local middle school. At the new school, there is a group of girls who have begun to taunt and torment Stella, calling her a variety of disparaging names stemming from Stella's obesity, her mixed race, and socioeconomic status. One girl has begun to send text messages and tweets that are filled with cruel comments about Stella. Not wanting to further burden her grandmother, Stella retreats into herself. An astute English teacher has noticed that something is wrong with Stella, she keeps her head down in class and seems to be literally shutting down and hiding in an effort to be un-noticed. The teacher is very friendly with the OTA who sees some children at the school. The teacher arranges a meeting with the OTA and mentions Stella. The OTA has just started a group for children who are victims of bullying. At the teacher's recommendation, she invites Stella to join the group. Stella accepts. ■

Internet Resources

American Academy of Child and Adolescent Psychiatry—http://www.aacap.org/cs/root/facts_for_families/bullying
Centers for Disease Control and Prevention—www.cdc.gov
Nemours Foundation—http://kidshealth.org/teen/your_mind/problems/bullies.html
Obesity Society—http://www.obesity.org/
US Census Bureau—http://www.census.gov

References

Centers for Disease Control and Prevention. *Obesity rates among all children in the United States*; 2012. Retrieved from http://www.cdc.gov/obesity/data/adult.html

Coleman A, Andrews M, Carlson S. Household food security in the United States in 2010. Economic Research Report No. ERR-125; 2011. Retrieved from http://www.ers.usda.gov/publications/err-economic-research-report/err125.aspx

Klomek AB, Sourander A, Gould MS. Bullying and suicide: detection and intervention. *Psychiatr Times* 2011;28(2):1–13. Retrieved from http://www.psychiatrictimes.com/pdf?p_p_id=PDF_CONTENT&articleId=1795797&groupId=10168

McKernan S-M, Caroline Ratcliffe C, Cellini SR. *Transitioning in and out of poverty.* Fact Sheet Number 1; 2009. Retrieved from http://www.urban.org/uploaded-pdf/411956_transitioningpoverty.pdf

Ogden C, Carroll M. *NCHS Health E-Stat. Prevalence of obesity among children and adolescents: United States, trends 1963–1965 through 2007–2008*; 2012. Retrieved from http://www.cdc.gov/nchs/data/hestat/obesity_child_07_08/obesity_child_07_08.htm

United States Census Bureau. Poverty; 2011. Retrieved from http://www.census.gov/hhes/www/poverty/about/overview/index.html

World Hunger. *Hunger in America: 2012 United States hunger and poverty facts*; 2012. Retrieved from http://www.worldhunger.org/articles/Learn/us_hunger_facts.htm

Young SK, Leventhal B. Bullying and suicide. A review. *Int J Adolesc Med Health* 2008;20(2):133–154.

CASE STUDY 5

CHAPTER 45

Service Members Returning from Combat Missions: The Implications of PTSD, TBI, and Traumatic Limb Loss on Function

Amy Wagenfeld, PhD, OTR/L, SCEM, CAPs

Background Information

For injured soldiers returning from battle, rehabilitation is complex and poses multiple physical and emotional challenges, including diagnosis and treatment for posttraumatic stress disorder (PTSD), traumatic brain injury (TBI), and traumatic limb loss.

Increasing evidence suggests that PTSD is one of the most prevalent mental health disorders impacting veterans returning from war combat in the recent Iraq/Afghanistan War eras, ranging from 10% to 18% (Buchanan et al., 2011; Dougherty et al., 2010). According to the *DSM-IV TR*, symptoms associated with PTSD include intense feelings of fear and anxiety, which may lead to avoidance of people, places, or situations that could trigger a reexperience of the trauma (American Psychiatric Association, 2013). People with PTSD commonly experience self-regulation issues and subsequently are challenged to prioritize, set, and meet goals and to deal with environmental demands (Tangney et al., 2004). Suicidal behaviors are higher for people with PTSD than those with depression (Chan et al., 2009). In addition to PTSD, for veterans returning from conflict, there is significant risk for other mental health issues such as depression, substance abuse, and interpersonal issues. Psychological suffering aside, over a 2-year period, the cost of PTSD to society ranges from 4 to 6.2 billion dollars (Rosenthal et al., 2011). Because of the perceived stigma associated with being diagnosed with PTSD, including threat to future military service and obstacles to seeking adequate services, many veterans do not receive the care that they need (Hoge et al., 2004).

The U.S. Veterans Administration finds that the primary causes of TBI in present day combat missions are blasts, blast plus motor vehicle accidents (MVAs), MVAs alone, and gunshot wounds (2011). According to the Department of Defense Report, "*Report to Congress in Accordance with Section 1634 (b) of the National Defense Authorization Act for Fiscal Year 2008*," the Military Health Congressional Research Service United States Military Casualty Statistics System (MHS) has "recorded 43,779 patients who have been diagnosed with a TBI in calendar years 2003 through 2007. The MHS has spent an estimated $100.0 million on direct and purchased care for TBI patients and $10.1 million on prescription costs for all prescriptions filled after a diagnosis of TBI" (Fischer, 2009, pp. 1–2).

Typically, people with a traumatic limb loss respond to their injury with shock, followed by denial, fear, distress, depression, grief, acknowledgment overlaid with hostility and frustration and drudging acceptance to participate in rehabilitation, and then early acceptance and reorganization or reframing of life (Bradway et al., 1984). Those with traumatic limb loss commonly use avoidance as a coping strategy more often than do those whose limb loss stems from disease (Reiber et al., 2010). Improved psychological adjustment to lower limb loss includes time since amputation, strong social supports, satisfaction with prosthesis devices, strong sense of coherence, increased resilience, lower level amputations, and less pain (Reiber et al., 2010). Qualities associated with limited adjustment include increased rate of depression and concurrent activity restriction, increased sense of vulnerability, poor sense of health, body image issues, and social discomfort (Reiber et al., 2010).

According to the Army Office of the Surgeon General, between September 2001 and January 12, 2009, there were 1,286 amputations in the Iraq/Afghanistan wars and unaffiliated conflicts. This figure includes 935 major limb amputations and 351 minor amputations. 643 (50%) were wounded by improvised explosive devices (IEDs) (US Veteran's Administration, 2011). Pain management as well as mental health is an issue of great concern to health care professionals treating veterans with traumatic limb loss. In fact, 38% of Iraq/Afghanistan war veterans with traumatic limb amputation are also diagnosed with PTSD (Dougherty et al., 2010). Current treatments to address pain issues, beyond traditional medication regimens, include mirror box therapy (amputations), acupuncture, and virtual reality (Reiber et al., 2010). Reiber and colleagues reported, a "recent Department of Defense (DOD) Rehabilitation Directive is facilitating the return of service members with major traumatic limb loss from OIF/OEF to their highest possible functional level so that major limb loss does not prevent [these service members] from maximizing their [future] career options in either the military or civilian sectors" (2010, p. 276).

Traditional Practice Areas: Rehabilitation, Disability, and Participation; Mental Health; Health and Wellness

Emerging Practice Area: Veteran and Wounded Warrior Care

Cross References: Chapter 16, *Working Together: Clinical Reasoning and Collaboration*; Chapter 21, *Adaptive Equipment*; Chapter 22, *Assistive Technology*; Chapter 23, *Activities of Daily Living*; Chapter 24, *Orthotics and Orthotic Fabrication*; Chapter 29, *Psychological Conditions*; Chapter 30, *Physical Disabilities*; Chapter 34, *Rehabilitation, Disability and Participation*; Chapter 34, *Mental Health*; Chapter 35, *Health and Well-Being*; Chapter 38, *Work and Industry*; Chapter 40, *Emerging Practice Areas*

CLINICAL PRESENTATION

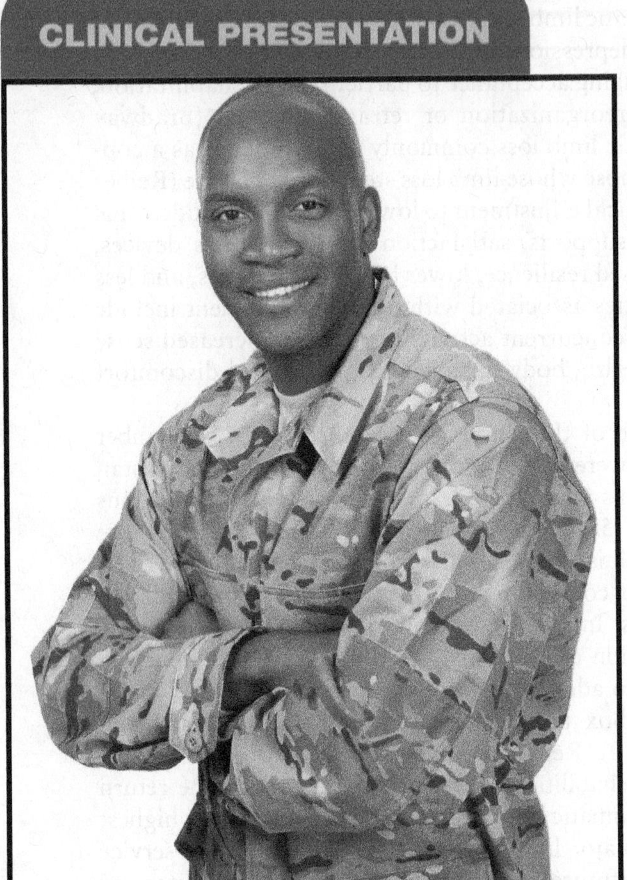

Sgt. Travis Long was on his second tour of duty in 18 months in Operation Enduring Freedom (OEF), when his convoy was hit by an IED. Several of his platoon members were killed, a few were uninjured, but most were injured. Sgt. Long's best friend was killed. In the blast explosion, Sgt. Long's left leg and right arm were blown off. He was immediately triaged, and the end result was an above the knee amputation of the left leg and an above the elbow amputation of the right arm (his dominant). When he was stable, Sgt. Long was flown stateside for a long rehabilitative process at a military medical facility in Texas.

Sgt. Long is 25 years old and married to high school sweetheart Rachel. They live in a small town in the Midwest. They have a 3-year-old son, Justin, and Rachel is pregnant with their second child. Rachel and Sgt. Long are both from large and supportive families who live close by and are actively engaged with the young family. Rachel and Sgt. Long are practicing Episcopalians, and Rachel teaches the preschool Sunday school class.

Prior to enlisting, Sgt. Long attended a technical college, where he took a certification course in cooling and refrigeration. Rachel completed a culinary program, specializing in baking. Since having children, Rachel works on an as-needed basis for a local bakery. Rachel and Sgt. Long and the children live on the third story of a walkup apartment building. They have one bathroom with a tub/shower unit.

Following Sgt. Long's transfer to the rehabilitation hospital in Texas, Rachel's parents helped Rachel pack and then drove her and the children to Texas. They flew home to enable Rachel to have a car, as she was told Sgt. Long was going to be in rehabilitation for many months. When Rachel and the children arrived, Sgt. Long was elated to see them. Rachel was relieved that despite his traumatic amputations, he seemed just like his old self, happy, and eager to wake up and enjoy each day. She breathed a silent breath of relief and got busy settling in to the on-site housing provided to wounded warriors and their families. Between watching the children, meeting other families, and being with Sgt. Long during occupational and physical therapies, the days were full. She was happy to be together again. Sgt. Long received upper and lower extremity prosthetics. In occupational therapy, he was learning to use the upper extremity prosthetic to do ADLs and was ready for ongoing just right challenges involving his new arm. Task-oriented activities focused on proximal and distal activities to improve skill in his right arm as well as to improve skilled use of the left. He had begun to walk with the prosthetic leg using a straight cane in physical therapy. Sgt. Long really liked his therapists and spent long hours in the clinic, determined to return home without requiring any assistance. He had even begun to think about Paralympic training as a hand cyclist.

Always at the periphery of his thoughts, Sgt. Long was plagued with guilt that his best friend had died and he survived. He became hyperalert and loud, and unexpected noises sent him into a panic attack. Reoccurring nightmares shaped his sleep; he often awoke screaming. Gradually, Sgt. Long began to withdraw from Rachel and was short tempered with the children. Rachel was worried. She had always taken Sgt. Long's sense of coherence, his "make lemonade out of lemons" attitude for granted. This was the man she knew, not one who was withdrawn and isolating. He no longer spent his days in the rehab clinic, instead preferring to stay in the apartment and watch crime shows on television and to go to therapies only as he was scheduled to do, nothing extra.

Sgt. Long became disinterested in social events on the base and just wanted to be alone. He was also experiencing daily debilitating headaches. Sgt. Long was having trouble remembering details and could not sit still for more than a few seconds. Further testing revealed that Sgt. Long had polytrauma; traumatic amputations, PTSD, and mild traumatic brain injury (MTBI). The new diagnosis entailed bringing a new discipline into Sgt. Long's care plan. He still received intense occupational and physical therapy services. Occupational therapy expanded their scope of service to address the memory and perceptual issues associated with the MTBI and also to support his psychosocial issues. Reluctantly, he began seeing a social worker with Rachel. His goal remained to go home and to be independent, but there was still a long road to travel before his goal was realized. ■

Internet Resources

American Psychiatric Association—www.psych.org
American Psychological Association—www.apa.org
Brain Line—www.brainline.org
Centers for Disease Control and Prevention—www.cdc.gov
National Amputation Foundation—www.nationalamputation.org
Veteran's Administration—www.va.gov

References

American Psychiatric Association. *Diagnostic and Statistical Manual of Mental Disorders DSM-V Fifth Edition.* Text Revision. Washington, DC: American Psychiatric Publishing, Inc.; 2013.

Bradway JK, Malone JM, Racy J, et al. Psychological adaptation to amputation: an overview. *Orthot Prosthet* 1984;38:46–50.

Buchanan C, Kemppainen J, Smith S, et al. Awareness of posttraumatic stress disorder in veterans: a female spouse/intimate partner perspective. *Mil Med* 2011;176(7):743–751.

Chan D, Cheadle AD, Reiber G, et al. Health care utilization and its costs for depressed veterans with and without comorbid PTSD symptoms. *Psychiatr Serv* 2009;60(12):1612–1617.

Dougherty PJ, McFarland LV, Smith DG, et al. Multiple traumatic limb loss: a comparison of Vietnam veterans to OIF/OEF service members. *J Rehabil Res Dev* 2010;47(4):333–348.

Fischer H. United States military casualty statistics: operation Iraqi Freedom and Operation Enduring Freedom. *CRS Report for Congress-7-5700 www.crs.gov RS22452.* Congressional Research Service; 2009, March.

Hoge CW, Castro CA, Messer SC, et al. Combat duty in Iraq and Afghanistan, mental health problems, and barriers to care. *N Engl J Med* 2004;351(1):13–22.

Reiber GE, McFarland LV, Hubbard S, et al. Service members and veterans with major traumatic limb loss from Vietnam War and OIF/OEF conflicts: survey methods, participants, and summary findings. *J Rehabil Res Dev* 2010;47(4):275–297.

Rosenthal JZ, Grosswald S, Ross R, et al. Effects of transcendental meditation in veterans of Operation Enduring Freedom and Operation Iraqi Freedom with posttraumatic stress disorder: a pilot study. *Mil Med* 2011;176(6):626–630.

Tangney JP, Baumeister RF, Boone, AL. High self-control predicts good adjustment, less pathology, better grades, and interpersonal success. *J Pers* 2004;72:271–322.

US Veterans Administration. *Mental Health Effects of Serving in Afghanistan and Iraq*; 2011. Retrieved from http://www.ptsd.va.gov/public/pages/overview-mental-health-effects.asp

CASE STUDY 6

CHAPTER 46

Developmental Disabilities and Cognitive Functioning: A Young Adult with Down Syndrome

Amy Wagenfeld, PhD, OTR/L, SCEM, CAPs

Background Information

Developmental disabilities are a diverse group of severe chronic conditions that result from either genetic or environmental factors. Many people with developmental disabilities present with cognitive and/or physical impairments. Developmental disabilities begin anytime during development up to 22 years of age (CDÇ, 2011; HHS, 2012). More than six million people in the United States have developmental disabilities (HHS, 2012). The lifetime cost of care, social support, education, and medical treatment for persons with developmental disabilities is substantial. Examples of developmental disabilities include, but are not limited to, autism, brain injury, fetal alcohol syndrome, cerebral palsy, mental retardation, behavioral disorders, spina bifida, and Down syndrome (HHS, 2012). Based on 2003 dollars, the approximate lifetime cost for those born in 2000 with a developmental disability was

$51.2 billion for people with mental retardation
$11.5 billion for people with cerebral palsy
$2.1 billion for people with hearing loss
$2.5 billion for people with vision impairment (CDC, 2011)

Most people with developmental disabilities experience significant challenges with major life activities including language, mobility, learning, self-help, independent living, and self-care.

Individuals with developmental disabilities often benefit from long-term comprehensive services in order to lead more productive lives. In adulthood, part of leading a healthy and productive life entails work. It is widely understood that people with developmental disabilities often struggle with and experience difficulties with employment including both obtaining and maintaining jobs (Stephens et al., 2005, p. 469). Results of *the Survey of Income and Program Participation* showed that a majority of adults with developmental disabilities were not only overwhelmingly under- or unemployed, even with support from government income assistance programs, their economic resources are extremely limited (Kiyoshi & Fujiura, 2002). Further, results of a survey of 200 individuals with developmental disabilities noted that those who were un- or underemployed had a lessor sense of control and quality of life than their counterparts who were competitively employed (Wehmeyer, 1994). Choice and control are critically important when setting up programming for people with developmental and cognitive disabilities.

Traditional Practice Area—Rehabilitation, Disability, and Participation

Cross Reference—Chapter 25, *Group Dynamics: Planning and Leading Effective Therapeutic Groups;* Chapter 26, *Workplace Safety;* Chapter 27, *Developmental Disabilities;* Chapter 33, *Rehabilitation, Disability, and Participation*

CLINICAL PRESENTATION

Rory is 30 years old. He has Down syndrome and currently lives at home with his parents, Ruth and Donald. Ruth is 70 years old, and Donald is 75 years old. Ruth is a retired nurse, and Donald is a retired train conductor. Both have health issues that limit their mobility. They rely on Rory's older sister Kathy to drive them to appointments. Kathy lives with her husband in the top floor of the family's double decker home.

Rory was born after the IDEA was signed into law so he received the benefit of a public education. Rory has a cognitive (intellectual) disability. His IQ is estimated to be 70, putting him in the moderately impaired or trainable range. His capacity for learning is impaired. As is typical for individuals with Down syndrome, Rory has cardiac as well as vision issues and has been diagnosed with hypothyroidism. Rory has been complaining of hip pain, which is noteworthy because hip dislocation commonly occurs in individuals with Down syndrome.

Rory has always been a very pleasant person. He is affable, polite, and easy going. He enjoys spending time with his family, taking walks, and watching television. He competes in Special Olympics tennis and attends a weekly training program. Rory enjoys eating, but his parents know that people with Down syndrome have a tendency toward obesity so as much as possible, monitor his caloric intake. Rory is verbal, yet many people have a difficult time understanding him because his articulation is poor. Rory is unable to read. He can write his name and recognizes road and restaurant/store signs.

Since Rory transitioned out of the public education system at age 22, he has had several simple jobs at sheltered workshops. For about 6 months, he was a bagger at the local grocery store, but tough economic times led to his termination. Rory often tells his parents that he misses working and getting "money." Lately, he has been attending an adult day training program (ADT) in the community. The occupational therapist employed at the ADT has been evaluating Rory's skills and interests in an attempt to help him develop specific skills to seek more consistent and permanent employment. She has learned that Rory has a keen interest in cars, so is in the process of seeking a donated car for Rory to work with on skills that are appropriate to his capabilities. Rory is looking forward to this opportunity and often reminds the OT that this is what he wants to do, forever. ■

Internet Resources

Administration on Intellectual and Developmental Disabilities—http://www.acf.hhs.gov/programs/add/

National Council on Disability—http://www.ncd.gov/

National Institute on Disability and Rehabilitation Research (NIDRR)—http://www2.ed.gov/about/offices/list/osers/nidrr/index.html

Office of Special Education Programs—http://www2.ed.gov/about/offices/list/osers/osep/index.html

Office of Special Education and Rehabilitative Services—http://www2.ed.gov/about/offices/list/osers/rsa/index.html

References

CDC. *Monitoring Developmental Disabilities*; 2011. Retrieved from http://www.cdc.gov/ncbddd/dd/ddsurv.htm

Kiyoshi Y, Fujiura GT. Employment and income status of adults with developmental disabilities living in the community. *Ment Retard* 2002;40(2):132–141.

Stephens DL, Collins MD, Dodden RA. A longitudinal study of employment and skill acquisition among individuals with developmental disabilities. *Res Dev Disabil* 2005;26(5):469–486.

US Department of Health and Human Services. Developmental Disabilities Assistance and Bill of Rights Act 2000; 2012. Retrieved from http://www.acf.hhs.gov/programs/add/ddact/DDACT2.html

Wehmeyer ML. Employment status and perceptions of control of adults with cognitive and developmental disabilities. *Res Dev Disabil* 1994;15(2):119–131.

CASE STUDY 7

CHAPTER 47

Recovering from Substance Abuse: A 35-Year-Old Woman with Alcoholism

Amy Wagenfeld, PhD, OTR/L, SCEM, CAPs

Background Information

Substance abuse is the harmful use of substances for mood altering purposes or in ways that they are unintended to be used (About.com, 2012). Engaging in substance abuse of any kind increases a person's risk of acquiring sexually transmitted diseases and is known teratogen for pregnant women. Abusing drugs and alcohol can also lead to significant physical and psychological problems. Common categories of substance abuse include alcohol, illicit, and prescription drug (abuse). The costs associated with substance abuse extend beyond the health of the individual with abuse issues. Societal issues, including medical costs, loss of productivity, incarceration, crime, motor vehicle accidents, and fires, are some secondary effects that are associated with substance abuse (Harwood et al., 1998). There appears to be a familiar pattern of substance abuse, particularly with alcohol. Alcohol abuse is on the rise; one in six people in the United States have a drinking problem (NIH, 2011). That is, if you have a parent with an alcohol abuse issue, there is a higher probability that you will develop this problem, but it is not inevitable. Other factors that increase a person's risk of substance abuse include the following:

Being a young adult under peer pressure
Having easy access to alcohol or drugs
Having identified psychological disorders
Having low self-esteem
Having problems with relationships
Living a stressful lifestyle (NIH, 2011)

Treatment for substance abuse can range from medical intervention, in- or outpatient rehabilitation, social support groups, holistic natural interventions, or a combination of all of these. Recovery from substance abuse involves complete abstinence or cessation of ingesting the substance. It is imperative that a person with an identified substance abuse issue take responsibility for their actions and acknowledge that they must change their behaviors in order to cease abusing. While researchers acknowledge that attention must be placed on reducing prescription drug abuse, at the same time, care must be taken to ensure that appropriate use of these drugs are not compromised (Cicero et al., 2005, p. 672).

Traditional Practice Area(s)—Mental Health

Emerging Practice Area—Recovery and Peer Support Model

Cross Reference—Chapter 19, *Spirituality*; Chapter 20, *Arts and Crafts*; Chapter 23, *Activities of Daily Living*; Chapter 25, *Group Dynamics: Planning and Leading Effective Therapeutic Groups*; Chapter 29, *Psychological Conditions*; Chapter 34, *Mental Health*; Chapter 35, *Health and Wellness*; Chapter 40, *Emerging Practice Areas*

CLINICAL PRESENTATION

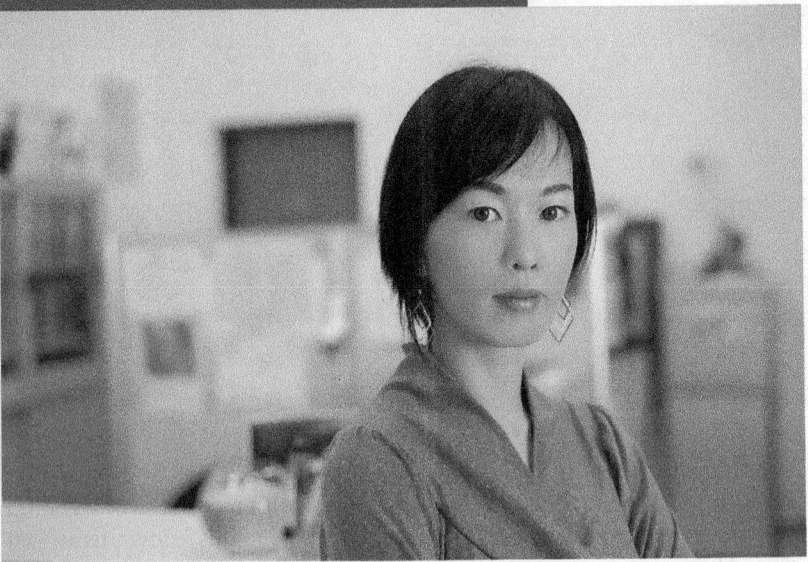

Talia M. is a 35-year-old Asian woman. She is married to Eldon, who is also Asian, and they have three children, ranging in age from 10 to 3. Mrs. M. is a stay-at-home mom, and Eldon works two jobs, as a data entry clerk at a local health club and as a night manager at a hotel. Eldon's mother lives with them. She has recently been diagnosed with lung cancer and is undergoing chemotherapy and experiencing many of the side negative associated with chemotherapy. Mrs. M. is the primary caregiver for the children and her mother-in-law.

Mrs. M. has been complaining to her husband recently about the extra burden of caring for and transporting her mother-in-law to chemotherapy sessions. She herself has been feeling tired and lethargic and in need of some pleasant diversion outside the house. At Eldon's urging, she invites several friends to join her for dinner at the local diner. Dinner is very pleasant, and although she makes it a habit to never drink because her mother was an alcoholic, she decides that with all she has been dealing with, one glass of wine would be fine. Mrs. M. enjoys the drink and feels more relaxed than she has in a long time.

As time goes by, Mrs. M. begins to drink on a more regular basis, rationalizing that it makes her more relaxed and a better person to be with. She finds herself hiding bottles of alcohol in the house and starts drinking as soon as the children are on their way to school. Gradually, her drinking increases and she starts to take less interest in doing the IADL and ADL tasks that comprised her daily life and instead watches old movies all day while she drinks.

Because her husband works so much, they seldom see each other so she is able to cover-up her drinking. One day, after consuming more alcohol than she ever had, Mrs. M. went to the kitchen to prepare a can of soup. She put the pot of soup on the stove, turned it on, and promptly passed out. Fortunately, just after the soup boiled down and the pot caught fire, her mother-in-law, now hypersensitive to smell (side effect of chemotherapy) knew something was wrong. She went to the kitchen and found a fire on the stove and her daughter-in-law on the floor. She was able to extinguish the fire and then called 911 for help. Then she called her son, who followed the ambulance to the hospital. Mrs. M. was diagnosed with extreme alcohol poisoning. After she was detoxed and as part of the decision-making team, Mrs. M. decided to enter an inpatient alcohol rehabilitation facility. It was there, during her 6-week stay, that she began an occupational therapy program that focused on nurturing spiritual development and fostering resilience as a means to reconnect with oneself as well as addressing impaired the effects of impaired executive functioning. The occupational therapy team focused on using meaningful and reflective activities such as working with clay and doing yoga and Tai Chi. Mrs. M. learned a great deal about herself during rehab and determined that her self-defeating behavior was not going to stop until she took positive steps to change her life. After discharge, Mrs. M. took a parttime job at the health club, began to exercise regularly, and attended daily AA meetings.

Internet Resources

National Institutes of Health—www.nih.gov
Alcoholics Anonymous—www.aa.org
Mayo Clinic—www.mayoclinic.com/health/alcoholism/DS00340

References

About.com. *What is substance abuse?* 2012. Retrieved from: http://alcoholism.about.com/cs/drugs/a/aa030425a.htm

Cicero TJ, Inciardi JA, Muniz A. Trends in abuse of oxycontin and other opioid analgesics in the United States: 2002–2004. *J Pain* 2005;6(10):662–672.

Harwood H, Fountain D, Livermore G. *Economic Costs of Alcohol and Drug Abuse in the United States*. Bethesda, MD: National Institute on Drug Abuse; 1998.

National Institutes of Health. Alcoholism and alcohol abuse; 2011. Retrieved from: http://www.ncbi.nlm.nih.gov/pubmedhealth/PMH0001940/

CASE STUDY 8

CHAPTER 48

Bariatrics and Implications for Healthy Living

Amy Wagenfeld, PhD, OTR/L, SCEM, CAPs

Background Information

Obesity rates have been rising over the past two decades at an alarming pace (cdc.gov, 2012). Extreme obesity, which is defined by a body mass index (BMI) ≥40 kg/m^2, positively correlates with increased risk of depression and with impairments in health-related quality of life (HRQoL), such as physical functioning, physical role limitations, and bodily pain (Fabricatore et al., 2005). It is imperative that people with extreme obesity be evaluated for depression and HRQoL factors (Annis, 2002; Fabricatore et al., 2005). Under the ADA, the U.S. Equal Employment Opportunity Commission (EEOC) finds reason to qualify obesity as a disability, and accordingly that accommodations must be made (EEOC, 2012).

The cost of obesity on human and financial capital is enormous. Approximately 37.5% of all adults in the United States are obese, and in 2008, the medical costs associated with obesity were approximately $147 billion (cdc.gov, 2012). Medical costs paid by health insurance providers for individuals who are obese were $1,429 higher than those of normal weight (cdc.gov, 2012). Some people for whom diet and exercise have proven to be ineffective or for whom excess weight has led to serious health concerns, such as cardiac, skeletal, or endocrine related, turn to gastric bypass or other weight loss surgeries. Collectively, these procedures are called bariatric surgeries. Gastric bypass or other types of weight loss surgeries change an individual's digestive system so that they can lose weight by limiting how much can be eaten or by reducing nutrient absorption, or a combination of both (Mayo Clinic, 2012). Because bariatric surgery is a major procedure, there are significant risks associated with it as well as side effects that some people will experience (Mayo Clinic, 2012). A very important adjunct to bariatric surgery is making permanent healthy lifestyle changes, including diet and regular exercise (Mayo Clinic, 2012). An interdisciplinary approach is most effective in addressing and remediating these issues.

Traditional Practice Area(s)—Rehabilitation, Disability, and Participation and Health and Wellness

Emerging Practice Area(s)—Obesity

Cross Reference—Chapter 16, *Working Together: Clinical Reasoning and Collaboration*; Chapter 21, *Adaptive Equipment*; Chapter 22, *Assistive Technology*; Chapter 23, *Activities of Daily Living*; Chapter 26, *Workplace Safety*; Chapter 30, *Physical Disabilities*; Chapter 33, *Rehabilitation, Disability and Participation*; Chapter 34, *Mental Health*; Chapter 35, *Health and Well-Being*; Chapter 38, *Work and Industry*; Chapter 39, *Management and Education*; Chapter 40, *Emerging Practice Areas*

CLINICAL PRESENTATION

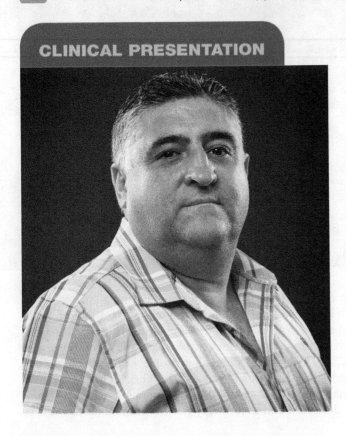

Brad is a Hispanic male, 42 years old, and recently divorced. His 20-year-old son James lives with him in a single story home. Brad, an electrical engineer, is morbidly obese, meaning that his weight is double that of what is considered ideal for him. Brad uses a scooter to get around and is having increasing difficulty doing his job because he cannot fit under his desk any longer. His ADL skills are in decline, toileting is very difficult, and he cannot stand to take a shower. He relies on James to help him don and doff his shoes and socks. James also does all of the meal preparation. His doctor continues to urge Brad to lose weight, as his blood pressure is very high, even with medication. He has developed diabetes and is getting peripheral neuropathy. Brad is feeling increasingly depressed as he finds himself less able to take care of himself. Ultimately, Brad decides to have bariatric surgery. While in the hospital, the discharge planner suggests that Brad allow an occupational therapy team come to his home and evaluate him and his house once he is home. Not knowing what occupational therapy is, he does an online search for AOTA on his tablet computer and realizes that occupational therapy is just what he has been in need of. Once home, the OT and OTA arrive and work together on Brad's personal and home (safety) evaluations. The OTA suggests several changes to the bathroom to make Brad's life easier and to help him regain independence with toileting. The OT's evaluation results indicate that Brad is very deconditioned, dependent in most ADLs, and also depressed. She and the OTA work with Brad to develop a meaningful therapy program. Brad's goals include regaining independence in ADL skills, to be able to work at his desk, and to return to a more productive and meaningful lifestyle. ■

Internet Resources

Centers for Disease Control and Prevention—http://www.cdc.gov/obesity/data/adult.html

Equal Employment Opportunity Commission—www.eeoc.gov

Mayo Clinic—http://www.mayoclinic.com

References

Annis TD. The interdisciplinary team across the continuum of care. *Crit Care Nurse* 2002;22(5):76–79.

Centers for Disease Control and Prevention. *Overweight and obesity facts*; 2012. Retrieved from http://www.cdc.gov/obesity/data/adult.html

Fabricatore AN, Wadden TA, Sarwer DB, et al. Health-related quality of life and symptoms of depression in extremely obese persons seeking bariatric surgery. *Obes Surg* 2005;15(3):304–309.

Mayo Clinic. Bariatrics; 2012. Retrieved from http://www.mayoclinic.com/health/gastric-bypass/MY00825

US Equal Employment Opportunity Commission. *EEOC sues resources for Human Development, Inc. for disability discrimination*; 2012. Retrieved from http://www.eeoc.gov/eeoc/newsroom/release/9-30-10u.cfm

CASE STUDY 9

CHAPTER 49

Improving the Workplace Environment: Ergonomics and the Built Environment

Amy Wagenfeld, PhD, OTR/L, SCEM, CAPs

Background Information

About 3.1 million nonfatal workplace-related accidents and illnesses were reported by employers in the private sector in 2010 (Bureau of Labor Statistics, U.S. Department of Labor, 2011a). Differentially, about 820,300 state and local governmental injury and illness cases were reported in 2010, or a rate of 5.7 cases per 100 full-time workers, which is "significantly higher than the rate among private industry workers (3.5 cases per 100 workers)" (Bureau of Labor Statistics, U.S. Department of Labor, 2011a). According to the U.S. Bureau of Labor Statistics (2011), the total number of fatal work injuries in the United States rose was 4,690. This number was the second lowest since the fatal injury census began recording data in 1992 and represents 3.6 fatal workplace injuries per 100,000 full-time equivalent workers (Bureau of Labor Statistics, U.S. Department of Labor, 2011b). The economic and personal costs for workplace-related injury, illness, and fatality take an enormous toll on society.

Changing workplace behaviors and safety outcomes, including making changes to how workers work and the built environment, can reduce work-related injuries, illnesses, and fatalities. This entails in part, understanding and using sound ergonomic techniques and creating environments that are conducive to rather than harm the worker. A recent meta-analysis of work place behaviors and safety outcomes showed that safety knowledge and safety motivation correlated most closely with safety performance behaviors (Christian et al., 2009, p. 1122). This was followed closely by psychological safety climate and group safety climate. Interestingly, and with respect to on the job accidents and injuries, the strongest association was found with group safety climate (Christian et al., 2009, p. 1122).

Traditional Practice Area(s)—Health and Wellness and Work and Industry

Cross Reference—Chapter 21, *Adaptive Equipment*; Chapter 22, *Assistive Technology*; Chapter 24, *Orthotics and Orthotic Fabrication*; Chapter 26, *Workplace Safety*; Chapter 29, *Psychological Conditions*; Chapter 30, *Physical Disabilities*; Chapter 33, *Rehabilitation, Disability and Participation*; Chapter 38, *Work and Industry*

CLINICAL PRESENTATION

Tyler, a 35-year-old single black male, works as a pastry chef at a high-end restaurant in a major city. This is a second (plus) career for Tyler. Although he always dreamed of being a pastry chef, it wasn't until about 6 years ago that he had the financial resources to attend pastry school full time. Prior to going to school, Tyler worked at various jobs in factories, as a salesperson in retail, and as a stocker in a food warehouse. Tyler is very committed to giving back to his community and volunteers twice weekly at the local soup kitchen and food pantry. When he is not at the restaurant or volunteering, Tyler enjoys playing cards with his poker buddies, going to the gym, singing in his church choir, and reading.

Tyler is the middle child in a family of seven. He is the only child to have ventured far from home. While he speaks with most of his family, including his parents, several times a week, it is just not the same as being close by. He gets home two or three times a year and usually a sibling or two and their families come to visit him each year. Tyler thoroughly enjoys showing his family around his adopted city.

When Tyler worked as a stocker at the warehouse in his early 20s, he was expected to lift and place items weighing up to 60 pounds throughout his day. He was also responsible for driving a forklift truck. Many days, he woke up in the mornings and thought to himself, "I feel so much older than 23; my back is really sore." After a few years of this heavy work, he sought out a job that was not as physically taxing, or so he thought. At the factory, he worked a line job that involved riveting. Although he was grateful to no longer be lifting and placing for much of the day, standing and riveting with few breaks during his shift was taxing on his body. His feet hurt, and flexing and extending his wrists and fingers was painful. Sometimes his elbows hurt. His days in retail sales were better. The job was varied as he floated within the store, some days in clothing and others in groceries or electronics. Being a people person, Tyler really enjoyed this job and the almost daily changes in assignments felt good on his body and mind. All the while he was working, Tyler managed to save enough money to attend school. He lived at home and was frugal with spending.

The 2-year pastry course flew by. Tyler thrived in school, and despite twinges in his low back and pain in his wrists and hands after whisking cream or using a torch to caramelize sugar, he was on top of the world. His tendency was to simply shake off the pain. His specialty was cakes; the more detailed the better, as far as Tyler was concerned. After graduation, he was recruited to apprentice under a master pastry chef at a nearby restaurant. It was an unprecedented learning experience and prepared him well for his current job as the master pastry chef in the high-end restaurant. It was very difficult to pack up and leave his family, and move nearly half across the country, pulling a trailer with his possessions and then setting up his fourth floor apartment was taxing. His back felt sorer than it had in years, and sometimes he could not grasp boxes and bags; they simply slipped out of his hands.

Undaunted, Tyler began his job. The hours are excruciatingly long, and Tyler is on his feet working for sometimes 12 hours a day. The atmosphere in the kitchen can be very stressful, as the pace is fast and customer satisfaction is of utmost importance to the owner and manager of the restaurant. Tyler takes great pride in his work and receives many accolades for his amazing cakes. All was well, until one day, while rushing to take a cake from the oven, he twisted his body to avoid running into another staff person, and felt an intense pain travel through his low back. Tyler fell onto the floor writhing in pain. He went via ambulance to the hospital emergency room, where he was treated and released but found he could not return to his former job without tremendous pain. Because the accident happened at work, Tyler went through a worker compensation hearing and was deemed eligible for rehabilitation. Tyler was adamant and determined to get back to work as quickly as he could safely do so; participation in his role as a pastry chef was his self-defining feature. He was provided with occupational therapy as well as physical therapy services. An OT performed a functional capacity evaluation and spent a great deal of time talking with Tyler about his past work history and his present job. With the OTA on staff, the three of them did a site visit to the restaurant kitchen. The site visited enable to OT practitioners to see what Tyler's roles were and then to recreate it back in the clinic. They also referenced the *Dictionary of Occupational Titles* as well as *O*NET* to better understand the general characteristics and physical job demands of being a pastry chef. The site visit also enabled them to see the layout of the kitchen in order to make informed recommendations for environmental modifications to promote better ergonomics and safety. He began a customized work hardening program. The team developed a graded program that in conjunction with the physical therapy program enabled Tyler to regain his functional capacity to be ready to return to work. The OT practitioners also worked with Tyler and the restaurant owner and manager to make changes to the kitchen to improve the safety of all the kitchen staff, Tyler not withstanding. Tyler checks in with the rehabilitation team twice yearly, but 2 years following the accident, Tyler is now very careful to use good body mechanics, practice energy conservation techniques, and to do his daily home program of stretching and strengthening exercises. For the most part, he is pain free and has resumed his regular routine of work, leisure, and volunteer work. It never fails that when Tyler comes for a follow-up appointment, the staff are treated to a delicious dessert. ■

Internet Resources

Bureau of Labor Statistics—www.bls.gov
Center for the Built Environment—www.cbe.berkeley.edu
Occupational Safety and Health Administration—http://www.osha.gov/SLTC/ergonomics/

References

Bureau of Labor Statistics, US Department of Labor. *Occupational injuries and illnesses*; 2011a. Retrieved from http://www.bls.gov/news.release/osh.toc.htm

Bureau of Labor Statistics, US Department of Labor. *Revisions to the 2010 census of fatal occupational injuries (CFOI) counts*; 2011b. Retrieved from http://www.bls.gov/iif/oshwc/cfoi/cfoi_revised10.pdf

Christian MS, Bradley JC, Wallace J, et al. Workplace safety: a meta-analysis of the roles of person and situation factors. *J Appl Psychol* 2009;94(5):1103–1127.

CASE STUDY 10

CHAPTER 50

Coping with Stress and Anxiety Disorder

Amy Wagenfeld, PhD, OTR/L, SCEM, CAPs

Background Information

Everyone experiences stress in different ways, and no person can live a completely stress-free life (APA, 2012b). In fact, a certain degree of stress helps to keep our lives in balance. When stress gets out of control and becomes chronic, that is cause for concern. There appears to be a connection between chronic stress and depressive symptoms in adults, depressive disorders in children and adolescents, and anxiety disorders in adolescents (Uliaszek et al., 2012). Stress can be looked at from two dimensions, independent/dependent and interpersonal/noninterpersonal (Uliaszek et al., 2012, p. 5). Independent stressors are beyond a person's control and include events such as hurricanes or the death of a friend. Dependent stress occurs in part because of a person's actions, such as failing an exam because of not studying. Interpersonal stress involves challenges with friends and family, and noninterpersonal stress is viewed as work or health issues (Uliaszek et al., 2012, p. 5). People with depression experience a higher rate of interpersonal stress than those without depression (Uliaszek et al., 2012, p. 5).

Anxiety disorders are characterized by excessive fear and avoidance with regard to "specific objects or situations and in the absence of true danger and are very common in the general population" (APA, 2012a; Shin & Liberzon, 2010, p. 169). Individuals with anxiety disorders frequently report "reoccurring thoughts or concerns" (APA, 2012a). Physical symptoms commonly associated with anxiety disorders include sweating, rapid heart rate, trembling, or dizziness (APA, 2012a). There is a connection between anxiety disorder, stress, and depression.

Traditional Practice Area(s): Mental Health and Health and Wellness

Emerging Practice Area—Depression

Cross Reference—Chapter 19, *Spirituality*; Chapter 20, *Arts and Crafts*; Chapter 25, *Group Dynamics: Planning and Leading Effective Therapeutic Groups*; Chapter 29, *Psychological Conditions*; Chapter 34, *Mental Health*; Chapter 40, *Emerging Practice Areas*

CLINICAL PRESENTATION

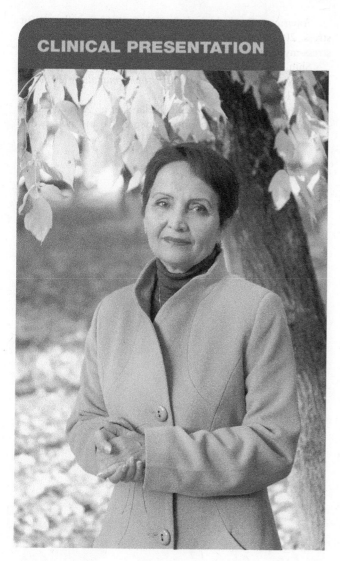

Diana is 55 years old. She is white and lives with her twin sister Lucie in their family home. Both parents are deceased. Neither Diana nor Lucie ever married. Diana and Lucie are vegetarians and grow much of their produce. When the harvest is abundant, they enjoy canning tomatoes to eat during the long winter months. Lucie has been involved in several long-term relationships, but Diana has not. Diana spends her time outside of work painting, reading, or quilting. Diana appears to all who know her as a quiet and unassuming person, one that may be easily lost in a group.

Diana is a pathologist and works in the laboratory at a hospital. She graduated from medical school with honors. After completing medical school, she put internship and residency on hold for several years, telling anyone who asked that she was simply unsure of what she wanted to do next. The truth is, Diana could not face the thought of more training. Too many times, the experience of being put on the spot during rounds and not knowing the answer well or fast enough had taken its toll on Diana. The thought of just more of the same was overwhelming. In fact, when she thought about it her heart would begin to race and she broke out into hives. Between the medical school stress and her ongoing inability to reach out to others in friendship, as well as losing her mother with whom she was very close to breast cancer while she was in medical school, life has been terribly hard for her. She often felt as if a weight was crushing her chest. She tried counseling for a while and found it to be helpful, especially to understand that she was experiencing chronic stress. She did not follow through on the breathing exercises that the therapist recommended.

After working for 2 years in a pathology lab as a technician, Diana realized that this was the medical specialty that best suited her and decided to finish her medical school training. Many days during her final years of training, Diana woke up feeling sad and tired. Her body hurt. Going up and down the stairs at home made her knees ache. She also woke up frequently during the night, her heart racing, thoughts running through her head, and sometimes even felt dizzy. Nonetheless, she did well in internship and residency and was rewarded with a well-paying job when she completed her training.

It wasn't until the past few years that Diana has been aware that between the stress of her demanding job, where nothing less than excellence is tolerated, her lack of social interaction, and her general lack of energy and desire to anything more than she has to, which never fully resolved after her training was completed, something had to be done. Diana decided to once again seek out the help of a mental health practitioner. At the outpatient psychiatric clinic where Diana's therapist practices, there happens to be an occupational therapy department. Diana's therapist recommends that Diana have an occupational therapy evaluation. She agrees and after obtaining a physician referral, goes forward with it. The OT does a series of psychosocial and ADL evaluations, as well as spends a great deal of time learning about Diana's wishes and goals, and in accordance with Diana's goals, develops an intervention treatment plan. She recommends that Diana participate in a psychosocial wellness group run by an OTA whose specialty is therapeutic yoga and meditation. Diana is somewhat reluctant, having never done yoga before but gives it a try. The group comprised eight middle-aged men and women, all with similar diagnoses of anxiety and depression. Within several months of attending the twice weekly group, Diana wakes up one morning and realizes that she had no nightmares and slept peacefully. She does not dread the thought of going to the lab, and in fact, looks forward to doing so. ■

Internet Resources

American Institute of Stress—http://www.stress.org/
American Psychological Association—www.apa.org
National Institute of Health–Medline Plus—http://www.nlm.nih.gov/medlineplus/stress.html
National Institute of Mental Health—http://www.nimh.nih.gov/health/topics/anxiety-disorders/index.shtml

References

American Psychological Association. *Anxiety*; 2012a. Retrieved from http://www.apa.org/topics/anxiety/index.aspx

American Psychological Association. Six myths about stress; 2012b. Retrieved from http://www.apa.org/helpcenter/stress-myths.aspx

Shin LM, Liberzon I. The neurocircuitry of fear, stress, and anxiety disorders. *Neuropsychopharmacology* 2010;35:169–191.

Uliaszek AA, Zinbarg RE, Mineka S, et al. A longitudinal examination of stress generation in depressive and anxiety disorders. *J Abnormal Psychol* 2012;121(1):4–15.

CASE STUDY 11

CHAPTER 51

Oh My Aching Back—Gardening for a Lifetime Despite Physical Challenges

Amy Wagenfeld, PhD, OTR/L, SCEM, CAPs

Background Information

Our bodies were built to move, which is why lack of physical activity can prematurely age our musculoskeletal and organ systems. A study of 8,800 adults found that each daily hour of television viewing was associated with an 18% increase in death from heart disease and an 11% increase in overall mortality (Veerman et al., 2011). There are many options for engaging in an active lifestyle, one of which is gardening. Gardening is, for many, a meaningful and purposeful activity that strengthens bones, muscles, and cardiovascular systems and elevates mood. Gardening can play a significant role in the fight against obesity. General gardening tasks burn approximately 270 calories per hour, while the heavy-duty activities like digging can burn up to 500 calories per hour (Calorie Calculator, n.d.). Gardening has been shown to reduce the incidence of osteoporosis, which is second only to cardiac disease as a worldwide health issue (National Osteoporosis Foundation, 2012). The National Osteoporosis Foundation reports that in the United States some 12 million people over the age of 50 have osteoporosis, while another 40 million have low bone mass. Researchers at the University of Arkansas found that regularly doing some of the heavy-duty gardening tasks such as digging, hauling, and edging had a positive influence on bone health (Turner et al., 2002).

Traditional Practice Area—Health and Wellness and Work and Industry

Cross Reference—Chapter 18, *Ensuring Purposeful and Meaningful Interventions*; Chapter 21, *Activities of Daily Living*; Chapter 21, *Adaptive Equipment*; Chapter 22, *Assistive Technology*; Chapter 23, *Activities of Daily Living*; Chapter 30, *Physical Disabilities*; Chapter 26, *Workplace Safety*; Chapter 35, *Health and Well-Being*; Chapter 40 *Emerging Practice Areas.*

CLINICAL PRESENTATION

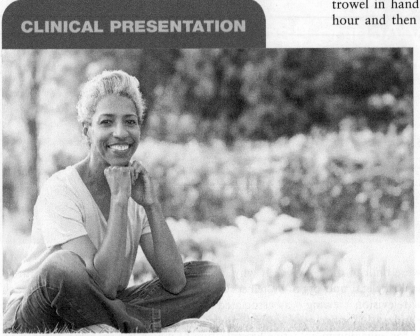

Jolene W. is a black 63-year-old female. She and her husband live in a two-story home on a quiet tree-lined street. She was diagnosed with osteoarthritis when she was 55 and has kyphosis. She also has osteopenia, so is monitored for potential osteoporosis. On the days when she feels at her worst, when her knees, hips, and fingers ache, she takes the anti-inflammatory medication her rheumatologist prescribed. Mainly, Mrs. W. just feels discomfort, and not intense pain. Her greatest passion is gardening. With the initial sign of spring, she has always been the first on her block to be outside, readying her many gardens for the growing season. In the winter, she spends lots of chilly evenings pouring over gardening catalogs and making wish lists for what to buy in the spring. Her husband, Coleman likes to tease Mrs. W. and tell her that her passion has turned to obsession. She just laughs it off and tells him that her so-called obsession feeds them all summer long and sometimes even in the winter.

Recently retired from her job as a 4th grade teacher, Mrs. W. is thrilled at the prospect of long days in the garden, uninterrupted by papers to grade, staff meetings, and the likes. Work has prevented Mrs. W. from ever spending more than an hour or two in the garden on any given day. But that hour or two is the best of the day, she has always thought. Time spent in the garden relaxes her and allows her to clear her mind and to feel a good sense of tired. In her retirement, Mrs. W. is even thinking about finally taking the master gardener course at the local cooperative extension service.

On a particularly balmy June day, Mrs. W. donned her hat and applied sunscreen and was out the door, trowel in hand at 6 AM. She planned to work for an hour and then come in for breakfast. She completely lost track of time, and when Cole came to the back door to ask if she was planning to join him for lunch, she was amazed. How had six hours passed so quickly? There was much to be done in the vegetable garden and it was going to get done, today. And, there was the perennial bed on the south side of the house that needed some attention. Reluctantly, she came in for lunch and then headed back outside as quickly as she could. Her knees were beginning to scream, and admittedly, her hands were very sore from gripping a trowel and pulling weeds. But she fared on, knowing that she had to still dig some holes to plant a few new perennials that she bought on sale at the garden shop. Tired and thirsty, she came inside for the day at 4 PM. She sat down to take off her garden boots and realized she could not bend over to do so. Calling for help, Coleman rushed in to assist her. With help from Coleman, Mrs. W. doffed her boots, went upstairs, showered (although stepping in and out of the bathtub was extremely painful), and lay down to rest. At Coleman's urging, she made an appointment with her rheumatologist for the next day.

The pain in Mrs. W.'s knees and back had significantly intensified overnight. Her hands throbbed with pain and were swollen at the joints. Dr. Martin carefully examined Mrs. W. and asked her what had changed in her daily life since the last visit. She told the doctor that now that she was retired, she was working pretty much full time in the garden. Instead of telling Mrs. W. that her gardening days were over, he recommended that she make an appointment with an occupational therapist in the outpatient unit of the local hospital. He referred many patients to occupational therapy, especially those whose functional skills were at serious risk. Not knowing what an occupational therapist does beyond working with children on fine motor skills, she was curious, but skeptical. At the first appointment, Mrs. W.'s OT did a complete evaluation and determined that Mrs. W. would benefit from a meaningful task-oriented rehabilitation program focused on rethinking how to garden safely. Not wanting to ever have to give up gardening, Mrs. W. agreed. The OT introduced Mrs. W. to Meredith, an OTA who had recently taken the local master gardener class. They quickly established a nice rapport with each other. Meredith was eager to work with Mrs. W. The feeling was mutual. ■

Internet Resources

American Society of Landscape Architects—www.asla.org
National Gardening Association—www.garden.org
American Occupational Therapy Association—http://www.aota.org/-/media/Corporate/Files/AboutOT/consumers/Health-and-Wellness/Gardening-tip-sheet.pdf

References

Calorie Calculator. Calories burned per activity—Calorie Calculator; n.d. Retrieved from www.thecaloriecalculator.net/calories-burned

National Osteoporosis Foundation. Learn about osteoporosis; 2012. Retrieved from nof.org/learn

Turner LW, et al. Influence of yard work and weight training on bone mineral density among older U.S. women. *J Women Aging* 2002;14(3–4):139–148.

Veerman JL, et al. Television viewing time and reduced life expectancy: a life table analysis. *Br J Sports Med* 2011;10: 1136.

CHAPTER 52

Function and Intervention for CVA

Amy Wagenfeld, PhD, OTR/L, SCEM, CAPs

Background Information

A cerebral vascular accident or stroke occurs when arteries supplying blood to specific regions of the brain are blocked or bursts. When the brain does not receive the blood it needs, it begins to die (National Stroke Association, 2012). There are three types of strokes, transient ischemic attacks (TIAs), ischemic strokes, and hemorrhagic strokes. A TIA is often called a ministroke and occurs when blood flow to the brain is briefly interrupted (NIH.gov, 2012). A TIA is not to be ignored, as it could be a warning sign for future ischemic or hemorrhagic stroke. An ischemic stroke is caused by a blood clot that either blocks or stops up a vessel in the brain (NIH.gov, 2012). A hemorrhagic stroke occurs when a blood vessel breaks and bleeds into the brain (NIH.gov, 2012). For those who have had a stroke, there are frequently significant physical and cognitive challenges to overcome.

Traditional Practice Area(s)—Rehabilitation, Disability, and Participation, Health and Wellness, Productive Aging

Emerging Practice Area—Chronic Disease Management and Aging in Place and Home Modifications

Cross Reference—Chapter 16, *Working Together: Clinical Reasoning and Collaboration*; Chapter 18, *Ensuring Purposeful and Meaningful Interventions*; Chapter 21, *Adaptive Equipment*; Chapter 22, *Assistive Technology*; Chapter 23, *Activities of Daily Living*; Chapter 24, *Orthotics and Orthotic Fabrication*; Chapter 30, *Physical Disabilities*; Chapter 31, *Vision*; Chapter 33, *Rehabilitation, Disability, and Participation*.

CLINICAL PRESENTATION

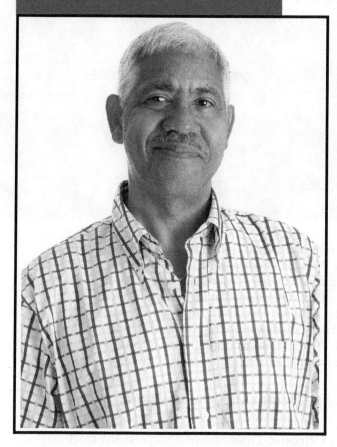

Mr. Jules R. is a 68-year-old Hispanic male. He is a widower, having recently lost his wife, Marie after 45 years of marriage. He deeply misses her, but his family is tight knit; five children and multiple grandchildren make sure that he is seldom lonely. Sometimes, he feels as if his split-level house is a revolving door for family visits. His children make sure that there is a healthy, low-fat meal ready for him to heat up in the microwave, as Marie prepared all the meals when she was alive. Mr. R. is learning to make simple breakfasts and lunches but often defaults to things such as canned soups and frozen meals.

Mr. R. is right handed and according to him was a top-notch pool player in his youth. What with family and work, he has not taken the cover off the family pool table located in the lower level of the house in years. Mr. R. was diagnosed with high blood pressure and elevated cholesterol in the past 10 years and takes medication for both. Lately, he has been having trouble sleeping and last week he just felt "off"—he couldn't really explain it to his eldest son; he was tired, felt a bit dizzy, and had a headache and a bit of pain in his left arm. His son urged him to see his doctor, but Mr. R. insisted it was just a passing thing and he was fine.

Mr. R. was an attorney and spent much of his career as a public defender. He retired 3 years ago. Mr. R. was proud of his work and his record, but could not deny that the demands of the job were at times, overwhelming. He worked hard to leave his work at the office, but often, he found himself angry and frustrated and short tempered with Marie and the children. For many years, Mr. R. smoked a pack of cigarettes a day, but 10 years ago, at the urging of his doctor and family, he quit. It was a very difficult thing to do. He was very proud of this accomplishment and became an antismoking activist, speaking out about the health risks of smoking at his church, the local schools, and community center. When he quit smoking, Mr. R. gained 30 pounds that first year, which, in the ensuing decade, has crept up to a total weight gain of 55 pounds. Mr. R. knows he needs to shed those excess pounds, but has not. He takes daily strolls in the neighborhood, often pushing his youngest granddaughter's stroller, where he stops at the local bakery for a sweet and cup of coffee with cream.

Five days after his episode of feeling "off," during a recent morning walk, the symptoms returned, but this time, Mr. R. felt significant weakness in his left arm. He could not think clearly and, at the bakery, he had trouble placing his order. His speech was garbled and unintelligible. An alert clerk trained in CPR recognized the potential warning signs of a stroke and immediately got Mr. R. a chair and called 911. Mr. R. was rushed to the hospital, where along the route, experienced a right ischemic stroke. As a result of the stroke, he lost significant function in his left upper and lower extremities, cannot stand without assistance or walk, and is unable to actively move his left upper extremity; there is evidence of spasticity in the right hand, and he has hemianopsia and difficulties with expressive language and short-term memory. Now that Mr. R. is stabilized, he has begun an inpatient rehabilitation program involving occupational, physical, and speech and language therapy. As part of his occupational therapy rehabilitation, and because of his expressed desire to return home, he is learning to operate appliances like an electric razor with a switch. Social work is also actively engaged in the rehabilitation process. With help from his eldest son, Mr. R. is able to convey to the OT practitioners that he wants to go home and with the exception of doing extensive meal prep, to take care of himself and not go to an assisted living facility. ■

Internet Resources

National Institutes of Health—www.nih.gov
National Stroke Association—www.stroke.org

References

National Institutes of Health. *Stroke*; 2012. Retrieved from http://www.nlm.nih.gov/medlineplus/stroke.html

National Stroke Association. *Explaining Stroke*; 2012. Retrieved from http://www.stroke.org/site/DocServer/Explaining Stroke_web.pdf?docID=3321

CASE STUDY 13

CHAPTER 53

Aging in Place and Community, Aging with Dignity

Amy Wagenfeld, PhD, OTR/L, SCEM, CAPs

Background Information

Over 28% of the US population is aged 50+ and comprises what is known as the baby-boomer generation. Nearly 90% of boomers with or without physical or other challenges indicate a strong desire to age in place in their homes and communities (AARP, 2012) and remain actively engaged in life. Returning home after illness or an accident or remaining at home depends in large part on the physical status of the home environment. Home modifications of both interior and exterior environments can go a long way to help those who need them to be safe and to enjoy and continue to participate in activities that are meaningful to them.

Traditional Practice Area(s)—Health and Wellness and Productive Aging

Emerging Practice Area—Chronic Disease Management and Aging in Place and Home Modifications

Cross Reference—Chapter 16, *Working Together: Clinical Reasoning and Collaboration*; Chapter 21, *Adaptive Equipment*; Chapter 22, *Assistive Technology*; Chapter 23, *Activities of Daily Living*; Chapter 35, *Health and Well-Being*; Chapter 37, *Productive Aging*; Chapter 40, *Emerging Practice Areas*

CLINICAL PRESENTATION

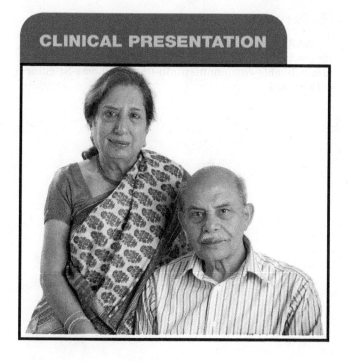

Mr. and Mrs. Stan and Lois F. have lived in their historic mission bungalow for the past 40 years. Mr. F. is 70 and Mrs. F is 74. They are Eastern Indian and maintain close ties to the local Indian community. They love their home and always have. Many happy memories were made in the house. Over the years, they have put many personal touches on the house. They cannot imagine ever leaving it. They chose the home because of the neighborhood. When their family was young, they dreamed of providing their children with a home in a neighborhood that would allow them to simply go outside to play and be with friends. When they found their home, they were thrilled. Mrs. F., being a self-professed home architecture enthusiast, had long been a fan of mission style architecture and understood that the underlying principles of a mission style home was to bring the family together, which closely aligned with their value system. Designed to stay in for a lifetime, most mission homes were one or one and a half story structures. Mrs. F. especially liked the coziness associated with mission bungalows.

The bungalow was somewhat unusual in that it was two full stories, but when they purchased the house, Mr. and Mrs. F. did not give a thought to the fact that the largest bedroom was upstairs. The pitch of the steps was steep, which, with having young children, worried Mrs. F, but they carpeted the steps and installed gates to reduce the risk of having a child tumble down the steps. With the laundry located in the basement, Mrs. F. got a great deal of exercise running up and down the stairs doing laundry when the children were young. Lately, there is no running up and down the stairs. Located on a hilly street, the house has seven steps up to the walkway, and then another four up to the porch. The porch was a huge selling point. It was so appealing as it spanned the width of the house and many evening were spent outside, watching the children play, rocking in the porch swing. The dark wooden floors located throughout the house still gleam. There are several treasured oriental rugs throughout the house that the couple purchased on a trip to India. The house has two full bathrooms, each equipped with a tub/shower combination and the original pedestal sinks. The upstairs bathroom has the original claw-foot tub, with a shower that was added after the family moved into the house. Built at the turn of the 20th century, the doorways are barely wide enough for Mr. F to fit through these days, as he has gained a significant amount of weight. He has learned to step sideway through doorframes. The kitchen has some of the original features, including a working fireplace and built-in table and benches. The over counter cabinets have small knobs, which, with Mrs. F.'s advancing arthritis, are increasingly hard to open. Not to mention, putting dishes away and getting food out of the pantry are daily challenges, as is carrying items from the refrigerator to the stove. Sometimes, although he is loath to admit it, Mr. F. has forgotten to turn the stove off after heating up water for a cup of tea, and secretly, he worries that he may be developing dementia. Mr. F. has spent many nights sleeping on the coach in the den as by nighttime he is simply too tired to climb the steps to their bedroom.

Like many turn of the 20th-century homes, the garage is located behind the house in an alley. It is getting to be a challenge to bring groceries into the house from the garage. Walking 65' through the backyard and up four steps to the back door is difficult but manageable, barely. Maintaining the rambling flowerbeds and yard no longer hold the appeal they used to for Mr. and Mrs. F. At a recent dinner party, the talk turned to who was planning to sell their home and move in with their children or to go to a continuing care retirement community (CCRC) or who wanted to stay in their home, forever. While many of their friends were interested in moving to CCRCs, Mr. and Mrs. F. were adamant in saying that no matter what, they wanted to stay in their bungalow forever. Later that evening, they recounted this conversation and began to wonder if, in fact, staying in the bungalow was feasible after all. They were not getting any younger and it was getting hard to be there on their own. When Mrs. F. went to her aerobics class at the local senior center, she noticed that an OT was going to be presenting a talk about a topic called aging in place and aging in community next week. She also noticed that the OT had several letters after her name, including CAPS, which, after attending the meeting, she learned it meant certified aging in place specialist. As a result of attending the meeting, Mr. and Mrs. F. engaged the services of the OT, who, along with her OTA and an OTA student on her second level fieldwork experience, came to their home to conduct a thorough home evaluation. Results of the evaluation showed that despite numerous challenges, it would be possible to develop an intervention plan to implement in order to modify their home in an aesthetically pleasing way to enable the couple to remain safely at home and to age in place with dignity. ■

Internet Resources

American Association of Retired Persons—www.aarp.org
National Association of Home Builders—www.nahb.org

Reference

AARP Oregon. *Focusing on your home—Get the Home Fit guide*; 2012. Retrieved from: http://www.aarp.org/home-family/livable-communities/info-06-2012/home-fit-guide-or1859.html

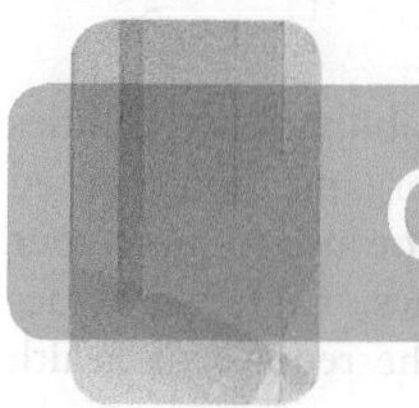

Glossary

Note: Each definition followed by numbers within the parentheses referred as chapter number.

A

academia the community of faculty and students within higher-level educational (39).

accommodation changes that individuals make in interaction style, task demand, or environmental conditions to function in a specific environment or under specific conditions (28).

Accreditation Council for Occupational Therapy Education (ACOTE) the organization that accredits occupational therapy and occupational therapy assistant educational programs (2).

active through experiences, people are active participants in shaping their course of development (8).

activities of daily living (ADL) activities oriented toward taking care of one's body (4, 23).

activity a specific deed, action, or function (11).

activity analysis an analysis of what is required of the client to participate in a chosen activity, and the relationship of the activity's requirements to engagement in occupation (10, 11, 16, 18, 27).

activity synthesis changing the activity demands of a task to match the skills and ability of the client (27).

acute hospital a hospital that provides inpatient medical care and other related services for surgery, acute medical conditions, or a short-term illness (33).

adaptation any alteration or modification in the structure or function of something or any of its parts by which that "thing" or "activity" becomes better fitted to suit the needs of the client (11).

adaptive behavior age-appropriate performance of self-care, social, and other daily living skills (27).

adaptive equipment and/or assistive devices products, apparatus, and occasionally services that make it possible for a person with a disability to perform everyday activities, preferably without assistance from another person (21).

adaptive response an appropriate action in which an individual responds successfully to an environmental demand (28).

administrative controls safety measures that are put in place through action of supervisors such as a change in job pacing or job rotation (26).

aging in place living in the same environment, typically one's home, as one ages (37).

agnosia difficulty interpreting visual, auditory, and/or sensory stimuli even though the sensory system is intact (32).

aide (technician) a therapy personnel member who is trained by an occupational therapist or an occupational therapy assistant to perform specifically delegated tasks. These nonskilled and nonbillable tasks are to be performed only after competency has been determined (13).

akinesia no movement (30).

American Occupational Therapy Association (AOTA) the national organization that represents the interests and concerns of occupational therapy practitioners and students and seeks to improve the quality of occupational therapy services (1).

Americans with Disabilities Act (ADA) the 1990 landmark federal legislation that provides civil rights to people with disabilities (1).

amputation cutting off of (e.g., a limb) (30).

analysis of occupational performance the end result of a client being able to complete an occupation based on the relationship between him/her, the environment and contexts, and the activity itself (10).

anterior front (30).

AOTF American Occupational Therapy Foundation; "serves the public interest by supporting occupational therapy research [education], and increasing public understanding of the important relationship between everyday activities (occupations) and health. It accomplishes its aims primarily through grants and scholarships, through programs, and through publications" (17).

apraxia the inability to formulate the plan needed to carry out movements or tasks that are needed to participate in daily living (32).

arousal level an individual's overall level of alertness and responsiveness to environmental stimuli (28).

arts and crafts movement emerged as a reaction to the industrial revolution and mass production of products. Reed (1989) posited in her Slagle Lecture that the Arts and Crafts movement revitalized the tenets of moral treatment into a new rationale, which the founders and early leaders of occupational therapy were quick to understand and embrace (20).

assessment specific tools, instruments, or procedures used to obtain data during the evaluative process (23).

assisted living facility a long-term care option that combines housing, support services, and health care, as needed. Assisted living is designed for individuals who require assistance with everyday activities such as meals, medication management or assistance with bathing, dressing, and transportation (33).

assistive technology adaptive devices that can range from simple to complex equipment that allows a person with a disability to engage in an activity (22, 27).

astigmatism an irregular shape of the eye that causes light to focus improperly on the retina (31).
attention the "ability to focus on a particular sensory stimulus to the exclusion of others" (32).
autonomy and confidentiality respecting the right of the individual to self determination (12).
axiology a philosophy that is concerned with the study of values and aesthetics (3).

B

balance maintaining upright standing position during stationary and movement activities (30).
barrier an obstacle that impedes completion of a task (23).
beliefs and practices center on trusting in a higher power to cope with an illness or crisis and/or connecting with something greater than ourselves (19).
beneficence demonstration of a concern for the well-being and safety of the recipients of their services (12).
bradykinesia slow movement (30).
bursa protect muscles and tendons from irritation (30).

C

CANIS a genus of carnivorous mammals, of the family Canidae, including the dogs and wolves (21).
centennial vision we envision that occupational therapy is a powerful, widely recognized, science-driven, and evidence-based profession with a globally connected and diverse workforce meeting society's occupational needs (1).
cephalocaudal physical development pattern that proceeds from head down toward toes (8).
cervical relating to the neck (30).
client-centered an orientation that honors the desires and priorities of clients in designing and implementing interventions (23).
client-centered approach service delivery that acknowledges, respects, and incorporates client wishes into the therapy plan (10).
client-centered practice a collaborative treatment approach based on the principle of empowering the client as an active partner in the treatment process rather than a passive recipient (34).
clinical reasoning the comprehensive cognitive process that practitioners use to make decisions about intervention based on the judgments made about the person receiving the therapy (16).
clot a coagulated mass of blood (30).
cognition the mental process of knowing; that which comes to be known; and processes and systems through perception, awareness, attention, memory, intuition, and knowledge (32).
cognitive development thinking and language development (8).
cognitive impairment (CI) the inability to remember, to formulate ideas, and/or to organize and recall information that impacts the person's safety and overall ability to complete everyday tasks (32).
collaboration a process of working cooperatively to achieve a goal (11).
collagen protein constituent of connective tissue (30).
Commission on Accreditation of Rehabilitation Facilities (CARF) an independent, nonprofit organization focused on advancing the quality of services you use to meet your needs for the best possible outcomes. CARF provides accreditation services worldwide at the request of health and human service providers (15).
compensation changes that individuals make in interaction style, approach, and task execution in response to loss or absence of needed abilities (28).
competency an individual's actual performance in a specific situation refers to one's capacity to perform job responsibilities (13).
Comprehensive Outpatient Rehabilitation Facilities (CORF) a facility that is primarily engaged in providing outpatient rehabilitation for the treatment of Medicare beneficiaries who are injured, disabled, or recovering from illness (33).
concavities hollowed inward (30).
conditional reasoning understanding the whole condition of the client including the family, social, and physical contexts that the client is engaged and imaging future possibilities for the client (16).
context the physical, social, emotional, and cultural environment in which a task is performed (28).
continuity development proceeds as a gradual and ongoing process (8).
contractures decreased range of motion in a joint due to shortened muscles (27).
convexities bulging outward (30).
core values (document) an official AOTA document originally published in 1993 whose purpose is to express the values and attitudes that are foundational to occupational therapy (3).
cosignature a signature on a document that indicates that more than one individual was responsible for the information in the document. In the field of occupational therapy, the term is often used when a supervisor signs a document to identify that there was oversight by him or her in the work done (13).
COTA Award of Excellence recognizes the unique role of an OTA through clinical practice, education, administrative education, publication, or presentation (2).
craft an activity involving skill in making things by hand (20).
critically appraised papers (CAPs) stand-alone summaries of single studies (5).
critically appraised topics (CATs) summarizes evidence on specific topics—less rigorous than a systematic review (5).
culturally responsive care understanding and appreciating cultural differences between people and its application to treatment (16).
cultural sensitivity considering specific behaviors and beliefs related to practice and the client (19).

D

delusions cognitive distortions that lead the client to believe in facts that are not real and can take on a variety of characteristics such as grandiose, religious, paranoid, or persecutory depending upon the content of the beliefs not likely to improve with reality testing and orientation (29).
deontological (ethical) theory focuses on idea that the action is right unto itself (12).

depressive episode defined by some configuration of the following depressive symptoms: feeling unhappy, sad, or blue; insomnia; anxiety; hopelessness; despair; irritability; feeling worthless; poor concentration and slowed mentation; preoccupation with death, dying, or suicide; feeling tired and fatigued; decreased libido (sex drive), changes in appetite; and unexplained physical symptoms (e.g., pain) (29).

developmental delay condition where a child (up to 9 years old) does not meet expected developmental milestones; usually requires at least 20% delay or one or more standard deviations below the mean on a standardized test of development; each state in the United States has its own definition of what constitutes developmental delay in order to qualify for services under IDEA (27).

developmental disability conditions that exist prior to age 22, are expected to remain throughout life, and affect cognitive development, physical development, or both (27).

developmental milestones expectations about what a person should be able to do at a specified age (often associated with children) (27).

diagnosis the art or act of identifying a disease from its signs and symptoms (23).

***Diagnostic and Statistical Manual of Mental Disorders* (DSM-5)** a diagnostic manual published by the American Psychiatric Association to standardize psychiatric diagnostic categories (34).

Dictionary of Occupational Titles (DOT) a two-volume set that describes the general characteristics and physical job demands in relation to lifting weight requirements and frequency ratings (38).

differential diagnosis a process of first eliminating all possible explanations for a client's symptom configuration before settling on a psychiatric diagnosis (29).

diplopia double vision, which can be caused by deficits in an individual's binocular visual status or neurological insult (31).

disability an umbrella term for impairments, activity limitations, and participation restrictions (30, 33).

discontinuity development occurs in distinct steps or stages (8).

discussion-oriented groups type of group that focuses on connections and communication (25).

disposition planning the plan for continuing health care of a patient following discharge from a given health care facility (29).

distal with regard to the human body, that which is furthest from the center of the body (i.e., fingers and toes) (8).

doff to take off or remove (23).

domain a concept that explains the purpose of occupational therapy and the areas in which occupational therapy helps clients (6).

don to put on (23).

dualism idea that the mind and body are separate parts or entities (3).

durable medical equipment equipment that can withstand repeated use, is primarily and customarily used to serve a medical purpose, and is generally not useful to a person in the absence of illness or injury (23).

duration refers to an amount of time (29).

dynamic orthosis an orthosis with moving parts, typically used to apply constant tension or force to a body part or mobilize a joint in a controlled manner (24).

E

early intervention (EI) program created in 1986 to provide services for families with young children who are developmentally delayed or at risk for delays from birth until age 2 (36).

education the act of receiving information, knowledge, or skills through a learning process (39).

emerging practice a multifaceted concept [that] encompasses diverse professional roles, a variety of contexts for the provision of services, as well as the development of innovative business models (40).

engineering controls safety measures that make changes to tools and/or environment (26).

entrepreneur a person who brings resources together that are needed to start a business (40).

epistemology a philosophy that examines the nature, origin, and limits of human knowledge (3).

equipment devices used to promote independence including adaptive equipment (e.g., reacher, sock aide, dressing stick) or durable medical equipment (e.g., tub seat, tub bench, commode) (23).

ethical actions a manifestation of moral character and mindful reflection... a commitment to benefit others, to virtuous practice of artistry and science, to genuinely good behaviors, and to noble acts of courage (12).

ethical behavior involves several concepts including universalism, disinterestedness, and cooperation (12).

ethical practice identify, analyze, and clarify ethical issues or dilemmas to make responsible decisions (12).

ethical reasoning understanding and making decisions about intervention approaches when there are resulting ethical considerations and conflicts (12, 16).

ethics the study of standards of conduct and moral judgment (12).

evaluation (occupational therapy) the process of establishing a profile of the client and analysis of client's occupational performance (11).

evidence the available facts and circumstances indicating whether or not something is true or valid (5).

evidence-based medicine applying the best existing evidence to help make decisions about individualized patient care (5).

evidence-based practice using theory and research to substantiate the approaches used in practice (5, 16).

evidence-based research research standard based on evidence *versus* anecdotal information. There are six levels of evidence-based research (5).

executive functions the brain's ability to execute and regulate complex cognitive functions such as motor planning, organizing information, time management, safety awareness, and regulate behaviors (32).

extinction occurs when a behavior diminishes because there is no positive response or a negative response is stopped (9).

F

fascia dense tissue surrounding bones (30).

fibrous resembling fibers (30).

fidelity treating colleagues and other professionals with respect, fairness, discretion, and integrity (12).

fine motor skills tasks that rely primarily on the small muscles and joints of the wrists and hands (8).

flow a state of being when an activity becomes so gratifying that it becomes spontaneous and automatic (4, 19).

forensic mental health the field of mental health practice provided within the legal system. Occupational therapy practitioners working in forensic mental health provide services to individuals accused or convicted of crimes, assisting them in developing life skills for coping with mental illness and/or transitioning back into the community following a period of incarceration (34).

Founding Vision the 1917 founding document of the profession, which states "The particular objects for which the corporation is formed are as follows: The advancement of occupation as a therapeutic measure for the study of the effect of occupation upon the human being for the scientific dispensation of this knowledge" (1).

frame of reference an organizer that provides overarching direction on how to provide treatment (7).

frontal plane divides the body into front and back segments (30).

functional capacity evaluation (FCE) a systemized, intensive, short-term evaluation that focuses on major physical tolerance abilities related to musculoskeletal strength, endurance, speed, and flexibility (38).

functional maintenance programs programs that are often developed for clients who have been discharged from therapy but will remain in a skilled nursing facility. The programs facilitate skills that are present but not utilized unless compensations or adaptations are provided (14).

functional vision refers to an individual's ability to use vision for functional activities (23, 31).

G

grading degree of change in an activity demand that occurs on a continuum from simple to complex. The change can be in one or all aspects of the activity (11).

gross motor skills tasks that rely primarily on the larger muscles and joints in the body (8).

H

HAAT Human Activity Assistive Technology (22).

habilitation services designed to help individuals establish skills that they have not previously developed (27).

habituation to become accustomed or acclimated to something (7).

hallucinations sensory experiences that are not linked to an actual stimulus and may be experienced along any sensory pathway auditory, visual, tactile, olfactory, or gustatory (29).

health collective physical, mental, and social well-being; not just absence or lack of disease or infirmity (AOTA, 2002). The components of health and health-related states include body functions and structures, engagement in activities, and participation in life situations and environmental factors (11, 35).

health promotion a plan or program that facilitates a person taking control of and improving his/her health (35).

hemopoiesis formation of blood or blood cells (30).

holism idea that the mind and body are a single integrated system (3).

home health care home health care services are provided by home health agencies to clients who are homebound and need skilled care (33).

horizontal plane divides the body in upper and lower segments (30).

humanism in clinical work represents that clients should be treated as a person and not an object, and people are capable of change (3).

hyperactivity higher level of activity (motor or verbal) than expected based on age and developmental level (27).

hypercoagulability tendency for blood to form blood clots (30).

hypothesis testable assumptions or predictions (8).

I

ICF *International Classification of Functioning, Disability and Health* (22).

impulsivity acting prior to considering consequence of actions to a greater extent than expected for age and developmental level (27).

inattention lower level of attention to task or shorter attention span than would be expected for age and developmental level (27).

Individualized Educational Plan (IEP) a written document that is developed after a child has been evaluated and found eligible for services in a school environment (36).

Individualized Family Service Plan (IFSP) a written document that is developed after a child has been evaluated and found eligible for services through early intervention (36).

Individuals with Disabilities Education Act (IDEA) a federal law requiring that all students with disabilities be educated in the least restrictive environment possible, mandating that students with disabilities be educated alongside those without disability (1).

Individual with Disabilities Educational Act Part B legislative Act that is part of the Americans with Disabilities Act (ADA) that legislates and regulates school-based services (36).

Individual with Disabilities Educational Act Part C legislative Act that is part of the Americans with Disabilities Act (ADA) that legislates and regulates early intervention services (36).

inflammation localized tissue reaction to irritation (30).

informed consent a legal and ethical communication process between client (or authorized agent) and clinician that results in the client's authorization or permission to participate in evaluation and treatment (14).

inpatient rehabilitation facility (IRF) a freestanding facility or a rehabilitation unit in an acute care hospital that provides intensive rehabilitation services to patients after an injury, illness, or surgery (33).

instrumental activities of daily living (IADL) activities to support daily life within the home and community that often require more complex interactions than self-care used in ADL (23).

intellectual disability condition that started prior to age 18 with significantly lower than normal IQ scores (below 70) and considerable issues meeting performance standards expected for their age and culture in two or more areas of occupation, learning, or social participation (27).

intensity the strength or severity of (with regard to this textbook) the presenting symptom(s) (29).

interactive reasoning understanding the client as an individual or demonstrating connected knowledge (16).

interoception awareness of sensation that originates inside the body, particularly the viscera (28).

interrater reliability the level at which two or more individuals arrive at the same results following the administration of the same process (13).

intervention the process and skilled actions taken by OT practitioners in collaboration with the client to facilitate engagement in occupation related to health and participation (18).

intervention approaches specific strategies selected to direct the process of interventions that are based on the client's desired outcome, evaluation data, and evidence (18).

intervention implementation putting the treatment plan into action (10).

intervention plan the action plan for the occupational therapist and occupational therapy assistant to follow to provide intervention (10).

intervention review ongoing means of reassessing the treatment plan, how it is being implemented, whether it is working, and how the client is making progress toward meeting his/her goals (10).

intervertebral discs material located between vertebrae of the spine (30).

intuitive reasoning a way of thinking and being with clients that entailed sensitivity to the practitioner's own emotions and those of the clients (16).

involvement taking part, being included or engaged in an area of life, being accepted, or having access to needed resources and gauged through performance (11).

ischemia tissue death (30).

J

Joint Commission on Accreditation of Healthcare Organizations (JCAHO) is an independent, not-for-profit organization that accredits and certifies more than 19,000 health care organizations and programs in the United States. Joint Commission accreditation and certification is recognized nationwide as a symbol of quality that reflects an organization's commitment to meeting certain performance standards (15).

just right challenge the balance between the challenge of the activity and the skills of the person (4).

K

kinesthesia the ability to sense the direction and extent of joint movement (28).

kyphosis spine bows posterior (backward) (30).

L

leadership the act of leading others through influence and guidance for a common purpose. Leadership requires one to create energy and motivation in such a way that others choose to follow (39).

learning the process of transforming experience into knowledge (9).

learning styles the myriad ways humans adapt and manage life events (9).

licensure within occupational therapy, recognition from a state or territory that a practitioner has met the requirements to practice in the field of occupational therapy for the time indicated by the license. Each state or territory determines these criteria as well as disciplinary action for those individuals not meeting the required standards (13).

life meaning the underlying beliefs and assumptions about the reason(s) for our existence, the reason(s) we are living and part of this world (19).

lifting index measurement of risk calculated by comparing the recommended weight limit to the actual weight being lifted (26).

ligaments dense non-elastic tissue that provide bone-to-bone (joint) support (30).

long-term acute care hospital (LTCH) hospital-based inpatient care (certified as an acute care hospital) for those who require a longer than the usual hospital stay (usually more than 25 days) because of the severity of illness or the chronic nature of the disease process (33).

lordosis spine bows anterior (forward) (30).

lumbar relating to area between lowest ribs and the pelvis (30).

M

mainstreaming placement of children with identified disabilities or delays in a regular classroom settings with peers who are typically developing (36).

maladaptive behavior the client's inability to adjust or adapt to a particular situation (38).

malpractice the breach by a member of a profession of either a standard of care or a standard of conduct usually results in damage to a client (13).

management the act or system of governing, directing, or controlling individuals in a work environment in order to achieve objectives (13, 39).

manager someone who is responsible for staff or employees and directs and supervises a business or enterprise and plans, directs, monitors, and takes corrective action of individuals or groups of people (15).

manic episode a period of predominant mood elevation, expansiveness, or irritation. These episodes are paired together with some combination of hyperarousal and diminished sleep, heightened self-esteem or grandiosity, talkativeness, flight of ideas, distractibility and poor concentration, hyperactivity, sexual promiscuity and possible unsafe sex practices, and impulsivity and recklessness (29).

meaningful making sense of what is being done in an occupation (4, 18).

meaningful activity activities that have an intrinsic value to an individual (11).

medical model the traditional approach to assessment and treatment, focused on remediation of pathology. In a medical model approach, the physician or other health care provider is generally regarded as the expert, while the client, usually referred to as a "patient," is a recipient of services (34).

medical necessity the intervention or treatment is consistent with the diagnosis, and failure to provide the treatment could jeopardize or significantly compromise the client's condition or quality of medical care (14).

Medicare a federal program that pays for certain health expenses for people 65 years of age or older; people under age 65 with certain disabilities; and people of all ages with end-stage renal disease (33).

mentoring the interaction that takes place between individuals with the goal of elevating a less experienced individual through the sharing of skills, knowledge, and perspectives (39).

meta-analysis like a systematic review; relies on multiple methods to search and consolidate findings from multiple studies on similar topics (5).

metabolic biochemical processes required for normal functioning (30).

metaphysical philosophy concerned with the mind–body relationship and whether there is a dualistic or holistic connection between the two (3).

milieu the therapeutic environment, including the group setting that provides opportunities for development of social skills and peer support (34).

model a means to organize thinking and intervention around the philosophical basis of a profession (7).

moral treatment respect for human individuality and a fundamental perception of the individual's need to engage in creative activity (1, 20).

motor development movement, reflex, and sensory development (8).

MPT model an assessment tool that encompasses Matching Person and Technology (22).

MSIPT a systematic motor access assessment that looks at movement, control site, input method, position, and targeting (22).

muscle tone the amount of tension in a skeletal muscle at rest (27).

myelin insulation surrounding nerve cells that speeds up conduction (30).

myopia nearsightedness, a refractive state where light is focused in front of the retina (31).

N

narrative reasoning the use of storytelling and story creation in order to share the client's story (16).

National Society for the Promotion of Occupational Therapy (NSPOT) the predecessor organization of the American Occupational Therapy Association (1).

nature development proceeds because of internal, biological factors (8).

NBCOT National Board for Certification in Occupational Therapy; "a not-for-profit credentialing agency that provides certification for the occupational therapy profession" (17).

negative prognostic indicators signs that indicate barriers inhibiting rehab potential (14).

negative reinforcement a strategy for strengthening a desired behavior by causing a negative condition to be stopped or avoided as a consequence of the desired behavior (9).

negative symptoms withdrawal of a trait that would normally be present such as when a range of affective states is replaced with flat affect (29).

neoplasm new or abnormal growth (30).

neuron specialized kind of cell located in the central nervous system (32).

neuropathy abnormal condition of the nerve (30).

nonmaleficence intentionally refraining from actions that cause harm (12).

nontraditional or emerging areas of practice areas of practice that are not typically reimbursed by the traditional health care system and/or are new areas of practice for occupational therapy practitioners (37).

normative aging changes changes that are an accepted part of aging. If you live to a certain age, you will experience these changes (37).

nursing facility (NF) a nursing home or nursing facility is a residence facility that provides room and meals and helps with activities of daily living and recreation. Generally, nursing home residents require 24-hour care for an indefinite period of time and have impairments that keep them from living on their own (33).

nurture development proceeds because of external, environmental factors (8).

nystagmus a rapid, rhythmic, involuntary motion of the eye usually caused by congenital visual impairment or neurological insult (31).

O

occupation an activity in which a person is engaged, usually indicating a purpose that is goal directed, extends over time, is composed of multiple tasks, and has meaning to their performer. Often described as the activities people engage in throughout their daily lives to fulfill their time and give life meaning (1, 4, 11).

occupational adaptation a lifelong transformation process that suggests that what we have done influences what we are to become (4).

occupational choice the conscious decision to engage in an occupation (4).

occupational deprivation lack of participation in occupation due to factors including injury, disability, prejudice, poverty, and employment (4).

occupational form the contextual information or meaning system of occupation (4).

occupational imbalance when the balance of habits, routines, and activities are negatively impacted by life-changing or stressful situations such as loss of a job, loss of a loved one, an illness, or injury (35).

Occupational Information Network (O*NET) online resource for obtaining information about job requirements (38).

occupational integrity integrating into one's occupational choices what matters most (19).

occupational justice the component of occupational participation that meets individual needs and embraces social equity (4).

occupational participation engagement in work, leisure, self-care, or sleep (4).

occupational performance a dynamic of occupation through which a person can literally change his or her own nature by engaging in occupation (11).

occupational performance analysis the observational evaluation of a person's task performance to identify discrepancies between the demands of a task and the skill of the person (11, 16).

occupational performance and function the doing component of occupation (4).

ocupational profile summation of a client's occupational history and experiences, patterns of daily living, interests, values, and needs (10, 18).

occupational role the occupations that a person ascribes to a role—they are individual and situational specific (11).

occupational science the formal study of occupation (4).

occupational therapist initially certified practitioner who is responsible for all aspects of occupational therapy service delivery and who is accountable for the safety and effectiveness of the occupational therapy service delivery process (13).

occupational therapy a profession that helps people do what they need and want to do through the use of therapeutic daily activities (1).

occupational therapy assistant a credentialed professional who works under the supervision of and in partnership with an occupational therapist to deliver safe and effective therapy services (2, 13).

***Occupational Therapy Practice Framework:* Domain and Process (I, II, III)** an official AOTA document that articulates "occupational therapy's contribution to promoting the health and participation of people, organizations, and populations through engagement in occupation" (6).

occupational value the selection of and engagement in occupations that hold importance (19).

occupation as ends situations when the end goal to be achieved is the occupation itself (4).

occupation as means simple and repetitive purposeful behaviors (4).

occupations of spirit select activities that may specifically elicit spiritual awareness and practice (19).

ophthalmologist a medical doctor who specializes in the care of the eye and diagnosis and management of eye disease (31).

optometrist a doctor of optometry who is trained in the diagnosis and management of eye disease and refractive error (31).

organismic philosophical perspective that recognizes that a person's behaviors influence the physical and social environment and, in turn, a person is impacted by changes in the environment (3).

orthosis a rigid or semirigid device applied externally to a body part for support or immobilization (24).

OT Connections AOTA's online community (17).

overresponsivity exhibition of a more intense, more rapid, and/or longer lasting response to sensory input than is typical (28).

P

panic attack a discrete period in which there is the sudden onset of intense fear or terror (29).

paralysis loss of the ability to move (30).

participation an outcome that "naturally occurs when clients are actively involved in carrying out occupations or daily life activities they find purposeful and meaningful in desired contexts" (33).

passive the environment shapes people "doing" is not the explanation for development (8).

peer reviewed evaluation of creative work or performance by other people in the same field in order to maintain or enhance the quality of the work or performance in that field (17).

PEOM Person–Environment–Occupation Model (22).

personal philosophy a way of life that sets the course for all thoughts and actions (3).

philosophy the study of why people think and act the way that they do (3).

PICO a way to organize a well-written question to research and then apply the results to an evidence-based process. The acronym stands for P (patient problem or population), I (intervention), C (comparison), and O (outcome) (5).

play activities performed for their simple intrinsic value with the focus on participation to create feeling of happiness (36).

positive prognostic indicators the indicators that the client has good rehab potential, which is essential for third-party reimbursement (14).

positive reinforcement a strategy for strengthening a desired behavior through experiences that are pleasant and appealing (9).

positive symptoms when describing behaviors associated with a psychotic disorder, "positive symptoms" are the addition of a symptom(s) such as hallucinations or delusions (29).

posterior back (30).

posture a position of the body or of the body parts in standing or sitting (30).

practitioner an occupational therapist or an occupational therapy assistant (13).

pragmatic reasoning understanding the practical limitations in the delivery of therapy (16).

praxis the process of conceiving of, organizing, and carrying out intentional, goal-directed actions (27, 28).

presbyopia loss of accommodation of the eye, typically begins around age 40 (31).

pressure area a place on the skin that becomes red or irritated because a part of an orthosis is too tight or rough (24).

private practices private clinics in which therapy services are typically provided in an outpatient setting and typically funded by third-party payers (insurance companies) and are not legislated (36).

procedural justice compliance with institutional rules, local, state, federal, and international laws and AOTA documents applicable to the profession of occupational therapy (12).

procedural reasoning understanding the client's underlying problem and then setting goals and planning intervention accordingly (16).

process the ways in which client-centered occupational therapy treatment is implemented in occupational therapy services (6, 10).

productive aging used to describe the societal contributions of older adults, including paid employment, volunteer activities, caring for others, and daily activities (37).

professional philosophy a collection of beliefs, attitudes, and thoughts that frames the way one engages in his or her work (3).

proprioception the ability to sense the position and location of a joint or body part (27, 28).

proximal with regard to the human body—that which is closest to the center of the body (i.e., shoulders and thighs) (8).

psychoeducation a form of verbal therapy that involves providing the client with information about their condition and/or tools for managing related life challenges (34).

psychosocial development psychological and emotional development (8).

psychotic symptoms signs or behaviors that a client is experiencing disruption of thought processes such that the individual may not maintain a complete connection with reality (29).

psychotropic medication medications that are used to treat mental and emotional disorders and behavior (34).
punishment weakens a behavior because negative conditions are imposed on a behavior (9).
purpose the desire to do something about a situation (18).
purposeful the intention part of an occupation (4).
purposeful activity an activity that has significance to the client; tends to be goal directed (11).

Q

qualitative research a type of research such as case studies or findings of interviews and self-report measures that looks to gain a deeper understanding of a problem and to understand relationships rather than causation (5).
quality of life a client's dynamic appraisal of life satisfactions (perceptions of progress toward identified goals), self-concept (the composite of beliefs and feelings about themselves), health and functioning (including health status, self-care capabilities), and socioeconomic factors (e.g., vocation, education, income) (23).
quantitative research a type of research that aims to determine causation or causal relationships; data are analyzed via statistical analyses and are reported as experimental studies (5).

R

randomized controlled trials quantitative, comparative research that involves randomly assigning participants to one or more groups, one of which is a control and the others are experimental. Researchers measure and compare the outcomes or results of the different groups through statistical analyses (5).
reach envelope primary, secondary, and tertiary ranges that identify how far a person is reaching and therefore what items or tasks should be completed in each range (26).
recommended weight limit a calculation of a safe weight that can be lifted in specified situations (26).
recovery model an approach to treatment of mental illness or substance dependence that focuses on supporting the individual in his/her journey of recovery. Key concepts include client empowerment, a collaborative partnership between the therapist and client, and a goal of facilitating social participation and client-driven goal attainment (34).
rehabilitation a set of measures that assist individuals who experience, or are likely to experience, disability to achieve and maintain optimal functioning in interaction with their environments (33).
reliability extent to which a research tool yields the same outcomes each time it is used (5)
representative assembly the body composed of representatives from identified constituencies (election areas) whose function is to legislate and establish policy for the association (2).
research gathering or collecting information about a topic (5).
resilience the ability of a person to persevere in extreme situations (8, 19).
RESNA Rehabilitation Engineering and Assistive Technology Society of North America (22).
restorative programs programs that facilitate the learning of new skills in an attempt to "restore" the client's previous abilities (14).
resume a document intended to construct a professional identity in order to get a job interview (17).
rigidity quality of being stiff or inflexible (30).
root cause analysis a systematic process of identifying method of injury as well as the context surrounding injuries (26).
Roster of Honor recognizes the contribution of an OTA to AOTA and the profession (2).

S

sacral relating to a triangular bone at distal end of spine (30).
sagittal plane divides the body into left and right segments (30).
scoliosis abnormal curving of the spine (30).
scope of practice the range of professional duties and abilities as defined by the profession's guidelines, regulatory bodies, and licensure statues and rules (13).
screening the process of determining if a client requires the skilled services of an occupational therapy practitioner. It helps to identify changes in functional status such as improvements or declines in physical or cognitive abilities (14).
self-determination process of making things happen in one's own life; higher levels involve knowing one's needs and advocating to get those needs met (27).
sense of coherence an overarching and fluid representation of confidence (4, 8).
sensitivity analysis a way to predict outcomes if the results are different than what were initially predicted (5).
sensory diet an individualized program of regularly scheduled and as-needed activities that facilitate an individual's ability to self-regulate arousal level and achieve a functional state of homeostasis (28).
sensory discrimination the ability to sense similarities and differences between sensations (28).
sensory integration the organization of sensation for use (28).
sensory modulation sensory responses that match the nature and intensity of the sensory input (28).
sensory processing reception and interpretation of sensory input for use (28).
sensory processing disorder difficulty receiving, processing, and appropriately responding to sensory information from the environment and our body (28).
sensory seeking a persistent craving for sensory input that is difficult to satiate, often in ways that are socially unacceptable (28).
sensory underresponsivity exhibition of less of a response to sensory input than the situation requires, longer response time to react to input, and/or the requirement of more intense or longer sensory input to generate a response (28).
serious mental illness classes of illness that are most intense and persistent in their presentation, resulting in often chronic impairment of functional performance (29).
SETT framework Student Environment Tasks Tools (22).
severe mental illness (SMI) diagnosed disorders with serious and persistent symptoms such as psychotic, mood, anxiety, and autism spectrum disorders. Symptoms of SMI can be life threatening if not treated and can significantly impact occupational performance (34).

skilled nursing facility (SNF) skilled nursing facilities or skilled nursing units (SNUs) are "primarily engaged in providing skilled nursing care and related services for residents who require medical or nursing care; or rehabilitation services for rehabilitation of injured, disabled, or sick persons" (33).
slope and rise the steepness or angle of a slope is dependent on the length of a ramp and the height of the rise (21).
social justice provision of services in a fair and equitable manner (12).
spiritual development overarching worldview development seeking answers to questions such as "who am I" and "what is my purpose" (8).
spirituality personal quest for understanding answers to ultimate questions about life, meaning, and the sacred or transcendent; a pervasive life force, manifestation of a higher self, source of will and self-determination; sensitivity to the presence of spirit; gives meaning to occupations (19).
staff evaluation review of staff performance usually completed during a predetermined time frame and including informal and formal assessment strategies. The goal of staff evaluation is to identify staff strengths, areas for improvement, and professional development plans (13).
standardized assessments methods used for data collection that have established reliability and validity (14).
State Regulatory Boards entity that has legal jurisdiction over occupational therapy practitioners (12).
static orthosis an orthosis that typically is composed of one nonmoving part, typically used to immobilize and/or stabilize joints (24).
static progressive orthosis an orthosis that can be incrementally changed for slow progressive tissue and joint adjustments that usually have movable parts, such as turnbuckles or hinges (24).
subcortical unconscious—not within voluntary control (32).
supervision the process of overseeing the work of others. This often includes the acknowledgement of responsibility for those individuals who are under one's care (13, 39).
synovial pertaining to a membrane located in joints (30).
systematic review a research tool that consolidates and summarizes many research findings on particular topics in order to provide evidence on that topic (5).

T

tachykinesia fast movement (30).
tactile sensation within skin about touch and pressure input (27).
task the smaller components, parts, or steps of an activity or occupation (11).
task analysis a systematic method of identifying the physical, cognitive, and psychosocial demands of a given task (11, 26).
task groups type of group that focuses on performing various types of tasks (25).
task-oriented activity an activity that has inherent meaning and purpose for a client (23).
taxonomy classification into ordered categories (6).
teaching the act of imparting knowledge or skills to others (39).
teleological (ethical) theory focuses on the consequences of actions (12).
tendon tissue that attaches muscles to bones (30).
teratogens any disease, drug, or other environmental agents that can harm a developing embryo or fetus (8).
Terry Brittell COTA/OTR Partnership Award recognizes outstanding partnership and collaboration between the roles within occupational therapy (2).
theory a set of related ideas that describe and explain specific concepts (7, 8).
therapeutic milieu the structure within a mental health unit that ensures patient safety, fosters agency, and enhances cohesion of the community (29).
therapeutic use of self the manner in which the occupational therapy practitioner uses his/her personality, life experiences, intuition, knowledge, and skills to develop therapeutic relationships with clients in order to encourage, inspire, communicate, and be effective in leading them to achieve meaningful therapy goals (25).
thermoplastic a polymer that becomes soft or moldable above a certain temperature and solid when cooled (24).
thoracic relating to the chest (30).
tone muscle tension (30).
transactional leader leads by exception (15).
transformational leader inspires, energizes, and stimulates employees (15).
transient ischemic attack (TIA) mini stroke (30).
trauma an injury to living tissue (30).
treatment planning process in which activities are chosen with goals established and modified to enhance functional performance toward an outcome (23).

U

Uniform Terminology predecessor document to the *Framework* whose purpose was to set forth a uniform reporting system to be used for reimbursement of occupational therapy services (6).
universal design the design of products and environments to be usable by all people, to the greatest extent possible, without the need for specialized design (21, 35).

V

validity degree to which an instrument measures what it is intended to measure (5).
values ideas and beliefs that an individual determines to be important (3).
veracity provision of comprehensive, accurate, and objective information when representing the profession (12).
vestibular sensation within the inner ear providing information about linear and circular movement of the head through space (27).
vestibular input information from the vestibular system about one's position in and movement through space (28).
vision therapy exercises or treatment with lenses to enhance visual development, typically used for binocular visual deficits in children (31).
visual acuity level of visual clarity or how well one can see (31).

visual field the area or perimeter of one's vision or how much one can see (31).

visual function function of the ocular system, usually described as visual acuity, visual field, and contrast sensitivity measurements (31).

volition the act of willing or choosing—making choices (7).

W

well-being an emotional satisfaction with life in general (35).

wellness taking control of choices to increase satisfaction in life and improve overall health (35).

WFOT World Federation of Occupational Therapists (WFOT) is an international organization that promotes "occupational therapy as an art and science internationally" (17).

work a task that requires physical, cognitive, and/or psychosocial effort (26).

work conditioning (WC) an "intensive, work-related, goal orientated conditioning program designed specifically to restore systemic neuromusculoskeletal functions, motor function, range of motion, and cardiovascular/pulmonary functions" to help the client return to work (38).

work hardening (WH) a "highly structured, goal-orientated, individualized intervention program designed" to return the client back to work (38).

Index

Note: Page numbers followed by *f* denote figures, those followed by *t* denote tables, and those followed by *b* denote boxes.

A

D

E

F

P

T